Books are to be returned
the last

KU-276-971

7–DAY
LOAN

3 0 MAR 2006

LIVERPOOL
JOHN MOORES UNIVERSITY
AVRIL ROBARTS LRC
TITHEBARN STREET
LIVERPOOL L2 2ER
TEL. 0151 231 4022

and
Assistant Professor
University of Cincinnati College of Medicine
Cincinnati, Ohio

Judith A. Aberg, MD
Assistant Clinical Professor of Medicine
AIDS and Oncology Division
University of California, San Francisco
San Francisco, California

LEXI-COMP, INC
Hudson (Cleveland), OH

**AMERICAN
PHARMACEUTICAL
ASSOCIATION** APhA

This handbook is intended to serve the user as a handy reference and not as a complete infectious disease resource. The publication covers common diseases with empiric treatment recommendations, common microorganisms, testing procedures necessary for diagnosis, and the majority of anti-infective agents available in the United States. The individual sections of this handbook are specifically designed to present certain important aspects of the disease states, the organisms, laboratory tests, and antimicrobial therapy in a more concise format than is typically found in medical literature or infectious disease texts.

The nature of infectious diseases and their diagnosis and treatment is that it is constantly evolving because of ongoing research and clinical experience and is often subject to interpretation. While great care has been taken to ensure the accuracy of the information presented, the reader is advised that the authors, editors, reviewers, contributors, and publishers cannot be responsible for the continued currency of the information or for any errors, omissions, or the application of this information, or for any consequences arising therefrom. Therefore, the author(s) and/or the publisher shall have no liability to any person or entity with regard to claims, loss, or damage caused, or alleged to be caused, directly or indirectly, by the use of information contained herein. Because of the dynamic nature of infectious disease as a discipline, readers are advised that decisions regarding the diagnosis and treatment of specific organisms and disease states must be based on the independent judgment of the clinician, changing information regarding drug therapy (eg, as reflected in the literature and drug manufacturer's most current product information), and changing medical practices. The editors are not responsible for any inaccuracy of quotation or for any false or misleading implication that may arise due to the text or formulas used or due to quotation of revisions no longer official.

The editors, authors, and contributors have written this book in their private capacities. No official support or endorsement by any federal or state agency or pharmaceutical company is intended or inferred.

The publishers have made every effort to trace the copyright holders for borrowed material. If they have inadvertently overlooked any, they will be pleased to make the necessary arrangements at the first opportunity.

If you have suggestions or questions regarding any information presented in this handbook, please contact our drug information pharmacist at

1-800-837-LEXI (5394)

Copyright ©9 by Lexi-Comp, Inc. All rights reserved.

Copyright ©Lexi-Comp, Inc: 1996, 2nd edition; 1995, reprint of 1st edition with additions; 19 1st edition

Printed in Canada. No part of this publication may be reproduced, stored in a retrieval system, or transmitted, in any form or by any means, electronic, mechanical, photocopying, recording, or otherwise, without the prior written permission of the publisher.

This manual was produced using the FormuLex™ and Pathfinder™ Programs — complete publishing services of Lexi-Comp, Inc.

Lexi-Comp, Inc
1100 Terex Road
Hudson, Ohio 44236
(330) 650-6506

ISBN 0-916589-81-1 (North American Edition)

ISBN 0-916589-89-7 (International Edition)

Infectious Diseases Handbook

— *including* —

Antimicrobial Therapy & Diagnostic Tests/Procedures

3rd Edition

LIVERPOOL JMU LIBRARY

3 1111 00880 9640

LIVERPOOL JOHN MOORES UNIVERSITY LEARNING SERVICES			
Accession No BM 272573 K			
Class No Q 616.9 ISA			
Aldham Robarts 0151-231-3701		By... of 0151-231-2329	✓
I M Marsh 0151-231-5216		Trueman Street 0151-231-4022	

TABLE OF CONTENTS

1

TABLE OF CONTENTS *(Continued)*

ABOUT THE AUTHORS

Carlos M. Isada, MD

Dr Isada received his undergraduate training and medical degree from the State University of New York at Buffalo. After completing his residency and chief residency in Internal Medicine at the Cleveland Clinic, he stayed on to pursue fellowship training in Infectious Diseases.

Along with his current duties as Staff Physician in the Department of Infectious Disease at the Cleveland Clinic Foundation, Dr Isada also serves as Director of the Infectious Diseases Fellowship Training Program and is Assistant Program Director for the Internal Medicine Residency Training. Dr Isada has developed a special interest in clinical virology and frequently participates in presentations and abstracts on this topic. In addition to these and other presentations and publications, Dr Isada is a major contributor to the *Diagnostic Procedures Handbook* published by Lexi-Comp, Inc, and a member of Lexi-Comp's editorial board.

Dr Isada is a member of the Infectious Diseases Society of America, American Society of Microbiology, American College of Physicians, and the American Medical Association.

Bernard L. Kasten, Jr, MD, FCAP

Dr Kasten is Vice President and Chief Laboratory Officer of Quest Diagnostics Inc. He is a graduate of Miami University, Oxford, Ohio and the Ohio State University College of Medicine. He interned at the University of Miami, Florida and served his residency in Clinical Pathology at the National Institute of Health Clinical Center. A fellowship at the National Cancer Institute Laboratory of Pathology followed. He is a Diplomate of American Board of Pathology certified in Anatomic and Clinical Pathology and Medical Microbiology. His staff appointments have included service in the Division of Laboratory Medicine at the Cleveland Clinic and as Associate Director of Pathology and Laboratory Services at Bethesda Hospitals in Cincinnati. Dr Kasten is active as a fellow of the College of American Pathologists, in which he participates in the Inspection and Accreditation Program, as an advisor to the Management Resource Committee, and as chair of the CAP's Worldwide Web Editorial Board. He was Chairman of the Publications Committee for 8 years and Chairman of the Editorial Board of *CAP Today* from its inception in 1987 until 1995. In 1993, he received the Frank W. Hartman Award in recognition of his service to the College of American Pathologists.

Dr Kasten is a principal author of the fourth edition of the *Laboratory Test Handbook* and the author of the *Physicians DRG Handbook*. He has presented numerous lectures and seminars on the subjects of improving workflow in the laboratory, total quality management, six sigma medical quality, and the appropriate use of laboratory tests. He is a member of Lexi-Comp, Inc's medical publishing editorial board.

Morton P. Goldman, PharmD

Dr Goldman received his bachelor's degree in pharmacy from the University of Pittsburgh, College of Pharmacy and his Doctor of Pharmacy degree from the University of Cincinnati, Division of Graduate Studies and Research. He completed his concurrent 2-year hospital pharmacy residency at the VA Medical Center in Cincinnati. Dr Goldman is presently the Assistant Director of Pharmacotherapy Services for the Department of Pharmacy at the Cleveland Clinic Foundation (CCF) after having spent over 3 years at CCF as an Infectious Disease pharmacist and 4 years as Clinical Manager. He holds faculty appointments from Case Western Reserve University, College of Medicine; The University of Toledo, College of Pharmacy; and The University of Cincinnati, College of Pharmacy. Dr Goldman is a board-certified Pharmacotherapy Specialist and is a fellow of the American College of Clinical Pharmacy.

In his capacity as Assistant Director of Pharmacotherapy Services at CCF, Dr Goldman remains actively involved in patient care and clinical research with the Department of Infectious Disease, as well as the continuing education of the medical and pharmacy staff. He is an editor of CCF's *Guidelines for Antibiotic Use* and participates in their annual Antimicrobial Review retreat. He is a member of the

ABOUT THE AUTHORS *(Continued)*

Pharmacy and Therapeutics Committee and many of its subcommittees. Dr Goldman has authored numerous journal articles and lectures locally and nationally on infectious diseases topics and current drug therapies. He is currently a reviewer for the *Annals of Pharmacotherapy* and the *Journal of the American Medical Association*, an editorial board member of the *Journal of Infectious Disease Pharmacotherapy*, and coauthor of the *Drug Information Handbook* and the *Drug Information Handbook for the Allied Health Professional* produced by Lexi-Comp, Inc. He also provides technical support to Lexi-Comp's Clinical Reference Library™ publications.

Dr Goldman is an active member of Cleveland's local clinical pharmacy society, the Ohio College of Clinical Pharmacy, the Society of Infectious Disease Pharmacists, the American College of Clinical Pharmacy, and the American Society of Health-Systems Pharmacy.

Larry D. Gray, PhD

Dr Gray received his bachelor's degree from the University of North Carolina at Chapel Hill and his master's and doctorate degrees from Wake Forest University (Bowman Gray School of Medicine). He received his postdoctoral training in Clinical Microbiology and Infectious Diseases at the Mayo Clinic.

Dr Gray has been the Director of Microbiology at Bethesda Hospitals in Cincinnati, Ohio for the last 5 years. He is a Volunteer Associate Professor of Pathology and Laboratory Medicine at the University of Cincinnati College of Medicine, is a Diplomate of the American Board of Medical Microbiology, and is on the editorial board of the *Journal of Clinical Microbiology*. In addition, he is an active member of the American Society for Microbiology, the American Board of Medical Microbiology, and the South Central Association for Clinical Microbiology. Dr Gray is also the president of Clinical Microbiology Laboratory Consultants, LLC.

Dr Gray's background includes 12 years of research in the pathogenesis of infectious diseases (ocular and pulmonary bacterial infections, electron microscopy) and the publication of many research, review, chapter, and book publications.

Judith A. Aberg, MD

Dr Aberg received a degree in Laboratory Technology from Norfolk General Hospital in 1975 and worked in medical microbiology, where she was responsible for the Mycology Laboratory and curriculum. After 11 years of laboratory experience, Dr Aberg graduated from Millersville University of Pennsylvania, Magna Cum Laude, BSMT. Dr Aberg then graduated from Pennsylvania State University College of Medicine.

During Dr Aberg's medical school training, she was a research technologist in neuroimmunology, resulting in publication of her work with multiple sclerosis. After medical school, Dr Aberg completed her internal medicine residency at the Cleveland Clinic, during which time she worked as a limited clinical practitioner in the Emergency Department and was involved in research projects in the Department of Infectious Disease. Dr Aberg then held a joint position as both Chief Medical Resident and Clinical Associate in Immunology at the Cleveland Clinic. As a Clinical Associate, she was involved in the HIV Center AIDS education in both the hospital and the community, and clinical trials for HIV-positive individuals.

Dr Aberg completed a fellowship in Infectious Disease at the Washington University School of Medicine in the Department of Infectious Disease. She is currently an Assistant Clinical Professor of Medicine in the AIDS and Oncology Division at the University of California, San Francisco where she is also Co-Investigator in the AIDS Clinical Trials Group. She is a member in many professional societies including the American Medical Association, American College of Physicians, American Society for Microbiology, American Society of Clinical Pathologists, and Infectious Diseases Society of America.

EDITORIAL ADVISORY PANEL

Lora L. Armstrong, RPh, BSPharm
Director of Drug Information Services
University of Chicago Hospitals
Chicago, Illinois

Verna L. Baughman, MD
Associate Professor
Anesthesiology
University of Illinois
Chicago, Illinois

Judith L. Beizer, PharmD
Clinical Associate Professor
College of Pharmacy and Allied Health Professions
St John's University
Jamaica, New York

Mark F. Bonfiglio, BS, PharmD, RPh
Director of Pharmacotherapy Resources
Lexi-Comp, Inc
Hudson, Ohio

Linda R. Bressler, PharmD
Department of Pharmacy Practice
University of Illinois
Chicago, IL

Marcelline Burns, PhD
Research Psychologist
Director, Southern California Research Institute
Los Angeles, California

Harold L. Crossley, DDS, PhD
Associate Professor
Pharmacology
Dental School
University of Maryland at Baltimore
Baltimore, Maryland

Francesca E. Cunningham, PharmD
Associate Professor
Pharmacy Practice/Anesthesiology
University of Illinois
Chicago, Illinois

Wayne R. DeMott, MD
Pathologists Chartered
Overland Park, Kansas

Andrew J. Donnelly, PharmD, MBA
Clinical Pharmacist
Operating Room/Anesthesia
Assistant Director of Pharmacy
Rush-Presbyterian-St Luke's Medical Center
Chicago, Illinois

Matthew A. Fuller, PharmD, MBA
Clinical Pharmacy Specialist
Psychiatry
Cleveland Department of Veterans Affairs Medical Center
Brecksville, Ohio

5

EDITORIAL ADVISORY PANEL *(Continued)*

Mark Geraci, PharmD
Department of Pharmacy Practice
University of Illinois
Chicago, Illinois

Harold J. Grady, PhD
Director of Clinical Chemistry
Truman Medical Center
Kansas City, Missouri

Martin D. Higbee, PharmD
Associate Professor
Department of Pharmacy Practice
The University of Arizona
Tucson, Arizona

Jane Hurlburt Hodding, PharmD
Supervisor, Children's Pharmacy
Miller Children's Hospital at Long Beach Memorial
Long Beach, California

Rebecca T. Horvat, PhD
Assistant Professor of Pathology and Laboratory Medicine
University of Kansas Medical Center
Kansas City, Kansas

David S. Jacobs, MD
President, Pathologists Chartered
Overland Park, Kansas

Polly E. Kintzel, PharmD
Clinical Pharmacy Specialist
Bone Marrow Transplantation, Detroit Medical Center
Harper Hospital
Detroit, Michigan

Donna M. Kraus, PharmD
Assistant Professor of Pharmacy Practice
Departments of Pharmacy Practice and Pediatrics
Clinical Pharmacist
Pediatric Intensive Care Unit
University of Illinois at Chicago
Chicago, Illinois

Charles Lacy, RPh, PharmD
Drug Information Pharmacist
Cedars-Sinai Medical Center
Los Angeles, California

Brenda R. Lance, RN, MSN
Nurse Coordinator
Ritzman Infusion Services
Akron, Ohio

Leonard L. Lance, RPh, BSPharm
Clinical Pharmacist
Lexi-Comp Inc
Hudson, Ohio

Jerrold B. Leikin, MD
Associate Director
Emergency Services
Rush Presbyterian-St Luke's Medical Center
Chicago, Illinois

6

Timothy F. Meiller, DDS, PhD
Professor
Department of Oral Medicine and Diagnostic Sciences
Baltimore College of Dental Surgery
Professor of Oncology
Greenebaum Cancer Center
University of Maryland at Baltimore
Baltimore, Maryland

Eugene S. Olsowka, MD, PhD
Pathologist
Institute of Pathology PC
Saginaw, Michigan

Thomas E. Page, MA
Drug Recognition Expert and Instructor
Officer in Charge, DRE Unit
Los Angeles Police Department
Los Angeles, CA

Frank P. Paloucek, PharmD
Clinical Associate Professor
University of Illinois
Chicago, Illinois

Christopher J. Papasian, PhD
Director of Diagnostic Microbiology and Immunology Laboratories
Truman Medical Center
Kansas City, Missouri

Martha Sajatovic, MD
Assistant Professor of Psychiatry
Case Western Reserve University
Cleveland, Ohio

Todd P. Semla, PharmD
Department of Clinical Pharmacy
Project Coordinator and Clinical Pharmacist
Evanston Hospital
Evanston, Illinois

Dominic A. Solimando, Jr, MA
Oncology Pharmacy Manager
Lombardi Cancer Center
Georgetown University Medical Center
Washington, DC

Carol K. Taketomo, PharmD
Pharmacy Manager
Children's Hospital of Los Angeles
Los Angeles, California

Lowell L. Tilzer MD
Associate Medical Director
Community Blood Center of Greater Kansas City
Kansas City, Missouri

Beatrice B. Turkoski, RN, PhD
Professor, Advanced Pharmacology and Applied Therapeutics
Kent State University School of Nursing
Kent, Ohio

Richard L. Wynn, PhD
Professor and Chairman of Pharmacology
Baltimore College of Dental Surgery
Dental School
University of Maryland at Baltimore
Baltimore, Maryland

PREFACE

"All disease is infectious disease". Although that may not be completely accurate, infectious disease crosses every discipline of medicine and surgery. With few exceptions, all physicians will diagnose and/or treat infectious diseases in their day-to-day practices. Infectious diseases are becoming more complicated to diagnose and treat. We are making many of our patients more immunocompromised and are performing more invasive procedures. There are more sophisticated diagnostic tests including serologies, probes, and polymerase chain reaction (PCR). The infecting organisms are becoming smarter - more resistant to routine therapies; and the number of antimicrobial agents available to us is staggering. Billions of dollars are spent each year on antimicrobial agents in the United States with billions more spent on office visits, hospitalization, and diagnostic procedures related to infection.

It is safe to say that infectious disease as a discipline is not easy, nor can it be made easy. This handbook is not, therefore, intended as a simplification of infectious disease. Instead, we wish to make the most pertinent aspects of infectious disease readily available to all practitioners as an aid in their infectious disease endeavors. The disease syndromes chapter provides concise, straightforward information on the clinical presentation, differential diagnosis, diagnostic tests, and drug therapy recommended for treatment of the more common diseases. The organism chapter provides descriptions of the microbiology, epidemiology, diagnosis, and treatment of each organism. The laboratory diagnosis chapter describes the performance of specific tests and procedures including preparation of the patient. The antimicrobial therapy chapter provides what we believe are the most important facts and considerations regarding each drug product. In addition, the appendix offers a compilation of tables, guidelines, and conversion information which can be helpful in consideration of patient care. Finally, an alphabetical index offers convenient cross-referencing by page number to each item found in every section of the book.

A unique feature of this handbook is that entries in each of the four sections of the book (disease syndromes, organisms, laboratory diagnosis, and antimicrobial therapy) contain relative information and cross-referencing to one or more of the other three sections. For example, an entry regarding a particular organism will also provide a cross-reference to the appropriate laboratory tests to detect the organism and appropriate antimicrobial agents used against the organism.

The authors envision this handbook to be a useful tool for physicians, residents, students, dentists, nurses, pharmacists, and anyone who has the opportunity to diagnose, treat, or care for patients with infectious diseases.

Accuracy, completeness, and timeliness of each fact or recommendation presented were major goals of the authors of this handbook. The authors hope these goals have been met. Users of the handbook, however, are strongly encouraged to offer suggestions for improvement, additional entries, and corrections to current entries. Such suggestions will be sincerely welcome and considered for future editions.

ACKNOWLEDGMENTS

The *Infectious Diseases Handbook* exists in its present form as the result of the concerted efforts of the following individuals: Robert D. Kerscher, publisher and president of Lexi-Comp Inc; Lynn D. Coppinger, managing editor; Diane M. Harbart, MT (ASCP), Medical Editor; David C. Marcus, director of information systems; and Julian I. Graubart, American Pharmaceutical Association (APhA), Director of Books and Electronic Products.

Other members of the Lexi-Comp staff whose contributions deserve special mention include Barbara F. Kerscher, production manager; Jeanne E. Wilson, production/ systems liaison; Leslie J. Ruggles, Julie A. Katzen, Jennifer L. Rocky, Stacey L. Hurd, and Linda L. Taylor, project managers; Alexandra J. Hart, composition specialist; Jackie L. Mizer, Ginger S. Conner, Kathleen E. Schleicher, and Kathy Smith, production assistants; Tracey J. Reinecke, graphic designer; Cynthia A. Bell, CPhT, imaging product manager; Edmund A. Harbart, vice-president, custom publishing division; Jack L. Stones, vice-president, reference publishing division; Jay L. Katzen, director of marketing and business development; Jerry M. Reeves, Marc L. Long, and Patrick T. Grubb, regional sales managers; Brad F. Bolinski, Kristin M. Thompson, Matthew C. Kerscher, Tina L. Collins, Kelene A. Murphy, and Leslie G. Rodia, sales and marketing representatives; Paul A. Rhine and Jason M. Buchwald, academic account managers; Kenneth J. Hughes, manager of authoring systems; Sean M. Conrad and James M. Stacey, system analysts; Thury L. O'Connor, vice-president of technology; David J. Wasserbauer, vice-president, finance and administration; Elizabeth M. Conlon and Rebecca A. Dryhurst, accounting; and Frederick C. Kerscher, inventory and fulfillment manager.

Special thanks goes to Chris Lomax, PharmD, director of pharmacy, Children's Hospital, Los Angeles, who played a significant role in bringing APhA and Lexi-Comp together.

Much of the material contained in the book was a result of pharmacy contributors throughout the United States and Canada. Lexi-Comp has assisted many medical institutions to develop hospital-specific formulary manuals that contains clinical drug information as well as dosing. Working with these clinical pharmacists, hospital pharmacy and therapeutics committees, and hospital drug information centers, Lexi-Comp has developed an evolutionary drug database that reflects the practice of pharmacy in these major institutions.

In addition, the authors wish to thank their families, friends, and colleagues who supported them in their efforts to complete this handbook.

Dr Kasten would like to acknowledge the assistance of Michael A. Lewinski, PhD, Scientific Director, Infectious Diseases, Quest Diagnostics Inc Nichols Institute, Patricia M. Venedly, MS, Director Medical Education, Quest Diagnostics Inc Nichols Institute, and Delbert A. Fisher, MD, Chief Science Officer, Quest Diagnostics Inc Nichols Institute for their invaluable support in the preparation of this book.

DESCRIPTION OF SECTIONS AND FIELDS USED IN THIS HANDBOOK

The *Infectious Diseases Handbook including Antimicrobial Therapy and Diagnostic Tests/Procedures* is organized into four major chapters, an appendix, a Classification of Organisms Index, and an alphabetical index. Information is presented in a consistent format with extensive cross-referencing between chapters. Each chapter will provide the following.

DISEASE SYNDROMES

Disease Syndrome Name	Common nomenclature for the disease
Related Information	Cross-references to other parts of the book including the Appendix information that may be helpful to the user
Synonyms	Other names or abbreviations for the disease state
Clinical Presentation	Signs, symptoms, and findings from physical and laboratory examination
Differential Diagnosis	A wide differential diagnosis of the disease
Likely Pathogens	Possible organisms causing the disease syndrome. Organisms listed in order of probability. Cross-references to the organism chapter.
Diagnostic Tests/ Procedures	Appropriate tests necessary for diagnosis. Bulleted tests are more diagnostic. Cross-references to diagnostic tests/ procedures chapter.
Drug Therapy Comment	Comment about the treatment
Empiric Drug Therapy	Appropriate empiric therapy in the opinion of the authors. Definitive therapy should be used when microbiologic diagnosis is made. Cross-reference to antimicrobial therapy chapter.
Selected Reading	General references are provided

ORGANISMS

Organism Name	Genus and species name
Synonyms	Other names or abbreviations for the organism
Applies To	Other organisms included in the named genus
Microbiology	A description of the organism by morphology, stain, biochemistry, serological differences, etc.
Epidemiology	May include the natural habitat and mode of transmission of the organism. May also include information on outbreaks and transmission prevention.
Clinical Syndromes	Specific disease states that can be caused by the organism
Diagnosis	Methods for determining that the organism is causing disease
Diagnostic Tests/ Procedures	Appropriate tests useful for diagnosis. Cross-references to diagnostic tests/procedures chapter.
Duration of Therapy	Length of treatment needed
Treatment	Description of treatment modalities including nondrug therapies
Drug Therapy Comment	Comment about the treatment
Drug Therapy	Drugs of choice and alternatives for treatment of disease caused by these organisms. Cross-reference to antimicrobial therapy chapter.
Selected Reading	General references are provided

(continued)

DIAGNOSTIC TESTS/PROCEDURES

Name	Common name for the test
Related Information	Cross-references to other information in the book that are related to the named test and may be helpful to the user
Synonyms	Other names or abbreviations for the laboratory test/ procedure
Applies To	Refers to various sample sites or specimen types that follow the same procedure
Replaces	Previous test/procedure that has been replaced by this more current test/procedure
Test Includes	All laboratory tests or procedures that may occur when the named test is performed
Abstract	A brief description of the test and its use
Patient Preparation	Any special preparation that the patient must undergo prior to the procedure being performed
Aftercare	Special instructions or warnings for medical personnel for the care of the patient after the procedure is performed
Special Instructions	Specific instructions for the acquisition and handling of specimens
Complications	Problems that may arise for the patient due to testing
Equipment	All equipment needed to perform the named procedure
Technique	Explanation of how procedure is performed
Data Acquired	Data obtained from the performed procedure
Specimen	All possible specimens that can be used for testing
Container	Type of container that specimen must be collected in to acquire and maintain a usable specimen
Sampling Time	The time frame a specimen should be collected
Collection	General and specific collection instructions that should be followed to obtain a proper and usable specimen
Storage Instructions	The appropriate storage of the specimen after collection but prior to testing
Causes for Rejection	Possible reasons why a specimen may be rejected by the laboratory
Turnaround Time	Time it takes for testing to be performed and results to be reported
Reference Range or Normal Findings	Serves as a general guideline. See specific testing facility for their ranges.
Critical Values	Values that alert the medical staff that the patient has reached a value that may be hazardous to the patient
Use	Common uses for the test/procedure
Limitations	Limits of the test/procedure
Contraindications	Reasons why this test should not be performed
Methodology	Testing methodologies available
Additional Information	Additional information about the test/procedure and its uses
Selected Reading	General references are provided

DESCRIPTION OF SECTIONS AND FIELDS USED IN THIS HANDBOOK *(Continued)*

ANTIMICROBIAL THERAPY

Generic Name	U.S. adopted name
Pronunciation	
Related Information	Cross-references to other pertinent drug information found in other areas of the book or the Appendix
U.S. Brand Names	Common U.S. trade names
Canadian Brand Names	Trade names found in Canada
Synonyms	Other names or accepted abbreviations for the generic drug
Generic Available	Drugs available in generic form
Use	Information pertaining to appropriate indications of the drug
Drug of Choice or Alternate For	Cross-references to organism or disease syndromes chapter for which this drug is indicated
Restrictions	The controlled substance classification from the Drug Enforcement Agency (DEA). U.S. schedules are I-V. Schedules vary by country and sometimes state (ie, Massachusetts uses I-VI).
Pregnancy Risk Factor	Five categories established by the FDA to indicate the potential of a systemically absorbed drug for causing birth defects
Pregnancy/Breast-Feeding Implications	Information pertinent to or associated with the use of the drug as it relates to clinical effects on the fetus, breast-feeding/lactation, and clinical effects on the infant
Contraindications	Information pertaining to inappropriate use of the drug
Warnings/Precautions	Hazardous conditions related to use of the drug and disease states or patient populations in which the drug should be cautiously used
Adverse Reactions	Side effects are grouped by percentage of incidence
Overdosage/Toxicology	Comments and/or considerations offered when appropriate
Drug Interactions	
Stability	
Mechanism of Action	How the drug works in the body to elicit a response
Pharmacodynamics/Kinetics	Pharmacokinetics are expressed in terms of absorption, distribution (including appearance in breast milk and crossing of the placenta), metabolism, bioavailability, half-life, time to peak serum concentration, and elimination. Additional pharmacokinetic data can be found in the appendix.
Usual Dosage	The amount of the drug to be typically given or taken during therapy
Dietary Considerations	Information is offered, when appropriate, regarding food, nutrition, and/or alcohol
Administration	Information regarding the recommended final concentrations, rates of administration for parenteral drugs, or other guidelines when giving the medication
Monitoring Parameters	Laboratory tests and patient physical parameters that should be monitored for safety and efficacy of drug therapy are listed when appropriate
Test Interactions	Listing of assay interferences when relevant; (B) = Blood; (S) = Serum; (U) = Urine

(continued)

Reference Range	Therapeutic and toxic serum concentrations listed when appropriate
Patient Information	Comments and/or considerations are offered when appropriate
Nursing Implications	
Additional Information	Information about sodium content and/or pertinent information about specific brands
Dosage Forms	Information with regard to form, strength, and availability of the drug
Extemporaneous Preparations	Directions for preparing liquid formulations from solid drug products. May include stability information and references.
Selected Readings	General references are provided

Appendix

The appendix offers a compilation of tables, guidelines, nomograms, and conversion information which can often be helpful when considering patient care.

Classification of Organisms Index

All organisms found in the handbook are listed according to their major classification.

Alphabetical Index

All disease syndromes, organisms, diagnostic tests/procedures, and antimicrobial therapy names, along with the brand names (including Canadian and Mexican), and synonyms are listed alphabetically with the page number on which the monograph may be found.

FDA PREGNANCY CATEGORIES

Throughout this book there is a field labeled Pregnancy Risk Factor (PRF) and the letter A, B, C, D, or X immediately following which signifies a category. The FDA has established these five categories to indicate the potential of a systemically absorbed drug for causing birth defects. The key differentiation among the categories rests upon the reliability of documentation and the risk:benefit ratio. Pregnancy Category X is particularly notable in that if any data exists that may implicate a drug as a teratogen and the risk:benefit ratio is clearly negative, the drug is contraindicated during pregnancy.

These categories are summarized as follows:

A   Controlled studies in pregnant women fail to demonstrate a risk to the fetus in the first trimester with no evidence of risk in later trimesters. The possibility of fetal harm appears remote.

B   Either animal-reproduction studies have not demonstrated a fetal risk but there are no controlled studies in pregnant women, or animal-reproduction studies have shown an adverse effect (other than a decrease in fertility) that was not confirmed in controlled studies in women in the first trimester and there is no evidence of a risk in later trimesters.

C   Either studies in animals have revealed adverse effects on the fetus (teratogenic or embryocidal effects or other) and there are no controlled studies in women, or studies in women and animals are not available. Drugs should be given only if the potential benefits justify the potential risk to the fetus.

D   There is positive evidence of human fetal risk, but the benefits from use in pregnant women may be acceptable despite the risk (eg, if the drug is needed in a life-threatening situation or for a serious disease for which safer drugs cannot be used or are ineffective).

X   Studies in animals or human beings have demonstrated fetal abnormalities or there is evidence of fetal risk based on human experience, or both, and the risk of the use of the drug in pregnant women clearly outweighs any possible benefit. The drug is contraindicated in women who are or may become pregnant.

DRUGS IN PREGNANCY

Analgesics
Acceptable: Acetaminophen, meperidine, methadone
Controversial: Codeine, propoxyphene
Unacceptable: Nonsteroidal anti-inflammatory agents, salicylates, phenazopyridine

Antimicrobials
Acceptable: Penicillins, 1st and 2nd generation cephalosporins, erythromycin (base and EES), clotrimazole, miconazole, nystatin, isoniazid*, lindane
Controversial: 3rd generation cephalosporins, aminoglycosides, nitrofurantoin†
Unacceptable: Erythromycin estolate, chloramphenicol, sulfa, metronidazole, tetracyclines, acyclovir

ENT
Acceptable: Diphenhydramine*, dextromethorphan
Controversial: Pseudoephedrine
Unacceptable: Brompheniramine, cyproheptadine, dimenhydrinate

GI
Acceptable: Trimethobenzamide, antacids*, simethicone, other H_2-blockers, psyllium, bisacodyl, docusate
Controversial: Metoclopramide, prochlorperazine

Neurologic
Controversial: Phenytoin, phenobarbital
Unacceptable: Carbamazepine, valproic acid, ergotamine

Pulmonary
   Acceptable: Theophylline, metaproterenol, terbutaline, inhaled steroids
   Unacceptable: Epinephrine, oral steroids

Psych
   Acceptable: Hydroxyzine*, lithium*, haloperidol
   Controversial: Benzodiazepines, tricyclics, phenothiazines

Other
   Acceptable: Heparin, insulin
   Unacceptable: Warfarin, sulfonylureas

*Do not use in first trimester
†Do not use in third trimester

SAFE WRITING

Health professionals and their support personnel frequently produce handwritten copies of information they see in print; therefore, such information is subjected to even greater possibilities for error or misinterpretation on the part of others. Thus, particular care must be given to how drug names and strengths are expressed when creating written health-care documents.

The following are a few examples of safe writing rules suggested by the Institute for Safe Medication Practices, Inc.*

1. There should be a space between a number and its units as it is easier to read. There should be no periods after the abbreviations mg or mL.

Correct	Incorrect
10 mg	10mg
100 mg	100mg

2. Never place a decimal and a zero after a whole number (2 mg is correct and 2.0 mg is **incorrect**). If the decimal point is not seen because it falls on a line or because individuals are working from copies where the decimal point is not seen, this causes a tenfold overdose.

3. Just the opposite is true for numbers less than one. Always place a zero before a naked decimal (0.5 mL is correct, .5 mL is **incorrect**).

4. Never abbreviate the word unit. The handwritten U or u, looks like a 0 (zero), and may cause a tenfold overdose error to be made.

5. IU is not a safe abbreviation for international units. The handwritten IU looks like IV. Write out international units or use int. units.

6. Q.D. is not a safe abbreviation for once daily, as when the Q is followed by a sloppy dot, it looks like QID which means four times daily.

7. O.D. is not a safe abbreviation for once daily, as it is properly interpreted as meaning "right eye" and has caused liquid medications such as saturated solution of potassium iodide and Lugol's solution to be administered incorrectly. There is no safe abbreviation for once daily. It must be written out in full.

8. Do not use chemical names such as 6-mercaptopurine or 6-thioguanine, as sixfold overdoses have been given when these were not recognized as chemical names. The proper names of these drugs are mercaptopurine or thioguanine.

9. Do not abbreviate drug names (5FC, 6MP, 5-ASA, MTX, HCTZ, CPZ, PBZ, etc) as they are misinterpreted and cause error.

10. Do not use the apothecary system or symbols.

11. Do not abbreviate microgram as µg; instead use mcg as there is less likelihood of misinterpretation.

12. When writing an outpatient prescription, write a complete prescription. A complete prescription can prevent the prescriber, the pharmacist, and/or the patient from making a mistake and can eliminate the need for further clarification. The legible prescriptions should contain:

    a. patient's full name

    b. for pediatric or geriatric patients: their age (or weight where applicable)

    c. drug name, dosage form and strength; if a drug is new or rarely prescribed, print this information

    d. number or amount to be dispensed

    e. complete instructions for the patient, including the purpose of the medication

    f. when there are recognized contraindications for a prescribed drug, indicate to the pharmacist that you are aware of this fact (ie, when prescribing a potassium salt for a patient receiving an ACE inhibitor, write "K serum level being monitored")

*From "Safe Writing" by Davis NM, PharmD and Cohen MR, MS, Lecturers and Consultants for Safe Medication Practices, 1143 Wright Drive, Huntington Valley, PA 19006. Phone: (215) 947-7566.

DISEASE SYNDROMES

see Brain Abscess *on next page*

Immunodeficiency Syndrome *see* Human Immunodeficiency Virus *on*

...sis *see Actinomyces* Species *on page 61*

...angitis *see* Cholangitis, Acute *on page 21*

Acute ...tive Valve Infective Endocarditis *see* Endocarditis, Acute Native Valve *on page 26*

Acute Obstructive Cholangitis *see* Cholangitis, Acute *on page 21*

Acute Sinusitis, Community-Acquired *see* Sinusitis, Community-Acquired, Acute *on page 48*

Acute Suppurative Cholangitis *see* Cholangitis, Acute *on page 21*

Acute Suppurative Otitis *see* Otitis Media, Acute *on page 41*

Amebiasis *see Entamoeba histolytica on page 132*

Animal and Human Bites Guidelines *see page 1061*

Animal Bites *see* Animal and Human Bites Guidelines *on page 1061*

Anthrax *see Bacillus anthracis on page 73*

Antibiotic-Associated Colitis *see Clostridium difficile on page 105*

Antibiotic Treatment of Adults With Infective Endocarditis *see page 1064*

Arthritis, Septic

Synonyms Septic Arthritis

Clinical Presentation The onset of septic arthritis is usually abrupt. Symptoms include chills, fever, and a monarthritis with warmth, swelling, erythema, and tenderness. Ten percent present with polyarthritis. Most commonly affects large joints, especially knees, ankles, and wrists. Presentation may be more indolent in patients with rheumatoid arthritis. Gonococcus is the most common cause of septic arthritis in adults.

Differential Diagnosis Crystal induced; palindromic rheumatism; other infections (ie, tubercular, fungal, viral); tendonitis, bursitis, juvenile rheumatoid arthritis

Likely Pathogens
Neisseria gonorrhoeae on page 215
Staphylococcus aureus, Methicillin-Susceptible *on page 258*

Diagnostic Tests/Procedures
- Aerobic Culture, Body Fluid *on page 310*
- Arthrocentesis *on page 330*
- Biopsy Culture, Routine *on page 337*
- Gram's Stain *on page 426*
  Lyme Disease Serology *on page 481*
  Mycobacteria Culture, Biopsy or Body Fluid *on page 493*
  Neisseria gonorrhoeae Culture *on page 501*

Empiric Drug Therapy
  Recommended
    Oxacillin *on page 849*
      or
    Oxacillin *on page 849*
      used in combination with
    Ceftriaxone *on page 655*
        Note: Ceftriaxone should be used if there is a high suspicion of gonococcal infection from the clinical setting.

Selected Readings
Donatto KC, "Orthopedic Management of Septic Arthritis," *Rheum Dis Clin North Am*, 1998, 24(2):275-86.

Goldenberg DL, "Septic Arthritis," *Lancet*, 1998, 351(9097):197-202.

Pioro MH and Mandell BF, "Septic Arthritis" *Rheum Dis Clin North Am*, 1997, 23(2):239-58.

Shetty AK and Gedalia A, "Septic Arthritis in Children," *Rheum Dis Clin North Am*, 1998, 24(2):287-304.

Athlete's Foot *see Dermatophytes on page 127*
Babesiosis *see Babesia microti on page 71*
Bacillary Angiomatosis *see Bartonella Species on page 76*
Bacterial Vaginosis *see Vaginosis, Bacterial on page 54*
Bilharziasis *see Schistosoma mansoni on page 249*
Blastomycosis *see Blastomyces dermatitidis on page 78*
Blennophthalmia *see Conjunctivitis on page 25*
Botulism *see Clostridium botulinum on page 103*

Brain Abscess

Synonyms Abscess, Brain

Clinical Presentation Brain abscess is an uncommon, serious, life-threatening infection. May originate from a contiguous site of infection (eg, chronic otitis media, mastoiditis, sinusitis, dental infections), from hematogenous spread or trauma, or cryptogenic. Occurs more frequently in males and mid-age. Twenty-five percent occurs in children <15 years of age. Occurs more frequently in children with a history of cyanotic congenital heart disease. Signs and symptoms vary depending on the size and location of abscess. Moderate to severe headache, frequently hemicranial is the most common complaint. Altered mental status, fever, focal neurological deficits, nausea, and vomiting occur approximately in 50%. Papilledema, nuchal rigidity, and seizures occur in 25% to 35%. Children are more likely to experience fever. Duration of symptoms is usually 2 weeks prior to diagnosis. Frontal lobe abscesses are more likely to present with headache, drowsiness, and altered mental status, whereas cerebellar abscesses are more likely to present with ataxia, nystagmus, dysmetria, and vomiting. May have leukocytosis and elevated sedimentation rate. A lumbar puncture is contraindicated due to its poor diagnostic yield and significant morbidity (eg, potential for herniation).

Differential Diagnosis Subdural empyema, epidural abscess, pyogenic meningitis, neoplasm, viral encephalitis, hemorrhagic leukoencephalopathy, CNS vasculitis, infarction, mycotic aneurysm, subdural hematoma

Likely Pathogens
Non-AIDS:
  Streptococcus, Viridans Group *on page 279*
  Staphylococcus aureus, Methicillin-Resistant *on page 256*
  Staphylococcus aureus, Methicillin-Susceptible *on page 258*
  Streptococcus pneumoniae on page 268
  Gram-negative rods and/or polymicrobial infections more common postoperatively or secondary to trauma.
Immunocompromised hosts without AIDS:
  Pseudomonas aeruginosa on page 235
  Nocardia Species *on page 218*
  Mycobacterium kansasii on page 204
  Mycobacterium tuberculosis on page 207
  Mycobacterium Species, Not MTB or MAI *on page 205*
  Mycobacterium avium-intracellulare on page 201
AIDS: The most common cause of a CNS mass lesion:
  Toxoplasma gondii on page 283
  Other etiologies include CNS lymphoma, progressive multifocal leukoencephalopathy, HIV encephalopathy, fungal, mycobacteria, viral, other malignancies

Diagnostic Tests/Procedures
Computed Transaxial Tomography, Appropriate Site *on page 374*
Electroencephalography *on page 397*
Magnetic Resonance Scan, Brain *on page 485*

Drug Therapy Comment Antimicrobials used should have acceptable penetration into brain abscess. Penicillins, cephalosporins, and vancomycin have reasonable penetration into the CSF with inflamed meninges. Chloramphenicol, metronidazole, and sulfonamides penetrate well, with or without inflammation. This information may be moot because alteration of blood-brain barrier occurs in abscess, and brain tissue levels have not been extensively studied.

Empiric Drug Therapy
  Recommended
    Penicillin G, Parenteral, Aqueous *on page 860*
    Cefotaxime *on page 642*
  (Continued)

Brain Abscess *(Continued)*

    used in combination with
    Metronidazole *on page 817*
    Chloramphenicol *on page 667*
AIDS patients:
    Pyrimethamine *on page 886*
    Sulfadiazine *on page 929*
    Folinic Acid
        all 3 used in combination
        or
    Pyrimethamine *on page 886*
    Clindamycin *on page 684*
    Folinic Acid
        all 3 used in combination

Selected Readings
Mathisen GE and Johnson JP, "Brain Abscess," *Clin Infect Dis*, 1997, 25(4):763-79.

Bronchitis

Synonyms Tracheobronchitis

Clinical Presentation Chronic bronchitis may be present in as many as 15% of all adults. Characterized by cough, hypersecretion of mucus, and expectoration of sputum for at least 3 months of the year for more than 2 consecutive years. Acute exacerbations may be either bacterial or viral. Bacterial exacerbations are characterized by increased frequency and severity of cough, increased sputum production, purulent sputum, chest discomfort and congestion, dyspnea and wheezing. Acute bacterial exacerbation in chronic bronchitis is the most common cause of hemoptysis. Patients may experience loss of appetite and feelings of fever and chills; however, true fever, rigors, or pleuritic pain suggest pneumonia. Physical exam may be misleading as some patients with chronic bronchitis always have abnormal breath sounds, and it is helpful to know patient's baseline lung exam.

Differential Diagnosis Chronic bronchitis; chronic obstructive pulmonary disease; emphysema; pneumonia; acute bronchitis

Likely Pathogens
    Influenza Virus *on page 181*
    Respiratory Syncytial Virus *on page 239*
    Adenovirus *on page 62*
    Parainfluenza Virus *on page 220*
    Streptococcus pneumoniae on page 268
    Haemophilus influenzae on page 157
    Moraxella catarrhalis on page 196

Diagnostic Tests/Procedures
    Aerobic Culture, Sputum *on page 312*
    Gram's Stain *on page 426*

Drug Therapy Comment For severe exacerbations of bronchitis in hospitalized patients, intravenous forms of antimicrobial therapy should be used. For mild to moderate recurrent episodes, the various recommended oral antibiotics may be cycled. Symptomatic therapy should be initiated such as cough suppressants and analgesics.

Empiric Drug Therapy
  Recommended
    Amoxicillin *on page 592*
    Co-Trimoxazole *on page 692*
    Doxycycline *on page 713*
    Cephalosporins, 2nd Generation *on page 662*
    Amoxicillin and Clavulanate Potassium *on page 593*

Selected Readings
Grossman RF, "Guidelines for the Treatment of Acute Exacerbations of Chronic Bronchitis," *Chest*, 1997, 112(6 Suppl):310S-3.

Heath JM and Mongia R, "Chronic Bronchitis: Primary Care Management," *Am Fam Physician*, 1998, 57(10):2365-72, 2376-8.

Hueston WJ and Mainous AG 3d, "Acute Bronchitis," *Am Fam Physician*, 1998, 57(6):1270-6, 1281-2.

Isada CM, "Pro: Antibiotics for Chronic Bronchitis With Exacerbations," *Semin Respir Infect*, 1993, 8(4):243-53.

Isada CM and Stoller JK, "Chronic Bronchitis: The Role of Antibiotics," *Respiratory Infections: A Scientific Basis for Management,* Niederman MS, Sarosi GA, and Glassroth J, eds, Orlando FL: WB Saunders, 1994, 621-33.

Wilson R and Rayner CF, "Bronchitis," *Curr Opin Pulm Med,* 1995, 1(3):177-82.

Brucellosis *see Brucella* Species *on page 85*

Bubonic Plague *see Yersinia pestis on page 300*

Candidiasis *see Candida* Species *on page 91*

Catheter Infection, Intravascular

Synonyms Line Sepsis

Clinical Presentation Catheter-related infection refers to an obvious sign of infection at the catheter site such as erythema, induration, or purulence. Catheter-related bacteremia refers to isolation of an organism in a catheter segment culture and in the peripheral blood without any clinical signs of sepsis. Less than 1% of patients go on to develop sepsis; however, if sepsis occurs, there is a 10% to 20% mortality rate. Use of triple-lumen central venous catheters coated with chlorhexidine and silver sulfadiazine appear to offer no benefit over uncoated catheters.

Likely Pathogens
Staphylococcus aureus, Methicillin-Susceptible *on page 258*
Staphylococcus epidermidis, Methicillin-Susceptible *on page 263*
Gram-Negative Bacilli *on page 154*
Enterococcus Species *on page 137*
Candida Species *on page 91*

Diagnostic Tests/Procedures
- Blood Culture, Aerobic and Anaerobic *on page 337*
- Blood Culture, Fungus *on page 341*
- Gram's Stain *on page 426*
- Intravenous Line Culture *on page 464*

Empiric Drug Therapy
Recommended
Vancomycin *on page 967*
used in combination with
Gentamicin *on page 747*
Alternate
Cefazolin *on page 632*
Penicillins, Penicillinase-Resistant *on page 864*

Selected Readings

Clarke DE, Raffin TA, "Infectious Complications of Indwelling Long-Term Central Venous Catheters", *Chest,* 1990, 97(4):966-72.

Cook D, Randolph A, Kernerman P, et al, "Central Venous Catheter Replacement Strategies: A Systematic Review of the Literature," *Crit Care Med,* 1997, 25(8):1417-24.

Farkas JC, Liu N, Bleriot JP, "Single-versus Triple-Lumen Central Catheter-Related Sepsis: A Prospective Randomized Study in a Critically Ill Population," *Am J Med,* 1992, 93(3):277-82.

Groeger JS, Lucas AB, Thaler HT, et al, "Infectious Morbidity Associated With Long-Term Use of Venous Access Devices in Patients With Cancer," *Ann Intern Med,* 1993, 119(12):1168-74.

Heard SO, Wagle M, Vijayakumar E, et al, "Influence of Triple-Lumen Central Venous Catheters Coated With Chlorhexidine and Silver Sulfadiazine on the Incidence of Catheter-Related Bacteremia," *Arch Intern Med,* 1998, 158(1):81-7.

Press OW, Ramsey PG, Larson EB, "Hickman Catheter Infections in Patients With Malignancies," *Medicine (Baltimore),* 1984, 63(4):189-200.

Cat Scratch Disease *see Bartonella* Species *on page 76*

Cellulitis *see* Skin and Soft Tissue *on page 50*

CFS *see* Chronic Fatigue Syndrome *on page 23*

Chancroid *see Haemophilus ducreyi on page 156*

Chickenpox *see* Varicella-Zoster Virus *on page 294*

Cholangitis, Acute

Synonyms Acute Cholangitis; Acute Obstructive Cholangitis; Acute Suppurative Cholangitis; Toxic Cholangitis

Clinical Presentation Caused by infection in an obstructed (most frequently by stones) biliary system. Fifty percent to 100% of patients with Charcot's triad; fever and chills, right upper quadrant pain, and jaundice. Less than 14% present with Reynolds pentad; Charcot's triad plus altered mental status and shock. Fever occurs in 90%, jaundice >60%, abdominal pain >70%, and peritoneal signs 14% to 45%. Majority of patients have leukocytosis and abnormal liver function tests consistent with cholestasis (elevated bilirubin, 2-5 times normal (Continued)

Cholangitis, Acute *(Continued)*

alkaline phosphatase, and mildly elevated transaminases). Bacteremia is common.

Differential Diagnosis Cholecystitis, recurrent cholangitis, AIDS cholangiopathy, sclerosing cholangitis, pancreatitis, right pyelonephritis, right lower lobe pneumonia, perforated duodenal ulcer, pulmonary infarcts

Likely Pathogens

Escherichia coli, Nonenterohemorrhagic *on page 147*
Klebsiella Species *on page 183*
Enterococcus Species *on page 137*
Most often polymicrobial including anaerobes especially:
Bacteroides Species *on page 75*
Clostridium perfringens on page 105
Rarely true pathogen:
Candida Species *on page 91*

Diagnostic Tests/Procedures

Computed Transaxial Tomography, Abdomen Studies *on page 373*
Ultrasound, Abdomen *on page 560*
Laboratory tests should include complete blood count with differential, liver function tests, and coagulation studies. Plain film radiograph of abdomen is abnormal in approximately 15% of patients. Abdominal ultrasound should be performed initially. If cause or site of obstruction is not seen on ultrasound, abdominal CT scan is warranted. If no dilated ducts are noted on ultrasound, then a cholescintigraphy may be needed.

Drug Therapy Comment Given the significant mortality seen in cholangitis, surgery and gastroenterology should be consulted specially if the patient has not responded to medical management within the first 24 hours. Approximately 45% patients will not respond to medical management of I.V. hydration and antibiotics. Percutaneous drainage, endoscopic retrograde cholangiopancreatography for possible endoscopic sphincterotomy, stone extraction and/or placement of indwelling prosthesis, or surgical intervention may be needed.

Empiric Drug Therapy

Recommended

Piperacillin *on page 869*
Aminoglycosides *on page 590*
Metronidazole *on page 817*
  all 3 used in combination
Mezlocillin *on page 820*
Aminoglycosides *on page 590*
Metronidazole *on page 817*
  all 3 used in combination
Ampicillin and Sulbactam *on page 607*
  used in combination with
Aminoglycosides *on page 590*
Ticarcillin and Clavulanate Potassium *on page 950*
  used in combination with
Aminoglycosides *on page 590*
Piperacillin and Tazobactam Sodium *on page 871*
  used in combination with
Aminoglycosides *on page 590*

Alternate

Cephalosporins, 2nd Generation *on page 662*
  or
Cephalosporins, 3rd Generation *on page 662*
  used in combination with
Aminoglycosides *on page 590*
  with or without
Metronidazole *on page 817*
Ciprofloxacin *on page 678*
Aminoglycosides *on page 590*
Metronidazole *on page 817*
  all 3 used in combination

Selected Readings

Hanau LH and Steigbigel NH, "Cholangitis: Pathogenesis, Diagnosis, and Treatment," *Curr Clin Topics Infect Dis*, 1995, 15:153-78.

van den Hazel SJ, Speelman P, Tytgat GN, et al, "Role of Antibiotics in the Treatment and Prevention of Acute and Recurrent Cholangitis," *Clin Infect Dis*, 1994, 19(2):279-86.

Cholera *see Vibrio cholerae on page 297*

Chromoblastomycosis *see* Dematiaceous Fungi *on page 125*

Chromomycosis *see* Dematiaceous Fungi *on page 125*

Chronic Fatigue Syndrome

Synonyms CFS

Clinical Presentation Chronic fatigue syndrome (CFS) is defined clinically as a syndrome characterized by chronic fatigue and a constellation of other symptoms and physical findings. In 1988, the Centers for Disease Control (CDC) developed and published a research case definition. See table.

Chronic Fatigue Syndrome: Case Definition for Researchers

Criteria	Description
Major	Persistent or relapsing fatigue or easy fatigability that does not resolve with bedrest and is severe enough to reduce average daily activity by ≥50%
	Satisfactory exclusion of other chronic conditions, including pre-existing psychiatric diseases
Minor	Mild fever (37.5°C to 38.6°C oral if documented by patient) or chills
	Sore throat
	Lymph node pain in anterior or posterior cervical or axillary chains
	Unexplained, generalized muscle weakness
	Muscle discomfort, myalgia
	Prolonged (≥24 h) generalized fatigue after previously tolerable levels of exercise
	New, generalized headaches
	Migratory, noninflammatory arthralgia
	Neuropsychologic symptoms: photophobia, transient visual scotomata, forgetfulness, excessive irritability, confusion, difficulty thinking, inability to concentrate, or depression
	Sleep disturbance
	Patient's description of initial onset of symptoms as acute or subacute
Physical findings (documented by physician at least twice ≥1 month apart)	Low-grade fever (37.6°C to 38.6°C oral or 37.8°C to 38.8°C rectal)
	Nonexudative pharyngitis
	Palpable or tender anterior or posterior cervical or axillary lymph nodes (<2 cm diameter)

Both major criteria and either ≥6 minor symptom criteria plus ≥2 minor physical criteria or ≥8 minor symptom criteria must occur to fulfill the Centers for Disease Control and Prevention case definition.

Adapted from Holmes GP, Kaplan JE, Gantz NM, et al, "Chronic Fatigue Syndrome: A Working Case Definition," *Ann Intern Med*, 1988, 108:387-9, with permission.

An NIH conference in 1991 further clarified the case definition. In 1995, Lapp and Cheney (see Selected Readings) offered the following case definition for practitioners.

Chronic Fatigue Syndrome: Case Definition for Practitioners

Step 1. Exclude alternative diagnoses and other causes of chronic fatigue.

    a. Alternative diagnoses and other causes of chronic fatigue have been excluded by history, physical examination, exclusionary laboratory tests, and mental status examination.

    b. There is no evidence of major depression or psychosis, an active medical condition, or substance abuse that could explain the presence of fatigue.

Step 2. Does the patient meet two inclusion criteria?

    a. A perception of diminished and finite energy that, when exceeded, demands a substantial change in the usual work- or lifestyle. This fatigue is typically new in onset, evolved over hours or days, and has been persisting or relapsing for at least 6 months. This fatigue is typically brought on by minimal exertion (exertional), and with overexertion fatigue may persist for 24 hours or longer (latent).

    b. The new onset of cognitive dysfunction characterized by short-term memory loss (frequently cannot recall recent conversations or events),

(Continued)

23

Chronic Fatigue Syndrome *(Continued)*

occasional confusion or disorientation, word searching or recall difficulties, diminished comprehension or oral or written information, new difficulty in processing, maintaining or expressing thoughts, difficulty with sequencing of events or numbers (do this, then that, then that, then that), or dyscalculia (difficulty in making change, doing simple mental math, or keeping a checkbook accurately).

Step 3. Does the patient show at least four of eight classic symptoms which have been present chronically or intermittently for at least 6 months, make up a significant component of the illness, but have not predated the fatigue?

- feverish feelings or chills or chilliness
- pharyngitis: nonexudative, "scratchy" or sore throat, frequent or relapsing in nature
- lymphatic soreness or swelling: lymphodynia or lymphadenopathy in at least two sites: lingual, anterior cervical, posterior cervical, supraclavicular, axillary, or inguinal
- muscle discomfort of a generalized nature: flu-like myalgias or tenderness to touch (allodynia or "touch-me-not")
- generalized weakness: may be just a weighty or "rag doll" feeling or may actually be physical weakness manifested, for example, by decreased grip strength, difficulty in going up stairs, or outstretched arms tiring quickly
- joint discomfort (arthralgias): usually migratory and involving large joints such as knees, hips, and elbows more than small joints such as fingers and toes
- new-onset pressure-like headaches: frequently retro-orbital or occipital and worsening with stress or exertion
- difficulty in initiating and maintaining sleep ("exhausted but cannot sleep") or hypersomnolence (at least 12 hours per night plus daily naps)

Subcategorization

Onset of illness (when did the illness start - date or period of time?)
   a. Abrupt onset over hours or days
   b. Gradual or insidious onset

Severity of symptoms
   a. Minimal: some symptoms, especially with effort; usually able to work
   b. Mild: mild symptoms with limitations, even at rest; may be able to work
   c. Moderate: moderate symptoms at rest, worse with effort; unable to work
   d. Severe: often housebound or bedbound

Final Clinical Impression

   a. Patient meets criteria for the chronic fatigue syndrome (CFS)
   b. CFS is probable or possible but confounded by a concurrent medical or psychiatric condition or lacks sufficient criteria
   c. Idiopathic chronic fatigue: chronic fatigue syndrome unlikely or excluded by ....

The relationship between chronic fatigue syndrome and defined neuropsychiatric syndromes is particularly important. Anxiety disorders, somatoform disorders, major depression, and other symptomatically defined syndromes are characterized by profound fatigue. Some of the features of chronic fatigue may represent deconditioning due to physical inactivity associated commonly with a diverse group of illnesses.

Whether chronic fatigue syndrome is viral, postviral, immune, allergic, psychological, or idiopathic remains to be determined. The high incidence of concurrent psychiatric symptoms compounds the difficulties encountered in the diagnosis and management of CFS.

The diagnosis of chronic fatigue syndrome is one of exclusion. It is established only after other medical and psychiatric causes of chronic fatigue illness have been ruled out.

Diagnostic Tests/Procedures No specific tests or pathognomonic signs for CFS have been validated. Bates et al observed statistically significant differences from control populations for the following analytes.

- Immune complexes ≥0.23 g/L
- Immunoglobulin G ≥12.5 g/L

- Antinuclear antibody titer ≥1:40
- Alkaline phosphatase ≥89 units/L
- Cholesterol ≥200 mg/dL (≥5.17 mmol/L)
- Lactic dehydrogenase ≥196 units/L
- Atypical lymphocyte count ≥2%

Other tests which are commonly performed include ALT, AST, CBC, sedimentation rate, and TSH. The immunologic abnormalities are consistent with the concept that a chronic low level activation of the immune system is a common finding in CFS. Pursuit of both objective physical and laboratory abnormalities in more loosely defined cases of fatigue has been relatively nonrewarding.

Drug Therapy Comment No specific therapy has been defined for CFS. Clinical care integrating medical and psychological management concepts, as well as symptomatic management, may prevent significant secondary impairment.

Selected Readings

Bates DW, Buchwald D, Lee J, et al, "A Comparison of Case Definitions of Chronic Fatigue Syndrome," *Clin Infect Dis*, 1994, 18(Suppl 1):S11-5.

Bates DW, Buchwald D, Lee J, et al, "Clinical Laboratory Test Findings in Patients With Chronic Fatigue Syndrome," *Arch Intern Med*, 1995, 155(1):97-103.

Fukuda K, Straus SE, Hickie I, et al, "The Chronic Fatigue Syndrome: A Comprehensive Approach to Its Definition and Study," *Ann Intern Med*, 1994, 121(12):953-9.

Holmes GP, Kaplan JE, Gantz NM, et al, "Chronic Fatigue Syndrome: A Working Case Definition," *Ann Intern Med*, 1988, 108(3):387-9.

Katon W and Russo J, "Chronic Fatigue Syndrome Criteria. A Critique of the Requirement for Multiple Physical Complaints," *Arch Intern Med*, 1992, 152(8):1604-9.

Kim E, "A Brief History of Chronic Fatigue Syndrome," *JAMA*, 1994, 272(13):1070-1.

Lane TJ, Matthews DA, and Manu P, "The Low Yield of Physical Examinations and Laboratory Investigations of Patients With Chronic Fatigue," *Am J Med Sci*, 1990, 299(5):313-8.

Lapp CW and Cheney PR, "The Chronic Fatigue Syndrome," *Ann Intern Med*, 1995, 123(1):74-5.

Manu P, Lane TJ, and Matthews DA, "Chronic Fatigue and Chronic Fatigue Syndrome: Clinical Epidemiology and Aetiological Classification," *Chronic Fatigue Syndrome*, Ciba Foundation Symposium 173, Wiley, Chichester, 1993, 23-42.

Schlueberberg A, Straus SE, Peterson P, et al, "Chronic Fatigue Syndrome Research: Definition and Medical Outcome Assessment," *Ann Intern Med*, 1992, 117(4):325-31.

Straus SE, Komaroff AL, and Wedner HJ, "Chronic Fatigue Syndrome: Point and Counterpoint," *J Infect Dis*, 1994, 170(1):1-6.

Wilson A, Hickie I, Lloyd A, et al, "The Treatment of Chronic Fatigue Syndrome: Science and Speculation," *Am J Med*, 1994, 96(6):544-50.

Chronic Sinusitis, Community-Acquired *see* Sinusitis, Community-Acquired, Chronic *on page 49*

Clinical Syndromes Associated With Foodborne Diseases *see page 1068*

Coccidioidomycosis *see Coccidioides immitis on page 109*

Colorado Tick Fever *see* Arboviruses *on page 67*

Community-Acquired Pneumonia in Adults *see page 1070*

Community-Acquired Sinusitis, Acute *see* Sinusitis, Community-Acquired, Acute *on page 48*

Community-Acquired Sinusitis, Chronic *see* Sinusitis, Community-Acquired, Chronic *on page 49*

Conjunctivitis

Synonyms Blennophthalmia; Koch-Weeks; Pink Eye; Red Eye

Clinical Presentation Inflammation of the conjunctiva associated with marked hyperemia and mucopurulent or watery discharge. The hyperemia is less intense in the perilimbal region as compared to ciliary flush.

Differential Diagnosis Conjunctivitis - allergic, viral, bacterial, granulomatous; iritis/iridocyclitis; herpes simplex keratitis; acute angle-closure glaucoma; episcleritis; scleritis; subconjunctival hemorrhage; pterygium; foreign body/abrasions

Likely Pathogens
Adenovirus *on page 62*
Chlamydia trachomatis *on page 99*
Herpes Simplex Virus *on page 170*
Staphylococcus aureus, Methicillin-Susceptible *on page 258*
Neisseria gonorrhoeae *on page 215*
Haemophilus influenzae *on page 157*
Streptococcus pneumoniae *on page 268*

Diagnostic Tests/Procedures
Aerobic Culture, Appropriate Site *on page 310*
(Continued)

Conjunctivitis *(Continued)*

Adenovirus Culture *on page 309*
Chlamydia Culture *on page 359*
Gram's Stain *on page 426*
Herpes Simplex Virus Culture *on page 446*
Ocular Cytology *on page 505*

Drug Therapy Comment Treatment should be based on suspected organism diagnosed. Many of the ophthalmic anti-infective agents are combined with steroids for their anti-inflammatory activity.

Selected Readings
Gausas RE and Rapoza PA, "Red Eye: Serious or Not?" *Hosp Med,* December, 1992, 63-72.

Croup *see Parainfluenza Virus on page 220*

Cryptococcosis *see Cryptococcus neoformans on page 117*

Cryptosporidiosis *see Cryptosporidium on page 119*

Darling's Disease *see Histoplasma capsulatum on page 173*

Dermatomycoses *see Dermatophytes on page 127*

Desert Rheumatism *see Coccidioides immitis on page 109*

Diphtheria *see Corynebacterium diphtheriae on page 111*

Dysentery *see Shigella Species on page 251*

Ehrlichiosis *see Ehrlichia Species on page 130*

Endocarditis, Acute, I.V. Drug Abuse

Related Information

Antibiotic Treatment of Adults With Infective Endocarditis *on page 1064*
Prevention of Bacterial Endocarditis *on page 1096*

Clinical Presentation In acute left-side bacterial endocarditis, patients typically present with high fever and rapid valvular dysfunction resulting in congestive heart failure or arrhythmias. In acute right-sided endocarditis, patients appear ill with fever, have pulmonary infiltrates, and have the murmur of tricuspid or pulmonary insufficiency. Patients that "wash" needles with fresh lemon are at risk of *Candida* endocarditis.

Likely Pathogens

Pseudomonas aeruginosa on page 235
Staphylococcus aureus, Methicillin-Susceptible *on page 258*
Staphylococcus aureus, Methicillin-Resistant *on page 256*
Candida Species *on page 91*

Diagnostic Tests/Procedures

- Blood Culture, Aerobic and Anaerobic *on page 337*
- Chest Films *on page 359*
- Gram's Stain *on page 426*
  Blood Culture, Fungus *on page 341*
  C-Reactive Protein *on page 378*
  Echocardiography, M-Mode *on page 395*
  Sedimentation Rate, Erythrocyte *on page 532*
  Serum Bactericidal Test *on page 533*
  Transesophageal Echocardiography *on page 553*

Empiric Drug Therapy

Recommended

Vancomycin *on page 967*
used in combination with
Gentamicin *on page 747*

Selected Readings
Chambers HF, "Short-Course Combination and Oral Therapies of *Staphylococcus aureus* Endocarditis," *Infect Dis Clin North Am,* 1993, 7(1):69-80.
Cherubin CE and Sapira JD, "The Medical Complications of Drug Addiction and the Medical Assessment of the Intravenous Drug User: 25 Years Later," *Ann Intern Med,* 1993, 119(10):1017-28.

Endocarditis, Acute Native Valve

Related Information

Antibiotic Treatment of Adults With Infective Endocarditis *on page 1064*
Prevention of Bacterial Endocarditis *on page 1096*

Synonyms Acute Native Valve Infective Endocarditis

Clinical Presentation Between 60% and 80% of patients have a pre-existing cardiac lesion such as rheumatic valvular disease, congenital heart disease, or degenerative heart disease.

In acute left-side bacterial endocarditis, patients typically present with high fever and rapid valvular dysfunction resulting in congestive heart failure or arrhythmias. In acute right-sided endocarditis, patients appear ill with fever, have pulmonary infiltrates, and have the murmur of tricuspid or pulmonary insufficiency.

Likely Pathogens
Staphylococcus aureus, Methicillin-Susceptible *on page 258*
Streptococcus pneumoniae on page 268
Neisseria gonorrhoeae on page 215

Diagnostic Tests/Procedures
- Blood Culture, Aerobic and Anaerobic *on page 337*
- Echocardiography, M-Mode *on page 395*
- Gram's Stain *on page 426*
  C-Reactive Protein *on page 378*
  Sedimentation Rate, Erythrocyte *on page 532*
  Serum Bactericidal Test *on page 533*
  Transesophageal Echocardiography *on page 553*

Empiric Drug Therapy
Recommended
  Penicillins, Penicillinase-Resistant *on page 864*
    used in combination with
  Gentamicin *on page 747*
Alternate
  Vancomycin *on page 967*
    used in combination with
  Gentamicin *on page 747*

Selected Readings

Bansal RC, "Infective Endocarditis," *Med Clin North Am*, 1995, 79(5):1205-40.

Dajani AS, Taubert KA, Wilson W, et al, "Prevention of Bacterial Endocarditis. Recommendations by the American Heart Association," *JAMA*, 1997, 277(22):1794-801.

Durack DT, Lukes AS, and Bright DK, "New Criteria for Diagnosis of Infective Endocarditis: Utilization of Specific Echocardiographic Findings. Duke Endocarditis Service," *Am J Med*, 1994, 96(3):200-9.

Lamas CC and Eykyn SJ, "Suggested Modifications to the Duke Criteria for the Clinical Diagnosis of Native Valve and Prosthetic Valve Endocarditis: Analysis of 118 Pathologically Proven Cases," *Clin Infect Dis*, 1997, 25(3):713-9.

Wilson WR, Karchmer AW, Dajani AS, et al, "Antibiotic Treatment of Adults With Infective Endocarditis Due to Streptococci, Enterococci, Staphylococci and HACEK Microorganisms. American Heart Association," *JAMA*, 1995, 274(21):1706-13.

Endocarditis, Prosthetic Valve, Early

Related Information
  Antibiotic Treatment of Adults With Infective Endocarditis *on page 1064*
  Prevention of Bacterial Endocarditis *on page 1096*

Synonyms Prosthetic Valve Endocarditis, Early; PVE, Early

Clinical Presentation Occurs within 60 days of surgery and is a consequence of valve contamination or bacteremia perioperatively. This usually presents as an acute event. In left sided early prosthetic valve endocarditis, patients typically present with high fever and rapid valvular dysfunction resulting in congestive heart failure or arrhythmias. In right sided disease, patients appear ill with fever, have pulmonary infiltrates, and have insufficiency murmurs.

Likely Pathogens
Staphylococcus epidermidis, Methicillin-Susceptible *on page 263*
Staphylococcus epidermidis, Methicillin-Resistant *on page 261*
Staphylococcus aureus, Methicillin-Susceptible *on page 258*
Staphylococcus aureus, Methicillin-Resistant *on page 256*
Gram-Negative Bacilli *on page 154*
Candida Species *on page 91*

Diagnostic Tests/Procedures
- Blood Culture, Aerobic and Anaerobic *on page 337*
- Gram's Stain *on page 426*
  Blood Culture, Fungus *on page 341*
  C-Reactive Protein *on page 378*
  Echocardiography, M-Mode *on page 395*
(Continued)

Endocarditis, Prosthetic Valve, Early *(Continued)*

Sedimentation Rate, Erythrocyte *on page 532*
Serum Bactericidal Test *on page 533*
Transesophageal Echocardiography *on page 553*

Empiric Drug Therapy

Recommended

Vancomycin *on page 967*
used in combination with
Gentamicin *on page 747*

Selected Readings

Bansal RC, "Infective Endocarditis," *Med Clin North Am*, 1995, 79(5):1205-40.

Lamas CC and Eykyn SJ, "Suggested Modifications to the Duke Criteria for the Clinical Diagnosis of Native Valve and Prosthetic Valve Endocarditis: Analysis of 118 Pathologically Proven Cases," *Clin Infect Dis*, 1997, 25(3):713-9.

Wilson WR, Karchmer AW, Dajani AS, et al, "Antibiotic Treatment of Adults With Infective Endocarditis Due to Streptococci, Enterococci, Staphylococci, and HACEK Microorganisms. American Heart Association," *JAMA*, 1995, 274(21):1706-13.

Endocarditis, Prosthetic Valve, Late

Related Information

Antibiotic Treatment of Adults With Infective Endocarditis *on page 1064*
Prevention of Bacterial Endocarditis *on page 1096*

Synonyms Prosthetic Valve Endocarditis, Late; PVE, Late

Clinical Presentation Occurs more than 60 days after valve surgery. This usually presents as an acute event. In left sided late prosthetic valve endocarditis, patients typically present with high fever and rapid valvular dysfunction resulting in congestive heart failure or arrhythmias. In right sided disease, patients appear ill with fever, have pulmonary infiltrates, and have insufficiency murmurs.

Likely Pathogens

Streptococcus, Viridans Group *on page 279*
Staphylococcus epidermidis, Methicillin-Susceptible *on page 263*
Staphylococcus epidermidis, Methicillin-Resistant *on page 261*

Diagnostic Tests/Procedures

- Blood Culture, Aerobic and Anaerobic *on page 337*
- Gram's Stain *on page 426*
C-Reactive Protein *on page 378*
Echocardiography, M-Mode *on page 395*
Sedimentation Rate, Erythrocyte *on page 532*
Serum Bactericidal Test *on page 533*
Transesophageal Echocardiography *on page 553*

Empiric Drug Therapy

Recommended

Vancomycin *on page 967*
used in combination with
Gentamicin *on page 747*

Selected Readings

Bansal RC, "Infective Endocarditis," *Med Clin North Am*, 1995, 79(5):1205-40.

Lamas CC and Eykyn SJ, "Suggested Modifications to the Duke Criteria for the Clinical Diagnosis of Native Valve and Prosthetic Valve Endocarditis: Analysis of 118 Pathologically Proven Cases," *Clin Infect Dis*, 1997, 25(3):713-9.

Wilson WR, Karchmer AW, Dajani AS, et al, "Antibiotic Treatment of Adults With Infective Endocarditis Due to Streptococci, Enterococci, Staphylococci, and HACEK Microorganisms. American Heart Association," *JAMA*, 1995, 274(21):1706-13.

Endocarditis, Subacute Native Valve

Related Information

Antibiotic Treatment of Adults With Infective Endocarditis *on page 1064*
Prevention of Bacterial Endocarditis *on page 1096*

Clinical Presentation Symptoms generally begin approximately 2 weeks after precipitating event. Onset is gradual with low-grade fever, malaise, and arthralgias. Cardiac murmur is usually present. May present with splenomegaly, petechia, splinter hemorrhages, Roth spots, Osler nodes, Janeway lesions, and clubbing. Embolic events, mycotic aneurysms, brain abscesses, meningitis, and renal disease may occur.

Differential Diagnosis Acute rheumatic fever; lupus erythematosus and other collagen vascular diseases; sickle cell; nonbacterial thrombotic endocarditis; malignancy; tuberculosis

Likely Pathogens
Streptococcus, Viridans Group on page 279
Enterococcus Species on page 137
HACEK Group on page 155
Streptococcus bovis on page 267

Diagnostic Tests/Procedures
- Blood Culture, Aerobic and Anaerobic on page 337
- Gram's Stain on page 426
  Chest Films on page 359
  C-Reactive Protein on page 378
  Echocardiography, M-Mode on page 395
  Q Fever Serology on page 525
  Sedimentation Rate, Erythrocyte on page 532
  Serum Bactericidal Test on page 533
  Transesophageal Echocardiography on page 553

Empiric Drug Therapy
Recommended
Gentamicin on page 747
  used in combination with
Penicillin G, Parenteral, Aqueous on page 860
Alternate
Vancomycin on page 967
  used in combination with
Gentamicin on page 747
  or
Penicillin G, Parenteral, Aqueous on page 860
  used in combination with
Gentamicin on page 747
  or
Ampicillin on page 604
  used in combination with
Gentamicin on page 747

Selected Readings
Bansal RC, "Infective Endocarditis," Med Clin North Am, 1995, 79(5):1205-40.
Dajani AS, Taubert KA, Wilson W, et al, "Prevention of Bacterial Endocarditis. Recommendations by the American Heart Association," JAMA, 1997, 277(22):1794-801.
Durack DT, Lukes AS, and Bright DK, "New Criteria for Diagnosis of Infective Endocarditis: Utilization of Specific Echocardiographic Findings. Duke Endocarditis Service," Am J Med, 1994, 96(3):200-9.
Lamas CC and Eykyn SJ, "Suggested Modifications to the Duke Criteria for the Clinical Diagnosis of Native Valve and Prosthetic Valve Endocarditis: Analysis of 118 Pathologically Proven Cases," Clin Infect Dis, 1997, 25(3):713-9.
Wilson WR, Karchmer AW, Dajani AS, et al, "Antibiotic Treatment of Adults With Infective Endocarditis Due to Streptococci, Enterococci, Staphylococci and HACEK Microorganisms. American Heart Association," JAMA, 1995, 274(21):1706-13.

Epiglottitis

Synonyms Supraglottitis

Clinical Presentation Acute epiglottitis is a rapidly progressive inflammation/ cellulitis of the epiglottis which may cause airway obstruction. Small children typically present with fever and dysphagia, while older children and adults complain of sore throat. Inspiratory stridor and hoarseness occur frequently, and patients may present with drooling. Diagnosis is confirmed by the presence of an edematous "cherry red" epiglottis which should be visualized in a controlled environment in which one should be able to secure the airway.

Differential Diagnosis Croup; diphtheria; allergic laryngeal edema; foreign body aspiration; abscess - retropharyngeal, peritonsillar

Likely Pathogens
Children:
  Haemophilus influenzae on page 157
Adults:
  Streptococcus pyogenes on page 274

Diagnostic Tests/Procedures
Aerobic Culture, Appropriate Site on page 310
(Continued)

Epiglottitis *(Continued)*

Group A *Streptococcus* Antigen Test *on page 428*
Throat Culture for Group A Beta-Hemolytic *Streptococcus on page 550*
Empiric Drug Therapy
Recommended
Children:
Cephalosporins, 2nd Generation *on page 662*
Cephalosporins, 3rd Generation *on page 662*
Adults:
Cephalosporins, 2nd Generation *on page 662*

Erythema Infectiosum *see* Parvovirus B19 *on page 222*

European Blastomycosis *see Cryptococcus neoformans on page 117*

Exanthem Subitum *see* Human Herpesvirus-6 *on page 175*

Fasciitis *see* Skin and Soft Tissue *on page 50*

Fever, Neutropenic

Clinical Presentation Classically, patients present with absolute neutropenia and fever without evidence of source either by history or physical examination. Generally lack symptoms of sweats and rigors.

Differential Diagnosis Infections - bacterial, viral, fungal, parasitic; drug associated; malignancy, especially lymphoma, leukemia

Likely Pathogens
Gram-Negative Bacilli *on page 154*
Staphylococcus aureus, Methicillin-Susceptible *on page 258*
Staphylococcus epidermidis, Methicillin-Susceptible *on page 263*
Candida Species *on page 91*
Streptococcus Species *on page 279*
Enterococcus Species *on page 137*

Diagnostic Tests/Procedures
• Aerobic Culture, Sputum *on page 312*
• Blood Culture, Aerobic and Anaerobic *on page 337*
• Blood Culture, Fungus *on page 341*
• Intravenous Line Culture *on page 464*
• Gram's Stain *on page 426*
• Urine Culture, Clean Catch *on page 565*

Empiric Drug Therapy
Recommended
Vancomycin *on page 967*
used in combination with
Ceftazidime *on page 651*
Cefepime *on page 634*
Ceftazidime *on page 651*
Imipenem and Cilastatin *on page 766*
Meropenem *on page 812*
Aminoglycosides *on page 590*
used in combination with
Piperacillin *on page 869*

Selected Readings
Hughes WT, Armstrong D, Bodey GP, et al, "1997 Guidelines for the Use of Antimicrobial Agents in Neutropenic Patients With Unexplained Fever. Infectious Diseases Society of America," *Clin Infect Dis*, 1997, 25(3):551-73.

Fifth Disease *see* Parvovirus B19 *on page 222*

Food Poisoning Table *see page 1068*

Gardener's Disease *see Sporothrix schenckii on page 253*

Gastroenteritis, Bacterial

Clinical Presentation Patients with bacterial gastroenteritis frequently present with lower gastrointestinal symptoms (diarrhea) with or without fever. Patients less likely present with primary upper gastrointestinal symptoms (ie, vomiting). The presence of bloody diarrhea suggests a bacterial pathogen, although *C. difficile* is usually nonhemorrhagic. It is impossible to separate different pathogens based on clinical diagnosis alone.

Differential Diagnosis Gastroenteritis, viral; drug toxicity; inflammatory bowel disease; parasitic gastroenteritis (eg, *Giardia*, cryptosporidia, microsporidia)

Likely Pathogens
Campylobacter jejuni on page 90
Salmonella Species *on page 245*
Shigella Species *on page 251*
Escherichia coli, Enterohemorrhagic *on page 143*
Clostridium difficile on page 105

Diagnostic Tests/Procedures
Stool Culture *on page 540*
Stool Culture, Diarrheagenic *E. coli on page 542*
Stool Culture, Uncommon Organisms *on page 543*
Clostridium difficile Toxin Assay *on page 367*

Drug Therapy Comment Drug therapy based on identification of the causative agent.

Selected Readings
Boone JH and Carman RJ, "*Clostridium perfringens*: Food Poisoning and Antibiotic-Associated Diarrhea," *Clin Microbiol Newslett*, 1997, 19(9):65-7.

Guerrant RL, Shields DA, Thorson SM, et al, "Evaluation and Diagnosis of Acute Infectious Diarrhea," *Am J Med*, 1985, 78(6B):91-8.

Kaspar CW and Weiss R, "Bacterial Foodborne Illness - The Unwanted Dinner Guest," *Clin Microbiol Newslett*, 1998, 20(19):161-4.

Novak SM, "Foodborne Illness - Chemical Fish and Shellfish Poisoning," *Clin Microbiol Newslett*, 1998, 20(3).

Siegel DL, Edelstein PH, Nachamkin I, "Inappropriate Testing for Diarrheal Diseases in the Hospital," *JAMA*, 1990, 263(7):979-82.

Gastroenteritis, Viral

Clinical Presentation Patients with viral gastroenteritis may present with upper gastrointestinal symptoms (vomiting), lower gastrointestinal symptoms (diarrhea), or both. Stools tend to be nonhemorrhagic. Viral gastroenteritis is much more common than bacterial gastroenteritis.

Differential Diagnosis Gastroenteritis, bacterial; drug toxicity; inflammatory bowel disease; parasitic gastroenteritis (eg, *Giardia*, cryptosporidia, microsporidia)

Likely Pathogens
Rotavirus *on page 244*

Diagnostic Tests/Procedures
Viral Culture, Stool *on page 573*
Rotavirus, Direct Detection *on page 529*
Enterovirus Culture *on page 405*

Drug Therapy Comment No antiviral agents have been proven to be effective in the treatment of rotavirus infections. Supportive therapy is recommended.

Selected Readings
Guerrant RL, Shields DA, Thorson SM, et al, "Evaluation and Diagnosis of Acute Infectious Diarrhea," *Am J Med*, 1985, 78(6B):91-8.

Hedberg CW and Osterholm MT, "Outbreaks of Food-Borne and Waterborne Viral Gastroenteritis," *Clin Microbiol Rev*, 1993, 6(3):199-210.

Kapikian AZ, "Overview of Viral Gastroenteritis," *Arch Virol*, 1996, 12:7-19.

Lifschitz CH, "Treatment of Acute Diarrhea in Children," *Curr Opin Pediatr*, 1997, 9(5):498-501.

Siegel DL, Edelstein PH, Nachamkin I, "Inappropriate Testing for Diarrheal Diseases in the Hospital," *JAMA*, 1990, 263(7):979-82.

Genital HSV *see* Herpes Simplex Virus *on page 170*

Giardiasis *see* Giardia lamblia *on page 153*

Gilchrist's Disease *see* Blastomyces dermatitidis *on page 78*

Gonorrhea *see* Neisseria gonorrhoeae *on page 215*

Granuloma Inguinale *see* Calymmatobacterium granulomatis *on page 89*

Hepatitis

Clinical Presentation See individual organisms for clinical presentation information.

Likely Pathogens
Hepatitis A Virus *on page 161*
Hepatitis B Virus *on page 162*
Hepatitis C Virus *on page 164*
Hepatitis D Virus *on page 168*
Hepatitis E Virus *on page 169*
Epstein-Barr Virus *on page 141*
(Continued)

Hepatitis *(Continued)*

Cytomegalovirus *on page 122*

Diagnostic Tests/Procedures

Hepatitis A Profile *on page 434*
Hepatitis B Profile *on page 435*
Hepatitis C Serology *on page 437*
Hepatitis D Serology *on page 442*
Epstein-Barr Virus Serology *on page 406*
Cytomegalovirus Serology *on page 392*

Drug Therapy Comment Drug therapy based on identification of the causative agent.

Histoplasmosis *see Histoplasma capsulatum on page 173*

Human Bites *see Animal and Human Bites Guidelines on page 1061*

Impetigo

Clinical Presentation Impetigo is a contagious superficial pyoderma caused by staphylococci and/or streptococci that typically begins as a solitary vesicle ruptures and forms a thick, yellow, honey-colored crust. Patients usually present after multiple lesions occur, most frequently on the face. A superficial glistening base is seen under the crust and no ulcerations are present.

Differential Diagnosis Secondary bacterial infection; ecthyma; herpes simplex, late stage; inflammatory fungal infections

Likely Pathogens

Streptococcus pyogenes on page 274
Staphylococcus aureus, Methicillin-Susceptible *on page 258*

Diagnostic Tests/Procedures

Aerobic Culture, Appropriate Site *on page 310*

Empiric Drug Therapy

Recommended

Penicillin V Potassium *on page 865*
Erythromycin *on page 722*
Cephalosporins, 1st Generation *on page 661*
Mupirocin *on page 825*

Influenza *see Influenza Virus on page 181*

Jock Itch *see Dermatophytes on page 127*

Joint Replacement, Early Infection

Clinical Presentation Most patients present with a long indolent course characterized by progressive increase in joint pain and occasional draining sinuses. May present with acute joint sepsis characterized by high fever, severe joint pain with localized warmth, swelling, and edema.

Differential Diagnosis Hemarthrosis; gout; bland loosening; dislocation

Likely Pathogens

Staphylococcus epidermidis, Methicillin-Resistant *on page 261*
Staphylococcus epidermidis, Methicillin-Susceptible *on page 263*
Staphylococcus aureus, Methicillin-Susceptible *on page 258*
Pseudomonas aeruginosa on page 235

Diagnostic Tests/Procedures

• Aerobic Culture, Body Fluid *on page 310*
• Arthrocentesis *on page 330*
• Biopsy Culture, Routine *on page 337*
• Blood Culture, Aerobic and Anaerobic *on page 337*
• Gram's Stain *on page 426*
Arthrogram *on page 334*
C-Reactive Protein *on page 378*
Sedimentation Rate, Erythrocyte *on page 532*

Empiric Drug Therapy

Recommended

Vancomycin *on page 967*

Alternate

Penicillins, Penicillinase-Resistant *on page 864*
Ceftriaxone *on page 655*

Selected Readings
Berbari EF, Hanssen AD, Duffy MC, et al, "Prosthetic Joint Infection Due to *Mycobacterium tuberculosis*: A Case Series and Review of the Literature," *Am J Orthop*, 1998, 27(3):219-27.

Berbari EF, Hanssen AD, Duffy MC, et al, "Risk Factors for Prosthetic Joint Infection: Case-Control Study," *Clin Infect Dis*, 1998, 27(5):1247-54.

Gillespie WJ, "Prevention and Management of Infection After Total Joint Replacement," *Clin Infect Dis*, 1997, 25(6):1310-7.

Joint Replacement, Late Infection

Clinical Presentation Most patients present with a long indolent course characterized by progressive increase in joint pain and occasional draining sinuses. May present with acute joint sepsis characterized by high fever, severe joint pain with localized warmth, swelling, and edema.

Differential Diagnosis Hemarthrosis; gout; bland loosening; dislocation

Likely Pathogens
> *Staphylococcus epidermidis*, Methicillin-Resistant *on page 261*
> *Staphylococcus epidermidis*, Methicillin-Susceptible *on page 263*
> *Staphylococcus aureus*, Methicillin-Susceptible *on page 258*

Diagnostic Tests/Procedures
- Aerobic Culture, Body Fluid *on page 310*
- Arthrocentesis *on page 330*
- Biopsy Culture, Routine *on page 337*
- Blood Culture, Aerobic and Anaerobic *on page 337*
- Gram's Stain *on page 426*
  Arthrogram *on page 334*
  C-Reactive Protein *on page 378*
  Sedimentation Rate, Erythrocyte *on page 532*

Empiric Drug Therapy
Recommended
> Vancomycin *on page 967*
Alternate
> Penicillins, Penicillinase-Resistant *on page 864*

Selected Readings
Berbari EF, Hanssen AD, Duffy MC, et al, "Prosthetic Joint Infection Due to *Mycobacterium tuberculosis*: A Case Series and Review of the Literature," *Am J Orthop*, 1998, 27(3):219-27.

Berbari EF, Hanssen AD, Duffy MC, et al, "Risk Factors for Prosthetic Joint Infection: Case-Control Study," *Clin Infect Dis*, 1998, 27(5):1247-54.

Gillespie WJ, "Prevention and Management of Infection After Total Joint Replacement," *Clin Infect Dis*, 1997, 25(6):1310-7.

Koch-Weeks *see* Conjunctivitis *on page 25*

Legionellosis *see* Legionella pneumophila *on page 185*

Legionnaires' Disease *see* Legionella pneumophila *on page 185*

Leptospirosis *see* Leptospira interrogans *on page 186*

Line Sepsis *see* Catheter Infection, Intravascular *on page 21*

Listeriosis *see* Listeria monocytogenes *on page 189*

Lumpy Jaw Syndrome *see* Actinomyces Species *on page 61*

Lyme Borreliosis *see* Borrelia burgdorferi *on page 84*

Lyme Disease *see* Borrelia burgdorferi *on page 84*

Lymphadenitis

Clinical Presentation Can be regional or diffuse depending on the causative organism. Lymph nodes are usually swollen and tender.

Differential Diagnosis Depends on the site of the enlarged node.

Generalized lymphadenopathy: HIV; scarlet fever (group A *Streptococcus*); miliary tuberculosis; brucellosis; syphilis; cat scratch disease; histoplasmosis; lymphogranuloma venereum (LGV); virus (CMV, EBV); toxoplasmosis; Whipple's disease; lymphoma

Inguinal adenopathy: Syphilis; LGV; chancroid; bacterial

Cervical adenopathy: Bacterial (*Streptococcus*); *Staphylococcus aureus*; tuberculosis; MAI; cat scratch disease; lymphoma; Kawasaki syndrome; sarcoidosis kikuchi's; others

Likely Pathogens
> *Toxoplasma gondii on page 283*
> *Mycobacterium* Species, Not MTB or MAI *on page 205*
> *Bartonella* Species *on page 76*
> (Continued)

Lymphadenitis *(Continued)*

Human Immunodeficiency Virus *on page 177*
Staphylococcus aureus, Methicillin-Susceptible *on page 258*
Epstein-Barr Virus *on page 141*

Diagnostic Tests/Procedures Diagnostic tests should be obtained based on clinical suspicion since not all tests are necessary.

Abscess Aerobic and Anaerobic Culture *on page 304*
Epstein-Barr Virus Serology *on page 406*
HIV-1 Serology *on page 454*
Lymph Node Biopsy *on page 482*
Mycobacteria Culture, Biopsy or Body Fluid *on page 493*
Toxoplasma Serology *on page 552*

Drug Therapy Comment Drug therapy based on identification of the causative agent.

Maduromycosis *see Dematiaceous Fungi on page 125*

Malaria *see Plasmodium Species on page 227*

Measles *see Measles Virus on page 193*

Meningitis, Community-Acquired, Adult

Clinical Presentation Patients present with fever, headache, nausea, vomiting, and nuchal rigidity. Focal neurologic abnormalities and papilledema are uncommon.

Differential Diagnosis Bacterial, viral, or other infectious agents; drug-induced; neoplastic; granulomatous; infectious endocarditis; collagen-vascular diseases; subdural hemorrhage; subarachnoid hemorrhage

Likely Pathogens

Haemophilus influenzae on page 157
Neisseria meningitidis on page 217
Streptococcus pneumoniae on page 268
Listeria monocytogenes(elderly, immunocompromised) *on page 189*

Diagnostic Tests/Procedures

- Blood Culture, Aerobic and Anaerobic *on page 337*
- Cerebrospinal Fluid Analysis *on page 354*
- Gram's Stain *on page 426*
- Lumbar Puncture *on page 477*
  Computed Transaxial Tomography, Head Studies *on page 374*
  Cryptococcal Antigen Serology, Serum or Cerebrospinal Fluid *on page 379*
  Enterovirus Culture *on page 405*
  Magnetic Resonance Scan, Brain *on page 485*

Empiric Drug Therapy

Recommended

Ampicillin *on page 604*
  used in combination with
Cephalosporins, 3rd Generation *on page 662*
    except cefoperazone which does not have reliable CSF penetration and should not be used in meningitis
  or
Penicillin G, Parenteral, Aqueous *on page 860*
  used in combination with
Cephalosporins, 3rd Generation *on page 662*
    except cefoperazone which does not have reliable CSF penetration and should not be used in meningitis
  with or without
Vancomycin *on page 967*
    (dependent on prevalence of penicillin-resistant *S. pneumoniae*)

Alternate

Chloramphenicol *on page 667*
Used only in patients with a history of anaphylaxis to penicillin.

Selected Readings

Askari S and Cartwright CP, "The Changing Epidemiology of Bacterial Meningitis: Implications for the Clinical Laboratory," *Clin Microbiol Newslett*, 1998, 20(5):33-6.

Butler JC, Hofmann J, Cetron MS, et al, "The Continued Emergence of Drug-Resistant *Streptococcus pneumoniae* in the United States: An Update From the Centers for Disease Control and Prevention Pneumococcal Sentinel Surveillance System," *J Infect Dis*, 1996, 174(5):986-93.

Tunkel AR and Scheld WM, "Acute Bacterial Meningitis," *Lancet*, 1995, 346(8991-8992):1675-80.

Tunkel AR and Scheld WM, "Acute Bacterial Meningitis in Adults," *Curr Clin Topics Infect Dis*, 1996, 16:215-39.

Meningitis, Neonatal (<2 months of age)

Clinical Presentation Baby is feeding poorly, has fever or is hypothermic, has seizure, sleepiness, irritability, or any other unusual behavior. A full fontanelle indicates progressive disease.

Differential Diagnosis Bacterial, viral, or other infectious agents; neoplasm; metabolic disorders; central nervous system hemorrhage

Likely Pathogens
Escherichia coli, Enterohemorrhagic *on page 143*
Klebsiella Species *on page 183*
Listeria monocytogenes *on page 189*
Streptococcus agalactiae *on page 266*

Diagnostic Tests/Procedures
- Blood Culture, Aerobic and Anaerobic *on page 337*
- Cerebrospinal Fluid Analysis *on page 354*
- Gram's Stain *on page 426*
- Lumbar Puncture *on page 477*
  Computed Transaxial Tomography, Head Studies *on page 374*
  Cryptococcal Antigen Serology, Serum or Cerebrospinal Fluid *on page 379*
  Enterovirus Culture *on page 405*
  Magnetic Resonance Scan, Brain *on page 485*

Empiric Drug Therapy
Recommended
Ampicillin *on page 604*
   used in combination with
Gentamicin *on page 747*
   if hospital acquired add
Vancomycin *on page 967*
Alternate
Chloramphenicol *on page 667*
   used in combination with
Gentamicin *on page 747*
   if hospital acquired add
Vancomycin *on page 967*

Selected Readings
Arango CA and Rathore MH, "Neonatal Meningococcal Meningitis: Case Reports and Review of Literature," *Pediatr Infect Dis J*, 1996, 15(12):1134-6.

Roos KL, Tunkel AR, Scheld WM, "Acute Bacterial Meningitis in Children and Adults," *Infections of the Central Nervous System*, Scheld WM, Whitley RJ, and Durack DT, eds, New York, NY: Raven Press, 1991, 335-410.

Meningitis, Pediatric (>2 months of age)

Clinical Presentation Patients present with fever or hypothermia, seizure, sleepiness, irritability, full fontanelle, and stiff neck. Focal neurologic abnormalities and papilledema are uncommon. The incidence of *H. influenzae* has markedly decreased due to the recommended vaccination of all children.

Differential Diagnosis Bacterial, viral, or other infectious agents; neoplasm; metabolic disorders; central nervous system hemorrhage

Likely Pathogens
Haemophilus influenzae *on page 157*
Neisseria meningitidis *on page 217*
Streptococcus pneumoniae *on page 268*

Diagnostic Tests/Procedures
- Blood Culture, Aerobic and Anaerobic *on page 337*
- Cerebrospinal Fluid Analysis *on page 354*
- Gram's Stain *on page 426*
- Lumbar Puncture *on page 477*
  Bacterial Antigens, Rapid Detection Methods *on page 335*
  Computed Transaxial Tomography, Head Studies *on page 374*
  Cryptococcal Antigen Serology, Serum or Cerebrospinal Fluid *on page 379*
  Enterovirus Culture *on page 405*
(Continued)

Meningitis, Pediatric (>2 months of age) *(Continued)*

Magnetic Resonance Scan, Brain *on page 485*

Empiric Drug Therapy

Recommended

Ceftriaxone *on page 655*
used in combination with
Vancomycin *on page 967*

Alternate

Chloramphenicol *on page 667*
used in combination with
Vancomycin *on page 967*
Meropenem *on page 812*

Selected Readings

Booy R and Kroll JS, "Bacterial Meningitis and Meningococcal Infection," *Curr Opin Pediatr*, 1998, 10(1):13-8.

Odio CM, Faingezicht I, Paris M, et al, "The Beneficial Effects of Early Dexamethasone Administration in Infants and Children With Bacterial Meningitis," *N Engl J Med*, 1991, 324(22):1525-31.

Roos KL, Tunkel AR, Scheld WM, "Acute Bacterial Meningitis in Children and Adults," *Infections of the Central Nervous System*, Scheld WM, Whitley RJ, and Durack DT, eds, New York, NY: Raven Press, 1991, 335-410.

Meningitis, Postsurgical

Clinical Presentation Patients present with fever, headache, nausea, vomiting, and nuchal rigidity. Focal neurologic abnormalities and papilledema are uncommon.

Differential Diagnosis Bacterial, viral, or other infectious agents; drug-induced; neoplastic; granulomatous; infectious endocarditis; collagen-vascular diseases; subdural hemorrhage; subarachnoid hemorrhage

Likely Pathogens

Pseudomonas aeruginosa on page 235
Gram-Negative Bacilli *on page 154*
Staphylococcus aureus, Methicillin-Susceptible *on page 258*
Staphylococcus epidermidis, Methicillin-Susceptible *on page 263*
Candida Species *on page 91*

Diagnostic Tests/Procedures

- Blood Culture, Aerobic and Anaerobic *on page 337*
- Gram's Stain *on page 426*
- Lumbar Puncture *on page 477*
  Computed Transaxial Tomography, Head Studies *on page 374*
  Magnetic Resonance Scan, Brain *on page 485*
  Wound Culture *on page 577*

Empiric Drug Therapy

Recommended

Vancomycin *on page 967*
used in combination with
Ceftazidime *on page 651*
with or without
Tobramycin *on page 953*

Alternate

Vancomycin *on page 967*
used in combination with
Penicillins, Extended Spectrum *on page 864*
with or without
Tobramycin *on page 953*
Candida infection:
Amphotericin B (Conventional) *on page 597*
used in combination with
Flucytosine *on page 734*

Selected Readings

Nazzaro JM and Craven DE, "Successful Treatment of Postoperative Meningitis Due to *Haemophilus influenzae* Without Removal of an Expanded Polytetrafluoroethylene Dural Graft," *Clin Infect Dis*, 1998, 26(2):516-8.

Nguyen MH and Yu VL, "Meningitis Caused by *Candida* Species: An Emerging Problem in Neurosurgical Patients," *Clin Infect Dis*, 1995, 21(2):323-7.

van Aken MO, de Marie S, van der Lely AJ, et al, "Risk Factors for Meningitis After Transsphenoidal Surgery," *Clin Infect Dis*, 1997, 25(4):852-6.

Venes JL, "Infections of CSF Shunts and Intracranial Pressure Monitoring Devices," *Infect Dis Clin North Am*, 1989, 3(2):289-99.

Meningitis, Post-traumatic

Clinical Presentation Patients present with fever, headache, nausea, vomiting, and nuchal rigidity. Focal neurologic abnormalities and papilledema are uncommon.

Differential Diagnosis Bacterial, viral, or other infectious agents; drug-induced; neoplastic; granulomatous; infectious endocarditis; collagen-vascular diseases; subdural hemorrhage; subarachnoid hemorrhage

Likely Pathogens

Haemophilus influenzae on page 157
Staphylococcus aureus, Methicillin-Susceptible on page 258
Streptococcus pneumoniae on page 268

Diagnostic Tests/Procedures

- Aerobic Culture, Cerebrospinal Fluid on page 311
- Blood Culture, Aerobic and Anaerobic on page 337
- Computed Transaxial Tomography, Head Studies on page 374
- Gram's Stain on page 426
- Lumbar Puncture on page 477
- Magnetic Resonance Scan, Brain on page 485

Empiric Drug Therapy

Recommended

Vancomycin on page 967
used in combination with
Cephalosporins, 3rd Generation on page 662
except cefoperazone which does not have reliable CSF penetration and should not be used in meningitis.

Alternate

Vancomycin on page 967
used in combination with
Penicillins, Extended Spectrum on page 864

Microsporidiosis see Microsporidia on page 195

Middle Ear Infection see Otitis Media, Acute on page 41

Moniliasis see Candida Species on page 91

Mononucleosis

Likely Pathogens

Epstein-Barr Virus on page 141
Cytomegalovirus on page 122
Toxoplasma gondii on page 283

Mucormycosis see Mucor Species on page 198

Mumps see Mumps Virus on page 199

Mycotic Vulvovaginitis see Candida Species on page 91

Myocarditis

Clinical Presentation May be acute or chronic. Most commonly is the result of an infectious process but may be secondary to rheumatologic diseases, toxins, radiation, and drugs. Almost all infectious agents are capable of causing myocarditis, the vast majority of acute myocarditis in the United States is secondary to a viral infection. Patients typically present with an antecedent upper respiratory tract infection 1-2 weeks prior to the development of dyspnea and chest pain with fever. Approximately 50% will have evidence of a pericardial effusion or cardiac dilatation on chest radiograph. Congestive heart failure occurs in 20%. EKG may show evidence of pericarditis, arrhythmias, or heart block. May develop dilated cardiomyopathy.

Differential Diagnosis The differential diagnosis for chest pain is quite exhaustive and for this text will be broken into four major systems: cardiovascular, pulmonary, gastrointestinal, and skeletal-muscular.

Likely Pathogens

Viruses:
Coxsackieviruses on page 116
Echovirus on page 129
Influenza Virus on page 181
Measles Virus on page 193
Rubella
Poliovirus on page 230

(Continued)

Myocarditis *(Continued)*

Adenovirus *on page 62*

HIV-associated Pathogens

Human Immunodeficiency Virus *on page 177*

Pyogenic: (usually a complication from endocarditis)

Staphylococcus aureus, Methicillin-Resistant *on page 256*

Staphylococcus aureus, Methicillin-Susceptible *on page 258*

Cryptococcus neoformans on page 117

Mycobacterium tuberculosis on page 207

Parasitic:

Trypanosoma cruzi

Toxoplasma gondii on page 283

Borrelia burgdorferi on page 84

Diagnostic Tests/Procedures Clinically diagnosed. Pathogens may be implicated by specific cultures or serological tests.

Drug Therapy Comment Recommended drug therapy is antimicrobial therapy directed against specific pathogen and supportive care. Most viral myocarditis is self-limiting.

Selected Readings

Anandasabapathy S and Frishman WH, "Innovative Drug Treatments for Viral and Autoimmune Myocarditis," *J Clin Pharmacol*, 1998, 38(4):295-308.

Brown CA and O'Connell JB, "Implications of the Myocarditis Treatment Trial for Clinical Practice," *Curr Opin Cardiol*, 1996, 11(3):332-6.

Caforio AL and McKenna WJ, "Recognition and Optimum Management of Myocarditis," *Drugs*, 1996, 52(4):515-25.

Pawsat DE and Lee JY, "Inflammatory Disorders of the Heart. Pericarditis, Myocarditis, and Endocarditis," *Emerg Med Clin North Am*, 1998, 16(3):665-81.

NGU *see* Urethritis, Nongonococcal *on page 51*

Nocardiosis *see Nocardia* Species *on page 218*

Nongonococcal Urethritis *see* Urethritis, Nongonococcal *on page 51*

"Nonspecific Vaginosis" *see* Vaginosis, Bacterial *on page 54*

Osteomyelitis, Diabetic Foot

Clinical Presentation Usually involves small bones of the feet and toes. Patients present with pain, swelling, and/or erythema of the involved bones with or without presence of ulcer. Most common x-ray finding is mottled lytic lesions.

Differential Diagnosis Charcot foot; fracture; cellulitis

Likely Pathogens

Staphylococcus aureus, Methicillin-Susceptible *on page 258*

Streptococcus-Related Gram-Positive Cocci *on page 278*

Gram-Negative Bacilli *on page 154*

Diagnostic Tests/Procedures

- Bone Films *on page 343*
- Bone Scan *on page 348*
- C-Reactive Protein *on page 378*
- Gram's Stain *on page 426*
- Sedimentation Rate, Erythrocyte *on page 532*
- Biopsy Culture, Routine *on page 337*

Anaerobic Culture *on page 316*

Bone Biopsy *on page 342*

Gallium Scan *on page 422*

Indium Leukocyte Scan *on page 461*

Empiric Drug Therapy

Recommended

Ticarcillin and Clavulanate Potassium *on page 950*

Ampicillin and Sulbactam *on page 607*

Piperacillin and Tazobactam Sodium *on page 871*

Cefoxitin *on page 646*

Cefotetan *on page 644*

Alternate

Imipenem and Cilastatin *on page 766*

or

Clindamycin *on page 684*

used in combination with

Cephalosporins, 3rd Generation *on page 662*

Meropenem *on page 812*

Selected Readings

Bamberger DM, Daus GP, and Gerding DN, "Osteomyelitis in the Feet of Diabetic Patients: Long-Term Results, Prognostic Factors, and the Role of Antimicrobial and Surgical Therapy," *Am J Med*, 1987, 83(4):653-60.

Lipsky BA, "Osteomyelitis of the Foot in Diabetic Patients," *Clin Infect Dis*, 1997, 25(6):1318-26.

Osteomyelitis, Healthy Adult

Clinical Presentation Usually occurs in the face of trauma with surrounding cellulitis; may be hematogenously spread in the face of bacteremia with or without endocarditis (often vertebral) osteomyelitis. Presents with point tenderness, fever, mild leukocytosis, and increased C-reactive protein and erythrocyte sedimentation rate. May be acute or chronic.

Differential Diagnosis Septic arthritis; skin/soft tissue infections; bursitis; tendonitis; fracture; malignancy; diskitis; epidural abscess

Likely Pathogens

Staphylococcus aureus, Methicillin-Susceptible *on page 258*

Diagnostic Tests/Procedures

- Biopsy Culture, Routine *on page 337*
- Bone Films *on page 343*
- Bone Scan *on page 348*
- C-Reactive Protein *on page 378*
- Gram's Stain *on page 426*
- Sedimentation Rate, Erythrocyte *on page 532*
  Anaerobic Culture *on page 316*
  Bone Biopsy *on page 342*
  Gallium Scan *on page 422*
  Indium Leukocyte Scan *on page 461*
  Teichoic Acid Antibody *on page 545*

Empiric Drug Therapy

Recommended

Penicillins, Penicillinase-Resistant *on page 864*
Fluoroquinolones *on page 736*

Alternate

Vancomycin *on page 967*
Cephalosporins, 1st Generation *on page 661*
Clindamycin *on page 684*

Selected Readings

Hass DW and McAndrew MP, "Bacterial Osteomyelitis in Adults: Evolving Considerations in Diagnosis and Treatment," *Am J Med*, 1996, 101(5):550-61.

Laughlin RT, Wright DG, Mader JT, et al, "Osteomyelitis," *Curr Opin Rheumatol*, 1995, 7(4):315-21.

Rissing JP, "Antimicrobial Therapy for Chronic Osteomyelitis in Adults: Role of the Quinolones," *Clin Infect Dis*, 1997, 25(6):1327-33.

Osteomyelitis, Pediatric

Clinical Presentation The child will not be using that extremity, may be limping, etc. Pain, fever, leukocytosis, and increased C-reactive protein and erythrocyte sedimentation rate. Is often hematogenously spread but can also be traumatic. May be acute or chronic.

Differential Diagnosis Septic arthritis; skin/soft tissue infections; bursitis; tendonitis; fracture; malignancy; diskitis; epidural abscess

Likely Pathogens

Staphylococcus aureus, Methicillin-Susceptible *on page 258*
Streptococcus pyogenes on page 274
<2 years old:
Haemophilus influenzae *on page 157*
HACEK Group *(Kingella* in particular) *on page 155*

Diagnostic Tests/Procedures

- Bone Films *on page 343*
- Bone Scan *on page 348*
- C-Reactive Protein *on page 378*
- Gram's Stain *on page 426*
- Sedimentation Rate, Erythrocyte *on page 532*
  Biopsy Culture, Routine *on page 337*
  Bone Biopsy *on page 342*
  Gallium Scan *on page 422*
  Indium Leukocyte Scan *on page 461*
  (Continued)

Osteomyelitis, Pediatric *(Continued)*

Teichoic Acid Antibody *on page 545*

Empiric Drug Therapy

Recommended

Penicillins, Penicillinase-Resistant *on page 864*

Alternate

Vancomycin *on page 967*

Cephalosporins, 1st Generation *on page 661*

Clindamycin *on page 684*

Selected Readings

Birgisson H, Steingrimsson O, and Gudnason T, "*Kingella kingae* Infections in Paediatric Patients: 5 Cases of Septic Arthritis, Osteomyelitis and Bacteremia," *Scand J Infect Dis*, 1997, 29(5):495-8.

Wall EJ, "Childhood Osteomyelitis and Septic Arthritis," *Curr Opin Pediatr*, 1998, 10(1):73-6.

Otitis Externa, Mild

Synonyms Swimmer's Ear

Clinical Presentation Acute localized otitis externa may present as a pustule, furuncle, or cellulitis within the external auditory canal. Hemorrhagic bullae may be present, as well as localized adenopathy. Gram-positive cocci are usually responsible.

Acute diffuse otitis externa (swimmer's ear) initially presents with itching and becomes painful as the canal swells and reddens. Gram-negative bacilli, particularly *Pseudomonas aeruginosa*, are the most likely pathogens.

Chronic otitis externa is characterized by intense itching secondary to the chronic irritation of drainage from chronic otitis media or granulomatous infections.

Malignant otitis externa is a severe necrotizing infection that spreads to adjacent tissue and bone. Associated with intense pain, tenderness, and pus in the canal.

Likely Pathogens

Pseudomonas aeruginosa on page 235

Diagnostic Tests/Procedures

Aerobic Culture, Appropriate Site *on page 310*

Gram's Stain *on page 426*

Empiric Drug Therapy

Recommended

Neomycin *on page 833*

Polymyxin B *on page 877*

Otitis Externa, Severe (Malignant)

Clinical Presentation Acute localized otitis externa may present as a pustule, furuncle, or cellulitis within the external auditory canal. Hemorrhagic bullae may be present, as well as localized adenopathy. Gram-positive cocci are usually responsible.

Acute diffuse otitis externa (swimmer's ear) initially presents with itching and becomes painful as the canal swells and reddens. Gram-negative bacilli, particularly *Pseudomonas aeruginosa*, are the most likely pathogens.

Chronic otitis externa is characterized by intense itching secondary to the chronic irritation of drainage from chronic otitis media or granulomatous infections.

Malignant otitis externa is a severe necrotizing infection that spreads to adjacent tissue and bone. Associated with intense pain, tenderness, and pus in the canal.

Likely Pathogens

Pseudomonas aeruginosa on page 235

Diagnostic Tests/Procedures

Aerobic Culture, Appropriate Site *on page 310*

Computed Transaxial Tomography, Paranasal Sinuses *on page 375*

Gram's Stain *on page 426*

Drug Therapy Comment Topical otic suspensions or solutions may also be indicated.

Empiric Drug Therapy

Recommended

Gentamicin *on page 747*

used in combination with

Ceftazidime *on page 651*
or
Gentamicin *on page 747*
    used in combination with
Penicillins, Extended Spectrum *on page 864*
Alternate
Ciprofloxacin *on page 678*

Otitis Media, Acute

Synonyms Acute Suppurative Otitis; Middle Ear Infection

Clinical Presentation Most commonly occurs in children. Present with otalgia and fever with or without purulent discharge. Infants may present with irritability. Diagnosis is confirmed by examination of the tympanic membrane which is full or bulging, opaque, and has little or no mobility.

Likely Pathogens
Streptococcus pneumoniae on page 268
Haemophilus influenzae on page 157
Moraxella catarrhalis on page 196
Staphylococcus aureus, Methicillin-Susceptible *on page 258*

Diagnostic Tests/Procedures
Aerobic Culture, Body Fluid *on page 310*
Gram's Stain *on page 426*

Empiric Drug Therapy
Recommended
Amoxicillin *on page 592*
Co-Trimoxazole *on page 692*
Cephalosporins, 2nd Generation *on page 662*
Alternate
Erythromycin and Sulfisoxazole *on page 725*

Selected Readings
Bluestone CD, "Epidemiology and Pathogenesis of Chronic Suppurative Otitis Media: Implications for Prevention and Treatment," *Int J Pediatr Otorhinolaryngol*, 1998, 42(3):207-23.
Conrad DA, "Should Acute Otitis Media Ever Be Treated With Antibiotics?" *Pediatr Ann*, 1998, 27(2):66-7, 70-4.
Heikkinen T and Ruuskanen O, "Otitis Media," *Curr Opin Pediatr*, 1998, 10(1):9-12.

PCP *see Pneumocystis carinii on page 228*

Pelvic Inflammatory Disease

Synonyms PID

Clinical Presentation Pelvic inflammatory disease (PID) is an infection of the pelvic organs usually by bacteria and its associated inflammatory response. Typically begins as an ascending infection from the vagina or cervix but may occur via hematogenous or lymphatic spread. Patients present with fever, chills, nausea, vomiting, anorexia, vaginal bleeding, and mucopurulent vaginal discharge. Endometritis usually develops postpartum or postabortal, whereas, salpingo-oophoritis with or without abscess is most associated with sexually transmitted diseases.

Differential Diagnosis Intestinal tract disease; urinary systems disease

Likely Pathogens
Chlamydia trachomatis on page 99
Neisseria gonorrhoeae on page 215
Escherichia coli, Nonenterohemorrhagic *on page 147*
Streptococcus, Viridans Group *on page 279*
Bacteroides Species *on page 75*

Diagnostic Tests/Procedures
Abscess Aerobic and Anaerobic Culture *on page 304*
Aerobic Culture, Body Fluid *on page 310*
Anaerobic Culture *on page 316*
Gram's Stain *on page 426*

Empiric Drug Therapy
Recommended
Cefotetan *on page 644*
    or
Cefoxitin *on page 646*
    used in combination with
Doxycycline *on page 713*
(Continued)

41

Pelvic Inflammatory Disease *(Continued)*

Clindamycin *on page 684*
  used in combination with
Gentamicin *on page 747*

Alternate

Ofloxacin *on page 847*
  used in combination with
Metronidazole *on page 817*
Ampicillin and Sulbactam *on page 607*
  used in combination with
Doxycycline *on page 713*
Ciprofloxacin *on page 678*
Doxycycline *on page 713*
Metronidazole *on page 817*
  all 3 used in combination

Selected Readings

Centers for Disease Control and Prevention, "1997 Sexually Transmitted Diseases Treatment Guidelines," *MMWR Morb Mortal Wkly Rep*, 1997, 47(RR-1):1-119.

Hensell DL, Little BB, Faro S, et al, "Comparison of Three Regimens Recommended by the Centers For Disease Control and Prevention for the Treatment of Women Hospitalized With Acute Pelvic Inflammatory Disease," *Clin Infect Dis*, 1994, 19(4):720-7.

Pericarditis

Clinical Presentation Acute: Pleuritic pain may vary from a slow progressive pain to a sharp inspiratory pain to a more subtle deep ache which radiates down the arms. Characteristically, the pain is alleviated by sitting up and leaning forward. Dyspnea is common. The pericardial friction rub is the cardinal feature. The EKG typically reveals widespread elevation of the ST segments. The presence of a paradoxical pulse should alert the physician for possible cardiac tamponade although a paradoxical pulse may be seen in other diseases. Viral pericarditis occurs more frequently in young adults and is characterized by an antecedent upper respiratory tract infection by about 1-2 weeks. Patients typically have constitutional symptoms including fever. Clinical classification is defined by duration of symptoms; acute is <6 weeks, subacute is 6 weeks to 6 months, and chronic is >6 months. It is further classified by either fibrinous, effusive, or constrictive. It may also be classified according to the etiology such as infectious, autoimmune including rheumatic fever, collagen-vascular diseases, drug-induced, and post cardiac injury, and a broad category of noninfectious which includes neoplasia, uremia, acute myocardial infarction, cholesterol, myxedema, trauma, structural cardiac defects, and others.

Differential Diagnosis The differential diagnosis for chest pain is quite exhaustive and for this text will be broken into four major systems: cardiovascular, pulmonary, gastrointestinal, and skeletal-muscular.

Likely Pathogens

Viruses:
  Coxsackieviruses *on page 116*
  Echovirus *on page 129*
  Herpes Simplex Virus *on page 170*
  Adenovirus *on page 62*
Pyogenic
Mycobacterial:
  Mycobacterium tuberculosis on page 207
  Mycobacterium avium-intracellulare on page 201
Fungal:
  Histoplasma capsulatum on page 173
  Blastomyces dermatitidis on page 78
  Aspergillus Species *on page 70*
Treponema pallidum on page 285
Parasitic
  Amebiasis
  Toxoplasma gondii on page 283
  Echinococcus
  Trichinella spiralis on page 289

Diagnostic Tests/Procedures

Culture (see specific organisms)

EKG
Echocardiography, M-Mode *on page 395*
Pericardiocentesis

Drug Therapy Comment Recommended drug therapy is antimicrobial therapy directed against specific pathogen and supportive care. Anti-inflammatory drugs such as NSAIDs and prednisone may be helpful.

Selected Readings
Pawsat DE and Lee JY, "Inflammatory Disorders of the Heart. Pericarditis, Myocarditis, and Endocarditis," *Emerg Med Clin North Am*, 1998, 16(3):665-81.

Perinephric Abscess *see* Urinary Tract Infection, Perinephric Abscess *on page 52*

Peritonitis, Spontaneous Bacterial

Clinical Presentation Patients with primary peritonitis present with abrupt onset of fever, abdominal pain, nausea, vomiting, diarrhea, diffuse abdominal tenderness, rebound tenderness, and hypoactive or absent bowel sounds. Patients with cirrhosis may have an atypical presentation with an insidious onset and lack of peritoneal signs. Most cirrhotics present with fever. Patients with secondary peritonitis present as the primary process with peritoneal signs being the most prominent. More than 60% of the cases of spontaneous bacterial peritonitis (SBP) are caused by gram-negative enteric bacteria. Gram-positive cocci, predominantly streptococcal species, are implicated in approximately 25% of the cases of SBP.

Differential Diagnosis Pneumonia; sickle cell anemia; herpes zoster; diabetic ketoacidosis; tabes dorsalis; porphyria; familial Mediterranean fever; plumbism; lupus erythematosus; uremia; other intra-abdominal infections

Likely Pathogens
Klebsiella Species *on page 183*
Escherichia coli, Nonenterohemorrhagic *on page 147*
Streptococcus Species *on page 279*

Diagnostic Tests/Procedures
Paracentesis *on page 509*
Abscess Aerobic and Anaerobic Culture *on page 304*
Aerobic Culture, Body Fluid *on page 310*
Anaerobic Culture *on page 316*
Gram's Stain *on page 426*

Empiric Drug Therapy
Recommended
Cefotaxime *on page 642*
Alternate
Cefoxitin *on page 646*
Cefotetan *on page 644*
Piperacillin and Tazobactam Sodium *on page 871*
Ticarcillin and Clavulanate Potassium *on page 950*
Ampicillin and Sulbactam *on page 607*
Imipenem and Cilastatin *on page 766*
Meropenem *on page 812*
Trovafloxacin *on page 960*

Selected Readings
Johnson CC, Baldessarre J, and Levison ME, "Peritonitis: Update on Pathophysiology, Clinical Manifestations, and Management,"*Clin Infect Dis*, 1997, 24(6):1035-47.
McClean KL, Sheehan GJ and Harding GK, "Intra-Abdominal Infection: A Review," *Clin Infect Dis*, 1994, 19(1):100-16.
Such J and Runyon BA, "Spontaneous Bacterial Peritonitis," *Clin Infect Dis*, 1998, 27(4):669-74.

Pertussis *see Bordetella pertussis on page 81*

Phaeohyphomycosis *see* Dematiaceous Fungi *on page 125*

Pharyngitis

Clinical Presentation Acute pharyngitis is an inflammatory syndrome of the pharynx caused by multiple organisms, predominantly viral. Patients complain of soreness, scratching, or irritation of the throat along with signs of congestion, malaise, and headaches. Patients with EBV or strep typically present with fever and an exudative pharyngitis.

Differential Diagnosis Retropharyngeal abscess; epiglottitis; Lemierre's disease
(Continued)

Pharyngitis *(Continued)*

Likely Pathogens
Streptococcus pyogenes on page 274
Respiratory Syncytial Virus *on page 239*
Influenza Virus *on page 181*
Parainfluenza Virus *on page 220*
Adenovirus *on page 62*
Epstein-Barr Virus *on page 141*

Diagnostic Tests/Procedures Viral detection studies indicated for severe or unusual cases and are not routine.

Group A *Streptococcus* Antigen Test *on page 428*
Throat Culture for Group A Beta-Hemolytic *Streptococcus* on page 550
Virus Detection by DFA *on page 576*
Viral Culture, Throat *on page 574*
Infectious Mononucleosis Serology *on page 462*

Drug Therapy Comment Drug therapy indicated is for *Streptococcus pyogenes* infections only.

Empiric Drug Therapy
Recommended
Penicillin V Potassium *on page 865*
Penicillin G Procaine *on page 862*
Alternate
Erythromycin *on page 722*
Cephalosporins, 1st Generation *on page 661*
Amoxicillin *on page 592*

Phycomycosis see Mucor Species *on page 198*

PID see Pelvic Inflammatory Disease *on page 41*

Pink Eye see Conjunctivitis *on page 25*

Plague see Yersinia pestis *on page 300*

***Pneumocystis carinii* Pneumonia** see *Pneumocystis carinii* on page 228

Pneumonia, Aspiration, Community-Acquired

Clinical Presentation Major symptoms are cough, fever, production of sputum, chest pain, and dyspnea. Although aspiration is a common cause of community-acquired pneumonia, it classically occurs in patients who have difficulty swallowing, no gag reflex, who are at high risk for aspirating.

Differential Diagnosis Congestive heart failure; pulmonary embolism; aspiration of gastric contents; neoplasm; adult respiratory distress syndrome; hypersensitivity pneumonitis; radiation pneumonitis; drug reactions

Likely Pathogens
Streptococcus-Related Gram-Positive Cocci *on page 278*
Streptococcus pneumoniae on page 268
Bacteroides Species *on page 75*

Diagnostic Tests/Procedures
- Aerobic Culture, Sputum *on page 312*
- Blood Culture, Aerobic and Anaerobic *on page 337*
- Chest Films *on page 359*
- Gram's Stain *on page 426*
Computed Transaxial Tomography, Thorax *on page 376*

Empiric Drug Therapy
Recommended
Penicillin G, Parenteral, Aqueous *on page 860*
Clindamycin *on page 684*
Alternate
Ampicillin and Sulbactam *on page 607*

Selected Readings
Bartlett JG, "Anaerobic Bacterial Infections of the Lung," *Chest*, 1987, 91(6):901-9.
Bartlett JG, Breiman RF, Mandell LA, et al, "Community-Acquired Pneumonia in Adults: Guidelines for Management. The Infectious Diseases Society of America," *Clin Infect Dis*, 1998, 26(4):811-38.
Leroy O, Vandenbussche C, Coffinier C, et al, "Community-Acquired Aspiration Pneumonia in Intensive Care Units. Epidemiological and Prognosis Data," *Am J Respir Crit Care Med*, 1997, 156(6):1922-9.

Pneumonia, Community-Acquired

Related Information

Community-Acquired Pneumonia in Adults *on page 1070*

Clinical Presentation Major symptoms are cough, fever, production of sputum, chest pain, and dyspnea. Viral or *Mycoplasma* pneumonia typically has prodromal upper respiratory tract phase associated with malaise, headache, sore throat, and nonproductive cough.

Differential Diagnosis Congestive heart failure; pulmonary embolism; aspiration of gastric contents; neoplasm; adult respiratory distress syndrome; hypersensitivity pneumonitis; radiation pneumonitis; drug reactions

Likely Pathogens

Streptococcus pneumoniae on page 268
Mycoplasma pneumoniae on page 211
Legionella pneumophila on page 185
Chlamydia pneumoniae on page 95
Haemophilus influenzae on page 157

Immunocompromised
  Pneumocystis carinii on page 228

Diagnostic Tests/Procedures

Severe Infection
  • Aerobic Culture, Sputum *on page 312*
  • Blood Culture, Aerobic and Anaerobic *on page 337*
  • Chest Films *on page 359*
  • Gram's Stain *on page 426*
    Legionella Serology *on page 471*
    Mycoplasma Serology *on page 499*
    Mycoplasma/Ureaplasma Culture *on page 499*

Mild Infection
  • Aerobic Culture, Sputum *on page 312*
  • Gram's Stain *on page 426*

Drug Therapy Comment Therapy should be directed at the specific pathogen when the pathogen is detected. Empiric treatment and in the setting when no

---

Empirical Antibiotic Selection for Patients With Community-Acquired Pneumonia

Outpatients
Generally preferred: Macrolides,* fluoroquinolones,† or doxycycline
Modifying factors
Suspected penicillin-resistant *Streptococcus pneumoniae*: fluoroquinolones†
Young adult (>17-40 y): Doxycycline
Hospitalized patients
General medical ward
Generally preferred: Beta-lactam‡ with or without a macrolide* or a fluoroquinolone† (alone)
Alternatives: Cefuroxime with or without a macrolide* or azithromycin (alone)
Hospitalized in the intensive care unit for serious pneumonia
Generally preferred: Erythromycin, azithromycin, or a fluoroquinolone† plus cefotaxime, ceftriaxone, or a beta-lactam - beta-lactamase inhibitor§
Modifying factors
Structural disease of the lung: Antipseudomonal penicillin, a carbapenem, or cefepime plus a macrolide* or a fluoroquinolone† plus an aminoglycoside
Penicillin allergy: A fluoroquinolone† with or without clindamycin
Suspected aspiration: A fluoroquinolone plus either clindamycin or metronidazole or a beta-lactam - beta-lactamase inhibitor§

*Azithromycin, clarithromycin, or erythromycin

†Levofloxacin, sparfloxacin, grepafloxacin, trovafloxacin, or another fluoroquinolone with enhanced activity against *S. pneumoniae*

‡Cefotaxime, ceftriaxone, or a beta-lactam - beta-lactamase inhibitor

§Ampicillin/sulbactam, or ticarcillin/clavulanate, or p iperacillin/tazobactam (for structural disease of the lung, ticarcillin/clavulanate or piperacillin)

(Continued)

Pneumonia, Community-Acquired *(Continued)*

etiologic agent is identified, the recommendations for outpatient care are a macrolide, a fluoroquinolone with good activity against *S. pneumoniae*, or doxycycline. The recommendation for the hospitalized patient is a β-lactam with or without a macrolide or a fluoroquinolone with good activity against *S. pneumoniae*. See table on previous page.

Empiric Drug Therapy

Recommended

Outpatients:

Azithromycin *on page 613*

Clarithromycin *on page 681*

Erythromycin *on page 722*

Levofloxacin *on page 795*

Sparfloxacin *on page 921*

Grepafloxacin *on page 752*

Doxycycline *on page 713*

Hospitalized patients:

Cefotaxime *on page 642*

Ceftriaxone *on page 655*

Erythromycin *on page 722*

Azithromycin *on page 613*

Clarithromycin *on page 681*

Levofloxacin *on page 795*

Ampicillin and Sulbactam *on page 607*

Ticarcillin and Clavulanate Potassium *on page 950*

Piperacillin and Tazobactam Sodium *on page 871*

Selected Readings

Bartlett JG, Breiman RF, Mandell LA, et al, "Community-Acquired Pneumonia in Adults: Guidelines for Management. The Infectious Diseases Society of America," *Clin Infect Dis*, 1998, 26(4):811-38.

Fine MJ, Smith MA, Carson CA, et al, "Prognosis and Outcomes of Patients With Community Acquired Pneumonia. A Meta-Analysis," *JAMA*, 1995, 275(2):134-41.

Pneumonia, Hospital-Acquired

Clinical Presentation Major symptoms are cough, fever, production of sputum, chest pain, and dyspnea. Although aspiration is a common cause of community-acquired pneumonia, it classically occurs in patients who have difficulty swallowing, no gag reflex, and who are at high risk for aspirating.

Differential Diagnosis Congestive heart failure; pulmonary embolism; aspiration of gastric contents; neoplasm; adult respiratory distress syndrome; hypersensitivity pneumonitis; radiation pneumonitis; drug reactions

Likely Pathogens

Pseudomonas aeruginosa on page 235

Enterobacter Species *on page 134*

Klebsiella Species *on page 183*

Serratia Species *on page 250*

Staphylococcus aureus, Methicillin-Susceptible *on page 258*

Diagnostic Tests/Procedures

• Aerobic Culture, Sputum *on page 312*

• Chest Films *on page 359*

• Gram's Stain *on page 426*

Drug Therapy Comment

Vancomycin added only if evidence of gram-positive infection.

Empiric Drug Therapy

Recommended

Vancomycin *on page 967*

Ceftazidime *on page 651*

Gentamicin *on page 747*

    all 3 used in combination

      or

Penicillins, Extended Spectrum *on page 864*

Aminoglycosides *on page 590*

Vancomycin *on page 967*

    all 3 used in combination

Selected Readings
Chastre J, Fagon JY, and Trouillet JL, "Diagnosis and Treatment of Nosocomial Pneumonia in Patients in Intensive Care Units," *Clin Infect Dis*, 1995, 21(Suppl 3):S226-37.

Joshi N, Localio AR, Hamory BH, "A Predictive Risk Index for Nosocomial Pneumonia in the Intensive Care Unit," *Am J Med*, 1992, 93(2):135-42.

Mandell LA and Campbell GD Jr, "Nosocomial Pneumonia Guidelines, an International Perspective," *Chest*, 1998, 113(3 Suppl):188S-93S.

Pneumonic Plague *see Yersinia pestis on page 300*

Poliomyelitis *see Poliovirus on page 230*

Related Information
Recommended Poliovirus Vaccination Schedule *on page 1044*

Pontiac Fever *see Legionella pneumophila on page 185*

Posadas-Wernicke's Disease *see Coccidioides immitis on page 109*

Prevention of Bacterial Endocarditis *see page 1096*

Primary Atypical Pneumonia
Likely Pathogens
Mycoplasma pneumoniae on page 211
Chlamydia pneumoniae on page 95
Legionella pneumophila on page 185

Prostatitis
Clinical Presentation Acute prostatitis typically occurs in young males but may be associated with indwelling urethral catheters. Characterized by fever, chills, dysuria, and a tense or extremely tender prostate on palpation. Chronic form may present as asymptomatic bacteriuria with a normal palpable prostate. May have intermittent symptoms of frequency, urgency, and dysuria.

Differential Diagnosis Bacterial; nonbacterial; prostatodynia; malignancy

Likely Pathogens
Escherichia coli, Nonenterohemorrhagic *on page 147*
Neisseria gonorrhoeae on page 215
Chlamydia trachomatis on page 99
Staphylococcus aureus, Methicillin-Susceptible *on page 258*

Diagnostic Tests/Procedures
- Genital Culture *on page 423*
- Gram's Stain *on page 426*
- *Neisseria gonorrhoeae* Culture *on page 501*
- Urine Culture, Clean Catch *on page 565*

Drug Therapy Comment Alpha-blockers may be helpful in the setting of chronic prostatitis.

Empiric Drug Therapy
Recommended
Co-Trimoxazole *on page 692*
Fluoroquinolones *on page 736*

Selected Readings
Barbalias GA, Nikiforidis G, and Liatsikos EN, "Alpha-Blockers for the Treatment of Chronic Prostatitis in Combination With Antibiotics," *J Urol*, 1998, 159(3):883-7.

Pewitt EB and Schaeffer AJ, "Urinary Tract Infection in Urology, Including Acute and Chronic Prostatitis," *Infect Dis Clin North Am*, 1997, 11(3):623-46.

Roberts RO, Lieber MM, Rhodes T, et al, "Prevalence of a Physician-Assigned Diagnosis of Prostatitis: The Olmsted County Study of Urinary Symptoms and Health Status Among Men," *Urology*, 1998, 51(4):578-84.

Prosthetic Valve Endocarditis, Early *see Endocarditis, Prosthetic Valve, Early on page 27*

Prosthetic Valve Endocarditis, Late *see Endocarditis, Prosthetic Valve, Late on page 28*

Pseudomembranous Colitis *see Clostridium difficile on page 105*

Psittacosis *see Chlamydia psittaci on page 97*

PVE, Early *see Endocarditis, Prosthetic Valve, Early on page 27*

PVE, Late *see Endocarditis, Prosthetic Valve, Late on page 28*

Q Fever *see Coxiella burnetii on page 115*

Rabies *see Rabies Virus on page 237*

Recommendations for Measles Vaccination *see page 1044*

Recommended Poliovirus Vaccination Schedule *see page 1044*

Red Eye *see Conjunctivitis on page 25*

Reticuloendotheliosis *see Histoplasma capsulatum on page 173*

Rheumatic Fever *see Streptococcus pyogenes on page 274*

Rheumatic Fever Criteria (Jones Criteria) *see Streptococcus pyogenes on page 274*

Ringworm *see Dermatophytes on page 127*

RMSF *see Rickettsia rickettsii on page 243*

Rocky Mountain Spotted Fever *see Rickettsia rickettsii on page 243*

Roseola Infantum *see Human Herpesvirus-6 on page 175*

Rubeola *see Measles Virus on page 193*

Salmonellosis *see Salmonella Species on page 245*

San Joaquin Fever *see Coccidioides immitis on page 109*

Scabies *see Sarcoptes scabiei on page 247*

Scarlet Fever *see Streptococcus pyogenes on page 274*

Schistosomiasis *see Schistosoma mansoni on page 249*

Sepsis

Clinical Presentation The patient may have fever or hypothermia, may be tachycardiac and tachypneic, may have altered mental status, hypoxia, increased plasma lactate levels, oliguria, or coagulopathy. Septic patients may also go into shock which is characterized by significant drop in blood pressure in the face of fluid challenges.

Likely Pathogens
Gram-Negative Bacilli *on page 154*
Staphylococcus aureus, Methicillin-Susceptible *on page 258*
Candida Species *on page 91*
Enterococcus Species *on page 137*

Diagnostic Tests/Procedures
- Aerobic Culture, Sputum *on page 312*
- Blood Culture, Aerobic and Anaerobic *on page 337*
- Gram's Stain *on page 426*
- Intravenous Line Culture *on page 464*
- Urine Culture, Clean Catch *on page 565*
  Computed Transaxial Tomography, Abdomen Studies *on page 373*

Empiric Drug Therapy
Recommended
Ceftazidime *on page 651*
Aminoglycosides *on page 590*
Vancomycin *on page 967*
all 3 used in combination
or
Penicillins, Extended Spectrum *on page 864*
Aminoglycosides *on page 590*
Vancomycin *on page 967*
all 3 used in combination

Septic Arthritis *see Arthritis, Septic on page 18*

Septic Thrombophlebitis *see Thrombophlebitis, Suppurative on page 50*

Shigellosis *see Shigella Species on page 251*

Shingles *see Varicella-Zoster Virus on page 294*

Sinusitis, Community-Acquired, Acute

Synonyms Acute Sinusitis, Community-Acquired; Community-Acquired Sinusitis, Acute

Clinical Presentation Symptoms depend on the site of involvement. Patients with maxillary sinusitis typically have pain over the canine/molar teeth and malar area. Patients with anterior ethmoid sinusitis present with temporal or retro-orbital headaches. Posterior ethmoid sinusitis presents with pain in the distribution of the trigeminal nerve and sphenoid sinusitis typically causes pain in the frontal, retro-orbital, or facial area. Patients usually complain of nasal congestion rhinitis, as most often acute sinusitis follows a viral upper respiratory tract infection. Initial treatment should consist of symptomatic relief with analgesia, topical, or systemic decongestants and steam inhalation.

Likely Pathogens
Streptococcus pneumoniae on page 268

Haemophilus influenzae on page 157
Moraxella catarrhalis on page 196
Note: Unusual organisms should be considered in immunosuppressed patients.

Diagnostic Tests/Procedures
Aerobic Culture, Appropriate Site *on page 310*
Gram's Stain *on page 426*

Empiric Drug Therapy
Recommended
Co-Trimoxazole *on page 692*
Cephalosporins, 2nd Generation *on page 662*
Amoxicillin *on page 592*
Alternate
Amoxicillin and Clavulanate Potassium *on page 593*
Azithromycin *on page 613*
Clarithromycin *on page 681*
Fluoroquinolones *on page 736*
Macrolides *on page 803*

Selected Readings
Evans KL, "Recognition and Management of Sinusitis," *Drugs*, 1998, 56(1):59-71.
Low DE, Desrosiers M, McSherry J, et al, "A Practical Guide for the Diagnosis and Treatment of Acute Sinusitis," *CMAJ*, 1997, 156(Suppl 6):S1-14.

Sinusitis, Community-Acquired, Chronic

Synonyms Chronic Sinusitis, Community-Acquired; Community-Acquired Sinusitis, Chronic

Clinical Presentation Patients generally complain of intermittent pain, nasal congestion, and rhinitis. Patients frequently have a chronic cough secondary to postnasal drip.

Differential Diagnosis Granulomatous disease

Likely Pathogens
Bacteroides Species *on page 75*
Streptococcus-Related Gram-Positive Cocci *on page 278*

Diagnostic Tests/Procedures
Aerobic Culture, Appropriate Site *on page 310*
Anaerobic Culture *on page 316*
Gram's Stain *on page 426*

Drug Therapy Comment Antibiotics are usually not effective. Use of decongestant and steroid nasal spray recommended.

Empiric Drug Therapy
Recommended
Clindamycin *on page 684*
Alternate
Macrolides *on page 803*

Selected Readings
Evans KL, "Recognition and Management of Sinusitis," *Drugs*, 1998, 56(1):59-71.
Orlandi RR and Kennedy DW, "Surgical Management of Rhinosinusitis," *Am J Med Sci*, 1998, 316(1):29-38.

Sinusitis, Hospital-Acquired

Clinical Presentation Common nosocomial infection in the intensive care units secondary to prolonged intubation with a nasal tracheal or nasal gastric tube. Patients may present with fever and/or leukocytosis. Unexplained fever or leukocytosis with a nasal tube warrants simple CT of the sinuses.

Likely Pathogens
Staphylococcus aureus, Methicillin-Resistant *on page 256*
Staphylococcus aureus, Methicillin-Susceptible *on page 258*
Pseudomonas aeruginosa on page 235

Diagnostic Tests/Procedures
Aerobic Culture, Appropriate Site *on page 310*
Gram's Stain *on page 426*
Computed Transaxial Tomography, Paranasal Sinuses *on page 375*

Empiric Drug Therapy
Recommended
Vancomycin *on page 967*
Gentamicin *on page 747*
Ceftazidime *on page 651*
(Continued)

49

Sinusitis, Hospital-Acquired *(Continued)*

    all 3 used in combination
      or
    Vancomycin *on page 967*
    Gentamicin *on page 747*
    Penicillins, Extended Spectrum *on page 864*
      all 3 used in combination
  Alternate
    Macrolides *on page 803*

Selected Readings
  Talmor M, Li P, and Barie PS, "Acute Paranasal Sinusitis in Critically Ill Patients: Guidelines for Prevention, Diagnosis, and Treatment," *Clin Infect Dis*, 1997, 25(6):1441-6.
  Westergren V, Lundblad L, Hellquist HB, et al, "Ventilator-Associated Sinusitis: A Review," *Clin Infect Dis*, 1998, 27(4):851-64.

Skin and Soft Tissue

Synonyms Cellulitis; Fasciitis

Clinical Presentation Erythema, warmth, and edema around the involved area. Patient may be febrile with leukocytosis. In patients with cellulitis of the extremities, deeper infections must be ruled out. (Patients with necrotizing fasciitis experience hyperesthesia in the face of an unimpressive lesion. Necrotizing disease is a surgical emergency; broad spectrum antimicrobial coverage including anaerobic must be administered.)

Differential Diagnosis Malignancy; osteomyelitis

Likely Pathogens
  Staphylococcus aureus, Methicillin-Resistant *on page 256*
  Staphylococcus aureus, Methicillin-Susceptible *on page 258*
  Streptococcus Species *on page 279*
  Clostridium perfringens on page 105

Diagnostic Tests/Procedures
  Anaerobic Culture *on page 316*
  Biopsy Culture, Routine *on page 337*
  Blood Culture, Aerobic and Anaerobic *on page 337*
  Gram's Stain *on page 426*
  Skin Biopsy *on page 535*

Empiric Drug Therapy
  Recommended
    Penicillins, Penicillinase-Resistant *on page 864*
    Cephalosporins, 1st Generation *on page 661*
  Alternate
    Clindamycin *on page 684*
    Vancomycin *on page 967*

Slapped Cheek *see* Parvovirus B19 *on page 222*

Sporotrichosis *see* Sporothrix schenckii *on page 253*

Strep Throat *see* Pharyngitis *on page 43*

Strongyloidiasis *see* Strongyloides stercoralis *on page 281*

Supraglottitis *see* Epiglottitis *on page 29*

Surgical Wound Infection *see* Wound Infection, Surgical *on page 54*

Swimmer's Ear *see* Otitis Externa, Mild *on page 40*

Syphilis *see* Treponema pallidum *on page 285*

Tetanus *see* Clostridium tetani *on page 107*

Thrombophlebitis, Septic *see* Thrombophlebitis, Suppurative *on this page*

Thrombophlebitis, Suppurative

Synonyms Septic Thrombophlebitis; Thrombophlebitis, Septic

Clinical Presentation Frequently associated with thrombosis and bacteremia. Upper extremity suppurative thrombophlebitis usually shows signs of local inflammation and fever. The majority of patients have an implicated catheter left in place for ≥5 days. Local inflammation is less prominent in lower extremity disease. Pelvic suppurative thrombophlebitis typically develops 1-2 weeks postpartum or postoperatively presenting with fever, chills, anorexia, nausea, vomiting, and abdominal pain. Majority of pelvic suppurative thrombophlebitis occurs unilaterally.

Differential Diagnosis Septic nonsuppurative thrombophlebitis

Likely Pathogens

Staphylococcus epidermidis, Methicillin-Susceptible *on page 263*
Staphylococcus aureus, Methicillin-Susceptible *on page 258*
Staphylococcus epidermidis, Methicillin-Resistant *on page 261*
Staphylococcus aureus, Methicillin-Resistant *on page 256*

Diagnostic Tests/Procedures

Blood Culture, Aerobic and Anaerobic *on page 337*
If deep venous thrombosis is suspected:
Ultrasound, Peripheral Arteries and Veins *on page 561*

Empiric Drug Therapy
Recommended

Penicillins, Penicillinase-Resistant *on page 864*
Vancomycin *on page 967*

Thrush *see Candida* Species *on page 91*

Tinea *see* Dermatophytes *on page 127*

Toxic Cholangitis *see* Cholangitis, Acute *on page 21*

Toxic Shock Syndrome

Clinical Presentation See individual organisms for clinical presentation information.

Likely Pathogens

Staphylococcus aureus, Methicillin-Resistant *on page 256*
Staphylococcus aureus, Methicillin-Susceptible *on page 258*
Streptococcus pyogenes on page 274

Diagnostic Tests/Procedures

Blood Culture, Aerobic and Anaerobic *on page 337*

Empiric Drug Therapy
Recommended

Vancomycin *on page 967*
Penicillins, Penicillinase-Resistant *on page 864*

Selected Readings

Davis D, Gash-Kim TL, and Heffernan EJ, "Toxic Shock Syndrome: Case Report of a Postpartum Female and a Literature Review," *J Emerg Med*, 1998, 16(4):607-14.

Holm C and Mühlbauer W, "Toxic Shock Syndrome in Plastic Surgery Patients: Case Report and Review of the Literature," *Aesthetic Plast Surg*, 1998, 22(3):180-4.

Kiska DL, "Staphylococcal and Streptococcal Toxic Shock Syndrome," *Clin Microbiol Newslett*, 1997, 19(5):33-7.

Stevens DL, "Streptococcal Toxic-Shock Syndrome: Spectrum of Disease, Pathogenesis, and New Concepts in Treatment," *Emerg Infect Dis*, 1995, 1(3):69-78.

Toxoplasmosis *see Toxoplasma gondii on page 283*

Tracheobronchitis *see* Bronchitis *on page 20*

Trachoma *see Chlamydia trachomatis on page 99*

Trichinosis *see Trichinella spiralis on page 289*

Trichomoniasis *see Trichomonas vaginalis on page 290*

Tuberculosis *see Mycobacterium tuberculosis on page 207*

Tularemia *see Francisella tularensis on page 148*

Uncomplicated Urinary Tract Infection *see* Urinary Tract Infection, Uncomplicated *on page 53*

Upper Urinary Tract Infection *see* Urinary Tract Infection, Pyelonephritis *on page 53*

Urethritis, Nongonococcal

Synonyms NGU; Nongonococcal Urethritis

Clinical Presentation Urethral discharge is more prominent in men than women and is less seen in NGU than gonococcal urethritis. The discharge may vary from a scant clear mucopurulent to frank pus. Men typically complain of pain at the meatus or distal portion of the penis and may have dysuria. Rarely, men complain of discomfort during ejaculation. Women may complain of dysuria and usually have symptoms of cervicitis although they may be asymptomatic.

Differential Diagnosis Gonococcal urethritis; prostatitis; epididymitis; cervicitis; salpingitis; urinary tract infection, cystitis; noninfectious urethritis

Likely Pathogens

Chlamydia trachomatis on page 99
Trichomonas vaginalis on page 290
Herpes Simplex Virus *on page 170*
(Continued)

51

Urethritis, Nongonococcal *(Continued)*

Ureaplasma urealyticum on page 292

Diagnostic Tests/Procedures

Chlamydia Culture *on page 359*
Chlamydia trachomatis by DNA Probe *on page 364*
Genital Culture for *Ureaplasma urealyticum on page 424*
Herpes Simplex Virus Culture *on page 446*
Trichomonas Preparation *on page 555*

Empiric Drug Therapy

Recommended

Doxycycline *on page 713*
Tetracycline *on page 944*
Azithromycin *on page 613*

Alternate

Erythromycin *on page 722*

Urinary Tract Infection, Catheter-Associated

Clinical Presentation Patient may have low-grade fever, chills, hematuria, pyuria, and peripheral leukocytosis.

Differential Diagnosis Colonization; trauma; infection - bacterial, fungal

Likely Pathogens

Escherichia coli, Nonenterohemorrhagic *on page 147*
Enterococcus Species *on page 137*
Pseudomonas aeruginosa on page 235
Candida Species *on page 91*

Diagnostic Tests/Procedures

- Blood Culture, Aerobic and Anaerobic *on page 337*
- Gram's Stain *on page 426*
- Urine Culture, Clean Catch *on page 565*
  Complete Blood Count *on page 369*
  Fungus Culture, Urine *on page 421*
  Leukocyte Esterase, Urine *on page 473*
  Nitrite, Urine *on page 503*

Empiric Drug Therapy

Recommended

Ampicillin *on page 604*
  used in combination with
Aminoglycosides *on page 590*

Alternate

Vancomycin *on page 967*
  used in combination with
Aminoglycosides *on page 590*

Selected Readings

Warren JW, "Catheter-Associated Urinary Tract Infections," *Infect Dis Clin North Am*, 1997, 11(3):609-22.

Urinary Tract Infection, Perinephric Abscess

Synonyms Perinephric Abscess

Clinical Presentation Often a complication of untreated (or insufficiently treated) urinary tract infection or pyelonephritis. Patient may have fever, flank pain, leukocytosis. Pain may be severe or dull and chronic.

Differential Diagnosis Kidney stones; staghorn calculi; malignancy; infection - bacterial, fungal

Likely Pathogens

Escherichia coli, Nonenterohemorrhagic *on page 147*
Staphylococcus aureus, Methicillin-Susceptible *on page 258*

Diagnostic Tests/Procedures

- Computed Transaxial Tomography, Abdomen Studies *on page 373*
- Ultrasound, Kidneys *on page 561*
- Urine Culture, Clean Catch *on page 565*
  Cystometrogram, Simple *on page 382*

Empiric Drug Therapy

Recommended

Cefazolin *on page 632*
Co-Trimoxazole *on page 692*

Selected Readings

Dembry LM and Andriole VT, "Renal and Perirenal Abscesses," *Infect Dis Clin North Am*, 1997, 11(3):663-80.

Urinary Tract Infection, Pyelonephritis

Synonyms Upper Urinary Tract Infection

Clinical Presentation Most commonly occurs in young females but may occur in any population. Patients may have fever, frequency, dysuria, urgency, hesitancy, plus flank pain. Leukocytosis, pyuria, and hematuria is common.

Differential Diagnosis Kidney stones; staghorn calculi, malignancy, infection - bacterial, fungal.

Likely Pathogens

Escherichia coli, Nonenterohemorrhagic *on page 147*

Proteus Species *on page 232*

Diagnostic Tests/Procedures

- Blood Culture, Aerobic and Anaerobic *on page 337*
- Urine Culture, Clean Catch *on page 565*

  Computed Transaxial Tomography, Abdomen Studies *on page 373*

  Gram's Stain *on page 426*

Empiric Drug Therapy

Recommended

Ampicillin *on page 604*

used in combination with

Gentamicin *on page 747*

or

Co-Trimoxazole *on page 692*

Alternate

Cephalosporins, 3rd Generation *on page 662*

Fluoroquinolones *on page 736*

Nitrofurantoin *on page 842*

Selected Readings

Barnett BJ and Stephens DS, "Urinary Tract Infection: An Overview," *Am J Med Sci*, 1997, 314(4):245-9.

Friedman AL, "Urinary Tract Infection," *Curr Opin Pediatr*, 1998, 10(2):197-200.

Hooton TM and Stamm WE, "Diagnosis and Treatment of Uncomplicated Urinary Tract Infection," *Infect Dis Clin North Am*, 1997, 11(3):551-81.

Urinary Tract Infection, Uncomplicated

Synonyms Uncomplicated Urinary Tract Infection; UTI, Uncomplicated

Clinical Presentation Patients with only lower tract disease (cystitis) present with dysuria, frequency, urgency, and suprapubic tenderness. Patients with both lower and upper tract disease present with cystitis, fever, and flank pain. Urinalysis reveals pyuria with or without hematuria. Elderly and diabetic patients may be asymptomatic.

Differential Diagnosis Urethritis; pyelonephritis; prostatitis; cervicitis

Likely Pathogens

Escherichia coli, Nonenterohemorrhagic *on page 147*

Klebsiella Species *on page 183*

Proteus Species *on page 232*

Staphylococcus saprophyticus on page 264

Diagnostic Tests/Procedures

Urinalysis *on page 562*

Urine Culture, Clean Catch *on page 565*

Empiric Drug Therapy

Recommended

Co-Trimoxazole *on page 692*

Alternate

Amoxicillin *on page 592*

Selected Readings

Barnett BJ and Stephens DS, "Urinary Tract Infection: An Overview." *Am J Med Sci*, 1997, 314(4):245-9.

Friedman AL, "Urinary Tract Infection," *Curr Opin Pediatr*, 1998, 10(2):197-200.

Hooton TM and Stamm WE, "Diagnosis and Treatment of Uncomplicated Urinary Tract Infection," *Infect Dis Clin North Am*, 1997, 11(3):551-81.

UTI, Uncomplicated *see* Urinary Tract Infection, Uncomplicated *on this page*

Vaginosis, Bacterial

Synonyms Bacterial Vaginosis; "Nonspecific Vaginosis"

Clinical Presentation Patients complain of vaginal odor, and a majority note a mild to moderate clear, gray discharge. Patients rarely complain of dysuria or dyspareunia. Physical exam of vagina and cervix are unremarkable except for presence of thin, homogeneous, gray, bubbly discharge.

Differential Diagnosis Other vaginal infections; noninfectious vulvovaginitis

Likely Pathogens
Gardnerella vaginalis on page 151
Bacteroides Species *on page 75*
Streptococcus-Related Gram-Positive Cocci on page 278

Diagnostic Tests/Procedures The pH of the vaginal discharge should be tested.

Genital Culture *on page 423*
Trichomonas Preparation *on page 555*

Drug Therapy Comment Clindamycin as a vaginal cream; metronidazole as a vaginal gel.

Empiric Drug Therapy
Recommended
Clindamycin *on page 684*
Metronidazole *on page 817*

Valley Fever *see Coccidioides immitis on page 109*

Vulvovaginitis, Mycotic *see Candida* Species *on page 91*

Whooping Cough *see Bordetella pertussis on page 81*

Wound Infection, Surgical

Synonyms Surgical Wound Infection

Clinical Presentation The Centers for Disease Control case definition of an incisional surgical wound infection is one that occurs at the incision site within 30 days of surgery and involves skin or subcutaneous tissue above muscle fascia. Infection should not be diagnosed by only the isolation of organisms from the wound site alone as this may represent colonization. The site should show signs of infection as manifested by purulence and breakdown of tissue. A deep surgical wound is one that occurs within 30 days of surgery if no implant is left in place or one that occurs within 1 year of placement of nonhuman-derived implantable foreign device. Infection must be related to site and involve tissues at or beneath the muscle fascia. The wound may spontaneously dehisce or require surgical opening especially if the patient has fever, localized pain, or tenderness.

Likely Pathogens
Staphylococcus epidermidis, Methicillin-Susceptible *on page 263*
Staphylococcus aureus, Methicillin-Susceptible *on page 258*
Staphylococcus epidermidis, Methicillin-Resistant *on page 261*
Staphylococcus aureus, Methicillin-Resistant *on page 256*
Gram-Negative Bacilli *on page 154*

Diagnostic Tests/Procedures
Aerobic Culture, Appropriate Site *on page 310*
Anaerobic Culture *on page 316*
Gram's Stain *on page 426*

Drug Therapy Comment If gram-negative bacilli seen on Gram's stain, use extended spectrum penicillins with or without aminoglycoside.

Empiric Drug Therapy
Recommended
Penicillins, Penicillinase-Resistant *on page 864*
Vancomycin *on page 967*

Zygomycosis *see Mucor* Species *on page 198*

ORGANISMS

Acanthamoeba Species

Microbiology *Acanthamoeba* is a unicellular, free-living, nonparasitic ameba. There are four genera of ameba which have been identified as pathogenic for humans: *Acanthamoeba*, *Entamoeba*, *Naegleria*, and *Vahlkampfia*. *Acanthamoeba* is a small organism, about 10-40 μm in diameter. The life cycle consists of an active trophozoite and a dormant cystic stage. The trophozoites are about 40 μm in diameter and have a single nucleus and characteristic fine cytoplasmic projections called acanthapodia. The cyst forms are also uninucleate but smaller (12 μm in diameter) and have a distinctive external wall surrounding a stellate endocyst (double wall).

Epidemiology The organism is present in many geographic areas and is associated with water and soil. Data from serologic studies and nasopharyngeal cultures of soldiers suggest that environmental exposure to *Acanthamoeba* appears to be common in the normal population. The organism has also been cultured from the nares of normal individuals being studied for respiratory virus infection. It is thought that *Acanthamoeba* is inhaled in the cyst phase, but it is unclear whether this organism is a part of the normal respiratory flora. Despite this common exposure, disease is uncommon. *Acanthamoeba* keratitis (see Clinical Syndromes) is a condition seen in healthy individuals who are contact lens wearers. Disease occurs following direct corneal inoculation. Risk factors for corneal infection with *Acanthamoeba* include wearing contact lenses while swimming and use of homemade saline for contact lens cleaning and storage. In contrast, *Acanthamoeba*-associated granulomatous encephalitis occurs mainly in persons who are debilitated and immunocompromised, including persons with AIDS, diabetes, transplant recipients, and persons undergoing chemotherapy. *Acanthamoeba* granulomatous encephalitis is not associated with fresh-water exposure, unlike primary amebic encephalitis caused by *Naegleria*. Because of the limited numbers of reported cases, the epidemiology of *Acanthamoeba* in AIDS patients remains to be defined. However, it appears that persons with AIDS may be predisposed to this infection of the central nervous system since in one series 7 of the reported 60 cases of *Acanthamoeba* encephalitis occurred in persons with AIDS. Most recently, a disseminated form of *Acanthamoeba* has been described in immunocompromised persons which appears distinct from granulomatous encephalitis.

Clinical Syndromes

- **Granulomatous amebic encephalitis:** This is a rare disease (less than 200 reported cases). It can be caused by either *Acanthamoeba* or *Naegleria*. The vast majority of patients are immunocompromised. Pathologically, there are areas of necrotizing granulomatous inflammation in the brain parenchyma, with cerebral edema. Both trophozoites and cysts are seen in areas of inflammation. Multinucleated giant cells may be present. Invasion of blood vessel walls by the trophozoites may be seen. Gross lesions tend to involve the posterior structures such as the brain stem, cerebellum, and midbrain. It is believed that this central nervous system infection is a result of hematogenous dissemination; *Acanthamoeba* organisms have been identified in other tissues outside the CNS including skin and lung. Clinically, patients present with the gradual onset of headaches, mental status changes, and focal neurologic deficits. Other symptoms reported include fever and seizures. Skin lesions have been reported in some cases and have been nodular or ulcerative. Head CT scans may show nonenhancing cortical mass lesions.
- **Disseminated *Acanthamoeba*:** This is a rare, but well-documented, form of *Acanthamoeba* infection. In general, disseminated infection is rapidly fatal although there are now several reports of successful treatment using multiple antibiotic agents. Disseminated disease has been described only in immunosuppressed patients such as advanced AIDS and bone marrow and renal transplant recipients. Infection is characterized by multiple nodular skin lesions although a variety of other skin lesions have been reported including plaques, papules, pustules, ulcers, and cellulitis. Organisms have been isolated from a variety of other sites including liver, gastrointestinal tract, and lung. The brain is not involved in many of the reported cases.
- ***Acanthamoeba* keratitis:** This serious infection is an important cause of corneal infection in the United States. It is associated with the use of soft contact lenses in healthy persons. Pathologically, cysts and trophozoite forms are seen in the cornea with an associated inflammatory reaction

which may contain giant cells. As the infection progresses, sometimes there is a characteristic ring-shaped infiltrate in the cornea which can be seen by an ophthalmologist. Inflammation of the anterior chamber (anterior uveitis) is also often present on ophthalmologic examination, and organisms may be present in the aqueous humor. Clinically, patients present with tearing in the eye, progressive pain and photophobia, and decreased visual acuity. The symptoms are nonspecific and often the condition is misdiagnosed as herpes or bacterial conjunctivitis/iritis for many weeks before the diagnosis of amebic keratitis is entertained.

Diagnosis *Acanthamoeba* can be detected in routine cytology preparations (eg, from corneal epithelial scrapings) and in histologic sections of tissue biopsy specimens (eg, skin, liver). Some authors have emphasized the limited sensitivity of routine laboratory methods, and in some cases, multiple tissue biopsies were required to identify the organism. In addition, specialized cytologic techniques have been described to improve the sensitivity. The organisms may also be misidentified on biopsy specimens with necrotic debris, histiocytes, and macrophages; the pathologist should be alerted to the possibility of *Acanthamoeba*. It may be difficult to distinguish *Acanthamoeba* from other pathogenic ameba solely on the basis of morphology, and culture confirmation may be necessary. The organism will not grow on routine culture media. The Microbiology Laboratory should be consulted prior to biopsy if *Acanthamoeba* culture is desired, since the specimen will require special media preparation (or may need to be sent to a reference laboratory). *Acanthamoeba* has been isolated from fresh tissue planted on non-nutrient agar plates (seeded with *Escherichia coli* broth to encourage the growth of *Acanthamoeba*) and cell culture systems. In general, tissue specimens submitted for *Acanthamoeba* culture should **not** be placed in any fixative (such as formalin) and should **not** be frozen. Some authors have recommended the use of Page's media for transportation of specimens to the laboratory for culture rather than sterile saline to increase the yield.

Acanthamoeba granulomatous encephalitis is difficult to diagnose antemortem, and most cases have been identified only at autopsy. This entity should be considered in immunocompromised persons presenting with a mass lesion of the brain of unknown etiology, particularly if skin lesions are present. Biopsy of concomitant skin lesions may reveal the organism. Lumbar puncture is not useful in diagnosing this infection because *Acanthamoeba* has never been identified in the CSF; the lumbar puncture may be useful in excluding other infectious etiologies. Definitive diagnosis usually requires a brain biopsy with identification of the organism in histologic sections.

Acanthamoeba keratitis: This should be considered in any patient with a persistent keratitis not responding to antibacterial or antiviral topical therapy, especially if associated with contact lens use. Early referral to an ophthalmologist is essential since dendriform epithelial changes may be identified prior to the development of the ring infiltrates in the cornea. Definitive diagnosis requires corneal scrapings and/or biopsies. Tissue material should be submitted for wet mount, cytology and histologic staining (hematoxylin-eosin, Wright-Giemsa stain, periodic acid Schiff, and others), and for specialized culture. Indirect fluorescent antibody examination of fixed slides has also been used successfully. Spray fixation if felt to be necessary prior to air-drying of smears to preserve the trophozoites. In many cases, culture of the contact lens solution has yielded the organism. Submit lens, case, and fluid in case to the laboratory.

Diagnostic Tests/Procedures

Brain Biopsy *on page 352*
Histopathology *on page 448*
Ocular Cytology *on page 505*

Treatment There are no established therapies for *Acanthamoeba* encephalitis or disseminated infection. The organism demonstrates *in vivo* resistance to a number of agents including amphotericin B and sulfonamides; pentamidine and related agents show activity against the organism but the clinical efficacy is unclear. In the few cases of successful therapy of disseminated infection reported thus far, multidrug antibiotic therapy has been used including a regimen of itraconazole, pentamidine, 5-flucytosine (5-FC), and topical chlorhexidine gluconate and ketoconazole cream.

Acanthamoeba keratitis may respond to a combination of surgical debridement of abnormal epithelium and topical antimicrobial agents. The optimal medical
(Continued)

Acanthamoeba Species *(Continued)*

and/or surgical regimen remains under study. Some authorities have recommended the combination of topical miconazole nitrate, propamidine isethionate, and Neosporin® ophthalmics. In a recent prospective study, propamidine isethionate 0.1% solution administered concomitantly with neomycin-polymyxin B-gramicidin ophthalmic solution (Neosporin®) resulted in an 83% success rate. Others have reported success with bacitracin and polymyxin B with or without neomycin. Oral antibiotics that have been used successfully have included paromomycin, ketoconazole, and itraconazole. Experimental infections with *Acanthamoeba* have responded to sulfadiazine, but the clinical efficacy is still unclear. Many patients may require corneal grafting; the role of keratoplasty is still controversial. Vision may remain significantly limited even with aggressive intervention.

Selected Readings

Gardner LM, Mathers WD, and Folberg R, "New Technique for the Cytologic Identification of Presumed *Acanthamoeba* From Corneal Epithelial Scrapings," *Am J Ophthalmol*, 1999, 127(2):207-9.

Gordon SM, Steinberg JP, Du Puis MH, et al "Culture Isolation of *Acanthamoeba* Species and Leptomyxid Amebas From Patients With Amebic Meningoencephalitis, Including Two Patients With AIDS," *Clin Infect Dis*, 1992, 15(6):1024-30.

Hargrave SL, McCulley JP, and Husseini Z, "Results of a Trial of Combined Propamidine Isethionate and Neomycin Therapy for *Acanthamoeba* Keratitis. Brolene Study Group," *Ophthalmology*, 1999, 106(5):952-7.

Marciano-Cabral F and Petri WA, "Free-Living Amebae," *Principles and Practice of Infectious Diseases*, 4th ed, Mandell GL, Bennett JE, and Dolin R, eds, New York, NY: Churchill Livingstone, 1995, 2408-15.

Migueles S and Kumar P, "Primary Cutaneous *Acanthamoeba* Infection in a Patient With AIDS," *Clin Infect Dis*, 1998, 27(6):1547-8.

Oliva S, Jantz M, Tiernan R, et al, "Successful Treatment of Widely Disseminated Acanthamoebiasis," *South Med J*, 1999, 92(1):55-7.

Achromobacter xylosoxidans see Alcaligenes Species *on page 65*

Acinetobacter Species

Microbiology *Acinetobacter* is a strictly aerobic, gram-negative coccobacillus which is an important cause of nosocomial colonization and disease. Microbiologically, *Acinetobacter* is related to *Neisseria* and *Moraxella* and can sometimes be confused with these organisms on Gram's stain. The organism is readily identified biochemically. All members of the genus *Acinetobacter* are lactose nonfermenters (ie, lactose-negative), oxidase-negative, nonmotile, and catalase-positive. The negative oxidase test is a rapid means of distinguishing *Acinetobacter* from many other gram-negative nonfermenters commonly isolated from hospitalized patients. Taxonomic systems for the classification of the genus *Acinetobacter* have undergone a number of changes over the years, in large part due to new molecular typing methods which clarify the relatedness of the various species. This has led to considerable confusion for clinicians. In the 1980s, only a single species of *Acinetobacter* was recognized (*A. calcoaceticus*) which was subdivided into different biovars (biologically distinct varieties or subspecies), such as *A. calcoaceticus* var *anitratus* and *A. calcoaceticus* var *lwoffii*. More recently, DNA sequencing studies have led to a new classification scheme where a number of genomic species have been identified and some have been formally named. The main human pathogens are *A. calcoaceticus* and *A. baumannii*. Because of the close relationship of several of these species, many microbiologists refer to genomic species number 1 (*A. calcoaceticus*), 2 (*A. baumannii*), 3, and 13 TU as the *A. calcoaceticus-A. baumannii* complex. Because of the similarities of these four genomic species, clinical microbiology laboratories may group them together as the "*A. calcoaceticus-A. baumannii* complex" without evaluating the isolates further. This complex approximates the older designation of *calcoaceticus* var *anitratus*. Additional changes in the various classification schemes in the future are likely.

Of the various genomic species, *A. baumannii* causes the majority of significant human infection and is the species most associated with nosocomial outbreaks of *Acinetobacter* spp. Other *Acinetobacter* species have sporadically been associated with nosocomial disease including *A. lwoffii*, *A. johnsonii*, and others. Recovery of the less common *Acinetobacter* spp from clinical specimens can be difficult to interpret since many of these species are natural commensals on the skin or can be environmental contaminants, and are not common causes of disease.

Epidemiology *Acinetobacter* is ubiquitous in nature and can be isolated in nearly 100% of soil and water samples tested. The organism is commensal in the human respiratory tract, skin, and urinary tract. It is estimated that up to 25% of healthy adults are colonized with *Acinetobacter* on the skin and >5% in the pharynx. Patients requiring tracheostomies for long-term mechanical ventilation have a much higher rate of respiratory colonization. Within the hospital environment, *Acinetobacter* is frequently found in areas of moisture such as humidifiers, bedside commodes, and ventilator tubing. In some series, it is the most common gram-negative organism carried on the hands of hospital workers.

Despite the prevalence of this organism in the environment, *Acinetobacter* is a relatively uncommon cause of bacteremia. The great majority of significant *Acinetobacter* infections are nosocomial and not community acquired. *Acinetobacter* species have been well described as a sporadic cause of hospital outbreaks, frequently in intensive care unit settings. However, in one of the largest studies reported, 52 episodes of *Acinetobacter* bacteremia were examined over a 6-year period and found to occur at a constant rate with no notable outbreaks or clusters.

Risk factors for hospital-acquired *Acinetobacter* bacteremia include the following.

- Malignancies: Some studies suggest a strong association with leukemia and breast cancer, in particular. Neutropenia itself does not seem to be a significant risk factor.
- Trauma patients: Particularly young men in motor vehicle accidents. The source of bacteremia in these cases is more likely from nosocomial pneumonia than from wound infection.
- Burn patients: The portal of entry for *Acinetobacter* is most likely from extensive soft tissue infection. In burn patients, *Acinetobacter* may be present as part of a polymicrobial bacteremia.
- Presence of an intravenous catheter: In some series, the presence of an indwelling central venous catheter appears to be an important risk factor for bacteremia, but in other series, the association is weak or absent. Some authors have speculated that an intravascular catheter should be regarded more as a marker of severity of illness rather than as a risk factor per se for bacteremia.

Clinical Syndromes *Acinetobacter* is an organism of relatively low virulence and is mainly a nosocomial pathogen. In the debilitated hospital patient, the severity of infection may range from mild to life-threatening. It is important to realize that many isolates of *Acinetobacter* from clinical specimens may represent benign colonization, especially when such isolates are reported from the respiratory tract in intubated patients. For this reason, the true *Acinetobacter* nosocomial infection rate is difficult to know with certainty. Surveillance studies in the United States have estimated that 0.3% to 1.4% of all nosocomial infections are caused by *Acinetobacter* spp.

Common nosocomial infections include:

- pneumonia, usually ventilator-associated and multilobar. Data from the National Nosocomial Infection Study estimates that 4% of all nosocomial pneumonias are caused by *Acinetobacter* spp. Several studies have examined *Acinetobacter* infection rates in the highest risk group for nosocomial pneumonia, namely mechanically ventilated patients in an intensive care unit. Using specimens obtained by bronchoscopy to minimize upper airway contamination, *Acinetobacter* spp were found to be the cause of ventilator-associated pneumonia in 15% to 20% of episodes. Estimates of crude mortality associated with *Acinetobacter* pneumonia varies between 30% to 75%. Some studies have suggested that the mortality associated with *Acinetobacter* pneumonia is higher than nosocomial pneumonia caused by other gram-negative organisms (55%) with the exception of *Pseudomonas aeruginosa*. Outbreaks of multidrug-resistant *Acinetobacter* pneumonias are becoming more common
- bacteremia, most commonly from a pulmonary focus but also secondary to intravenous catheters. Again, the most common species is *A. baumannii*. Immunocompromised patients are at highest risk. Outbreaks of bacteremia have been described in neonatal intensive care units. Bacteremias also may be polymicrobial, particularly when associated with intravascular catheter infection.

(Continued)

Acinetobacter Species *(Continued)*

- meningitis, following neurosurgical procedures or associated with ventricular shunt devices
- urinary tract infections, including cystitis or pyelonephritis associated with indwelling bladder catheters or renal stones. This is a relatively uncommon *Acinetobacter* spp infection.
- intra-abdominal sepsis, usually as part of a polymicrobial infection
- soft tissue infections, particularly with postoperative wound dehiscence or extensive burn injuries

Community-acquired *Acinetobacter* infections are unusual but have been reported in certain situations:

- tracheobronchitis in healthy children
- community-acquired pneumonia in alcoholics

Diagnosis The diagnosis of *Acinetobacter* species infections is made by identification of the organism through Gram's stain and culture in a patient with a relevant clinical syndrome. No special media or conditions are necessary to grow these organisms, although selective media are available (media which contain antibiotics which suppress the growth of other organisms).

Diagnostic Tests/Procedures

Aerobic Culture, Appropriate Site *on page 310*
Gram's Stain *on page 426*

Treatment Since the mid 1970s, isolates of *Acinetobacter* have steadily become resistant to antibiotics of a variety of classes. Some authors feel that *Acinetobacter* develops drug resistance much more rapidly than other gram-negative bacilli. Resistance to multiple antibiotics has been demonstrated by a number of mechanisms including the production of high levels of beta-lactamase enzymes, either plasmid-mediated resistance and/or chromosomally-mediated resistance; alterations in penicillin-binding proteins; alterations in cell permeability; and production of aminoglycoside-inactivating enzymes.

Resistance to β-lactam antibiotics in many isolates of *Acinetobacter* is mediated by the production of the TEM-1 and TEM-2 plasmid-mediated β-lactamases, enzymes which are involved in resistance with other gram-negative bacilli. However, β-lactam resistance is not the only factor involved in penicillin resistance since in some studies, β-lactamases were not identified in the majority of clinical isolates which were ticarcillin-resistant. These other factors include cell permeability changes and alterations of penicillin-binding proteins. Of note, *A. baumannii* commonly produces cephalosporins (four enzymes termed ACE1-ACE4), which are chromosomally-mediated mutations. Cephalosporinases seem to account for most of the high level cephalosporin resistance. Aminoglycoside resistance of *Acinetobacter* spp has been increasing as well, and all of the three common aminoglycoside-modifying enzymes have been reported, namely acetylating, adenylating, and phosphorylating enzymes. Quinolone resistance has also been reported in increasing numbers. The mechanism for this resistance is probably mutation in DNA gyrase (as has been reported in other gram-negative bacilli), but this has been more difficult to prove in *Acinetobacter*. Serious infections caused by multiple-drug resistant species are often quite difficult to treat and may require the use of newer, alternative agents.

Acinetobacter species resistant to cephalosporins and extended spectrum penicillins may be susceptible to either imipenem and/or ampicillin/sulbactam, but the clinician must carefully review the antibiogram. One author has described a decreasing susceptibility to ampicillin/sulbactam with only 61% of *Acinetobacter* isolates now susceptible *in vitro*. In addition, *Acinetobacter* species are no longer uniformly susceptible to imipenem, as they once were in many hospitals prior to 1990. Outbreaks of imipenem-resistant *A. baumannii* have recently been described (see Selected Readings). A new β-lactamase termed ARI-1 has been identified in some imipenem-resistant isolates and has become a great concern; it appears to be plasmid-mediated and easily transferable between strains. In such cases of imipenem-resistant, β-lactam-resistant *Acinetobacter*, there may be no proven alternative therapy.

Because of these considerations, the optimal therapy of *Acinetobacter* infection depends on the specific antibiotic-susceptibility pattern of the isolate. Empiric therapy for *Acinetobacter* infection (ie, before susceptibility data is known) is difficult and should be based on known drug-resistance patterns in the hospital.

Drug Therapy
Recommended
   Cephalosporins, 3rd Generation *on page 662*
   Penicillins, Extended Spectrum *on page 864*
Alternate
   Imipenem and Cilastatin *on page 766*
   Ampicillin and Sulbactam *on page 607*
   Aztreonam *on page 615*
   Meropenem *on page 812*

Selected Readings

Bergogne-Berezin E and Towner KJ, "*Acinetobacter* spp. as Nosocomial Pathogens: Microbiological, Clinical, and Epidemiological Features," *Clin Microbiol Rev*, 1996, 9(2):148-65.

Husni RN, Goldstein LS, Arroliga AC, et al, "Risk Factors for an Outbreak of Multi-Drug-Resistant *Acinetobacter* Nosocomial Pneumonia Among Intubated Patients," *Chest*, 1999, 115(5):1378-82.

Smego RA Jr, "Endemic Nosocomial *Acinetobacter calcoaceticus* Bacteremia. Clinical Significance, Treatment, and Prognosis," *Arch Intern Med*, 1985, 145(12):2174-9.

Tilley PA and Roberts FJ, "Bacteremia With *Acinetobacter* Species: Risk Factors and Prognosis in Different Clinical Settings," *Clin Infect Dis*, 1994, 18(6):896-900.

Urban C, Go E, Mariano N, et al, "Effect of Sulbactam on Infections Caused by Imipenem-Resistant *Acinetobacter calcoaceticus* Biotype *anitratus*," *J Infect Dis*, 1993, 167(2):448-51.

Wood CA and Reboli AC, "Infections Caused by Imipenem-Resistant *Acinetobacter calcoaceticus* Biotype *anitratus*," *J Infect Dis*, 1993, 168(6):1602-3.

Actinomyces Species

Microbiology *Actinomyces* species are gram-positive, "higher order" bacteria and are related to *Nocardia* species. The most common *Actinomyces* species to cause disease is *Actinomyces israelii*, accounting for about 75% of all cases. These organisms are normal residents of the oral flora and are of low virulence. In the laboratory, *Actinomyces* species grow optimally under anaerobic conditions; growth may also occur in a microaerophilic environment (and sometimes aerobically). When stained, the organism appears thin, with filamentous branches, and may be difficult to distinguish from *Nocardia* species. Growth is slow even under optimal conditions, and the laboratory should be notified if *Actinomyces* is suspected. If a patient receives antibiotics, the organism will only rarely grow in culture because of its susceptibility to a number of agents.

In clinical specimens, *Actinomyces israelii* is often found associated with characteristic **sulfur granules**. These granules are irregularly shaped, mineralized masses consisting of calcium phosphate, inflammatory cells, and masses of *Actinomyces* filaments. Occasionally, sulfur granules may be caused by other organisms but are most commonly associated with *Actinomyces israelii*.

Epidemiology *Actinomyces* species are commensal organisms found in the oral cavity and may be cultured from tooth cavities, gingival creases, dental plaque, tonsils, and related areas; they are harmless saprophytes and do not cause disease when mucous membranes are intact. These organisms also may be part of the normal gastrointestinal flora and can be cultured from the female genital region in the absence of disease. The majority of patients who develop *Actinomyces* infections are immunocompetent. Actinomycosis is not considered an opportunistic infection, although it has been reported occasionally with malignancies and AIDS. Infection usually results from breakdown in the normal mucosal barrier with spread of the organism into deeper sites, such as after dental extractions, trauma, etc.

Clinical Syndromes
- **Cervicofacial actinomycosis:** This is the most common syndrome produced by this organism. Also known as the "lumpy jaw syndrome", patients may present with subacute or acute soft tissue swelling in the head or neck. In chronic cases, progression of localized abscesses may lead to draining sinuses and fistulas. Often a history of a preceding dental procedure can be obtained. In some cases, cervicofacial involvement may be dramatic and rapid, with trismus.
- **Pulmonary actinomycosis:** Patients may develop pulmonary *Actinomyces* infection, usually following an aspiration event or as a complication of head and neck actinomycosis. Clinical symptoms may be mild with only a minor cough and no fever. With serious disease, lung cavitation resembling *M. tuberculosis* may be seen. Other potential chest x-ray or CT scan findings include alveolar pneumonia, upper lobe infiltrates, a lung mass with or without invasion into the chest wall, mediastinal mass, rib destruction, and others. Occasionally, a sinus tract may develop from the lung to the chest wall which is highly suggestive of this organism.

(Continued)

Actinomyces Species *(Continued)*

- **Abdominal actinomycosis:** Following abdominal surgery or rupture of an abdominal viscus (eg, perforated duodenal ulcer), patients may develop abdominal actinomycosis. This may be a very difficult diagnosis to establish. The development of sinus tracts is suggestive of this organism.
- **Pelvic actinomycosis:** Actinomycosis has been well-known as a potential complication of intrauterine devices (IUDs). There is a wide spectrum of presentations, including pelvic inflammatory disease. It should be noted that since *Actinomyces* species may be harmless residents of the female genital tract, positive cervical cultures or Pap smears for *Actinomyces* species may or may not represent an infectious disease.
- **Brain abscess:** This may occur as a result of direct extension from a cervicofacial site or hematogenously.
- **Human bite wounds:** Local actinomycosis may occur as a complication of a human bite.
- **Disseminated disease:** On rare occasions, *Actinomyces* can disseminate hematogenously and deposit on skin and other organs.

Diagnosis The clinician should consider *Actinomyces* in any patient presenting with a painful subcutaneous swelling in the head and neck. Draining sinus tracts are highly suggestive of actinomycosis, whether in the head and neck, or the thorax. Recurrent infections are the hallmark of this chronic infection, and patients empirically given oral antibiotics for mandibular or neck swelling may show a partial response followed by relapse.

At times, sulfur granules may be found in purulent fluid from abscesses or sinus tracts when the patient is examined at the bedside. These granules are about 2 mm in size and are hard, yellow to white in color, and round in appearance. They should be sent for histopathologic analysis and culture, since other organisms can produce similar-appearing granules. The absence of sulfur granules in no way excludes actinomycosis. Every effort should be made to isolate the organism in the Microbiology Laboratory. Since *Actinomyces* is fastidious, multiple aspirations or biopsies may be necessary.

As noted above, the finding of a positive culture for *Actinomyces* does not always indicate significant disease since it is part of the normal oral and gastrointestinal flora of many persons.

Treatment Penicillin G remains the drug of choice. For cervicofacial actinomycosis, penicillin G given at 10-20 million units daily I.V. has been effective and well tolerated by most. Surgical debridement may often be necessary in addition to antibiotics and treatment failures with antibiotics alone may occur. After several weeks of parenteral penicillin, oral penicillin at high doses may be substituted, such as penicillin V potassium up to 4 g daily. Some clinicians may use probenecid in combination with oral penicillin. For the penicillin-allergic, several antibiotics may be used including erythromycin, tetracycline, and clindamycin. Quinolones and cephalosporins should be avoided.

Drug Therapy
Recommended
Penicillin G, Parenteral, Aqueous *on page 860*
Ampicillin *on page 604*
Alternate
Doxycycline *on page 713*

Selected Readings
Burden P, "Actinomycosis," *J Infect*, 1989, 19(2):95-9.
Russo TA, "Agents of Actinomycosis," *Principles and Practice of Infectious Diseases*, 4th ed, Mandell GL, Bennett JE, and Dolin R, eds, New York, NY: Churchill Livingstone, 1995, 2280-8.

Adenovirus

Microbiology Adenovirus is a double-stranded DNA virus which can cause several infectious syndromes in both adults and children. Exposure to this virus is common, and serologic studies suggest that by 10 years of age most children have experienced either clinical or subclinical infection. The symptoms associated with adenovirus infection are likely due to lysis of infected host cells coupled with a brisk host immune response. Most cases of symptomatic disease are associated with the initial infection in a nonimmune host. However, some evidence suggests that adenovirus can enter a latent (asymptomatic) phase in some individuals and can reactivate later in life, particularly if the host becomes immunosuppressed (organ transplantation, corticosteroids, etc).

Epidemiology With humans providing the only known reservoir for adenoviruses, 5% to 10% of all viral respiratory illnesses in civilians are caused by these viruses. Epidemics are usually restricted to the military with small outbreaks among children. Person-to-person transmission through respiratory and ocular secretions is thought to be the major route of transmission. Adenoviruses associated with infantile gastroenteritis are probably transmitted by the fecal-oral route.

Clinical Syndromes

- **Respiratory tract infection, at all ages:** This is the most common manifestation of adenovirus infection and is responsible for approximately 10% of infant and childhood ambulatory respiratory infections. In boarding schools or military camps, outbreaks of influenza-like respiratory infections have been well described. Adenovirus has also been implicated as a common cause of atypical pneumonia in adults, characterized by low-grade fever, subacute onset, prominent constitutional symptoms (headache, myalgias, malaise), and an absence of purulent sputum.
- **Asymptomatic infection of the tonsils and adenoids (usually adenovirus types 1,2,5) in infants**
- **Pharyngitis in infants**
- **Infantile diarrhea**
- **Pharyngoconjunctival fever in older children:** Especially in summer camps or schools. This is manifested by the acute onset of conjunctivitis, sore throat, fever, and rhinitis, and tends to be a self-limited illness.
- **Hemorrhagic cystitis in adults:** Usually caused by types 11 and 21
- **Keratoconjunctivitis:** Adenovirus is an important cause of epidemic keratoconjunctivitis. Patients present with inflamed conjunctivae (often bilateral) with preauricular adenopathy.
- **Adenovirus and HIV infection:** Persons infected with the human immunodeficiency virus may be carriers of adenovirus. Despite this, there appears to be a very low incidence of recognized adenovirus in persons with AIDS. Case reports have described disseminated adenovirus with hepatic necrosis, adenovirus colitis, and necrotizing adenovirus infection of the renal tubules.
- **Infections in other immunosuppressed patients:** Fatal adenovirus infections due to disseminated disease have been described in transplant recipients (bone marrow, renal transplant), as well as other chronically immunosuppressed patients (see Selected Readings).

Diagnosis Laboratory studies can confirm suspected cases of adenovirus infection, but the turnaround time can exceed 1 week. Serologic studies demonstrating a fourfold or greater rise in specific IgG titer to adenovirus strongly supports the diagnosis of recent infection. Direct cultures for the virus are available in many laboratories, but the time for viral isolation is variable and highly dependent on the amount of virus in the clinical specimen.

Diagnostic Tests/Procedures

Adenovirus Antibody Titer *on page 309*
Adenovirus Culture *on page 309*
Virus Detection by DFA *on page 576*

Treatment No antiviral agents have been proven to be effective in the treatment of adenovirus infections. Supportive care is the treatment of choice.

Selected Readings

Baum SG, "Adenovirus," *Principles and Practice of Infectious Diseases*, 4th ed, Mandell GL, Bennett JE, and Dolin R, eds, New York, NY: Churchill Livingstone, 1995, 1382-7.

Flomenberg P, Babbitt J, Drobyski WR, et al, "Increasing Incidence of Adenovirus Disease in Bone Marrow Transplant Recipients," *J Infect Dis*, 1994, 169(4):775-81.

Green WR, Greaves WL, Frederick WR, et al, "Renal Infection Due to Adenovirus in a Patient With Human Immunodeficiency Virus Infection," *Clin Infect Dis*, 1994, 18(6):989-91.

Hierholzer JC, "Adenoviruses in the Immunocompromised Host," *Clin Microbiol Rev*, 1992, 5(3):262-74.

Klinger JR, Sanchez MP, Curtin LA, et al, "Multiple Cases of Life-Threatening Adenovirus Pneumonia in a Mental Health Center," *Am J Respir Crit Care Med*, 1998, 157(2):645-9.

Krilov LR, Rubin LG, Frogel M, et al, "Disseminated Adenovirus Infection With Hepatic Necrosis in Patients With Human Immunodeficiency Virus Infection and Other Immunodeficiency States," *Rev Infect Dis*, 1990, 12(2):303-7.

Lukashok SA and Horwitz MS, "New Perspectives in Adenoviruses," *Curr Clin Top Infect Dis*, 1998, 18:286-305.

Shields AF, Hackman RC, Fife KH, et al, "Adenovirus Infections in Patients Undergoing Bone-Marrow Transplantation," *N Engl J Med*, 1985, 312(9):529-33.

Aeromonas Species

Microbiology *Aeromonas* species are gram-negative bacilli which can be recovered from a variety of fresh water sources. They belong to the family Vibrionaceae and several species are important for human disease including *A. caviae* and *A. hydrophila*. The organisms can also be recovered from the stool of some healthy individuals. *Aeromonas* species are lactose-variable (either lactose-positive or lactose-negative) and oxidase-positive, which helps distinguish the organism from other enteric gram-negative bacilli found in the stool. Growth is supported on several routine solid media although special techniques are often necessary to isolate the organism from stool samples. The Microbiology Laboratory should be notified if *Aeromonas* is suspected.

Epidemiology Cases of *Aeromonas* have been reported worldwide. Since *Aeromonas* is found in fresh and brackish waters, human infections have been reported to follow injuries related to contaminated water exposure. *Aeromonas* infections have also been associated with the medical use of leeches since the organism is part of the normal flora of the leech. Cases of diarrhea secondary to *Aeromonas* have been reported from a variety of countries and tends to be sporadic. Day care outbreaks of *Aeromonas*-associated diarrhea have been well described.

Clinical Syndromes

- **Diarrheal illness**: *Aeromonas* has recently been recognized as a cause of a nonbloody diarrhea. The illness tends to be self resolving but sometimes the patient may be ill with fever and bloody diarrhea. Occasionally, a protracted diarrhea may develop.

- **Soft tissue infection**: *Aeromonas hydrophila* is known to cause a rapidly progressive cellulitis following exposure of wounds or traumatized body areas to fresh water. Deeper infections such as myositis and osteomyelitis have been described. Necrosis with gas formation is a serious complication. Surgical site infections may be infected without a history of water exposure.

- **Bloodstream infection**: Mainly seen in patients with leukemia and lymphoma, although other immunosuppressed individuals are at risk. Mortality rates are high.

Diagnosis *Aeromonas* infection should be suspected in persons presenting with a soft tissue infection following exposure to water. *Vibrio* species are also in the differential diagnosis. *Aeromonas* should also be considered in persons with an acute diarrheal illness where other more common pathogens have been excluded. Laboratory confirmation of *Aeromonas* is necessary. Appropriate samples of stool, wound discharge, and/or blood should be submitted for special *Aeromonas* culture.

Diagnostic Tests/Procedures

Blood Culture, Aerobic and Anaerobic *on page 337*
Stool Culture *on page 540*
Wound Culture *on page 577*

Treatment A number of antibiotics are effective. *Aeromonas* is susceptible to third generation cephalosporins, fluoroquinolones, co-trimoxazole, gentamicin, and tobramycin. It is less susceptible or resistant to the extended spectrum penicillins (ticarcillin, ampicillin, piperacillin). Multidrug-resistant isolates have been isolated from clinical specimens and therapy should be based on formal antibiotic susceptibility testing.

Drug Therapy

Recommended
Cephalosporins, 3rd Generation *on page 662*

Alternate
Fluoroquinolones *on page 736*
Co-Trimoxazole *on page 692*

Selected Readings

Barillo DJ, McManus AT, Cioffi WG, et al, "*Aeromonas* Bacteraemia in Burn Patients," *Burns*, 1996, 22(1):48-52.

Deutsch SF and Wedzina W, "*Aeromonas sobria*-Associated Left-Sided Segmental Colitis," *Am J Gastroenterol*, 1997, 92(11):2104-6.

Janda JM and Abbott SL, "Evolving Concepts Regarding the Genus *Aeromonas*: An Expanding Panorama of Species, Disease Presentations, and Unanswered Questions," *Clin Infect Dis*, 1998, 27(2):332-44.

Jones BL and Wilcox MH, "*Aeromonas* Infections and Their Treatment," *J Antimicrob Chemother*, 1995, 35(4):453-61.

AIDS Virus *see* Human Immunodeficiency Virus *on page 177*

Alcaligenes Species

Synonyms *Achromobacter xylosoxidans*

Microbiology *Alcaligenes* species are aerobic, gram-negative bacilli which are increasingly important in nosocomial infections. They are considered "nonfermenters", meaning the organisms do not utilize (ferment) glucose. Growth in culture is easily supported on common solid media including blood agar plates; special culture techniques are not necessary. The organism is oxidase-positive. There are several important *Alcaligenes* species: *Alcaligenes xylosoxidans* subspecies *xylosoxidans* (also called *Achromobacter xylosoxidans*), *Alcaligenes xylosoxidans* subspecies *dentrificans*, *Alcaligenes piechaudii*, and *Alcaligenes faecalis*. These organisms may be difficult to treat in some patients because of the organisms' ability to produce several β-lactamase enzymes which inactivate commonly used antibiotics. Some strains produce very high levels of β-lactamase and may be particularly difficult to treat.

Epidemiology Like other nonfermenting gram-negative bacilli, *Alcaligenes* species may be recovered from a variety of environmental sources including water and soil. *A. xylosoxidans* also appear to be part of the normal flora of the gastrointestinal tract and of the ear. In hospitalized patients, the organism can be recovered from some additional sites including the airways of intubated patients and the skin. Contamination of hospital equipment by *Alcaligenes* has been reported, including ventilatory tubing, saline flushes, intravenous fluids, hemodialysis equipment, and others. Risk factors for infection appear to be prolonged hospitalization and perhaps underlying malignancy. Outbreaks of *Alcaligenes* may occur.

Clinical Syndromes

- **Community-acquired infection:** This remains unusual. *Alcaligenes xylosoxidans* can be a cause of recurrent otitis in some individuals. The organism has also been isolated from children with chronic otitis media. Some authors feel that *Alcaligenes* should not be considered a colonizer or contaminant if isolated from ear fluid, particularly in the presence of clinical signs and symptoms of ear infection. In addition, occasional cases of community-acquired prosthetic joint infections have been reported.

- **Nosocomial infection:** Infection with *Alcaligenes* species generally is seen in debilitated patients who have been hospitalized for a prolonged period of time. There is no single distinctive clinical syndrome characteristic of *Alcaligenes*. Some sites of infection include:

  pneumonia, especially in patients requiring mechanical ventilation; empyema may be seen as a complicating feature

  bloodstream infections, often primary infections or catheter-related. In one review of the literature (Duggan et al), 77 cases of bacteremia due to *Achromobacter xylosoxidans* were analyzed. Nosocomial bacteremia occurred in 70%, and in 36% the bacteremia was part of an outbreak or acquired from a discrete point source. The most common underlying illnesses were malignancies (30%) and cardiac disease. Primary bacteremias accounted for 19% of cases, catheter-associated bacteremia 19%, and pneumonia accounted for 16%. The case-fatality rate was 30%. The case-fatality rate of persons with primary or catheter-associated bacteremia was very low (3%), but a much higher mortality rate was found in patients with meningitis, endocarditis, and pneumonia (65%). The case-fatality rate in neonates was extremely high, almost 80%.

  postoperative wound infections, especially after gastrointestinal tract surgery

  postoperative neurosurgical infections, including meningitis

- ***Alcaligenes* infection in persons with AIDS:** This is an uncommon infection in persons with HIV, although several series of *Alcaligenes* bloodstream infection have been reported. In one series, seven cases of *Alcaligenes xylosoxidans* bacteremia and/or respiratory disease in patients infected with HIV were described. This complication occurred during different phases of HIV infection and was associated with leukopenia in four patients and a central vascular catheter in two. Although the majority of cases were diagnosed after day 3 of hospitalization, a specific source of infection was never identified. In four patients with advanced HIV infection, *Alcaligenes* was present as part of a polymicrobial infection. *In vitro* resistance to several classes of antibiotics was present, but treatment with fluoroquinolones,

(Continued)

Alcaligenes Species *(Continued)*

piperacillin, or an aminoglycoside in combination with either ceftazidime or pefloxacin was successful in all cases.

Diagnosis Since the clinical syndromes caused by *Alcaligenes* are nonspecific and may be caused by other organisms, laboratory diagnosis is important. Routine cultures from appropriate sites are adequate for isolating *Alcaligenes*. It should be emphasized that the recovery of *Alcaligenes* from some body sites does not necessarily mean significant clinical disease. Positive cultures from respiratory secretions in intubated patients may or may not be clinically significant since colonization may occur without disease. Recovery of *Alcaligenes* from sterile body fluids such as cerebrospinal fluid, pleural fluid, and bloodstream nearly always indicates disease.

Diagnostic Tests/Procedures

Aerobic Culture, Appropriate Site *on page 310*
Blood Culture, Aerobic and Anaerobic *on page 337*

Treatment *Alcaligenes* species may become resistant to a variety of antibiotics because of the production of high levels of β-lactamase. Generally, *Alcaligenes* are susceptible to third generation cephalosporins and ureidopenicillins, and imipenem. The organisms are often less susceptible or variably susceptible to quinolones, aminoglycosides, and aztreonam. It is important to obtain antibiotic susceptibility results on clinical isolates of *Alcaligenes* to help direct appropriate therapy, particularly in patients who have been receiving antibiotics.

In the series of 77 patients with *Alcaligenes* bacteremia described above, susceptibility studies showed that all strains were resistant to aminoglycosides, most were resistant to quinolones, and all were susceptible to broad-spectrum penicillins, imipenem, ceftazidime, and trimethoprim-sulfamethoxazole. Time-kill studies showed synergy or additive effects for the combination of gentamicin and piperacillin against most strains.

Drug Therapy

Recommended

Cephalosporins, 3rd Generation *on page 662*
Piperacillin *on page 869*
Imipenem and Cilastatin *on page 766*
Meropenem *on page 812*

Alternate

Fluoroquinolones *on page 736*
Aminoglycosides *on page 590*
Aztreonam *on page 615*

Selected Readings

Decre D, Arlet G, Danglot C, et al, "A Beta-Lactamase Overproducing Strain of *Alcaligenes denitrificans* Subspecies *xylosoxidans* Isolated From a Case of Meningitis," *J Antimicrob Chemother*, 1992, 30(6):769-79.

Duggan JM, Goldstein SJ, Chenoweth CE, et al, "*Achromobacter xylosoxidans* Bacteremia: Report of Four Cases and Review of the Literature," *Clin Infect Dis*, 1996, 23(3):569-76.

Mandell WF, Garvey GJ, and Neu HC, "*Achromobacter xylosoxidans* Bacteremia," *Rev Infect Dis*, 1987, 9(5):1001-5.

Manfredi R, Nanetti, Ferri M, et al, "Bacteremia and Respiratory Involvement by *Alcaligenes xylosoxidans* in Patients Infected With the Human Immunodeficiency Virus," *Eur J Clin Microbiol Infect Dis*, 1997, 16(12):933-8.

McGown J and Steinberg JP, "Other Gram-Negative Bacilli," *Principles and Practice of Infectious Diseases*, 4th ed, Mandell GL, Bennett JE, and Dolin R, eds, New York, NY: Churchill Livingstone, 1995, 2111-2.

Mensah K, Philippon A, Richard C, et al, "Susceptibility of *Alcaligenes denitrificans* Subspecies *xylosoxidans* to Beta-Lactam Antibiotics," *Eur J Clin Microbiol Infect Dis*, 1990, 9(6):405-9.

Wintermeyer SM and Nahata MC, "*Alcaligenes xylosoxidans* Subsp *Xylosoxidans* in Children With Chronic Otorrhea," *Otolaryngol Head Neck Surg*, 1996, 114(2):332-4.

Anaerobic *Streptococcus* *see Streptococcus-Related Gram-Positive Cocci on page 278*

Ancylostoma duodenale

Synonyms Hookworm

Applies to *Necator americanus*

Microbiology *Ancylostoma duodenale* is an intestinal roundworm. Often called "Old World hookworm," this parasite is one of two common hookworms causing human disease. The second hookworm, *Necator americanus* ("New World hookworm"), is structurally related to *Ancylostoma duodenale* and differs mainly in geographic distribution. Hookworms have been estimated to infect nearly 25% of the world's population.

Like all other nematodes (roundworms), *Ancylostoma duodenale* is visible to the naked eye, although the adult tends to be only 1 cm long. The infectious cycle begins when filariform larvae penetrate intact skin of the host. The most common portal of entry is the human foot, usually associated with walking barefoot on contaminated soil. Once through the skin, the larvae are carried via the venous circulation into the right heart and pulmonary circulation. The larvae then migrate through the alveoli of the lungs, in a fashion similar to *Ascaris lumbricoides.* Later, the parasites move into the trachea and pharynx and are then swallowed by the host. Within the small bowel, the adult hookworms attach to the mucosa and can remain there for years. The worms suck blood continuously from the intestinal tissue and can ultimately cause an iron deficiency anemia, with an estimated blood loss of 0.2 mL per day. Thousands of eggs are laid each day by the adult worm and are passed into the feces of the host. When contaminated human feces are mixed into the soil, larvae are released. Under the appropriate environmental conditions, these noninfective larvae become infective (filariform larvae), and the cycle begins again.

Epidemiology Hookworm infection is most common in tropical or subtropical regions and has been reported worldwide. Warm climates favor hookworm infection, since the ova do not tolerate cold soil temperatures. Prevalence is highest in areas where sanitation is poor and human feces are mixed with topsoil. Efforts to control hookworm infection in the United States have been generally successful, although cases still occur in the southeastern states.

Clinical Syndromes
- **Iron deficiency anemia:** Caused by the adult hookworm parasitizing blood in the upper small intestine
- **Pneumonitis:** Occurring during the lung migration phase. This is characterized by wheezing, eosinophilia, and diffuse pulmonary infiltrates, resembling Löffler's syndrome.
- **Ground itch:** An allergic reaction to the hookworm localized to the area of initial skin penetration. The individual may present with erythema, pruritus, and a papular rash in the lower extremity.
- **Abdominal pain, diarrhea, weight loss, and malabsorption:** In developing countries, mental retardation can result from chronic nutritional deficiencies caused by the hookworm.

Diagnosis The clinical suspicion of hookworm infection is confirmed by direct examination of stool specimens for the presence of the characteristic eggs.

Diagnostic Tests/Procedures
Ova and Parasites, Stool *on page 505*

Treatment Mebendazole is the drug of choice with cure rates exceeding 90%. The anemia caused by *Ancylostoma duodenale* usually responds to standard iron supplementation.

Drug Therapy
Recommended
Mebendazole *on page 808*
Alternate
Thiabendazole *on page 947*
Pyrantel Pamoate *on page 883*

Selected Readings
Grencis RK and Cooper ES, "Enterobius, Trichuris, Capillaria, and Hookworm Including Ancylostoma caninum," *Gastroenterol Clin North Am,* 1996, 25(3):579-97.
Juckett G, "Common Intestinal Helminths," *Am Fam Physician,* 1995, 52(7):2039-48, 2051-2.
Mahmoud AA, "Intestinal Nematodes (Roundworms)," *Principles and Practice of Infectious Diseases,* 4th ed, Mandell GL, Bennett JE, and Dolin R, eds, New York, NY: Churchill Livingstone, 1995, 2526-31.
Miller TA, "Hookworm Infection in Man," *Adv Parasitol,* 1979, 17:315-84.
Warren KS, "Hookworm Control," *Lancet,* 1988, 2(8616):897-8.

Animal and Human Bites Guidelines *see page 1061*

Arboviruses

Microbiology The group of viruses commonly known as arboviruses (arthropod-borne viruses) is composed of approximately 500 viruses which have in common the fact that the vectors which transmit these viruses to humans are arthropods (mosquitos, ticks, and certain blood-sucking flies). Mosquitos are the most common vectors. Arboviruses are morphologically diverse and can be either (Continued)

Arboviruses *(Continued)*

enveloped or nonenveloped, and either icosahedral or helical; however, most arboviruses are 40-110 nm and contain RNA. Some of the more commonly discussed and encountered arbovirus infections in the United States are shown in the table.

Arboviruses

Disease	Virus	Vector	Clinical Syndrome	Geographical Location	Mortality (%)
Colorado tick fever*	Orbivirus	Tick	F, M, H	West U.S.	<1
Congo-Crimean hemorrhagic fever	Nariovirus	Tick, infected blood	H	Africa, Europe, Asia	10-50
Dengue	Flavivirus	Mosquito	F, H	Tropical, world-wide	5 (H)
Eastern equine encephalitis*	Alphavirus	Mosquito	M	East U.S., Central & South America	30
LaCrosse encephalitis*	Bunyavirus	Mosquito	M	East U.S.	<1
Powassan encephalitis*	Flavivirus	Tick, mosquito	M	U.S., Russia, China, Canada	
Rift Valley fever	Phlebovirus	Mosquito, infected blood	F, M, H	Africa, Middle East	<1
St Louis encephalitis*	Flavivirus	Mosquito	M	North, Central, & South America	7
Tick-borne encephalitis	Flavivirus	Tick	F, M, H	Europe, Asia	1-10
Western equine encephalitis*	Alphavirus	Mosquito	M	West U.S., South America, Canada, Mexico	5
Yellow fever	Flavivirus	Mosquito	F, H	South America, Africa	15

*One of the six significant arbovirus diseases in the United States.

F: Febrile illness; M: Meningoencephalitis; H: Hemorrhagic fever.

Information in this table is adapted from the publications by Tsai TF. See Selected Readings.

Epidemiology Arboviruses are found worldwide but are more common in tropical than in temperate climates. Only about 150 of the ~500 arboviruses cause disease in humans. Generally, arboviruses are transmitted between small mammals and birds. The aforementioned arthropod vectors transmit the arboviruses from these small animals to humans who are dead-end hosts for these viruses.

Clinical Syndromes Most arbovirus infections in humans are mild viral infections which often are indistinguishable from many other viral infections. Acute arbovirus infections often are characterized by sudden onset of headache, fever, muscle and joint pain, and other constitutional symptoms. If disease progresses beyond these symptoms, the disease can be extremely serious and usually manifests as a severe febrile illness (with or without rash, with or without arthritis), meningoencephalitis, or hemorrhagic fever. In more severe cases, more than one of these three conditions can be present (see table).

Diagnosis The basis of a definitive diagnosis of an arbovirus infection is a thorough physical examination and an extremely close examination of the exposure, travel, work, and socioeconomic history of the patient. Enzyme immunoassay, immunofluorescence, and nucleic acid hybridization with or without polymerase chain reaction amplification methods can be used to detect virus antigens in throat and blood specimens and paraffin-embedded tissues. However, these tests are not widely available and are applicable to only a few arboviruses. The test of choice in the laboratory diagnosis of an arbovirus infection is serology. Acute and convalescent sera must be collected if an accurate diagnosis is sought. Immunofluorescence, enzyme immunoassay, hemagglutination inhibition, complement fixation, and antibody neutralization tests are generally available at reference laboratories and the Centers for Disease Control and Prevention. Contact the local laboratory for details on specimen collection, availability of tests, turnaround time, and discussions regarding the most likely virus to cause the disease of a particular infection.

Diagnostic Tests/Procedures

Encephalitis Viral Serology *on page 404*

Treatment Treatment for specific arbovirus infections usually is supportive and directed toward making the patient comfortable and reducing symptoms.

Drug Therapy Comment There is no specific antiviral agent(s) for arboviruses.

Selected Readings

"Arboviral Infections of the Central Nervous System--United States, 1996-1997," *MMWR Morb Mortal Wkly Rep*, 1998, 47(25):517-22.

Calisher CH, "Medically Important Arboviruses of the United States and Canada," *Clin Microbiol Rev*, 1994, 7(1):89-116.

Griffin DE, "Arboviruses and the Central Nervous System," *Springer Semin Immunopathol*, 1995, 17(2-3):121-32.

Johnson RT, "Acute Encephalitis," *Clin Infect Dis*, 1996, 23(2):219-24.

Lowry PW, "Arbovirus Encephalitis in the United States and Asia," *J Lab Clin Med*, 1997, 129(4):405-11.

Nelson JA, "Tickborne Illnesses: United States," *Clin Microbiol Newslett*, 1992, 14(14):105-8.

Tsai TF, "Arboviruses," *Manual of Clinical Immunology*, 4th ed, Rose NR, de Macario, Fahey JL, et al, eds, Washington DC: American Society for Microbiology, 1992, 606-18.

Tsai TF, "Arboviruses," *Manual of Clinical Microbiology*, 6th ed, Murray PR, Baron EJ, Pfaller MA, et al, eds, Washington DC: American Society for Microbiology, 1995, 980-96.

Ascaris

Microbiology Over 4 million individuals in the United States are infected with the intestinal parasite *Ascaris lumbricoides*, commonly referred to as "the giant roundworm." Ascariasis is the term used to describe human infection with *A. lumbricoides*. With a worldwide prevalence over 1 billion, ascariasis is the single most common worm infection of humans.

Ascaris lumbricoides is a nematode (roundworm) which passes through several developmental stages: egg (ova), larva, and mature adult. The infectious cycle for the human begins with ingestion of *Ascaris* eggs by the host; these eggs are found most often in contaminated food or soil. In the small intestine, the larvae are released from the egg and penetrate through the intestinal mucosa. After entering the venous circulation, the larvae migrate into the pulmonary vessels. For a period of 10-14 days, the larvae grow within the alveoli of the lungs, the so-called "pulmonary phase." The larvae then pass up the trachea and are coughed up and swallowed by the host. The worms return to the jejunum where they mature into adult forms. During this "intestinal phase" which can last several months, the adult worm attains a length of over 15 cm. Thousands of fertilized eggs are passed into the feces of the host and eventually into the environment, where the cycle begins again.

Epidemiology *Ascaris* infections occur worldwide, although more commonly in tropical climates. In the United States, ascariasis is most prevalent in the southeastern states. Poor sanitation is a predisposing factor to infection. The eggs of *Ascaris lumbricoides* are hardy and can survive cold temperatures and dry environments. In communities where human feces contaminate both the food and water supply, ascariasis is endemic because of its fecal-oral transmission. School-age children are at particularly high risk of parasitism.

Clinical Syndromes The clinical presentation depends to some degree on the worm burden and the specific host organ involved.

- **Asymptomatic infection:** This is the most common manifestation, and usually occurs when only a small number of eggs are ingested.
- **Pneumonitis, caused by migration of large numbers of larvae through the lungs:** The individual presents with bronchospasm, pulmonary infiltrates on the chest radiograph, and peripheral blood eosinophilia. This may be mistaken for an asthmatic attack or Löffler's syndrome.
- **Intestinal obstruction, especially when the worm burden is high:** Appendicitis has also been described when a tangled mass of worms obstructs the lumen of the appendix.
- **Common bile duct obstruction, usually caused by a single adult worm:** Characteristically, the individual has nausea, vomiting, abdominal pain, and sometimes jaundice.
- **Nutritional deficiencies, particularly in children**

Diagnosis The clinical suspicion of ascariasis is confirmed by direct examination of stool specimens. Because of the enormous numbers of eggs which are shed in the feces each day, in most cases there is little difficulty identifying the fertilized and unfertilized eggs. Less commonly, the adult worm may be passed (Continued)

Ascaris (Continued)

in the stool as well. In rare cases, the diagnosis of ascariasis may be suspected or confirmed by using radiographic contrast studies of the bowel or biliary tract; the outline of the worm may be seen as a filling defect.

Diagnostic Tests/Procedures
Ova and Parasites, Stool *on page 505*

Treatment Mebendazole is considered the drug of choice for intestinal ascariasis. Piperazine citrate is indicated for cases of intestinal or biliary obstruction. **Note**: In cases of dual or multiple infections with *Ascaris* and other intestinal parasites, *Ascaris* must be treated first. Some antiparasitic agents not directed toward *Ascaris* can antagonize *Ascaris* and cause the large worms to react violently to the point of damaging or even penetrating the bowel.

Drug Therapy
Recommended
Mebendazole *on page 808*
Alternate
Pyrantel Pamoate *on page 883*

Selected Readings
Khuroo MS, Zargar SA, Mahajan R, et al, "Sonographic Appearances in Biliary Ascariasis," *Gastroenterology*, 1987, 93(2):267-72.

Mahmoud AA, "Intestinal Nematodes (Roundworms)," *Principles and Practice of Infectious Diseases*, 4th ed, Mandell GL, Bennett JE, and Dolin R, eds, New York, NY: Churchill Livingstone, 1995, 2526-31.

Sarinas PS and Chitkara RK, "Ascariasis and Hookworm," *Semin Respir Infect*, 1997, 12(2):130-7.

Stephenson LS, "The Contribution of *Ascaris lumbricoides* to Malnutrition in Children," *Parasitology*, 1980, 81(1):221-33.

Aspergillus Species

Microbiology *Aspergillus* is a potentially pathogenic fungus found throughout the environment. Aspergillosis is the term used to describe human infection caused by any one of the 900 reported species of this mold. Infection with *Aspergillus* can range from benign colonization of the respiratory tract to lethal blood vessel invasion and remains a major cause of morbidity and mortality in neutropenic patients.

Aspergillus is a mold and is composed of hyphae which grow by extension and branching. The fungus is recognized in tissue specimens by its septate hyphae and its dichotomous, acute angle branching. A definitive diagnosis of *Aspergillus* is quite difficult from histopathologic sections alone unless characteristic sporulation is seen. Confirmation of *Aspergillus* requires growth of the mold on appropriate culture media, but it is well recognized clinically that fungal cultures may still be negative despite positive tissue sections.

Epidemiology *Aspergillus* is ubiquitous in the environment but is not considered part of the normal flora of humans. Although there is no specific reservoir for this fungus, it tends to grow heavily in hay, dung, soil (including the soil of potted plants), grain, and compost piles; occasionally, a history of a massive inhalational exposure can be obtained from individuals with overwhelming infection. Well-documented studies have shown that *Aspergillus* can be recovered from the air of hospital wards, and outbreaks in susceptible patients have been associated with heavily colonized hospital air-ventilation systems. *Aspergillus* outbreaks have also been reported following hospital renovation projects.

Although *Aspergillus* is universally present in the environment, it causes disease in relatively few individuals. Life-threatening acute infection is nearly always limited to immunocompromised patients. *Aspergillus* infections of a more chronic and indolent nature are often seen in individuals with less debilitating underlying diseases (eg, asthma, chronic bronchitis, sarcoidosis). Acquisition of *Aspergillus* is exclusively via inhalation of airborne spores; person-to-person transmission does not occur.

Clinical Syndromes There are three major manifestations of an *Aspergillus* infection which can overlap in an individual patient.

- **Allergic bronchopulmonary aspergillosis (ABPA):** This is a specific form of hypersensitivity pneumonitis. It is characterized by asthma, eosinophilia, immediate skin reactivity to *Aspergillus* antigen, elevated immunoglobulin E (IgE), and positive *Aspergillus* precipitins in the serum. This is considered an allergic response to *Aspergillus* and is not truly infectious in nature. Treatment is with corticosteroids in selected cases, rather than antifungal therapy.

- **_Aspergillus_ colonization:** This is the most common scenario, in which _Aspergillus_ exists as a fungus ball in a lung cavity such as an old tuberculosis cavity. This fungus ball is a mass of hyphal elements which elicits little inflammatory response. A patient can be colonized for years without symptoms or tissue damage, except for hemoptysis. However, serious complications can occur such as empyema or bronchopleural fistula.
- **Invasive fungal infection:** This occurs almost exclusively as an opportunistic infection in the severely immunocompromised patient. Prolonged neutropenia is a well recognized risk factor. Rarely, invasive disease has been described in otherwise healthy hosts. Systemic aspergillosis is an often lethal infection with fever, progressive pneumonitis with or without cavitation, and widespread dissemination to almost any organ system. _Aspergillus_ characteristically invades blood vessels in the lungs and other tissues.
- **Miscellaneous:** Other manifestations of _Aspergillus_ have been described, including cerebral infarction, endocarditis, gastrointestinal ulcerations in immunocompromised hosts, necrotizing skin ulcers, and bone lesions. Meningitis has been described rarely.

Diagnosis _Aspergillus_ requires identification of the fungus in biopsy samples and/or appropriate body fluids. It should be noted that the recovery of _Aspergillus_ from clinical specimens such as expectorated sputum or bronchial lavage fluid does not necessarily imply clinically significant infection. In some cases, _Aspergillus_ may be present as a colonizer without damage to surrounding tissues; this does not warrant specific therapy. Demonstration of tissue invasion on histopathologic specimens is the gold standard for diagnosing invasive aspergillosis. In all cases, a positive culture for _Aspergillus_ must be viewed in the context of the individual case.

Diagnostic Tests/Procedures

Cytology, Body Fluids _on page 386_
Fungus Culture, Appropriate Site _on page 414_
KOH Preparation _on page 467_

Treatment Surgical excision of sequestered foci of _Aspergillus_ infection may be the treatment of choice for diseases such as brain lesions, sinus involvement, infections on prosthetic material, and some lung lesions, with subsequent drug therapy with amphotericin B. As the drug of choice for _Aspergillus_ infections, amphotericin B is administered in doses as high as 1 mg/kg/day. Although agents such as flucytosine, rifampin, and clindamycin have been added to amphotericin B in hopes of increasing antifungal activity, these combinations have not been proven to be superior to amphotericin B alone. Itraconazole may be an alternative for long-term maintenance or suppression but has no track record for this or in the treatment of acute _Aspergillus_ infection.

Drug Therapy

Recommended

Amphotericin B (Conventional) _on page 597_

Alternate

Itraconazole _on page 785_
Amphotericin B Cholesteryl Sulfate Complex _on page 596_
Amphotericin B (Conventional) _on page 597_
Amphotericin B, Lipid Complex _on page 600_

Selected Readings

Cockrill BA and Hales CA, "Allergic Bronchopulmonary Aspergillosis," _Annu Rev Med_, 1999, 50:303-16.
Denning DW and Stevens DA, "Antifungal and Surgical Treatment of Invasive Aspergillosis: Review of 2,121 Published Cases," _Rev Infect Dis_, 1990, 12(6):1147-201.
Latge JP, "_Aspergillus fumigatus_ and Aspergillosis," _Clin Microbiol Rev_, 1999, 12(2):315-50.
Robinson LA, "_Aspergillus_ and Other Fungi," _Chest Surg Clin N Am_, 1999, 9(1):193-225, x.
Talbot GH, Huang A, and Provencher M, "Invasive _Aspergillus_ Rhinosinusitis in Patients With Acute Leukemia," _Rev Infect Dis_, 1991, 13(2):219-32.

Babesia microti

Microbiology _Babesia microti_ is an intracellular protozoan which causes a febrile illness in the northeastern United States. The illness, babesiosis, resembles malaria. _Babesia microti_ primarily infects animals; humans are incidental hosts. In the United States, rodents are the primary animal reservoir, including the white-footed deer mouse, rats, and field mice. The vector for transmission of the organism from the rodent to the human is the tick _Ixodes dammini_, the hard-shelled tick also responsible for the transmission of Lyme disease. Following the (Continued)

Babesia microti (Continued)

bite of an infected tick, *Babesia microti* invade the human circulation and enter erythrocytes. The trophozoites of *Babesia microti* divide within erythrocytes into two or four daughter cells, sometimes forming a characteristic tetrad ring which can be recognized on a blood smear. The organisms eventually leave the red blood cells, perforating the membrane and causing asynchronous cell lysis. With the merozoites being released, other host erythrocytes are at risk for infection, and the infectious cycle is maintained.

Epidemiology Babesiosis occurs most commonly along the northeastern seaboard of the United States in states such as Massachusetts, New York, and Rhode Island. In particular, Martha's Vineyard, Cape Cod, Shelter Island, Fire Island, and Nantucket Island report a high prevalence. Infections mainly occur from May to September when the nymph form of *Ixodes dammini* is feeding. Epidemiologic studies suggest that most infections with *Babesia microti* are subclinical or asymptomatic. A seroprevalence rate of 3% to 4% was found in endemic areas, with many individuals unaware of past infection. Less commonly, babesiosis has been transmitted by transfusion from an asymptomatic donor.

Clinical Syndromes The incubation period following the bite of the infected tick is 1-3 weeks. The majority of patients are not able to recall a recent tick bite. Most infections with *Babesia microti* are either asymptomatic or mild. In severe cases, symptoms include fever up to 40°C, chills, sweats, myalgias, malaise, and headache. Some individuals may experience photophobia, sore throat, and cough. Hepatosplenomegaly may be observed less commonly, but generalized lymphadenopathy is not seen. The most fulminant cases of babesiosis occur in patients who are asplenic, emphasizing the important role of the spleen in the host defense against this protozoan.

Diagnosis The diagnosis of babesiosis is suspected when there is a characteristic clinical presentation in an individual from an endemic area. The diagnosis is confirmed microbiologically by examination of Wright-Giemsa stained thick and thin blood smears. The parasite is visualized within the erythrocytes. At times it may be difficult to distinguish *Babesia* sp from other intracellular parasites such as *Plasmodium falciparum* (one of the causative agents of malaria). The finding of intracellular merozoites in a tetrad configuration is pathognomonic for babesiosis but frequently is absent. Other laboratory aids include the classic findings of an intravascular hemolytic anemia with hemoglobinuria, elevated reticulocyte count, and depressed haptoglobin level. The diagnosis can also be confirmed by using an indirect immunofluorescent antibody titer against *Babesia microti*, but serum must be sent to the Centers for Disease Control.

Diagnostic Tests/Procedures

Peripheral Blood Smear, Thick and Thin *on page 519*

Treatment Many patients with babesiosis recover without specific therapy. When infection is severe or the patient is known to be asplenic, the drugs of choice are clindamycin intravenously and quinine orally. Chloroquine, which is effective in some cases of malaria, has no efficacy in treating babesiosis; thus, it is important to distinguish babesiosis from malaria on the peripheral blood smear. Life-threatening infections may respond to exchange transfusions in combination with antimicrobial therapy, in an effort to decrease the degree of parasitemia.

Drug Therapy

Recommended

Clindamycin *on page 684*

   used in combination with

Quinine *on page 890*

Selected Readings

Gelfand JA and Callahan MV, "Babesiosis," *Curr Clin Top Infect Dis*, 1998, 18:201-6.

Gorenflot A, Moubri K, Precigout E, et al, "Human Babesiosis," *Ann Trop Med Parasitol*, 92(4):489-501.

Rosner F, Zarrabi MH, Benach JL, et al, "Babesiosis in Splenectomized Adults: Review of 22 Reported Cases," *Am J Med*, 1984, 76(4):696-701.

White NJ and Breman JG, "Malaria and Babesiosis," *Harrison's Principles of Internal Medicine*, 13th ed, Isselbacher KJ, Braunwald E, Wilson JD, et al, eds, New York, NY: McGraw-Hill, 1994, 887-96.

Woolley I, "Piroplasmosis," *Clin Microbiol Newslett*, 1998, 20(4):25-8.

Bacillus anthracis

Microbiology Bacillus anthracis is an aerobic, gram-positive bacillus with a large polypeptide capsule. Some isolates may appear gram-variable rather than gram-positive. On Gram's stain, there is a characteristic "box car" appearance to these organisms, a feature common to the genus Bacillus. The organism forms spores when grown aerobically in the laboratory, but spores are not seen in clinical specimens. Virulence factors for this organism include anthrax toxin (made up of three components) and a capsule (which protects against host antibodies).

Epidemiology Bacillus anthracis causes the disease anthrax. The organism is ubiquitous in the environment, being found in soil and decaying vegetation. The spores of the organism are hardy and survive for years under adverse conditions. These spores contaminate the hide of herbivores such as cattle, sheep, and goats. Animals consume the spores and ultimately expire. In this way, anthrax is a zoonosis. Humans are only incidentally exposed. Direct contact with the contaminated hides or hair of these herbivores leads to human disease. Cases still occur in the United States but are rare. In 1992, there was only one case of anthrax in the United States reported to the Centers for Disease Control. The disease is more common in the Middle East (Iran, Turkey).

Clinical Syndromes

- **Cutaneous anthrax:** This form of human infection results from direct inoculation of Bacillus anthracis spores into the skin. Exposure results from handling insulation made from animal hair (usually commercial buildings), infected animal hides, clothing products, or wool. Less commonly, spores come from contaminated soil. Spores enter intact or exposed skin in an extremity such as the forearm. A papule develops locally at the site of inoculation of the spores and later ulcerates and turns into a black eschar. Systemic symptoms of fever, chills, and total body edema can result from the effects of anthrax toxin. The disease is often rapidly fatal if the diagnosis and treatment are delayed.

- **Inhalation anthrax:** Also known as Woolsorter's disease, inhalational anthrax presents as a rapidly progressive pneumonitis. Widening of the mediastinum is a common finding on chest x-ray and may be a clue to the diagnosis. Meningeal involvement is common. Mortality is high.

- **Gastrointestinal anthrax:** This is a rare presentation of the disease in humans.

Diagnosis Because of the rarity of anthrax in the United States, diagnosis is difficult to make in a timely fashion. It is important to obtain an occupational history for all patients who present with an infectious disease, and it is particularly important with anthrax. A history of exposure to animal products may be the only clue to this disease. Patients who present with unusual necrotic ulcerations of the extremities should be questioned along these lines. Notify laboratory of suspected organism.

Diagnostic Tests/Procedures

Aerobic Culture, Appropriate Site on page 310
Aerobic Culture, Sputum on page 312
Gram's Stain on page 426

Treatment The antibiotic of choice for Bacillus anthracis is penicillin. The organism has remained sensitive to penicillin but may not always be responsive to therapy, particularly if initiated late in the disease course. Adults with cutaneous anthrax can be treated with intravenous penicillin G, 2 million units every 6 hours for several days. Little data is available for inhalation anthrax or gastrointestinal anthrax; high doses of penicillin are recommended since the mortality of inhalation anthrax approaches 100%. Alternative agents include tetracycline or chloramphenicol.

Drug Therapy

Recommended

Penicillin G, Parenteral, Aqueous on page 860

Alternate

Tetracycline on page 944
Chloramphenicol on page 667

Selected Readings

Brachman PS, "Anthrax," Bacterial Infections of Humans, 2nd ed, Evans AS and Brachman PS, eds, New York, NY: Plenum Medical Book Company, 1991, 75-86.

Brachman PS, "Inhalation Anthrax," Ann N Y Acad Sci, 1980, 353:83-93.

Lew D, "Bacillus anthracis (Anthrax)," Principles and Practice of Infectious Diseases, 4th ed, Mandell GL, Bennett JE, and Dolin R, eds, New York, NY: Churchill Livingstone, 1995, 1885-9.

(Continued)

Bacillus anthracis (Continued)

"Summary of Notifiable Diseases, United States 1992," *MMWR Morb Mortal Wkly Rep*, 1992, 41:1-73.

Tuazon CU, "Other *Bacillus* Species," *Principles and Practice of Infectious Diseases*, 4th ed, Mandell GL, Bennett JE, and Dolin R, eds, New York, NY: Churchill Livingstone, 1995, 1890-4.

Weber DJ and Rutala WA, "*Bacillus* Species," *Infect Control Hosp Epidemiol*, 1988, 9(8):368-73.

Bacillus, Calmette-Guérin *see Mycobacterium bovis on page 203*

Bacillus cereus

Related Information

Timing of Food Poisoning *on page 1069*

Microbiology *Bacillus cereus* is an aerobic, gram-positive bacillus associated with a variety of disease states including food poisoning, ocular infections, bacteremia, and septicemia. *Bacillus cereus* is a spore-forming aerobe which stains gram-positive or gram-variable. It grows readily on standard laboratory media and does not need special culturing techniques.

Epidemiology *Bacillus cereus* is ubiquitous in the environment, growing readily in such diverse areas as soil, water, vegetables, decaying matter, and dust. In certain individuals, it can be part of the normal human flora, explaining in part its tendency to colonize surgical wounds and serious burn injuries. The needles and syringes of heroin addicts in the United States have also been found to be contaminated with this bacterium. *Bacillus cereus* food poisoning, caused by ingestion of a toxin elaborated by this organism, has been reported from several countries around the world, including the United States and Canada.

Clinical Syndromes

- **The "emetic form" of *Bacillus cereus* food poisoning:** This results from the ingestion of a preformed toxin produced by this organism. Nausea, vomiting, and abdominal cramping usually occur soon (1-6 hours) following the ingestion of contaminated foods. In particular, this emetic toxin has been associated with fried rice served in Chinese food restaurants. The spores of *B. cereus* can survive the process of boiling rice followed by quick frying.

- **The "diarrheal form" of *Bacillus cereus* food poisoning:** This results from ingestion of a different, heat-labile enterotoxin. The incubation period is longer than for the emetic form, usually more than 9 hours. Profuse watery diarrhea is the predominant symptom, along with abdominal cramping.

- **Ocular infection, including endophthalmitis:** *Bacillus cereus* is a leading pathogen in post-traumatic endophthalmitis. Other common settings include ophthalmitis in farm workers and intravenous drug users. In the latter case, infection can be fulminant. Several toxins have been identified which may play a role in this often rapidly destructive panophthalmitis: cerelysin, necrotic toxin, and phospholipase C.

- **Bacteremia:** Isolation of *Bacillus cereus* from the blood may have little clinical significance (as in the transient *Bacillus* bacteremia commonly seen in the intravenous drug user or in blood culture contamination) or may represent life-threatening septicemia. Clinically significant bacteremias tend to occur most often in patients with indwelling intravascular catheters and may warrant treatment.

- **Miscellaneous infections:** *Bacillus cereus* can be a cause of pneumonia in the compromised host (rare), endocarditis in the intravenous drug user, necrotizing fasciitis, acute or chronic osteomyelitis, meningitis (often in the setting of disseminated infection), ventricular shunt infection, and can be a part of a polymicrobial wound infection (eg, surgical wounds, tumor, breast prostheses).

Diagnosis *Bacillus cereus* is readily identified in the laboratory from cultures of blood and other sterile body fluids. In cases of suspected *Bacillus* food poisoning, the implicated foods should be cultured for this organism. There is little benefit in culturing the patient's stool since gastrointestinal tract colonization is not uncommon. As mentioned previously, isolation of *Bacillus cereus* from the blood need not be treated in every case, and clinical judgment is required.

Diagnostic Tests/Procedures

Aerobic Culture, Appropriate Site *on page 310*

Gram's Stain *on page 426*

Treatment *Bacillus cereus* food poisoning does not respond to antimicrobial therapy. Attention should instead be focused on supportive measures such as hydration and electrolyte balance. Clinically significant infections with this organism should be treated with vancomycin intravenously. Unlike other *Bacillus* species (eg, *Bacillus alvei, B. subtilis, B. circulans*, etc), *Bacillus cereus* is often resistant to beta-lactam antibiotics such as the penicillins and cephalosporins. Vancomycin should be used until the antimicrobial susceptibility pattern is finalized; limited data suggests the addition of an aminoglycoside to vancomycin may have some minor benefit in s erious infections.

Drug Therapy
Recommended
Vancomycin *on page 967*

Selected Readings
"Bacillus cereus Food Poisoning Associated With Fried Rice at Two Child Day Care Centers - Virginia, 1993," *MMWR Morb Mortal Wkly Rep,* 1994, 43(10):177-8.

Davey RT Jr and Tauber WB, "Post-traumatic Endophthalmitis: The Emerging Role of *Bacillus cereus* Infection," *Rev Infect Dis,* 1987, 9(1):110-23.

Schricker ME, Thompson GH, and Schreiber JR, "Osteomyelitis Due to *Bacillus cereus* in an Adolescent: Case Report and Review," *Clin Infect Dis,* 1994, 18(6):863-7.

Sliman R, Rehm S, and Shlaes DM, "Serious Infections Caused by *Bacillus* Species," *Medicine (Baltimore),* 1987, 66(3):218-23.

Terranova W and Blake PA, "*Bacillus cereus* Food Poisoning," *N Engl J Med,* 1978, 298(3):143-4.

Tuazon CU, "Other *Bacillus* Species," *Principles and Practice of Infectious Diseases,* 4th ed, Mandell GL, Bennett JE, and Dolin R, eds, New York, NY: Churchill Livingstone, 1995, 1890-4.

Bacteroides Species

Microbiology *Bacteroides* species are gram-negative, anaerobic, pleomorphic rods some of which are aerotolerant. Gram's staining is pale. The organisms stain irregularly. *B. fragilis* grows as a nonhemolytic glistening colony on blood agar. *B. melaninogenicus* appears as pigmented, brown to black colonies which fluoresce under UV light. *B. fragilis* will grow in 20% bile; *B. melaninogenicus* will not. Catalase positivity and resistance to kanamycin, vancomycin, and colistin are used for preliminary speciation. Biochemical testing utilizing carbohydrate fermentation and gas-liquid chromatography (GLC) are used for definitive speciation. DNA homology has allowed clarification of the taxonomy of the *Bacteroides* species. *Bacteroides* species have a broad spectrum of resistance to antimicrobial agents.

Epidemiology *Bacteroides* species are normal flora of the oral cavity, gastrointestinal tract, and female genital tract. They are the organism most frequently isolated from suppurative anaerobic infections. Nosocomial colonization by virulent strains of *B. fragilis* may occur. Although *B. fragilis* makes up only a small fraction of the oral and colonic flora, it accounts for a disproportionate percentage of infections due to *Bacteroides* species.

Clinical Syndromes
- **Abscess infection:** *Bacteroides* species infections are associated with closed abscesses and are frequently present in mixed or polymicrobic infections. The most common are intra-abdominal abscesses which result from diverticulitis, rupture of the appendix, surgical procedures, and abdominal trauma or tumor. The liver and subdiaphragmatic space are frequent sites for abscess formation. Splenic, kidney, and perinephric abscesses are also well known. Liver abscess may occur as the result of peritoneal seeding or by spread from the portal or biliary system. *B. fragilis* may be isolated from more than 50% of intra-abdominal abscesses, and anaerobes may be isolated in more than 90%. Most infections are mixed, with aerobic and facultative organisms also being present. Sixty percent to 70% of pelvic abscesses involve *B. fragilis*. *B. melaninogenicus* is more often implicated in lung abscesses than is *B. fragilis*. In most cases, lung abscesses are polymicrobic.
- **Bacteremia:** Usually heralds a localized site of infection.
- **Endocarditis:** Rare but has been observed in patients without underlying valvular disease.
- **Skin infection:** Often associated with trauma surgery, decubitus ulcers, diabetic foot ulcers, and human bites. Contamination by feces, saliva, and oropharyngeal secretions may allow anaerobic organisms to become established and cause infection.
- **Gangrene, synergistic cellulitis, necrotizing fascitis, and crepitant cellulitis:** May also be frequently attributed to infection with *Bacteroides* species.

Diagnostic Tests/Procedures
Anaerobic Culture *on page 316*
Gram's Stain *on page 426*
(Continued)

Bacteroides Species *(Continued)*

Duration of Therapy 7-10 days

Treatment Drainage is the treatment of choice for infections with *Bacteroides* species. This can be accomplished either by surgical intervention or by needle aspiration under ultrasound or CT control. Although there are differences of opinion, coverage for anaerobes is usually included in the therapy of polymicrobic abscesses. Specific therapy for *Bacteroides* infections include metronidazole, clindamycin, cefoxitin, piperacillin, ticarcillin, and imipenem. Cross-reactive resistance to β-lactam antimicrobials has been reported. Metronidazole resistance is rarely encountered. Clindamycin, cefoxitin, and cefotetan are effective alternatives. Selection of an antimicrobial agent may be influenced by susceptibility testing if available.

Drug Therapy Comment Most patients with HTLV-I disease will respond to some degree to chemotherapeutic agents used for non-Hodgkin's lymphoma. Nucleotide analogs might be effective during early (but not late) stages of ATL.

Drug Therapy
Recommended
Metronidazole *on page 817*
Clindamycin *on page 684*
Alternate
Cefoxitin *on page 646*
Cefotetan *on page 644*
Imipenem and Cilastatin *on page 766*
Meropenem *on page 812*
Piperacillin and Tazobactam Sodium *on page 871*
Ticarcillin and Clavulanate Potassium *on page 950*
Ampicillin and Sulbactam *on page 607*

Selected Readings

Edwards R, "Resistance to Beta-Lactam Antibiotics in Bacteroides Spp," *J Med Microbiol*, 1997, 46(12):979-86.

Patrick S, "The Virulence of Bacteroides fragilis," *Rev Med Microbiol*, 1993, 4:40-9.

Styrt B and Gorbach SL, "Recent Developments in the Understanding of the Pathogenesis and Treatment of Anaerobic Infections," *N Engl J Med*, 1989, 321(5):298-302.

Wexler HM, "Susceptibility Testing of Anaerobic Bacteria - State of the Art," *Clin Infect Dis*, 1993, 16(Suppl 4):S328-33.

Bartonella Species

Synonyms *Rochalimaea* Species

Microbiology *Bartonella* species are small, pleomorphic gram-negative bacilli which have received considerable attention over recent years because of their role in two important diseases: cat scratch disease and bacillary angiomatosis. Until recently, *Bartonella henselae* and *Bartonella quintana* species were considered *Rochalimaea* species. *Bartonella henselae* was first isolated and described in 1992, when it was cultured from the blood of an HIV-infected individual. *Bartonella* species are slow-growing and difficult to isolate in the laboratory. The organisms have occasionally been recovered from blood cultures, skin biopsies, spleen tissue, and lymph node biopsies. However, because of the fastidious nature of these organisms, clinical specimens may often be culture-negative. Of note, *Bartonella* species are best visualized in clinical specimens (such as lymph nodes) using a Warthin-Starry stain; the finding of Warthin-Starry staining bacteria in lymph node tissue is suggestive of cat scratch disease.

Epidemiology Cat scratch disease: For years, the cause of cat scratch disease was unknown. Although the epidemiology, clinical manifestations, and therapies of cat scratch disease have been described in the past, only within the past 2 years has *B. henselae* been implicated as the major causative agent of cat scratch disease (CSD).

The exact distribution of *Bartonella* in the environment is not known, but the organism can be found in soil. Cats appear to be an important reservoir of this organism. In the United States, there are approximately 22,000 cases of cat scratch disease diagnosed each year with about 10% requiring hospitalization. Most cases of CSD occur in children and adolescents who are otherwise healthy (ie, immunocompetent). Family outbreaks have been reported. The majority of cases seem to occur in the fall and winter. Transmission is from direct animal contact. Nearly all patients (90% to 99%) report a recent exposure to a cat, and a history of a cat scratch or bite can be elicited in many (75% to 90%). In some series, kittens appear more likely to transmit disease than older cats. Most animals who transmit CSD are otherwise healthy. Rarely, the picture of CSD has been described in individuals without an animal exposure.

Bacillary angiomatosis: Unlike cat scratch disease, bacillary angiomatosis usually is seen in the immunocompromised, particularly in persons with AIDS. This infection usually occurs late in HIV infection; in one study the average CD4+ cell count was 57/μL. Both *B. henselae* and *B. quintana* can cause this disease. A history of a recent cat scratch from a patient with bacillary angiomatosis is uncommon, in some series <20%. *B. henselae* has been isolated from the blood of pet cats in some AIDS patients with bacillary angiomatosis. Limited evidence suggests that fleas of infected cats may also become infected with *B. henselae*, although the importance of insect transmission is unknown. Since many cases of bacillary angiomatosis cannot be linked to a feline source, other modes of acquisition are likely and are currently being studied.

Clinical Syndromes

- **Cat scratch disease:** Typically, patients with CSD present with fever and painful lymphadenopathy. In 60% to 90% of cases an "inoculation lesion" is present, consisting of an erythematous pustule or papule at the site of the initial cat scratch or bite. These are most commonly found on the arms, head, and neck. The hallmark of CSD is regional adenopathy which develops within 2 weeks proximal to the initial site of the bite or inoculation lesion. Common nodes involved are the axillary, cervical, and supraclavicular nodes, but others have been described. Other symptoms include headache, malaise, arthralgias, and conjunctivitis. In 1% to 2% of cases, there may be unusual complications such as encephalopathy, Parinaud's oculoglandular syndrome, erythema nodosum, thrombocytopenic purpura, pneumonia, osteomyelitis, hepatosplenomegaly, and others.

- **Bacillary angiomatosis:** Bacillary angiomatosis can be either cutaneous or extracutaneous. Patients with cutaneous bacillary angiomatosis present with bright red round papules on the skin. Often they are multiple but occasionally may be solitary. These lesions are highly vascular and blanch on pressure. Often there are associated constitutional symptoms such as fever and malaise. The lesions may be difficult to distinguish from Kaposi's sarcoma in HIV-infected persons (see Selected Readings).

Diagnosis A variety of methods are available to help diagnose *Bartonella* infection. The organism can be recovered from blood cultures and from tissue biopsy specimens. However, since the organism is fastidious, other methods may be helpful including:

- histologic examination of tissue (ie, lymph nodes) with Warthin-Starry staining
- serologic methods - indirect fluorescence antibody for *B. henselae* or enzyme immunoassay
- cat scratch skin test (not widely available)
- polymerase chain reaction

Diagnostic Tests/Procedures

Polymerase Chain Reaction *on page 523*

Treatment Successful therapy of cat scratch disease has been reported with a variety of antimicrobial agents including erythromycin, doxycycline, co-trimoxazole, ciprofloxacin, gentamicin, and rifampin. No controlled trials are available to determine the most beneficial therapy as each of these agents has also been associated with significant failure rates. The macrolides are considered first-line agents as are the tetracyclines.

Drug Therapy

Recommended

Erythromycin *on page 722*

Doxycycline *on page 713*

Alternate

Co-Trimoxazole *on page 692*

Selected Readings

Anderson BE and Neuman MA, "*Bartonella* Spp as Emerging Human Pathogens," *Clin Microbiol Rev*, 1997, 10(2):203-19.

Hensel DM and Slater LN, "The Genus *Bartonella*," *Clin Microbiol Newslet*, 1995, 17(2):9-13.

Margileth AM, "Antibiotic Therapy for Cat-Scratch Disease: Clinical Study of Therapeutic Outcome in 268 Patients and a Review of the Literature," *Pediatr Infect Dis J*, 1992, 11(6):474-8.

Maurin M and Raoult D, "*Bartonella (Rochalimaea) quintana* Infections," *Clin Microbiol Rev*, 1996, 9(3):273-92.

BCG see Mycobacterium bovis on page 203

BK Virus see JC Virus and BK Virus on page 183

Black Molds see Dematiaceous Fungi on page 125

Black Piedra see Dematiaceous Fungi on page 125

Blastocystis hominis

Microbiology Blastocystis hominis is an anaerobic protozoan that reproduces by binary fission. Bacteria must be present for the organisms to grow and replicate. Three morphological types have been described: ameboid, granular, and vacuolated. Its exact taxonomic position as a parasite or fungus has not been established.

Epidemiology The role of B. hominis as an intestinal pathogen is unclear because it may be found in stool specimens of both asymptomatic and symptomatic persons. Although the concentration of B. hominis in stools of symptomatic patients tends to be higher than in asymptomatic patients, some asymptomatic patients may have larger numbers of organisms present. B. hominis is frequently isolated in the presence of other intestinal pathogens. Endoscopic examination has failed to reveal any intestinal injury in symptomatic patients with B. hominis. In addition, fecal leukocytes are not usually seen. Intestinal permeability is not altered. May be more pathogenic in children and patients with AIDS. Contaminated drinking water is thought to be the reservoir.

Clinical Syndromes Symptoms that may be associated with B. hominis include abdominal pain, bloating, flatus, diarrhea, constipation, anorexia, nausea, vomiting, weight loss, and fatigue. May be associated with chronic urticaria and/or eosinophilia.

Diagnosis B. hominis is easily detected in iodine wet mount or trichrome. May be detected on touch prep (imprint from endoscopic biopsy specimen) stained with Giemsa. Acridine orange stain differentiates the cystic and central body forms.

Diagnostic Tests/Procedures

Ova and Parasites, Stool on page 505

Treatment The treatment of Blastocystis remains controversial, and the efficacy of antibiotics is unclear. Symptomatic patients without evidence of another intestinal pathogen may be treated with metronidazole for eradication of B. hominis. An apparent therapeutic response may be related to treatment of an undetected pathogen or may be coincidental, as nearly 60% of untreated symptomatic patients will have resolution of symptoms.

Drug Therapy

Recommended

Metronidazole on page 817

Selected Readings

Albrecht H, Stellbrink HJ, Koperski K, et al, "Blastocystis hominis in Human Immunodeficiency Virus-Related Diarrhea," Scand J Gastroenterol, 1995, 30(9):909-14.

O'Gorman MA, Orenstein SR, Proujansky R, et al, "Prevalence and Characteristics of Blastocystis hominis Infection in Children," Clin Pediatr (Phila), 1993, 32(2):91-6.

Stenzel DJ and Boreham PF, "Blastocystis hominis Revisited," Clin Microbiol Rev, 1996, 9(4):563-84.

Udkow MP and Markell EK, "Blastocystis hominis: Prevalence in Asymptomatic Versus Symptomatic Hosts," J Infect Dis, 1993, 168(1):242-4.

Zuckerman MJ, Watts MT, Ho H, et al, "Blastocystis hominis Infection and Intestinal Injury," Am J Med Sci, 1994, 308(2):96-101.

Blastomyces dermatitidis

Microbiology Blastomyces dermatitidis is a dimorphic fungus uncommonly seen in the immunocompromised population. In the mold form, it has round to pyriform 4-5 µm conidia attached directly on the hyphae or on short stalks. Initially the colony appears yeast-like at room temperature then develops hyphal projections eventually becoming a fluffy white mold. The spores are difficult to isolate from the soil or bird droppings but have been recovered from wet soil.

The yeast form grows as a brown, wrinkled, folded colony at 37°C. Microscopically, the yeasts appear as round, budding, thick-walled yeast cells with a daughter cell forming a single bud that has a broad base 5-15 µm in diameter and which may be found extra- or intracellular in macrophages.

Epidemiology Blastomyces usually occurs in healthy hosts and is associated with point-source exposure; more commonly in men than women which may be secondary to more male occupational exposures. Immunosuppressed patients typically develop infection following exposure but may be secondary to reactivation. It is uncommon in the AIDS population and is not recognized as an AIDS-defining illness. When an AIDS patient does develop blastomycosis, it is usually more severe with multiple visceral involvement plus CNS infection and progresses to a fatal course rapidly.

It is endemic in the south-central and midwestern United States. After inhalation of the spores, which are taken up by bronchopulmonary macrophages, there is an approximate 45-day incubation period. The initial response is suppurative and progresses to granuloma formation (also referred to as a pyogranulomatous response). *Blastomyces* most commonly infects the lungs followed by skin, bone, prostate, and CNS.

Clinical Syndromes

- **Subclinical:** Approximately 60% of people living in an endemic area with occupational exposure have laboratory evidence via immune markers of *Blastomyces* but no clinical disease.
- **Acute blastomycosis:** Typically presents as a flu-like illness with fever, malaise, fatigue, weight loss, and pulmonary involvement. Occurs more commonly in men 25-50 years of age with occupational/environmental exposure. Rarely infects children except in epidemics.
- **Acute pneumonia:** Self-limited. Presents with fever, chills, purulent sputum, and sometimes hemoptysis. Chest radiograph reveals alveolar or mass-like infiltrates. May be associated with erythema nodosum.
- **Chronic pneumonia:** Symptoms last 2-6 months, and patient presents with weight loss, night sweats, fever, chest pain, and productive cough.
- **Cutaneous:** Verrucous or ulcerative lesions. Mimics squamous cell cancer and keratoacanthoma. May be found in the brain, skeletal system, prostate, myocardium, pericardium, sinuses, pituitary, or adrenal glands. May invade reticuloendothelial system.
- **Osteomyelitis:** Up to 25% of extrapulmonary cases. Noncaseating granulomas, suppuration or necrosis in the bone may occur. May require surgical debridement as well as antifungal treatment.
- **Genitourinary:** Prostatitis and epididymo-orchitis. Has been isolated in the urine after prostatic massage. Female tract complications have been reported transmitted by male sexual partner with cutaneous form of disease.
- **CNS:** Five percent to 10% disseminated disease may cause epidural or cranial abscesses, as well as meningitis.

No matter where the infection exists, always obtain a chest x-ray because there is almost always a simultaneous pulmonary infection. Infrequent complication is adult respiratory distress syndrome.

Diagnosis Skin test and serological markers are useful epidemiological tools but have too low sensitivity and specificity to be diagnostic. Diagnosis depends on direct examination of tissue or the isolation of *Blastomyces* in culture.

Diagnostic Tests/Procedures

Fungus Culture, Appropriate Site *on page 414*
Fungus Culture, Biopsy *on page 414*
Fungus Culture, Body Fluid *on page 415*
Fungus Culture, Skin *on page 417*
Fungal Serology *on page 410*

Treatment Therapy is determined by the severity of the clinical presentation and presentation and consideration of the toxicities of the antifungal agent. Typically pneumonia is self-limited to 1-2 weeks and does not require therapy. If the pneumonia persists and develops respiratory insufficiency or pleural disease, treatment with ketoconazole, 400-800 mg/day orally is recommended. Amphotericin B, up to 2 g, is recommended in life-threatening systemic disease. There is a 97% cure rate with amphotericin B as opposed to 89% with ketoconazole. Itraconazole, 200-400 mg/day orally may prove to have a higher cure rate than ketoconazole. Fluconazole at doses of 400-800 mg/day for at least 6 months is effective therapy for nonlife-threatening disease. Neither ketoconazole nor itraconazole penetrate the blood-brain barrier so they are not recommended for CNS involvement. Fluconazole, itraconazole, and ketoconazole are all used as suppressive therapy.

Drug Therapy

Recommended

Severe infection:
Amphotericin B (Conventional) *on page 597*
(Continued)

Blastomyces dermatitidis (Continued)

Chronic infection:
Ketoconazole *on page 791*
Alternate
Itraconazole *on page 785*
Fluconazole *on page 732*

Selected Readings
Bradsher RW, "Blastomycosis," *Clin Infect Dis*, 1992, 14(Suppl 1):S82-90.
Bradsher RW, "Histoplasmosis and Blastomycosis," *Clin Infect Dis*, 1996, 22(Suppl 2):S102-11.
Pappas PG, Bradsher RW, Kauffman CA, et al, "Treatment of Blastomycosis With Higher Doses of Fluconazole. The National Institute of Allergy and Infectious Diseases Mycoses Study Group," *Clin Infect Dis*, 1997, 25(2):200-5.
Pappas PG, Pottage JC, Powderly WG, et al, "Blastomycosis in Patients With the Acquired Immunodeficiency Syndrome," *Ann Intern Med*, 1992, 116(10):847-53.
Saccente M, Abernathy RS, Pappas PG, et al, "Vertebral Blastomycosis With Paravertebral Abscess: Report of Eight Cases and Review of the Literature,"*Clin Infect Dis*, 1998, 26(2):413-8.

Blood Fluke *see Schistosoma mansoni on page 249*

Bordetella bronchiseptica

Synonyms Kennel Cough; Snuffles

Microbiology *B. bronchiseptica* is an aerobic gram-negative coccobacillus that distinguishes itself from *B. pertussis* by its ability to grow readily on MacConkey agar, possess peritrichous flagella for motility, reduces nitrate, and is urea-positive. See table. Although it does possess the pertussis toxin, only *B. pertussis* can elaborate the toxin. The dermonecrotic toxin of *B. bronchiseptica* is thought to contribute to inflammation and destruction of the bony and cartilaginous tissues in the upper respiratory tract of animals, but its role in human disease is unknown.

Bordetella bronchiseptica Properties

Test	*B. pertussis*	*B. bronchiseptica*
Growth on MacConkey agar	No	Yes
Urease	No	Yes
Nitrate reduction	No	Yes
Oxidase	Yes	Yes
Motility	No	Yes

Epidemiology *B. bronchiseptica* is predominantly an animal pathogen that causes respiratory infections such as kennel cough in dogs, snuffles in rabbits, atrophic rhinitis in swine, and pneumonia in koala bears. Most patients have a history of exposure to animals. Immunocompromised patients are at a higher risk than immunocompetent hosts. It is recommended that patients with AIDS avoid exposure to sick animals and exposure to known environmental sources such as kennels.

Clinical Syndromes
- **Respiratory:** Most often presents as bronchitis or pneumonia characterized by fever and cough. May have paroxysmal cough similar to whooping cough.
- **Other:** Sinusitis, bacteremia, endocarditis, and meningitis have been reported.

Diagnosis Confirmatory diagnosis made by isolation of organism in infected source, most commonly respiratory cultures.

Diagnostic Tests/Procedures
Aerobic Culture, Appropriate Site *on page 310*
Gram's Stain *on page 426*

Treatment May have variable susceptibility to beta-lactams, macrolides, and sulfonamides. Treatment failures are common and treatment usually requires a prolonged course of therapy to eradicate the organism. For patients with AIDS, a two-drug therapy such as antipseudomonal penicillin or fluoroquinolones with an aminoglycoside is recommended.

Drug Therapy
Recommended
Penicillins, Extended Spectrum *on page 864*
or

Fluoroquinolones *on page 736*
  plus
Aminoglycosides *on page 590*
Alternate
Cephalosporins, 3rd Generation(if susceptible) *on page 662*
  or
Imipenem and Cilastatin *on page 766*
  plus
Aminoglycosides *on page 590*

Selected Readings

Gomez L, Grazziutti M, Sumoza D, et al, "Bacterial Pneumonia Due to *Bordetella bronchiseptica* in a Patient With Acute Leukemia," *Clin Infect Dis*, 1998, 26(4):1002-3.

Woodard DR, Cone LA, and Fostvedt K, "*Bordetella bronchiseptica* Infection in Patients With AIDS," *Clin Infect Dis*, 1995, 20(1):193-4.

Bordetella pertussis

Microbiology *Bordetella pertussis* is a fastidious, nonmotile, gram-negative coccobacillus which tends to arrange itself singly and in pairs. "Pertussis" means violent cough, an appropriate name for the etiologic agent of whooping cough. *B. pertussis* is difficult to grow in culture. The starch-blood-agar medium described by Bordet and Gengou in 1900 was first used to isolate this organism *in vitro*. Some modern microbiology laboratories still use the Bordet and Gengou medium, but others have adopted a synthetic medium with growth factors which supports the growth of this fastidious organism equally well. It is important to notify the Microbiology Laboratory promptly if infection with *B. pertussis* is suspected since the organism usually cannot grow on routine agar used for planting sputum and other respiratory specimens.

Several virulence factors for *Bordetella pertussis* have been identified.

- Filamentous hemagglutinin - promotes attachment of *Bordetella* to the respiratory epithelium.
- Tracheal cytotoxin - causes ciliostasis in the respiratory epithelium and direct tracheal cell damage. This interferes with the "first line of defense".
- Adenylate cyclase toxin - causes accumulation of cyclic AMP in leukocytes leading to impairment of phagocyte functions such as chemotaxis.
- Dermonecrotic toxin - causes ischemic necrosis of the soft tissue in mice and likely causes local damage to the tracheal mucosa.
- Pertussis toxin - causes a sustained impairment in phagocytosis by a variety of different biological mechanisms and is thought to account for many of the systemic manifestations of pertussis.

Epidemiology Despite the introduction of the pertussis vaccine in many countries, there are still an estimated 51 million cases of pertussis annually worldwide with 600,000 fatalities. In most populations, pertussis is endemic (ie, there is a relatively constant background level of disease), but superimposed epidemics occur at 3- to 4-year intervals. For example, recent peaks in pertussis in the United States occurred in 1983, 1986, and 1990.

The whole-cell pertussis vaccine became available in the United States in the early 1940s. Prior to this, pertussis was most common in children 1-5 years of age. Maternally-acquired antibodies provided passive protection in the first year of life. After the whole-cell pertussis vaccine was licensed as DTP in 1949, there was a steady decrease in the number of pertussis cases in the U.S., reaching a nadir of about 1000 cases in 1976. However, since 1976 there has been a steady increase in the number of pertussis cases in the U.S. with 1990 being a 20-year peak. It is not clear whether this represents a true increase in the incidence of pertussis in the community or whether there is only improved reporting of cases. In addition, there has been a shift in the population at highest risk. Infants younger than 1 year of age now account for half the reported cases; many of these infants were never vaccinated or did not receive vaccinations as recommended (2, 4, 6, and 15-18 months). Vaccination coverage in school-aged children has been relatively broad, accounting for much of the decline in pertussis in this older group.

Pertussis is a highly contagious infection with an attack rate estimated at 50% to 100%. Transmission is via the respiratory route with the organism being carried for several feet in aerosolized droplets. Humans are the only natural reservoir for *B. pertussis*. It is likely that infected adults with undiagnosed pertussis are the
(Continued)

Bordetella pertussis (Continued)

major (and perhaps only) reservoir for the organism, which is then transmitted by cough to a susceptible infant.

About 10% to 15% of pertussis cases now involve persons older than 15 years of age. Large outbreaks of pertussis are rare in adolescents and young adults. However, in Massachusetts during 1992, there was an unusual increase in the number of adult pertussis cases. In that year, 78% of reported cases involved people 10-19 years of age, with only 9% involving infants. Many of the cases involved an outbreak in a high school and nearby middle school. A similar outbreak was reported in a Maryland high school the same year. It is clear that vaccine immunity decreases over time and is estimated to last about 12 years. Thus, pertussis can occur in adolescents and adults, regardless of vaccination status as a child. Adults lacking immunity cannot offer passive immunity to infants, who are at the greatest risk for morbidity and mortality.

Clinical Syndromes

- **Pertussis or whooping cough:** The presentation of pertussis can be divided into three phases: catarrhal phase, paroxysmal (cough) phase, and recovery phase. The catarrhal stage of pertussis begins with symptoms of the common cold (rhinorrhea, conjunctivitis, coryza, and low-grade fever). Infants may present with apneic spells. This phase generally lasts from several days to 1 or more weeks and is indistinguishable from any other upper respiratory infection. After this, the patient develops a mild cough which escalates to severe, violent coughing, or the paroxysmal stage. The typical "whooping cough" is characterized by several brief expiratory coughs in succession followed by a rapid inspiration of air past a swollen glottis (which produces the classic "whoop"). Many patients will not present with the classic "whoop," particularly infants and adults. Vomiting after a paroxysm of coughing is common. The paroxysmal state may last for 1-4 weeks. Coughing paroxysms may continue for up to 6 months after infection. (In China, pertussis has been called the "cough of 100 days".) Potential complications of the paroxysmal state include severe vomiting with subsequent weight loss, dehydration, and malnutrition. Other complications include those related to high intrathoracic pressures (eg, subconjunctival hemorrhages, pneumothorax, hernias, etc). Secondary bacterial infections, such as aspiration pneumonia during vomiting and coughing, are the leading cause of death. Central nervous system manifestations are relatively common in pertussis. These include seizures and encephalopathy in up to 2% of hospitalized pertussis cases. During the recovery or convalescent phase, the cough and frequency of paroxysms slowly decreases. Apparent "relapses" of cough are not uncommon during the recovery phase but are most likely due to common respiratory viruses rather than relapses of *B. pertussis.*

- **"Atypical" pertussis:** The clinical picture described above may be altered in infants and in older individuals who are partially immunized. The catarrhal phase may be shortened or absent in some cases. Adults often do not have a typical "whoop", and thus, the diagnosis of pertussis is often not even considered. In HIV-infected persons, *B. pertussis* has been reported to cause a chronic, paroxysmal cough with dyspnea but otherwise negative cultures.

Diagnosis Pertussis is often difficult to diagnose, particularly if the typical whooping cough is absent. Pertussis should be considered in the differential diagnosis of any person with a prolonged cough illness, regardless of the childhood DTP vaccination status. The laboratory diagnosis of *B. pertussis* is important, but many of the available laboratory tests suffer from poor sensitivity, specificity, or both. Thus, a clinical case definition for pertussis has been used. For reporting purposes, the Centers for Disease Control have defined a clinical case of endemic or sporadic pertussis as any cough illness lasting 14 days or more (without apparent cause) with any of the following: paroxysms of coughing, inspiratory "whoop", or post-tussive vomiting.

In situations where an outbreak of pertussis is occurring, a clinical case has been defined as a cough illness lasting 14 days or more.

Laboratory confirmation of *B. pertussis* should be attempted in all suspected cases. Techniques include:

- Nasopharyngeal culture: This is considered the gold standard for diagnosing pertussis. If possible, a nasopharyngeal wash should be performed to maximize the yield, although a nasopharyngeal swab (calcium alginate swab) is acceptable. Despite careful specimen collection, *B. pertussis* may fail to grow in culture. This is considered a relatively insensitive technique.

- Direct fluorescent antibody (DFA): DFA systems for detection of *B. pertussis* are widely used but are also insensitive and have the additional problem of variable specificity. The CDC has recommended that DFA should not be used as the criterion for laboratory confirmation of pertussis.

- Serologic tests: Antibody tests for *B. pertussis* are only available on a research basis.

- Other techniques: Polymerase chain reaction (PCR) amplification of *B. pertussis* nucleic acid sequences appears promising but has not been standardized and is still considered a research tool.

Individuals with a prolonged cough and a nasopharyngeal culture positive for *B. pertussis* are considered to have a confirmed case of clinical pertussis (although *B. pertussis* can sometimes be cultured from asymptomatic contacts who never develop disease). Those with a positive DFA and cough for more than 14 days without culture confirmation still have a high likelihood of pertussis. Persons with a cough for longer than 14 days but with a negative DFA and negative culture may have pertussis to a variable degree of certainty, since other organisms can occasionally cause an acute respiratory illness followed by prolonged cough. Persons with a positive DFA, negative culture, and a cough less than 14 days have a much lower likelihood of pertussis. Persons with a cough less than 14 days and a negative DFA and culture probably do not have pertussis.

Diagnostic Tests/Procedures

Bordetella pertussis Direct Fluorescent Antibody *on page 349*
Bordetella pertussis Nasopharyngeal Culture *on page 349*
Bordetella pertussis Serology *on page 351*

Treatment Although a variety of antibiotics appear to be effective against *B. pertussis in vitro*, the drug of choice is erythromycin, given at a dose of 50 mg/kg/day, up to about 2 g/day. Erythromycin has been shown to decrease symptoms even if started after the catarrhal phase. Treatment should be at least 14 days, and longer courses may be necessary. Ampicillin has been associated with clinical failures and should not be used. Alternative agents include tetracycline, co-trimoxazole, and chloramphenicol, but the data regarding clinical efficacy of these agents is limited. Hospitalization of infants may be warranted to avoid complications. Adjunctive therapies such as corticosteroids and beta-adrenergic agonists are either controversial or unwarranted and should be reserved for severe disease at physician discretion.

Prevention of *B. pertussis* remains the cornerstone for containment of this infection. There are two vaccines available, the whole-cell vaccine and the acellular vaccine. The whole-cell vaccine is used most frequently throughout the world with an efficacy of >80% in most series. The main drawback of the whole-cell vaccine is its reactogenicity (local pain and swelling, systemic symptoms). The Centers for Disease Control recommends the whole-cell vaccine be administered as part of the diphtheria-tetanus-pertussis combination vaccine at 6-8 weeks, 4 months, 6 months, 15 months, and 4-6 years (before school entry). The acellular pertussis vaccine was developed to minimize the problems of reactogenicity of the whole-cell vaccine. Acellular pertussis vaccine is available in combination with diphtheria and tetanus toxoids (DTaP). DTaP is currently recommended only for use as the fourth and/or fifth doses of the DTP series among children aged 15 months to 6 years. The new acellular pertussis vaccines appear to be immunogenic in adults and less reactogenic (see Selected Readings).

Drug Therapy
Recommended
Erythromycin *on page 722*
Alternate
Tetracycline *on page 944*
Co-Trimoxazole *on page 692*
Chloramphenicol *on page 667*
(Continued)

Bordetella pertussis (Continued)

Selected Readings

Edwards KM, "Pertussis in Older Children and Adults," *Adv Pediatr Infect Dis*, 1997, 13:49-77.

Edwards KM, Decker MD, Graham BS, et al, "Adult Immunization With Acellular Pertussis Vaccine," *JAMA*, 1993, 269(1):53-6.

Farizo KM, Cochi SL, Zell ER, et al, "Epidemiological Features of Pertussis in the United States, 1980-89," *Clin Infect Dis*, 1992, 14(3):708-19.

Herwaldt LA, "Pertussis in Adults. What Physicians Need to Know," *Arch Intern Med*, 1991, 151(8):1510-2.

Hewlett EL, "*Bordetella* Species," *Principles and Practice of Infectious Diseases*, 4th ed, Mandell GL, Bennett JE, and Dolin R, eds, New York, NY: Churchill Livingstone, 1995, 2078-84.

Marcon M, "Clinical and Laboratory Diagnostic Features of *Bordetella* spp - Pertussis and Beyond," *Clin Microbiol Newslett*, 1997, 19(24):185-91.

Muller FM, Hoppe JE, and Wirsing von Konig CH, "Laboratory Diagnosis of Pertussis: State of the Art in 1997," *J Clin Microbiol*, 1997, 35(10):2435-43.

"Pertussis Outbreaks: Massachusetts and Maryland, 1992," *MMWR Morb Mortal Wkly Rep*, 1993, 42(11):197-200.

Borrelia burgdorferi

Related Information

Lyme Disease Vaccine Guidelines *on page 1053*

Microbiology *Borrelia burgdorferi* is a tickborne spirochete which causes Lyme disease.

Epidemiology Lyme disease (more properly, Lyme borreliosis) is the most commonly reported vectorborne illness in the United States. The spirochete is transmitted by the bite of the tick *Ixodes dammini*. These ticks are endemic in the northeast coastal regions of the U.S., the midwest, and the west coast. Nine states account for 90% of the cases: Massachusetts, New York, New Jersey, Connecticut, Rhode Island, Pennsylvania, Minnesota, Wisconsin, and California. In very endemic areas, 30% to 75% of *Ixodes dammini* ticks are infected with *B. burgdorferi*. Lyme disease is most common in individuals living near wooded areas with abundant deer, especially transitional zones of woods to brush. Peak seasons for Lyme disease are May to September, in particular June, July, and August.

There are two insect vectors that can transmit *B. burgdorferi*, *Ixodes dammini* and *Ixodes pacificus* (found on the west coast). *Ixodes dammini* is much more efficient in transmitting the disease. The tick has three stages. The larva hatches from eggs during the spring and ingests a blood meal from the white-footed mouse host (*Peromyscus leucopus*) later in the summer. An infected mouse then transmits the infection (*B. burgdorferi*) to the larva. The larva detach from the mouse and develop into nymphs during the following spring. The nymphal ticks feed during the late spring/summer on other white-footed mice and on human hosts. The nymphal ticks mature into adult male and female ticks and feed on white-tailed deer (*Odocoileus virginianus*) in the fall, winter, and early spring. Females lay eggs which will hatch to larva, and the cycle starts again.

Infection can be transmitted during any stage, but the nymphs are the most efficient. Since the nymph is the size of a poppy seed, it is easily missed or just brushed off. When the nymph bites, it secretes a cement-like substance to keep it attached to the host and secretes a coumarin-like substance which maintains the blood capillary feeding lesion. It feeds to engorgement over about 3 days. Approximately 10% of people bitten by infected ticks will acquire Lyme disease.

Clinical Syndromes The clinical manifestations of Lyme disease were originally divided into three stages: stage I, II, III. More recently, manifestations have been divided into early Lyme disease (stage I and II) and late (III).

Stage I: 3-32 days after the tick bite, a rash develops. A papule appears at the site of the bite followed by an annular (ring-like) rash which spreads outwardly. There is often an area of central clearing. This rash is termed erythema chronicum migrans (ECM). The rash usually resolves in time, even if untreated. Patients may complain of additional symptoms such as headache, malaise, and myalgias. In some, the infection progresses.

Stage II: This stage involves the heart and nervous system primarily. Cardiac symptoms begin about 5 weeks after the bite (range 4 days to 7 months). Atrioventricular heart block is the most common finding and is usually self-limited. From 10% to 20% of people will develop neurologic disease weeks to months after the bite. This includes aseptic meningitis, cranial nerve palsy, peripheral radiculopathy, and Bell's palsy. Examination of the cerebrospinal fluid may show a lymphocytic pleocytosis. Intrathecal production of IgG directed against *B. burgdorferi* can be shown in some patients.

Stage III: Arthritis is the hallmark of stage III Lyme disease. The large joints are generally involved (knees, hips, etc). Joint symptoms begin from several days to over 2 years after the erythema chronicum migrans rash.

Diagnosis Lyme disease is a clinical diagnosis, not a laboratory diagnosis. Laboratory tests are not standardized and **never** should be used alone.

Diagnostic Tests/Procedures
Lyme Disease Serology *on page 481*
Lyme Disease Serology by Western Blot *on page 482*
Polymerase Chain Reaction *on page 523*

Treatment The treatment for Lyme disease depends in large part on the stage of the disease.
- Erythema chronicum migrans: Doxycycline is the drug of choice, but also effective are amoxicillin, penicillin, and erythromycin.
- Carditis: Ceftriaxone or penicillin
- Neurologic: Ceftriaxone or penicillin
- Arthritis: Ceftriaxone or penicillin

Lyme disease virus vaccine is available for prevention of Lyme disease in high-risk individuals or individuals living in endemic areas.

Pediatric Drug Therapy
Recommended
Ceftriaxone *on page 655*
Alternate
Ampicillin *on page 604*
Penicillin G, Parenteral, Aqueous *on page 860*

Adult Drug Therapy
Recommended
Ceftriaxone *on page 655*
Doxycycline *on page 713*

Prophylaxis:
Lyme Disease Vaccine *on page 801*
Alternate
Ampicillin *on page 604*
Penicillin G, Parenteral, Aqueous *on page 860*

Selected Readings
Evans J, "Lyme Disease," *Curr Opin Rheumatol*, 1998, 10(4):339-46.
Haass A, "Lyme Neuroborreliosis," *Curr Opin Neurol*, 1998, 11(3):253-8.
Nadelman RB and Wormser GP, "Lyme Borreliosis, *Lancet*, 1998, 352(9127):557-65.
Rahn DW, Malawista SE, "Lyme Disease: Recommendation for Diagnosis and Treatment," *Ann Intern Med*, 1991, 114(6):472-81.
Schmidt BL, "PCR in Laboratory Diagnosis of Human *Borrelia burgdorferi* Infections," *Clin Microbiol Rev*, 1997, 10(1):185-201.
Sigal LH, "Musculoskeletal Manifestations of Lyme Arhritis," *Rheum Dis Clin North Am*, 1998, 24(2):323-51.
Sigal LH, "The Polymerase Chain Reaction Assay for *Borrelia burgdorferi* in the Diagnosis of Lyme Disease," *Ann Intern Med*, 1994, 120(6):520-1.
Spach DH, Liles WC, Campbell GL, et al, "Tick-Borne Diseases in the United States," *N Engl J Med*, 1993, 329(13):936-47.
Steere AC, "Lyme Disease," *N Engl J Med*, 1989, 321(9):586-96.

Branhamella catarrhalis see Moraxella catarrhalis *on page 196*

Brucella Species

Microbiology *Brucella* species are small, aerobic, gram-negative coccobacilli which primarily cause disease in domestic animals. There are four species which cause human disease:
- *B. abortus* (cattle)
- *B. melitensis* (goats and sheep)
- *B. suis* (swine)
- *B. canis* (dogs)

The organism is nonmotile and does not form spores. All species tend to be slow-growing and fastidious. Supplemental carbon dioxide is required for optimal growth of *B. abortus*. The cell walls of *B. abortus*, *B. suis*, and *B. melitensis* contain endotoxin and two major surface antigens (A and M). The endotoxin is structurally and biologically different from endotoxins produced by many other enteric gram-negative bacilli.
(Continued)

Brucella Species *(Continued)*

Epidemiology Human brucellosis occurs worldwide. Approximately 500,000 cases are reported annually. The incidence has declined following mandatory pasteurization of dairy products and immunization of cattle with live-attenuated *Brucella abortus* vaccine. Endemic areas include the Mediterranean basin, South America, and Mexico. In the United States, more than half the cases of human brucellosis occur in Texas, California, Virginia, and Florida. A small number of cases (1% to 2%) result from exposure to *Brucella* in the microbiology or research laboratory.

Transmission to humans occurs by one of three routes:
- Direct contact of infected tissue, blood, or lymph with broken skin or conjunctivae
- Ingestion of contaminated meat or dairy products
- Inhalation of infected aerosols

Clinical Syndromes *Brucella* species enter the human via breaks in the skin or mucous membranes or via inhalation. Normal human serum has good bactericidal activity against *B. abortus* but not *B. melitensis*. Organisms not killed by polymorphonuclear leukocytes travel to regional lymph nodes, then enter the circulation, and localize in organs of the reticuloendothelial system where they are ingested by macrophages. Some will survive intracellularly and multiply, but when the macrophage is activated, the intracellular organisms are killed and release endotoxin. The host response to endotoxin can result in the signs and symptoms of acute brucellosis.

The clinical manifestations depend on both the immune status of the patient and the species of *Brucella* involved.
- **Asymptomatic infection**
- **Acute brucellosis, or "Malta fever":** Acute symptoms appear 1 week to several months following exposure. Symptoms include fever, sweats, chills, weakness, malaise, headache, and anorexia. In 25% to 50% of cases, there is weight loss, myalgias, arthralgias, and back pain. Epididymis is common in some series. Splenomegaly occurs in 20% to 30% of cases and lymphadenopathy in 10% to 20%.

  A number of complications of acute brucellosis have been reported. When infection is present for more than 2 months without therapy, the complication rate can approach 30%.
- **Musculoskeletal:** Sacroiliitis, arthritis, osteomyelitis, paraspinal abscess
- **Neurologic:** Meningoencephalitis, myelitis, others
- **Genitourinary:** Epididymo-orchitis, prostatitis
- **Endocarditis**
- **Granulomatous hepatitis**
- **Caseating or noncaseating granulomatous disease**
- **Splenic abscess**
- **Nodular lung lesions; lung abscess**
- **Erythema nodosum; other skin manifestations**
- **Ocular lesions**
- **Localized disease:** Can occur in any of the sites listed above
- **Subclinical infection**

Diagnosis The clinician should suspect brucellosis in any individual presenting with fever and who has a history of travel to endemic areas; exposure to livestock; a history of consuming unpasteurized milk, cheese, or other dairy products; or suggestive occupational risk factors (veterinarians, laboratory workers, etc). Laboratory confirmation is essential since the signs and symptoms of human brucellosis may be nonspecific. The diagnosis is established by recovery of the organism from blood, fluid, or other tissues (bone, abscesses, etc). In patients with *B. melitensis* infections, cultures of blood will be positive in 70% of cases. Bone marrow biopsy for histopathology and culture may be positive when other specimens are negative. In many laboratories, blood cultures for *Brucella* sp are processed using the Castañeda technique which utilizes biphasic media in a bottle. The Microbiology Laboratory should always be informed if *Brucella* sp are highly suspected.

Serologic techniques for diagnosing brucellosis include a standard tube agglutination test. A *Brucella* titer ≥1:160 or a fourfold rise in titer is considered presumptive evidence of recent infection with *Brucella* sp.

Diagnostic Tests/Procedures
Aerobic Culture, Appropriate Site *on page 310*
Blood Culture, *Brucella on page 340*
Gram's Stain *on page 426*

Treatment The recommendation from the World Health Organization for the treatment of acute brucellosis is doxycycline 200 mg/day with rifampin 600-900 mg/day for 6 weeks. Longer courses may be required in severe infections or if focal suppurative complications are present. Single agent therapy with tetracycline, streptomycin, rifampin, or trimethoprim are associated with a high relapse rate. For relapsed infection or central nervous system infection, the suggested regimens are third generation cephalosporin and rifampin or tetracycline, streptomycin, and rifampin, in combination. A consultation with an Infectious Disease specialist is recommended for suspected cases in the United States.

Pediatric Drug Therapy
  Recommended
    Co-Trimoxazole *on page 692*
      used in combination with
    Gentamicin *on page 747*

Adult Drug Therapy
  Recommended
    Doxycycline *on page 713*
      used in combination with
    Rifampin *on page 902*
  Alternate
    Co-Trimoxazole *on page 692*
      used in combination with
    Gentamicin *on page 747*

Selected Readings
Ariza J, Gudiol F, Pallares R, et al, "Treatment of Human Brucellosis With Doxycycline Plus Rifampin or Doxycycline Plus Streptomycin," *Ann Intern Med*, 1992, 117(1):25-30.

"Brucellosis Outbreak at a Pork Processing Plant - North Carolina, 1992," *MMWR Morb Mortal Wkly Rep*, 1994, 43(7):113-6.

Kaye D, "Brucellosis," *Harrison's Principles of Internal Medicine*, 13th ed, Isselbacher KJ, Braunwald E, Wilson JD, et al, eds, New York, NY: McGraw-Hill, 1994, 685-7.

Shehabi A, Shakir K, el Khateeb M, et al, "Diagnosis and Treatment of 106 Cases of Human Brucellosis," *J Infect*, 1990, 20(1):5-10.

Wise RI, "Brucellosis in the United States. Past, Present, and Future," *JAMA*, 1980, 244(20):2318-22.

Young EJ, "Serologic Diagnosis of Human Brucellosis: Analysis of 214 Cases by Agglutination Tests and Review of the Literature," *Rev Infect Dis*, 1991, 13(3):359-72.

Burkholderia cepacia

Microbiology The genus *Burkholderia* (formerly *Pseudomonas*) is composed of two species, *B. cepacia* and *B. pseudomallei. Burkholderia* spp are motile, gram-negative, nonspore-forming rods. *B. cepacia* is not difficult to grow and isolate in a clinical laboratory because the bacterium grows readily on most standard media. However, physicians should notify the laboratory whenever *B. cepacia* is suspected or whenever pulmonary specimens from cystic fibrosis patients are submitted for culture because *B. cepacia* can require up to 3 days of incubation before colonies of the bacterium are able to be observed on selective media, and technologists need to be especially aware of the potential presence of *B. cepacia.*

Epidemiology *Burkholderia* spp are found worldwide in water and soil, and on many plants, including vegetables and fruit. In agriculture, *B. cepacia* is most known for causing "slippery skin" rot in onions; in humans, *B. cepacia* is most known for being an opportunistic nosocomial pathogen. *B. cepacia* was first described as an opportunistic pathogen in a cystic fibrosis patient in 1972. By the mid 1980s, up to 40% of patients who were attending cystic fibrosis clinics in the United States, Canada, and the United Kingdom were reported to be colonized with *B. cepacia.* In hospitals, *B. cepacia* has been found on equipment and in medications, lotions, and disinfectants. Highly efficient person-to-person transmission of certain molecular types of *B. cepacia* is well documented, especially among cystic fibrosis patients. This high efficiency of transmission is especially important because it occurs not only nosocomially but also in social settings such as cystic fibrosis support groups, conferences, and camps. Sadly, patients with documented *B. cepacia* colonization often are subjected to social isolation.

(Continued)

Burkholderia cepacia (Continued)

Clinical Syndromes

- *Burkholderia cepacia*, in immunocompetent persons, can cause nosocomially-acquired septicemia, urinary tract infections, and respiratory tract infections. Such infections usually are not life-threatening in immunocompetent persons because *B. cepacia* is not especially virulent. However, in immunocompromised persons and persons with cystic fibrosis or chronic granulosis disease, pulmonary infections caused by *B. cepacia* can be fulminant and severe. In cystic fibrosis patients who have undergone lung transplants, *Burkholderia cepacia* can cause life-threatening pulmonary infections with a mortality rate as high as 80%.

- *Burkholderia pseudomallei* is the etiological agent of melioidosis, a disease with protean manifestations which range from asymptomatic infection to soft tissue abscesses to fulminant septicemia. Melioidosis is mostly in southeast Asia and Australia.

Diagnosis In gram-stained specimens, *Pseudomonas* spp and *Burkholderia cepacia* usually are not distinguishable. The suggestion of *B. cepacia* in a gram-stained specimen or the growth of *B. cepacia* in culture is not automatically indicative of *B. cepacia* being an etiological agent of an infectious process. The Gram's stain and culture information must be interpreted in the context of an appropriate clinical presentation (eg, cystic fibrosis or an association with a nosocomial setting). **Note:** The laboratory should be notified of the diagnosis when a pulmonary specimen (including sputum) is collected from a cystic fibrosis patient and submitted for culture.

Diagnostic Tests/Procedures

Aerobic Culture, Sputum *on page 312*
Gram's Stain *on page 426*

Treatment Many strains of *B. cepacia* are resistant to multiple antibacterial agents, especially in the setting of patients with cystic fibrosis (CF). The extended spectrum penicillins, quinolones, carbapenems, third generation cephalosporins, tobramycin, co-trimoxazole, minocycline, and chloramphenicol have all shown activity against this organism. Susceptibility testing is imperative, especially in CF patients who have received multiple antimicrobial regimens and have exacerbations of their disease. These patients also have altered pharmacokinetics of many antibacterials including cephalosporins and aminoglycosides. This along with potentially higher MICs for infecting organisms often necessitates higher doses of standard therapies. Some authors suggest combination drug therapy that would show synergy such as aminoglycoside/beta-lactam or ciprofloxacin/beta-lactam combinations. There is also a suggestion that amiloride may be synergistic with tobramycin *in vitro*.

Drug Therapy

Recommended

Tobramycin *on page 953*
  plus
Ceftazidime *on page 651*
Tobramycin *on page 953*
  plus
Penicillins, Extended Spectrum *on page 864*
Ciprofloxacin *on page 678*
  plus
Ceftazidime *on page 651*
  or
Penicillins, Extended Spectrum *on page 864*

Alternate

Chloramphenicol *on page 667*
Ciprofloxacin *on page 678*
Minocycline *on page 823*
Co-Trimoxazole *on page 692*

Selected Readings

Goldmann DA and Klinger JD, "*Pseudomonas cepacia*: Biology, Mechanisms of Virulence, and Epidemiology," *J Pediatr*, 1986, 108(5 Pt 2):806-12.

LiPuma JJ, "*Burkholderia cepacia*, Management Issues and New Insights," *Clin Chest Med*, 1998, 19(3):473-86.

Pujol M, Corbella X, Carratala J, et al, "Community-Acquired Bacteremic *Pseudomonas cepacia* Pneumonia in an Immunocompetent Host," *Clin Infect Dis*, 1992, 15(5):887-8.

Reed R, "Community-Acquired *Burkholderia cepacia* Sepsis in Children," *Clin Microbiol Newslett*, 1998, 20(17):147-8.

Sanford J, "*Pseudomonas* Species (Including Melioidosis and Glanders)," *Principles and Practice of Infectious Diseases*, 4th ed, Mandell GL, Bennett JE, and Dolin R, eds, New York, NY: Churchill Livingstone, 1995, 2003-9.

Calymmatobacterium granulomatis

Microbiology *Calymmatobacterium granulomatis* is the causative agent of granuloma inguinale, a sexually transmitted disease. The organism is an encapsulated gram-negative bacillus found within vacuoles of large histiocytic cells. The bacteria multiply within these vacuoles (about 30 organisms per vacuole), mature, and eventually rupture the cell.

Epidemiology Granuloma inguinale, also referred to as donovanosis, is quite rare in the United States, but in many developing countries, it is one of the most prevalent sexually transmitted diseases. Granuloma inguinale is common in India, the Caribbean, and Africa. In 1984, an outbreak of 20 cases was recognized in Texas (Rosen et al). The epidemiology and pathogenesis of donovanosis in the United States (and endemic countries as well) are poorly characterized. The precise role of sexual transmission is unclear, but repeated anal intercourse appears to be a risk factor for rectal and penile lesions in homosexual couples. Available data suggest that the infection is only mildly contagious and repeated exposures to an infected partner are necessary for transmission.

Clinical Syndromes

- **Granuloma inguinale:** The major disease associated with *Calymmatobacterium granulomatis* is granuloma inguinale, an infection characterized by genital ulceration and regional lymphadenopathy. As such, it must be differentiated from other classic STDs which can cause genital ulceration with regional adenopathy, such as primary syphilis, genital herpes simplex virus, chancroid, and lymphogranuloma venereum.

- **Genital ulcers:** The incubation period for granuloma inguinale varies from 8-80 days. Genital lesions initially appear as subcutaneous nodules (either single or multiple) which later erode. The ulcerations that form above the nodules are painless, clean, granulomatous, and often "beefy-red" with occasional contact bleeding. The lesions are most common on the glans or prepuce of the male and labial area in the female. The ulcers progressively enlarge in a chronic, destructive fashion. The ulcerations of donovanosis may be misidentified as carcinoma of the penis, chancroid, condyloma lata of secondary syphilis (when perianal lesions are present), and others.

- **Inguinal enlargement:** Infection with *Calymmatobacterium granulomatis* does not produce true regional lymphadenopathy. Instead, the granulomatous process in the genitals may extend into the inguinal region causing further fibrosis and granulation tissue, termed "pseudobuboes." These are present in only 10% of patients with donovanosis and are variably painful.

- **Constitutional symptoms:** In most cases of granuloma inguinale, constitutional symptoms are usually absent.

Diagnosis The diagnosis of granuloma inguinale can be confirmed by finding the characteristic **"Donovan bodies"** in a crush preparation. Fresh granulation tissue from a genital ulcer is spread over a clean microscope slide, air-dried, and stained with Wright or Giemsa stain. "Donovan bodies" are multiple, darkly-staining intracytoplasmic bacteria (*Calymmatobacterium granulomatis*) found within the vacuoles of large mononuclear cells. Donovan bodies can also be identified in formal biopsy specimens using standard light microscopy.

Treatment Granuloma inguinale responds well to the following first-line oral antibiotics (used singly): tetracycline 500 mg orally 4 times/day, ampicillin 500 mg 4 times/day, or co-trimoxazole (Bactrim™ DS) twice daily. Antibiotics are continued until the lesions are completely healed, usually 21 days or more; shorter courses are associated with relapses. Alternative therapies include chloramphenicol 500 mg orally 3 times/day or gentamicin 1 mg/kg twice daily. In pregnancy, erythromycin 500 mg orally 4 times/day is recommended. The treatment for HIV-infected individuals with granuloma inguinale is the same.

Drug Therapy
Recommended
Tetracycline *on page 944*
Ampicillin *on page 604*
Co-Trimoxazole *on page 692*
(Continued)

LIVERPOOL
JOHN MOORES UNIVERSITY
AVRIL ROBARTS LRC
TEL. 0151 231 4022

Calymmatobacterium granulomatis *(Continued)*

Alternate
Chloramphenicol *on page 667*
Gentamicin *on page 747*
Erythromycin *on page 722*

Selected Readings
Holmes KK, "Donovanosis (Granuloma Inguinale)," *Harrison's Principles of Internal Medicine*, 13th ed, Isselbacher KJ, Braunwald E, Wilson JD, et al, eds, New York, NY: McGraw-Hill, 1994, 694-5.

Krockta WP and Barnes RC, "Sexually Transmitted Diseases. Genital Ulceration With Regional Adenopathy," *Infect Dis Clin North Am*, 1987, 1(1):217-33.

Rosen T, Tschen JA, Ramsdell W, et al, "Granuloma Inguinale," *J Am Acad Dermatol*, 1984; 11(3):433-7.

"1998 Guidelines for Treatment of Sexually Transmitted Diseases. Centers for Disease Control and Prevention," *MMWR Morb Mortal Wkly Rep*, 1998, 47(RR-1):1-111.

Campylobacter jejuni

Microbiology *Campylobacter jejuni* is a curved, gram-negative bacillus which is the most common cause of bacterial diarrhea in the United States. On Gram's stain, *Campylobacter jejuni* appears as a curved, comma-shaped, gram-negative rod which often has a distinctive "seagull wing" appearance.

Campylobacter jejuni is a microaerophilic organism and fails to grow under routine aerobic and anaerobic conditions. The laboratory should be informed that *C. jejuni* is suspected clinically and a special request made for *Campylobacter* culture. A 5% to 10% oxygen, 5% to 10% carbon dioxide, and 80% to 90% nitrogen atmosphere is generally used to facilitate growth.

Epidemiology Infection with this agent occurs worldwide. With over 2 million cases per year in the U.S., *Campylobacter*-induced enteritis is more common than *Salmonella* and *Shigella* combined. The organism is found in the gastrointestinal flora of a number of wild and domestic animals, most notably in chickens. Transmission to humans generally occurs by consumption of the meat or milk of an infected animal, consumption of water contaminated with the feces of infected animals (eg, mountain streams), or fecal-oral transmission from an infected human or household pet. Undercooked chicken is notorious for transmission of *C. jejuni*, accounting for >50% of the cases of campylobacteriosis. Outbreaks have been linked to unpasteurized goat's cheese, clams, and untreated stream water in Wyoming. Infection occurs year round but is most common in the summer months.

Clinical Syndromes

- **Acute enteritis:** The organism can cause destructive, ulcerative changes in the mucosal surfaces of the small intestine (especially jejunum and distal ileum) and colon. Invasion of the organism causes inflammation of the lamina propria, bowel wall edema, and crypt abscesses. Patients initially present with nonspecific symptoms such as fever, headache, and myalgias. One to 2 days later, there is crampy abdominal pain and diarrhea. The quality and severity of the diarrhea is variable (although usually mild), and stools may be frequent and watery or visibly bloody. Most cases resolve spontaneously without antimicrobial therapy within 1 week. Less commonly, a fulminant acute colitis may occur. Again, a nonspecific prodrome of fever and malaise precedes any gastrointestinal complaints. However, the diarrhea which follows is voluminous and bloody with large amounts of mucous. Tenesmus is common and further suggests involvement of the colon. Fevers can reach 40°C, and occasionally the patient can appear in extremis. This syndrome may be confused with bacillary dysentery from *Shigella* species, severe salmonellosis, or even the initial presentation of inflammatory bowel disease (particularly if it is in a young adult). Toxic megacolon may complicate the hospital course.

- **Appendicitis-like syndrome:** Occasionally, *C. jejuni* can cause right lower quadrant pain mimicking appendicitis, without diarrhea. This "pseudoappendicitis" has been seen in association with other enteric pathogens including *Yersinia enterocolitica*.

- **Bacteremia:** This is an unusual finding in *C. jejuni* infection (even when the patient is febrile), unlike *Campylobacter fetus* which is commonly recovered from the blood. Blood cultures may turn positive several days after a mild diarrheal illness has already resolved; in such cases, antibiotic therapy is usually unnecessary. In other cases, bacteremia may be sustained, particularly in immunocompromised hosts, and this may suggest a deep focus of infection. Consultation with an Infectious Disease specialist is appropriate in such cases since prolonged antimicrobial therapy may be necessary.

- **Septic abortion:** *C. jejuni* infection in the pregnant female may lead to this complication. However, *Campylobacter* bacteremia during pregnancy does not automatically justify a therapeutic abortion since the outcome is not uniformly poor.
- **Reactive arthritis:** Following *Campylobacter* enteritis, a reactive arthritis may be seen, particularly in patients who are HLA-B27 positive.
- **Miscellaneous:** Guillain-Barré syndrome, hepatitis, and the hemolytic-uremic syndrome have been associated with *C. jejuni*.

Diagnosis *Campylobacter jejuni* should be suspected in any case of acute gastroenteritis or fulminant colitis. The findings of fecal leukocytes and occult blood in the stool is suggestive of campylobacteriosis and other gastrointestinal infections such as those caused by *Salmonella* sp, *Shigella* sp, enteroinvasive *E. coli*, enterohemorrhagic *E. coli* (O157:H7), Crohn's disease or ulcerative colitis, and others. The diagnosis is confirmed by a positive stool culture for *C. jejuni* or positive blood cultures for the organism.

Diagnostic Tests/Procedures
Blood Culture, Aerobic and Anaerobic *on page 337*
Stool Culture *on page 540*

Treatment The organism is sensitive *in vitro* to many common antimicrobial agents including erythromycin, ciprofloxacin, tetracyclines, aminoglycosides, and others. Ampicillin or penicillin should usually be avoided, and the susceptibility to co-trimoxazole is variable. Most patients with *Campylobacter* enteritis do not require antibiotics; they recover quickly without sequelae. Antimicrobial therapy should be targeted towards the more acutely ill patient. Limited clinical trials suggest that the following groups may benefit from the prompt use of antibiotics: children with severe dysentery, adults with severe bloody diarrhea and fever, individuals with worsening symptoms when seeking medical attention, and prolonged diarrhea (more than 1 week). Treatment with antibiotics does not prolong the fecal carriage of *C. jejuni* (as opposed to *Salmonella*). The drug of choice is erythromycin. For the toxic patient, combination therapy may be useful, but consultation should be made with an Infectious Disease specialist.

Drug Therapy
Recommended
Erythromycin *on page 722*
Doxycycline *on page 713*
Alternate
Fluoroquinolones *on page 736*

Selected Readings
Blaser MJ, "*Campylobacter* and Related Species," *Principles and Practice of Infectious Diseases*, 4th ed, Mandell GL, Bennett JE, and Dolin R, eds, New York, NY: Churchill Livingstone, 1995, 1948-56.

Blaser MJ, Wells JG, Feldman RA, et al, "*Campylobacter* enteritis in the United States. A Multicenter Study," *Ann Intern Med*, 1983, 98(3):360-5.

Johnson RJ, Nolan C, Wang SP, et al, "Persistent *Campylobacter jejuni* Infection in an Immunocompromised Patient," *Ann Intern Med*, 1984, 100(6):832-4.

Peterson MC, Farr RW, and Castiglia M, "Prosthetic Hip Infection and Bacteremia Due to *Campylobacter jejuni* in a Patient With AIDS," *Clin Infect Dis*, 1993, 16(3):439-40.

Sorvillo FJ, Lieb LE, and Waterman SH, "Incidence of Campylobacteriosis Among Patients With AIDS in Los Angeles County," *J Acquir Immune Defic Syndr*, 1991, 4(6):598-602.

Campylobacter pylori see Helicobacter pylori *on page 160*

Candida Species

Microbiology *Candida* species are normal host saprophyte yeasts found commonly in the gastrointestinal tract, genitourinary tract, and oropharynx. On direct mounts of infected material, they appear as small, oval, thin-walled, budding cells 2-5 μm in diameter with or without the presence of pseudohyphae. They stain gram-positive.

C. albicans is identified by the ability to produce germ tubes and/or chlamydospores in cornmeal agar. All *Candida* species may be distinguished by sugar fermentation and assimilation tests.

Epidemiology *Candida* species are found worldwide. Seventy percent of nosocomial candidal infections are due to *Candida albicans*. The other 30% are due to *C. glabrata*, *C. guilliermondii*, *C. krusei*, *C. pseudotropicalis*, *C. stellatoidea*, and *C. tropicalis*. According to the National Nosocomial Infections Surveillance
(Continued)

Candida Species *(Continued)*

System, *Candida* is now the fifth most common blood pathogen isolated from hospitalized patients and the fourth most common in ICU patients.

Risk factors for candidiasis include age extremes, central venous catheters, TPN, burns, exogenous hormone therapy, prosthetic devices, malnourishment, metabolic disease, concurrent infections with other pathogens, antibiotic therapy, uncontrolled diabetes mellitus, GI surgery, AIDS, mechanical disruption of epithelial surfaces, and physiological impairment of epithelial barrier function.

Clinical Syndromes

- **Cutaneous:** Intertriginous infection occurs most commonly in diabetes and obesity. Patients present with pain, burning and/or itching. Skin appears uniformly erythematous and inflamed with small papules and pustules. May have satellites distal to the border of the lesion. Follicular candidiasis usually occurs in areas that are occluded (ie, under bandages). Paronychial infection is characterized by swelling, tenderness, and redness around the nail.

- **Oral candidiasis:** Early premonitory sign of HIV. Presents as pseudomembranous, hyperplastic, atrophic, or angular cheilitis. Most commonly appears as erythematous patches with white discharge on the buccal mucosa with complaints of burning. The most efficient and cost-effective method of diagnosis is direct microscopic detection of *Candida* in a scraped sample of the oral lesion.

- **Candiduria:** Significance and natural history of progression are not known. Colony count not predictive of severity of infection or location. Treatment based on clinical judgment of severity of illness and risk factors. Symptoms include nocturia, frequency, and dysuria. Associated with urethritis, cystitis, and primary renal candidiasis.

- **Disseminated:** Requires pathological identification of organism (yeast) in tissues and growth of the yeast in culture. Thirty percent of patients with fungemia have endophthalmitis. Rarely occurs early postoperatively. It is indistinguishable from bacterial sepsis and can occur simultaneously with bacterial pathogens. Only 25% of the patients with extensive invasive organ infection will have positive blood cultures. Mortality exceeds 80%. Ten percent to 13% will have cutaneous manifestations. Other foci include septic arthritis, osteomyelitis, pericarditis (especially status post open heart surgery), suppurative phlebitis, and abscesses. Dissemination is likely if three or more colonized sites are present. *Candida* meningitis should be in the differential in patients with a history of intravenous drug abuse especially in the setting of HIV infection.

- **Vulvovaginitis:** Second most common cause of vaginal infections. Seventy-five percent childbearing age women will acquire this infection, and 40% will have a second occurrence. Less than 5% experience recurrent disease defined as more than four infections in a 12-month period. Eighty-five percent are due to *C. albicans*. Associated with pregnancy, high estrogen oral contraceptives, uncontrolled diabetes mellitus, tight-fitting clothes, antibiotic therapy, dietary factors, intestinal colonization, and sexually transmitted disease. The relationship between HIV infection and the risk of vulvovaginitis remains unclear. Human to human transmission is questionable, although male sexual partners may experience a transient rash, erythema, pruritus or burning sensation of the penis minutes to hours after unprotected sexual intercourse. May cause balanitis. Present with marked itching, watery to cottage cheese thick discharge, vaginal erythema with adherent white discharge, dyspareunia, external dysuria, erythema, and swelling of labia and vulva with discrete pustulopapular peripheral lesions. Cervix appears normal. Symptoms exacerbate the week preceding menses with some relief once menstrual flow begins.

Diagnosis Diagnosis is dependent on visualization of budding yeast with or without pseudohypha and the presence of clinical symptoms. If wet mounts, KOH, or histological stains are negative, need growth of yeast in culture. Endophthalmitis diagnosed by vitrectomy or anterior chamber aspiration (presumptive diagnosis by indirect fundoscopic exam). Serological tests such as nonspecific antigen tests vary in sensitivity and specificity. Serological detection of mannan, beta-1,3-glucan, and enolase are still investigational.

Diagnostic Tests/Procedures

Fungus Culture, Appropriate Site *on page 414*

Gram's Stain *on page 426*
KOH Preparation *on page 467*
Skin Biopsy *on page 535*

Treatment

- **Cutaneous:** Requires drying. Nystatin powder or imidazole (butoconazole, clotrimazole, miconazole, tioconazole) powder. Topical steroids may be used to reduce inflammation for the first 5-7 days of therapy. Paronychia infections may require topical imidazole up to 3 months.
- **Oral candidiasis:** Nystatin 100,000 units 3-5 times/day for 14 days versus azoles topically or orally.
- **Candiduria:** Remove predisposing factors, (ie, Foley catheter). Recommend amphotericin B irrigation 50 mg in 1 L sterile water continuous for 5 days. Alternate therapy includes flucytosine or azoles (fluconazole 50-100 mg/day for 7 days).
- **Disseminated:** Drainage or debridement of accessible sites. Recommended therapy is amphotericin B 0.5 mg/kg/day for 14 days. Fluconazole at doses 200-400 mg/day has been shown to be effective but not against *C. krusei* or *C. glabrata.* Endophthalmitis may require subtenonian or intracameral injection of amphotericin B.
- **Vulvovaginitis:** Imidazole derivatives (butoconazole, clotrimazole, miconazole, tioconazole) and triazole derivative (terconazole) (85% to 90%) are better than polyene preparations (nystatin) (75%). Extensive vulvar inflammation usually requires topical cream. For resistant or recurrent infections, oral agents are preferred (ketoconazole 400 mg orally 5-14 days, fluconazole 150 mg orally one dose, or itraconazole 200 mg orally 3 days). Both ketoconazole and fluconazole are effective prophylactic agents.

Drug Therapy

Recommended

Amphotericin B (Conventional) *on page 597*
Fluconazole *on page 732*
Ketoconazole *on page 791*
Antifungal, Topical *on page 610*

Alternate

Itraconazole *on page 785*
Amphotericin B, Lipid Complex *on page 600*

Selected Readings

Burchard, KW, "Fungal Sepsis," *Infect Dis Clin North Am,* 1992, 6(3):677-92.
Casado JL, Quereda C, Oliva J, et al, "Candidal Meningitis in HIV-Infected Patients: Analysis of 14 Cases," *Clin Infect Dis,* 1997, 25(3):673-6.
Darouiche RO, "Oropharyngeal and Esophageal Candidiasis in Immunocompromised Patients: Treatment Issues," *Clin Infect Dis,* 1998, 26(2):259-74.
Fichtenbaum CJ and Aberg JA, "Candidiasis," *The AIDS Knowledge Base,* 3rd ed, Chapter 57, Philadelphia, PA: Lippincott Williams & Wilkins, 1999, 659-68.
Fichtenbaum CJ and Powderly WG, "Refractory Mucosal Candidiasis in Patients With Human Immunodeficiency Virus Infection," *Clin Infect Dis,* 1998, 26(3):556-65.
Gubbins PO, Piscitelli SC, and Danziger LH, "Candidal Urinary Tract Infections: A Comprehensive Review of Their Diagnosis and Management," *Pharmacotherapy,* 1993, 13(2):110-27.
Pariser DM, "Cutaneous Candidiasis. A Practical Guide for Primary Care Physicians," *Postgrad Med,* 1990, 87(6):101-3, 106-8.
Peterson DE, "Oral Candidiasis," *Clin Geriatr Med,* 1992, 8(3):513-27.
Saiman L, "Neonatal Candidiasis," *Clin Microbiol Newslett,* 1998, 20(18):149-52.
Sobel JD, "Candidal Vulvovaginitis," *Clin Obstet Gynecol,* 1993, 36(1):153-65.
Walsh TJ, "Supplement of Presentations From the Ninth International Symposium on Infections in the Immunocompromised Host," *Int J Infect Dis,* 1997, 1(Suppl 1):S1-59.
White MH, "Is Vulvovaginal Candidiasis an AIDS-Related Illness?" *Clin Infect Dis,* 1996, 22(Suppl 2):S124-7.

Capnocytophaga Species

Synonyms DF-2

Microbiology *Capnocytophaga* is a thin, fusiform gram-negative rod. The long fusiform appearance of this organism is characteristic and helps to distinguish it from other gram-negative organisms. It is a pleomorphic organism and is facultatively anaerobic. There are three species that colonize the oral cavity of normal adults: *C. ochracea, C. sputigena, C. gingivalis.* Two species colonize the oral flora of dogs (the "dog bite" organism): *C. canimorsus* and *C. cynodegmi.* Growth of *Capnocytophaga* is supported by routine media such as blood agar. However, the organism may be fastidious and optimal growth requires 5% to 10% CO_2. The Microbiology Laboratory should be notified if *Capnocytophaga* is being considered (such as after a dog bite).
(Continued)

Capnocytophaga Species *(Continued)*

Epidemiology The species of *Capnocytophaga* that are part of the oral flora of adults have been recently recognized as a cause of disease in immunocompromised individuals, especially patients with neutropenia and mucositis. A wide spectrum of illness has also been described in otherwise healthy individuals, mainly infections in the oral cavity but also keratoconjunctivitis, lung abscess, osteomyelitis, and others. Other species of *Capnocytophaga* are part of the oral flora of canines (and some other animals including cats). Serious human infections including sepsis have been well described following dog-bite injuries. Cases of *C. canimorsus* tend to occur in older men.

Clinical Syndromes

- **"Dog bite sepsis":** *C. canimorsus* has caused a fulminant, life-threatening infection after a dog bite injury in immunocompromised patients. Patients present with septic shock, disseminated intravascular coagulopathy, and local necrosis at the site of inoculation. Pneumonitis, meningitis, and endocarditis may occur. Most notably, fulminant disease occurs in patients who are asplenic. Other groups at risk for the sepsis syndrome include alcoholics and other immunocompromised individuals. Not all patients with sepsis have a history of a recent dog exposure. Rapid diagnosis is essential because there is a high fatality rate of this syndrome.

- **Localized infection following dog bites:** A mild form of *Capnocytophaga* infection can occur in both healthy and immunocompromised persons.

- **Sepsis in immunocompromised patients:** This can result from those *Capnocytophaga* species normally inhabiting the oral cavity of humans. Patients tend to be neutropenic and blood cultures are often positive. The portal of entry is presumed to be odontogenic or via defects in the oral mucosa especially in patients with mucositis.

- **Miscellaneous:** Wound infections, abdominal abscesses, lung disease, and others have been reported.

Diagnosis *Capnocytophaga* infection should be considered in any patient who has a dog bite injury, especially if the person is asplenic or otherwise immunocompromised. It should also be considered in neutropenic patients with fever. Laboratory confirmation is required and cultures of appropriate wound sites, blood, or other appropriate body fluids should be submitted.

Diagnostic Tests/Procedures

Aerobic Culture, Appropriate Site *on page 310*

Gram's Stain *on page 426*

Wound Culture *on page 577*

Treatment Most isolates of *Capnocytophaga* are susceptible to penicillin and this is considered the antibiotic of choice. For asplenic patients with sepsis, consultation with an Infectious Disease specialist is strongly recommended. Recommended drug therapy in immunocompromised hosts includes clindamycin, erythromycin, ciprofloxacin, or imipenem.

Drug Therapy

Recommended

Penicillin V Potassium *on page 865*

Alternate

Amoxicillin and Clavulanate Potassium *on page 593*

Cestodes

Synonyms Tapeworms

Microbiology Cestodes (tapeworms; segmented worms) are intestinal and tissue parasites of mammals and some fish and are found worldwide. Cestodes have complex life cycles which involve intermediate hosts, in which the worms develop into only a larvae, and definitive hosts, in which worms have sexual reproduction and develop into adults. Humans can serve as both kinds of hosts. Cestodes can be divided into two groups according to the common sites they infect in humans, intestinal and tissue cestodes (see table). Cestodes cause illness in humans in two stages of their life cycles, larvae and adults. If larvae are ingested, the larvae mature into adults which attach by their heads to the intestinal mucosa, grow, lay eggs, and usually produce only minimal damage and discomfort to the host. If eggs are ingested, stomach acid releases larvae from eggs, larvae migrate to specific organs, and encyst. Cysts can grow and damage surrounding tissue. The form of the cyst (cysticercus, coenurus, hydatid cyst, etc) depends on the type of cestode.

Cestodes

Cestode	Ingested Infectious Form and Source
Intestinal	
Diphyllobothrium latum	Larvae in freshwater fish
Taenia solium	Larvae in undercooked pork or eggs in soil or feces
Taenia saginata	Larvae in undercooked beef or eggs in soil or feces
Hymenolepis nana	Larvae in arthropods or eggs in human feces
Hymenolepis diminuta	Larvae in arthropods or eggs in human feces
Dipylidium caninum	Larvae in dog fleas
Tissue	
Echinococcus granulosus	Eggs in dog feces
Echinococcus multilocularis	Eggs in fox and cat feces
Spirometra mansonoides	Larvae in freshwater fish
Diphyllobothrium latum	Larvae in freshwater fish
Multiceps sp	Eggs in dog fleas

Epidemiology Cestodes are parasites of humans, wild animals, domestic animals, and fish. Cestodes and cestode diseases have been recognized since the time of Hippocrates and continue to occur worldwide. Infections occur almost invariably because of poor sanitation habits, carelessness, ingestion of poorly cooked meat, or letting infected animals lick oral membranes (eg, child being licked by dog or cat which has crushed infected fleas in its mouth).

Clinical Syndromes The presentation of someone infected with cestodes is astonishingly varied and includes but is not limited to the following: unusual "things" in stools, "uncomfortable" intestinal symptoms, change in mental status, abdominal cramps, "hunger pains", etc. In addition CNS symptoms (headache, hemiparesis, altered vision, seizures, etc) can suggest cystic disease.

Diagnosis Diagnosis is most commonly made by ova and parasite examination (for eggs and proglottids) of stool. Cystic disease is visualized best by CT or MRI of suspected infected organs (often, brain and liver). Sensitive and specific serological tests (enzyme immunoassay and Western blot) are available for detecting antibody to *Echinococcus*.

Diagnostic Tests/Procedures
Brain Biopsy *on page 352*
Computed Transaxial Tomography, Appropriate Site *on page 374*
Magnetic Resonance Scan, Brain *on page 485*
Ova and Parasites, Stool *on page 505*

Drug Therapy
Recommended
Praziquantel *on page 880*
Alternate
Niclosamide *on page 841*

Selected Readings
Garcia LS and Bruckner DA, *Diagnostic Medical Parasitology*, Washington DC: American Society for Microbiology, 1993, 266-301.

King CH, "Cestodes (Tapeworms)," *Principles and Practice of Infectious Diseases*, 4th ed, Mandell GL, Bennett JE, and Dolin R, eds, New York, NY: Churchill Livingstone, 1995, 2544-53.

Maddison SE, "Serodiagnosis of Parasitic Diseases," *Clin Microbiol Rev*, 1991, 4(4):457-69.

Chlamydia pneumoniae

Synonyms Chlamydia TWAR; TWAR

Microbiology *Chlamydia pneumoniae*, like all *Chlamydia*, is an obligate intracellular bacterium, which stains gram-negative. This newly described agent was originally named *Chlamydia* TWAR, named after the first two clinical isolates (TW-183 from the eye of a child in a trachoma vaccine study, and AR-39 from a throat swab of a student with pharyngitis). Both names are used interchangeably. *Chlamydia pneumoniae* is one of three distinct species within the genus *Chlamydia*. The two other species of *Chlamydia* are *C. psittaci* (the cause of psittacosis) and *C. trachomatis* (a cause of nongonococcal urethritis and the eye infection called trachoma). *C. pneumoniae* shares about 5% DNA sequence homology with *C. trachomatis* and about 10% with *C. psittaci*. *Chlamydia* species are unique in having two separate forms with separate functions: the elementary body (EB), which is well-suited for extracellular life but lacks the (Continued)

Chlamydia pneumoniae (Continued)

ability to replicate and the reticulate body (RB), which is adapted to intracellular life and can divide by binary fission.

The life cycle of *Chlamydia pneumoniae* is as follows:
1. Elementary bodies attach to the host cell,
2. EBs enter the cell by inducing their own phagocytosis,
3. EBs transform into larger reticulate bodies,
4. the RBs grow and replicate by binary fission within vacuoles; these vacuoles become filled with EBs and appear as inclusion bodies in the host cytoplasm,
5. vacuoles rupture and release infectious organisms, and the cycle begins again.

Epidemiology There is no known animal reservoir for *C. pneumoniae*, unlike *C. psittaci* which is highly associated with birds. Transmission is person-to-person. Seroprevalence studies have shown that infection is uncommon in early childhood and increases during the teenage years (prevalence 25% to 50%). Many adults are seropositive, and some believe that nearly all adults are infected at least once.

Clinical Syndromes
- **Atypical pneumonia:** *C. pneumoniae* has been recognized as an important cause of community-acquired pneumonia. Approximately 10% of both outpatient and inpatient pneumonias are caused by this agent. Patients present with subacute malaise, cough, and low-grade fever. Hoarseness and pharyngitis are prominent. Chest x-ray show a single subsegmental infiltrate in most cases. The disease is usually mild to moderate in severity, but symptoms may be prolonged.
- **Bronchitis:** *C. pneumoniae* is also a frequent cause of bronchitis, accounting for about 45% of bronchitis cases in young adults. Typically, patients present with pharyngitis followed by dry cough. Chest x-rays are clear.
- **Pharyngitis:** Cases may be quite severe, with prolonged hoarseness. Some cases progress to lower respiratory tract infections.
- **Sinusitis:** The spectrum of *C. pneumoniae* sinusitis is becoming better recognized. In young adults, about 5% of cases of primary sinusitis are due to *C. pneumoniae*.
- **Other:** Fever of unknown origin, influenza-like illness

Diagnosis *Chlamydia pneumoniae* should be suspected in any case of atypical pneumonia, particularly if there is pharyngitis and hoarseness. Other diagnostic considerations for atypical pneumonia should include *Mycoplasma pneumoniae*, *Legionella* infections, viral lower respiratory infections, and others. The diagnosis can be confirmed primarily with serologic studies. The antigens which are used for antibody tests include lipopolysaccharide antigens and major outer membrane protein antigens. Lipopolysaccharide antigen is common to all members of the *Chlamydia* genus. This antigen is measured using complement fixation. Thus, positive studies are not specific for *C. pneumoniae* and can be positive during *C. trachomatis* and *C. psittaci* infections. Major outer membrane proteins (MOMPs) are specific for the different species of *Chlamydia*. These proteins are the basis for microimmunofluorescence (MIF) studies.

There are two patterns of antibody response with Chlamydial infections. Primary infection: Early on, complement fixation antibody is positive; 10 days to 1 month, MIF IgM is positive; 6 weeks, IgG is positive. Secondary infection: Complement fixation antibody is negative, IgM is positive in low titer; IgG response is more prompt. *C. pneumoniae* can also be isolated in cell culture systems but is difficult to do. The organism grows in HeLa cell culture, and identification has been enhanced by development of monoclonal antibodies specific for *C. pneumoniae*.

Diagnostic Tests/Procedures
Chlamydia Culture *on page 359*
Chlamydia pneumoniae Serology *on page 361*
Chlamydia Species Serology *on page 362*
Polymerase Chain Reaction *on page 523*

Treatment Large controlled studies comparing different antimicrobial agents have not been performed. Available data suggest that tetracycline and doxycycline are clinically effective. Failure with erythromycin has been reported. Therapy is usually continued for 10-14 days.

Pediatric Drug Therapy
Recommended
Erythromycin *on page 722*
Adult Drug Therapy
Recommended
Doxycycline *on page 713*
Tetracycline *on page 944*
Alternate
Erythromycin *on page 722*
Fluoroquinolones *on page 736*
Selected Readings
Gaydos CA, "*Chlamydia pneumoniae*: A Review and Evidence for a Role in Coronary Artery Disease," *Clin Microbiol Newslet*, 1995, 17(7):49-54.

Grayston JT, "Infections Caused by *Chlamydia pneumonia* Strain TWAR," *Clin Infect Dis*, 1992, 15:757-63.

Grayston JT, Campbell LA, Kuo CC, et al, "A New Respiratory Tract Pathogen: *Chlamydia pneumoniae*, Strain TWAR," *J Infect Dis*, 1990, 161(4):618-25.

Kauppinen M and Saikku P, "Pneumonia Due to *Chlamydia pneumoniae*: Prevalence, Clinical Features, Diagnosis, and Treatment," *Clin Infect Dis*, 1995, 21:S244-52.

Saikku P, Leinonen M, Tenkanen L, et al, "Chronic *Chlamydia pneumoniae* Infection as a Risk Factor for Coronary Heart Disease in the Helsinki Heart Study," *Ann Intern Med*, 1992, 116(4):273-8.

Chlamydia psittaci

Microbiology *Chlamydia psittaci* is an obligate intracellular bacterium and is the causative agent of psittacosis, or parrot fever. In the past, *Chlamydia* was classified as a virus, in part because of its nature as a cellular parasite. However, the organism also has many bacteria-like characteristics and is now regarded as a specialized bacterium. *Chlamydia psittaci* is one of three distinct species within the genus *Chlamydia*. *Chlamydia pneumoniae* (also called *Chlamydia* TWAR) and *Chlamydia trachomatis*, the cause of trachoma (an eye infection) and a cause of urethritis, are the other two. All *Chlamydia* species are obligate parasites of eukaryotic cells and are unable to replicate extracellularly. *Chlamydia* species are unique in having two separate forms with separate functions; the elementary body (EB), which is well-suited for extracellular life but lacks the ability to replicate, and the reticulate body (RB), which is adapted to intracellular life and can divide by binary fission.

Epidemiology Infections from *C. psittaci* occur sporadically. Approximately 50 cases are reported annually in the United States, with 50% occurring in individuals who own pet birds. High risk groups include pigeon collectors, employees of pet shops, and veterinarians. Outbreaks of psittacosis have been reported in turkey processing plants. Psittacosis has been traditionally associated with psittacine birds such as parrots, and this group remains an important reservoir for infection. However, it is clear that many other bird species can act as reservoirs, such as pigeons, turkeys, canaries, cockatiels, ducks, and many others. *C. psittaci* can be harbored in several sites within an infected bird including the bloodstream, feathers, liver, spleen, and feces. The organisms remain viable for prolonged periods of time within bird excreta. Some infected birds appear only mildly ill (anorexia, diarrhea), and the sympathetic pet owner may deliberately increase the amount of physical contact and time spent with the bird. Transmission can take place by several routes such as inhalation of dried, infected bird feces (this appears to be the most common route of human infection), touching contaminated bird feathers, physical intimacy with a highly infected bird, and person-to-person spread (very rare).

Prolonged, intimate contact with an infected bird is not necessary for transmission. Cases have been reported following brief avian contact. Birds can also be infected but show no signs of clinical disease; viable organisms continue to be shed in the feces for weeks.

Clinical Syndromes
- **Psittacosis (parrot fever):** Infection occurs in two stages. In the first stage, the organisms enter the host via the respiratory tract and travel to the liver and spleen. The organisms replicate in these sites. In the second stage, the organisms disseminate via the bloodstream to various sites, especially the lungs. Patients present with the sudden onset of high fevers and a severe headache. The presence of a severe headache, although nonspecific, is important in suggesting psittacosis and is highly characteristic of this infection. A variable number of days into the illness, patients frequently develop a
(Continued)

Chlamydia psittaci (Continued)

nonproductive cough which can be paroxysmal and severe. Other symptoms include chills, muscle aches, gastrointestinal upset, and anorexia. On physical examination, the patient presentation can range from comfortable to acutely ill. As with other infections from intracellular pathogens, there may be a pulse-temperature dissociation (ie, the pulse is slow relative to the degree of fever). Lung examination usually shows localized inspiratory rales. Signs of lung consolidation can occur with severe disease. An important physical finding is the presence of hepatomegaly and/or splenomegaly which frequently develop in psittacosis. Routine laboratory studies are usually not helpful and Gram's stain of sputum reveals no predominant microorganisms and few polymorphonuclear leukocytes. A variety of chest x-ray findings have been reported including a patchy interstitial lower lobe infiltrate (most common), a miliary pattern resembling tuberculosis, and occasionally a densely consolidated lobar pneumonia.

- **Endocarditis:** *C. psittaci* is a rare but reported cause of endocarditis. The diagnosis may be entertained in difficult cases of "culture-negative endocarditis" where multiple blood cultures properly collected are negative for pathogens. An Infectious Disease specialist may be useful in approaching this problem.

Diagnosis *Chlamydia pneumoniae* should be suspected in any case of atypical pneumonia, particularly if there is pharyngitis and hoarseness. The other diagnostic considerations for atypical pneumonia should include *Mycoplasma pneumoniae*, *Legionella* infections, viral lower respiratory infections, and others. The diagnosis can be confirmed primarily with serologic studies. The two major antigens which are used for antibody tests are lipopolysaccharide antigens and major outer membrane protein antigen. Lipopolysaccharide antigen, which is common to all members of the *Chlamydia* genus. This antigen is measured using complement fixation. Thus, positive studies are not specific for *C. pneumoniae* and can be positive during *C. trachomatis* and *C. psittaci*. Major outer membrane proteins (MOMPs), which are specific for the different species of *Chlamydia*. These proteins are the basis for microimmunofluorescence (MIF) studies.

There are two patterns of antibody response with chlamydial infections. Primary infection: Early, complement fixation antibody is positive; 10 days to 1 month, MIF IgM is positive; 6 weeks, IgG is positive. Secondary infection: Complement fixation antibody is negative; IgM is positive in low titer; IgG response is more prompt. *C. pneumoniae* also can be isolated in cell culture systems, but can be difficult. The organism grows in HeLa cell culture and identification has been enhanced by development of monoclonal antibodies specific for *C. pneumoniae*.

Diagnostic Tests/Procedures
Chlamydia psittaci Serology *on page 362*

Treatment Large controlled studies comparing different antimicrobial agents have not been performed. Available data suggest that tetracycline and erythromycin are clinically effective. Failure with erythromycin have been reported. Therapy is usually continued for 10-14 days.

Pediatric Drug Therapy
Recommended
Erythromycin *on page 722*

Adult Drug Therapy
Recommended
Doxycycline *on page 713*

Alternate
Erythromycin *on page 722*

Selected Readings
Barnes RC, "Laboratory Diagnosis of Human Chlamydial Infections," *Clin Microbiol Rev*, 1989, 2(2):119-36.

Kuritsky JN, Schmid GP, Potter ME, et al, "Psittacosis. A Diagnostic Challenge," *J Occup Med*, 1984, 26(10):731-3.

Potter ME, Kaufmann AK, and Plikaytis BD, "Psittacosis in the United States 1979," *MMWR CDC Surveill Summ*, 1983, 32(1):27SS-31SS.

Schlossberg D, "*Chlamydia psittaci* (Psittacosis)," *Principles and Practice of Infectious Diseases*, 4th ed, Mandell GL, Bennett JE, and Dolin R, eds, New York, NY: Churchill Livingstone, 1995, 1693-6.

Yung AP and Grayson ML, "Psittacosis - A Review of 135 Cases," *Med J Aust*, 1988, 148(5):228-33.

Chlamydia trachomatis

Microbiology *Chlamydia trachomatis* is a bacterium-like obligate intracellular organism. There are at least 15 recognized serotypes (immunotypes, serovars, biovars) of *C. trachomatis* which can be distinguished by immunofluorescent techniques. Certain serotypes are highly associated with disease syndromes. For example, *C. trachomatis* types L1, L2, and L3 are found only in patients with the disease lymphogranuloma venereum; whereas types A, B, and C are associated with trachoma, an infection of the eye.

C. trachomatis is one of three distinct species within the genus *Chlamydia*. The two other species are *Chlamydia psittaci* (the cause of psittacosis) and *Chlamydia pneumoniae* (a cause of community-acquired tracheobronchitis and pneumonia). *Chlamydia* species are unique in having two separate forms with separate functions: the **elementary body (EB)**, which is well-suited for extracellular life but lacks the ability to replicate and the **reticulate body (RB)**, which is adapted to intracellular life and can divide by binary fission.

The life cycle of *Chlamydia trachomatis* is as follows:
1. Elementary bodies attach to the host cell,
2. EBs enter the cell by inducing their own phagocytosis,
3. EBs transform into larger reticulate bodies,
4. the RBs grow and replicate by binary fission within vacuoles; these vacuoles become filled with EBs and appear as inclusion bodies in the host cytoplasm,
5. vacuoles rupture and release infectious organisms, and the cycle begins again.

C. trachomatis is difficult to identify on a Gram's stain. The Giemsa stain can be used for staining elementary bodies, reticulate bodies, and intracellular inclusion bodies but should not be trusted for definitive diagnosis.

Epidemiology Is specific for each disease state and clinical syndrome for which it is responsible. This information is included below.

Clinical Syndromes

Infections in Adults:
- **Nongonococcal urethritis (NGU) in men:** *Chlamydia trachomatis* accounts for about 50% of the cases of NGU. The organism is usually sexually acquired and is harbored in the urethra. About 25% of infected men are asymptomatic but are still able to transmit the organism. When symptoms such as dysuria and/or penile discharge occur, they tend to be mild. This is in contrast to gonococcal urethritis, which tends to be more severe. The characteristic watery or mucoid urethral discharge should be examined under Gram's stain to rule out *Neisseria gonorrhoeae*. Serious complications from chlamydial NGU are rare in males.
- **Mucopurulent cervicitis:** This is the female counterpart of NGU in the male. *Chlamydia trachomatis* is an important cause of mucopurulent cervicitis, usually acquired through sexual intercourse. The differential diagnosis of acute cervicitis includes *C. trachomatis*, *Neisseria gonorrhoeae*, herpes simplex virus, and others, making accurate diagnosis important. Many patients with chlamydial infections of the cervix remain asymptomatic. The diagnosis is further suggested by a positive "swab test" (ie, endocervical mucous appearing yellow-green when collected on a white cotton-tipped swab). Gram's staining of endocervical secretions is essential to confirm the presence of inflammatory cells (>10 polymorphonuclear cells per high power field correlates well with infectious cervicitis) and to exclude *Neisseria gonorrhoeae*. Complications of chlamydial cervicitis include pelvic inflammatory disease.
- **Pelvic inflammatory disease (PID):** This is probably the most important manifestation of *C. trachomatis* infection with respect to morbidity, permanent sequelae, and cost. In some women, chlamydial infection ascends from the cervix to the upper reproductive tract. The incidence and predisposing factors for this are unclear. Symptoms may be mild, with only nonspecific abdominal discomfort, but at laparoscopy, inflammation can be severe. Salpingitis, endometritis, and peritonitis can occur. Perihepatitis due to *C. trachomatis* has been described (the **Fitz-Hugh Curtis syndrome**).

    Complications of PID include involuntary infertility, chronic and recurrent pelvicoabdominal pain, and ectopic pregnancy. PID is also commonly
(Continued)

Chlamydia trachomatis (Continued)

caused by *Neisseria gonorrhoeae*. The number of cases due to either *Neisseria* or *Chlamydia* varies widely depending on the population studied.

- **Lymphogranuloma venereum (LGV):** Several serotypes of *C. trachomatis* cause LGV, a rare sexually transmitted disease in the United States (170 cases reported in the U.S. in 1984). LGV is an important cause of the syndrome of genital lesions with regional adenopathy. The incubation period for LGV ranges from 3-21 days. The LGV genital lesion is not striking and may be missed by the patient or the physician. The lesion is usually single and painless; it may be a papule, vesicle, or an ulcer. It resolves within several days. The key to the diagnosis of LGV is the nature of the regional adenopathy, not the genital lesion. The inguinal nodes in LGV develop 2-6 weeks after the primary lesion. The nodes are matted, fluctuant, and large. They tend to be unilateral (66% of the cases) and painful. Fistulas have been described, especially after diagnostic needle aspiration. Constitutional symptoms are very prominent, with complaints of fever, headache, myalgias, and malaise.

- **Acute urethral syndrome:** *C. trachomatis* may play an important role in a subgroup of young women who present with recurrent dysuria and pyuria but who have repeatedly sterile urine cultures.

- **Ocular infections:** Worldwide, *C. trachomatis* is one of the leading causes of blindness. Over 400 million people suffer from trachoma, a chronic keratoconjunctivitis caused by *C. trachomatis*. Trachoma is an ancient disease described thousands of years ago. Initial infection occurs in childhood: a gradual onset of epithelial keratitis, infiltrates in the subepithelium, and invasion of blood vessels into the cornea (pannus formation). Bacterial coinfection and scarring of the conjunctiva are common. Trachoma is endemic in Africa, Asia, and the Mediterranean basin. Sporadic cases still occur in the U.S.

  C. trachomatis can also cause inclusion conjunctivitis, an ocular infection different from trachoma (but possibly related). This is most commonly seen in sexually active young adults. The pathogenesis of this ocular infection is either self-inoculation with infected genital secretions or exposure of the eye to infected secretions during orogenital contact.

- **Proctocolitis:** An acute proctocolitis can be caused by *C. trachomatis*, particularly in homosexual males who practice receptive anal intercourse. Symptoms include tenesmus, watery rectal discharge, and rectal pain, but many patients remain asymptomatic.

- **Epididymitis:** *C. trachomatis* accounts for nearly 50% of cases of epididymitis in adolescents and young adults. *Neisseria gonorrhoeae* usually makes up the remainder of cases in this age group.

- **Reiter's syndrome (conjunctivitis, reactive arthritis, and urethritis):** The majority of cases of Reiter's syndrome appear to be related to *C. trachomatis*, although a "postdiarrheal" Reiter's syndrome is well recognized. *C. trachomatis* can be cultured from the urethra in the majority of cases of Reiter's syndrome. Untreated chlamydial urethritis appears to be a risk factor. Although *C. trachomatis* has not been isolated from synovial fluid from patients with Reiter's syndrome, elementary bodies suggestive of *Chlamydia* have been found in joint fluid.

Infections in infants: Newborns acquire *C. trachomatis* infection usually during passage through an infected birth canal. About 66% of those exposed during vaginal delivery ultimately become infected.

- **Pneumonia in infants:** *C. trachomatis* is one of the leading causes of pneumonia in infants 1-6 months of age. About 16% of neonates exposed to *C. trachomatis* during delivery will develop pneumonia. Infants present subacutely with rhinitis and a characteristic "staccato cough" followed by tachypnea and inspiratory rales. Fever is absent. Many have had a preceding conjunctivitis or will develop it during the course of the pneumonia. Chest radiographs show a diffuse interstitial pneumonitis. There is an increased incidence of pulmonary function test abnormalities later in childhood.

- **Conjunctivitis in infants:** Approximately 25% of newborns exposed to *C. trachomatis* during delivery will develop *Chlamydia* conjunctivitis. *C. trachomatis* remains the most common cause of neonatal conjunctivitis, despite prophylaxis with ophthalmic silver nitrate. Newborns present with a mucopurulent ocular discharge and inflamed conjunctivae 2 days to 3 weeks after birth. Most cases resolve spontaneously within several months without long-term sequelae, but some may develop a chronic ocular infection resembling a mild case of trachoma.

Diagnosis Recent recommendations by the Centers for Disease Control (1993) have emphasized the importance of more aggressive testing for the confirmation of *Chlamydia*. A variety of newer, more accurate tests are available, and the CDC now recommends laboratory testing of clinically suspected cases, sex partners of known or suspected cases, and certain asymptomatic individuals in high risk groups (sexually active women younger than 20 year of age, women 20-24 years of age who do not use barrier contraceptives and who have a new sex partner in the previous 3 months, and others).

Diagnostic tests can be classified as follows:
1. Cell culture
2. Nonculture tests:
   • Direct fluorescent antibody (DFA) tests
   • Enzyme immunoassays (EIA) tests
   • Nucleic hybridization (DNA probe) tests

For further information regarding the different tests, see the Laboratory Diagnosis section and the referenced article by the Centers for Disease Control and Prevention.

For the diagnosis of lymphogranuloma venereum (LGV), serologic titers for LGV may be useful. The complement fixation (CF) test is positive in most cases of active LGV at titers ≥1:64. Such titers become positive between 1 and 3 weeks postinfection. Occasionally, high CF titers have been found in individuals with other chlamydial infections and in asymptomatic patients. Titers <1:64 are suggestive but not diagnostic of LGV. It is difficult to demonstrate a classical fourfold rise in specific antibody titer in LGV due to the late presentation of many patients. Microimmunofluorescent tests are more sensitive than CF for the detection of LGV-producing *C. trachomatis* strains. However, the microimmunofluorescent antibody test is available only in a select number of research laboratories. Finally, *Chlamydia* species can be isolated in cell culture systems in some laboratories. The rate of recovery of LGV *Chlamydia* from buboes or genital lesions is about 30% or less.

Diagnostic Tests/Procedures
Chlamydia Culture *on page 359*
Chlamydia trachomatis by DNA Probe *on page 364*
Chlamydia trachomatis by DFA *on page 363*
Chlamydia trachomatis DNA by LCR *on page 365*
Ocular Cytology *on page 505*

Treatment Current treatment recommendations: Oral: Doxycycline 100 mg twice daily for 21 days. Alternatives: Tetracycline 500 mg 4 times/day for 21 days or erythromycin 500 mg 4 times/day for 21 days. In pregnancy, use erythromycin 500 mg 4 times/day. Treatment is the same in HIV-infected individuals.

Pediatric Drug Therapy
Recommended
Erythromycin *on page 722*
Adult Drug Therapy
Recommended
Doxycycline *on page 713*
Tetracycline *on page 944*
Alternate
Erythromycin *on page 722*

Selected Readings
Batteiger BE and Jones RB, "Chlamydial Infections," *Infect Dis Clin North Am*, 1987, 1(1):55-81.
Caliendo AM, "Diagnosis of *Chlamydia trachomatis* Infection Using Amplification Methods: Can We Afford It?" *Clin Microbiol Newslett*, 1998, 20(9):75-8.
Peeling RW and Brunham RC, "Chlamydiae as Pathogens: New Species and New Issues," *Emerg Infect Dis*, 1996, 2(4):307-19.
"Recommendations for the Prevention and Management of *Chlamydia trachomatis* Infections, 1993. Centers for Disease Control and Prevention," *MMWR Morb Mortal Wkly Rep*, 1993, 42(RR-12):1-39.
Smith TF, Brown SD, and Weed LA, "Diagnosis of *Chlamydia trachomatis* Infections by Cell Cultures and Serology," *Lab Med*, 1982, 13:92-100.
"1998 Guidelines for Treatment of Sexually Transmitted Diseases. Centers for Disease Control and Prevention," *MMWR Morb Mortal Wkly Rep*, 1998, 47(RR-1):1-111.

Chlamydia **TWAR** *see Chlamydia pneumoniae on page 95*

Citrobacter Species

Microbiology *Citrobacter* species are gram-negative rods which are important causes of nosocomial infection and are only rarely associated with community-acquired infections in normal hosts. *Citrobacter* species are moderate-sized, aerobic, gram-negative bacilli which belong to the large family Enterobacteria-ceae. The organism cannot be identified on the basis of its morphologic appearance on Gram's stain alone, and is morphologically indistinguishable from other Enterobacteriaceae. *Citrobacter* species are closely related to such gram-negative bacilli as *Klebsiella*, *Serratia*, *Salmonella*, and *E. coli* (about 40% DNA sequence homology with *Citrobacter*). Currently recognized *Citrobacter* species are *C. diversus*, *C. freundii*, and *C. amalonaticus*, all of which are potential human pathogens. Laboratory identification is generally straightforward. Special requests for isolation of *Citrobacter* are not necessary.

Citrobacter shares several potential virulence factors with other Enterobacteria-ceae, including endotoxin, the lipopolysaccharide (LPS) associated with the outer membrane of the bacteria. When cell lysis occurs (as with antibiotic therapy), the LPS is released into the host and can lead to such inflammatory responses as fever, leukopenia or leukocytosis, hypotension, and disseminated intravascular coagulation. Thus, LPS is regarded as an important mediator of the sepsis syndrome.

Epidemiology Because *Citrobacter* commonly inhabits the human gastrointestinal tract, it is considered one of the "enteric bacteria." In hospitalized patients, *Citrobacter* can asymptomatically colonize the urine, respiratory tract, abdominal wounds, decubitus ulcers, and others. Community-acquired infection is rare.

Clinical Syndromes

- **Lower respiratory tract infection:** Nosocomial *Citrobacter* infections are often seen in debilitated and ventilator-dependent patients. It should be noted that *Citrobacter* and other gram-negative bacilli can asymptomatically colonize the upper respiratory tract of hospitalized patients. Thus, the recovery of *Citrobacter* in a sputum or tracheal aspirate culture does not necessarily indicate a significant infectious disease. The diagnosis of a pneumonia still rests on standard criteria such as the presence of purulence (many leukocytes) on the Gram's stain of sputum, the presence of a pulmonary infiltrate, and signs of systemic inflammation in the patient. A positive sputum culture alone is not sufficient justification for initiating antimicrobial therapy.

- **Urinary tract infection:** Seen in hospitalized patients, often in those with indwelling Foley catheters. However, *Citrobacter* may harmlessly colonize the urine of patients with chronic bladder catheters without causing disease. The decision to initiate antibiotics in such patients should be based on the clinical situation (the presence of pyuria on urinalysis, suprapubic pain, fever, etc). Even the finding of large numbers of *Citrobacter* in a urine culture ($>10^5$ colony forming units/mL) by itself does not automatically indicate antibiotic therapy.

- **Hospital-associated bacteremias:** *Citrobacter* may be recovered from blood cultures in association with a known focus of infection (eg, pneumonia or catheter infection) or may be a "primary bacteremia" with no clear source. *Citrobacter* may also be cultured as part of a polymicrobial bacteremia, usually from an intravascular catheter or intra-abdominal sepsis. Endocarditis has rarely been reported.

- **Neonatal central nervous system infections:** *Citrobacter diversus* is a recognized cause of meningitis and brain abscesses in this age group.

Diagnosis The clinical presentations of the various nosocomial infections caused by *Citrobacter* are not distinctive, and laboratory isolation is necessary.

Diagnostic Tests/Procedures

Aerobic Culture, Appropriate Site *on page 310*
Gram's Stain *on page 426*

Treatment *Citrobacter* species present a challenging therapeutic problem, especially with nosocomial infection. High level drug resistance has been described in some isolates. Preliminary data suggest that the popular third generation cephalosporins may act to select mutants of *Citrobacter* that are resistant to a wide variety of antibiotics, including both cephalosporins and extended spectrum penicillins. These "stably derepressed mutants" are becoming more common in intensive care units and pose a significant and growing problem. Consultation with an Infectious Disease specialist may be useful in such cases.

Drug Therapy

Recommended

Cephalosporins, 3rd Generation *on page 662*
Penicillins, Extended Spectrum *on page 864*

Alternate

Imipenem and Cilastatin *on page 766*
Meropenem *on page 812*
Fluoroquinolones *on page 736*

Selected Readings

Drelichman V and Band JD, "Bacteremia Due to *Citrobacter diversus* and *Citrobacter freundii*: Incidence, Risk Factors, and Clinical Outcome," *Arch Intern Med*, 1985, 145(10):1808-10.

Lipsky BA, Hook EW 3d, Smith AA, et al, "*Citrobacter* Infections in Humans: Experience at the Seattle Veterans Administration Medical Center and a Review of the Literature," *Rev Infect Dis*, 1980, 2(5):746-60.

Samonis G, Ho DH, Gooch GF, et al, "*In Vitro* Susceptibility of *Citrobacter* Species to Various Antimicrobial Agents," *Antimicrob Agents Chemother*, 1987, 31(5):829-30.

Williams WW, Mariano J, Spurrier M, et al, "Nosocomial Meningitis Due to *Citrobacter diversus* in Neonates: New Aspects of the Epidemiology," *J Infect Dis*, 1984, 150(2):229-55.

Clostridium botulinum

Related Information

Timing of Food Poisoning *on page 1069*

Microbiology The etiologic agent of botulism is *Clostridium botulinum*. The organism is a gram-positive, anaerobic bacillus. The natural reservoir is soil and sediment where the organism survives by forming spores. Most foodborne epidemics are associated with home canned foods. Restaurants and commercially canned products are also the source of outbreaks.

As the bacteria grow and undergo autolysis, a powerful polypeptide neurotoxin is released. The toxin is heat labile and thus, is destroyed by appropriate heating in commercial canning processes. An acidic pH inhibits spore germination. This is the basis for adding ascorbic acid to home-canned products. Ingestion of even a small amount of contaminated food may cause severe clinical symptoms.

Epidemiology *Clostridium botulinum* is found in soil worldwide. Incidence of reported botulism is increasing. Most cases are individual or occur as a small cluster. If the outbreak is the result of contaminated commercially distributed food, the cases may occur in a widespread area. Early consultation with the State Health Department in conjunction with the Center for Disease Control is imperative for case management and epidemic control. Botulism is almost always caused by *C. botulinum* types A, B, and E in the western U.S., eastern U.S., and Alaska, respectively.

Clinical Syndromes

- **Infant botulism:** The most commonly reported form of botulism in the United States is infant botulism. *C. botulinum* toxin is released from organisms colonizing the intestinal tract. The toxin binds to synaptic membranes of cholinergic nerves and prevents the release of acetylcholine. Transmission of nerve fiber impulses to muscle is interrupted with resultant autonomic nerve dysfunction which progresses to motor weakness (flaccid paralysis).

  Subsequently, cranial and peripheral nerve weakness, constipation, and autonomic instability is the result of toxin effect on the ganglionic and postganglionic parasympathetic synapses. Typically, infants 1 week to 1 year of age present with progressive descending weakness following a period of constipation. Weak suck and poor feeding are frequent complaints.

- **Foodborne botulism:** Symptoms of botulism begin as descending paralysis or weakness within a few hours to 1-2 days following ingestion of contaminated food. Symptoms may commence as late as 1 week. Dizziness, lassitude, and weakness are common. Nausea and vomiting are less common. Blockage of autonomic nerve impulse transmission causes dry tongue, mouth, and pharynx which is unrelieved by fluids. Urinary retention, ileus, and constipation frequently follow. Paralysis descends from cranial nerves to extremities and the respiratory muscles. Speech and vision are often impaired. Key clinical observations include the fact that the patients are oriented, alert, or easily roused and afebrile. They may demonstrate postural hypotension and dilated unreactive pupils.

(Continued)

Clostridium botulinum *(Continued)*

- **Wound botulism:** Botulism may result from germination of spores contaminating traumatic wounds. Wounds caused by intravenous drug and nasal cocaine abuse have also been reported as sources. The clinical syndrome resembles that of foodborne botulism. Toxin can be recovered from the serum and wound drainage of affected patients. *C. botulinum* may be recovered from debrided tissue and drainage.

Diagnosis Outbreaks of botulism may be documented by identifying toxin in the stool or serum of symptomatic patients or from suspected food. Isolation of *C. botulinum* from stool or demonstration of the toxin by the mouse neutralization test establishes the diagnosis. Toxin is difficult to recover from serum; therefore, toxin recovery from stool may be more productive, but acquiring a stool specimen may be difficult because of the constipation. A low volume, normal saline, colonic irrigation may yield a useful specimen. Electromyography and repetitive nerve stimulation may yield corroborative evidence. The electromyographer should be alerted to the suspicion of botulism so that the study can be directed toward the diagnosis. A cerebrospinal fluid analysis to exclude meningitis, poliomyelitis, and Fisher Guillain-Barré syndrome is a useful part of the work-up.

Diagnostic Tests/Procedures
Botulism, Diagnostic Procedure *on page 351*
Cerebrospinal Fluid Analysis *on page 354*

Treatment

Infant botulism: The primary modes of treatment for infant botulism are supportive involving rehydration, nutritional supplementation, and respiratory support. Nasogastric tube feedings have been used relatively early in the course; however, the patients should be monitored for ileus. Oral feeding should not be reinstituted until ileus is gone, a gag reflex is present, and swallowing is normal. Intubation is required in the majority of cases for airway protection and, in about 25%, for ventilation. These patients have a significant risk of atelectasis and aspiration. Antitoxin is usually not used because the level of circulating toxin available to be bound is very low. In addition, there are significant complications of antitoxin therapy which include serum sickness, anaphylaxis, and life-long sensitivity to horse serum. Aminoglycoside antimicrobial therapy is contraindicated because aminoglycosides can cause neuromuscular blockade. Since sepsis is a key differential diagnosis, alternatives to aminoglycosides such as third generation cephalosporins should be considered in cases where botulism is in the differential. Therapy directed at eradication of *C. botulinum* toxin from the bowel has not been shown to produce objective clinical benefit.

Hospitalizations have a mean of about 50 days with complications including atelectasis, inappropriate antidiuretic hormone, autonomic instability, urinary tract infection, pneumonia sepsis, seizures, and subglottic stenosis as a complication of intubation. Despite the complications, mortality is very low (<3%), and prognosis for complete recovery is good.

Foodborne botulism: In cases of foodborne botulism, administration of equine antitoxin should be considered. In conjunction with the State Department of Health, consultation with the Foodborne Diseases branch of the Center for Disease Control is available, (404) 639-2206. The electromyogram, cerebrospinal fluid analysis, summary of the clinical syndrome, and chronology of the patient's illness should be available to facilitate the consultation. The main principle of therapy for botulism is respiratory support.

Wound botulism: Treatment is similar to the therapy for foodborne botulism. Incision and debridement of the wound should also be considered.

Drug Therapy
Recommended
Botulinum Toxoid, Pentavalent Vaccine (Against Types A, B, C, D, and E Strains of *C. botulinum*) *on page 623*

Selected Readings
Domachowske JB, "Infant Botulism," *Clin Microbiol Newslett*, 1998, 20(23):189-91.
Hurst DL and Marsh WW, "Early Severe Infantile Botulism," *J Pediatr*, 1993, 122(6):909-11.
McDonald TD and Lange DJ, "Botulism: Diagnosis and Treatment," *Hosp Med*, March, 1992, 42-57.
Midura TF, "Update: Infant Botulism," *Clin Microbiol Rev*, 1996, 9(2):119-25.
Schmidt RD and Schmidt TW, "Infant Botulism: A Case Series and Review of the Literature," *J Emerg Med*, 1992, 10(6):713-8.
Wigginton JM and Thill P, "Infant Botulism. A Review of the Literature," *Clin Pediatr (Phila)*, 1993, 32(11):669-74.

Clostridium difficile

Microbiology *Clostridium difficile* is a spore-forming, gram-positive, anaerobic rod which is the most frequent cause of antibiotic-associated colitis. This organism can be cultured from the stool of about 3% of normal adults. The percentage of hospitalized patients who are colonized with this agent is higher. The bacterium is capable of producing several toxins within the intestinal lumen, the best characterized being toxins A and B.

Epidemiology *C. difficile* colitis is most frequent in elderly persons and in hospitalized patients. The organism causes disease when antibiotics cause an alteration in the normal intestinal flora allowing the bacterium to colonize and ultimately produce toxins. *C. difficile* has been isolated from several sources besides stool, including the hands of healthcare workers, fomites, endoscopy equipment, and other instruments.

Clinical Syndromes *C. difficile* colitis: The range of severity of symptoms is broad, ranging from mild diarrhea to a more profuse, watery, and mucoid diarrhea. In general, symptoms begin several days after receiving antibiotics. In most cases, the stool is guaiac-negative, although bloody stools can occur. A more severe, sepsis-like presentation has been well-described, in which patients present with high fevers, marked abdominal pain, hypotension, hypoalbuminemia, and evidence of serositis. In some cases, patients may present with a syndrome resembling a toxic megacolon and have little or no diarrhea.

Diagnosis Some cases of antibiotic-associated colitis caused by *C. difficile* are associated with the formation of pseudomembranes in the colon. These are recognized by sigmoidoscopy with or without biopsy. More commonly the condition is confirmed by obtaining stool samples for the toxin produced by *C. difficile*, rather than culture of the stool for this organism.

Diagnostic Tests/Procedures

Clostridium difficile Toxin Assay *on page 367*

Fecal Leukocyte Stain *on page 408*

Treatment The mainstay of treatment for *C. difficile* colitis is discontinuation of all offending antibiotics, whenever feasible. Oral vancomycin is very effective in this condition, but its high cost is almost prohibitive. Metronidazole is also effective in antibiotic-associated colitis and is considerably less expensive.

Drug Therapy

Recommended

Metronidazole *on page 817*

Alternate

Vancomycin *on page 967*

Selected Readings

Bartlett JG, "Antibiotic-Associated Diarrhea," *Clin Infect Dis*, 1992, 15(4):573-81.

Bartlett JG, "*Clostridium difficile*: Clinical Considerations," *Rev Infect Dis*, 1990, 12(Suppl 2):S243-51.

Johnson S and Gerding DN, "*Clostridium difficile*-Associated Diarrhea," *Clin Infect Dis*, 1998, 26(5):1027-36.

Kelly CP, Pothoulakis C, and LaMont JT, "*Clostridium difficile* Colitis," *N Engl J Med*, 1994, 330(4):257-62.

McFarland LV, Mulligan ME, and Kwok RY, "Nosocomial Acquisition of *Clostridium difficile* Infection," *N Engl J Med*, 1989, 320(4):204-10.

Clostridium perfringens

Related Information

Timing of Food Poisoning *on page 1069*

Microbiology *Clostridium perfringens* is an anaerobic gram-positive rod; occasionally it can appear gram-negative or gram-variable. It is a spore-forming organism, but the spores are not usually seen on Gram's stain. It has been termed "aerotolerant" because of its ability to survive when exposed to oxygen for limited periods of time.

The organism produces 12 toxins active in tissues and several enterotoxins which cause severe diarrhea. Four toxins can be lethal. The toxins separate the species into five types, A-E.

- Alpha toxin: A lecithinase which damages cell membranes. It is produced by *C. perfringens* type A. It is the major factor causing tissue damage in *C. perfringens*-induced gas gangrene (myonecrosis). The toxin is a phospholipase which hydrolyzes phosphatidylcholine and sphingomyelin and leads to increased vascular permeability, myocardial depression, hypotension, bradycardia, and shock.

(Continued)

Clostridium perfringens (Continued)

- Enterotoxin: Produced mainly by *C. perfringens* type A but also by types C and D. This toxin is responsible for the diarrheal syndromes classically ascribed to this organism. The enterotoxin binds to intestinal epithelial cells after the human ingests food contaminated with *C. perfringens*. The small bowel (ileum) is primarily involved. The toxin inhibits glucose transport and causes protein loss.
- Beta toxin: Produced by *C. perfringens* type B and C. This toxin causes enteritis necroticans or pigbel. This disease is seen in New Guinea where some natives ingest massive amounts of pork at feasts after first gorging on sweet potatoes. The sweet potatoes have protease inhibitors which prevent the person from degrading the beta toxin which is ingested in the contaminated pork.

Epidemiology *C. perfringens* is ubiquitous in the environment, being found in soil and decaying vegetation. The organism has been isolated from nearly every soil sample ever examined except in the sand of the Sahara desert. In the human, *C. perfringens* is common in the human gastrointestinal tract. In one study, it was found in 28 of 40 adults. It can also be commonly recovered from many mammals including cats, dogs, whales, and others.

Clinical Syndromes The organism can be pathogenic, commensal, or symbiotic. Important diseases caused by *C. perfringens* include the following.

- **Food poisoning:** *C. perfringens* is one of the most common causes of food poisoning in the United States. Foods commonly contaminated with *C. perfringens* are meat, poultry, and meat products such as gravies, hash, and stew. Human disease is caused by ingestion of heat-labile toxin. The highest risk comes from meats which are partially cooked, cooled, then reheated. Spores present in the food germinate during the reheating process. Symptoms include watery diarrhea and abdominal cramps, which occur about 12 hours after the meal. Fever is generally not part of this illness. Vomiting is unusual. Duration of symptoms is about 24 hours. The diagnosis is made by culturing the stools and, for epidemiological purposes, the food.
- **Pigbel:** See description under Microbiology above. This follows massive ingestion of contaminated pork and sweet potatoes. Incubation period is 24 hours. There is intense abdominal pain, bloody diarrhea, vomiting, shock, and intestinal perforation in some cases. A vaccine is available for travelers.
- **Gynecologic infections:** *C. perfringens* has been isolated in association with septic abortions, tubo-ovarian abscesses, and uterine gas gangrene. Interestingly, *C. perfringens* has been isolated from the blood of healthy females in the immediate postnatal period; the organism appeared to be a commensal in the blood since the patients remained well without antibiotic therapy. This underscores the often enigmatic nature of *C. perfringens*.
- **Skin and soft tissue infection colonization:** Many wounds can be contaminated with *C. perfringens*, particularly when there is an open wound exposed to soil. The organism may or may not be causing disease, and its relevance should be based on clinical findings; a superficial wound growing *C. perfringens* can often be treated using local care alone.
- **Anaerobic cellulitis:** *C. perfringens* alone or in a mixed infection causes a local tissue invasion with some necrosis. Patients are afebrile, and there is little pain or swelling. Gas may be quite noticeable in the infected tissues. Anaerobic cellulitis is seen in patients with infected diabetic foot ulcers and patients with perirectal abscesses. Localized infection can spread if not appropriately treated.
- **Fasciitis:** Patients with *C. perfringens* fasciitis present with rapidly progressive infection through soft tissue planes. **This is a medical emergency.** Anaerobic organisms cause pain, swelling, and gas formation; and patients frequently present in a florid sepsis syndrome. The classic setting for this is the patient with known colonic cancer with presumed abdominal fascial metastases; this is the nidus for colonic contamination, followed by rapid movement along the fascial planes. Although the muscle is not involved, the mortality of anaerobic cellulitis remains very high even with early surgical intervention.
- **Clostridial myonecrosis:** This entity has been described after traumatic wounds, especially during war time when wounds are grossly contaminated with soil. In World War II, 30% of battlefield wounds were associated with this, but in Vietnam only 0.02%. Clostridial myonecrosis can also be seen

with crush injury, colon resections, septic abortions, and other conditions. Clinically, there is systemic toxicity, with tissue hypoxia and vascular insufficiency. The involved muscles appear black and gangrenous. Often there is abundant gas felt as crepitance in the wound. Treatment is surgical removal of devitalized tissue and, often, amputation.

Diagnosis The diagnosis of infection by *C. perfringens* begins with a high index of suspicion when a patient presents with one of the clinical syndromes described above. One important caveat is that the laboratory isolation of *C. perfringens* from a necrotic wound does not necessarily imply disease from this organism; many wounds can be colonized. In the right clinical setting, however, a positive *C. perfringens* culture and a compatible clinical presentation are highly suggestive of disease caused by this agent. Gram's stain preparations of wound material, uterine tissue, cervical discharge, muscle tissues, and other relevant materials should be made; a predominance of gram-positive rods should bring anaerobic infection, including *C. perfringens*, to mind.

In patients with clostridial septicemia, accompanying abnormalities may be a clue to clostridial disease before culture confirmation is made. Patients may have disseminated intravascular coagulation with a brisk hemolysis, hemoglobinuria, and proteinuria. X-rays of diseased areas may reveal the presence of gas in muscle or soft tissue; this is suggestive of clostridial infection, although other anaerobes (and aerobes) can cause gas formation. If clostridial myonecrosis is suspected, a muscle biopsy usually performed at the time of tissue debridement, can be diagnostic.

Diagnostic Tests/Procedures
Anaerobic Culture *on page 316*
Gram's Stain *on page 426*
Skin Biopsy *on page 535*

Treatment In general, the treatment of clostridial infection is high-dose penicillin G, to which the organism has remained susceptible. For skin and soft tissue infections, the extent of infection determines the need for surgical debridement. When wounds are simply colonized with clostridia, neither antibiotics nor surgery are indicated. Localized soft tissue infections can often be managed by surgical debridement alone, without antibiotics. When systemic symptoms are present and there is extension of infection into deeper tissues, antibiotics and surgical intervention are required. In fulminant cases of gas gangrene with myonecrosis, immediate surgical intervention (debridement, amputation) is the primary treatment of choice, and antibiotics have little effect.

Drug Therapy
Recommended
Penicillin G, Parenteral, Aqueous *on page 860*
Metronidazole *on page 817*
Alternate
Imipenem and Cilastatin *on page 766*
Clindamycin *on page 684*
Meropenem *on page 812*

Selected Readings
"*Clostridium perfringens* Gastroenteritis Associated With Corned Beef Served at St Patrick's Day Meals - Ohio and Virginia, 1993," *MMWR Morb Mortal Wkly Rep*, 1994, 43(8):137, 143-4.

Lorber B, "Gas Gangrene and Other *Clostridium*-Associated Diseases," *Principles and Practice of Infectious Diseases*, 4th ed, Mandell GL, Bennett JE, and Dolin R, eds, New York, NY: Churchill Livingstone, 1995, 2182-95.

Shandera WX, Tacket CO, and Blake PA, "Food Poisoning Due to *Clostridium perfringens* in the United States," *J Infect Dis*, 1983, 147(1):167-70.

Clostridium tetani
Related Information
Immunization Guidelines *on page 1041*

Microbiology *Clostridium tetani* is a strictly anaerobic, gram-positive, motile, spore-forming rod. Bacteria in very young or very old cultures can be gram-negative. Under adverse conditions, vegetative cells form polar ("drumstick" or "tennis racquet" appearance) spores which are extremely resistant to drying, boiling for 1 hour, and chemical disinfectants; the spores are killed by autoclaving. *C. tetani* is the etiological agent of tetanus, a strikingly dramatic infectious disease which has been recognized for many centuries. *C. tetani* was first isolated in pure culture in 1889 by Kirtasato, and the tetanus toxoid was first prepared the following year.
(Continued)

Clostridium tetani (Continued)

Epidemiology *Clostridium tetani* and its spores are found in the soil (especially manured soil) worldwide; the spores can survive in soil for many years. Sometimes *C. tetani* is also found in the lower intestinal tracts of humans and animals. In the United States since the mid 1970s, the number of cases of tetanus per year has remained at about 0.5 per 100,000 persons. Tetanus is most prevalent in the older age group (>60 years of age) and, in all populations, is directly related to an absence of immunization or to inadequate immunization. Tetanus is not uncommon (1 million cases per year) in developing countries, where mortality rates are high, probably because of a lack of intensive and proper supportive care. In developing countries, most cases occur in mothers with incompletely removed and subsequently infected placentas and in their newborns with unclean and infected umbilical cord stumps.

The portal of entry of *C. tetani* is usually a traumatized site (eg, piercing wound, burn, parenteral drug abuse, implantation of infected soil, war, and traumatic motor vehicle accident). Predisposing wounds often are quite small (eg, prick of a rose thorn or small splinter) and not recognized. Resulting traumatized or deep necrotic tissue environment is conducive to germination of implanted spores and the subsequent production of tetanospasmin, the potent neurotoxin of *C. tetani*. The vegetative cells produce the neurotoxin at the site of trauma and do not invade. Tetanospasmin circulates through the blood and lymphatic systems, attaches strongly to ganglioside receptors of presynaptic inhibitory neuron synapses, and inhibits the release of glycine, an inhibitory transmitter. The result of this binding and inhibition is simultaneous contraction of opposing flexor and extensor muscle groups and subsequent, often extremely violent, local and generalized muscle spasms.

Clinical Syndromes Tetanus: The incubation period for tetanus can be from a few days to several months. Shorter incubation periods are associated with more severe disease. The initial presentation of tetanus usually is characterized by general weakness, cramping, stiffness, and/or difficulty swallowing or chewing. "Lockjaw" can be an early sign. During the first week, spasms occur more frequently and become more generalized. Later, spasms can become intensely painful and more severe to the point of affecting breathing, speech, swallowing, and cardiac function. Cardiac, respiratory, and renal failure are the major causes of death. Mortality rates for mild, moderate, severe, and neonatal tetanus have been reported to be 0%, 9%, 44%, and 75%, respectively.

Diagnosis The diagnosis of tetanus is made by clinical judgment and patient history. Culture of specimens is not productive and not clinically useful. A history of appropriate immunization against tetanus almost always eliminates the possibility of tetanus. A differential diagnosis can include rabies, meningitis, peritonitis, antipsychotic drugs, poisoning, and epilepsy.

Treatment Supportive therapy with emphasis on appropriate ventilation should be the major consideration in the treatment of patients with tetanus. The neuromuscular symptoms and spasms from tetanus may be managed with benzodiazepines. Additional sedation may also be necessary. Tetanus immune globulin (TIG) should be administered immediately in a dose of 500-3000 units. Intrathecal TIG (250 units) may be administered, but its use is still investigational.

Tetanus Prophylaxis in Wound Management

Number of Prior Tetanus Toxoid Doses	Clean, Minor Wounds		All Other Wounds	
	Td*	TIG†	Td*	TIG†
Unknown or fewer than 3	Yes	No	Yes	Yes
3 or more‡	No#	No	No¶	No

*Adult tetanus and diphtheria toxoids; use pediatric preparations (DT or DTP) if the patient is younger than 7 years old.

†Tetanus immune globulin.

‡If only three doses of fluid tetanus toxoid have been received, a fourth dose of toxoid, preferably an adsorbed toxoid, should be given.

#Yes, if more than 10 years since last dose.

¶Yes, if more than 5 years since last dose.

Adapted from Report of the Committee on Infectious Diseases, American Academy of Pediatrics, Elk Grove Village, IL: © American Academy of Pediatrics, 1986.

Equine antiserum has also been used but is associated with significantly more adverse reactions than TIG.

Patients should also be treated with antimicrobial therapy. Although intravenous penicillin is often used, metronidazole is at least as effective. Theoretically, TIG should be administered prior to antibiotic therapy to abate any increase in toxin release caused by antibiotic administration. Local wound care is also important.

Other clinical manifestations that may require therapeutic intervention include autonomic instability, increased risk of pulmonary embolus, increased risk of stress ulceration, decubitus ulcers, fluid and electrolyte imbalance, and nutritional imbalance.

Tetanus can be prevented by appropriate immunization. Immunization guidelines can be found in the appendix.

Drug Therapy
Recommended
Tetanus Immune Globulin (Human) *on page 941*
used in combination with
Metronidazole *on page 817*
or
Tetanus Immune Globulin (Human) *on page 941*
used in combination with
Penicillin G, Parenteral, Aqueous *on page 860*

Selected Readings
Bleck TP, "*Clostridium tetani*," *Principles and Practice of Infectious Diseases*, 4th ed, Mandell GL, Bennett JE, and Dolin R, eds, New York, NY: Churchill Livingstone, 1995, 2173-8.
"Tetanus Fatality - Ohio, 1991," *MMWR Morb Mortal Wkly Rep*, 1993, 42(8):148-9.

CMV see Cytomegalovirus *on page 122*

Coccidioides immitis

Microbiology *Coccidioides immitis* is a dimorphic fungus. In the mycelial form on culture, the mold grows relatively fast producing a flat, moist, gray colony in 3-5 days and then developing fluffy white aerial mycelium. Wet mount reveals branching septate hyphae and chains of thick-walled, barrel-shaped arthrospores (up to 10 μm) separated by "ghost" spaces (remnants of empty cells). **Arthrospores are highly infectious to laboratory workers.** The yeast form can be seen on direct examination of infected material as round, thick-walled spherules 20-80 μm with many small endospores.

Epidemiology *Coccidioides immitis* is a normal inhabitant of the sandy, salty, dry soil of the lower Sonora Desert. It is found only in the western hemisphere and has been isolated in specific areas of Argentina and Central America, as well as the southwestern United States. The warm, dry environment facilitates the growth of arthroconidia that break from the parent mycelium and become airborne. The infectious arthroconidia are inhaled and within the pulmonary acinus convert to spherules and reproduce by endosporulation.

Coccidioides infects more than 50,000 people each year and is increasing in incidence. In 1991, there was a threefold increase followed by a tenfold increase in 1992 in California as compared to the previous 5 years. Most cases occur in late childhood and early middle age. Epidemics are typically associated with dust storms, construction, archaeological digs, and exploration for oil. Infections in persons residing outside endemic areas arise from travel exposure, laboratory exposure, or inhalation of contaminated fomites.

Impaired T-cell immunity is associated with severe pulmonary and disseminated disease. Approximately 33% of AIDS patients have no focal lesion or only focal pulmonary lesions despite evidence of systemic disease. *Coccidioides* is an AIDS-defining illness.

Risk factors for dissemination include infants and elderly, male sex, race (Filipinos > Blacks > Native Americans > Hispanic > Oriental), negative skin test, serum complement fixation >1:64, immunosuppression, second half of pregnancy, and postpartum.

Clinical Syndromes
- **Asymptomatic:** Subclinical infection. Positive skin test without clinical evidence of disease. Occurs in approximately 60% of cases.
- **Primary pulmonary:** Acute respiratory illness characterized by fever, cough, headache; often associated with malaise, myalgias, and fatigue. Self-limited. Approximately 25% develop more severe disease associated

(Continued)

Coccidioides immitis (Continued)

with pleuritic chest pain, yet very few will progress. May have erythema nodosum or erythema multiforme. May develop arthritis, most commonly in the knee, which is an immune complex reaction and not dissemination (referred to as Desert Rheumatism).

- **Pulmonary sequelae:** Characterized by pulmonary infiltrates that are frequently subpleural with overlying pleural effusions (12%), which is usually self-limited. Hilar adenopathy is common, but paratracheal or superior-mediastinal adenopathy suggests dissemination as does diffuse miliary infiltrates. Five percent develop persistent cavities or thin-walled coccidioidal abscesses or nodules (coccidioidoma). Thirty-three percent of the cavities will close within 2 years while the rest may rupture, bleed, or develop secondary infections which may require surgical excision.

- **Chronic persistent fibrocavitary disease:** Associated with pre-existing bronchopulmonary disease.

- **Disseminated disease:** In approximately 1% of infected individuals. Spreads beyond pulmonary parenchyma or hilar nodes. Found in every organ except GI. Most common site of spread is the skin (granulomas) followed by subcutaneous abscesses, synovitis, and osteomyelitis. Majority of deaths secondary to meningitis which occurs 2-3 weeks to years after initial infection. Hydrocephalus is frequent and is a severe complication. Direct cranial nerve involvement is secondary to a vasculitis that may present as a stroke-like syndrome or transverse myelitis.

Diagnosis Skin tests and serological markers are useful epidemiologic, as well as prognostic tools. More than 50% of the population in endemic areas are skin test positive. The presence of substantial or prolonged infection in the presence of negative skin test is a poor prognostic marker. Similarly, high complement fixation titers (>1:64) are associated with extrapulmonic spread and poor prognosis. Serial rising titers are significant.

Diagnosis is made by biopsy material revealing granulomatous response with characteristic spherules with evidence of endosporulation or isolation in culture.

Diagnostic Tests/Procedures

Fungal Serology *on page 410*
Fungus Culture, Appropriate Site *on page 414*
KOH Preparation *on page 467*

Treatment Severe infection requires 1-3 g amphotericin B. Mild to moderate pulmonary disease may be treated with ketoconazole, 400 mg, or fluconazole, 400 mg. There is approximately a 33% relapse when treated with azoles. Primary disease in immunocompetent hosts typically requires no treatment. Mounting clinical evidence indicates that fluconazole is at least as effective as amphotericin B independent of whether patients are HIV-infected or not. Given the practical difficulties of administering amphotericin B intrathecally and the high frequency of associated adverse effects, initiation of fluconazole treatment (800 mg/day orally) in patients with coccidiodal meningitis has become the preferred initial treatment. Itraconazole may also be effective. Only in patients who do not respond clinically after 1-2 months of therapy should intrathecal amphotericin B be considered. As with other forms of disseminated disease, lifelong therapy is necessary in patients with meningitis.

Drug Therapy

Recommended

Amphotericin B (Conventional) *on page 597*

Alternate

Fluconazole *on page 732*
Itraconazole *on page 785*
Ketoconazole *on page 791*

Selected Readings

Centers for Disease Control and Prevention, "Coccidioidomycosis - Arizona, 1990-1995," *MMWR Morb Mortal Wkly Rep*, 1996, 45(49):1069-73.

Galgiani JN, Catanzaro A, Cloud GA, et al, "Fluconazole Therapy for Coccidioidal Meningitis. The NIAID-Mycoses Study Group," *Ann Intern Med*, 1993, 119(1):28-35.

Singh VR, Smith DK, Lawerence J, et al, "Coccidioidomycosis in Patients Infected With Human Immunodeficiency Virus: Review of 91 Cases at a Single Institution," *Clin Infect Dis*, 1996, 23(3):563-8.

Stevens DA, "Coccidioidomycosis," *N Engl J Med*, 1995, 332(16):1077-82.

Tauber MG, Lee BL, and Aberg JA, "Coccidioidomycosis," *The AIDS Knowledge Base*, 3rd ed, Chapter 60, Philadelphia, PA: Lippincott Williams & Wilkins, 1999, 685-9.

Tucker RM, Denning DW, Dupont B, et al, "Itraconazole Therapy for Chronic Coccidioidal Meningitis," *Ann Intern Med*, 1990, 112(2):108-12.

Corynebacterium diphtheriae

Microbiology *Corynebacterium diphtheriae* is the causative agent of the once common disease human diphtheria. On Gram's stain, the organism appears as a pleomorphic, gram-positive rod (bacillus) and has a characteristic appearance resembling "Chinese characters" or "Chinese letters". The organism has a clubbed appearance at both ends and does not form spores. Although it can be grown in culture using a variety of solid media, optimal isolation of *C. diphtheriae* from clinical specimens requires special selective media which inhibits the growth of other bacterial species; this is especially true if the specimen is submitted from the throat which is often colonized with other nonpathogenic bacteria. Thus, the laboratory should be notified if diphtheria is suspected. The organism itself is not considered highly virulent, despite its ability to cause lethal disease. An asymptomatic carrier state was recognized as far back as the late 19th century. Even in patients with diphtheria, the organism generally does not invade the host tissues and does not cause local tissue destruction. Instead, the virulence of *C. diphtheriae* comes from the ability of some strains to elaborate a potent exotoxin. These strains carry a lysogenic β-phage which is integrated into the bacterial DNA. The mechanism of action of this important toxin has been well studied. Diphtheria toxin binds to the membrane of the host cell, enters the cytoplasm, inactivates elongation factor 2, which ultimately leads to termination of polypeptide production within the host cell. The diphtheria toxin is a potent cardio- and neurotoxin although damage to almost any organ can be seen.

Epidemiology Diphtheria was once a leading cause of death in children. Over the past 75 years there has been a relatively steady decline in the number of cases in the United States and is considered a rare disease. No significant outbreaks have been reported in the U.S. in the 1990s but sporadic cases continue. Worldwide, the incidence of diphtheria has also generally decreased although less consistently, and the disease remains endemic in some developing countries and in some urban areas in Eastern Europe. The epidemiology of diphtheria has changed. Diphtheria was thought to be primarily a disease of childhood but more contemporary epidemics have involved adults. Groups at risk include the urban poor, injection drug users, and minority groups. Cases usually involve persons who have not been adequately immunized with the diphtheria vaccine, although diphtheria has been reported in fully immunized individuals.

Transmission of *C. diphtheriae* occurs primarily person-to-person by the respiratory route. Some cases have been reported transmitted by other routes such as ingestion of milk. Skin disease due to *C. diphtheriae* can occur, and spread via exposure to infected skin has been well described.

Clinical Syndromes

- **Asymptomatic infection:** Asymptomatic carriage of *C. diphtheriae* is rare in the U.S. but occurs in a low percentage of the population in endemic areas. The organism usually colonizes the upper respiratory tract. This is felt to be the main reservoir of the organism in the community since there are no recognized animal sources.

- **Respiratory tract:** *C. diphtheriae* causes local inflammation in a variety of areas in the upper respiratory tract, including the nares, pharynx, larynx, and/or tracheobronchial tree. Disease of the pharynx is the most common manifestation and is characterized by a thick "pseudomembrane" covering the tonsils, uvula, palate, and other areas of the pharynx. The membrane is usually gray often with areas of necrosis. It consists of respiratory epithelium, fibrin, inflammatory cells, and organisms. The membrane can also involve the nasopharynx, and there may be purulent discharge from the nares. Although the pharyngeal membrane is the hallmark of diphtheria, it may be absent in 50% of culture-proven cases. Regional adenopathy in the cervical area is common, and in severe cases, the patient may present with a "bull neck". The voice may be hoarse. The spectrum of disease is wide and patients may present with localized pharyngeal disease without fever, and others may have significant constitutional symptoms with respiratory compromise with stridor.

- **Systemic disease:** Diphtheria toxin is an extremely potent peptide and can cause a wide range of systemic disease. Studies have shown that these systemic complications are unusual when the local respiratory tract disease

(Continued)

Corynebacterium diphtheriae (Continued)

is mild and are much more likely to occur when the local disease is advanced, diagnosis is delayed, and diphtheria antitoxin is given late. Complications include myocarditis, both subclinical and fulminant cardiac involvement; cranial nerve palsies, especially paralysis of the palate; motor neuron dysfunction, ranging from mild weakness to paralysis; renal failure with acute tubular necrosis.

- **Skin disease:** *C. diphtheriae* has been associated with nonhealing cutaneous ulcers, sometimes associated with a membrane on the skin lesion. This form of diphtheria has been primarily seen in tropical climates but has recently been described in homeless and indigent adults in the United States. Individuals with chronic skin ulcers caused by *C. diphtheriae* represent another reservoir for the organism in the population and transmission from an infected skin lesion can occur. However, some controversy exists regarding the significance of isolating *C. diphtheriae* from a chronic skin lesion; some experts feel it may sometimes be a harmless colonizer and should not be automatically considered the cause of the lesion.

Diagnosis The diagnosis of diphtheria may be quite difficult in the United States due to the rarity of the disease and lack of clinical experience. Clearly, there are a number of etiologies of tonsillitis and pharyngitis, but the unusual case of diphtheria should be considered if a membrane is seen on examination (although the membrane may be absent in many cases). Other clues include the presence of toxin-mediated complications such as neuropathies or myocarditis, and the presence of stridor in an adult. Laboratory diagnosis is important for confirmation. Throat swabs and membrane material should be planted on selective culture media. It should be noted that other diseases may cause tonsillar membranes, including infectious mononucleosis.

Diagnostic Tests/Procedures

Throat Culture for *Corynebacterium diphtheriae* on page 549

Treatment Diphtheria antitoxin is recommended for pharyngeal and laryngeal diphtheria. This neutralizing agent has been shown to improve outcome and is derived from horse antiserum. Thus, a hypersensitivity reaction to horse-derived products may be seen. Antitoxin should be administered as soon as feasible (within 48 hours if possible) since it does not act on toxin which has already entered the cells. Antibiotic therapy against *C. diphtheriae* is also recommended to decrease the organism burden (and thus decrease toxin production) and improve local disease such as pharyngitis. The organism is sensitive to a variety of agents but generally procaine penicillin G or erythromycin is recommended.

The cornerstone of disease control remains the use of the diphtheria vaccine (diphtheria toxoid). This is included in the standard recommendations for vaccination issued by the Centers for Disease Control and Prevention, both as part of the diphtheria-pertussis-tetanus (DPT) vaccine for children and the tetanus-diphtheria (Td) toxoid in older children and adults.

Drug Therapy

Recommended

Treatment:
Penicillin G Procaine on page 862
Erythromycin on page 722
Prevention:
Diphtheria and Tetanus Toxoid on page 707
Diphtheria, Tetanus Toxoids, and Acellular Pertussis Vaccine on page 708
Diphtheria, Tetanus Toxoids, Whole-Cell Pertussis, and *Haemophilus influenzae* Type b Conjugate Vaccines on page 711

Selected Readings

Harnisch JP, Tronca E, Nolan CM, et al, "Diphtheria Among Alcoholic Urban Adults. A Decade of Experience in Seattle," *Ann Intern Med*, 1989, 111(1):71-82.

MacGregor RR, "*Corynebacterium diphtheriae*," *Principles and Practice of Infectious Diseases*, 4th ed, Mandell GL, Bennett JE, and Dolin R, eds, New York, NY: Churchill Livingstone, 1995, 1865-72.

Millar OS, Cooper On, Kakkar VV, et al, "Invasive Infection With *Corynebacterium diphtheriae* Among Drug Users," *Lancet*, 1992, 339(8805):1359-63.

Wilson AP, Efstratiou A, Weaver E, et al, "Unusual Non-Toxigenic *Corynebacterium diphtheriae* in Homosexual Men," *Lancet*, 1992, 339(8799):998.

Corynebacterium equi see *Rhodococcus* Species on page 242

***Corynebacterium* Group JK** see *Corynebacterium jeikeium* on next page

Corynebacterium jeikeium

Synonyms *Corynebacterium* Group JK

Microbiology *Corynebacterium jeikeium* was only recently described as a human pathogen in 1976. Like other *Corynebacterium* species, it is a gram-positive, aerobic bacterium but tends to have a more coccobacillary (rather than bacillary) appearance and must be distinguished from streptococci. It is considered one of the "diphtheroids," a term which encompasses several similarly-appearing gram-positive bacilli or coccobacilli which morphologically resemble *Corynebacterium diphtheriae*.

Epidemiology *Corynebacterium jeikeium* can colonize the skin of many hospitalized patients. *Corynebacterium jeikeium* has been cultured from the skin of 50% of hospitalized oncology patients. Sites of colonization include the rectum, axilla, and inguinal areas. Oncology patients who have received broad-spectrum antibiotics are at risk for colonization. Healthy individuals living in the community are less likely to be colonized with this organism.

Clinical Syndromes

- **Septicemia:** *Corynebacterium jeikeium* has been increasingly recognized as a cause of bloodstream infections, particularly in those with underlying malignancies. There are also reports of bacteremias in cardiac surgery patients. In many cases, the portal of entry appears to be a skin defect, and often a bloodstream infection is associated with an indwelling vascular catheter. Risk factors also include neutropenia, lengthy hospitalization, and multiple prior antibiotics.
- **Endocarditis:** Several cases of early prosthetic valve endocarditis from *Corynebacterium jeikeium* have been described.
- **Other infections:** Infected peritoneal dialysis catheters, prosthetic central nervous system shunt infections, prosthetic orthopedic implant infections, pneumonitis, and others.

Diagnosis *Corynebacterium jeikeium* diagnosis is made by identification of the organism by Gram's stain and culture in a patient with a relevant clinical syndrome. No special media or conditions are necessary for growth. Any *Corynebacterium* isolated from the blood or catheter of an immunocompromised patient should be examined to determine if the isolate is *Corynebacterium jeikeium*.

Diagnostic Tests/Procedures

Aerobic Culture, Appropriate Site *on page 310*
Anaerobic Culture *on page 316*
Gram's Stain *on page 426*

Treatment *Corynebacterium jeikeium* is unique in that it is highly resistant to antimicrobial therapy. The clinically-isolated strains of JK tend to be resistant to cephalosporins and penicillins; some data suggest that antibiotic-susceptible strains of *C. jeikeium* are replaced by resistant strains during prolonged hospitalization. The antibiotic of choice is vancomycin.

Drug Therapy

Recommended

Vancomycin *on page 967*

Alternate

Penicillin G, Parenteral, Aqueous *on page 860*
used in combination with
Gentamicin *on page 747*

Selected Readings
Holmes RK, "Diphtheria, Other Corynebacterial Infections, and Anthrax," *Harrison's Principles of Internal Medicine*, 13th ed, Isselbacher KJ, Braunwald E, Wilson JD, et al, eds, New York, NY: McGraw-Hill, 1994, 623-30.

Rozdzinski E, Kern W, Schmeister T, et al, "*Corynebacterium jeikeium* Bacteremia at a Tertiary Care Center," *Infection*, 1991, 19(4):201-4.

Spach DH, Opp DR, and Gabre-Kidan T, "Bacteremia Due to *Corynebacterium jeikeium* in a Patient With AIDS," *Rev Infect Dis*, 1991, 13(2):342-3.

Corynebacterium Species, Other Than C. jeikeium

Microbiology *Corynebacterium* species are gram-positive bacteria which are part of the normal flora of humans. They are important members of a larger group of loosely related organisms referred to as "coryneform bacteria" or "diphtheroids" because they morphologically resemble the organism *Corynebacterium diphtheriae*. All members of the diphtheroid group (including *Corynebacterium* species) are aerobic, gram-positive bacilli or coccobacilli that
(Continued)

Corynebacterium Species, Other Than *C. jeikeium* (Continued)

often appear pleomorphic in clinical samples. Medically important coryneform bacteria include *Corynebacterium jeikeium* (see entry *Corynebacterium jeikeium on page 113*), *Corynebacterium* CDC group D-2, *Corynebacterium ulcerans*, *Arcanobacterium haemolyticum* (formerly *Corynebacterium haemolyticum*), and *Corynebacterium minutissimum*. A number of additional *Corynebacterium* species are potential pathogens.

Epidemiology Many *Corynebacterium* species are part of the normal flora of humans and are thus common isolates in a clinical microbiology laboratory. Various sites that are commonly colonized by *Corynebacterium* species include the skin of healthy persons (eg, *C. pseudodiphtheriticum*, *C. xerosis*), the skin of hospitalized patients (eg, *Corynebacterium* CDC group D-2), and the nasopharynx (several species). It may be difficult to determine the significance of a single isolate of *Corynebacterium* from a clinical specimen since it may represent colonization, skin contamination, or true disease.

Clinical Syndromes As noted above, the isolation of *Corynebacterium* species from a clinical specimen (eg, wound culture, vascular catheter culture, blood culture) requires careful interpretation by the physician. Serious disease has been associated with some *Corynebacterium* species, and the finding of a positive culture does not necessarily imply skin contamination or colonization. *Corynebacterium* species are considered organisms of low pathogenicity, and patients may present with a mild or chronic illness. Some species have been associated with specific illnesses as follows:

- **Urinary tract infections:** *Corynebacterium* CDC group D-2 has recently been recognized as a potential cause of urinary tract infections. This organism is similar to *Proteus mirabilis* in its ability to use the enzyme urease to hydrolyze urea; this leads to alkalinization of the urine and formation of struvite kidney stones which can become chronically infected. Complications include chronic cystitis secondary to infected stones and pyelonephritis. Again, the finding of a positive urine culture for "diphtheroids" or corynebacteria should be interpreted cautiously since this could also represent contamination of the urine sample from normal flora in the urethral region.

- **Erythrasma:** This common infection of the skin has been associated with *Corynebacterium minutissimum*, although the precise etiology of erythrasma is still unknown. Patients with erythrasma present with a patchy, erythematous rash often in the groin region. Under the fluorescent light of a Wood's lamp, the rash of erythrasma characteristically appears coral red. Cultures for *C. minutissimum* from patients with suspected erythrasma are not usually necessary since the diagnosis can usually be made clinically.

- **Pharyngitis:** *Arcanobacterium haemolyticum* (formerly *Corynebacterium haemolyticum*) can cause a pharyngitis associated with a scarlatiniform skin rash, particularly in young adults. The organism *C. ulcerans* (part of the flora of cows and horses) has occasionally been associated with a diphtheria-like pharyngitis in humans.

- **Pneumonia:** *Corynebacterium* species only rarely have been associated with pneumonia. There are case reports describing pneumonia in AIDS patients from *C. pseudodiphtheriticum*.

- **Bacteremia:** Since many *Corynebacterium* species are part of the normal skin flora, they may contaminate blood cultures (reported as "diphtheroids" in many laboratories). However, these organisms have been reported to cause both true bacteremia and endocarditis.

Diagnosis Most of the clinical manifestations of *Corynebacterium* species (with the exception of erythrasma) are nonspecific and isolation of the organism in the laboratory is necessary. The organisms, in general, grow readily on standard media. At times, *Corynebacterium* CDC group D-2 may be more difficult to grow from urine cultures, and the laboratory should be notified that this organism is suspected (alkaline urine, gram-positive bacilli on Gram's stain, presence of stones, etc).

Diagnostic Tests/Procedures

Aerobic Culture, Appropriate Site *on page 310*
Anaerobic Culture *on page 316*
Gram's Stain *on page 426*

Treatment Treatment of *Corynebacterium* depends on the severity of the infection and to some extent on the species involved. *Corynebacterium* CDC Group

D-2 tends to be somewhat more antibiotic resistant than other species, and some isolates are resistant to the quinolones, which are commonly used for urinary tract infections. *Corynebacterium* species are generally susceptible to erythromycin, vancomycin, and to most beta-lactam antibiotics. If serious infections are documented, full susceptibility testing of the organism should be performed. Note that *Corynebacterium jeikeium* (see entry *on page 113*) is often resistant to multiple antibiotics.

Drug Therapy

Recommended

Erythromycin *on page 722*

Alternate

Penicillin G, Parenteral, Aqueous *on page 860*

Selected Readings

Cohen Y, Force G, Gros I, et al, "*Corynebacterium pseudodiphtheriticum* Pulmonary Infection in AIDS Patients," *Lancet*, 1992, 340(8811):114-5.

Coyle MB and Lipsky BA, "Coryneform Bacteria in Infectious Diseases: Clinical and Laboratory Aspects," *Clin Microbiol Rev*, 1990, 3(3):227-46.

George MJ, "Clinical Significance and Characterization of *Corynebacterium* Species," *Clin Microbiol Newslet*, 1995, 17(23):177-180.

Holmes RK, "Diphtheria, Other Corynebacterial Infections, and Anthrax," *Harrison's Principles of Internal Medicine*, 13th ed, Isselbacher KJ, Braunwald E, Wilson JD, et al, eds, New York, NY: McGraw-Hill, 1994, 623-30.

Soriano F, Aguado JM, Ponte C, et al, "Urinary Tract Infection Caused by *Corynebacterium* Group D-2: Report of 82 Cases and Review," *Rev Infect Dis*, 1990, 12(6):1019-34.

Coxiella burnetii

Microbiology *Coxiella burnetii* is an obligately intracellular, gram-negative coccobacillus and a member of the group of organisms known as rickettsiae (*Rickettsia, Ehrlichia, Rochalimaea,* and *Coxiella*). *C. burnetii* survives extracellularly probably in spore form and can survive weeks to years in adverse environmental conditions. *C. burnetii* exists in two antigenic forms or "phases". Phase I organisms are avirulent, exist in nature and in laboratory animals, and react serologically with convalescent sera. Phase II organisms are virulent and react with acute sera. If phase I organisms are passed through chicken eggs, the phase I organisms become phase II organisms. *C. burnetii* is extremely infectious to humans; a single organism can cause infection.

Epidemiology Q fever was first described in Australia in 1937 (Q: "query"), occurs worldwide, and is not uncommon. Cattle, goats, sheep, and ticks are natural reservoirs. Persons at high risk for Q fever are persons associated with slaughter houses, persons who work with the aforementioned animals, persons who work with hides and wool, farmers, veterinarians, and researchers. The most common causes of infection are inhalation of organisms, handling of infected birth products (especially cat and cattle placentas), skinning infected animals, and transport of infected animals. *C. burnetii* is not transmitted person-to-person and only rarely by blood products.

Clinical Syndromes The most common form of Q fever is a self-limited febrile illness. Humans are the only known animals which regularly develop infection with *C. burnetii*. Incubation period is 2-4 weeks. Pneumonia, hepatitis, and endocarditis are the most common manifestations. Q fever usually presents as an atypical pneumonia; Q fever can also present as a rapidly progressive disease or as a secondary finding in someone with fever of unknown origin. The hepatitis form can present as infectious hepatitis. Endocarditis is the primary manifestation of chronic Q fever.

Diagnosis Typical signs and symptoms include headache, usually high fever, chills, fatigue, and myalgia. Other symptoms depend on which organ is affected. A rash can occur in the chronic endocarditis form of Q fever; a rash occurs only rarely in acute Q fever. Isolation of *C. burnetii* is an extremely dangerous laboratory procedure and is not practical. The most practical and clinically relevant method is serology. Complement fixation (CF) and immunofluorescence (IF) are the two most commonly used serological methods. CF is widely available and can demonstrate a fourfold rise in titer; however, CF does not separate IgG from IgM. Immunofluorescence uses separate phase I and II antigens and is more clinically useful. Phase II and I antibody titers are usually high in acute and convalescent disease, respectively. IgM antibody can persist for more than a year in some cases, but this is not a common finding. Some laboratories offer enzyme immunoassay (EIA) serology. EIA probably is the most sensitive of the three tests.

(Continued)

Coxiella burnetii *(Continued)*

Diagnostic Tests/Procedures
Q Fever Serology *on page 525*

Pediatric Drug Therapy
Recommended
Chloramphenicol *on page 667*

Adult Drug Therapy
Recommended
Doxycycline *on page 713*
Tetracycline *on page 944*
Alternate
Chloramphenicol *on page 667*

Selected Readings
Feld RD, "Q Fever," *Diag Clin Test,* 1990, 28:30-2.
Marrie TJ, *"Coxiella burnetii* (Q Fever)," *Principles and Practice of Infectious Diseases,* 4th ed, Mandell GL, Bennett JE, and Dolin R, eds, New York, NY: Churchill Livingstone, 1995, 1727-35.
Marrie TJ, *"Coxiella burnetii* (Q Fever) Pneumonia," *Clin Infect Dis,* 1995, 21(Suppl 3):S253-64.
Reimer L, "Q Fever," *Clin Microbiol Rev,* 1993, 6(3):193-8.

Coxsackieviruses

Microbiology The name "Coxsackievirus" is derived from the town where this agent was first isolated: Coxsackie, New York. These viruses are composed of single-stranded RNA and have a positive-sense linear genome. They belong to the genus Enterovirus and the family Picornaviridae. The name "Picornaviridae" summarizes the nature of the family: pico (small), -rna (ribonucleic acid), - viruses. Coxsackieviruses are related to poliovirus, echovirus, and rhinovirus. There are two major types of Coxsackieviruses, types A and B. These are further subdivided into numbered serotypes.

Epidemiology Coxsackieviruses can infect all age groups. The virus is found worldwide and predominantly during the summer months. Transmission is mainly by the fecal-oral route, but droplet infection by the respiratory route is also possible. Infection rates are higher in communities with poor sanitation and crowding.

Clinical Syndromes

Diseases caused by Coxsackieviruses, group A:
- **Herpangina:** Patients present with sore throat, fever, and sometimes nausea and vomiting. On examination, there are vesicles present on the soft palate, a location unusual for other agents. Lesions are also seen on the uvula, and less commonly on the hard palate. Cultures of active ulcerating vesicles will yield the organism. Symptoms resolve spontaneously over several days.
- **Hand-foot-and-mouth syndrome**
- **Epidemic conjunctivitis**
- **Pharyngitis**

Diseases caused mainly by Coxsackieviruses, group B:
- **Epidemic pleurodynia:** Group B Coxsackieviruses cause this syndrome of fever, sharp pleuritic pain in the rib cage or upper abdomen. Patients describe this as a "stitch" in the side and is caused by disease of the muscle (not pleura or ribs). The pain is spasmodic in nearly all cases. The diagnosis can be confirmed by obtaining cultures of the throat and/or stool for this virus, or by demonstrating a rise in antibody titer.
- **Myocarditis, pericarditis**
- **Overwhelming infection of the newborn**

Diseases caused by either group A or B Coxsackieviruses:
- **Acute aseptic meningitis**
- **Undifferentiated febrile illness**
- **Fever with upper respiratory infection**
- **Encephalitis**
- **Asymptomatic infection**

In addition, the Coxsackieviruses have been linked with such diverse diseases as the Guillain-Barré syndrome, hemolytic uremic syndrome, diarrheal illnesses, myositis, Reye's syndrome, and a syndrome similar to infectious mononucleosis.

Diagnosis Coxsackievirus infection is suspected when an individual presents with one of the syndromes mentioned above. The differential diagnosis of these syndromes is wide, and laboratory confirmation is often necessary. Appropriate specimens of cerebrospinal fluid, rectal swabs, conjunctival swabs, or throat swabs should be promptly submitted to the Microbiology Laboratory. A special request for a Coxsackievirus (or enterovirus) culture should be made.

Diagnostic Tests/Procedures

Coxsackie A Virus Serology *on page 377*

Coxsackie B Virus Serology *on page 377*

Enterovirus Culture *on page 405*

Drug Therapy Comment

No antiviral agents have been proven effective.

Selected Readings

Kaplan MH, Klein SW, McPhee J, et al, "Group B Coxsackievirus Infections in Infants Younger Than Three Months of Age: A Serious Childhood Illness," *Rev Infect Dis*, 1983, 5(6):1019-32.

Modlin JF, "Coxsackieviruses, Echoviruses, and Newer Enteroviruses," *Principles and Practice of Infectious Diseases*, 4th ed, Mandell GL, Bennett JE, and Dolin R, eds, New York, NY: Churchill Livingstone, 1995, 1620-36.

Cryptococcus neoformans

Microbiology *Cryptococcus neoformans* is an encapsulated round to oval yeast 4-6 μm with a surrounding polysaccharide capsule ranging in size from 1 to over 30 μm. In its natural environment, it is smaller and poorly encapsulated.

In its perfect state (*Filobasidiella neoformans*), mycelia are produced bearing basidiospores 1-3 μm. This state has never been isolated in nature nor patients, although it has been postulated that it may be in this state that route of transmission occurs via inhalation of the basidiospores or unencapsulated forms leading to colonization of the airways and subsequently respiration infection.

It is distinguished from other yeasts by its ability to assimilate urea and possesses membrane-bound phenoloxidase enzymes that convert phenolic compounds to melanin as demonstrated on certain agars (ie, birdseed agars).

Epidemiology There are four serotypes designated A, B, C, and D. Serotypes A and D (*C. neoformans* var *neoformans*) is the most common cause of infection and usually occurs in immunocompromised hosts. Serotypes B and C (*C. neoformans* var *gattii*) is typically seen in normal hosts and has a predilection for CNS invasion.

Cryptococcus is found worldwide. *C. neoformans* var *gattii* is endemic in the tropical and subtropical regions (Southern California, Australia, Southeast Asia, Brazil, Central America), particularly in the soils under eucalyptus trees. *Cryptococcus* grows readily from soil contaminated with avian excreta, particularly pigeon droppings but also has been isolated from nonavian sources such as fruits, vegetables, and dairy products. There have been no outbreaks attributable to environmental sources.

Cryptococcosis is the most common life-threatening meningitis in AIDS. Prior to the introduction of potent antiretroviral therapy, approximately 5% to 8% of AIDS patients developed a cryptococcal infection. The incidence of AIDS-related cryptococcal disease is decreasing presumably due to the use of potent antiretroviral therapy and the increased use of azoles. Prior to AIDS, 50% of patients had no known underlying immune defect. Risk factors prior to AIDS include diabetes, rheumatoid arthritis, cirrhosis, leukopenia, and malignancy. It was rarely seen in children, and the incidence in men was three times that of women.

Mortality risk factors include positive India ink, increased opening CSF pressure, decreased CSF glucose, CSF leukocyte count <20 cells/μL, extraneural site, absent *Cryptococcus* antibody, *Cryptococcus* antigen >1:32, and steroids or lymphoreticular malignancy. Good prognostic indications include headache as a symptom, normal mental status, and CSF leukocytes >20 cells/μL. Most important prognostic factor is patient's underlying disease process. Morbidity, mortality, and relapse are all increased in immunocompromised hosts.

Clinical Syndromes

- **Asymptomatic:** Solitary or multiple nodules found on plain chest x-ray.
- **Pulmonary cryptococcosis:** Most common infection. Present with cough, fever, and lobar infiltrates or mass. May see diffuse interstitial pattern or pleural effusion. If positive serum *Cryptococcus* antigen, look for disseminated disease.
- **CNS:** Second most common site of infection. Presents as either acute (headache, fever, nuchal rigidity) or chronic (headache, altered mental

(Continued)

Cryptococcus neoformans (Continued)

status) meningitis. May see cryptococcomas on CT or MRI. Usually secondary to lung but may represent reactivation similar to *Histoplasma* and tuberculosis.

- **Cutaneous:** Wide variation, may appear as papules, tumors, vesicles, plaques, abscesses, cellulitis, purpura, draining sinus, ulcers, bullae, or subcutaneous swelling. Usually a sign of dissemination.
- **Other:** Rarely invades eyes, bones, joints, liver, kidneys, or adrenal.

Diagnosis *Cryptococcus* skin test is not standardized as it is not completely characterized; therefore, its sensitivity and specificity is unknown and not used as a diagnostic aid. Diagnosis is confirmed by isolation from sterile body fluids including blood or histopathology revealing encapsulated yeast cells by alcian blue or mucicarmine. The India ink stain is positive in only approximately 50% of the time in normal hosts and >80% of the time in AIDS patients.

Cryptococcal antigen has >95% sensitivity and specificity but does cross react with *Trichosporon beigelii*. It is difficult to interpret a persistently high titer but has been associated with poor prognosis. Cryptococcal antigen in the CSF is produced locally in the subarachnoid space by the invading yeast and not by passive or active diffusion from the serum into the CNS. **Serial monitoring of the serum cryptococcal antigen in patients with AIDS-related cryptococcal disease on treatment does not provide any useful clinical data and should not be repeated after the initial diagnosis is made.** CSF findings include a pleocytosis lasting 6-12 months, low glucose concentrations, and high protein concentrations.

All AIDS patients with a positive serum cryptococcal antigen **must** have a lumbar puncture performed to exclude CNS disease.

Diagnostic Tests/Procedures

Cryptococcal Antigen Serology, Serum or Cerebrospinal Fluid *on page 379*
Cryptococcus Serology *on page 380*
Fungus Culture, Appropriate Site *on page 414*
India Ink Preparation *on page 460*
KOH Preparation *on page 467*

Treatment Current standard of practice for treatment of *Cryptococcus neoformans* in patients without AIDS is amphotericin B, 0.3 mg/kg/day given in combination with flucytosine, 150 mg/kg/day, based on the earlier pre-AIDS clinical trials. Many clinicians choose to use amphotericin B, 0.7 mg/kg/day, plus flucytosine, 100 mg/kg/day, for 6 weeks based on clinical trials in HIV-infected patients. The clinical efficacy of the triazoles in the primary management of cryptococcal meningitis in non-AIDS patients is unknown. Azoles may be used for cutaneous and pulmonary cryptococcosis, however, CNS infection must be excluded.

AIDS-related cryptococcosis:

1. Pulmonary disease: Mild to moderate disease may be treated with fluconazole, 200-400 mg/day. Moderate to severe disease should be treated as disseminated disease with amphotericin B.
2. Positive serum cryptococcal antigen: Search for disseminated disease. All AIDS patients should be treated with fluconazole, 200 mg/day, for chronic suppressive therapy.
3. Acute cryptococcal meningitis in AIDS patients should be treated with amphotericin B, 0.7 mg/kg/day, in combination with flucytosine, 100 mg/kg/day, for 2 weeks, followed by fluconazole, 400 mg/day for 8-10 weeks. Itraconazole, 200 mg twice daily, may be used as alternative consolidation therapy but is not ideal for chronic suppressive therapy due to an associated higher relapse rate than with fluconazole. Fluconazole, 200 mg/day, has proven to be the maintenance drug of choice for life-long suppression of cryptococcosis in AIDS.

HIV-infected patients absolutely intolerant of amphotericin B may be treated with high doses of fluconazole, 800-2000 mg/day, for 10 weeks in combination with flucytosine, 100 mg/kg/day, for the first 4 weeks followed by chronic suppressive therapy.

All patients should have measurement of intracranial pressure (ICP). If opening pressure is >240 mm/H_2O, remove 30 mL CSF. Repeat daily measurements of ICP should be done. If ICP remains elevated for 3 days, then a lumbar drain or shunt is recommended.

4. Prophylaxis: Although fluconazole and itraconazole have been shown to reduce the incidence of systemic fungal disease, primary prophylaxis for cryptococcosis is not recommended due to no survival benefit, drug-drug interactions, potential for resistance, and adverse drug effects.

Drug Therapy

Recommended

Amphotericin B (Conventional) *on page 597*

or

Amphotericin B (Conventional) *on page 597*
used in combination with
Flucytosine *on page 734*

Alternate

Fluconazole *on page 732*
Itraconazole *on page 785*

Selected Readings

Aberg JA and Powderly WG, "Cryptococcosis," *Adv Pharmacol*, 1997, 37:215-51.

Aberg JA and Powderly WG, "Cryptococcosis," *The AIDS Knowledge Base*, 3rd ed, Chapter 58, Philadelphia, PA: Lippincott Williams & Wilkins, 1999, 669-77.

Mitchell TG and Perfect JR, "Cryptococcosis in the ERA of AIDS - 100 Years After the Discovery of *Cryptococcus neoformans*," *Clin Microbiol Rev*, 1995, 8(4):515-48.

Saag MS, Cloud GA, Graybill JR, et al, "A Comparison of Itraconazole Versus Fluconazole as Maintenance Therapy for AIDS-Associated Cryptococcal Meningitis. National Institute of Allergey and Infectious Diseases Mycoses Study Group," *Clin Infect Dis*, 1999, 28(2):291-6.

van der Horst CM, Saag MS, Cloud GA, et al, "Treatment of Cryptococcal Meningitis Associated With the Acquired Immunodeficiency Syndrome. The National Institute of Allergy and Infectious Diseases Mycoses Study Group and the AIDS Clinical Trials Group," *N Engl J Med*, 1997, 337(1):15-21.

Cryptosporidium

Microbiology Although *Cryptosporidium* was identified as early as 1907, it was not recognized as a human pathogen until 1976. *Cryptosporidium* is classified as a protozoan and is structurally related to *Toxoplasma* and *Plasmodium* species. Several species of *Cryptosporidium* have been found; the species most associated with human disease is *C. parvum*. The organism is approximately 2.5 μm in diameter and is about the same size and shape as many yeasts. *Cryptosporidium* can be identified by use of an acid-fast stain or an immunofluorescence test of a fresh stool specimen.

The parasite has four spores (sporozoites) within an oocyst. Its life cycle occurs within a single host. Human infection begins when the mature oocyst form of *Cryptosporidium* is ingested or perhaps inhaled. The four sporozoites excyst and divide asexually into meronts which release merozoites which can either reinvade the human or develop sexually into meronts. The sexual cycle ends in the formation of oocysts. The oocysts then can exit the body of the host through the feces to begin the infectious cycle in a new human or in the same host (autoinfection).

Epidemiology Cryptosporidial infections occur worldwide. In the United States, the organism is most prevalent in persons with AIDS, with infection rates ranging from 3% to 20%. In such countries as Africa and Haiti, *Cryptosporidium* can infect over 50% of the AIDS population. The organism is also a cause of sporadic diarrheal illness in normal individuals. Outbreaks of cryptosporidiosis have been well-described in the U.S. and include a recent outbreak in Wisconsin related to a contaminated metropolitan water supply.

The modes of transmission are as follows:
- Person-to-person: Accounts for spread of infection within day care centers, households, and hospitals. Transmission is usually by a fecal-oral route.
- Environmental contamination: The oocyst can be found in rivers and other natural water supplies, and thus, the traveler and camper is at risk. *Cryptosporidium* resists standard chlorination procedures in many areas and thus, can initiate major outbreaks of diarrheal illness when water supplies are contaminated.
- Animal-to-human
- Foodborne illness

Clinical Syndromes
- **Acute diarrhea in the normal host:** The most common manifestation of human cryptosporidiosis is a syndrome characterized by profuse, watery diarrhea, malaise, and abdominal cramping or pain. Fevers to the 39°C to 40°C range have occurred even in immunologically competent individuals.

(Continued)

Cryptosporidium *(Continued)*

The incubation period is estimated to be 2-14 days following exposure to the parasite. The diarrhea often has an acute onset and symptoms can last 2 weeks or more.

- **Acute diarrhea in the immunocompromised host:** Cryptosporidiosis can be more subacute in onset. However, it is still characterized by voluminous diarrhea and weight loss over a several-week period can occur.
- **Cryptosporidial cholecystitis:** This has been described in immunocompromised patients. Symptoms include right upper quadrant abdominal pain, nausea, vomiting, and fever. There can be a concomitant diarrheal illness.

Diagnosis The symptoms of human cryptosporidiosis are nonspecific and cannot be distinguished from other causes of acute diarrheal illnesses. A high level of suspicion must be maintained because the organism cannot be readily identified using standard fecal smears.

Standard laboratory studies are not helpful in establishing the diagnosis. The leukocyte count may be normal, and there is usually not a peripheral blood eosinophilia to suggest a parasitic disease. Abnormalities in radiographic studies such as barium enemas and small bowel series have been described but again are not diagnostic of the organism. The only reliable means of identifying *Cryptosporidium* is to perform a direct exam (acid-fast stain) of a stool sample. This allows rapid identification of the organism. Because excretion of the parasite in the feces may be intermittent, it is recommended that two or more separate samples be submitted to the laboratory. Other techniques for identification of *Cryptosporidium* have been developed, including a direct immunofluorescence assay (DFA) and an enzyme immunoassay (EIA).

Diagnostic Tests/Procedures

Acid-Fast Stain *on page 305*

Cryptosporidium Diagnostic Procedures, Stool *on page 381*

Treatment At present, there is no widely accepted antimicrobial agent which is effective against *Cryptosporidium*. Some initial reports suggest the extended spectrum macrolides such as clarithromycin may have some use, but further studies are needed.

Drug Therapy Comment

Supportive care as treatment of choice.

Selected Readings

Adams RB, Guerrant RL, Zu S, et al, "*Cryptosporidium parvum* Infection of Intestinal Epithelium: Morphologic and Functional Studies in an *In vitro* Model," *J Infect Dis*, 1994, 169(1):170-7.

Bissuel F, Cotte L, Rabodonirina M, et al, "Paromomycin: An Effective Treatment for Crytosporidial Diarrhea in Patients With AIDS," *Clin Infect Dis*, 1994, 18(3):447-9.

Current WL, Reese NC, Ernst JV, et al, "Human Cryptosporidiosis in Immunocompetent and Immunodeficient Persons: Studies of an Outbreak and Experimental Transmission," *N Engl J Med*, 1983, 308(21):1252-7.

Danziger LH, Kanyok TP, and Novak RM, "Treatment of Cryptosporidial Diarrhea in an AIDS Patient With Paromomycin," *Ann Pharmacother*, 1993, 27(12):1460-2.

Goodgame RW, "Understanding Intestinal Spore-Forming Protozoa: Cryptosporidia, Microsporidia, *Isospora*, and *Cyclospora*," *Ann Intern Med*, 1996, 124(4):429-41.

Hayes EB, Matte TD, O'Brien TR, et al, "Large Community Outbreak of Cryptosporidiosis Due to Contamination of a Filtered Public Water Supply," *N Engl J Med*, 1989, 320(21):1372-6.

Jokipii L and Jokipii AM, "Timing of Symptoms and Oocyst Excretion in Human Cryptosporidiosis," *N Engl J Med*, 1986, 315(26):1643-7.

Kotler DP, Francisco A, Clayton F, et al, "Small Intestinal Injury and Parasitic Diseases in AIDS," *Ann Intern Med*, 1990, 113(6):444-9.

Newman RD, Zu SX, Wuhlib T, et al, "Household Epidemiology of *Cryptosporidium parvum* Infection in an Urban Community in Northeast Brazil," *Ann Intern Med*, 1994, 120(6):500-5.

Cyanobacterium-Like Body *see Cyclospora cayetanensis on this page*

Cyclospora cayetanensis

Synonyms Cyanobacterium-Like Body

Microbiology *Cyclospora cayetanensis* is a protozoal parasitic organism recently recognized as a cause of prolonged diarrhea in both immunocompromised and healthy individuals. Originally it was thought to be similar to blue-green algae and thus referred to as "Cyanobacteria-like bodies"; later the organism was found to be distinct from any known Cyanobacteria type. Based on characteristics such as excystation and sporulation, *Cyclospora* is now classified in the coccidian genus. *Cyclospora* is similar to but distinct from *Cryptosporidium* species, a related protozoal organism which causes infectious diarrhea. In the past *Cyclospora* has been referred to as "big cryptosporidia". The oocysts of

Cyclospora are 8-10 μm in diameter, approximately twice as large as *Cryptosporidium* species, an important distinguishing feature. After excretion in human feces, the oocysts are not immediately infectious and require some days to weeks under the proper conditions to sporulate.

Cyclospora is difficult to identify by conventional means. It cannot be recovered on routine stool culture and cannot be seen with a variety of stains including Gram's stain, hematoxylin-eosin (H & E), Giemsa, methylene blue, silver stain, and others. The organism can be identified by several techniques.

1. Modified acid-fast stain of stool, where organisms often stain deep red or pink.
2. Examination of fresh (unpreserved) stool under wet mount using phase microscopy, in order to identify the nonrefractile hyaline cysts.
3. Ultraviolet microscopy of either fresh or preserved stool, since *Cyclospora* autofluoresce (appear neon blue) under ultraviolet light.

Although the modified acid-fast stain is rapid and can establish the diagnosis in many cases, some *Cyclospora* oocysts are not acid-fast and may be missed. Some techniques may not be available in all laboratories and stool specimens in suspected cases should be referred to a specialized laboratory such as a state reference laboratory or the Centers for Disease Control and Prevention (CDC), Division of Parasitic Diseases (telephone 770-488-7760).

Epidemiology *Cyclospora* has only recently been recognized as a cause of human disease, with the first case diagnosed in 1977. Cases have been reported worldwide, particularly in Nepal during the rainy season. In one study, 11% of travelers and residents in Nepal who had gastrointestinal symptoms had *Cyclospora* in stool specimens as compared with 1% of healthy controls. Children from slum areas in Lima, Peru had a high rate of *Cyclospora* infection (up to 18%), although most were asymptomatic. Other at-risk areas include Mexico, Morocco, India, and Pakistan. Disease has been reported in U.S. travelers returning from all of these areas. The true prevalence of this disease globally is unknown and is under study. Transmission is by the fecal-oral route, with human to human transmission unlikely. Disease is primarily waterborne and usually follows ingestion of contaminated food or water. Cases are clustered in the spring and summer.

The majority of *Cyclospora* infections have been reported in otherwise healthy children and adults. However, it also appears to be a cause of some cases of significant diarrhea in HIV-infected persons especially in persons from Haiti. A cohort of HIV-infected Haitian patients was studied from 1990-1993. Of 450 persons with chronic diarrhea, 51 were diagnosed with *Cyclospora* in fecal samples.

The first outbreak of *Cyclospora* in the United States was reported in 1995 from 11 persons working in a Chicago hospital. The source of the *Cyclospora* was identified as tap water from a physicians' dormitory, probably as a result of stagnant water in a storage tank. Since then three other outbreaks have been reported in the United States. The most recent outbreak occurred in May, 1996 in Charlestown, South Carolina where 37 of 64 persons attending a luncheon developed *Cyclospora* infection. The offending food items were identified as raspberries and possibly strawberries. Cases have since been reported from 10 states associated with consumption of fresh fruits at social functions.

Clinical Syndromes

- **Asymptomatic infection:** Studies have suggested that *Cyclospora* may be identified in the stool of persons with no diarrheal symptoms.
- **Diarrhea in immunocompetent persons:** *Cyclospora* causes a nonspecific diarrheal illness characterized by cycles of exacerbations and remissions. The primary area of pathology appears to be the small bowel. The average incubation period is 1 week. Disease is characterized mainly by frequent watery stools; other symptoms include abdominal cramping, muscle aches, anorexia, fever, nausea, and vomiting. Symptoms may be prolonged, with an average of 6 weeks in some studies, although the diarrhea is usually self-limited.
- **Diarrhea in immunocompromised persons:** *Cyclospora* is a potential cause of prolonged diarrhea in persons with AIDS. The clinical course is similar to diarrhea in immunocompetent persons and is essentially the same as diarrhea caused by Cryptosporidia or *Isospora belli*. There appears to be

(Continued)

Cyclospora cayetanensis (Continued)

a high recurrence rate for *Cyclospora* diarrhea and antibiotic prophylaxis has been suggested.

Diagnosis *Cyclospora* is still infrequently identified but should be considered in the differential diagnosis of prolonged diarrhea in persons traveling to high risk areas, patients with AIDS and diarrhea of unknown origin, and in outbreak settings which appear to be food- or waterborne. Stool specimens should be submitted in suspected cases. The organism has also been identified in duodenal aspirates and small bowel biopsy. This organism may be missed on routine stool studies and thus should be considered in culture-negative and stain-negative cases. Specialized laboratory techniques are necessary for optimal identification (see Microbiology above). It is important to establish a proper diagnosis since treatment for *Cyclospora* is available.

Diagnostic Tests/Procedures

Acid-Fast Stain *on page 305*

Treatment The drug of choice is co-trimoxazole. Although only limited data is available concerning treatment options, co-trimoxazole for 7 days administered orally proved superior to placebo both in clinical symptoms and eradication of the organism from the stools. In persons with AIDS and *Cyclospora* infection, some authorities have recommended chronic prophylaxis with co-trimoxazole, given the high relapse rate. Alternative agents for persons who are sulfa-allergic are as yet unknown.

Drug Therapy

Recommended

Co-Trimoxazole *on page 692*

Selected Readings

Eberhard ML, Pieniazek NJ, and Arrowood MJ, "Laboratory Diagnosis of *Cyclospora* Infections," *Arch Pathol Lab Med*, 1997, 121(8):792-7.

Goodgame RW, "Understanding Intestinal Spore-Forming Protozoa: Cryptosporidia, Microsporidia, *Isospora*, and *Cyclospora*," *Ann Intern Med*, 1996, 124(4):429-41.

Hoge CW, Shlim DR, Ghimire M, et al, "Placebo-Controlled Trial of Co-Trimoxazole for *Cyclospora* Infections Among Travellers and Foreign Residents in Nepal," *Lancet*, 1995, 345:691-3.

Huang P, Weber JT, Sosin DM, et al, "The First Reported Outbreak of Diarrheal Illness Associated With *Cyclospora* in the United States," *Ann Intern Med*, 1995, 123(6):409-14.

Ortega YR and Sterling CR, "*Cyclospora cayetanensis*: Epidemiology and Diagnosis," *Clin Microbiol Newslett*, 1996, 18(22):169-72.

"Outbreaks of *Cyclospora cayetanensis* Infection - United States, 1996," *MMWR Morb Mortal Wkly Rep*, 1996, 45(25):549.

Pape JW, Verdier RI, Boncy M, et al, "*Cyclospora* Infection in Adults Infected with HIV: Clinical Manifestations, Treatment, and Prophylaxis," *Ann Intern Med*, 1994, 121(9):654-7.

Cytomegalovirus

Synonyms CMV

Microbiology As a member of the herpesvirus family, CMV is a DNA virus which replicates in the cell nucleus. Human CMV's are antigenically heterogeneous with differences expressed through endonuclease mapping. No serological distinctions are made. Although difficult to grow in experimental animals, it can be cultured (1-4 weeks) in human fibroblasts. Monoclonal antibody techniques can shorten the identification time to 48 hours.

Epidemiology CMV infections occur worldwide. About 50% of the general population is seropositive by the third decade of life. The incidence of CMV infection is more common in underdeveloped countries, lower socioeconomic groups, and in individuals who are sexually promiscuous. Virus can be isolated from several body fluids including saliva, feces, urine, and milk. Transmission requires repeated, prolonged contact. Spread is common in day care centers. In young adults, CMV is often a sexually transmitted disease, with asymptomatic carriage in the semen and cervical secretions. CMV may also be acquired from blood transfusions or organ transplantation.

Clinical Syndromes

- **Congenital CMV infection:** The fetus may become infected with CMV in two ways, primary CMV infection of the mother during pregnancy or reactivation of latent CMV in the mother during pregnancy. Primary maternal infection is much more likely to cause significant fetal infection. The manifestations of disease in the fetus are quite variable. Severe CMV disease is seen in only a small percentage of infected fetuses (5%). At birth, infants have hepatosplenomegaly, jaundice, microcephaly, and other abnormalities.

Prognosis depends on the severity of the disease. The majority of congenitally-infected neonates appear healthy at birth. Up to 25% of these asymptomatically infected infants will show developmental disorders later in childhood, such as deafness and mental retardation. Severe CMV infections are associated with a mortality approaching 30%.

- **Perinatal infection:** These infants are not infected in utero but instead acquire CMV during delivery. Seropositive mothers may shed virus into the birth canal due to CMV reactivation. Many infants infected in this manner remain healthy. In a small number of cases, neonates may develop pneumonia, lymphadenopathy, and rash. Infants excrete CMV for months. Neonatal infection can also be transmitted by breast milk.

- **CMV mononucleosis syndrome:** In normal adults, primary infection with CMV is usually asymptomatic. The most common form of clinically apparent disease in previously healthy adults is a febrile illness resembling Epstein-Barr virus mononucleosis. Typically, the patient presents with fever, chills, myalgias, and headache. Examination reveals an enlarged spleen and liver, but unlike EBV infection, adenopathy and pharyngitis are minimal. Most patients recover without incident but occasionally symptoms may persist for weeks. Laboratory studies show elevated liver function tests and circulating atypical lymphocytes on blood smear. Heterophil antibody tests are negative. CMV can be recovered in urine and saliva for an extended period of time. The physician must rely on serologic tests and appropriate viral cultures to distinguish CMV mononucleosis from similar syndromes caused by either EBV or *Toxoplasma gondii*.

- **CMV in the transplant recipient:** One of the most feared complications of transplantation is CMV infection, particularly pneumonia. The peak time for CMV disease occurs several weeks post-transplantation, the so-called "40-day fever". CMV pneumonitis carries a high morbidity. Patients present with dyspnea, fever, cough, and interstitial infiltrates on chest x-ray. Bronchoscopy is usually necessary for both culture and lung biopsy. The diagnosis of CMV pneumonia has been somewhat controversial; it is apparent that a bronchial lavage culture positive for CMV is not necessarily diagnostic of pneumonia. Many clinicians prefer to see the characteristic CMV "owl's eye" inclusion bodies on lung biopsy before diagnosing true pneumonia. Treatment of CMV pneumonia is with ganciclovir intravenously, but failures still occur. Some researchers advocate the use of CMV hyperimmune globulin (concentrated CMV immunoglobulins) in conjunction with ganciclovir, but results of such use have been mixed.

In an effort to decrease serious CMV infections, transplant centers have adopted a variety of strategies. One approach is to use ganciclovir prophylactically, that is, to give the drug prophylactically as a means of preventing CMV disease. This prophylactic treatment is based on the observation that patients who develop CMV pneumonia often do not have positive buffy coats for CMV (or other culture sites) consistently. Recent clinical trials have supported the prophylactic use of ganciclovir for bone marrow transplants at risk for CMV infection; ganciclovir is begun soon after transplantation and continued for 100 days. Another approach is to develop a reliable laboratory marker to detect CMV disease early. The CMV antigenemia assay appears to be promising. Detection of the pp65 matrix antigen in peripheral polymorphonuclear leukocytes may be a good predictor of impending clinical disease. Potentially, this would allow the "pre-emptive" use of ganciclovir, but clinical trials are needed to confirm this.

- **CMV in AIDS:** Several different organs may be infected with CMV in individuals with AIDS. CMV retinitis occurs in >10% of patients with AIDS. Patients typically complain of altered vision or "floaters" in one or both eyes. Examination reveals characteristic retinal lesions with exudates and hemorrhages ("cottage cheese and catsup"). Patients require lifetime antiviral therapy. Foscarnet or ganciclovir are usually given via a permanent indwelling catheter. Progression is inevitable, although the retinitis can be suppressed for extended periods of time. Other CMV infections are common in AIDS including CMV colitis, adrenalitis, and esophagitis. The incidence of CMV pneumonia in AIDS is unclear but is probably much less common than with the transplant population. Rare manifestations include CMV radiculopathy, encephalopathy, and myelopathy.

Diagnosis Cytomegalovirus-associated disease diagnosis is often very difficult because CMV can often be found in normal patients without the presence of any
(Continued)

Cytomegalovirus *(Continued)*

disease syndrome. Diagnosis depends on clinical symptoms consistent with CMV disease along with the appropriate cultures and serologies for CMV. Positive serologies should be confirmed by culture of the organism with the presence of CMV inclusion bodies from biopsy material of appropriate sites. A significant rise in serology titers also may be useful, but culture confirmation is always preferred. The presence of virus in the blood by buffy coat is also helpful. Presence of a positive culture from lung or gut for example, may not be sufficient to make the diagnosis of pulmonary or colonic CMV disease without confirmation by the presence of CMV inclusions. Some laboratories offer polymerase chain reaction (PCR) techniques to detect CMV DNA directly in specimens (most commonly, peripheral blood mononuclear cells). The test is extremely sensitive and specific but does not yield clinically relevant results in all situations and is neither cost-effective enough nor practical enough to be used routinely. PCR can detect the onset of CMV viremia 1-2 weeks earlier than culture or antigenemia tests and can detect CMV DNA in 30% of specimens which are culture- and antigenemia-negative. The clinical significance of such extreme sensitivity and early detection of CMV in asymptomatic patients who are not viremic and who do not show antigenemia has not been demonstrated. In addition, such results in these patients do not correlate with an indication for antiviral therapy. For most patients, PCR for CMV DNA appears to correlate best with seropositivity rather than active infection. The results of some studies suggest that detection of CMV DNA in blood, CSF, or tissue from immunocompromised persons might predict clinically significant disease. Recently, rapid and quantitative tests to detect CMV antigens in polymorphonuclear leukocytes (PMN) have been shown to be extremely sensitive and specific. The results of some studies show that there is clinically significant correlation between antigenemia (the number of circulating antigen-positive PMN) and the potential to develop active disease.

Diagnostic Tests/Procedures

Duration of Therapy Ganciclovir prophylaxis in solid organ transplant patients usually consists of 4 weeks of therapy with full doses (induction) (5 mg/kg twice daily) for the first 2 weeks and lower doses (maintenance) (5-6 mg/kg/day) for the last 2 weeks. Prophylaxis in allogeneic BMTs usually consists of 100 days of therapy. For treatment of colitis, pneumonitis, and hepatitis, a defined 2- to 3-week course is usually sufficient, even in patients with AIDS. Treatment for CMV retinitis in patients with AIDS typically consists of a 2-week course of induction therapy followed by life-long maintenance.

Treatment Ganciclovir is presently the treatment of choice for all CMV diseases including "CMV syndrome", retinitis, colitis, pneumonitis, and hepatitis. In patients with immunosuppressive agents, decreasing the amount of immunosuppressant may also be helpful. An alternative agent in failures or those patients who are intolerant to ganciclovir is foscarnet. Foscarnet is at least as active as ganciclovir against CMV but is more toxic. The addition of cytomegalovirus immune globulin (CMVIG) has not been proven to be any more effective than either of the antiviral agents alone. In bone marrow transplant patients with severe CMV infections, the addition of intravenous immune globulin (IVIG) to ganciclovir may be useful for CMV prophylaxis in transplant recipients, a variety of agents have been utilized including acyclovir, ganciclovir, IVIG, and CMVIG. CMVIG is effective in preventing primary disease in kidney transplant patients at highest risk for disease (patients who are CMV serology negative, receiving a serologically positive organ) but has not been proven to be effective in these high risk patients undergoing other organ transplants. Ganciclovir and CMVIG are each effective in preventing secondary CMV disease in transplant recipients who are already CMV serology positive. Acyclovir, which is not effective in treating CMV disease, has also been shown to be an effective prophylactic agent, but controversy remains.

Drug Therapy Comment Both ganciclovir and foscarnet are limited by their toxicities (mainly leukopenia and renal dysfunction, respectively). Resistance has been reported to both drugs. Occasionally, it may be necessary to use the combination of both drugs to minimize toxicity and improve efficacy in patients failing single-drug therapy. Ganciclovir commonly causes leukopenia to a variable degree. Filgrastim (G-CSF) has been used to elevate the WBC.

Drug Therapy
Recommended
    Ganciclovir *on page 745*
      separate or in combination with
    Foscarnet *on page 739*

Alternate
    Cidofovir *on page 676*

Selected Readings

Balfour HH Jr, "A Randomized, Placebo-Controlled Trial of Oral Acyclovir for the Prevention of Cytomegalovirus Disease in Recipients of Renal Allografts," *N Engl J Med*, 1989, 320(21):1381-7.

Hirsch MS, "Cytomegalovirus Infection," *Harrison's Principles of Internal Medicine*, 13th ed, Isselbacher KJ, Braunwald E, Wilson JD, et al, eds, New York, NY: McGraw-Hill, 1994, 794-7.

Hodinka RL and Friedman HM, "Human Cytomegalovirus," *Manual of Clinical Microbiology*, 6th ed, Murray PR, Baron EJ, Pfaller MA, et al, eds, Washington, DC: American Society for Microbiology, 1995, 545-8.

Kanj SS, Sharara AI, Clavien PA, et al, "Cytomegalovirus Infection Following Liver Transplantation: Review of the Literature," *Clin Infect Dis*, 1996, 22:537-49.

Mazzulli T, "Improved Diagnosis of Cytomegalovirus Infection by Detection of Antigenemia or Use of PCR Methods," *Clin Microbiol Newslet*, 1993, 15(13):97-100.

Schmidt GM, Horak DA, Niland JC, "A Randomized, Controlled Trial of Prophylactic Ganciclovir for Cytomegalovirus Pulmonary Infection in Recipients of Allogeneic Bone Marrow Transplants," *N Engl J Med*, 1991, 324(15):1005-11.

Yow MD, "CMV Infection in Young Women," *Hosp Prac (Off Ed)*, 1990, 25(3A):61-5, 69, 72-9.

Dematiaceous Fungi

Synonyms Black Molds; Black Piedra; Madura Foot; Phaeomycotic Cyst; Tinea Nigra

Microbiology There are over 100 species of dematiaceous fungi that are pathogenic. Dematiaceous fungi are those fungi that are darkly pigmented due to the presence of melanin in their cell wall. The McGinnis classification divides the dematiaceous fungi into two major distinct clinical entities: chromoblastomycosis and phaeohyphomycosis. Chromoblastomycosis is a cutaneous and subcutaneous infection characterized by hyperkeratosis and epidermal hyperplasia, intraepidermal microabscess formation, granulomatous inflammation in the dermis and presence of sclerotic bodies. Sclerotic bodies probably represent vegetative forms intermediate between yeast and hyphae. Yeast and hyphae are not seen. Phaeohyphomycosis is a group of diseases in which the involved tissue contains yeast forms, hyphae, and/or pseudohyphae. Sclerotic bodies are not seen. Phaeohyphomycosis is further subdivided into superficial, cutaneous and corneal, subcutaneous, and systemic phaeohyphomycosis. The most common dematiaceous fungi isolated are *Phialophora* species, *Fosecaea* species, *Cladosporium* species, *Exophilia* species, *Exserohilum* species, *Curvularia* species, *Alternaria* species, and *Bipolaris* species. Isolation of fungi may take 4-6 weeks of incubation at 25°C to 30°C. Species are distinguished from one another by morphology, biochemical properties, and DNA analysis.

Epidemiology The dematiaceous fungi are ubiquitous organisms found in the soil and vegetation. *Phialophora* species are common contaminants of wood and cause bluing of wood and paper products. The mode of acquisition is usually inoculation with subsequent formation of a subcutaneous granuloma or abscess. Invasive disease is unusual and most often seen in immunocompromised patients. The majority of patients cannot recall the inciting trauma probably due to the prolonged period after an inoculation injury to development of infection. Soils of cultivated indoor plants may serve as reservoirs of conidia within the hospital environment. Although the organisms may be dispersed throughout the environment by insects and animals, there have been no reported cases of insect or animal transmission to humans.

Clinical Syndromes
- **Chromoblastomycosis:** Most commonly seen in males secondary to occupational exposure in the tropical/subtropical regions of the Americas and Africa. Presents as chronic infection of skin and soft tissue. Initially may appear as scaly, pink to violaceous papule at site of traumatic inoculation.

(Continued)

Dematiaceous Fungi *(Continued)*

Lesions may appear as nodular, tumorous, verrucous, plaque-like, or cicatrical. May develop deformity at anatomic site.

- **Phaeohyphomycosis:** Systemic phaeohyphomycosis may present as either progressive localized disease or dissemination secondary to lower respiratory tract infection. Sinusitis is the most common invasive manifestation reported in immunocompromised hosts. Sinusitis due to dematiaceous fungi does not appear to be as aggressive as sinusitis caused by the more common opportunistic fungi such as *Aspergillus* species and *Mucor* species. Sinusitis due to the dematiaceous fungi presents as an indolent process in immunocompetent hosts that have a history of allergic rhinitis, nasal polyps, or recurrent bacterial infections. CNS lesions are most often secondary to a traumatic injury with inoculation of contaminated material; however *Cladosporium* species, *Xylohypha* species, and *Dactylaria* species have a predilection for CNS invasion with primary infection being the lung. Patients present with signs and symptoms of intracranial mass lesion such as headache, seizure, and focal neurological deficits without fever. The fungal abscess is usually limited to the cerebrum and rarely found invading the cerebellum or brainstem. Meningitis has been reported.

- **Phaeohyphomycotic cyst:** Is a distinct type of subcutaneous phaeohyphomycosis which presents as a solitary, well-encapsulated subcutaneous granuloma with necrosis. The overlying skin is normal. There is no regional lymphadenopathy. Usually secondary to subcutaneous inoculation with contaminated materials. It is associated with malnutrition, malignancy, hematologic or lymphoreticular malignancy, tuberculosis, leprosy, filariasis, syphilis, schistosomiasis, chronic renal failure, steroids, and diabetes mellitus. Lesions vary in size from 1-7 cm. May be present for months to years. *Exophilia* species and *Philophora* species predominate in normal hosts.

- **Mycetoma:** Chronic disease of the skin and underlying structures caused by a variety of actinomycetes and fungi including dematiaceous fungi. Most commonly occurs in feet secondary to inoculation trauma. Most often seen in farm workers in tropical/subtropical environment. Presents as a nodular mass with abscess or sinus tract formation draining seropurulent exudate containing granules or grains. The granules form a compact mass of organized hyphae.

Diagnosis Histopathology may be confused with other molds unless melanin-specific stain such as Fontanna-Masson is performed. Definitive diagnosis is made by identification of mold from culture of tissue.

Diagnostic Tests/Procedures

Fungus Culture, Biopsy *on page 414*

Treatment Flucytosine with or without amphotericin B plus surgical excision or incision and drainage is treatment of choice for chromoblastomycosis and mycetomas. Alternative therapy includes ketoconazole, itraconazole, or fluconazole. Flucytosine plus an azole may be effective. Phaeohyphomycotic cysts usually respond to excision alone. Phaeohyphomycosis responds best to itraconazole, however, the other azoles or amphotericin B may be effective. Antifungal susceptibility testing lacks correlation with clinical response.

Drug Therapy

Recommended

Flucytosine *on page 734*
with or without
Amphotericin B (Conventional) *on page 597*

Alternate

Ketoconazole *on page 791*
Itraconazole *on page 785*
Fluconazole *on page 732*

Selected Readings

Pitrak DL, Koneman EW, Estupinan RC, et al, "*Philophora richardsiae* Infections in Humans," *Rev Infect Dis*, 1988, 10(6):1195-203.

Sharkey PK, Graybill JR, Rinaldi MG, et al, "Itraconazole Treatment of Phaeohyphomycosis," *J Am Acad Dermatol*, 1990, 23(3 Pt 2):577-86.

Stracher AR and White MH, "Dematiaceous Fungal Infections in Patients With Cancer," *Infect Med*, 1995, 12(7):303-8.

Sutton DA, Slifkin M, Yakulis R, et al, "U.S. Case Report of Cerebral Phaeohyphomycosis Caused by *Ramichloridium obovoideum* (*R. mackenziei*): Criteria for Identification, Therapy, and Review of Other Known Dematiaceous Neurotropic Taxa," *J Clin Microbiol*, 1998, 36(3):708-15.

Tintelnot K, "Therapy of Infections Caused by Dematiaceous Fungi," *Mycoses*, 1997, 40(Suppl 1):91-6.

Dengue Virus

Microbiology Dengue virus is a member (species) of the genus *Flavivirus* which is a member of the family Flaviridiae. Dengue virions are 45-55 nm viruses which exist as a single strand of RNA enclosed in a protein capsid which is enclosed in a host cell membrane-derived envelope. There are four serologically distinct types of dengue virus.

Epidemiology Dengue fever is essentially an urban disease of most tropical countries, especially southeast Asia, India, and the American tropics. Dengue fever has been well documented to be occurring in epidemics for the last 200 years. Taken together, two factors suggest the distinct possibility that dengue fever can easily occur in epidemic form in the United States: increasing numbers of cases have been reported in the Caribbean, northern Mexico, and southern Texas, and vectors of dengue virus (*Ades aegypti* and *A. albopictus* mosquitoes) have been found in southern Texas and other Gulf Coast areas. The natural reservoirs of dengue virus are humans. The distribution of dengue fever is equivalent to that of malaria. As of 1995, dengue fever was the most important mosquitoborne disease in the world. Dengue virus infects and causes disease (often life-threatening) in millions of people worldwide each year.

Clinical Syndromes

- **Dengue fever ("breakbone fever"):** Is an acute febrile viral disease characterized by sudden onset, fever of less than 1 week, intense headache, myalgia, retro-orbital pain, arthralgia, anorexia, GI disturbances, and development of a general maculopapular rash as the fever subsides. Recovery is extremely gradual, and fatalities are rare.

- **Dengue hemorrhagic fever/shock syndrome:** Is the most severe form of dengue disease and is characterized by hypovolemia, dramatic internal and cutaneous bleeding disorders, and shock. The mortality rate of this severe form of dengue disease is ≥10%.

Diagnosis Dengue disease is difficult to distinguish from many arthropodborne and/or febrile diseases (eg, malaria, bacterial sepsis, numerous viral infections, and many viral hemorrhagic viral fevers). A complete and well-studied history of the patient's travel and lifestyle is imperative in the preparation of a differential diagnosis.

Diagnostic Tests/Procedures Serological tests for most diseases of viral etiology are available. Contact the clinical laboratory for details.

Encephalitis Viral Serology *on page 404*

Treatment Treatment for typical dengue fever is symptomatic and supportive. Treatment of dengue hemorrhagic fever/shock syndrome should be directed toward extremely early supportive care, intensive monitoring of vital signs, hydration, and control of bleeding.

Drug Therapy Comment No specific drugs or antiviral agents are available.

Selected Readings

"Dengue and Dengue Hemorrhagic Fever in the Americas," *Guidelines for Prevention and Control*, Washington, DC: Pan American Health Organization, 1994, 548.

"Dengue Fever" and "Dengue Hemorrhagic Fever/Dengue Shock Syndrome (DHF/DSS)", *Control of Communicable Diseases in Man*, 15th ed, Benenson AS, ed, Washington, DC: American Public Health Association, 1990, 117-23.

Diaz A, Kouri G, Guzman MG, et al, "Description of the Clinical Picture of Dengue Hemorrhagic Fever/Dengue Shock Syndrome (DHF/DSS) in Adults," *Bull Pan Am Health Organ*, 1988, 22(2):133-44.

Gubler DJ and Clark CG, "Dengue/Dengue Hemorrhagic Fever: The Emergence of a Global Health Problem," *Emerg Infect Dis*, 1995, 1(2):55-7.

Monath TP, "Flaviviruses (Yellow Fever, Dengue, Dengue Hemorrhagic Fever, Japanese Encephalitis, St Louis Encephalitis, Tick-Borne Encephalitis)," *Principles and Practice of Infectious Diseases*, 4th ed, Mandell GL, Bennett JE, and Dolin R, eds, New York, NY: Churchill Livingstone, 1995, 1465-74.

Dermatophytes

Microbiology Dermatophytes are fungi that invade the keratinized areas of the body (hair, nails, and skin) and are members of the genera *Epidermophyton*, *Microsporon*, or *Trichophyton*. Dermatophytes may be classified by the organism's name, their ecology (anthropophilic, geophilic, or zoophilic), or anatomical location of invasion.

(Continued)

Dermatophytes *(Continued)*

They are differentiated by their colonial morphology, microscopic appearance of conidia, hair perforation or fluorescence, and biochemical/nutritional requirements.

Epidemiology Dermatophytes are the most common fungal infections in humans. They are found worldwide with some species limited geographically. They colonize nonviable structures. Invasion occurs when the role of penetration of the dermatophyte into the keratin exceeds the role of keratin growth and shedding. Local trauma-altered primary host defenses and impaired cell-mediated immunity contribute to infection. *E. floccosum* is the only species of *Epidermophyton* that infects man. It only invades the skin and nails and not hair. *Microsporon* and *Trichophyton* have many species that infect humans. *M. gypseum* is the most important geophilic dermatophyte and typically causes infections secondary to occupational exposure from direct contact with the soil. *M. canis* may be transmitted from animals to their owners and handlers. *T. tonsurans* is the most common cause of tinea capitis worldwide.

Clinical Syndromes

- **Tinea barbae:** Occurs on the bearded areas of face and neck. Most frequently seen in farm workers. May occur as circinate spreading type, vesiculopustular border with central scaling or superficial type characterized by perifollicular involvement with fever, malaise, and regional adenopathy. Most common organism is *T. mentagrophytes.*

- **Tinea capitis:** More common in pediatrics. Present with erythema, marked scaling, and hair loss. Severe form associated with large, boggy pustules, fever, leukocytosis, and regional lymphadenopathy. Associated with erythema nodosum. Transmitted person to person. *T. mentagrophytes* is the most common organism, previously *M. audouinii.*

- **Tinea corporis:** Infection of the skin except groin, palms, scalp, or soles. Affects all ages and sexes. More frequent in hot, humid, tropical areas. Transmitted from other humans, animals, fomites, and, rarely, soil. Presents as erythematous papules with a red, pruritic, raised scaling border with central cleaning.

- **Tinea cruris:** Pruritic, erythematous eruption with circumscribed inflammatory margins that begins on inner thigh and spreads to groin, perineum, and perianal regions. Risk factors include obesity, diabetes, intertrigo, humidity, and tight-fitting clothes. Arthroconidia may survive for years, necessitating sterilization of clothes and linens.

- **Tinea pedis:** May occur as intertriginous involvement of toe webs or chronic hyperkeratotic form with minimal inflammation of soles and sides of feet or acutely as erythematous, clear vesicles which may become secondarily infected. Twenty-five percent to 75% of the normal population are culture positive and asymptomatic. Incidence increases with age. Most common organism is *T. rubrum.*

- **Tinea unguium:** Invasion of the nail; must be differentiated from onychomycosis which is a general term for any nail infection.

- **Deep local invasion:** Dissemination; uncommon; seen in immunosuppressed population.

Diagnosis Diagnosis is made by KOH examination of infected material or identification of characteristic macroconidia in culture. Up to 50% of KOH-positive samples may be culture-negative. Some of the organisms may be fluorescent under a Wood's lamp (ie, *M. canis* yellow and green, *T. schoenleinii* dull bluish white). Erythrasma caused by *Corynebacterium minutissimum* will be coral red under Wood's lamp. Other diagnostic tests employed are the hair perforation test and DTM (dermatophyte test media).

Diagnostic Tests/Procedures

Fungus Culture, Skin *on page 417*
KOH Preparation *on page 467*
Skin Biopsy *on page 535*

Treatment The most important aspect of therapy is educating patients for the need to continue therapy for a period of time after the infection appears resolved. Therapy is directed at anatomical location.

- **Tinea barbae:** Griseofulvin for 4-6 weeks
- **Tinea capitis:** Griseofulvin for 1-2 weeks after lesion cleared for a total of 4-8 weeks. Alternative therapy is ketoconazole.

- **Tinea corporis:** Imidazole creams or topical keratolytics. In severe infection, griseofulvin, or ketoconazole.
- **Tinea cruris:** Topical imidazole 3-4 weeks
- **Tinea pedis:** Topical imidazole 3-4 weeks. Chronic form requires griseofulvin, however, *T. rubrum* may develop resistance.
- **Tinea unguium:** Terbinafine 250 mg/day for 12 weeks. Alternate therapy:
  Itraconazole: Oral: 200 mg twice daily for 1 week every month for 4 months or 200 mg/day for 3 months
  Fluconazole: Oral: 150-300 mg 1 day a week for 3 months (non-FDA approved indication)
  Griseofulvin ultramicrosize: Oral: 330-750 mg/day for 3-6 months. Not recommended due to adverse drug effects especially hepatotoxicity.
- **Deep or disseminated:** Amphotericin B

Drug Therapy
Recommended
Superficial infection:
  Antifungal, Topical *on page 610*
  Terbinafine *on page 936*
  Itraconazole *on page 785*
  Fluconazole *on page 732*
  Griseofulvin *on page 753*
  Ketoconazole *on page 791*
Disseminated infection:
  Amphotericin B (Conventional) *on page 597*

Selected Readings
De Backer M, De Vroey C, Lesaffre E, et al, "Twelve Weeks of Continuous Oral Therapy for Toenail Onychomycosis Caused by Dermatophytes: A Double-Blind Comparative Trial of Terbinafine 250 mg/day Versus Itraconazole 200 mg/day," *J Am Acad Dermatol*, 1998, 38(5 Pt 3):S57-63.

Elewski BE and Hazen PG, "The Superficial Mycoses and the Dermatophytes," *J Am Acad Dermatol*, 1989, 21(4 Pt 1):655-73.

Gupta AK, Einarson TR, Summerbell RC, et al, "An Overview of Topical Antifungal Therapy in Dermatomycoses. A North American Perspective," *Drugs*, 1998, 55(5):645-74.

Salata RA, "Ringworm and Other Superficial Mycoses," *Tropical and Geographical Medicine Companion Handbook*, 2nd ed, Mahmoud AAF, ed, New York, NY: McGraw-Hill 1993, 371-7.

DF-2 *see* Capnocytophaga Species *on page 93*

Diarrheagenic *E. coli see* Escherichia coli, Enterotoxigenic *on page 145*

DRSP *see* Streptococcus pneumoniae, Drug-Resistant *on page 270*

Eaton's Agent *see* Mycoplasma pneumoniae *on page 211*

EBV *see* Epstein-Barr Virus *on page 141*

Echovirus

Microbiology Echoviruses are very small, single-stranded RNA viruses belonging to the family Picornavirdae which has recently been reclassified to comprise four groups based on genomic sequence information. One of these groups is the Enterovirus in which echoviruses are a subclass. The other subclasses are polioviruses, Coxsackieviruses, and newer enteroviruses. (See Poliovirus *on page 230*, Coxsackievirus *on page 116*, and Enterovirus *on page 139*). When these viruses were first isolated from stool specimens from children, they were noted to produce cytopathic effects in primate cell cultures but were nonpathogenic in mice and the primate central nervous system; hence they were called enteric cytopathic human orphan viruses or Echoviruses. There are now 31 serotypes of echoviruses recognized.

Epidemiology Infection rates vary with the season, geography, age, and socioeconomic status. In temperate climates, infections occur more frequently in the summer and autumn. The majority of echovirus infections occur in children younger than 15 years of age with the highest frequency occurring in infants younger than 1 year. An estimated 30 million nonpolio enterovirus infections occur annually in the United States. Of more than 3000 cerebrospinal fluid, nasopharyngeal swab, or stool isolates obtained from 1993 to 1996, echovirus 9 was the predominant serotype reported. Echoviruses 6, 7, 11, and 30 are among the most frequently detected serotypes associated with aseptic meningitis, encephalitis, and pneumonia. Echovirus 9 was the etiologic agent responsible for the aseptic meningitis outbreak that occurred in Whiteside County, Illinois in 1995. Although transmission of echoviruses usually is person-to-person, either through fecal-oral or oral-oral routes or communal contamination such as a (Continued)

Echovirus *(Continued)*

swimming facility, no point source contamination could be located in the White-side outbreak.

Clinical Syndromes

- **Acute aseptic meningitis:** Characterized by fever, headache, stiff neck and photophobia in the presence of cerebrospinal fluid pleocytosis and negative bacteria/fungal cultures. Pharyngitis and upper respiratory tract symptoms are common. The illness may be biphasic with fever and myalgias initially present for a few days followed by no symptoms for 2-10 days and then development of a sudden reappearance of headache and fever. Five percent to 10% of children may develop seizures, lethargy, coma, or other neurological disorders.
- **Encephalitis:** May or may not be associated with meningitis. Usually a generalized encephalitis characterized by lethargy but may occur more localized characterized by partial motor seizures or ataxia or paresis.
- **Exanthems:** Associated with little morbidity. Can present as rubelliform, roseoliform, vesicular or petechial.
- **Respiratory disease:** Characterized by sore throat, cough, and coryza. Echovirus 11 is the most common cause of upper respiratory tract disease and is associated with croup.
- **Myopericarditis:** More associated with Coxsackieviruses than echoviruses. Predilection for adolescents and young adults. An upper respiratory tract infection precedes the onset of cardiac manifestations by 1-2 weeks. Patients present with dyspnea, dull precordial pain, fever, and malaise. Sharp pleuritic pain may accompany pericarditis. Approximately 50% will have evidence of a pericardial effusion or cardiac dilatation on chest radiograph. Congestive heart failure occurs in 20%. EKG may show evidence of pericarditis, arrhythmias, or heart block.
- **Neonatal infections:** Echovirus 11 has been associated with fatal disease in the newborn. Mild and nonspecific symptoms such as listlessness, anorexia usually occur within the first 3-7 days of life. Fever may or may not be present. Approximately 33% will have a biphasic illness. While Coxsackieviruses are more associated with myocarditis, the echoviruses cause a fulminant hepatitis associated with hypotension, hemorrhage, and multiple organ failure. There are reports of fatal pneumonia secondary to echoviruses occurring within the first few days of life. Echoviruses particularly serotype 22 has been associated with gastroenteritis.

Diagnosis Isolation of virus in cell culture from infected source.

Diagnostic Tests/Procedures

Viral Culture, Central Nervous System Symptoms *on page 570*
Viral Culture, Stool *on page 573*
Viral Culture, Throat *on page 574*

Treatment Supportive care for symptoms. No known effective antivirals. Immuno-globulin prophylaxis may be useful during neonatal outbreaks. Avoidance of transmission via good handwashing and personal hygiene.

Selected Readings

"Nonpolio Enterovirus Surveillance - United States, 1993-1996," *MMWR Morb Mortal Wkly Rep*, 1997, 46(32):748-50.

"Outbreak of Aseptic Meningitis - Whiteside County, Illinois, 1995," *MMWR Morb Mortal Wkly Rep*, 1997, 46(10):221-4.

E. coli **O157:H7** *see Escherichia coli*, Enterohemorrhagic *on page 143*

EHEC *see Escherichia coli*, Enterohemorrhagic *on page 143*

Ehrlichia Species

Microbiology *Ehrlichia* species are small gram-negative bacteria (0.5 μm) which can cause fever and pancytopenia in several mammalian hosts. The genus *Ehrlichia* contains several species which are primarily pathogenic for animals (eg, dogs, horses, jackals, and others). *Ehrlichia canis* was first identified as the agent of ehrlichiosis in dogs in the 1930s and was found to be transmitted to the dog by a tick vector. Infection in humans was not identified in the United States until 1986. Although human ehrlichiosis was originally thought to be caused by *E. canis*, it is later became apparent that human disease is caused by a genetically distinct species which has recently been named *Ehrlichia chaffeensis*.

Ehrlichia species are aerobic, gram-negative bacilli which are related to *Rickettsia* in terms of DNA content, geographic distribution, and clinical disease.

Ehrlichia are obligate intracellular organisms which cluster within vacuoles of the infected cell; these intracellular inclusion bodies have been identified on light and electron microscopy and are called morulae (meaning mulberry-like). *Ehrlichia chaffeensis* infects the cytoplasm of macrophages. A newly described species of *Ehrlichia* distinct from *E. chaffeensis* (as yet unnamed) has recently been found to infect human granulocytes instead of macrophages. It has been called the agent of "human granulocytic ehrlichiosis". Morulae from *E. chaffeensis* can sometimes be identified on careful examination of peripheral blood smears (buffy coats) of infected patients using a Giemsa stain, but the sensitivity of this technique is very low. In contrast, the agent of human granulocytic ehrlichiosis is frequently seen as morulae in circulating leukocytes. The organisms do not grow on routine blood cultures. Special culture techniques utilizing cell culture systems have been occasionally successful in isolating the organism, but the sensitivity of culture is low.

Epidemiology *Ehrlichia* is spread to humans by the bite of a tick. The precise insect vector is still under study but *Dermacentor variabilis* (dog tick) and *Amblyomma americanum* (Lone Star tick) have been implicated, as have others. The peak incidence is from May to July. Infection is four times more common in men then women and cases are reported most commonly from rural areas. Geographic areas at highest risk are in the southern and south-central regions, as follows:

- South: South Carolina, North Carolina, Florida, Alabama, Kentucky, Tennessee, Georgia, Virginia, Maryland
- South-central/central: Arkansas, Oklahoma, Missouri, Texas, Louisiana
- Others: New Jersey, Wyoming, Vermont, Washington.

Over 300 cases of human ehrlichiosis have been reported to date, but this is likely an underestimate of the true prevalence of the disease.

Clinical Syndromes

- **Asymptomatic infection**: Studies have shown that many individuals with a demonstrable seroconversion to *E. chaffeensis* develop no symptoms.
- **Human ehrlichiosis**: The spectrum of human ehrlichiosis is very broad, ranging from a mild illness in many patients to a multiorgan system failure with protracted fever. After the tick bite, the organisms enter a number of host cells including the macrophage system. The incubation period between the tick bite and the onset of clinical symptoms is about 1 week. Infected persons typically present with the acute onset of nonspecific symptoms such as malaise, fever, headache and muscle pains. More severely ill persons may have additional symptoms such as nausea and vomiting, diarrhea, dyspnea, and cough. Serious complications have been reported in 40% of hospitalized patients. These include hypotension, neurologic abnormalities (ie, encephalitis, cerebrospinal fluid pleocytosis), coagulopathies, acute renal failure, hepatocellular necrosis, and death. It is important to note that a rash is present in only 33% of patients. Ehrlichiosis has been nicknamed "Rocky Mountain **spotless** fever" because of the similarities between ehrlichiosis and this common rickettsial illness. In general, the symptoms of ehrlichiosis are not unique and may be seen in a variety of other illnesses.

Diagnosis Laboratory abnormalities are common in ehrlichiosis and may be important clues to the disease. A mild leukopenia and thrombocytopenia are common. Elevated liver function tests are also common during the acute phase of the illness. The chest X-ray may show transient infiltrates. Anemia is seen after about 1 week of illness.

Human ehrlichiosis should be suspected in any patient with an unexplained febrile illness who resides in or has traveled to an area endemic for this disease. A history of a tick bite is useful but not necessary. The disease may be difficult to distinguish from Rocky Mountain spotted fever (RMSF) which has a similar geographic distribution. Several characteristics may be used to separate the two diseases: skin rash is less common in ehrlichiosis; when a skin rash is present in ehrlichiosis, it is less often petechial, as is the case with RMSF; leukopenia is more common in ehrlichiosis.

Laboratory confirmation of ehrlichiosis rests primarily on serologic studies. Indirect immunofluorescence assays (IFA) for *E. chaffeensis* are available from some specialty laboratories. A fourfold rise in titer between acute and convalescent samples is diagnostic. Although the direct visualization of ehrlicial morulae in host white blood cells has been reported in some cases, this appears to be a rare finding and is insensitive for the diagnosis of *E. chaffeensis*. Neither *E.* (Continued)

Ehrlichia Species *(Continued)*

chaffeensis nor the agent of human granulocytic ehrlichiosis can be cultured on routine aerobic blood culture media.

The differential diagnosis of human ehrlichiosis includes RMSF, viral syndromes, and bacterial septicemia. Because of the variable clinical presentation, consultation with an Infectious Diseases specialist may be useful if this infection is suspected.

Diagnostic Tests/Procedures

Ehrlichia Serology *on page 397*
Polymerase Chain Reaction *on page 523*

Treatment Tetracycline and doxycycline appear to be useful. Intravenous chloramphenicol also has been used successfully.

Pediatric Drug Therapy
Recommended
Chloramphenicol *on page 667*

Adult Drug Therapy
Recommended
Tetracycline *on page 944*
Doxycycline *on page 713*
Chloramphenicol *on page 667*

Selected Readings

Dumler JS, "Laboratory Diagnosis of Human Rickettsial and Ehrlichial Infections," *Clin Microbiol Newslet*, 1996, 18(8):57-61.

Eng TR, Harkess JR, Fishbein DB, et al, "Epidemiologic, Clinical, and Laboratory Findings of Human Ehrlichiosis in the United States, 1988," *JAMA*, 1990, 264(17):2251-8.

Everett ED, Evans KA, Henry RB, "Human Ehrlichiosis in Adults After Tick Exposure. Diagnosis Using Polymerase Chain Reaction," *Ann Intern Med*, 1994, 120(9):730-5.

Fishbein DB, Dawson JE, and Robinson LE, "Human Ehrlichiosis in the United States, 1985 to 1990," *Ann Intern Med*, 1994, 120(9):736-43.

"Human Ehrlichiosis - United States," *MMWR Morb Mortal Wkly Rep*, 1988, 37(17):270, 275-7.

Magnarelli LA and Dumler JS, "Ehrlichioses: Emerging Infectious Diseases in Tick-Infested Areas," *Clin Microbiol Newslet*, 1996, 18(11):81-3.

McDade JE, "Ehrlichiosis - A Disease of Animals and Humans," *J Infect Dis*, 1990, 161(4):609-17.

Rikihisa Y, "The Tribe Ehrlichieae and Ehrlichial Diseases," *Clin Microbiol Rev*, 1991, 4(3):286-308.

Walker DH and Dumler JS, "Emergence of the Ehrlichioses as Human Health Problems," *Emerg Infect Dis*, 1996, 2(1):18-29.

Walker DH and Dumler JS, "Human Monocytic and Granulocytic Ehrlichiosis. Discovery and Diagnosis of Emerging Tick-Borne Infections and the Critical Role of the Pathologist," *Arch Pathol Lab Med*, 1997, 121(8):785-91.

Entamoeba histolytica

Microbiology *Entamoeba histolytica* is an enteric protozoan that exists in two forms, cyst and trophozoite. The cyst ranges in size from 5-20 μm and contains one to four nuclei. The trophozoite is an ameba, ranges in size from 12-60 μm, and contains a single nucleus with a centrally located nucleolus with a uniformly distributed peripheral chromatin. Although all strains of *E. histolytica* are morphologically identical, there is epidemiological and biological evidence that there are pathogenic and nonpathogenic strains. Isoenzyme analysis reveal that there are four distinct zymodemes which appear to correlate with the virulence of the ameba.

Epidemiology It is estimated that 10% of the world is infected with *E. histolytica*, with 50,000-100,000 *E. histolytica*-associated deaths per year, making amebiasis the third leading parasitic cause of death in the world. It is endemic in Mexico, India, West and South Africa, and portions of Central and South America. It appears to be most virulent in the tropics. The vast majority (90%) of patients remain asymptomatic. High risk factors for invasive diseases in the United States include recent immigration, institutionalization, and homosexuality, although 30% to 40% of male homosexuals harbor a nonpathogenic strain. It is imperative to exclude other etiologies of diarrhea in patients with AIDS given the large number of asymptomatic carriers. Infection with *E. histolytica* begins with ingestion of the cyst via contaminated food or water or fecal-oral route. The ingested mature cyst excysts in the lower ileum and multiplies by binary fission producing eight trophozoites. The trophozoites may remain in the lumen of the colon and multiply or invade the wall of the colon and spread hematogenously. Trophozoites encyst in the colon, and both mature and immature cysts are excreted in the feces.

Clinical Syndromes
Intestinal:

- **Asymptomatic colonization:** Affects 90% of those infected. Also referred to as cyst passage.
- **Acute amebic colitis:** Present with lower abdominal pain and explosive bloody diarrhea. Approximately 30% to 40% will have fever. Onset over 7-10 days with a 1- to 4-week duration. More severe in children, pregnant women, and immunosuppressed individuals, especially those on steroids. Toxic megacolon associated with steroid use. Almost all patients will have heme-positive stools but few or no leukocytes presumably due to ability of ameba to lyse leukocytes hence the name "histolytica". Chronic colitis must be differentiated from inflammatory bowel disease.
- **Fulminant colitis:** More common in children. Diffuse abdominal pain and profuse bloody diarrhea. Seventy-five percent of children may develop colonic perforation.
- **Ameboma:** Develops in 1% of patients with colitis. Localized chronic amebic infection usually in cecum or ascending colon. Presents as a tender mass.

Extraintestinal:

- **Hepatic abscess:** Acute hepatic abscess presents with dull, pleuritic, right upper quadrant pain and fever. Subacute less likely to have fever. Ten percent to 15% may present with fever and no pain. Fifty percent acute presentations will have multiple hepatic lesions, whereas 80% subacute will have a single lesion located in the right lobe liver. Fifty percent will have no history of antecedent dysentery. Laboratory reveals leukocytosis without eosinophilia, alkaline phosphatase elevated >75%, transaminase elevated >50%.

  Other rare complications of hepatic abscess include genitourinary, skin, adrenal, and kidney invasion.
- **Pleuropulmonary:** Most common complication of hepatic abscess, occurring 20% to 35%. Typically associated with lesion from left lobe liver. Present with pleuritic pain, cough. May have serous effusions, consolidation, empyema, or hepatobronchial fistula.
- **Peritoneal:** Second most common complication of hepatic abscess is intra-peritoneal rupture in 2% to 7.5%. Indolent leaks much more common than rupture or abscess.
- **Pericardial:** Most serious complication of hepatic abscess. Perforation of abscess into the pericardium usually results in tamponade and/or shock. Greater than 60% have abscesses in left lobe liver. Mortality is 40%.
- **CNS:** Brain abscesses occur where intestinal amebiasis is endemic. Aggressive, multifocal disease known as secondary cerebral amebiasis (SCA). Must be differentiated from *Naegleria* and *Acanthamoeba* as treatment differs. Rapidly progressive disease with spreading abscesses with internal necrosis of gray-white junction of cerebral cortex. SCA occurs in 0.6% to 0.8% patients with hepatic abscess. Extremely rare without hepatic invasion. Presentation depends on size, location, and number of lesions. May present as chronic infection with fever, weight loss, hepatomegaly, abdominal pain, dyspnea, and pleuritic pain. Diarrhea may be absent. Less than 33% will have positive ova and parasite fecal exam. Incubation period is typically 2-5 months. Male to female ratio is 5:1. CSF examination reveals mononuclear cells with normal and low glucose. CT scan reveals ring enhancing lesions.

Diagnosis Eighty percent to 90% of patients with acute dysentery will have cysts or trophozoites on fecal examination after examining three samples. Trophozoites rapidly die after passage; therefore, feces must be examined within 20 minutes of collection. Serology titers are positive in 60% to 90% of the cases after 7 days, however 6% to 20% of patients in endemic areas will have positive serologies which may persist for years after acute infection. Sigmoidoscopy or colonoscopy with biopsy is recommended for patients with chronic colitis to differentiate between inflammatory bowel versus amebiasis. Extraintestinal disease should be diagnosed by aspiration of abscess or biopsies. Liver abscesses aspirate is classically chocolate colored or has an anchovy paste appearance. More than 90% will have positive serology. Absence of serology titer is strong evidence against amebiasis.

Entamoeba dispar is morphologically identical to *E. histolytica*, and most laboratories do not have the ability to distinguish them apart. Therefore, it is imperative (Continued)

Entamoeba histolytica (Continued)

that one consider the risk factors and likelihood that the organism reported is in fact *E. histolytica*. *E. dispar* is a gut commensal and is not associated with dysentery.

Diagnostic Tests/Procedures

Entamoeba histolytica Serology *on page 404*
Ova and Parasites, Stool *on page 505*
Ova and Parasites, Urine or Aspirates *on page 508*

Treatment

Dysentery: Metronidazole 750 mg three times/day for 10 days plus luminal amebicide either iodoquinol, diloxanide furoate (from CDC), or paromomycin. Fluid electrolyte support. May need surgical decompression if megacolon.

Hepatic: Metronidazole plus iodoquinol 650 mg three times/day for 10 days. May need percutaneous draining.

CNS: Metronidazole plus surgical drainage. If no surgical drainage, metronidazole 500 mg four times/day for 4 weeks, chloroquine 300 mg once daily for 4 weeks, tetracycline 500 mg four times/day for 4 weeks followed by dehydroemetine 80 mg once daily for 10 days.

Prevention: Boiling is only means of eradicating *E. histolytica* cysts in water. Vegetables must be cleansed in strong detergent soap and soaked in acetic acid or vinegar for 10-15 minutes. Travelers to endemic areas should be advised to avoid uncooked vegetables, salads, fruits that cannot be peeled, and ice cubes.

Drug Therapy

Recommended

Asymptomatic (cyst passers):
  Diloxanide Furoate *on page 706*
Invasive infection:
  Metronidazole *on page 817*
    followed by
  Diloxanide Furoate *on page 706*

Alternate

Invasive infection:
  Metronidazole *on page 817*
    followed by
  Paromomycin *on page 856*
    or
  Iodoquinol *on page 781*

Selected Readings

Aucott JN and Ravdin JI, "Amebiasis and "Nonpathogenic" Intestinal Protozoa," *Infect Dis Clin North Am*, 1993, 7(3):467-85.
Campbell S, "Amebic Brain Abscess and Meningoencephalitis," *Semin Neurol*, 1993, 13(2):153-60.
Jackson TF, "*Entamoeba histolytica* and *Entamoeba dispar* Are Distinct Species; Clinical, Epidemiological, and Serological Evidence," *Int J Parasitol*, 1998, 28(1):181-6.
Reed SL, "Amebiasis: An Update," *Clin Infect Dis*, 1992, 14(2):385-93.

Enterobacter Species

Microbiology *Enterobacter* species are gram-negative rods which are increasingly important causes of nosocomial infection, particularly because of the emergence of highly antibiotic-resistant isolates. *Enterobacter* species (formerly called *Aerobacter* species) are aerobic gram-negative bacilli which normally colonize the intestinal tract. The genus name "*Enterobacter*" should not be confused with the broader family name "Enterobacteriaceae;" the latter designation refers to many gram-negative bacteria including *Enterobacter* species, *E. coli*, *Klebsiella*, *Serratia*, and others. Based on studies of DNA relatedness, *Enterobacter* is most closely related to *Klebsiella*, with >50% DNA sequence homology. The organism cannot be distinguished from other related GNBs on the basis of Gram's stain alone, and culture identification is necessary. The major species of *Enterobacter* which are pathogenic for humans include *E. cloacae* (accounting for most infections), *E. aerogenes*, and *E. agglomerans*.

Enterobacter produces endotoxin, the lipopolysaccharide (LPS) component which is associated with the outer membrane of the bacteria. When cell lysis occurs (as with antibiotic therapy) the LPS is released into the host and can lead to such inflammatory responses as fever, leukopenia or leukocytosis, hypotension, and disseminated intravascular coagulation. Thus, LPS is regarded as an important mediator of the sepsis syndrome.

Epidemiology Because *Enterobacter* commonly inhabits the human gastrointestinal tract, it is considered one of the "enteric bacteria." In hospitalized patients, it often asymptomatically colonize the urine, respiratory tract, abdominal wounds, decubitus ulcers, and other sites. Community-acquired infection is rare, and *Enterobacter* is generally considered an opportunist of the hospitalized, debilitated individual.

Clinical Syndromes

- **Lower respiratory tract infection:** Nosocomial *Enterobacter* infections are seen in patients with extended hospitalizations, particularly those who are ventilator-dependent. Patients who have been on prolonged broad spectrum antibiotics seem at particular risk for *Enterobacter* infection. Lengthy courses of broad spectrum antibiotics do not "protect" the patient from opportunistic *Enterobacter* infections. It should be noted that *Enterobacter* and other gram-negative bacilli can asymptomatically colonize the upper respiratory tract of hospitalized patients. Thus, the recovery of a sputum or tracheal aspirate culture for *Enterobacter* does not necessarily indicate a significant infectious disease. The diagnosis of a pneumonia still rests on standard criteria such as the presence of purulence (many leukocytes) on the Gram's stain of sputum, the presence of a pulmonary infiltrate, and signs of systemic inflammation in the patient. A positive sputum culture alone is not sufficient justification for initiating, antibiotic therapy.

- **Burn wound infections:** Outbreaks of serious *Enterobacter* infections (primarily septicemias) have been reported in burn units.

- **Urinary tract infection:** Seen in hospitalized patients, often those with indwelling Foley catheters. However, *Enterobacter* may harmlessly colonize the urine of patients with chronic bladder catheters without causing disease. The decision to initiate antibiotics in such patients should be based on the clinical situation (the presence of pyuria on urinalysis, suprapubic pain, fever, etc). Even the finding of large numbers of *Enterobacter* in a urine culture ($>10^5$ colony forming units/mL) by itself does not automatically indicate antimicrobial therapy.

- **Hospital-associated bacteremias:** In 1975, *Enterobacter* strains were associated with a national epidemic of contaminated intravenous products. The organisms were found to grow in commercially available fluids used for intravenous infusions and were the cause of rapid-onset septicemia. There have been no nationwide *Enterobacter* outbreaks since then, but the organism is still recovered periodically from blood cultures.

Diagnosis The clinical presentations of the various nosocomial infections caused by *Enterobacter* are not distinctive, and laboratory isolation is necessary.

Diagnostic Tests/Procedures

Aerobic Culture, Appropriate Site *on page 310*
Gram's Stain *on page 426*

Treatment *Enterobacter* species present a challenging therapeutic problem, especially when isolates exhibit high level antibiotic resistance. Preliminary data suggest that the popular third generation cephalosporins may act to select naturally-occurring mutants of *Enterobacter* that are resistant to a wide variety of antibiotics. In the typical case, the cephalosporin is able to eradicate the vast majority of sensitive *Enterobacter* species. However, when the bacterial load is high (as in an abscess), these mutants may be present in small numbers along with the normally susceptible bacteria and continue to divide in the face of selective antibiotic pressure. In time, this resistant strain will dominate and often demonstrates complete resistance to all cephalosporins and all penicillins, even if penicillins were not given. This disturbing trend is particularly common in intensive care units, where prolonged courses of antibiotics are given empirically for fever without a clear focus of infection. Such "type I chromosomal mutants" may still remain susceptible to imipenem; infectious disease consultation may be helpful since imipenem-resistance can develop rapidly as well.

Drug Therapy

Recommended

Penicillins, Extended Spectrum *on page 864*
Cephalosporins, 3rd Generation *on page 662*

Alternate

Imipenem and Cilastatin *on page 766*
(Continued)

135

Enterobacter Species *(Continued)*

Meropenem *on page 812*
Fluoroquinolones *on page 736*

Selected Readings

Chow JW, Fine MJ, Shlaes DM, et al, "*Enterobacter* Bacteremia: Clinical Features and Emergence of Antibiotic Resistance During Therapy," *Ann Intern Med*, 1991, 115(8):585-90.

Quinn JP, DiVincenzo CA, and Foster J, "Emergence of Resistance to Ceftazidime During Therapy For *Enterobacter cloacae* Infections," *J Infect Dis*, 1987, 155(5):942-7.

Wolff MA, Young CL, and Ramphal R, "Antibiotic Therapy For *Enterobacter* Meningitis: A Retrospective Review of 13 Episodes and Review of the Literature," *Clin Infect Dis*, 1993, 16(6):772-7.

Enterobius vermicularis

Synonyms Pinworm

Microbiology *Enterobius vermicularis*, or pinworm, causes a form of perianal pruritus called enterobiasis, often seen in children. *Enterobius vermicularis* is a nematode, or roundworm, and is thus related to such parasites as *Ascaris lumbricoides*, *Ancylostoma duodenale* (hookworm), and *Strongyloides stercoralis*. *E. vermicularis* is a small, white worm with a cylindric unsegmented body. It is visible to the naked eye. The infectious cycle begins when the human host ingests the embryonated egg, which is infective within hours. The eggs hatch in the small intestine, and the emerging larval forms migrate to the large intestine. There, the larvae penetrate and develop within the mucosa and mature into male and female adult forms over a 2- to 6-week period. Fertilization takes place and the gravid female migrates to the perianal region of the host at night and lays its eggs in the perianal folds. The eggs mature rapidly and are infectious within hours.

Epidemiology Pinworm infection is most common in school children, although infection may occur at all ages. Infection is favored by close living conditions and is typically seen in institutions, schools, and day care centers. Cases frequently are clustered in families. All socioeconomic groups are at risk. Over 500 million cases occur worldwide, with about 40 million individual infections in the United States. Humans are the only known reservoir. Transmission occurs primarily via direct person-to-person spread. Eggs of the parasite frequently are carried beneath the fingernails of children who have been scratching the irritated perianal area. *E. vermicularis* eggs are relatively hardy and remain viable in dust, clothing, day care toys, furniture, and other fomites; infection can occur from inhalation of the eggs contained in infested dust.

Clinical Syndromes

- **Asymptomatic carriage:** Many infected individuals experience no symptoms from *E. vermicularis* but are still capable of spreading the worm.
- **Perianal pruritus:** This is the most common manifestation of pinworm infestation. Often there is severe local pruritus, interfering with sleep. Excessive scratching of the perianal region may lead to bacterial infection in severe cases.
- **Miscellaneous:** Unusual complications include appendicitis, salpingitis, granuloma formation, penetration through the intestinal wall, and bowel lesions.

Diagnosis Pinworm infestation is usually suspected in the individual who presents with refractory itching in the perianal area, particularly in children. The "Scotch tape test" is an accurate and inexpensive means of confirming the diagnosis. Clear adhesive tape is pressed to the perianal region early in the morning, prior to bathing or bowel movement . The eggs deposited overnight by the migrating adult readily adhere to the cellophane tape. This tape may be brought in later for examination by the physician. The thin-walled eggs are easily seen at low power under the microscope. Several examinations over consecutive days may be necessary since a single test may be falsely negative in 50% of cases. Commercial kits may be used in place of the less formal Scotch tape method; these kits utilize an adhesive paddle and follow the same general principles. Stool examinations are rarely diagnostic for pinworm. Peripheral eosinophilia is not characteristically seen.

Diagnostic Tests/Procedures

Pinworm Preparation *on page 520*

Treatment The drug of choice is mebendazole (Vermox®), which leads to a cure in >90% of the cases. Retreatment may be necessary in some cases, especially if reinfection occurs. Family members should be tested, even if asymptomatic, and treated as necessary.

Drug Therapy
Recommended
Mebendazole *on page 808*

Pyrantel Pamoate *on page 883*

Selected Readings
Mahmoud AA, "Intestinal Nematodes (Roundworms)," *Principles and Practice of Infectious Diseases*, 4th ed, Mandell GL, Bennett JE, and Dolin R, eds, New York, NY: Churchill Livingstone, 1995, 2526-31.

Wagner ED and Eby WC, "Pinworm Prevalence in California Elementary School Children, and Diagnostic Methods," *Am J Trop Med Hyg*, 1983, 32(5):998-1001.

Enterococcus Species

Microbiology Historically, the term *Enterococcus* was used to describe hardy, nonfastidious streptococci that were able to be cultured under a variety of conditions. The enterococci, *Streptococcus bovis* and *Streptococcus equinus* were classified as group D streptococci. Subsequently in 1984, the genus streptococci was divided into three genera, *Streptococcus*, *Lactococcus*, and *Enterococcus*. Enterococci, on Gram's stain, are gram-positive, oval cocci that occur in pairs or short chains. In culture, they can grow in 6.5% NaCl broth at 10°C to 45°C, can hydrolyze esculin in 4% bile, and hydrolyze L-pyrholidonyl β-napththylamide.

Epidemiology In the human host, the main reservoir for *Enterococcus* species is the intestinal tract. They are also commonly found in the oral cavity, urethra, and vagina. Infections may arise from endogenous flora and may be spread as nosocomial infections by hand and environmental contamination. *E. faecalis* and *E. faecium* are the species recovered in 80% to 90% of enterococcal infections. Isolates of enterococci from blood are generally considered pathogenic because 85% of these patients have clinical infections. Broad spectrum antibiotic therapy may suppress normal flora and allow enterococcal overgrowth of the intestinal flora. Wound colonization is common and superinfection in compromised hosts and those on antimicrobial therapy also occurs frequently. The organism is considered to have low intrinsic virulence and is considered to be primarily an opportunistic pathogen.

Clinical Syndromes The enterococci are recognized as causes of urinary tract infections, bacteremia, endocarditis, intra-abdominal infections, and osteomyelitis primarily in diabetic patients. Pneumonia and meningitis due to *Enterococcus* are rare in adult patients. Fifteen percent to 20% of bacterial endocarditis is caused by enterococci. *Streptococcus viridans* and *Staphylococcus* are the only organisms more frequently isolated. Enterococcal endocarditis occurs in the elderly more in association with urinary tract manipulation (ie, cystoscopy and catheterization); in young women associated with childbirth, cesarean sections, intrauterine devices (IUDs), curettage (D & Cs), and abortions. Intravenous drug abusers have a high incidence of enterococcal endocarditis which most frequently affects the mitral and/or aortic valves. Bacteremia is frequently detected in patients with serious underlying medical conditions including recent surgery, trauma, or burns. Enterococcal bacteremia is frequently nosocomial and often represents superinfection. Polymicrobic infections are frequently more fulminant with a higher incidence of shock, thrombocytopenia, and disseminated intravascular coagulation (DIC) than infections where enterococci are the sole pathogens. Gram-negative bacilli are the most frequently encountered copathogens. Prior antimicrobial therapy and long hospital stays are risk factors. The urinary tract is a frequent source of enterococcal bacteremia; however, because these cases are almost always associated with host factors enterococcal urinary tract infections (UTIs) are rarely encountered in office patients who are healthy otherwise. In intra-abdominal infections, enterococci are frequently present in part of a mixed infection where they may act synergistically with other bacteria. Neonatal meningitis may occur as nosocomial epidemics associated with prematurely low birth weight, previous antimicrobial therapy, arterial or venous catheterization, and nasogastric intubation.

Diagnostic Tests/Procedures
Aerobic Culture, Appropriate Site *on page 310*

Antimicrobial Susceptibility Testing, Aerobic and Facultatively Anaerobic Organisms *on page 323*

Blood Culture, Aerobic and Anaerobic *on page 337*

Gram's Stain *on page 426*

(Continued)

Enterococcus Species *(Continued)*

Duration of Therapy Enterococcal endocarditis is commonly treated with combination therapy for 4-6 weeks. Therapy for other enterococcal infections range from 7-14 days.

Treatment Appropriate treatment for enterococcal infections other than those of the urinary bladder includes a bactericidal combination of penicillin or glycopeptide (vancomycin) and an aminoglycoside. In uncomplicated cystitis, the achievable antimicrobial concentrations in urine generally greatly exceed the minimal inhibitory concentration thus monotherapy with a β-lactam (ampicillin) or glycopeptide (vancomycin) can be utilized. The American Heart Association (AHA) currently recommends treating enterococcal endocarditis with penicillin G 20 million units or ampicillin 12 g administered as a continuous infusion or in six equally divided doses in combination with gentamicin 1-2 mg every 8 hours to achieve a postdose peak of 3-5 mg/L. Streptomycin dosages are 7.5 mg/kg, not to exceed 500 mg, every 12 hours to achieve a postdose peak of 15-30 mg/L. Vancomycin dosages are 15 mg/kg every 12 hours to achieve a postdose concentration of 30-45 μg/L and a predose concentration <10 μg/L. If a vancomycin-resistant organism is encountered in a penicillin-sensitive patient, desensitization should be considered.

Typically enterococci have low level resistance to aminoglycosides. High level aminoglycoside resistance mediated by plasmids and transposons has become an increasing problem. *E. faecalis* frequently exhibits high level resistance to all currently available aminoglycosides. In serious infections, high level synergy testing is recommended for gentamicin and streptomycin. Because of β-lactamase production by some strains, β-lactamase testing (nitrocefin) also is performed by some laboratories. Vancomycin resistance is emerging; therefore, susceptibility testing for vancomycin is also indicated.

The resistance determinants of the enterococci reside on highly mobile genetic elements (plasmids and transposons) which have the potential to spread within the genus as well as to other gram-positive cocci. Thus the recognition, appropriate therapy, and awareness of the potential for nosocomial spread are of particular importance.

Co-trimoxazole frequently may appear to have a low minimal inhibitory concentration (MIC) against enterococci. This is due to low folate concentrations in the test medium. *In vivo*, folate from the host can be used by the enterococci to overcome the metabolic block of the co-trimoxazole thus co-trimoxazole should not be used in the therapy of enterococcal infections.

Cephalosporin *in vitro* susceptibility tests frequently suggest susceptibility; however, **cephalosporins are not effective *in vivo***.

Vancomycin-resistant enterococci (VRE): Several risk factors associated with VRE colonization, and infection are well recognized. Proximity to a VRE-colonized patient, length of stay (particularly in ICU), severity of illness, recent surgery, renal failure, previous nursing home stay, transplant recipient status, and immunosuppression are amongst the most common. Previous therapy with vancomycin, ceftazidime, ciprofloxacin, and metronidazole also may contribute. Usual nosocomial infection control procedures are appropriate. The efficacy of gowns in addition to gloves has been definitively established. Vancomycin should be used only when clearly indicated to help reduce the selective pressure favoring the emergence of VRE.

Drug Therapy
Recommended
Penicillin G, Parenteral, Aqueous *on page 860*
  used in combination with
Gentamicin *on page 747*
  or
Ampicillin *on page 604*
  used in combination with
Gentamicin *on page 747*
Vancomycin-resistant *Enterococcus*
Quinupristin/Dalfopristin *on page 891*
Chloramphenicol *on page 667*
Doxycycline *on page 713*

Alternate

Vancomycin *on page 967*
used in combination with
Gentamicin *on page 747*
or
Penicillin G, Parenteral, Aqueous *on page 860*
used in combination with
Streptomycin *on page 924*
or
Ampicillin *on page 604*
used in combination with
Streptomycin *on page 924*

Selected Readings

File TM Jr, "Overview of Resistance in the 1990s," *Chest*, 1999, 115(3 Suppl):3S-8S.

Leclercq R and Courvalin P, "Resistance to Glycopeptides in Enterococci," *Clin Infect Dis*, 1997, 24(4):545-56.

Linden PK and Miller CB, "Vancomycin-Resistant Enterococci: The Clinical Effect of a Common Nosocomial Pathogen," *Diagn Microbiol Infect Dis*, 1999, 33(2):113-20.

Maki DG and Agger WA, "Enterococcal Bacteremia: Clinical Features, the Risk of Endocarditis and Management," *Medicine (Baltimore)*, 1988, 67(4):248-69.

Megran DW, "Enterococcal Endocarditis," *Clin Infect Dis*, 1992, 15(1):63-71.

Moellering RC Jr, "Emergence of Enterococcus as a Significant Pathogen," *Clin Infect Dis*, 1992, 14(6):1173-6.

Moellering RC Jr, "Vancomycin-Resistant Enterococci," *Clin Infect Dis*, 1998, 26(5):1196-9.

Murray BE, "Vancomycin Resistant Enterococci," *Am J Med*, 1997, 102(3):284-93.

Namdari H, "Application of PCR for the Characterization of Enterococci," *Clin Microbiol Newslett*, 1998, 20(11):91-4.

Tailor SA, Bailey EM, and Rybak MJ, "Enterococcus, An Emerging Pathogen," *Ann Pharmacother*, 1993, 27(10):1231-42.

Weber DJ, Raasch R, and Rutala WA, "Nosocomial Infections in the ICU: The Growing Importance of Antibiotic-Resistant Pathogens," *Chest*, 1999, 115(3 Suppl):34S-41S.

Enterotoxigenic *E. coli* *see Escherichia coli*, Enterotoxigenic *on page 145*

Enterovirus

Microbiology Enteroviruses are small, single-stranded RNA viruses belonging to the family Picornaviridae. The term "enterovirus" may be a source of confusion since it may refer to either the genus Enterovirus (which includes echovirus, Coxsackieviruses A and B, poliovirus, and enterovirus) or the species enterovirus. The following discussion applies to the species enterovirus, which is further classified into enterovirus serotypes 68-71. These agents are sometimes referred to as the "newer enteroviruses" because of their recent recognition as agents of disease. The enteroviruses lack a lipid envelope. Important biophysical properties include the ability to survive in conditions of low pH and relatively high temperatures, and resistance to chlorine and alcohol decontamination. Enteroviruses grow best at body temperature. They replicate well in the upper respiratory and gastrointestinal tracts and can survive the acid environment of the stomach.

Epidemiology The newer enteroviruses are widely distributed throughout the world. Enteroviruses 70 and 71 are the two serotypes best characterized from an epidemiological and clinical standpoint. Enterovirus serotype 70 was first reported as a pathogen in 1969 during an outbreak of hemorrhagic conjunctivitis in Indonesia. This previously unrecognized virus has since spread throughout the globe and has been linked to millions of cases of hemorrhagic conjunctivitis. Pandemics are reported almost yearly. The majority of cases occur in the Far East, India, and Africa, generally in crowded urban areas with tropical climates. In the western hemisphere, most cases have been reported from Central America and the Caribbean, although an outbreak was reported from Florida in 1981 in an indigent population.

Enterovirus 71 was first isolated in 1969 from the stools of an infant in California with encephalitis. Over the next 10 years, a total of 8 epidemics were reported globally. The largest outbreak occurred in 1973 in Japan with over 3000 cases with hand-foot-and-mouth disease and aseptic meningitis. In 1975, an epidemic in Bulgaria involving 700 persons received worldwide attention. Over 20% of cases, mostly children, developed a polio-like paralysis with a significant number of fatalities; this was the first time a virus other than poliovirus was found to cause an epidemic paralytic disease. Small clusters of cases have been reported in the United States including a 1972 New York State outbreak characterized by meningitis and encephalitis in 11 cases and a similar small outbreak in 1977 in Rochester, New York, with two patients developing a self-resolving
(Continued)

Enterovirus *(Continued)*

paralysis. An additional 5 children developed a polio-like paralysis in the summer of 1987 in Philadelphia, which remains the largest series of Enterovirus 71-associated paralysis reported in the United States.

Infections caused by the genus Enterovirus most commonly involve infants and younger children. Although specific data regarding Enterovirus 71 is somewhat limited, infants and younger children are at highest risk for infection with this serotype, based on data derived from the major epidemics of Enterovirus 71. In addition, most of the serious complications of Enterovirus 71, such as muscle paralysis and encephalitis, were reported in young children. Infections caused by Enterovirus 70 seem to involve all age groups equally.

Less is known about the transmission of the newer enteroviruses than related Enteroviruses such as poliovirus or Coxsackievirus. In general, the fecal-oral route is felt to be the major route of spread for the genus Enterovirus. Live virus may be shed from the oropharynx for weeks after acute infection, and there may be persistent shedding of virus in the stools for months. Direct person-to-person spread via the fecal-oral route is likely in this setting. Enterovirus 70 is an exception to this rule in that spread most likely occurs directly from hand-to-eye or indirectly from fomites to the eye.

Clinical Syndromes Infections caused by the newer enteroviruses have a diverse clinical spectrum but tend to be neurovirulent. There is also some overlap in the types of illnesses caused by the newer enteroviruses, poliovirus, Coxsackievirus A and B, and Echovirus.

- **Asymptomatic infection:** Many of the infections caused by viruses of the genus Enterovirus are asymptomatic, with an estimated 90% or more of enteroviral infections resulting in a nonspecific febrile illness. This likely holds true for the newer enteroviruses.

- **Poliomyelitis-like paralysis:** As noted above, Enterovirus 71 is a potential cause of an epidemic, lower motor neuron paralysis similar to polio. Anterior horn cells in the spinal cord are involved, as in poliomyelitis. The disease is acute in onset and usually involves children. Patients present with asymmetric flaccid paralysis of the extremities with absent reflexes in the involved extremity. The sensory system is typically intact. This clinical syndrome is still rare in the United States but should be considered in the differential diagnosis of a child presenting with an unexplained paralytic disease.

- **Acute hemorrhagic conjunctivitis:** This disease, caused by Enterovirus serotype 70, tends to occur in an epidemic fashion and is highly contagious. Patients present with acute onset of a hemorrhagic conjunctivitis, with pain in the eye, photophobia, and periorbital swelling. Some may have constitutional symptoms such as fever and malaise. Nearly all will have subconjunctival bleeding, and this is distinctive. Complications include keratitis and occasionally neurologic complications such as motor paralysis have been reported following the conjunctivitis. Since only a limited number of cases have been reported from the western hemisphere, this diagnosis is unlikely in the United States but should be considered in immigrants or travelers.

- **Aseptic meningitis:** Like other enteroviruses, Enterovirus 71 has been associated with the syndrome of aseptic meningitis. Patients present with headache, neck stiffness, and a lymphocytic pleocytosis in the spinal fluid. Enterovirus 71 is a relatively uncommon cause of this syndrome, with many studies demonstrating Coxsackievirus as the major etiologic agent.

- **Hand-foot-and-mouth syndrome:** Like Coxsackievirus A16, Enterovirus 71 can cause this syndrome of vesicular lesions in the palms of the hands (exanthem) and the mucous membranes of the mouth (enanthem). This is a self-limited disease.

Diagnosis The clinical suspicion of enteroviral infection needs to be confirmed by viral culture. It is less important to differentiate the newer enteroviruses from Coxsackievirus or echovirus, than it is to differentiate it from bacterial causes of infection. The virus can be isolated in cell culture, particularly from rectal swabs or from throat secretions. In addition, it can be grown in cell culture from clinical specimens such as cerebrospinal fluid, skin lesions, or pericardial fluid.

Serologic studies are available to look for specific antibody responses to enterovirus. IgG antibody and IgM antibody against enteroviruses are available, and the finding of a fourfold increase in IgG or the presence of IgM antibody is helpful in establishing the diagnosis. However, it should be noted that recovery of enterovirus from a throat swab or a rectal swab does not necessarily establish enterovirus as the cause of an illness, since asymptomatic viral shedding may persist for periods of time. However, recovery of enterovirus from a site such as spinal fluid or a swab of a conjunctival lesion is confirmatory.

Diagnostic Tests/Procedures

Enterovirus Culture *on page 405*

Polymerase Chain Reaction *on page 523*

Drug Therapy Comment Currently, there are no antiviral agents available which are active *in vivo* against enterovirus.

Epstein-Barr Virus

Synonyms EBV

Microbiology EBV is a DNA virus and a member of the herpesvirus family. Two strains of EBV, differing in their B lymphocyte transformation and in viral gene sequence expression, infect humans. The structure of the viral DNA of EBV is unique as compared to other herpesvirus. The virus selectively infects human B lymphocytes and produces "immortalized" cell lives and usually causes latent infection.

Epidemiology Infection with EBV is common, with about 95% of the population demonstrating specific antibodies to this virus. In the U.S., the first peak of EBV infection occurs in children, with nearly 50% of 5 year olds seroconverting. There is a second peak of infection in the 20-30 year old age group.

EBV is transmitted by exchange of saliva containing live virus. EBV often persists in the throat of acutely infected individuals for months. Periodic asymptomatic shedding of virus is common. EBV may be cultured from the throat of 10% to 20% of healthy adults. Many with acute EBV are not aware of a sick contact who may have transmitted the disease. Prolonged intimate contact is necessary for spread. In general, the data suggest that EBV is widespread but is a virus of relatively low pathogenicity. Following the initial exposure to the virus, there is a 1-2 month incubation period prior to clinical disease. During this time, the virus disseminates through the reticuloendothelial system (liver, spleen, lymph nodes).

Clinical Syndromes

- **Infectious mononucleosis:** In the United States, "mono" occurs most commonly in individuals between 15-25 years of age. Characteristically, the patient presents with the "classic triad" of fever, sore throat, and lymphadenopathy. Rash is seen in only 5% of cases, but the rash is seen in nearly 100% of patients who mistakenly receive ampicillin for their symptoms. The tonsils are enlarged and the pharynx is inflamed, often with petechiae. Splenomegaly is an important physical finding in this setting and is present in nearly 50% of cases. Liver enlargement may also occur and liver function tests are frequently elevated. In many cases, the clinician must rely heavily on laboratory confirmation of suspected infectious mononucleosis, since both toxoplasmosis and cytomegalovirus can cause a similar syndrome. A compatible clinical syndrome, a positive heterophil test, and atypical lymphocytosis on blood smear are usually enough to establish the diagnosis of EBV mononucleosis. However, many cases may lack one or more of these findings; children are particularly prone to have heterophil-negative EBV mononucleosis. More detailed serologic testing is often necessary to confirm the diagnosis. Most patients recover completely from infectious mononucleosis over 2-3 weeks. However, a variety of complications have been reported: splenic rupture, hemolytic anemia, airway obstruction, profound thrombocytopenia, encephalitis, and the Guillain-Barré syndrome. Rare patients demonstrate objective evidence of ongoing EBV infection, with leukopenia, pulmonary infiltrates, and progressive neurologic disorders; this is in distinction to the "chronic EBV syndrome" described below. Although acyclovir inhibits EBV *in vitro* and probably *in vivo* as well, it appears to have minimal benefit in acute EBV mononucleosis. In large part, this is likely due to the observation that the clinical events in EBV mononucleosis result from the host's immune response rather than from direct viral invasion. Case reports have described the benefit of acyclovir in life-threatening EBV, but data are limited. The use of corticosteroids is controversial. Some have advocated corticosteroids only in complicated EBV infection (airway obstruction, thrombocytopenia, etc), but the benefits are unclear.

(Continued)

Epstein-Barr Virus *(Continued)*

- **Possible relationship with the chronic fatigue syndrome (CFS):** Persistent EBV infection has been theorized to cause the CFS. This controversial syndrome is characterized by overwhelming fatigue, muscle aches, poor concentration, low grade fevers, and minor lymphadenopathy. Initially, this symptom complex was termed the "chronic mononucleosis syndrome" due to its similarities with the prodromal symptoms of infectious mononucleosis. EBV was further implicated as an etiologic cause of "chronic mono" because many such individuals demonstrated high titers of EBV-specific antibody. Carefully controlled studies later showed that EBV titers were equivalent in patients with CFS and matched normal controls. In addition, clinical trials using acyclovir in CFS demonstrated no benefit. Currently, there is little objective evidence to link CFS and EBV.

- **EBV and malignancies:** EBV has been implicated as a cofactor in the development of Burkitt's lymphoma, a malignancy common in Africa. A direct causal relationship is suspected but has yet to be proven. EBV DNA sequences and virions have been identified in biopsy samples of Burkitt's lymphoma. EBV has also been strongly associated with nasopharyngeal carcinoma, a neoplasm most common in the Orient. Again, EBV nucleic acid has been found within malignant tissues.

- **EBV in transplant recipients:** In patients who have undergone solid organ or bone marrow transplantation, EBV has been reported to cause an unusual lymphoma-like syndrome called the "post-transplantation lymphoproliferative disorder." Patients receiving cyclosporin A, a medication used to prevent organ rejection, appear to be at increased risk. Biopsies of involved organs reveal a B-cell lymphoproliferative malignancy with identifiable EBV nucleic acid sequences. The spectrum of this disorder is still under study. In general, and unlike cytomegalovirus or herpes simplex virus, EBV is an unusual opportunistic pathogen in the transplant population.

- **EBV infection in patients with AIDS:** An EBV-related lymphoproliferative syndrome has also been reported in patients with advanced HIV infection. Another disease associated with EBV infection is oral hairy leukoplakia. This disease is a commonly seen lesion of the tongue and is frequently noted in advanced AIDS. EBV has been implicated as a possible etiologic cause (or cofactor) in this disorder.

Diagnostic Tests/Procedures

Epstein-Barr Virus Culture *on page 406*
Epstein-Barr Virus Serology *on page 406*
Immunofluorescent Studies, Biopsy *on page 460*
Infectious Mononucleosis Serology *on page 462*

Drug Therapy Comment No antiviral agents have been proven to be effective in the treatment of Epstein-Barr virus infections. Supportive care is the treatment of choice.

Selected Readings

Schooley RT, "Epstein-Barr Virus Infections, Including Infectious Mononucleosis," *Harrison's Principles of Internal Medicine*, 13th ed, Isselbacher KJ, Braunwald E, Wilson JD, et al, eds, New York, NY: McGraw-Hill, 1994, 790-3.

Straus SE, Cohen JI, Tosato G, et al, "Epstein-Barr Virus Infections: Biology, Pathogenesis, and Management," *Ann Intern Med*, 1993, 118(1):45-58.

Erysipelothrix rhusiopathiae

Microbiology *Erysipelothrix rhusiopathiae* is a thin, gram-positive rod that has been known to be an important animal pathogen since the late 1800s. More recently it has been recognized as a potentially serious cause of human disease. The organism is an aerobic bacillus (or facultatively anaerobic) that sometimes can appear as long nonbranching filaments. The organism can appear pleomorphic. *E. rhusiopathiae* can be distinguished from *Bacillus* species (another gram-positive rod) by the lack of spore formation in the former. *E. rhusiopathiae* grows on routine culture media where it has two distinctive forms on solid agar, one smooth and pinpoint, the other flat and rough and does not require specialized techniques for recovery from the blood.

Epidemiology The organism is ubiquitous in the environment and has a predilection for dead or decomposing nitrogenous substances. It can be found worldwide primarily as a colonizer of animals. The major reservoir of *E. rhusiopathiae* is probably domestic pigs, although the organism can be recovered from several species including birds, rats, and fowl. The slime that covers various species of fish also harbors the organism where it acts as a harmless commensal. Human infection generally occurs by direct inoculation from an infected animal to a human. The highest incidence of human disease occurs in those individuals with frequent exposures to animals, fish, poultry, grease, and fertilizer. Occupations at highest risk for *E. rhusiopathiae* infection are fish handlers, butchers, slaughterhouse workers, fisherman, and veterinarians.

Clinical Syndromes

- **Erysipeloid ("erysipelas-like"):** This is the most common clinical syndrome. Erysipeloid is a localized cellulitis which occurs as a result of cuts or abrasions to the hand followed by inoculation of the organism into the wounds from infected fish or animal meat. Clinically, patients present with severe pain, itching, and swelling of the finger or hand, often with discrete purplish erythema in the skin. These violaceous lesions are elevated and demarcated. Joint involvement may occur in the fingers. Left untreated, the infection often spreads proximally, and axillary adenopathy may develop. Vesicles are relatively uncommon, unlike true erysipelas caused by streptococci. This syndrome has been called the erysipeloid of Rosenbach, whale finger, seal finger, or fish poisoning. A more diffuse form of skin infection has also been described but is much less common; the violaceous skin lesions are more severe and progressive, and patients are more systemically ill.

- **Bacteremia and endocarditis:** This is a serious but uncommon complication, with about 60 reported cases. Skin lesions were seen in approximately 33% of bacteremic cases. Endocarditis has developed on previously normal valves and has a poorly understood tropism for the aortic valve. There is still a strong correlation with specific occupations. Mortality is high.

Diagnosis *Erysipelothrix* infection should be considered in any individual who presents with a significant hand or digital pain or swelling, particularly if there are occupational risk factors. Other considerations include staphylococcal or streptococcal infections, *Sporothrix* infection, mycobacterial infection, and lymphangitis. The violaceous lesions are distinctive for *Erysipelothrix* but are not always present. Laboratory confirmation is essential. The organism is best identified by deep soft tissue biopsy submitted for histopathology and culture. Blood cultures are negative in the erysipeloid form of the disease.

Diagnostic Tests/Procedures

Biopsy Culture, Routine *on page 337*
Blood Culture, Aerobic and Anaerobic *on page 337*
Gram's Stain *on page 426*
Histopathology *on page 448*
Skin Biopsy *on page 535*

Treatment *E. rhusiopathiae* is highly susceptible to penicillin but resistant to vancomycin. Other agents highly active against the organism *in vitro* include imipenem and the cephalosporins. Most authorities consider penicillin the drug of choice. It is important to note that the organism is resistant to vancomycin, an agent commonly used for empiric therapy of serious soft tissue infections. *E. rhusiopathiae* is also relatively resistant to trimethoprim-sulfamethoxazole and aminoglycosides and is only variably susceptible to erythromycin and tetracyclines.

Drug Therapy
Recommended
Penicillin V Potassium *on page 865*
Penicillin G, Parenteral, Aqueous *on page 860*
Alternate
Imipenem and Cilastatin *on page 766*
Cephalosporins, 1st Generation *on page 661*

Escherichia coli, **Enteroaggregative** *see Escherichia coli*, Enterotoxigenic *on page 145*

Escherichia coli, Enterohemorrhagic

Related Information
Escherichia coli, Enterotoxigenic *on page 145*

Synonyms *E. coli* O157:H7; EHEC

Microbiology Enterohemorrhagic *E. coli* causes a distinct form of hemorrhagic colitis in humans. Like other *E. coli* strains, enterohemorrhagic *E. coli* is a facultative, gram-negative bacillus. The most common serotype is O157:H7. (Continued)

Escherichia coli, Enterohemorrhagic *(Continued)*

Essentially all published information regarding enterohemorrhagic *E. coli* refers only to this serotype.

Epidemiology In 1982, the first large-scale outbreak of *E. coli* O157:H7 colitis was described. Multiple cases of severe bloody diarrhea were found to be epidemiologically linked to ingestion of contaminated hamburger meat. Since then, the organism has been recognized as an important cause of bloody diarrhea and the hemolytic uremic syndrome. Over 12 major outbreaks have been reported, along with numerous sporadic cases. The majority of cases have been traced to contaminated ground beef, although other potential sources have been cited, including unpasteurized milk, apple cider, municipal water, and roast beef. The organism inhabits the gastrointestinal tract of some healthy cattle and is thought to contaminate meat during slaughter and the processing of ground beef ("internal contamination"). If the ground beef is undercooked, the organism remains viable; undercooking of hamburger patties has proven important in several outbreaks.

In 1993, a well-publicized multistate outbreak of *E. coli* O157:H7 took place in the western United States (Washington, California, Idaho, and Nevada). Over 500 infections and four deaths were documented. The vast majority of cases were ultimately linked to contaminated hamburger meat from a particular restaurant chain. Further investigation by the Centers for Disease Control identified several slaughter plants in the United States and one in Canada as the probable source. Thousands of contaminated patties not yet consumed were discovered. In March, 1994, the USDA Food Safety and Inspection Service recommended that all raw meat should be cooked thoroughly, with an increase in the internal temperature for cooked hamburgers to 155°F.

A 2-year nationwide surveillance study by the Centers for Disease Control has found *E. coli* O157:H7 to be the most commonly identified pathogen associated with bloody diarrhea. In many parts of the U.S., *E. coli* O157:H7 is the second most common cause of bacterial diarrhea.

Acquisition of disease is usually by ingestion of contaminated food, but person-to-person transmission has been documented, especially in day care centers. Children and elderly individuals are at highest risk for severe infections. Simple and careful hand washing essentially eliminates the probability of person-to-person transmission.

Clinical Syndromes

- **Hemorrhagic colitis:** *E. coli* O157:H7 causes a bloody diarrhea associated with abdominal cramps. Pathologically, there is no invasion or inflammation of the intestinal mucosa, and thus fever is often absent. The diarrhea is caused by shiga-like toxins. In most cases, the illness resolves within 7 days, but death can occur in the elderly.

- **Hemolytic uremic syndrome:** Approximately 5% to 10% of patients with *E. coli* O157:H7 diarrhea develop a syndrome characterized by acute renal failure, thrombocytopenia, and evidence of hemolysis on a peripheral blood smear. Children are at high risk for this syndrome. The patient may be toxic-appearing, and the presentation may be confused with a variety of diseases including sepsis with disseminated intravascular coagulation, vasculitis, thrombotic thrombocytopenia purpura, and others. The estimated mortality is 3% to 5%.

Diagnosis Enterohemorrhagic *E. coli* should be strongly considered in any patient presenting with bloody diarrhea, whether or not hemolytic uremic syndrome is present. It is likely that many sporadic cases of *E. coli* O157:H7 diarrhea occur in the community and go unrecognized for two reasons: many clinicians do not order stool cultures for stable patients with diarrhea; many microbiology laboratories do not routinely culture stools for *E. coli* O157:H7 unless there is a specific order from the physician.

Diagnosis is confirmed by isolation of *E. coli* O157:H7 from stool specimens and subsequent serological confirmation. This requires special media in the Microbiology Laboratory (sorbitol-MacConkey medium). Other methods for the rapid detection of this organism are currently under study.

Diagnostic Tests/Procedures

Shiga Toxin Test, Direct *on page 534*

Stool Culture, Diarrheagenic *E. coli on page 542*

Treatment Treatment is supportive. Patients should be monitored for signs and symptoms of hemolytic uremic syndrome (HUS). O157:H7 strains of *E. coli* are sensitive to most common antimicrobial agents, but antimicrobials should be avoided. Some reports suggest that patients treated with antimicrobial agents may actually be more prone to develop HUS. Antimotility agents are always contraindicated in patients with bloody diarrhea.

Drug Therapy Comment No antibiotics proven effective.

Selected Readings
"*Escherichia coli* O157:H7 Outbreak Linked to Home-Cooked Hamburger - California, July 1993," *MMWR Morb Mortal Wkly Rep*, 1994, 43(12):213-6.

Griffin PM, Ostroff SM, Tauxe RV, et al, "Illnesses Associated With *Escherichia coli* O157:H7 Infections: A Broad Clinical Spectrum," *Ann Intern Med*, 1988, 109(9):705-12.

Riley LW, Remis RS, Helgerson SD, et al, "Hemorrhagic Colitis Associated With a Rare *Escherichia coli* Serotype," *N Engl J Med*, 1983, 308(12):681-5.

"Update: Multistate Outbreak of *Escherichia coli* O157:H7 Infections From Hamburgers - Western United States, 1992-1993," *MMWR Morb Mortal Wkly Rep*, 1993, 42(14):258-63.

***Escherichia coli*, Enteroinvasive** *see Escherichia coli*, Enterotoxigenic *on this page*

***Escherichia coli*, Enteropathogenic** *see Escherichia coli*, Enterotoxigenic *on this page*

Escherichia coli, Enterotoxigenic

Related Information
Escherichia coli, Enterohemorrhagic *on page 143*
Escherichia coli, Nonenterohemorrhagic *on page 147*

Synonyms Diarrheagenic *E. coli*; Enterotoxigenic *E. coli*; ETEC

Applies to *Escherichia coli*, Enteroaggregative; *Escherichia coli*, Enteroinvasive; *Escherichia coli*, Enteropathogenic

Microbiology ETEC is usually discussed, considered, and presented in the context of four other diarrheagenic *E. coli*: enterohemorrhagic *E. coli* (EHEC), enteroinvasive *E. coli* (EIEC), enteropathogenic *E. coli* (EPEC), and enteroaggregative *E. coli* (EAEC). See table.

Nondiarrheagenic *E. coli*: Nondiarrheagenic (typical or common) *E. coli* is a facultative gram-negative rod and is the most common bacterium isolated in the clinical microbiology laboratory and causes numerous types of extraintestinal infections.

Diarrheagenic *E. coli*: Like the typical *E. coli*, the four aforementioned diarrheagenic *E. coli* grow extremely well on commonly used laboratory media and are easily identified as *E. coli* by commonly used biochemical tests. In most cases, typical *E. coli* and diarrheagenic *E. coli* usually are indistinguishable when observed grossly on solid laboratory media and microscopically when stained with the Gram's stain. EHEC, ETEC, EIEC, EPEC, and EAEC have characteristic virulence factors which define each as a specific type of diarrheagenic *E. coli*.

Epidemiology The diarrheagenic *E. coli* are enteric pathogens which are found in different environments throughout the world: bowels of cattle, areas of poor sanitation, contaminated water supplies, slaughter houses where fresh meat contacts cattle fecal material, and agricultural areas where fresh vegetables and fruits contact cattle fecal material. The portal of entry for diarrheagenic *E. coli* is oral/ingestion. The organisms (and, thus, the diseases) are transmitted person-to-person extremely efficiently by hand contact. See table.

Clinical Syndromes Some strains of *E. coli* (the diarrheagenic strains) can cause severe and life-threatening diarrhea. There are five distinct groups of diarrheagenic *E. coli* which cause gastrointestinal illnesses ranging from mild diarrhea to cholera-like diarrhea to potentially fatal complications such as hemolytic uremic syndrome. These groups include EHEC, ETEC, EIEC, EPEC, and EAEC. EHEC causes (often bloody) diarrhea and hemorrhagic colitis usually in children and the elderly and is associated with contaminated beef (usually hamburger). ETEC causes a profuse watery diarrhea most commonly known as "traveler's diarrhea" (also tourista, deli belly, Montezuma's revenge, the hot galloping screamo's, etc). EPEC causes an acute diarrhea in children usually <2 years of age. EIEC causes diarrhea which, in some (rare) cases, is similar to the dysentery caused by *Shigella*. EAEC is not well characterized but has been reported to cause both chronic and acute watery diarrhea in all age groups. See table on next page.

(Continued)

Properties of *E. coli* Strains That Cause Enteric Infections

Diarrheagenic *E. coli*	Pathogenic Mechanisms	Enteric Infection(s)	Common Clinical Presentations	Common Age Group	Common Risk Factor	Diagnostic Tests‡
Enterotoxigenic *E. coli* (ETEC)	Heat-stable enterotoxin; Heat-labile enterotoxin	Diarrhea; traveler's diarrhea	Profuse watery diarrhea, cramps, nausea, dehydration	Children, adults	Foreign travel (usually Mexico)	EIA for enterotoxins; cell culture for cytotoxicity
Enteropathogenic *E. coli* (EPEC)	Adherence factor; attachment to and effacement of intestinal epithelium	Acute diarrhea	Watery diarrhea, fever, vomiting, mucus in stool	Children <2 years of age, adults	<2 years of age	Adherence to HEp-2 cell cultures
Enteroinvasive *E. coli* (EIEC)	Invasion and destruction of intestinal mucosal epithelium; enterotoxin?	Diarrhea; rarely dysentery similar to *Shigella* dysentery	Watery diarrhea; dysentery: scant stool, blood, mucus, and leukocytes in stool; fever; cramps	Adults	Foreign travel (usually Mexico)	Cytopathic effect of HeLa cell cultures
Enterohemorrhagic *E. coli* (EHEC)	Shiga-like toxins	Diarrhea; hemorrhagic colitis	Diarrhea (no leukocytes); abdominal cramps; blood in stool; fever, HUS†, and TTP* may or may not be present	Children, elderly	Consumption of undercooked ground beef	Isolation in culture; EIA for toxin in stool
Enteroaggregative *E. coli* (EAggEC)	Characteristic histopathologic lesion; cytotoxin?	Chronic and acute diarrheas	Watery diarrhea, vomiting	All ages	Unknown	Adherence pattern to HEp-2 cell cultures

*TTP: thrombocytopenic purpura

† HUS: hemolytic uremic syndrome

‡Many of the tests to confirm the identification of ETEC, EIEC, EPEC, and EAEC as etiological agents are relatively difficult to perform and are usually performed only in specialized reference laboratories.

Adapted from Larry D. Gray, "*Escherichia, Salmonella, Shigella,* and *Yersinia*," *Manual of Clinical Microbiology,* 6th ed, Murray PR, Baron EJ, Pfaller MA, et al. eds. Washington, DC: American Society for Microbiology, 1995, 451, with permission.

Diagnosis Attribution of diarrhea to one of the diarrheagenic *E. coli* depends on evaluation of the type of diarrhea, age of the patient, travel history, blood/mucus in the stool, duration of diarrhea, and the consideration that the diarrhea might be caused by more common causes of diarrhea (viruses, *Giardia*, *Salmonella*, *Shigella*, and *Campylobacter*). Diagnosis is confirmed by isolation of the particular pathogen and biochemical proof that the isolate is *E. coli*, and then subsequent demonstration of characteristic surface antigens by serologic agglutination with specific antisera (eg, EPEC and EIEC), the production of characteristic enterotoxins in culture (eg, ETEC), the ability to invade mammalian cell cultures (eg, EIEC), or the ability to adhere to certain mammalian cell cultures (eg, EAEC).

Diagnostic Tests/Procedures Many of the tests to confirm the identification of ETEC, EIEC, EPEC, and EAEC as etiological agents are relatively difficult to perform and are usually performed only in specialized reference laboratories. Some of the tests/reagents/kits are commercially available to standard clinical microbiology laboratories, and, therefore, are available to physicians locally. Contact the Microbiology Laboratory for advice regarding collection of specimens, isolation of the *E. coli*, which tests are available, the analyte (antigen, toxin, organism, etc) detected by each test, and which tests can and should be ordered. See table.

Shiga Toxin Test, Direct *on page 534*

Stool Culture, Diarrheagenic *E. coli on page 542*

Selected Readings

Boyce TG, Swerdlow DL, and Griffin PM, "*Escherichia coli* O157:H7 and Hemolytic Uremic Syndrome," *N Engl J Med*, 1995, 333(6):364-8.

Gray LG, "*Escherichia, Salmonella, Shigella*, and *Yersinia*," *Manual of Clinical Microbiology*, 6th ed, Murray PR, Baron EJ, Pfaller, et al, eds, Washington DC: American Society for Microbiology, 1995, 450-6.

Kay BA, Griffin PM, Strockbine NA, et al, "Too Fast Food: Bloody Diarrhea and Death From *Escherichia coli* O157:H7," *Clin Microbiol Newslett*, 1994, 16(3):17-9.

Nataro JP and Kaper JB, "Diarrheagenic *Escherichia coli*," *Clin Microbiol Rev*, 1998, 11(1):142-201.

Raj P, "Pathogenesis and Laboratory Diagnosis of *Escherichia coli*-Associated Enteritis," *Clin Microbiol Newslett*, 1993, 15(3):89-93.

Slutsker L, Ries AA, Greene KD, et al, "*Escherichia coli* O157:H7 Diarrhea in the United States: Clinical and Epidemiologic Features," *Ann Intern Med*, 1997, 126(7):505-13.

Su C and Brandt LJ, "*Escherichia coli* O157:H7 Infection in Humans," *Ann Intern Med*, 1995, 123(9):698-707.

Escherichia coli, Nonenterohemorrhagic

Related Information

Escherichia coli, Enterotoxigenic *on page 145*

Microbiology *Escherichia coli* is a lactose-positive, gram-negative, facultative bacillus with variable motility. A member of the Enterobacteriaceae family, *E. coli* is probably the most widely studied free-living organism. Most *E. coli* are nonpigmented, produce lysine decarboxylase, utilize acetate as a carbon source, and hydrolyze tryptophan to indole. Serologic typing is based on three surface antigens (O, H, K). The lipopolysaccharide of the cell wall is known as endotoxin and is a factor in sepsis and septic shock in infected individuals.

Epidemiology *E. coli*, as well as other Enterobacteriaceae, are normal colonizers of the human and animal gastrointestinal tract. It is often considered an opportunistic pathogen in hospitalized or debilitated patients but is the most common cause of urinary tract infections among "normal" hosts.

Clinical Syndromes

- **Urinary tract infections:** In the United States, *E. coli* is the most common cause of urinary tract infections both in normal hosts and immunocompromised or hospitalized patients. Although most common in sexually active young women, *E. coli* urinary tract infections occur in patients who are at increased risk of urinary tract infections in general (catheterized, obstructed, diabetic, prostatitis, etc).

- **Lower respiratory infections:** *E. coli* causes a significant number of nosocomial pneumonias in the United States and is an uncommon cause of community-acquired pneumonia or bronchitis. *E. coli* may also colonize the respiratory tract of hospitalized patients without causing disease, and its treatment in the absence of clinically relevant findings is usually unwarranted.

- **Neonatal meningitis:** Although uncommon in older populations, *E. coli* is a rare but important cause of meningitis and subsequent mortality in neonates.

(Continued)

Escherichia coli, Nonenterohemorrhagic *(Continued)*

- **Peritonitis:** *E. coli* is a major pathogen in polymicrobial intra-abdominal infections.
- **Sepsis and other infections:** *E. coli* is one of the leading causes of bacteremia, sepsis, and septic shock. It can also cause a variety of other infections including wound infections, cellulitis, and diarrhea.

Diagnosis *E. coli* infection diagnosis can be made by identification through Gram's stain and culture in patients with relevant clinical syndromes. No special media or conditions are necessary to grow this organism. *E. coli* should always be one of several suspected organisms in patients with peritonitis.

Diagnostic Tests/Procedures
Aerobic Culture, Appropriate Site *on page 310*
Gram's Stain *on page 426*

Treatment Although the majority of *E. coli* are still sensitive to ampicillin, amoxicillin, and first generation cephalosporins, increasing resistance is being noted, especially in nosocomial isolates. Most mild to moderate urinary tract infections can be treated with amoxicillin or co-trimoxazole until susceptibility confirmation. In more serious or nosocomial infections, more broad spectrum antibiotics, such as third generation cephalosporins, should be initiated until susceptibility data is available. In patients who are septic, supportive care will also be necessary along with appropriate antibiotics.

Drug Therapy
  Recommended
    Severe infection:
      Cephalosporins, 3rd Generation *on page 662*
    Mild to moderate infection:
      Ampicillin *on page 604*
      Co-Trimoxazole *on page 692*
  Alternate
    Cephalosporins, 1st Generation *on page 661*
    Cephalosporins, 2nd Generation *on page 662*
    Fluoroquinolones *on page 736*

Selected Readings
Eisenstein BI, "*Enterobacteriaceae*," *Principles and Practice of Infectious Diseases*, 4th ed, Mandell GL, Bennett JE, and Dolin R, eds, New York, NY: Churchill Livingstone, 1995, 1964-80.
Zwadyk P, "*Enterobacteriaceae*: General Characteristics," *Zinsser Microbiology*, 20th ed, Joklik WK, Willett HP, Amos DB, et al, eds, Norwalk, CT: Appleton & Lange, 1992, 538-43.
Zwadyk P, "Opportunistic Enterobacteriaceae," *Zinsser Microbiology*, 20th ed, Joklik WK, Willett HP, Amos DB, et al, eds, Norwalk, CT: Appleton & Lange, 1992, 544-55.

ETEC *see Escherichia coli*, Enterotoxigenic *on page 145*

Francisella tularensis

Microbiology *Francisella tularensis* is a nonmotile, pleomorphic, strictly aerobic, gram-negative rod. The bacterium possesses a lipid capsule which is a virulence factor and which might be responsible, at least in part, for the ability of the bacterium to survive weeks to months in adverse environmental conditions such as water, mud, and decaying animal carcasses. The bacterium is biochemically inert when grown (for identification purposes) *in vitro* on sugars or other substrates. The bacterium exists as two clinically significant biogroups. Biogroup *F. tularensis* (type A, mortality rate 5%) is found in North America and produces the most severe form of tularemia. Biogroup *Palearctica* (type B, extremely low mortality) is found only in the northern hemisphere (particularly Asia and Europe) and produces a milder form of tularemia. Biogroup *Francisella tularensis* causes tularemia (rabbit fever, deer fly fever), a zoonosis of wild animals and the third most common human tickborne illness in the United States.

Epidemiology *Francisella tularensis* is found throughout the United States (except the southeast, the northeast, and the Great Lakes areas). Tularemia is endemic in Missouri, Arkansas, and Oklahoma (together, 50% of all United States cases). The bacterium is strikingly absent from the United Kingdom, Africa, South America, and Australia. Hundreds of wild animal species and common house pets are hosts of the bacterium which is perpetuated freely and often in nature as it is passed from wild animal to wild animal by ectoparasites, poor environmental conditions, and less-than-respectable eating and culinary habits. The most common vectors which transmit *F. tularensis* to humans (incidental and dead-end hosts) are ticks and biting flies. In addition, humans who handle hides, woodland water, and animal carcasses can acquire the bacterium by the respiratory route. Occupations associated with a higher risk for tularemia are laboratory worker, veterinarian, sheep worker, hunter, trapper, and meat handler. Since 1965, the number of cases of tularemia in the United States has remained between 0.05 and 0.15 per 100,000.

Clinical Syndromes The severity of tularemia depends on the virulence of the biotype, portal of entry, inoculation dose, extent of dissemination, and immunocompetence of the host. After an incubation period of 2-10 days, flu-like symptoms usually occur. These symptoms can be chronic and debilitating. A nonhealing skin ulcer or lesion can develop at the cutaneous portal of entry and last for months. Tularemia usually presents in one or more of the following forms.

- **Ulceroglandular**: 21% to 87% of cases; obvious nonhealing, erythematous, eroding ulcers
- **Glandular**: 3% to 20% of cases; cutaneous ulcers are not found
- **Oculoglandular**: 0% to 5% of cases; severely painful, yellow, pinpoint conjunctival ulcers
- **Esophageal**: Severely painful sore throat; enlarged tonsils; white pseudomembrane
- **Systemic**: 5% to 30% of cases; "typhoidal form"; acute septicemia; classic ulcers and lymphadenopathy usually not present
- **Gastrointestinal**: consumption of contaminated food and water; persistent diarrhea; fulminating and often fatal
- **Pulmonary**: 7% to 20% of cases; usually presents as a nonproductive pneumonia which is observed radiographically but not clinically

The most common complaints of these forms of tularemia are lymphadenopathy and necrosis of infected lymph nodes (even with appropriate treatment). Severe cases of tularemia are complicated - dissemination of the bacterium, toxemia, DIC, renal failure, and hepatitis.

Diagnosis Physicians must take a complete physical, occupational, recreational, and travel history, and, preferably, be suspicious of tularemia. Cultures of blood, tissue, gastric washings, and sputum are possible and can yield the bacterium; however, culture is extremely nonproductive. Physicians must notify laboratory personnel when culture for *F. tularensis* is ordered because the bacterium is an extreme health hazard to laboratory workers. The most recommended, useful, and productive tests to help diagnose tularemia are serological methods (standard tube agglutination, haemagglutination, and enzyme immunoassay [the most sensitive tests]). Antibodies in sera from infected persons are detectable and are highest 2-5 weeks postinfection, respectively. A single titer ≥160 and a fourfold rise in titer are presumptive and diagnostic for tularemia, respectively. Titers ≥1024 are common late in the acute stage of disease. Both IgG and IgM titers of 20-80 can persist for years.

Diagnostic Tests/Procedures
Tularemia Serology *on page 559*

Treatment Treatment is directed toward the symptoms associated with gram-negative bacterial infection and, if present, septicemia.

Drug Therapy Comment Antimicrobial susceptibility testing cannot be performed with *F. tularensis* because the bacterium is too fastidious to be tested by standardized, reliable methods. Aminoglycosides (especially streptomycin) are the antimicrobial agents of choice. Fluoroquinolones are also effective. Generally, chloramphenicol, tetracycline, beta-lactams (except for imipenem), sulfonamides, and macrolides are not as effective as aminoglycosides. Relapses are more common with both tetracycline and chloramphenicol than the aminoglycosides probably due to its bacteriostatic action rather than cidal activity. Tetracycline should be administered at a minimum dose of 2 g/day to be effective. Chloramphenicol should be added to the aminoglycosides in the treatment of meningitis secondary to this organism. Tetracycline has also been used with some success in the treatment of tularemia. Erythromycin is also active but little clinical experience is available.

Drug Therapy
Recommended
  Streptomycin *on page 924*
  Gentamicin *on page 747*
For meningitis:
  Chloramphenicol *on page 667*
(Continued)

149

Francisella tularensis (Continued)
Alternate
Tetracycline on page 944
Cephalosporins, 3rd Generation on page 662

Selected Readings
Nelson JA, "Tickborne Illnesses: United States," Clin Microbiol Newslett, 1992, 14(14):105-8.

Penn RL, "Francisella tularensis (Tularemia)," Principals and Practice of Infectious Diseases, 4th ed, Mandell GL, Bennett JE, and Dolin R, eds, New York, NY: Churchill Livingston, 1995, 2060-8.

Stewart SJ, "Francisella," Manual of Clinical Microbiology, 6th ed, Murray PR, Baron EJ, Pfaller MA, et al, eds, Washington, DC: American Society for Microbiology, 1995, 545-8.

Fusarium Species

Microbiology Fusarium is a member of the hyalohyphomycosis, molds that are light-colored with branched or unbranched hyphae with nonpigmented cell walls. There are several different classification systems based on the morphology of the macroconidia, microconidia, and chlamydospores. F. solani, F. oxysporum, F. chlamydosporum, and F. moniliforme are the common species pathogenic to humans. F. sporotrichioides produce the mycotoxin T-2 resulting in toxic alimentary aleukia which was attributed to the poisoning of approximately 1 million people during World War II after ingesting contaminated grain. Other Fusarium species may produce similar fumonisins which cause significant morbidity and mortality to grazing animals. Its adherence properties especially to plastic catheters and contact lenses may enhance its pathogenicity. Fusarium grows readily on potato dextrose agar and blood culture medium. Identification is based on the conidia characteristics.

Epidemiology Fusarium species are ubiquitous soil organisms that are pathogenic to plants. Human infection most commonly results from traumatic inoculation of contaminated material; however, disseminated disease is becoming more common in neutropenic patients without clear evidence of inoculation. Disseminated disease in a normal healthy human host is exceedingly rare. More than 60% of the reported cases of invasive fusariosis have occurred in the United States; however, the organism has been found worldwide. The geographic discrepancy is unclear and may have to do with host factors and/or laboratory investigation rather than climatic differences.

Clinical Syndromes
- **Cutaneous:** Cutaneous lesions most often secondary to traumatic inoculation; may cause mycetoma. Also seen secondary to dissemination which initially appear as a maculopapular to vesicular rash, then develop into lesions with necrotic centers with surrounding induration. May present as cellulitis, onychomycosis, and keratitis.
- **Pulmonary:** Fusarium species may colonize the upper airway or cause an upper respiratory infection, particularly sinusitis. Approximately 40% of disseminated disease is attributed to a lower respiratory tract infection. Clinical presentation is similar to aspergillosis in that patients may develop a fungal ball or pneumonia. Allergic bronchopulmonary fusariosis has been described similarly to that seen with aspergillosis.
- **Gastrointestinal:** Alimentary toxic aleukia is caused by mycotoxins in infected grains. Presents as gastrointestinal illness characterized by nausea, vomiting, diarrhea, fever, and chills. Patients may develop headache, stomatitis, dermatitis, CNS disease, and suppression of the bone marrow leading to aplastic anemia and hemorrhaging. Urov or Kashin-Beck disease is also probably related to mycotoxins in infected grain resulting in a chronic, disabling, deforming, dystrophic osteoarthritis. Akakabi-byo is a disease of various grains in Japan that may cause gastrointestinal upset in humans.
- **Disseminated:** Most commonly seen in neutropenic patients secondary to cytotoxic therapy for hematologic malignancies. Most often presents as fever, myalgias, disseminated cutaneous lesions, and fungemia with multi-organ system failure although may present as neutropenic fever without localizing signs or symptoms. A mycotoxin may play a role in prolonging the aplasia initially induced by chemotherapy. Also seen in severe burn victims. Portals of entry include central-venous catheters, respiratory tract, gastrointestinal tract, and onychomycosis or cutaneous lesions. Blood cultures are positive in approximately 60% to 80%. Without recovery of neutrophils, mortality is essentially 100% except in cases of vascular catheter-related infections in which the catheter can be removed.

- **Miscellaneous:** Septic arthritis, catheter-related peritonitis, cystitis, endophthalmitis, and CNS lesions have been reported.

Diagnosis Histopathology may be confused with other molds especially aspergillosis given its propensity for vascular invasion. Definitive diagnosis is made by identification of the mold from tissue or blood culture.

Diagnostic Tests/Procedures
Blood Culture, Fungus *on page 341*
Fungus Culture, Biopsy *on page 414*
KOH Preparation *on page 467*

Treatment Treatment of disseminated disease is targeted at treatment of the underlying illness. Antifungal therapy including amphotericin B has remained ineffective without recovery of the neutrophils. Investigational agents are being studied. Surgical excision is warranted in localized infections. Catheter-related infections should have all catheters removed. Localized infections such as septic arthritis or osteomyelitis secondary to trauma may respond to amphotericin B.

Drug Therapy Comment Azoles are typically ineffective against *Fusarium*.

Drug Therapy
Recommended
Amphotericin B (Conventional) *on page 597*

Selected Readings
Anaissie E, Nelson P, Beremand M, et al, "*Fusarium*-Caused Hyalohyphomycosis: An Overview," *Curr Top Med Mycol*, 1992, 4:231-49.

Boutati EI and Anaissie EJ, "*Fusarium*, a Significant Emerging Pathogen in Patients With Hematologic Malignancy: Ten Years' Experience at a Cancer Center and Implications for Management," *Blood*, 1997, 90(3):999-1008.

Martino P, Gastaldi R, Raccah R, et al, "Clinical Patterns of *Fusarium* Infections in Immunocompromised Patients," *J Infect*, 1994, 28(Suppl 1):7-15.

Nelson PE, Dignani MC, and Anaissie EJ, "Taxonomy, Biology, and Clinical Aspects of *Fusarium* Species," *Clin Microbiol Rev*, 1994, 7(4):479-504.

Rombaux P, Eloy P, Bertrand B, et al, "Lethal Disseminated *Fusarium* Infection With Sinus Involvement in the Immunocompromised Host: Case Report and Review of the Literature," *Rhinology*, 1996, 34(4):237-41.

GABHS *see Streptococcus pyogenes on page 274*

Gardnerella vaginalis

Microbiology *Gardnerella vaginalis* is a small gram-negative rod which is part of the normal vaginal flora in many healthy women. It has been implicated as the cause of bacterial vaginosis, a common superficial infection of the vaginal mucosa. The organism is a nonmotile, pleomorphic, gram-negative (or gram-variable) rod. It lacks a capsule and does not form spores. Although *Gardnerella vaginalis* stains gram-negative in clinical specimens, the cell wall is morphologically more characteristic of gram-positive bacteria. Most isolates are facultatively anaerobic, and the organism can be isolated in the laboratory without anaerobic culture techniques. The organism tends to be fastidious in its growth and nutritional requirements. Specific enrichment media may be used in the laboratory to optimize its recovery in culture; these media are combinations of Columbia agar base and human blood.

Epidemiology *Gardnerella vaginalis* can be recovered from the vagina in up to 60% of asymptomatic females. In the condition called bacterial vaginosis, it can be cultured in 95% to 100% of women. Its role as the causative agent of bacterial vaginosis is controversial, since it is so frequently found in healthy individuals. Other organisms comprising the normal vaginal flora can also significantly increase in women with bacterial vaginosis, including the obligate anaerobes *Peptococcus*, *Eubacterium*, and *Mobiluncus*. Some believe these other bacteria work in combination with *Gardnerella* to alter the physiologic environment within the vagina which ultimately leads to bacterial vaginosis. This is not a sexually transmitted disease. Although *Gardnerella* may at times be cultured from the urethra of the male sexual partner of a woman with bacterial vaginosis, there is no clinical counterpart of this condition in men.

Clinical Syndromes
- **Bacterial vaginosis:** As noted above, the precise role of *Gardnerella vaginalis* in the pathogenesis of this condition is not known. In bacterial vaginosis, there is characteristically a new vaginal discharge with a "fishy odor." The woman may be otherwise asymptomatic or may have mild vaginal irritation. Vaginal pruritus or severe burning are not seen. Bacterial vaginosis may be diagnosed clinically if the following are present: 1. a thin, homogeneous vaginal discharge is present on pelvic examination; 2. the pH of the

(Continued)

Gardnerella vaginalis (Continued)

vaginal mucosa/discharge is >4.5 (normal is <4); 3. the vaginal discharge has a "fishy odor" when a drop of 10% KOH is added to the discharge on a microscope slide ("whiff test"); 4. "clue cells" are seen on a wet mount of the vaginal discharge. These distinctive cells are actually the normal large vaginal epithelial cells which have been covered by sheets of gram-negative *Gardnerella* organisms. Generally, the presence of three of these four criteria is sufficient to establish bacterial vaginosis and to separate this condition from the two other common causes of vaginitis, namely *Candida albicans* and *Trichomonas vaginalis*.

- **Urinary tract infections:** *Gardnerella* is a rare (<1%) cause of either lower or upper urinary tract infections. Since the organism so often colonizes the normal vaginal flora, it is often difficult to determine if a positive urine culture for *Gardnerella* represents vaginal contamination. However, case reports have argued that it may be truly pathogenic in the urinary tract in a small number of patients, particularly young women and men with underlying renal disease.

- **Bacteremia:** Isolation of *Gardnerella* in blood cultures has been reported following various obstetric and gynecologic manipulations, including septic abortion and postpartum endometritis. It has also been reported in men following transurethral resection of the prostate (TURP).

- **Miscellaneous infections:** Less commonly, *Gardnerella* has also been associated with salpingitis, vaginal abscesses, and infection following cesarian section. Preliminary studies have implicated bacterial vaginosis as a potential cause of premature delivery and premature rupture of membranes in pregnant women. It is hypothesized that *Gardnerella* has phospholipase A_2 activity which may initiate labor. This relationship is still under study.

Diagnosis The diagnosis of bacterial vaginosis is made clinically, based on the criteria outlined above. Routine laboratory studies such as the complete blood count or electrolyte panel are not necessary. The Gram's stain of vaginal discharge is helpful in identifying clue cells, which are pathognomonic for bacterial vaginosis. A striking decrease in the number of lactobacilli (gram-positive rods) normally dominant in the vaginal flora is also characteristic of bacterial vaginosis. A direct wet mount of vaginal secretions is useful in identifying clue cells and ruling out the presence of trichomonads (as seen in vaginal trichomoniasis) or yeast cells (as seen in candidal vaginitis). Although often obtained, cultures of the vagina for *Gardnerella* do little to establish the presence of bacterial vaginosis and are not indicated in the majority of cases. Vaginal Gram's stains have been shown to be as sensitive as vaginal cultures (including semiquantitative culture techniques), with greater specificity and positive predictive value. Cultures for *Gardnerella vaginalis* from extravaginal sites (such as blood) are appropriate in the proper clinical setting. *Gardnerella* can be grown in blood culture media which is free of sodium polyanetholsulfonate (SPS).

Diagnostic Tests/Procedures

Gram's Stain *on page 426*

KOH Preparation *on page 467*

Trichomonas Preparation *on page 555*

Treatment Unlike other gram-negative bacilli, *Gardnerella vaginalis* is susceptible to penicillin, ampicillin, vancomycin, and clindamycin. Most strains are resistant to nalidixic acid, sulfadiazine, and neomycin. The organism is resistant to metronidazole *in vitro*, but is effective *in vivo*, probably due to an active metabolite of metronidazole. Treatment guidelines are as follows:

1. For nonpregnant women with bacterial vaginosis, metronidazole (Flagyl®) is the drug of choice, 500 mg orally 2 times a day for 7 days. As an alternative, clindamycin may be used, 300 mg orally 2 times a day for 7 days. Since bacterial vaginosis is not a sexually transmitted disease, there is no need to routinely treat the male sexual partner.

2. For the pregnant female, treatment is at the physician's discretion. Limited data has linked bacterial vaginosis with premature delivery, but the benefits of antibiotic therapy, if any, are presently unknown. Metronidazole is contraindicated in the first trimester of pregnancy. The Centers for Disease Control have recommended clindamycin in this situation, should treatment be initiated.

3. For bacteremia with *Gardnerella*, a variety of antibiotics may be used including ampicillin.

Drug Therapy

Recommended

Metronidazole *on page 817*

Alternate

Ampicillin *on page 604*

Clindamycin *on page 684*

Selected Readings

Josephson S, Thomason J, Sturino K, et al, "*Gardnerella vaginalis* in the Urinary Tract: Incidence and Significance in a Hospital Population," *Obstet Gynecol*, 1988, 71(2):245-50.

Spiegel CA, "*Gardnerella vaginalis* and *Mobiluncus* Species," *Principles and Practice of Infectious Diseases*, 4th ed, Mandell GL, Bennett JE, and Dolin R, eds, New York, NY: Churchill Livingstone, 1995, 2050-3.

"1998 Guidelines for Treatment of Sexually Transmitted Diseases. Centers for Disease Control and Prevention," *MMWR Morb Mortal Wkly Rep*, 1998, 47(RR-1):1-111.

Gemella morbillorum *see Streptococcus*, Viridans Group *on page 279*

Giardia lamblia

Microbiology *Giardia lamblia* is an important intestinal parasite classified as a protozoan flagellate. It is related to other clinically relevant protozoans such as *Trichomonas vaginalis* and *Dientamoeba fragilis*. The organism exists as either a trophozoite or a cyst, and both can be detected in stool samples. Microscopically, *G. lamblia* trophozoites are characterized by long flagella at one end (which provide motility in fluid environments), a ventral adhesive disk (which attaches to the intestinal villi of humans), and two parabasal bodies located near the nucleus. These paired bodies give a characteristic and easily identifiable appearance of "two eyes" looking at the examiner. The cyst form of *Giardia* is somewhat smaller than the trophozoite and is considered the infective form of *Giardia*.

The infectious cycle for humans begins with ingestion of *Giardia lamblia* cysts (eg, from contaminated water or food). As few as 10 organisms can initiate human disease. In the stomach, excystation is promoted by gastric acid, and trophozoites are released in the duodenum and multiply by longitudinal binary fission. The trophozoites attach to the intestinal villi by means of the ventral sucking disk. Histologically, there is a mild to moderate inflammation of the small bowel mucosa. Both the cyst and trophozoite are passed into the human feces.

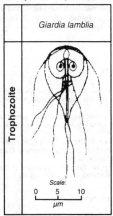

Giardia lamblia

Trophozoite

Scale:
0   5   10
μm

From Brooks MM and Melvin DM,
*Morphology of Diagnostic Stages
of Intestinal Parasites of Humans*,
2nd ed, Atlanta, GA: U.S. Department
of Health and Human Services,
Publication No. 84-8116, Centers for
Disease Control, 1984, with
permission.

(Continued)

Giardia lamblia (Continued)

Epidemiology Infection with *Giardia* occurs worldwide. In particular, it can be found in wilderness streams, lakes, and mountainous areas. Beavers, muskrats, and other wild animals serve as another reservoir for this organism. Common means of acquisition include:

- Ingestion of contaminated water. Outbreaks from contaminated water in mountain resorts have been described. *Giardia lamblia* cysts are not killed by the chlorine concentrations used in many water treatment facilities. It is important to obtain a travel history (including recent camping) in patients with acute giardiasis.
- Ingestion of contaminated food.
- Oral-anal sexual contact. This is an important means of person-to-person spread, particularly amongst male homosexuals.
- Fecal-oral spread, especially in children attending day care centers.

Clinical Syndromes

- **Asymptomatic carriage:** In almost 50% of cases, infection with *Giardia lamblia* occurs in the absence of symptoms. This state of carriage can persist indefinitely in some individuals.
- **Gastrointestinal disease:** The spectrum of symptomatic giardiasis is variable and ranges from a mild nonspecific diarrheal illness to a more severe illness characterized by abdominal pain, bloating, and profuse diarrhea. A chronic malabsorption syndrome has been described. The diarrhea tends to be watery and associated with abdominal cramping; stools are almost always guaiac-negative since *Giardia* does not invade the mucosal tissues. Patients at particular risk for severe or relapsing giardiasis are individuals with an underlying IgA deficiency or diverticulosis.

Diagnosis Diagnosis can be made by wet mount of liquid stool for cysts or trophozoites, or exam of fresh semiformed stool for cysts, preserved stool (formalin or PVA) can be stained with trichrome or iron hematoxylin. If stool as negative, duodenal biopsy aspiration or sting test can be performed. The sting test consists of a gelatin capsule or a nylon string that is swallowed. After a testing incubation period (at least 4-6 hours), the sting is removed and examined/stained for the organism.

Diagnostic Tests/Procedures

Giardia Specific Antigen (GSA65) *on page 426*
Ova and Parasites, Stool *on page 505*

Treatment Many cases of giardiasis are self-resolving without specific therapy. However, both symptomatic and asymptomatic *G. lamblia* infections should be treated. The drug of choice is metronidazole, with quinacrine being a good alternative.

Drug Therapy

Recommended

Metronidazole *on page 817*

Selected Readings

Adam RD, "The Biology of *Giardia* spp.," *Microbiol Rev*, 1991, 55(4):706-32.

Lengerich EJ, Addiss DG, and Juranek DD, "Severe Giardiasis in the United States," *Clin Infect Dis*, 1994, 18(5):760-3.

Ortega YR and Adam RD, "*Giardia*: Overview and Update," *Clin Infect Dis*, 1997, 25(3):545-50.

Overturf GD, "Endemic Giardiasis in the United States - Role of the Day Care Center," *Clin Infect Dis*, 1994, 18(5):764-5.

Pickering LK and Engelkirk PG, "*Giardia lamblia*," *Pediatr Clin North Am*, 1988, 35(3):565-77.

Pickering LK, Woodward WE, DuPont HL, et al, "Occurrence of *Giardia lamblia* in Children in Day Care Centers," *J Pediatr*, 1984, 104(4):522-6.

Steketee RW, Reid S, Cheng T, et al, "Recurrent Outbreaks of Giardiasis in a Child Day Care Center, Wisconsin," *Am J Public Health*, 1989, 79(4):485-90.

GNB *see* Gram-Negative Bacilli *on this page*

Gram-Negative Bacilli

Synonyms GNB

Refer to

Acinetobacter Species *on page 58*
Aeromonas Species *on page 64*
Alcaligenes Species *on page 65*
Bartonella Species *on page 76*

HACEK Group

Microbiology HACEK is a pneumonic which includes *Haemophilus aphrophilus*, *Actinobacillus actinomycetemcomitans*, *Cardiobacterium hominis*, *Eikenella corrodens*, and *Kingella* species. These organisms are pleomorphic, coccobacilli and bacilli and occur as chains or filamentous forms. These organisms are all fastidious, gram-negative bacteria which require specific types of growth conditions. These conditions include enhanced CO_2, specific growth factors (*Haemophilus*), growth only on chocolate and/or blood agar, and often increased time for incubation. Organisms in this group may be differentiated by reaction to oxidase and catalase, cell shape, indole positivity, nitrate to nitrite, and fermentation of carbohydrates. In a microbiology laboratory, these five bacteria are identified and reported separately.

Epidemiology Members of the HACEK group are normal flora of the mouth and respiratory tract and are opportunistic organisms that cause infections in patients with oral cavity disease or trauma and in immunocompromised hosts. *Eikenella* infections are often associated with other mouth flora organisms.

Clinical Syndromes Although many of the HACEK organisms have been know to cause disease in several organ systems and clinical settings, endocarditis is by far the most common. Endocarditis is usually subacute with a very insidious onset, often in patients with previously damaged or prosthetic valves. Although medical treatment is often successful, reporting bias must be considered.

Diagnosis The diagnosis of a HACEK group infection can only be made by identification of the specific pathogen through culture in a patient with a relevant clinical syndrome. Patients with seemingly culture-negative endocarditis should have their cultures held, as prolonged incubation time may be needed. Also, special media and conditions may be necessary as described above.

Diagnostic Tests/Procedures
Blood Culture, Aerobic and Anaerobic on page 337
(Continued)

HACEK Group *(Continued)*

Gram's Stain *on page 426*

Treatment Empiric therapy with ampicillin plus gentamicin or a third generation cephalosporin should be considered if a HACEK organism is suspected in patients with endocarditis. There are strains of these organism which have been shown to produce beta-lactamases that inactivate ampicillin. The final therapeutic decision should be based on clinical condition of the patient (especially while cultures are pending or negative) and sensitivity testing. Treatment should be maintained for 4-6 weeks.

Drug Therapy

Recommended

Cephalosporins, 3rd Generation *on page 662*

or

Ampicillin *on page 604*

used in combination with

Gentamicin *on page 747*

Selected Readings

Baron EJ and Finegold SM, eds, "Gram-Negative Facultatively Anaerobic Bacilli and Aerobic Coccobacilli," *Bailey & Scott's Diagnostic Microbiology*, St Louis, MO: CV Mosby Co, 1990, 408-30.

Berbari EF, Cockerill FR 3d, and Steckelberg JM, "Infective Endocarditis Due to Unusual or Fastidious Microorganisms," *Mayo Clin Proc*, 1997, 72(6):532-42.

Das M, Badley AD, Cockerill FR, et al, "Infective Endocarditis Caused by HACEK Microorganisms," *Annu Rev Med*, 1997, 48:25-33.

Ellner JJ, Rosenthal MS, Lerner PI, et al, "Infective Endocarditis Caused by Slow-Growing, Fastidious, Gram-Negative Bacteria," *Medicine (Baltimore)*, 1979, 58(2):145-58.

Meyer DJ and Gerding DN, "Favorable Prognosis of Patients With Prosthetic Valve Endocarditis Caused by Gram-Negative Bacilli of the HACEK Group," *Am J Med*, 1988, 85(1):104-7.

Murray PR, Drew WL, Kobayashi GS, et al, eds, "Miscellaneous Gram-Negative Bacilli," *Medical Microbiology*, St Louis, MO: CV Mosby Company, 1990, 175-9.

Haemophilus ducreyi

Microbiology *Haemophilus ducreyi* is a gram-negative coccobacillus which causes a sexually transmitted disease called chancroid. It is indistinguishable on Gram's stain from other *Haemophilus* species (such as *H. influenzae*).

Epidemiology In 1838, chancroid (soft chancre) was first differentiated from syphilis (or hard chancre) by the French microbiologist Ricord. Although chancroid has remained an uncommon sexually transmitted disease in the U.S., its worldwide incidence may exceed that of syphilis. In 1986, there were 3418 cases reported, the largest number since the 1950s.

From 1981 to 1987, nine major outbreaks of chancroid were reported in the U.S. Chancroid was seen mainly in Hispanic and black heterosexual men who patronized prostitutes. In Florida, chancroid was seen in highly sexually active men without clear prostitute exposure. In Boston, the outbreak may have been related to individuals who had been originally infected in endemic foreign countries, such as Haiti and the Dominican Republic.

Clinical Syndromes *H. ducreyi* is an important cause of the syndrome of **genital ulceration with regional adenopathy**. Other sexually transmitted diseases that can cause this syndrome include primary syphilis, genital herpes simplex virus, lymphogranuloma venereum, and others. The incubation period for *H. ducreyi* is 1-21 days with an average of 7 days. Chancroid ulcers are painful, deep, shaggy and friable. The borders of the ulcer are undermined. In men, ulcers are more commonly single, but in women, the ulcers are multiple. Regional adenopathy occurs simultaneously with the ulcer and is seen in 50% to 65% of cases. The nodes are quite tender and tend to be unilateral. In addition, they tend to be fluctuant and can easily fistulize. Constitutional symptoms are uncommon.

Diagnosis Isolation of *Haemophilus ducreyi* from an active genital ulcer is the only accurate means of confirming a case of chancroid. However, special media and culture techniques are required to culture this fastidious organism, and the Microbiology Laboratory must be alerted to the possibility of *H. ducreyi*. Cotton or calcium alginate swabs should be rolled over a purulent ulcer base. The Gram's stain of an ulcer specimen may be misleading because of the presence of polymicrobial flora colonizing genital ulcers. Isolation of *H. ducreyi* from active genital ulcers is variable (50% to 80% depending on the culture medium). *H. ducreyi* is almost never isolated from aspiration of inguinal buboes.

Unfortunately, it is difficult to diagnose chancroid on the basis of clinical suspicion alone. Chancroid is presumptively diagnosed in patients presenting with genital ulcers with a negative RPR/VDRL, darkfield-negative for *T. pallidum*, and negative for HSV (by clinical appearance). However, as pointed out by Salzman et al, many such presumptive cases are ultimately found not to be chancroid.

Treatment Chancroid is an unusual disease in the U.S., and consultation with an Infectious Disease specialist is appropriate. Suggested therapy is erythromycin 500 mg orally 4 times/day for 7 days or ceftriaxone 250 mg I.M. times 1. Alternatives include co-trimoxazole DS orally twice daily for 7 days, or amoxicillin and clavulanate potassium 500 mg orally 3 times/day for 7 days, or ciprofloxacin 500 mg orally twice daily for 3 days. The choice of antibiotics is the same in pregnancy.

Drug Therapy

Recommended

Erythromycin *on page 722*

Ceftriaxone *on page 655*

Alternate

Co-Trimoxazole *on page 692*

Amoxicillin and Clavulanate Potassium *on page 593*

Ciprofloxacin *on page 678*

Selected Readings

Hammond GW, Slutchuk M, Scatliff J, et al, "Epidemiologic, Clinical, Laboratory, and Therapeutic Features of an Urban Outbreak of Chancroid in North America," *Rev Infect Dis*, 1980, 2(6):867-79.

Ronald AR and Plummer FA, "Chancroid and *Haemophilus ducreyi*," *Ann Intern Med*, 1985, 102(5):705-7.

Schmid GP, Sanders LL Jr, Blount JH, et al, "Chancroid in the United States. Reestablishment of an Old Disease," *JAMA*, 1987, 258(22):3265-8.

"1998 Guidelines for Treatment of Sexually Transmitted Diseases. Centers for Disease Control and Prevention," *MMWR Morb Mortal Wkly Rep*, 1998, 47(RR-1):1-111.

Haemophilus influenzae

Related Information

Haemophilus influenzae Vaccine *on page 1051*

Microbiology *Haemophilus influenzae* are typically gram-negative, aerobic (facultatively anaerobic), coccobacilli; however, they are often pleomorphic, gram-variable, and filamentous. There are six types (a-f) based on polysaccharide capsular properties; type b is the most invasive. There are also nonencapsulated, nontypable *Haemophilus influenzae*. There are eight different biotypes (with different biochemical properties) of which biotype 1 is most prevalent as a pathogen.

Haemophilus influenzae grows on chocolate agar which has X and V factors necessary for growth. It can also grow on Levinthal and Fildes enriched agar which are useful in determining encapsulation properties.

Epidemiology The epidemiology of *Haemophilus influenzae* is changing in the 1990s because of successful early childhood immunization, which is dramatically decreasing the incidence of invasive disease caused by *Haemophilus influenzae* b. *Haemophilus influenzae* is often found in the nasopharynx of normal asymptomatic individuals. Most *Haemophilus influenzae* isolates in the United States are nonencapsulated and rarely are pathogenic. Historically, the frequency of invasive disease was based on age with meningitis most common in children 2 month to 2 years of age, epiglottitis in the 3-5 years of age range, and other infections having an increasing incidence in older adults. The total increase incidence over the past two decades may have been due in part to improved laboratory identification of organisms.

Clinical Syndromes Early *Haemophilus influenzae* b vaccination has decreased the incidence of serious *Haemophilus influenzae* b disease dramatically over the past few years. *Haemophilus influenzae* can cause a variety of clinical syndromes including meningitis, epiglottitis, cellulitis, otitis, respiratory tract infection, and other infections.

- **Meningitis:** Although not a high mortality when diagnosed early, *Haemophilus influenzae* meningitis often causes permanent neurologic sequelae even when "successfully" treated. Meningitis characteristically occurred in infants up to 2 years of age.
- **Epiglottitis (ages 3-5 years):** Is a medical emergency which often requires ventilatory support if not managed promptly.
- *Haemophilus influenzae* **otitis:** Common in children of various ages.

(Continued)

Haemophilus influenzae (Continued)

- **Respiratory tract infections:** More common in adults, especially those with chronic obstructive pulmonary disease and smokers.

Diagnosis Diagnosis can be made by Gram's stain and culture of specimens from appropriate sites. Gram's stain will reveal gram-negative coccobacilli but is neither sensitive nor specific enough to be diagnostic. *Haemophilus influenzae* grows well on chocolate agar supplemented by growth factors V and X. These factors differentiate it from other *Haemophilus* species. Satellite colonies may appear around *S. aureus* species. Antigen detection for the polyribophosphate capsule is available but is no more sensitive than Gram's stain or culture. Subgrouping may be performed for epidemiologic purposes.

Diagnostic Tests/Procedures

Aerobic Culture, Appropriate Site *on page 310*
Gram's Stain *on page 426*

Treatment Meningitis and epiglottitis should be treated with a third generation cephalosporin when *Haemophilus influenzae* is suspected, as these are medical emergencies. Up to 30% of *Haemophilus influenzae* b strains are resistant to ampicillin. Less serious infections may be treated with ampicillin or amoxicillin (when susceptible), co-trimoxazole, or a second generation cephalosporin. Most strains are also susceptible to chloramphenicol and quinolones (not first line agents). *Haemophilus influenzae* b vaccine is now a part of routine vaccinations administered in the first few months of life.

Prophylaxis may be desirable in *H. influenzae* outbreaks or in close contacts with invasive disease. Rifampin is the recommended agent for prophylaxis in a 4-day regimen of 600 mg daily for adults and 20 mg/kg daily for infants and children.

Drug Therapy

Recommended
Severe infection:
Cephalosporins, 3rd Generation *on page 662*
Mild infection:
Co-Trimoxazole *on page 692*

Alternate
Severe infection:
Cephalosporins, 2nd Generation *on page 662*
Chloramphenicol *on page 667*
Fluoroquinolones *on page 736*
Mild infection:
Ampicillin *on page 604*
Amoxicillin and Clavulanate Potassium *on page 593*
Cefaclor *on page 627*
Amoxicillin *on page 592*

Selected Readings

Adams WG, Deaver KA, Cochi SL, et al, "Decline of Childhood *Haemophilus influenzae* Type b (Hib) Disease in the Hib Vaccine Era," *JAMA*, 1993, 269(2):221-6.

Baron EJ and Finegold SM, eds, "Gram-Negative Facultatively Anaerobic Bacilli and Aerobic Coccobacilli," *Bailey & Scott's Diagnostic Microbiology*, St Louis, MO: CV Mosby Co, 1990, 408-30.

Mohammdkhani M and Ruoff KL, "A 29-Year-Old Man With *Haemophilus influenzae* in the Cerebrospinal Fluid: Case Report and Review of the Organism," *Clin Microbiol Newslett*, 1998, 20(5):36-9.

Neumann MA and Thompson KD, "Acute Bacterial Meningitis: Prevention and Treatment," *Clin Microbiol Newslett*, 1998, 20(22):181-4.

Quagliarello V and Scheld WM, "Bacterial Meningitis: Pathogenesis, Pathophysiology, and Progress," *N Engl J Med*, 1992, 327(12):864-72.

Haemophilus influenzae Vaccine *see page 1051*

Hantavirus

Microbiology The virus family Bunyaviridae is composed of more than 200 mostly arthropod-borne RNA viruses (arboviruses) such as California encephalitis virus, LaCrosse virus, Rift Valley fever virus, Congo-Crimean hemorrhagic fever virus, Hantaan virus, and the genus Hantavirus. Hantavirus is composed of several (hantaviruses) which usually cause one of two severe clinical syndromes: hemorrhagic fever with renal syndrome (HFRS) and hantavirus pulmonary syndrome (HPS). Hantavirus, as the term is being used in the United States, most commonly refers to Muerto Canyon/Sin Nombre virus and to Black

Creek Canal virus, both of which cause HPS. Muerto Canyon virus is the virus which was responsible for the infamous outbreak of HPS in the Four Corners area (the intersection of New Mexico, Utah, Arizona, and Colorado) of the southwest United States in May, 1993. Hantaviruses are single-strand RNA, 80-120 nm, spherical, pleomorphic, enveloped viruses which are susceptible to most disinfectants.

Epidemiology Hantaviruses occur almost worldwide (see table). Human infection by hantavirus became a public health concern in the United States in the 1950s when U.S. soldiers who served in the Korean War developed Korean hemorrhagic fever (Hantaan virus). Muerto Canyon virus has been found only in North America. As of July 27, 1994, 83 cases of HPS (54% mortality) had been reported to the CDC, including the cases in the 1993 Four Corners outbreak, during which the natural history of Muerto Canyon virus was elucidated. The reservoir of the virus is *Peromyscus maniculatus*, the deer mouse, which always remains asymptomatic. If high populations of *Peromyscus* experience times of drought, scarce food, and reduced natural cover, the mice will seek food and shelter in human dwellings and outbuildings and drastically increase their contact with humans. Muerto Canyon virus is easily transmitted to humans by inhalation of aerosolized droplets of mouse urine and feces and by saliva from the bites of mice. The virus can be acquired in a laboratory setting; however, the virus is not transmitted human to human.

Hantavirus

Hantavirus	Geographical Location	Disease	Mortality (%)
Hantaan (prototype) and Seoul	Asia	HFRS	1-15
Puumala	Scandanavia, Western Europe	HFRS	Rare
Belgrade/Dobrava	Central and Eastern Europe	HFRS	5-35
Prospect Hill	Eastern and Midwest United States	None	?
Muerto Canyon and Black Creek Canal	North America	HPS	50-70

Clinical Syndromes HPS usually occurs in healthy young adults, and the presentation of HPS can be considered to be similar to that of acute respiratory distress syndrome (ARDS). The incubation period of HPS is 10-30 days. HPS usually begins with a short period of general myalgia and fever which is followed by 1-10 days of fever, cough, tachycardia, and tachypnea. Mild pulmonary edema can follow. In some cases, fulminating severe pulmonary edema manifested as ARDS can develop and can lead to shock and death in only a few hours. The mortality rate of HPS is extremely high (56% to 70%); however, successful respiratory therapy is possible, and complete recovery can occur in a few days. Histopathologically, lung tissue from patients with HPS show interstitial infiltration of lymphocytes and severe alveolar edema. Necrosis and polymorphonuclear infiltration is not present. The complete pathogenesis of HPS has not been completely established. HPS should be considered in any healthy adult who presents with unexplained ARDS.

Diagnosis The diagnosis of HPS is clinical and depends on careful examination of the patient's travel, work, and social history, on the patients living conditions, and on timely recognition of ARDS. The laboratory diagnosis of HPS caused by Muerto Canyon virus can be accomplished by viral culture and serology. Culture is not practical and not widely available. Almost all patients with HPS will have anti-Muerto Canyon IgG and IgM antibodies at the time of presentation and acute disease. Therefore, serological methods (enzyme immunoassay, haemagglutination inhibition, indirect immunofluorescence, complement fixation, and antibody neutralization) are the methods of choice. Both acute and convalescent sera must be tested if an accurate diagnosis of HPS is sought. Polymerase chain reaction and nucleic acid hybridization have been used to amplify and detect, respectively, Muerto Canyon virus DNA in fixed and sectioned tissue from infected patients.

Diagnostic Tests/Procedures

Hantavirus Serology *on page 430*
Polymerase Chain Reaction *on page 523*

Treatment Treatment is supportive and should be given in an intensive care unit. (Continued)

Hantavirus *(Continued)*

Drug Therapy Comment Ribavirin has been used to treat HPS; however, reproducible success has not been documented. Ribavirin used for this purpose can be obtained from the CDC.

Selected Readings

Beebe JL, "Emerging Infections: Hantavirus Disease Outbreak," *Clin Microbiol Newslett*, 1994, 16(10): 73-6.

Butler JC and Peters CJ, "Hantaviruses and Hantavirus Pulmonary Syndrome," *Clin Infect Dis*, 1994, 19(3):387-95.

Yablonski T, "The Mystery of the Hantavirus," *Lab Med*, 1994, 25:557-60.

Zhao X, "The Epidemiology of Hantavirus Infections," *Clin Microbiol Newslett*, 1997, 19(7):49-52.

HBV *see* Hepatitis B Virus *on page 162*

HCV *see* Hepatitis C Virus *on page 164*

HDV *see* Hepatitis D Virus *on page 168*

Helicobacter pylori

Related Information

Helicobacter pylori Treatment *on page 1076*

Synonyms *Campylobacter pylori*

Microbiology Controversy surrounds *Helicobacter pylori*, a gram-negative bacillus recently implicated as a cause of duodenal and gastric ulcers and a potential cause of the nonulcer dyspepsia syndrome. Originally named *Campylobacter pyloridis*, then *Campylobacter pylori*, this organism was renamed *Helicobacter pylori* in 1989. It is a spiral-shaped gram-negative bacillus which is susceptible *in vitro* to a variety of antimicrobial agents including tetracycline, metronidazole, amoxicillin, and clarithromycin. Resistance to these antibiotics has been described in some isolates, including metronidazole-resistant strains which have been associated with treatment failures. The organism is unique in its ability to survive the acidic pH of gastric fluids, which is otherwise sterile in healthy individuals. *H. pylori* is most commonly recognized in histologic analysis of gastric biopsies. Cultures for the organism are available in many laboratories but have variable sensitivity.

Epidemiology *H. pylori* has been associated with infection in adults over the age of 20 years, with an increased incidence with aging. The natural reservoir appears to be in humans, although the precise source is unknown. Transmission has been theorized to be fecal-oral. In some studies, *H. pylori* has been recovered from nearly 100% of patients with duodenal ulcers and has thus stimulated much research concerning its role as a possible etiologic agent of peptic ulcer disease.

Clinical Syndromes

- **Duodenal ulcers:** *H. pylori* has been implicated as a cause of duodenal ulcers in patients who are not receiving nonsteroidal anti-inflammatory agents. This is based on a number of lines of evidence. The prevalence of *H. pylori* in duodenal ulcer cases is nearly 100%. Eradication of *H. pylori* decreases the relapse rate of duodenal ulcers when compared with patients with duodenal ulcers who have persistent infection with *H. pylori*. Other experts have strongly disagreed with these findings and conclusions and suggest that *H. pylori* is only a cofactor in causation of duodenal ulcers.

- **Gastric ulcers:** Again, epidemiologic evidence suggests a relationship between *H. pylori* and gastric ulcers. Studies have suggested a weaker relationship with gastric ulcers than with duodenal ulcers, with 60% of gastric ulcer cases positive for *H. pylori*. (Some studies has shown a higher rate of recovery, approaching 100%). Relapse rates in patients who have been successfully treated for *H. pylori* have been close to 0% at 1 year, as compared with 60% in controls.

- **Non-ulcer dyspepsia:** In this difficult to define entity, individuals complain of chronic symptoms of abdominal pain similar to peptic ulcer disease but have no objective disease on upper endoscopy. *H. pylori* has also been associated with this condition. The results of studies eradicating *H. pylori* in non-ulcer dyspepsia have been inconclusive to date. The data suggest a subgroup of patients may in fact benefit from eradication of the organism, but the difficulty has been identifying such individuals prior to therapy.

- **Gastric carcinoma:** Limited evidence has linked chronic *H. pylori* infection with some individuals with gastric cancer.

Diagnostic Tests/Procedures
Helicobacter pylori Antigen, Direct *on page 431*
Helicobacter pylori Culture and Urease Test *on page 432*
Helicobacter pylori Culture, Gastric Biopsy *on page 433*
Helicobacter pylori Serology *on page 433*

Treatment The decision to treat an individual for *H. pylori* infection should be made after review of the conflicting opinions and the published data. Recent reviews on both sides of the issue are referenced below. An increasing body of literature is supporting the practice of treating individuals with histologically proven *H. pylori* infection. Patients who appear to benefit the most from therapy are those with recurrent duodenal ulcers (endoscopically proven), duodenal ulcers resistant to conventional therapy, or perforated duodenal ulcers. The data do not suggest that all patients with peptic ulcer disease will benefit from antibiotics. Only patients who have chronic *H. pylori* infection associated with peptic ulcer disease benefit from therapy; those with other mechanisms to produce ulcers (such as nonsteroidal-induced ulcers or Zollinger-Ellison syndrome) are not likely to benefit. One currently accepted treatment is a three drug regimen for 10-14 days, such as tetracycline, bismuth subsalicylate (Pepto-Bismol®), and metronidazole. Other successful regimens have substituted amoxicillin for tetracycline. There is a significant incidence of minor side effects such as nausea, vomiting, and diarrhea with these oral regimens. Patient compliance may be low, and close monitoring and encouragement is necessary. Some regimens have combined an H_2-antagonist or omeprazole with a combination antibiotic regimen with good results.

Drug Therapy
Recommended
Amoxicillin *on page 592*
Tetracycline *on page 944*
Metronidazole *on page 817*
Alternate
Bismuth Subsalicylate *on page 622*

Selected Readings
Dubois A, "Spiral Bacteria in the Human Stomach: The Gastric Helicobacters," *Emerg Infect Dis*, 1995, 1(3):79-85.
Dunn BE, Cohen H, and Blaser MJ, "*Helicobacter pylori*," *Clin Microbiol Rev*, 1997, 10(4):720-41.
Perez-Perez GI, Cutler AF, and Blaser MJ, "Value of Serology as a Noninvasive Method for Evaluating the Efficacy of Treatment of *Helicobacter pylori* Infection," *Clin Infect Dis*, 1997, 25(5):1038-43.
Van Enk RA, "Serologic Diagnosis of *Helicobacter pylori* Infection," *Clin Microbiol Newslet*, 1996, 18(12):89-91.
Versalovic J, "*Helicobacter pylori* Update," *Clin Microbiol Newslett*, 1998, 20(13):107-13.

***Helicobacter pylori* Treatment** *see page 1076*
Hepatitis A Immunization *see page 1055*

Hepatitis A Virus
Related Information
Hepatitis A Immunization *on page 1055*
Immunization Guidelines *on page 1041*
Occupational Exposure to Bloodborne Pathogens (Universal Precautions) *on page 1088*

Microbiology Hepatitis A virus (HAV; enterovirus 72) is a member of the Picovirus family (poliovirus, Coxsackievirus, echovirus). Mature HAV virions are nonenveloped, have icosahedral capsids, and contain single-stranded RNA.

Epidemiology HAV caused "infectious" hepatitis which was observed and recorded by Hippocrates. Epidemics of infectious hepatitis have been recorded throughout modern history, especially during World Wars I and II. Today, infectious hepatitis occurs worldwide and is very common in areas with poor sanitation and in institutional settings such as facilities for the developmentally disabled, the military, prisons, and day care centers. In developing countries, almost all persons become infected with HAV (or at least become HAV antibody-positive) during childhood. In developed countries, the number of HAV antibody-positive persons is age-dependent and increases sharply with adulthood. The natural reservoir for HAV is humans. HAV is spread by the oral-fecal route. Transmission of HAV by blood and blood products occurs, but it is a rare event. Chronic excretion of HAV has not been documented.

Clinical Syndromes HAV causes acute infectious hepatitis which is usually mild in children and young patients, more severe in adults, and almost impossible to distinguish from acute hepatitis caused by other viruses. The incubation period
(Continued)

Hepatitis A Virus *(Continued)*

for infectious hepatitis is about 30 days (range, 10-50 days). Typically, infectious hepatitis is characterized by a 1- to 7-day prodrome phase (fever, headache, fatigue, vomiting, abdominal pain, elevated serum ALT and AST levels [especially ALT]). (In all types of hepatitis, ALT levels are higher than AST levels.) Subsequently, more specific characteristics develop (dark urine, light-colored stool, jaundice, right upper quadrant pain, enlarged liver and spleen). Infectious hepatitis usually is acute and self-limiting. Infectious hepatitis is not chronic.

Diagnosis Infectious hepatitis is diagnosed clinically and serologically. The most useful methods for the laboratory diagnosis of infectious hepatitis are enzyme immunoassays for HAV-specific antibody (total and IgM). Almost all patients have anti-HAV IgM by the time symptoms are observed; IgM levels usually are not detectable 3-6 months after infection.

Diagnostic Tests/Procedures

Hepatitis A Profile *on page 434*

Drug Therapy Comment

No antiviral agents active against hepatitis A, but for pre-exposure and postexposure, prophylaxis intravenous immunoglobulins may be appropriate.

Drug Therapy

Recommended

Immune Globulin, Intramuscular *on page 770*
used in combination with
Hepatitis A Vaccine *on page 759*

Selected Readings

Battegay M, Gust ID, and Feinstone SM, "Hepatitis A Virus," *Principles and Practice of Infectious Diseases*, 4th ed, Mandell GL, Bennett JE, and Dolin R, eds, New York, NY: Churchill Livingstone, 1995, 1636-56.

Hojvat SA, "Diagnostic Tests for Viral Hepatitis," *Clin Microbiol Newslett*, 1989, 11:33-9.

Hepatitis B Virus

Related Information

Immunization Guidelines *on page 1041*
Occupational Exposure to Bloodborne Pathogens (Universal Precautions) *on page 1088*
Postexposure Prophylaxis for Hepatitis B *on page 1054*

Synonyms HBV

Microbiology Hepatitis B virus (HBV) is the etiological agent of serum hepatitis. HBV (archaic term, Dane particle) is a nonenveloped, partially double-stranded DNA virus which is trophic for liver cells. HBV is composed of a surface protein coat, a nucleocapsid, and internal proteins and nucleic acid. HBV usually is referred to as being composed of three antigens, surface (HB$_s$Ag), core (HB$_c$Ag), and e (HB$_e$Ag). The surface of HBV is a complex antigen with many determinants/epitopes. The amount of HB$_s$Ag produced during an infection usually is excessive, extremely large, and out of proportion to the amount needed to assemble mature, complete circulating HBV virions produced during infection. The HB$_c$Ag (nucleocapsid) is found in the blood only as an internal part of the complete HBV virion; HB$_c$Ag has not been detected free in blood. The HB$_e$Ag is always associated with complete infectious HBV particles and, therefore, with infectivity.

Epidemiology Serum hepatitis is a common and serious endemic disease throughout the world. The prevalence of serum hepatitis depends on age and socioeconomic situation. At least 280 million cases and 1 million persons are chronic carriers of HBV worldwide and in the United States, respectively. The carrier rate in some parts of Asia is 15%. The natural reservoirs of HBV are humans and probably a few other primates, such as chimps and monkeys. HBV is transmitted parenterally by needles and intravenous equipment, sexually, in unscreened blood products, and perinatally. HBV is not transmitted by the fecal-oral route. One of the sequelae of HBV infection, hepatocellular carcinoma, is a major public health problem worldwide. HBV probably is the cause of 80% of all cases of hepatocellular carcinoma worldwide. HBV has been found in almost all body secretions, but only blood, serum, semen, and vaginal fluids have been shown to be infectious. Perinatal transmission in developing countries is believed to be the main reason HBV is so prevalent worldwide. Perinatal infection has a high incidence resulting in chronic hepatitis, cirrhosis, and hepatocellular carcinoma.

Clinical Syndromes Most primary HBV infections are subclinical, self-limiting, and resolve within 3-6 months. HBV can produce mild to fulminant acute hepatitis, chronic persistent hepatitis, chronic active hepatitis, and hepatocellular carcinoma. The incubation period for serum hepatitis is 4-28 weeks. Signs and symptoms of acute serum hepatitis are quite variable and often include insidious onset of serum sickness-like illness, rash, and fever for several days to weeks. Subsequently, liver disease and joint involvement become clinically apparent. The presence of jaundice and abdominal pain are variable. This clinical condition usually is not distinguishable from that of acute disease caused by hepatitis A virus. Several variant forms of serum hepatitis have been described.

Diagnosis Diagnosis usually is made clinically, and determination of the specific etiological agent is made by serological and specific viral tests. Serological tests for several HBV antigens (surface and core) and antibodies to those antigens (antisurface, anticore, and anti-e) are widely available and clinically useful. Results of these tests are interpreted by consulting widely available charts which correlate various results (antigen and antibody patterns) with stages of infection. See the following tables and the listing Hepatitis B Profile *on page 435* for interpretation of the results of serology testing.

Diagnostic Tests/Procedures
Hepatitis B Profile *on page 435*

Drug Therapy Comment
Alpha interferon for chronic active hepatitis only. No drug therapy for acute hepatitis B. Hepatitis B immune globulin for prophylaxis.

Hepatitis B Serological Profile
Core Window Identification

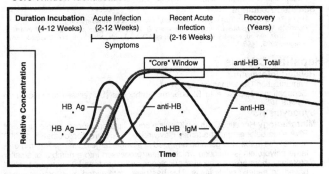

Hepatitis B Chronic Carrier
No Seroconversion

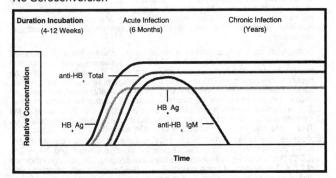

(Continued)

Hepatitis B Virus *(Continued)*

Hepatitis B Chronic Carrier
Late Seroconversion

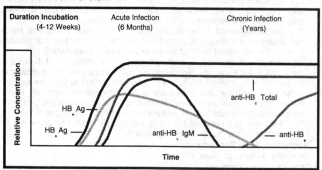

Duration Incubation (4-12 Weeks)	Acute Infection (6 Months)	Chronic Infection (Years)

Relative Concentration vs Time

HB_sAg, HB_eAg, anti-HB_c IgM, anti-HB_c Total, anti-HB_e

Drug Therapy
Recommended
    Interferon Alfa-2b *on page 778*
    Lamivudine *on page 793*
Prophylaxis:
    Hepatitis B Immune Globulin *on page 760*

Selected Readings
Hojvat SA, "Diagnostic Tests for Viral Hepatitis," *Clin Microbiol Newslett*, 1989, 11:33-9.

Robinson WS, "Hepatitis B Virus and Hepatitis D Virus," *Principles and Practice of Infectious Diseases*, 4th ed, Mandell GL, Bennett JE, and Dolin R, eds, New York, NY: Churchill Living-stone, 1995, 1406-39.

Hepatitis C Virus
Related Information
Immunization Guidelines *on page 1041*
Occupational Exposure to Bloodborne Pathogens (Universal Precautions) *on page 1088*

Synonyms HCV

Microbiology Hepatitis C virus (HCV) is a small, lipid-enveloped, single-stranded RNA virus belonging to the family Flaviviridae. There are approximately 10,000 nucleotides in the viral genome arranged in a single large open reading frame. A large polyprotein is encoded which is later processed into a number of smaller proteins. There are now six viral genotypes and more than 80 subtypes of HCV based on genetic relatedness. This has been determined by direct sequence analysis. Genotypes 1, 2, and 3 have a worldwide distribution, whereas geno-types 4, 5, and 6 are more localized. In the United States, about 66% of hepatitis C cases are due to genotype 1 (1a and 1b). The clinical significance of the various genotypes and subtypes is still under study, and it is not clear whether the natural history of the liver disease differs from one genotype to the other. However, response to antiviral therapy has been shown to be genotype-dependent.

During viral replication, a number of mutations occur which leads to substantial heterogeneity of the viral population. The RNA polymerase introduces random nucleotide errors at a high rate as it copies the viral RNA, particularly within the hypervariable region (HVR1) of one of the envelope proteins. For an individual patient infected with HCV, there exist a number of closely related, but heterogeneous, genome sequences termed "quasispecies". During the course of infection, antibodies develop against HVR1; but over a period of time, some of the evolving quasispecies may not be recognized by these neutralizing antibodies. This is one mechanism by which the virus can elude the immune system.

Epidemiology In the United States, HCV is the most common chronic blood-borne infection, according to the Centers for Disease Control and Prevention (CDC). Approximately 3.9 million Americans are infected with HCV, an incidence of 1.8%. The majority of these individuals are 30-50 years of age, asymptomatic, and unaware of their infection. The number of new cases of HCV in the U.S. has fallen considerably over the past decade, from 230,000 new cases per year in the late 1980s to 28,000 in 1998, an almost 90% decline. A number of factors have probably contributed to this decline, including the availability of laboratory assays for routine screening for HCV in blood donors, a decrease in the use of shared needles amongst injection drug users (primarily due to concerns for HIV transmission), and a decrease in the use of blood from paid donors. However, despite this recent decline in new cases, there is a large population who were infected during the HCV epidemic 10-20 years ago and will lead to a "cohort effect" in which the clinical impact of an epidemic 10-20 years ago will become apparent in the near future.

Routes of transmission:

Blood transfusions: HCV is the most common cause of transfusion-related hepatitis. Formerly termed non-A, non-B hepatitis, it is now clear that HCV is responsible for the majority of these cases. However, blood transfusion is not the most common route of transmission of HCV; in 1990, transfusions accounted for only 6% of new HCV cases. Aggressive screening of blood donors has helped decrease the incidence of HCV infection.

Intravenous drug use: Is the most commonly identified means of transmission. Up to 85% of I.V. drug users have serologic evidence of HCV infection. In 1990, about 40% of HCV cases appeared to be related to I.V. drug use.

Sexual transmission: Current data suggests that sexual transmission of HCV is inefficient. Some studies have shown no increased risk of HCV transmission between sex partners in a stable and monogamous relationship. Hepatitis B virus and HIV are much more easily acquired sexually.

Sporadic hepatitis: A number of individuals with serologic evidence of HCV infection have no obvious risk factor for acquisition. The extent of these "sporadic" cases has been debated with some estimates around 20% of all acute cases.

Miscellaneous: Other higher risk groups include healthcare workers, hemodialysis patients, individuals requiring multiple transfusions (hemophiliacs), and others.

Based on these considerations of the epidemiology of HCV, the CDC has made the following recommendations for screening for HCV.

Group 1: Patients who should be routinely tested for HCV (risk history - lifetime)
- Persons who injected illegal drugs, including those who injected even once many years ago and do not consider themselves as drug users
- Clotting factor recipients (before 1987)
- Transfusion or solid organ recipients (before July, 1992)
- Persons notified that they received blood from donor who later tested HCV-positive
- Long-term dialysis patients
- Persons with evidence of liver disease
- Healthcare workers exposed to anti-HCV antibody-positive blood
- Infants older than 12 months of age born to HCV-positive women

Group 2: Uncertain need for HCV testing
- Intranasal cocaine and other noninjection illegal drug users
- Persons with history of tatooing and body piercing
- Recipients of transplanted tissue (eg, corneal, musculoskeletal, skin, ova, sperm)
- Persons with a history of multiple sex partners or sexually transmitted diseases
- Long-term steady sexual partners of HCV-positive persons

Group 3: Routine HCV testing not recommended (risk history - lifetime)
- Men who have sex with men
- Healthcare, emergency medical, and public safety workers
- Pregnant women
- Household (nonsexual) contacts of HCV-infected persons

Clinical Syndromes
- **Asymptomatic infection:** The majority of cases (~75%) of HCV infection are asymptomatic. Some individuals are identified by serologic testing (eg, blood donor screening programs), but many remain undetected. This is particularly problematic for several reasons. The virus can be unknowingly

(Continued)

Hepatitis C Virus *(Continued)*

transmitted to others, liver damage occurs despite the absence of symptoms, and >50% will develop a chronic hepatopathy.

- **Acute HCV infection:** Following an initial incubation period (2 weeks to 6 months), the patient enters a "preicteric" phase. Symptoms tend to be nonspecific, with malaise and anorexia. In some cases, there is also right upper quadrant pain, nausea, and vomiting. This is followed by the "icteric" phase, where the patient presents with jaundice and dark urine. Systemic symptoms usually improve during the icteric phase. Several points should be noted: Infection with HCV cannot be accurately distinguished from other causes of viral hepatitis (including hepatitis B) on the basis of clinical presentation alone; the course of acute HCV tends to be more indolent than hepatitis B; clinical symptoms may be quite variable; a high clinical suspicion should be maintained since serologic tests for HCV may be negative early on. Fulminant hepatic failure secondary to acute HCV infection is a rare but important complication.

Although a serum sickness-like illness with fever, arthritis, and skin rash has been well recognized in acute hepatitis B infection, only rarely has this been reported with hepatitis C infection. Other extrahepatic complications of acute HCV include aplastic anemia and pancreatitis.

- **Chronic HCV infection:** Over 50% of individuals infected with HCV develop chronic liver disease (hepatitis B, 5% to 10%). Symptoms are usually mild and nonspecific, with the main complaint being fatigue. The diagnosis is often difficult since liver function tests may be normal or only minimally elevated much of the time. Liver abnormalities include chronic persistent hepatitis, chronic active hepatitis, and cirrhosis.

Chronic HCV infection has been associated with several syndromes, including membranoproliferative glomerulonephritis, type II cryoglobulinemia, hepatocellular carcinoma; growing evidence supports an epidemiologic link between chronic HCV and hepatocellular carcinoma, independent of hepatitis B infection or alcoholic liver disease.

Diagnosis As noted above, the diagnosis of HCV infection is quite difficult on clinical grounds alone and routine liver function tests may intermittently be normal. Thus, laboratory confirmation is essential.

Serologic tests: These assays are designed to detect host antibodies to HCV. Several caveats: antibodies to HCV remain undetectable until weeks or months after the initial infection; serologic studies may be needed at 6 months (90% of seroconverters identified) and possibly 12 months; in a few individuals, antibodies to HCV fail to develop for unclear reasons at any time postinfection. Available tests include:

- Enzyme-linked immunosorbent assay (ELISA) for detection of antibody against the C100-3 protein. One of the earlier tests made available, it has been found to have a high false-positive rate.
- ELISA for antibody to core protein C22. This "second generation" test is currently a popular screening test in many laboratories. False-negative reactions are still possible.
- Radioimmunoblot assay (RIBA) is used as a supplemental or confirmatory test for patients who are anti-HCV positive by ELISA. Currently the RIBA is designed to detect distinct antibodies to four different HCV proteins, including protein C100-3.

Molecular detection methods:
- Polymerase chain reaction for amplification and detection of small quantities of HCV RNA (target amplification) directly from blood specimens.
- Branched chain detection for detection of HCV RNA from blood without target amplification (signal amplification).
- Hepatitis C viral RNA genotyping

Diagnostic Tests/Procedures

Treatment The treatment of HCV infection is rapidly evolving and changes in recommended therapies occur often. A specialist in hepatology or infectious diseases should be consulted if therapy is being considered.

In 1991, interferon (IFN-alpha2b) became the first drug approved for use in hepatitis C. This was administered at 3 million units 3 times/week for a 6-month period. The sustained response rate was low, about 10% to 20%. (In clinical trials, a "sustained response" is defined as having normal ALT tests and undetectable HCV by PCR 6 months after discontinuing the therapy. Relapses after therapy usually occur within 6 months). Although the number of patients who demonstrated a sustained response was low, 90% of those who did respond were still in remission 5 years later, with undetectable HCV, normal ALTs, and improvements in the liver biopsy histology. Later, it was shown that treating for a longer period of time, 12-18 months, with IFN-alpha2b led to a modest increase in the sustained response rate.

More recently, studies have shown that the combination of IFN-alpha2b given in combination with ribavirin is about three times greater than monotherapy with IFN-alpha2b alone. Ribavirin as monotherapy is ineffective. The IFN-alpha2b and ribavirin combination has led to a 40% sustained response rate in clinical trials. The success of this combination depends in large part on the HCV genotype of the individual patient. Persons with genotype 1 (the most common in the United States) have a 28% sustained response compared with 66% of persons infected with genotypes 2 and 3. There are a number of side effects seen with this regimen including flu-like symptoms, psychiatric manifestations, and hemolytic anemia.

In one study, predictors of a sustained response with initial IFN-alpha2b/ribavirin therapy included:
- HCV genotype 2 or 3
- HCV RNA $<2 \times 10^4$ copies/mL
- liver fibrosis stage 0-1
- female sex
- age <40 years

The risks and benefits of combination therapy are under study in several groups with HCV infection including:
- Patients with normal liver function tests - earlier studies suggested that treatment might exacerbate liver disease and cause increased ALT (at least with IFN monotherapy)
- Persons with hemophilia - there has been a concern that IFN would stimulate anti-factor VIII antibody production
- Persons with renal disease - IFN may be poorly tolerated in this group with high dropout rates
- Persons with HIV and HCV

In 1997, the National Institutes of Health (NIH) consensus statement on management of HCV recommended the following:

Persons Recommended for Treatment (greatest risk for progression to cirrhosis):
- Patients with persistently elevated ALT levels,
- Detectable HCV RNA, and
- A liver biopsy indicating either portal or bridging fibrosis and at least moderate degrees of inflammation and necrosis.

Persons for Whom Treatment Is Unclear:
- Patients with compensated cirrhosis (without jaundice, ascites, variceal hemorrhage, or encephalopathy)
- Patients with persistent ALT elevations but with less severe histologic changes (ie, no fibrosis and minimal necroinflammatory changes). In these patients, progression to cirrhosis is likely to be slow, if at all. Therefore, observation and serial measurements of ALT and liver biopsy every 3-5 years are an acceptable alternative to treatment with interferon.
- Patients <18 years or >60 years of age

Persons for Whom Treatment Is Not Recommended:
- Patients with persistently normal ALT values
- Patients with advanced cirrhosis who might be at risk for decompensation with therapy
- Patients who are currently drinking excessive amounts of alcohol or who are injecting illegal drugs (treatment should be delayed until these behaviors have been discontinued for >6 months)

(Continued)

Hepatitis C Virus *(Continued)*

- Persons with major depressive illness, cytopenias, hyperthyroidism, renal transplantation, evidence of autoimmune disease, or who are pregnant

Drug Therapy

Recommended

Interferon Alfa-2b *on page 778*

Interferon Alfa-2b and Ribavirin Combination Pack *on page 780*

Selected Readings

Alter MJ, Mast EE, Moyer LA, et al, "Hepatitis C," *Infect Dis Clin North Am*, 1998, 12(1):13-26.

Bell H, Hellum K, Harthug S, et al, "Treatment With Interferon-Alpha2a Alone or Interferon-Alpha2a Plus Ribavirin in Patients With Chronic Hepatitis C Previously Treated With Interferon-Alpha2a. CONSTRUCT Group," *Scand J Gastroenterol*, 1999, 34(2):194-8.

Davis GL, Esteban-Mur R, Rustgi V, et al, "Interferon Alfa-2b Alone or in Combination With Ribavirin for the Treatment of Relapse of Chronic Hepatitis C. International Hepatitis Interventional Therapy Group," *N Engl J Med*, 1998, 339(21):1493-9.

Liang TJ, "Combination Therapy for Hepatitis C Infection," *N Engl J Med*, 1998, 339(21):1549-50.

Management of Hepatitis C," *NIH Consens Statement*, 1997, 15(3):1-41.

McHutchison JG, Gordon SC, Schiff ER, et al, "Interferon Alfa-2b Alone or in Combination with Ribavirin as Initial Treatment for Chronic Hepatitis C. Hepatitis Interventional Therapy Group," *N Engl J Med*, 1998, 339(21):1485-92.

Poynard T, Marcellin P, Lee SS, et al, "Randomised Trial of Interferon Alpha2b Plus Ribavirin for 48 Weeks or for 24 Weeks Versus Interferon Alpha2b Plus Placebo for 48 Weeks for Treatment of Chronic Infection With Hepatitis C Virus. International Hepatitis Interventional Therapy Group," *Lancet*, 1998, 352(9138):1426-32.

"Recommendations for Prevention and Control of Hepatitis C (HCV) Infection and HCV-Related Chronic Disease. Centers for Disease Control and Prevention," *MMWR Morb Mortal Wkly Rep*, 1998, 47(RR-19):1-39.

Hepatitis D Virus

Related Information

Occupational Exposure to Bloodborne Pathogens (Universal Precautions) *on page 1088*

Synonyms HDV

Microbiology Hepatitis D virus (HDV) is the etiological agent of delta hepatitis. HDV was first recognized in an Amazon tribe in 1969 and was first described in 1977. HDV is a small (35-40 nm) virus composed of only a circular single-strand RNA genome and a two-protein complex (the delta antigen) which surrounds and is intimately associated with the RNA. The RNA genome is the smallest of any animal virus. HDV can replicate on its own but requires the presence of HBV for transmission. Therefore, HDV is a defective/incomplete virus and invariably is found only in persons with acute or chronic HBV infection. During coinfection and when HBV and HDV are within the same cell, the HDV acquires a protein coat (envelope) composed of HBV surface antigen. This coat allows HDV to infect other cells. HDV will not be found in a HBV surface antigen-negative person.

Epidemiology HDV is present in extremely high numbers in circulating blood and usually is transmitted parenterally in ways similar to those of HBV (eg, by blood, blood products, and contaminated needles). In general, delta hepatitis is most prevalent in populations at high risk for hepatitis B (eg, multiply infused patients, intravenous drug users, hemophiliacs, inhabitants of underdeveloped countries, etc). Sexual transmission of HDV has been reported. Hepatitis D is a worldwide problem because the many millions of worldwide carriers of HBV surface antigen are potentially susceptible to HDV. Worldwide, HDV is present in about 5% of HBV carriers. Many epidemics of hepatitis D outside of the United States have been described, particularly in Africa and South America. In the United States, hepatitis B is a reportable disease, but hepatitis D is not reportable. This is probably because hepatitis D is not easy to diagnose, it is not common in the United States, and it is not yet a public health problem. HDV causes <1% of all viral hepatitis diseases.

Clinical Syndromes Acute viral hepatitis is a distinct clinical entity and usually is not too difficult to diagnose. In general, the diseases produced by hepatitis A, B, C, D, and E viruses are clinically indistinguishable. The clinical presentations of the diseases vary drastically from asymptomatic infections to icteric hepatitis to fulminant and fatal hepatitis.

Acute delta hepatitis occurs either as a coinfection at the same time as acute hepatitis B or as a superinfection during chronic hepatitis B. In both cases, the resulting disease is more severe than hepatitis B alone. A third type of hepatitis D has been suggested, a latent HDV infection which is active only after a subsequent HBV infection. Hepatitis D coinfection usually is clinically indistinguishable from acute hepatitis B, except the course is more severe. Less than 5% of patients with acute HDV coinfection develop chronic hepatitis D; however, most patients with hepatitis D acquired as a superinfection develop chronic hepatitis D. Patients who experience a superinfection can deteriorate rapidly and experience abrupt liver failure. Both acute and chronic hepatitis D are usually severe. Mortality rates for acute hepatitis D are 2% to 20%. Sixty percent to 70% of patients with chronic hepatitis D develop cirrhosis; most of these patients die of liver disease.

Diagnosis Viral hepatitis usually is diagnosed clinically, and determination of the specific etiological agent is made by serological and specific viral tests. Serological tests for anti-HDV IgG and IgM antibodies are widely available and clinically useful. Results of these tests are interpreted by consulting widely available charts which correlate various results (antigen and antibody patterns) with stages of infection. Tests for HDV antigen are available but are technically demanding and are not particularly diagnostically useful. Hepatitis A, B, C, D, and E viruses produce somewhat characteristic, but essentially indistinguishable, lesions in the liver. Polymerase chain reaction and associated nucleic acid probe tests for HDV RNA and HDV antigen have been reported.

Diagnostic Tests/Procedures

Hepatitis D Serology on page 442

Drug Therapy Comment Currently, no antiviral therapy effective against hepatitis D.

Selected Readings

Gupta S, Govindarajan S, Cassidy WM, et al, "Acute Delta Hepatitis: Serological Diagnosis With Particular Reference to Hepatitis Delta Virus RNA," Am J Gastroenterol, 1991, 86(9):1227-31.

Holt DA, Baran DA, Oehler RL, et al, "Delta Hepatitis: A Diagnostic Algorithm," Infect Med, 1993, 10:23-9.

Hsu HH, Feinstone SM, and Hoofnagle JH, "Acute Viral Hepatitis," Principles and Practice of Infectious Diseases, 4th ed, Mandell GL, Bennett JE, and Dolin R, eds, New York, NY: Churchill Livingstone, 1995, 1136-53.

Polish LB, Gallagher M, Fields HA, et al, "Delta Hepatitis: Molecular Biology and Clinical and Epidemiological Features," Clin Microbiol Rev, 1993, 6(3):211-29.

Hepatitis E Virus

Related Information

Occupational Exposure to Bloodborne Pathogens (Universal Precautions) on page 1088

Synonyms HEV

Microbiology Hepatitis E virus (HEV) is an unenveloped single-strand RNA virus, is structurally similar to caliciviruses, and is found in the stool of hepatitis E patients during incubation and early acute phase of the disease. HEV is the etiological agent of "epidemic" or "enterically transmitted" non-A, non-B hepatitis and is associated with epidemics and contaminated water. ("Classic" non-A, non-B hepatitis is caused by hepatitis C virus and is associated with parenteral exposure.)

Epidemiology HEV causes <1% of all viral hepatitis diseases. Hepatitis E is transmitted by the fecal-oral route, is found in stool, and has been reported to be the cause of several large outbreaks of hepatitis in India, China, Peru, Russia, Africa, and Mexico. None of these epidemics were associated with either HAV or HBV; most of these outbreaks were associated with fecally contaminated water supplies and poor sanitation. Hepatitis E is very rare in the United States. HEV has not caused outbreaks in the United States and western Europe. Hepatitis E occurs only rarely in the United States, where persons with hepatitis E are almost always immigrants from endemic areas. Mortality rates of pregnant females who acquire hepatitis E are very high (15% to 30%), and fetal wastage is common.

Clinical Syndromes Clinically, hepatitis E is similar to hepatitis A except for the following: early presentations tend to include pruritus and joint pain; cholestasis is common; concentrations of serum aminotransferase and alkaline phosphatase tend to be lower and higher, respectively.

Diagnosis Hepatitis E is diagnosed clinically. Antibody to HEV develops early in the disease. Laboratory tests to detect antibody to HEV (immune electron microscopy and inhibition of immunofluorescence) are available in only a few (usually research) laboratories.

Diagnostic Tests/Procedures

Hepatitis E Serology on page 443

(Continued)

Hepatitis E Virus (Continued)

Drug Therapy Comment Currently, no antiviral therapy effective against hepatitis E.

Selected Readings

"Hepatitis E Among U.S. Travelers, 1989-1992," *MMWR Morb Mortal Wkly Rep*, 1993, 42(1):1-4.

Hsu HH, Feinstone SM, and Hoofnagle JH, "Acute Viral Hepatitis," *Principles and Practice of Infectious Diseases*, 4th ed, Mandell GL, Bennett JE, and Dolin R, eds, New York, NY: Churchill Livingstone, 1995, 1136-53.

Yarbough PO, "Hepatitis E: Diagnosis of Infection," *Clin Microbiol Newslett*, 1993, 15(15):113-5.

Herpes Simplex Virus

Synonyms HSV

Microbiology Herpes simplex is a member of the DNA virus family herpesvirus. Herpes simplex 1 and 2 can be differentiated by neutralization titrations but often cross react. Differentiating the simplex virus from other members of the family is performed by antigenic analysis, and DNA, polypeptide, and molecular analysis.

Epidemiology Herpes simplex virus (HSV) infections occur worldwide. HSV 1 infection is common in childhood. By the fourth decade, approximately 90% of individuals will be seropositive for HSV 1. In lower socioeconomic groups, the incidence is even higher. HSV 2 is less common than HSV 1, and primary infections tend to occur in an older age group. The seroprevalence of HSV 2 in the U.S. is 10% to 40%. Clearly, HSV 2 is an important sexually transmitted disease (STD), and seroprevalence correlates well with increasing sexual activity. Up to 50% of young adults attending an STD clinic may demonstrate seropositivity for HSV 2. The general rule that HSV 1 causes "above the waist" infections and HSV 2 causes "below the waist" infections still holds true in many cases, but cross infections are increasingly common.

The incubation period following exposure to the virus is about 1 week (range 1-26 days). HSV transmission is most efficient in individuals with active ulcerations of the mucous membranes or genitalia but can still occur when virus is shed asymptomatically. HSV 1 can be cultured from the oropharynx of 2% to 9% of healthy adults and 5% to 8% of healthy children, indicating that asymptomatic shedding of the virus is common. Similarly, HSV 2 can be recovered from the genital tracts of asymptomatic, sexually active patients.

Clinical Syndromes

- **Genital herpes:** Herpes genitalis is still more commonly caused by HSV 2 (70% to 90% of cases), although there are a sizeable number of cases caused by HSV 1 (10% to 30%). Young adults and adolescents are most commonly infected. In males, vesicular lesions occur on the penile shaft or glans. In the female, similar lesions are seen in a variety of areas, including the cervix, perineum, vulva, and vagina. Symptoms are most severe during the primary infections, and patients may display fever and inguinal lymph node enlargement. The vesicles are typically tender and have an erythematous base. Lesions may persist for weeks with severe primary infections but eventually crust over. Recurrent genital lesions occur in both sexes. The systemic symptoms and severity of the lesions are diminished in comparison with primary infection. Patients will often complain of a prodrome of burning prior to an outbreak. Lesions typical for HSV develop during recurrences and heal over 7-10 days. Some patients experience frequent recurrences. Data suggests that chronic suppression with acyclovir may be useful in decreasing the number of outbreaks per year.

- **Oral HSV infections:** Primary herpes gingivostomatitis is seen mainly in children and is caused by HSV 1 in 90% of cases. Less commonly, primary infection occurs in the young adult; in such cases infection may be from either HSV 1 or 2. The incubation period following exposure is 2-12 days. Vesicles develop in the oral cavity, including the pharynx, palate, buccal mucosa, and/or tongue. The vesicles rapidly break down into small ulcers and are covered with an exudate. Lesions may extend to involve the lips and cheek. Severe primary lesions can be accompanied by high fevers, malaise, cervical lymphadenopathy, and dehydration. However, it is known that primary oral HSV infections are most commonly asymptomatic or mild. The lesions generally resolve without therapy in 2 weeks. HSV pharyngitis is probably under-recognized in the college-aged population, where it may be misdiagnosed as "strep throat." Recurrent HSV labialis (lip lesions) is problematic in some adults. Recent data suggest that chronic daily acyclovir may have some minor benefit in this group. In patients who are immunosuppressed, recurrences of HSV labialis can be quite severe.

- **Herpetic keratitis:** HSV 1 is one of the most common causes of corneal blindness. Patients typically present with unilateral eye pain, lacrimation, conjunctivitis, and blurred vision. It is important to identify HSV because topical corticosteroids can worsen the condition. Recurrences are common. Permanent visual damage may occur if there is significant corneal scarring. Other eye diseases associated with HSV infection include chorioretinitis (seen in HIV-infected individuals as a result of disseminated HSV) and the acute retinal necrosis syndrome (a rare cause of visual loss seen in healthy adults).

- **Herpetic whitlow:** This is the term used for HSV infection of the finger. It may result from occupational exposure, as in a respiratory technologist whose finger is inoculated with virus from a patient excreting the virus orally. Characteristically, there are vesicular lesions on the finger, with redness and edema. Recurrences are common. The lesions may be mistaken for bacterial pustules, especially when the patient presents with fever and regional lymphadenopathy. Many physicians mistake these lesions as being filled with pus and, subsequently, lance the lesions. The lesion can then develop a secondary bacterial infection.

- **HSV infections of the central nervous system:** HSV 1 is the most common cause of sporadic encephalitis in the United States. Encephalitis may result from primary HSV 1 infection, reactivation, or reinfection. It is theorized that the virus travels along the olfactory nerve of a susceptible host and reaches the temporal lobe of the brain. Patients present with the subacute onset of confusion. Other features include fever, headache, focal seizures, and olfactory hallucinations. It is difficult to distinguish encephalitis caused by HSV from other etiologies of encephalitis (such as arboviruses, tuberculosis, fungal infections, etc). Cerebrospinal fluid findings are usually nondiagnostic, and HSV 1 is only rarely isolated from spinal fluid culture. Electroencephalography (EEG) is helpful in localizing the area of inflammation to the temporal lobe. CT scan or MRI scan of the brain can reveal necrosis of the temporal lobe in some cases, a finding highly suggestive of HSV encephalitis. The definitive diagnostic test is the brain biopsy, with viral culture and histopathology. However, surgeons are becoming less willing to perform this invasive procedure and may suggest an empiric course of intravenous acyclovir instead.

- **HSV and AIDS:** Severe and recurrent HSV infections are frequently seen in AIDS. Progressive perianal ulcerations with proctitis may be due to either HSV 1 or 2. This infection may be quite debilitating, with anorectal pain, bloody stools, tenesmus, and fever. Such patients usually respond to I.V. or oral acyclovir. Since recurrences are the rule, these patients are often placed on chronic acyclovir suppression. This has led to the emergence of acyclovir-resistant HSV mutants and progressive rectal infection. HSV esophagitis may result from direct extension of oral HSV lesions into the esophagus or from reactivation of HSV in the vagus nerve which innervates the esophagus. The clinical presentation is indistinguishable from *Candida* esophagitis, another common condition in AIDS. Unfortunately, HSV esophageal lesions have a nonspecific appearance both on barium swallow and upper endoscopy, and tissue biopsy is required to rule out *Candida* (or cytomegalovirus) esophagitis.

- **HSV pneumonia:** This unusual manifestation of HSV is seen in the immunosuppressed. Cases have also been reported in burn unit patients. The pathogenesis is direct extension of herpetic tracheobronchitis into the lungs. A necrotizing pneumonia results, and bronchoscopy is usually required to confirm the diagnosis.

- **Neonatal infection:** HSV infection in newborns (younger than 6 weeks of age) is frequently devastating. Visceral dissemination of the virus and central nervous system infection are common. Untreated, the mortality exceeds 65%. Many who survive exhibit developmental disabilities. Infection occurs most commonly during delivery as the neonate passes through an infected birth canal. *In utero* infection, while reported, is much less common.

Diagnosis Diagnosis can be made by culture, stain and/or serology depending on the clinical setting. Culture is performed on cell culture, with cytopathic effects appearing as early as 24-48 hours after inoculation. Monoclonal antibodies are also used to identify and type HSV isolates. Direct examination of a lesion can
(Continued)

Herpes Simplex Virus *(Continued)*

be done, staining a scraping with Giemsa stain (Tzanck smear). A variety of serology tests are also available with a fourfold rise in convalescence titers necessary in primary disease. Some laboratories offer polymerase chain reaction (PCR) techniques to detect HSV DNA directly in body fluids (most commonly, urine, CSF, and vesicular fluid). PCR appears to be more sensitive than culture and enzyme immunoassays which detect HSV protein antigens. Unlike culture methods, PCR can detect viral DNA in herpetic lesions and body secretions several days after symptoms subside and after lesions no longer yield culturable virions. The clinical relevance of this ability to detect prolonged presence and shedding of virus is not known. On the other hand, PCR to detect HSV DNA probably yields the most clinically useful and relevant results when used to evaluate CSF from patients with HSV meningitis and/or encephalitis. Although the test is extremely sensitive and specific and can be extremely useful in carefully selected patients, it is not widely available, has not been described extensively in the literature, and should be neither offered nor used routinely.

Diagnostic Tests/Procedures

Electroencephalography *on page 397*
Herpes Cytology *on page 444*
Herpes Simplex Antibody *on page 445*
Herpes Simplex Virus Culture *on page 446*
Herpes Simplex Virus by Direct Immunofluorescence *on page 445*
Herpes Simplex Virus Isolation, Rapid *on page 447*
Polymerase Chain Reaction *on page 523*
Skin Biopsy *on page 535*

Treatment Acyclovir is the drug of choice for most herpes infections. For primary genital lesions, a 7-10 day course of oral acyclovir may decrease pain and viral shedding by several days. Topical acyclovir is less effective. Acyclovir is of limited utility in recurrences of genital herpes lesions, although long-term low dose oral acyclovir may be of benefit in preventing chronic recurrences (>6 per year). Herpes keratitis is often best treated with topical ophthalmic idoxuridine or trifluridine. Disseminated herpes simplex or HSV encephalitis should be treated aggressively with high-dose I.V. acyclovir. In patients who are failing therapy or who are intolerant to acyclovir, ganciclovir or foscarnet may be utilized. In immunocompromised patients, such as transplant or chemotherapy patients, HSV infection can be prevented with prophylactic administration of acyclovir or ganciclovir.

Drug Therapy Comment Famciclovir and valacyclovir, only, have the indications for treatment of varicella-zoster infections and recurrent HSV infections. These agents have not been studied in immunocompromised patients.

Drug Therapy

Recommended

Acyclovir *on page 581*

Alternate

Famciclovir *on page 729*
Foscarnet *on page 739*
Ganciclovir *on page 745*
Valacyclovir *on page 965*

Selected Readings

Corey L, Spear PG, "Infections with Herpes Simplex Viruses," *N Engl J Med*, 1986, 314(11):686-91 and 314(12):749-57.

Erlich KS, Mills J, Chatis P, et al, "Acyclovir-Resistant Herpes Simplex Virus Infections in Patients With the Acquired Immunodeficiency Syndrome," *N Engl J Med*, 1989, 320(5):293-6.

Field AK and Biron KK, "'The End of Innocence' Revisited: Resistance of Herpesvirus to Antiviral Drugs," *Clin Microbiol Rev*, 1994, 7(1):1-13.

Marcon MJ and Salamon D, "Traditional and Newer Approaches to Laboratory Diagnosis of Herpes Simplex Virus Infections," *Clin Microbiol Newslett*, 1997, 19(2):9-14.

Stone KM and Whittington WL, "Treatment of Genital Herpes," *Rev Infect Dis*, 1990, 12(Suppl 6):S610-9.

Whitley RJ, Kimberlin DW, and Roizman B, "Herpes Simplex Viruses," *Clin Infect Dis*, 1998, 26(3):541-55.

Herpes Zoster *see* Varicella-Zoster Virus *on page 294*

HEV *see* Hepatitis E Virus *on page 169*

HHV-6 *see* Human Herpesvirus-6 *on page 175*

Histoplasma capsulatum

Microbiology *Histoplasma capsulatum* is a dimorphic fungus of low pathoge-nicity. It differs from other pathogenic fungi in that it is primarily a parasite of the reticuloendothelial system and rarely is found extracellular.

In the mold form, it has microconidia (2-6 μm) on short lateral branches or sessile on the sides of hyphae and large round to pyriform tuberculate macroco-nidia (8-14 μm) . This mold form is found in the soil and grows best in humid, shady environments at modest temperatures. Bird droppings and bat guano facilitate its growth. The spores become airborne and are inhaled.

The yeast form may be seen in human infections by direct examination. The cells are ovoid, 1-2 μm by 3-3.5 μm, and proliferate in macrophages (and occasionally neutrophils) which can be seen intracellular throughout the reticulo-endothelial system including lymph nodes, bone marrow, spleen, liver, and adrenal glands.

Epidemiology Histoplasmosis is the most frequently diagnosed systemic fungal disease with approximately 500,000 cases per year in the United States. Endemic areas include the Mississippi and Ohio River Valleys, as well as some parts of Central America. Environmental sources include caves, chicken coops, bamboo canebrakes, bird roosts, school yards, prison grounds, decayed wood piles, dead trees, chimneys, and old buildings. Epidemics typically occur where contaminated soil is disturbed causing the spores to become airborne.

Clinical Syndromes

- **Asymptomatic:** Approximately 99% of all cases of histoplasmosis are asymptomatic and is an incidental finding on autopsy or seen as calcification on plain films of the lungs or spleen or noted as lymphadenopathy.
- **Acute histoplasmosis:** Typically presents as a flu-like syndrome with fever (95%), anorexia (85%), nonproductive cough (75%), and chest pain (75%). Retrosternal pain is a prominent feature and may be related to mediastinal adenopathy. Skin and joint involvement is more common in women. Phys-ical exam is typically normal except for pulmonary crackles and adenopathy. Chest x-ray may reveal hilar and mediastinal adenopathy with or without patchy or diffuse infiltrates. Rarely, patients present with pericarditis with or without tamponade. This syndrome is typically self-limited, lasting approxi-mately 2 weeks.
- **Histoplasmomas:** Granulomatous nodules form on the lungs, usually in the lower lobes and less than 3 cm. Usually associated with hilar lymph node calcification, and 75% are found to be solitary lesions.
- **Acute pulmonary histoplasmosis:** Self-limited interstitial pneumonitis.
- **Chronic histoplasmosis:** Chronic pulmonary disorder that typically occurs in older patients with emphysema. Mimics tuberculosis. Referred to as the "marching cavity" because, in >50% of the cases, the walls of the lung cavity gradually enlarge.
- **Mediastinal histoplasmosis:** Approximately 25% of patients who develop this syndrome present with SVC syndrome, pulmonary vessel or esopha-geal or large airway obstruction, which may require surgical intervention. Rarely, associated with fibrosing mediastinitis.
- **Disseminated:** Defined as extrapulmonic spread with progressive clinical illness (ie, intestinal or oral ulcers, endocarditis, adrenal involvement). Both reactivation of previously acquired infections and newly acquired infections can occur in immunocompromised individuals. Classified as an AIDS-defining illness. Ten percent to 20% of all HIV-infected patients with dissemi-nated histoplasmosis experience a rapid, fulminant course of the infection with findings of hypotension, respiratory insufficiency, multiple end-organ failure, disseminated intravascular coagulation, and mental status changes. In the remainder of the patients, the disease can be more chronic, mani-festing as fever, weight loss, dry cough, hepatomegaly, splenomegaly, and lymphadenopathy. Approximately 10% of AIDS patients with disseminated histoplasmosis have nonspecific skin manifestations. The chest radio-graphic findings of disseminated histoplasmosis in AIDS patients are varied and nonspecific. Over 50% of AIDS patients with disseminated histoplas-mosis will have normal chest radiographs. Unusual manifestations of disseminated histoplasmosis including chorioretinitis, meningitis, and brain abscesses have been observed in patients with HIV disease. Since the presence of CNS disease may influence the choice of antifungal therapy, a

(Continued)

Histoplasma capsulatum (Continued)

brain imaging study should be performed in AIDS patients with disseminated histoplasmosis and symptoms indicating possible CNS involvement.

Diagnosis Skin tests are usually not helpful. Over 50% of the population in endemic areas may have positive skin tests. Approximately 50% of patients that do have disseminated diseases may have negative skin tests secondary to impaired immunity. False-positive skin tests may occur secondary to other systemic fungal diseases. Similar results are found with the complement fixation tests, however, a fourfold rise in titer is significant. A radioimmunoassay that detects *H. capsulatum* polysaccharide antigen (HPA) demonstrated positivity in >90% of patients with disseminated infection. False-positive results have been noted in patients with other disseminated fungal infections. The level of HPA declines promptly with treatment and increases upon relapse. Results are interpreted as <1.0 is negative, 1.0-2.0 is weakly positive, and >2.0 is positive. Direct examination and isolation in culture is the preferred diagnostic procedure.

Diagnostic Tests/Procedures

Fungal Serology *on page 410*

Fungus Culture, Appropriate Site *on page 414*

Histoplasma capsulatum Antigen Assay *on page 450*

Histoplasmosis Serology *on page 450*

KOH Preparation *on page 467*

Treatment No antifungal treatment is necessary for mild or asymptomatic histoplasmosis. Acute, nondisseminated disease is self-limited and requires only symptomatic care unless it persists for more than 3 weeks, at which time ketoconazole may be initiated. Heavy exposure, acute diffuse pulmonary involvement with respiratory insufficiency, and disseminated disease requires treatment with amphotericin B.

Patients with erythema nodosum or erythema multiform and arthralgias/arthritis may be treated with NSAIDs or corticosteroids. Eighty percent of patients with chronic pulmonary histoplasmosis respond to ketoconazole but have a higher relapse than those treated with amphotericin B.

Although ketoconazole has been shown to be effective in normal hosts, ketoconazole is not recommended for use in patients with AIDS given its high failure rate in both acute management and suppressive therapy.

AIDS patients with moderate to severe disseminated histoplasmosis or with evidence of endocarditis or CNS involvement should be treated with amphotericin B 1 mg/kg/day for a minimum of 15 mg/kg total dose followed by consolidation therapy with itraconazole 200 mg twice daily for 12 weeks followed by itraconazole 200-400 mg/day for life.

AIDS patients with mild disease may be treated initially with itraconazole 300 mg twice daily for 3 days then 200 mg twice daily for 12 weeks followed by chronic suppressive therapy with itraconazole 200-400 mg/day.

High-dose fluconazole, 800 mg/day, is associated with a higher relapse rate compared with itraconazole. The role of liposomal amphotericin B products is unclear.

Life-long suppressive therapy is recommended in HIV-infected individuals due to the high frequency of relapse. Relapse rates of 50% to 90% have been reported in AIDS patients with disseminated histoplasmosis who have not received any maintenance therapy. Infusions of amphotericin B (50-80 mg weekly or biweekly) prevent relapse. Oral itraconazole is the preferred drug of choice for chronic suppressive therapy for histoplasmosis. Fluconazole 200-400 mg/day orally appears to be somewhat less effective than itraconazole as long-term suppressive therapy but may be used in patients who are unable to tolerate or absorb itraconazole.

Studies are currently in progress to examine whether chronic suppressive therapy may be discontinued in AIDS patients who have had presumed immune restoration following potent antiretroviral therapy.

Drug Therapy

Recommended

Severe infection:

Amphotericin B (Conventional) *on page 597*

Chronic pulmonary infection in immunocompetent hosts:
Ketoconazole *on page 791*
Itraconazole *on page 785*

Selected Readings

Bradsher RW, "Histoplasmosis and Blastomycosis," *Clin Infect Dis*, 1996, 22(2):S102-11.

Lee BL, Tauber MG, and Aberg JA, "Histoplasmosis," *The AIDS Knowledge Base*, 3rd ed, Chapter 59, Philadelphia, PA: Lipincott Williams & Wilkins, 1999, 679-84.

Sharkey-Mathis PK, Velez J, Fetchick R, et al, "Histoplasmosis in the Acquired Immunodeficiency Syndrome (AIDS): Treatment With Itraconazole and Fluconazole," *J Acquir Immune Defic Syndr*, 1993, 6(7):809-19.

Wheat LJ, Connolly-Stringfield PA, Baker RL, et al, "Disseminated Histoplasmosis in the Acquired Immune Deficiency Syndrome: Clinical Findings, Diagnosis and Treatment, and Review of the Literature," *Medicine*, 1990, 69(6):361-74.

Wheat J, Hafner R, Korzun AH, et al, "Itraconazole Treatment of Disseminated Histoplasmosis in Patients With the Acquired Immunodeficiency Syndrome. AIDS Clinical Trial Group," *Am J Med*, 1995, 98(4):336-42.

Wheat J, Hafner R, Wulfsohn M, et al, "Prevention of Relapse of Histoplasmosis With Itraconazole in Patients With the Acquired Immunodeficiency Syndrome. The National Institute of Allergy and Infectious Diseases Clinical Trials and Mycoses Study Group Collaborators," *Ann Intern Med*, 1993, 118(8):610-6.

HIV *see* Human Immunodeficiency Virus *on page 177*

HIV Therapeutic Information *see page 1008*

HLTV-I *see* Human T-Cell Lymphotropic Viruses *on page 180*

Hookworm *see* Ancylostoma duodenale *on page 66*

HSV *see* Herpes Simplex Virus *on page 170*

HTLV-II *see* Human T-Cell Lymphotropic Viruses *on page 180*

HTLV-III *see* Human Immunodeficiency Virus *on page 177*

Human Herpesvirus-6

Synonyms HHV-6

Microbiology In 1986, a novel cytopathic virus was isolated from peripheral blood cells from patients with lymphoproliferative disease. The virus was originally named human β-lymphotropic virus because of its ability to infect B cells *in vitro* but later was found to be tropic for primarily T lymphocytes. It has since been classified as one of the human herpesviruses. It is a double-stranded DNA virus with an icosahedral capsid and outer envelope. HHV-6 is indistinguishable from other herpesviruses by electron microscopy, with the same morphology and size. In addition to its T-lymphocyte tropism, HHV-6 can infect B cells, monocytes, macrophages, and other cell lines. CD4⁺ T cells, in particular, are targets for viral infection. The genome has been analyzed and sequenced for research purposes. A close homology between HHV-6 DNA and cytomegalovirus DNA has been found. The degree of relatedness of these two viruses remains to be seen since the gene products of HHV-6 are still being studied. There appear to be two general types of HHV-6, types A and B. The clinical significance of these two types is unknown, although most clinical isolates are type B.

Epidemiology Knowledge of the epidemiology of HHV-6 is still evolving. Much of the epidemiologic data for this virus will rest on the use of specific serologic tests. Unfortunately, serologic techniques are still being developed and have yet to be standardized. Earlier use of an immunofluorescence assay for antibody detection has been criticized on technical grounds and is probably too insensitive. To date there is no accepted gold standard for serologic tests and "borderline" positive specimens are difficult to interpret.

Available data indicate that HHV-6 infection occurs at an early age, between 6 months and 3 years most commonly. The seroprevalence is about 80% in the general population. It is likely to be as common as other herpesvirus infections. Newborns have a high level of antibody, probably from passive transfer from the mother. The titer of antibody rapidly decreases in the neonate as maternal antibody is lost; this is followed later by a second peak of antibody signifying primary infection in childhood.

Preliminary data suggest that asymptomatic HHV-6 shedding occurs in seropositive individuals. The virus has been isolated from the saliva of healthy children and adults who have had prior HHV-6 infection. Asymptomatic salivary excretion in the general population has been hypothesized as the main reservoir of the virus in the community and potentially could explain the large number of children who become infected. Initial studies reported very high salivary excretion rates, but later studies failed to confirm these results. Some experts have been critical
(Continued)

Human Herpesvirus-6 (Continued)

of the methodologies employed in the earlier studies, suggesting that some of the viral isolates could have been HHV-7 rather than HHV-6. At the present time, it is clear that salivary excretion does take place, but the precise incidence is still debatable.

The mechanism(s) of HHV-6 transmission have not been definitively established. It is also unclear whether the virus can be transmitted by transfusion of blood products or by transplantation of organs.

Clinical Syndromes

- **Exanthem subitum (roseola):** Also known as roseola infantum, exanthem subitum is a benign disease of childhood that is caused by HHV-6. The disease is most common in children aged 6 months to 3 years old. In typical cases, there is an abrupt onset of high fever (often 40°C), and in a variable number of cases there may be additional symptoms such as sore throat, otitis, or cervical adenopathy. After 3-5 days, the fever resolves completely. This is followed 24-48 hours later by a maculopapular rash involving the trunk and neck. Although the rash itself is nonspecific in appearance, the timing of the rash is distinctive for roseola. The rash also resolves spontaneously after several days. Roseola is nearly always a benign disease. More serious complications of acute HHV-6 infection have been described (meningoencephalitis, hepatitis). During the febrile phase of exanthem subitum, HHV-6 can be cultured from peripheral blood mononuclear cells. Seroconversion can also be documented.

- **Undifferentiated febrile illness:** Primary HHV-6 infection appears to be a common, identifiable cause of high fevers in children. In a recent study, 14% of children who presented to an emergency room for evaluation of fever were found to have HHV-6 viremia. Of note, the rash of classic roseola was absent in many children, and the most common presentation was irritability, inflamed tympanic membranes, and temperatures higher than 40°C. Although the full range of HHV-6 infection has yet to be determined, it is likely that many primary infections are either nonspecific, febrile syndromes or entirely asymptomatic.

- **HHV-6 in adults:** Primary infection with HHV-6 is probably uncommon in adults. The clinical course of such infections have been described in small numbers of adults with documented seroconversion. Symptoms included fever, headache, and fever lasting over 1 week. Cervical lymphadenopathy was noted in several cases and was persistent for months. Laboratory abnormalities included a minor elevation in liver function tests, leukopenia, and atypical lymphocytosis. Latent HHV-6 infection appears to take place following primary infection, as with other herpesviruses. Reactivation has also been reported in adults. Little is known about the incidence or mechanisms underlying either latency or reactivation.

- **HHV-6 in immunocompromised hosts:** The role of HHV-6 in transplant recipients is still largely unknown. The following observations have been made: 1. Many individuals are seropositive for HHV-6 prior to transplantation. 2. An increase in specific antibody against HHV-6 is commonly seen after transplantation. Viremia with HHV-6 also appears to be common at 2-3 weeks post-transplantation, earlier than the peak for cytomegalovirus. The importance of these findings has yet to be determined. 3. Primary infection with cytomegalovirus in the transplant patient is often associated with a significant rise in HHV-6 antibodies. The significance of this simultaneous seroconversion is unclear. 4. Some kidney biopsy specimens which have demonstrated acute rejection have stained positive for HHV-6. The relationship between HHV-6 and acute rejection is unknown.

HHV-6 has also been implicated by some as a possible cofactor in HIV infection. This is based on several observations, including the mutual tropism for the host's CD4+ T lymphocytes. Whether HHV-6 alters the natural course of HIV infection is still under study.

Diagnosis Viral isolation can be performed in specialized laboratories. HHV-6 can be cultured in peripheral blood mononuclear cells (with or without the addition of donor cells). Standard tissue culture used for isolation of other viruses is suboptimal for HHV-6. Even under optimal conditions, the cytopathic effect of HHV-6 in peripheral blood mononuclear cells can be subtle; multiple passages of the virus in culture may be necessary. Detection methods are then necessary to confirm the presence of this virus.

HHV-6 has been isolated from clinical samples of saliva and blood. Antigen detection methods, while still being perfected, have been used to identify the virus directly from biopsy samples. Polymerase chain reaction has been used successfully in limited reports. A serologic test has recently become available.

Diagnostic Tests/Procedures

Human Herpesvirus 6, IgG and IgM Antibodies, Quantitative *on page 458*

Treatment Most infections caused by HHV-6 are mild and self-limiting. Susceptibility to antiviral agents are probably similar to CMV, where acyclovir only inhibits the organism at high concentrations. Ganciclovir has been shown to inhibit HHV-6 at achievable concentrations, although this data is inconsistent.

Drug Therapy Comment No drug therapy is recommended.

Selected Readings

Agbede O, "Human Herpesvirus 6: A Virus in Search of a Disease," *Clin Microbiol Newslet*, 1993, 15(4):25-28.

Chou S, "Human Herpesvirus 6 Infection and Associated Disease," *J Lab Clin Med*, 1993, 121(3):388-93.

Pruksananonda P, Hall CB, Insel RA, et al, "Primary Human Herpesvirus-6 Infection in Young Children," *N Engl J Med*, 1992, 326(22):1445-50.

Rathore MH, "Human Herpesvirus 6," *South Med J*, 1993, 1197-1205.

Yamanishi K, "Pathogenesis of Human Herpesvirus 6 (HHV-6)," *Infect Agents Dis*, 1992, 1(3):149-55.

Human Immunodeficiency Virus

Related Information

HIV Therapeutic Information *on page 1008*

Synonyms AIDS Virus; HIV; HTLV-III; Human T-Cell Lymphotrophic Virus

Microbiology HIV is one of the four known pathogenic human retroviruses and a member of the Lentiviruses. There are two recognized subtypes of HIV; HIV-1 causes AIDS worldwide, and HIV-2 produces an AIDS-like illness but appears to be less pathogenic than HIV-1. HIV is an enveloped virus about 100 μm in diameter that forms by budding from cell membranes. HIV is diploid, meaning that an electron-dense central core surrounds two identical copies of a single-stranded viral RNA genome. Reverse transcriptase catalyzes the transcription of the RNA genome into a double-stranded DNA (known as the "provirus") that migrates from the cytoplasm to the nucleus, integrates into the host cell DNA, and remains integrated for the lifetime of the cell. HIV contains three essential genes for viral replication, "gag", "pol", and "env". "Gag" (glycosaminoglycan) refers to genes which code for group antigens associated with viral core proteins which include p24. "Pol" (polymerase) encodes reverse transcriptase. "Env" (envelope) encodes the envelope surface glycoproteins gp 120 and gp 41.

Epidemiology HIV is now the leading cause of death of men aged 25-40, the sixth leading cause of death of adolescent males 15-24 years of age, and the fourth leading cause of death in women 25-44 years of age. It is estimated that over 1 million U.S. residents are HIV infected; roughly 1 out of 250. By the year 2000, it is estimated by the World Health Organization that there will be 40 million HIV-infected individuals worldwide.

Male homosexuality continues to be the most common mode of transmission. HIV secondary to I.V. drug use and heterosexual transmission continues to rise. Approximately 14% of reported cases of AIDS in 1994 are women as compared to 5% in 1991. Nationally for both men and women, 7% of cases are secondary to heterosexual contact, however in Florida, New York, and California that number approaches 30%. Minorities account for a disproportionate amount of AIDS as expected by population statistics.

Clinical Syndromes During initial HIV infection, CD4 counts transiently decrease and HIV antigen (viremia) rises; antibody is detectable usually by 3 months. At 2-6 weeks after infection, patients may develop viral-like illness consisting of fever, sweats, fatigue, malaise, lymphadenopathy, sore throat, and sometimes splenomegaly. Patients may remain asymptomatic for months to years depending on the progression of their disease. In 1993, the Centers for Disease Control revised the previous classification of HIV (see table on next page).

(Continued)

Human Immunodeficiency Virus (Continued)

1993 Revised CDC HIV Classification System and Expanded AIDS Surveillance Definition for Adolescents and Adults
(MMWR Morb Mortal Wkly Rep, 1992, 41:RR-17.)

The revised system emphasizes the importance of CD4-lymphocyte testing in clinical management of HIV-infected persons. The system is based on three ranges of CD4 counts and four clinical categories giving a matrix of nine exclusive categories. The system replaces the 1986 classification.

Criteria for HIV Infection

Persons 13 years of age or older with repeatedly (2 or more) reactive screening tests (ELISA) plus specific antibodies identified by a supplemental test, eg, Western blot ["reactive" pattern = positive for any two of p24, gp41, or gp120/160 (MMWR, 1991, 40:681)]. Other specific methods of diagnosis of HIV-1 include virus isolation, antigen detection, and detection of HIV genetic material by PCR.

Classification System

CD4 Cell† Category	Clinical Category*		
	A	B	C
≥500/mm³	A1	B1	C1
200–499/mm³	A2	B2	C2
<200/mm³	A3	B3	C3

*See following clinical definitions. Italics indicate expansion of AIDS surveillance definition. Category C currently "reportable." Categories A3 and B3 are "reportable" as AIDS effective January 1, 1993.

†There is a diurnal variation in CD4 counts averaging 60/mm³ higher in the afternoon in HIV-positive individuals and 500/mm³ in HIV-negative persons. Blood for sequential CD4 counts should be drawn at about the same time of day each time (J AIDS, 1990, 3:144). The equivalence between CD4 counts and CD4 % of total lymphocytes: ≥500 = ≥29%, 200–499 = 14%-28%, <200 = <14%.

Clinical Category A
Asymptomatic HIV infection
Persistent generalized lymphadenopathy (PGL)*
Acute (primary) HIV illness
*Nodes in two more extrainguinal sites, at least 1 cm in diameter for ≥3 months.

Clinical Category B
Symptomatic, not A or C conditions
Examples include but not limited to:
> Bacillary angiomatosis
> Candidiasis, vulvovaginal: persistent >1 month, poorly responsive to therapy
> Candidiasis, oropharyngeal
> Cervical dysplasia, severe, or carcinoma in situ
> Constitutional symptoms (eg, fever >38.5°C or diarrhea >1 month)

The above must be attributed to HIV infection or have a clinical course or management complicated by HIV.

Clinical Category C†
Candidiasis: esophageal, trachea, bronchi
Coccidioidomycosis, extrapulmonary
Cryptococcosis, extrapulmonary
Cervical cancer, invasive†
Cryptosporidiosis, chronic intestinal (>1 month)
CMV retinitis, or other than liver, spleen, nodes
HIV encephalopathy
Herpes simplex with mucocutaneous ulcer >1 month, bronchitis, pneumonia
Histoplasmosis: disseminated, extrapulmonary
Isosporiasis, chronic (>1 month)
Kaposi's sarcoma
Lymphoma: Burkitt's, immunoblastic, primary in brain
M. avium or M. kansasii, extrapulmonary
M. tuberculosis,† pulmonary or extrapulmonary
Mycobacterium, other species disseminated or extrapulmonary
(Continued)

Pneumocystis carinii pneumonia
Pneumonia,† recurrent (≥2 episodes in 1 year)
Progressive multifocal leukoencephalopathy
Salmonella bacteremia, recurrent
Toxoplasmosis, cerebral
Wasting syndrome due to HIV

†These are the 1987 CDC case definitions (*MMWR*, 1987, 36:15). The 1993 CDC *Expanded Surveillance Case Definition* includes all conditions contained in the 1987 definition (above) plus persons with documented HIV infection and any of the following: (1) CD4 T-lymphocyte count <200/mm³ (or CD4 <14%), (2) pulmonary tuberculosis,† (3) recurrent pneumonia† (≥2 episodes within 1 year) or, (4) invasive cervical carcinoma.†

Diagnosis Is made serologically. Detection of HIV antibody by ELISA must be confirmed by Western blot. Alternate diagnosis may be made by viral culture, antigen detection, or HIV by polymerase chain reaction (PCR). Maternal antibodies may persist in infants until 18 months of age; therefore, CD4 counts, viral culture, and/or PCR followed by antibody detection after 18 months must be performed in order to diagnose HIV in infants.

Diagnostic Tests/Procedures
HIV Genotyping *on page 456*
HIV-1 RNA, Quantitative bDNA, 3rd Generation *on page 451*
HIV-1 RNA, Quantitative PCR, 2nd Generation *on page 452*
HIV-1 Serology *on page 454*
Human Immunodeficiency Virus Culture *on page 459*
p24 Antigen *on page 509*
T4/T8 Ratio *on page 545*

Treatment Currently, the optimal therapy for HIV infection is still being studied. Recent evidence suggests that a combination of antiretroviral agents is superior to monotherapy (ie, single antiretroviral agent). Several combinations of nucleoside analogs appear effective including zidovudine and epivir, didanosine and stavudine, and others. The protease inhibitors such as ritonavir, saquinavir, and indinavir represent a new class of antiretroviral agents with a different mechanism of action from the older nucleoside analogs. The role of the protease inhibitors is under intense study (see reference below). Available evidence strongly suggests that the protease inhibitors should not be used as monotherapy due to the development of viral resistance. Instead, combinations of nucleoside analogs and protease inhibitors appear to be superior in selected patients. However, the optimal time for initiation of a protease inhibitor is still under study. Most clinical trials have studied these agents in patients with moderate or advanced HIV.

Drug Therapy
Recommended
Indinavir *on page 773*
Lamivudine *on page 793*
Ritonavir *on page 909*
Do not take with carbonated colas as may cause emesis.
Saquinavir *on page 915*
Zidovudine *on page 977*
Didanosine *on page 704*
Nevirapine *on page 839*
Zalcitabine *on page 974*

Selected Readings
American College of Physicians and Infectious Diseases Society of America, "Human Immunodeficiency Virus Infection," *Clin Infect Dis*, 1994, 18(6):963-73.
Chaisson RE and Volberding PA, "Clinical Manifestations of HIV Infection," *Principles and Practice of Infectious Diseases*, 4th ed, Mandell GL, Bennett JE, and Dolin R, eds, New York, NY: Churchill Livingstone, 1995, 1217-52.
Cotton P, "Use of Antiretroviral Drugs in HIV Disease Declines Following Preliminary Results From Concorde Trial," *JAMA*, 1994, 271(7):488-9.
"Guidelines for the Use of Antiretroviral Agents in Pediatric HIV Infection," *MMWR Morb Mortal Wkly Rep*, 1998, 47(RR-4):16.
Isada CM, "Protease Inhibitors: Promising New Weapons Against HIV," *Cleve Clin J Med*, 1996, 63(4):204-8.
"Public Health Service Task Force Recommendations for the Use of Antiretroviral Drugs in Pregnant Women Infected With HIV-1 for Maternal Health and for Reducing Perinatal HIV-1 Transmission in the United States," *MMWR Morb Mortal Wkly Rep*, 1998, 47(RR-2):16-7.
"Report of the NIH Panel to Define Principles of Therapy of HIV Infection and Guidelines for the Use of Antiretroviral Agents in HIV-Infected Adults and Adolescents," *MMWR Morb Mortal Wkly Rep*, 1998, 47(RR-5).
U.S. Department of Health and Human Resources, *Evaluation and Management of Early HIV Infection*, Agency for Health Care Policy and Research Pub No. 94-0572, January 1994 (to obtain copy call 1-800-342-AIDS).

(Continued)

Human Immunodeficiency Virus *(Continued)*

"1997 USPHS/IDSA Guidelines for the Prevention of Opportunistic Infections in Persons Infected With Human Immunodeficiency Virus. USPHS/IDSA Prevention of Opportunistic Infections Working Group," *MMWR Morb Mortal Wkly Rep*, 1997, 46(RR-12):1-46. (Updated on website www.hivatis.org)

Watkins BA, Klotman ME, and Gallo RC, "Human Immunodeficiency Viruses," *Principles and Practice of Infectious Diseases*, 4th ed, Mandell GL, Bennett JE, and Dolin R, eds, New York, NY: Churchill Livingstone, 1995, 1590-1605.

Human T-Cell Lymphotrophic Virus *see* Human Immunodeficiency Virus *on page 177*

Human T-Cell Lymphotropic Viruses

Synonyms HLTV-I; HTLV-II

Microbiology Human retroviruses are members of the family *Retroviridae*: 100 nm, enveloped, single-strand RNA viruses which contain a reverse transcriptase used by the viruses to transcribe viral RNA into DNA. The newly formed DNA can integrate into host cell genome DNA. The family Retroviridae is composed of three genera: *Oncovirinae* (HTLV-I and -II), *Lentivirinae* (HIV-1 and HIV-2), and *Spumavirinae* (syncytial foamy viruses of cattle and cats). HTLV-I and -II are not related genetically, medically, or antigenically to HIV-1 and -2. However, the four viruses have similar routes of transmission and can have extremely long periods of latency prior to manifestation of disease. In addition, blood is screened for the presence of each of the four viruses.

Epidemiology HTLV-I is endemic in southern Japan (3% to 20%), the Carribean (2% to 5%), the U.S. Gulf Coast, and many other scattered populations throughout the world. Most of the persons infected with HTLV-I are asymptomatic. HTLV-II is endemic in some Native American populations in Florida and New Mexico but is detected mostly in intravenous drug users and their sexual partners. In the United States, seroprevalence of anti-HTLV in asymptomatic blood donors, and intravenous drug users and prostitutes is ~0.05% and 7% to 49%, respectively. Specific testing for separate antibodies to HTLV-I and HTLV-II is not routinely available, especially for large scale screening and epidemiological studies. HTLV-I and (probably) HTLV-II are transmitted transplacentally (extremely effective), parenterally (almost exclusively by sharing needles), by sexual contact (especially male to female), and by receipt of infected blood products.

Clinical Syndromes

- **Adult T-cell leukemia/lymphoma (ALT):** HTLV-I is the etiological agent of adult T-cell leukemia/lymphoma (ATL), a malignant proliferation of infected T cells. ATL can be extremely slow progressing or it can be fulminant and lead to death in a few months. ATL commonly is characterized by skin lesions, lymphadenopathy, splenomegaly, and hepatomegaly.

- **Tropical spastic paraparesis (TSP):** HTLV-I also causes most of the cases of tropical spastic paraparesis (TSP), more recently known as **HTLV-I-associated myelopathy (HAM)**. TSP/HAM is characterized by deficits such as weakness in the legs which progresses to spastic paraparesis and incontinence, in many ways not unlike the characteristics of multiple sclerosis. Approximately 5% and 0.25% of carriers of HTLV-I will develop ATL and HAM, respectively.

- HTLV-II has been detected in some patients with T-cell malignancies and in some patients with TSP/HAM-like illnesses, and it probably causes illnesses similar to those caused by HTLV-I. However, HTLV-II has not been conclusively shown to be the etiological agent of any specific disease.

CDC Guidelines for patients: The following advice from the CDC should be given to all patients who are seropositive for HTLV.

- HTLV is not HIV and does not cause AIDS.
- Inform your physician of your positive status if the physician does not know.
- Do not donate blood, semen, organs, or any other tissues.
- Do not share needles or syringes.
- Do not breast feed.
- Use latex condoms during sex (practice safe sex) if your monogamous partner is HTLV-negative or if you have multiple sex partners.

Diagnosis The diagnosis of HTLV-I and -II infections is a clinical diagnosis supported by laboratory diagnosis. HTLV nucleic acid in peripheral lymphocytes can be detected directly by Southern blot restriction mapping and by polymerase chain reaction amplification and subsequent nucleic acid hybridization. Peripheral leukocytes from persons suspected of having HTLV can be cultured *in vitro*, but culture is extremely specialized and not widely available. Serology is the routine method of choice. In the serological diagnosis of HTLV infection, most laboratories follow an algorithm to assure maximum sensitivity and specificity. Sera are screened for HTLV by use of an enzyme immunoassay which is repeated if a positive result is obtained. A second positive screen result is followed by confirmation by some combination of immunofluorescence, immunoblotting, and radioimmunoprecipitation methods.

Diagnostic Tests/Procedures HTLV-I/II Antibody

Selected Readings

Dobkin JF, "Update on HIV's Distant Cousins: HTLV-I and -II," *Infect Med*, 1993, 10(11).

Lee H, Burczak JD, and Shih J, "Human T-Cell Lymphotrophic Virus Type I and II," *Manual of Clinical Microbiology*, 6th ed, Murray PR, Baron EJ, Pfaller MA, et al, eds, Washington, DC: American Society for Mcrobiology, 1995, 1115-20, Progressive Multifocal.

Recommendations for Counseling Persons Infected With Human T-Lymphotropic Virus, Types I and II. Centers for Disease Control and Prevention and U.S. Public Health Service Working Group, *MMWR Morb Mortal Wkly Rep*, 1993, 42(RR-9):1-13.

Stoeckle W, "Introduction-Type C Oncoviruses Including Human T-Cell Lymphotrophic Viruses Types I and II," *Principals and Practice of Infectious Diseases*, 4th ed, Mandell GL, Bennett JE, and Dolin R, eds, New York, NY: Churchill Livingston, 1995, 1579-84.

Immunization Guidelines *see page 1041*

Influenza Virus

Related Information

Immunization Guidelines *on page 1041*

Microbiology Influenza virus is the etiological agent of influenza, is an enveloped, double-stranded (multi-segmented) RNA virus, and is the only member of the Orthomyxovirus family. Influenza virus is broadly classified into three groups (A, B, and C) which are based primarily on antigenic (serological) differences in internal proteins. The envelope of influenza virus contains transmembrane proteins H (three types) and N (two types) which are associated with hemagglutination and neuraminidase activities, respectively. Gradual and continual antigenic changes in the H and N proteins (usually the H) are called "antigenic drift" and are responsible for bypassing human immunity year to year. Sudden and major antigenic changes in the H and N proteins are called "antigenic shift" and are responsible for worldwide epidemics (pandemics) of influenza every 10-20 years or so. Strains of influenza are designated by the type of internal protein, host species (human if not designated), strain number, year of isolation, and H/N types (eg, A/California/10/78/H1N2). The natural reservoirs of influenza virus are as follows: type A, humans and many types of animals; type B, humans; type C, swine. Type A is by far the most prominent and important because of its association with pandemics of influenza.

Epidemiology Influenza virus causes influenza and is an important cause of worldwide respiratory disease. Recurrent episodes of influenza (due to antigenic drift and usually in isolated countries or regions of the world) have been observed every 1-3 years for the last 400 years. Worldwide pandemics of influenza occur every 10-20 years and have been responsible for an estimated 21 million deaths. Influenza virus is spread person to person by inhalation of the virus in aerosolized droplets and possibly by contaminated fomites.

Clinical Syndromes Signs and symptoms of influenza vary greatly and can range from a mild upper respiratory tract illness to rapidly fatal pneumonia. There are three basic clinical presentations of influenza virus infection:

- **Uncomplicated rhinotracheitis:** Abrupt onset of headache, myalgia, malaise, runny nose, chills, and cough. The course of this disease is usually 7-10 days.
- **Rhinotracheitis and subsequent bacterial pneumonia:** Typical rhinotracheitis, a brief period of feeling well, and subsequent secondary bacterial pneumonia typically caused by *Streptococcus pneumoniae*, *Staphylococcus*, or *Haemophilus influenzae*.
- **Frank viral pneumonia:** Can be fulminating and can lead to hypoxia and death in only a few days.

Diagnosis Influenza usually is diagnosed clinically, but laboratory diagnosis and confirmation is highly recommended because symptoms of influenza often are not readily distinguishable from those caused by other respiratory pathogens. Influenza virus is rather easily grown in cell culture, and positive cultures can be observed within 4 days. Some laboratories offer direct detection of influenza-
(Continued)

Influenza Virus *(Continued)*

infected cells obtained from nasopharyngeal aspirates or swabs, or from sputum. Serological tests for antibodies for influenza virus are easy to perform and are cost-efficient. Influenza-specific antibodies often can be detected as soon as 4-7 days after the onset of symptoms and can reach peak titers at 14-21 days after symptoms. However, serological tests are retrospective, and acute and convalescent sera must be examined for a fourfold rise in titer.

Diagnostic Tests/Procedures
Influenza A and B Serology *on page 463*
Influenza Virus Culture *on page 463*
Viral Culture, Throat *on page 574*
Virus Detection by DFA *on page 576*

Drug Therapy Comment
Use amantadine or rimantadine for influenza A infections only. No antiviral therapy for influenza B infections.

Drug Therapy
Recommended
Amantadine *on page 586*
Rimantadine *on page 908*

Selected Readings
Betts RF, "Influenza Virus," *Principles and Practice of Infectious Diseases*, 4th ed, Mandell GL, Bennett JE, and Dolin R, eds, New York, NY: Churchill Livingstone, 1995, 1546-67.

Greenberg SB, "Viral Pneumonia," *Infect Dis Clin North Am*, 1991, 5(3):603-21.

Shaw MW, Arden NH, and Maassab HF, "New Aspects of Influenza Viruses," *Clin Microbiol Rev*, 1992, 5(1):74-92.

"Update: Influenza Activity - United States, 1993-94 Season," *MMWR Morb Mortal Wkly Rep*, 1994, 43(1):1-3.

Isospora belli

Microbiology *Isospora belli* is a host-specific coccidian protozoan parasite. Both the asexual and sexual stages occur within the host's small intestine which results in the passage of an environmentally resistant cyst stage, the oocyst. The oocysts mature within a few days. Infections are acquired by the ingestion of infective oocysts in contaminated food or water.

Epidemiology Occurs more commonly in tropical and subtropical climates. In the United States, it is more commonly seen in patients with AIDS. Has been implicated in institutional outbreaks and as a cause of traveler's diarrhea.

Clinical Syndromes
- **Immunocompetent hosts:** Presents as a self-limiting diarrheal illness characterized by watery diarrhea without blood or fecal leukocytes, crampy abdominal pain, anorexia, weight loss, and occasionally fever.
- **Immunocompromised hosts including AIDS:** Symptoms as above but much more severe with profuse watery diarrhea resulting in dehydration. The disease is often chronic with detectable organisms in the stool or biopsy specimen for several months to years. Relapse is common. Rare cases of dissemination have been reported. May have peripheral eosinophilia.

Diagnosis Diagnosis is dependent on the identification of oocysts by wet mount or acid-fast stains in fecal material. Histopathologic examination of the small intestine reveals atrophic mucosa, shortened villi, hypertrophic cysts, and inflammation of the lamina propria including eosinophils.

Diagnostic Tests/Procedures
Ova and Parasites, Stool *on page 505*

Treatment Co-trimoxazole DS 4 times/day usually results in rapid clearance of *I. belli*. Immunocompromised hosts frequently require a long course such as 8 weeks and may require life-long suppression with either low-dose co-trimoxazole or sulfadoxine and pyrimethamine.

Drug Therapy
Recommended
Co-Trimoxazole *on page 692*
Alternate
Sulfadoxine and Pyrimethamine *on page 931*

Selected Readings
Lindsay DS, Dubey JP, and Blagburn BL, "Biology of *Isospora* spp From Humans, Nonhuman Primates, and Domestic Animals," *Clin Microbiol Rev*, 1997, 10(1):19-34.

JC Virus and BK Virus

Synonyms BK Virus

Microbiology The virus family Papovaviridae is composed of two genera: Polyomavirus (JC and BK viruses) and Papillomavirus (wart viruses). JC virus (JCV) and BK virus (BKV) are nonenveloped, slowly growing, icosahedral, 40 nm, double-stranded DNA viruses. JCV and BKV can be cultured *in vitro*; however, culture is not routinely performed in most clinical virology laboratories because the viruses grow slowly (weeks to months) and because susceptible cells are not readily available. JCV and BKV are serologically distinct. Little is known about the portal of entry, transmission, and primary infection of these viruses.

Epidemiology JCV and BKV are found worldwide. Humans appear to be the only animal reservoir for these viruses. Eighty percent of humans develop antibodies to JCV and BKV by the age of 8. Throughout their lives, many persons maintain detectable levels of antibodies to one or both viruses. Ten percent to 25% of healthy adults excrete BKV in their urine.

Clinical Syndromes The majority of JCV and BKV infections are asymptomatic. Most JCV and BKV infections occur in immunocompromised persons and probably are reactivations of latent infections. Asymptomatic shedding of JCV and/or BKV in the urine of transplant patients and pregnant females is common. JCV is associated with progressive multifocal leukoencephalopathy (PML). In PML, JCV infects oligodendrocytes in the brain, and elicits plaques of demyelination in the white matter. The clinical manifestations of PML are motor dysfunction, visual deficits, and progressive dementia or cognitive impairment. PML occurs in ~5% of AIDS patients. BKV is associated with renal infections, hemorrhagic cystitis, and ureteral stricture in bone marrow and renal transplant patients. The presence of BKV does not always predict poor prognosis or clinical illness of the transplant patients.

Diagnosis Before submitting a specimen, consult the Microbiology Laboratory to determine the availability of reference laboratory tests for JCV and BKV. Routine culture for the viruses is not practical and not routinely available. The results of serological tests for the viruses are not clinically relevant because of the high prevalence in infection and antibody in the population. Antigen detection and DNA hybridization tests are the most useful tests for the laboratory diagnosis of JCV and BKV infections. Immunofluorescence methods to detect JCV and BKV antigens in excreted renal cells and in brain (JCV), kidney (JCV and BKV), and bone marrow (JCV) are the methods of choice. DNA hybridization tests to detect JCV and BKV DNA in the aforementioned four specimens are reported to be more sensitive and specific than are immunofluorescence tests to detect antigen.

Diagnostic Tests/Procedures

Polymerase Chain Reaction *on page 523*

Treatment Most JCV and BKV infections are asymptomatic and do not require treatment. Cytosine arabinoside, interferon, 5-iodo-2′-deoxyuridine, and zidovudine have been anecdotally reported to improve the clinical progress of PML. However, a commonly accepted treatment for symptomatic JCV and BKV infections does not exist.

Selected Readings

Demeter LM, "JK, BK, and Other *Polyomaviruses*: Progressive Multifocal Leukoencephalopathy," *Principals and Practice of Infectious Diseases*, 4th ed, Mandell GL, Bennett JE, and Dolin R, eds, New York, NY: Churchill Livingston, 1995, 1400-4.

Major EO, "*Polyomaviruses*," *Manual of Clinical Microbiology*, 6th ed, Muffay PR, Baron EJ, Pfaller MA, et al, eds, Washington DC: American Society for Microbiology, 1995, 1090-6.

Kennel Cough *see Bordetella bronchiseptica on page 80*

Klebsiella Species

Microbiology *Klebsiella* species are aerobic gram-negative bacilli belonging to the tribe Klebsielleae and the family Enterobacteriaceae. The main species causing human disease are *K. pneumoniae* and *K. oxytoca*. A distinctive characteristic of most isolates of *Klebsiella* is the polysaccharide capsule which imparts a mucoid appearance of the organisms when growing on solid media. The prominent capsule also makes the organism appear large on Gram's stain. The presence of the capsule is a virulence factor. As with other gram-negative bacilli of this family, *Klebsiella* produces endotoxin, a mediator of the sepsis syndrome. (Continued)

Klebsiella Species *(Continued)*

Epidemiology *Klebsiella* sp are primarily nosocomial pathogens. However, the organism is associated with one important community-acquired infection, primary lobar pneumonia.

Clinical Syndromes

- **Primary lobar pneumonia:** This infection is community-acquired and is seen in alcoholics and other patients with chronic debilitating underlying illnesses (such as chronic obstructive pulmonary disease). It is rarely seen in the otherwise healthy individual and is considered a type of opportunistic infection. Characteristically, a patient with underlying alcoholism presents with the acute onset of fever, purulent sputum with a "currant jelly" appearance (reflecting lung necrosis and blood), and dyspnea. The classic x-ray finding is the "bowed fissure;" the lobe is swollen and the fissure appears to be sagging and widened. Complications include lung abscess, empyema, cavity formation, and progressive infiltrates. This form of pneumonitis is severe with extensive necrosis. Many patients expire, in part due to their comorbidity conditions.

- **Bronchitis and bronchopneumonia:** Not all forms of *Klebsiella* lung infection lead to the severe form of necrotizing pneumonia described above. Community-acquired *Klebsiella* bronchitis and bronchopneumonia do occur but are much less frequently seen than hospital-acquired respiratory infections.

- **Nosocomial pneumonia:** Hospital-acquired *Klebsiella* lower respiratory infections are seen in debilitated, ventilator-dependent patients. *Klebsiella* and other gram-negative bacilli can asymptomatically colonize the upper respiratory tract of hospitalized patients. Thus, the recovery of *Klebsiella* from a sputum or tracheal aspirate culture does not necessarily indicate a significant infection. The diagnosis of a nosocomial pneumonia still rests on standard criteria such as the presence of purulence (many leukocytes) on the Gram's stain of sputum, the presence of a pulmonary infiltrate, and signs of systemic inflammation in the patient. **A positive sputum culture alone is not sufficient justification for initiating antibiotic therapy.**

- **Nosocomial urinary tract infections:** Hospitalized patients with indwelling Foley catheters are at risk for cystitis or pyelonephritis from *Klebsiella*. *Klebsiella* may be recovered more frequently from the urine than from any other site, including the respiratory tract. However, the organism may also harmlessly colonize the urine of patients with chronic bladder catheters without causing disease. The decision to initiate antibiotics in such patients should be based on the clinical situation (the presence of pyuria on urinalysis, suprapubic pain, fever, etc). Even the finding of large quantity of *Klebsiella* in a urine culture ($>10^5$ colony forming units/mL) by itself does not automatically indicate antibiotic therapy.

- **Hospital-associated bacteremias:** *Klebsiella* is a common cause of primary bacteremia. In some series, it approaches *E. coli* as one of the most frequently recovered gram-negative bacillus from the bloodstream.

- **Surgical wound infections.**

- **Biliary tract infections, especially following instrumentation.**

Diagnosis The diagnosis of lobar pneumonia secondary to *Klebsiella* should be considered in any debilitated patient who presents with a necrotizing pneumonia. The history of "currant jelly" sputum and the finding of a "bowed fissure" on chest x-ray are highly suggestive but are not always present. The differential diagnosis of such cases should include anaerobic lung abscess, tuberculosis, *Pseudomonas* and other gram-negative bacilli, and mixed aspiration pneumonitis, among others. The presentation of nosocomial *Klebsiella* infections are more nonspecific and can be due to a variety of pathogenic gram-negative bacilli. Culture and Gram's stain of appropriate clinical specimens (sputum, urine, blood, catheter tips, etc) is necessary to make the diagnosis.

Diagnostic Tests/Procedures

Aerobic Culture, Appropriate Site *on page 310*
Gram's Stain *on page 426*

Treatment Like many other nosocomial pathogens, *Klebsiella* sp may be difficult to treat because of antimicrobial resistance. Although the organisms have been traditionally susceptible to cephalosporins, including the first generation agents, increasing problems with resistance are emerging. Isolates of *Klebsiella* which are resistant to cephalosporins and aminoglycosides have emerged because of widespread use of these antimicrobial agents. Resistance is spread bacterium to bacterium by plasmid-mediated resistance mechanisms. In all cases, the final selection of antibiotics must be based on the susceptibility pattern of the particular isolate because the organism is no longer predictably sensitive to all agents.

Drug Therapy

Recommended

Cephalosporins, 1st Generation *on page 661*
Cephalosporins, 2nd Generation *on page 662*
Cephalosporins, 3rd Generation *on page 662*

Alternate

Penicillins, Extended Spectrum *on page 864*
Imipenem and Cilastatin *on page 766*
Aztreonam *on page 615*
Fluoroquinolones *on page 736*
Meropenem *on page 812*

Selected Readings

Carpenter JL, "*Klebsiella* Pulmonary Infections: Occurrence at One Medical Center and Review," *Rev Infect Dis*, 1990, 12(4):672-80.

Garcia de la Torre M, Romero-Vivas J, Martinez-Beltran J, et al, "*Klebsiella* Bacteremia: An Analysis of 100 Episodes," *Rev Infect Dis*, 1985, 7(2):143-50.

Meyer KS, Urban C, Eagan JA, et al, "Nosocomial Outbreak of *Klebsiella* Infection Resistant to Late-Generation Cephalosporins," *Ann Intern Med*, 1993, 119(5):353-8.

Legionella pneumophila

Microbiology *Legionella pneumophila* is an aerobic, gram-negative rod first isolated in 1947 which causes a pneumonia called Legionnaires' disease (or legionellosis), as well as a distinct febrile illness called Pontiac fever. There are over 30 *Legionella* species, with *L. pneumophila* accounting for about 90% of human infections. The organism is very difficult to visualize on Gram's stain of clinical specimens. Other stains are more effective in identifying the organism, such as the silver stain (Dieterle or Warthin-Starry stains), Gimenez stain, and others. The organism also requires special medium for growth and cannot be cultured using standard bacteriologic media. Charcoal yeast extract is the medium most commonly used for culture isolation.

Epidemiology The importance of this organism was recently recognized in 1976 following an outbreak of pneumonia involving an American Legion convention in Philadelphia, Pennsylvania. The cause of this well-publicized outbreak which involved over 200 individuals was initially unknown. Only later was the bacterium *Legionella pneumophila* isolated from lung autopsy specimens by the Centers for Disease Control. Another epidemic of Legionnaires' disease had been described in 1965, where the diagnosis was established by serologic studies rather than identification of the organism. Since then, prospective studies have shown *L. pneumophila* to be one of the three most common causes of community-acquired pneumonia. The prevalence of *L. pneumophila* varies geographically. In some areas of the United States, it is the most common cause of community-acquired pneumonia.

The bacterium typically inhabits lakes, ponds, polluted waters, and hot water systems in buildings and homes. Evidence suggests that human disease is likely caused by aspiration of contaminated water. Airborne transmission by aerosolization has been theorized as well but cannot explain many cases.

Clinical Syndromes

- **Community-acquired pneumonia:** The incidence of *L. pneumophila* as a cause of community-acquired pneumonia has ranged from 1% to 15%. There is a well-recognized, broad spectrum of clinical symptoms. Patients may present with a minor cough or with a progressive five-lobe pneumonia with shock. Fever is almost always present, and often over 40°C. Typically, the cough is nonproductive although pleuritic chest pain may occur. Other accompanying features are shaking chills, relative bradycardia, diarrhea and other gastrointestinal symptoms (up to 50% of cases), and hyponatremia. No single symptom or constellation of symptoms is diagnostic of legionellosis. In one study, the extrapulmonary symptoms such as diarrhea and neurologic findings were not found more frequently with Legionnaires' disease in comparison with other forms of pneumonia. The chest radiograph classically shows unilateral patchy infiltrates early on, which progress over

(Continued)

Legionella pneumophila (Continued)

several days to consolidation. However, a very wide variety of x-ray abnormalities has been described with this infection. Pleural effusions are common.

- **Nosocomial pneumonia:** L. pneumophila is a sporadic cause of hospital-acquired pneumonias.
- **Pontiac fever:** This is a febrile illness caused by L. pneumophila which tends to be self-resolving without antibiotics. Patients present with fever, myalgias, headache and malaise, mimicking the flu, however, pneumonia is not present.
- **Miscellaneous:** L. pneumophila has been described rarely as a cause of endocarditis, sinusitis, pericarditis, peritonitis, pancreatitis, encephalopathy, and wound infections.

Diagnosis A high level of suspicion must be maintained by the clinician since the presentation of Legionnaires' disease is varied and notoriously nonspecific. Laboratory testing is essential in making the diagnosis since the organism cannot be reliably recovered in routine cultures of sputum, blood, or bronchoscopy specimens. The clinician must specify both special stains and cultures for L. pneumophila.

Diagnostic Tests/Procedures

Legionella Antigen, Urine on page 468
Legionella DNA Probe on page 469
Legionella pneumophila Culture on page 469
Legionella pneumophila Smear on page 470
Legionella Serology on page 471
Polymerase Chain Reaction on page 523

Treatment The antibiotic of choice is erythromycin, which has been shown to improve survival in several studies. The preferred regimen is erythromycin 2-4 g/day intravenously. Some authors recommend a combination of erythromycin and rifampin for known cases of Legionnaires' disease, based mainly on in vitro susceptibility data.

Drug Therapy

Recommended

Erythromycin on page 722
or
Erythromycin on page 722
used in combination with
Rifampin on page 902

Alternate

Clarithromycin on page 681
Azithromycin on page 613
Ciprofloxacin on page 678
Fluoroquinolones on page 736

Selected Readings

Bernstein MS, Locksley RM, "Legionella Infections," Harrison's Principles of Internal Medicine, 13th ed, Isselbacher KJ, Braunwald E, Wilson JD, et al, eds, New York, NY: McGraw-Hill, 1994, 654-8.

Blatt SP, Dolan MJ, Hendrix CW, et al, "Legionnaires' Disease in Human Immunodeficiency Virus-Infected Patients: Eight Cases and Review," Clin Infect Dis, 1994, 18(2):227-32.

Edelstein PH, "Legionnaires' Disease," Clin Infect Dis, 1993, 16(6):741-7.

Lowry PW, Blankenship RJ, Gridley W, et al, "A Cluster of Legionella Sternal-Wound Infections Due to Postoperative Topical Exposure to Contaminated Tap Water," N Engl J Med, 1991, 324(2):109-13.

Nguyen MH, Stout JE, and Yu VL, "Legionellosis," Infect Dis Clin North Am, 1991, 5(3):561-84.

Leptospira interrogans

Microbiology Leptospira interrogans is an aerobic spirochete which causes the febrile human disease leptospirosis. L. interrogans is the main pathogenic species of the genus Leptospira, which is divided into 170 serotypes. A second species, L. biflexa, is saprophytic. The organism is a finely coiled, motile, helical rod 0.1 μm in width and 6-20 μm in length. One or both ends of the rod are usually hooked, giving the appearance of a question mark (thus the name L. interrogans).

Epidemiology Leptospirosis is an unusual disease in the U.S., with 50-100 cases reported annually. It is primarily a disease of wild and domestic mammals. Humans are infected only occasionally through direct animal contact or through indirect contact with soil or water that is contaminated with infected urine. Groups at risk include farmers, veterinarians, abattoir workers, campers, and swimmers. Worldwide, rats are the most common source of human infection with a 90% carriage rate. In the U.S., the most important sources of infection are dogs, livestock, rodents, wild mammals, and cats. Person-to-person transmission is extremely rare. Most cases of leptospirosis occur in young adult men, and the peak incidence is in the summer and early fall.

Clinical Syndromes The organisms are capable of penetrating intact mucous membranes or abraded skin of the host. The leptospires enter the bloodstream and are rapidly disseminated even to "sequestered sites" such as the cerebrospinal fluid and the eye. The primary pathologic lesion is damage to the endothelium of small blood vessels.

- **Subclinical leptospirosis:** Some individuals may have minimal symptoms after infection with *L. interrogans*. This occurs most commonly in those who are frequently exposed to infected animals. Leptospires can establish a symbiotic relationship with many animal hosts, persisting for long periods in the renal tubules without producing disease or pathologic changes in the kidney.

- **Anicteric leptospirosis:** Among patients ill with leptospirosis, 90% have a mild anicteric disease. The incubation period is 7-12 days usually. Individuals with anicteric leptospirosis have an abrupt onset of remitting fever, headache, abdominal pain, nausea and vomiting, severe myalgias, and malaise. Prostration may persist for 4-7 days. The illness may be biphasic. Following this initial flu-like illness, the patient is then afebrile for several days. The second phase, called the "immune phase" occurs in some, but not all, patients and is characterized by low grade fever, throbbing headaches, and sometimes delirium without encephalitis. Up to 90% will have evidence of meningitis, with a cerebrospinal fluid pleocytosis. Although the CSF pressure is normal, characteristically the spinal tap will improve the headaches. Other symptoms include ocular manifestations, in particular suffusion of the bulbar conjunctiva, photophobia, ocular pain, and conjunctival hemorrhage; abdominal pain, with nausea and vomiting; myalgias; splenomegaly (15% to 25% of cases); lymphadenopathy; rash, with raised 1-5 cm erythematous lesions in the pretibial area (so-called Fort Bragg fever caused by *L. autumnalis*).

- **Icteric leptospirosis:** Also known as Weil syndrome, this severe form of leptospirosis is characterized by hepatic dysfunction, jaundice, impaired renal function, hemorrhage, vascular collapse, and severe mental status changes. Mortality is 5% to 10%. Jaundice is due to hepatocellular damage without necrosis. Marked elevation of the serum creatine phosphokinase, with only modest elevations of transaminases is seen. Severely jaundiced patients are the ones most likely to exhibit renal failure and subsequent loss of intravascular volume. Renal failure is primarily the result of tubular damage, with the leptospires visible in the tubular lumen. Immune complex glomerulonephritis may be seen. Urinalysis shows proteinuria, hematuria, and casts. Hemorrhagic myocarditis often contributes to fatal cases.

Diagnosis Definitive diagnosis can only be made by isolation of the organism as seroconversion (greater than 4 times rise in serologic titer) in patients with relevant clinical syndromes. There are a variety of serological tests available including a macroscopic slide agglutination test (killed antigen), microscopic agglutination test (live antigen), indirect hemagglutination test, an ELISA and a Dot-ELISA test.

Culture of organism requires special media (Tween® 80-albumin medium is preferred) and takes 5-6 weeks at 28°C to 30°C to grow (in the dark). A rapid method using the Bactec® 460 system may detect organisms from blood with 2-5 days. Organisms will be present in the blood only during the first 10 days of an acute illness and are present in urine during week two. These organisms can be seen by the experienced microbiologist upon darkfield examination.

Diagnostic Tests/Procedures

Darkfield Examination, Leptospirosis *on page 393*

Leptospira Culture *on page 472*

Leptospira Serology *on page 472*

Treatment Early studies suggested that penicillin or tetracycline might shorten the duration of fever and reduce the incidence of renal, hepatic, meningeal, and hemorrhagic complications, but only if therapy was started by the fourth day of illness. Recently it was found that therapy may be effective in severe disease (Continued)

Leptospira interrogans (Continued)

even when treatment was delayed. Administration of a single dose of doxycycline, 200 mg once a week, prevented infection in soldiers in Panama.

Treatment recommendations are for penicillin G, 1.5 million units every 6 hours or ampicillin, 1000 mg I.V. every 6 hours in severe disease. In less severe disease, oral therapy with doxycycline, 100 mg orally twice daily or ampicillin, 500-750 mg orally every 6 hours for 5-7 days.

In the U.S., there is no licensed human vaccine, but in other countries, human vaccine against leptospirosis has been reported to be useful.

Pediatric Drug Therapy
Recommended

Penicillin G, Parenteral, Aqueous *on page 860*

Ampicillin *on page 604*

Adult Drug Therapy
Recommended

Penicillin G, Parenteral, Aqueous *on page 860*

Ampicillin *on page 604*

Alternate

Tetracycline *on page 944*

Doxycycline *on page 713*

Selected Readings
Emmanouilides CE, Kohn OF, and Garibaldi R, "Leptospirosis Complicated by a Jarisch-Herxheimer Reaction and Adult Respiratory Distress Syndrome," *Clin Infect Dis*, 1994, 18(6):1004-6.

Farrar WE, "*Leptospira* Species (Leptospirosis)," *Principles and Practice of Infectious Diseases*, 4th ed, Mandell GL, Bennett JE, and Dolin R, eds, New York, NY: Churchill Livingstone, 1995, 2137-41.

Kennedy ND, Pusey CD, Rainford DJ, et al, "Leptospirosis and Acute Renal Failure - Clinical Experiences and a Review of the Literature," *Postgrad Med J*, 1979, 55(641):176-9.

O'Neil KM, Rickman LS, and Lazarus AA, "Pulmonary Manifestations of Leptospirosis," *Rev Infect Dis*, 1991, 13(4):705-9.

Takafuji ET, Kirkpatrick JW, Miller RN, et al, "An Efficacy Trial of Doxycycline Chemoprophylaxis Against Leptospirosis," *N Engl J Med*, 1984, 310(8):497-500.

Lice

Synonyms *Pediculus humanus; Phthirus pubis*

Microbiology Human lice are ectoparasites and thus tend to live on or in the skin of the host. They belong to the insect class *Hexapoda*. There are three species important in human infection. *Pediculus humanus* var *corporis* is the human body louse, *Pediculus humanus* var *capitis* is the human head louse, and *Phthirus pubis* is the crab louse. The body and head louse have similar appearances and are about 4 mm long. The pubic louse is much wider and has a crablike appearance from which its name is derived. The eggs adhere to human hair and to clothing and are termed nits.

Epidemiology Humans are the reservoir for lice. Infestations have been described worldwide especially in areas of overcrowding. The incubation period is about 1-4 weeks following exposure. Individuals are communicable until all the lice and eggs have been treated and destroyed. Pediculosis capitis is a particular problem with school-aged children, where the practice of sharing combs or brushes facilitates epidemic transmission. All socioeconomic backgrounds are at risk for head lice. In contrast, pediculosis corporis is seen mainly in areas of poor sanitation. The body louse resides almost exclusively in soiled clothing, rather than the skin, and only leaves the clothing for a blood meal from the host. Pediculosis corporis also transmits the rickettsial infection epidemic typhus, as well a several others. *Phthirus pubis* is usually sexually transmitted, although spread via infested bedding or clothing can occur.

Clinical Syndromes

- **Pediculosis corporis:** Typically, the patient complains of severe pruritus, and small, erythematous papules are found on the body. Often extensive self-induced excoriations across the trunk are noted. If left untreated for long periods, hyperpigmentation and scarring may occur, called "vagabond's disease."

- **Pediculosis capitis:** The most common presentation is intractable scalp pruritus. On examination there may be evidence of secondary bacterial infection of the scalp from excoriations. At times, an "id reaction" occurs, characterized by a dramatic skin eruption over the arms and trunk, felt to be a hypersensitivity reaction.

- **Pediculosis pubis:** Most patients present with pruritus in the region of the pubic hairs, but other areas may be involved including the eyelashes and hairs in the axilla. Secondary bacterial infections are less common.

Diagnosis The diagnosis of pediculosis is often suspected when an individual presents with severe pruritus. On some occasions, the patient may have identified lice themselves or have had a recent contact history. The diagnosis is confirmed by finding lice (1-4 mm long, depending on species) and/or the "nits" (usually 1 mm or less, attached to hairs).

Diagnostic Tests/Procedures
Arthropod Identification *on page 334*

Treatment General principles of treating pediculosis include discarding or carefully laundering clothing, discarding infested combs or hats, and laundering bedsheets. In general, clothes and bedsheets can be effectively decontaminated by dry cleaning or by machine washing and drying in a hot cycle. Secondary bacterial infections of the skin are common and generally respond to antibiotics effective against *Staphylococcus aureus* (dicloxacillin, erythromycin, and others). Pruritus is typically quite severe and may be alleviated by hydroxyzine (Atarax®), diphenhydramine (Benadryl®), and/or topical steroid creams. Treatment guidelines are as follows:

1. Pediculosis corporis: Since the louse resides mainly in the creases of clothes and not on the host, the infection can often be eradicated by delousing contaminated items and maintaining careful hygiene.
2. Pediculosis capitis. Several agents are effective: 1% lindane (Kwell®) shampoo to the scalp, pyrethrin liquid (RID), or permethrin creme rinse (Nix™). These insecticides are probably equal in efficacy. Only lindane requires a prescription. **Caution:** Lindane has been associated with seizures and other nervous system toxicities. However, the risk of serious adverse effects during treatment for pediculosis is small due to its minimal systemic absorption. Nevertheless, lindane should be avoided in pregnancy and in lactating women.
3. Pediculosis pubis: The treatment recommendations are the same as for pediculosis capitis. In addition, sexual partners should be identified and treated in the same manner. Pediculosis involving the eyelashes should **not** be treated with insecticides. Instead, occlusive ophthalmic ointment should be applied to the eyelashes twice daily for at least 8 days in an attempt to smother the parasites.

Patients should be seen in follow-up if symptoms persist 1 week after treatment. A second application may be necessary. Some clinicians routinely instruct patients to reapply the insecticide at the 1 week point.

Drug Therapy
Recommended
Pyrethrins *on page 885*
Permethrin *on page 868*
Malathion *on page 804*
Alternate
Lindane *on page 797*

Listeria monocytogenes

Microbiology *Listeria monocytogenes* is a gram-positive bacillus which causes sporadic cases of meningoencephalitis, neonatal infection, septicemia, and several less common syndromes. It is a leading cause of meningitis in immunocompromised individuals, especially renal transplant patients.

The organism is an aerobic, gram-positive rod which does not produce spores. At times it may assume a more coccoid appearance on Gram's stain of clinical samples (eg, cerebrospinal fluid) and may thus be mistaken for gram-positive cocci such as *Streptococcus pneumoniae*. *Listeria* can also be confused morphologically with the more commonly seen *Corynebacterium* species, which are also gram-positive bacilli (but are often contaminants). *Listeria* is primarily an intracellular pathogen, and tends to reside within mononuclear phagocytes of the host. This feature is thought to contribute to its pathogenicity, since the organism can spread from cell to cell in a somewhat protected fashion.

When *Listeria monocytogenes* meningitis is suspected, the clinician should try to submit at least 10 mL of cerebrospinal fluid for bacterial culture, since only a few
(Continued)

Listeria monocytogenes (Continued)

Listeria organisms may be present. The organism generally grows well on most routine media used in the laboratory, and special requests for selective or enrichment cultures for *Listeria* are usually not necessary. It is important that the clinician does not automatically dismiss a report of a "gram-positive rod" isolated from multiple blood or a sterile body site as a contaminant, particularly in an immunocompromised host in whom *Listeria* infection is possible.

Epidemiology The epidemiology of listeriosis can be important in certain cases, since clinical presentations may be nonspecific. The precise prevalence of human infection is unclear, but the attack rate appears to be increasing (perhaps due to better reporting or laboratory recognition). Asymptomatic carriage of *Listeria* in stools is relatively frequent; some studies suggest a fecal excretion rate of 1% or more in healthy humans. Humans may be exposed to *Listeria* by one of several routes: consumption of contaminated food, direct exposure to infected animals, or exposure to environmental reservoirs (soil, water, etc).

Cases of listeriosis tend to be sporadic and difficult to predict. Most infections occur in the summer months and are more common in urban than rural settings, despite its reputation as a zoonotic infection. Often, the source of the *Listeria* remains unknown. Increasing attention has been given to foodborne transmission, particularly in the setting of a traceable outbreak. Mexican-style cheese, coleslaw, undercooked chicken, hot dogs, dairy products, and other foods have caused outbreaks. The ability of the organism to survive (and even multiply) during refrigeration probably contributes to food-related transmission.

Infection with *Listeria* usually occurs in definable groups in the community. Cell mediated immunity is critically important in defense against *Listeria*, whereas neutropenia is not clearly a risk factor. Those at highest risk include patients with solid organ transplants, malignancies (particularly lymphoma), and patients receiving corticosteroids. Pregnant females, neonates, and alcoholics are additional groups at risk for infection. Interestingly, listeriosis does not appear to be a common pathogen in patients with AIDS, despite the deficiencies in T-cell function. Although uncommon, serious infections with *Listeria* have been described in otherwise healthy individuals.

Clinical Syndromes

- **Adult meningoencephalitis:** *Listeria* is the most common cause of community-acquired meningitis in immunosuppressed individuals. *Listeria* meningitis can be quite variable in its presentation and can range from a subacute course to a rapid and fulminant one. In some cases the diagnosis may be quite difficult when high fevers and nuchal rigidity are absent. There are no pathognomonic features of *Listeria* meningitis which allow diagnosis on clinical grounds alone. CSF chemical analysis is variable and frequently nondiagnostic. The degree of CSF pleocytosis can range from several cells to >12,000 cells/mm^3. Differential cell counts vary from nearly 100% polymorphonuclear cells to 100% mononuclear cells. Often a modest elevation of CSF protein is seen, along with a minor decrease in CSF glucose. The differential diagnosis of a subacute meningitis in an immunosuppressed host must also include *Cryptococcus neoformans*. The finding of focal brain lesions by CT scan or MRI broadens the differential to include toxoplasmosis, *Nocardia asteroides*, bacterial brain abscess, fungal meningitis, and others. Meningoencephalitis has also been sporadically reported in otherwise healthy individuals and should be considered in the differential diagnosis of any community-acquired meningitis.

- **Meningoencephalitis of the neonate:** This is a "late-onset" neonatal disease, occurring several days to weeks postpartum. As with adult cases, isolated neonatal meningitis from *Listeria* can be variable in its presentation. Fever may be low grade or absent, and irritability and failure to thrive may be the only clues. CSF findings in the neonate are similar to those in the adult. It is important to review the Gram's stain of CSF carefully to avoid confusing *Listeria* with Group B streptococci, a common cause of neonatal meningitis.

- **Cerebritis:** This form of nonmeningeal central nervous system infection is gaining increased recognition. Patients may complain of fever, cephalgia, and hemiparesis. This form of listeriosis may be mistaken for a stroke, vasculitis, brain tumor, or abscess. CT and MRI scans suggest focal inflammation without a discrete abscess or ring enhancement. Cerebrospinal fluid is usually normal and CSF cultures are negative for *Listeria*. The diagnosis is usually made when *Listeria* is isolated from blood cultures.

- **Listeriosis in pregnancy:** Unfortunately, this is often difficult to diagnose, since the woman may be asymptomatic or complain of only a mild fever and malaise. Other symptoms variably present include diarrhea and flank pain. The differential diagnosis is usually broad and listeriosis may be mistaken for pyelonephritis, lower urinary tract infection, and viral syndromes (eg, influenza). Blood cultures may be positive and should be performed. Complications include premature delivery, septic abortion, and *in utero* fetal infection.

- **Granulomatosis infantiseptica:** This unique, transplacentally acquired infection is severe and often lethal. It is an "early onset" neonatal infection apparent within hours of birth. Typically, the infants are seriously ill. There are widespread abscesses involving visceral organs such as the liver, spleen, lungs, intestinal tract, and brain. The lesions are usually abscesses with polymorphonuclear leukocytes, but granulomas have also been seen (referred to as "miliary granulomatosis"). Dark papular skin lesions may be present on the trunk and lower extremities, suggesting the diagnosis. Gram's stain and culture of meconium, amniotic fluid, conjunctival exudates, CSF, throat, blood, or skin lesions frequently are positive for *L. monocytogenes*. Antibiotic therapy should be started immediately if this diagnosis is suspected, since death may occur if treatment is withheld until cultures are finalized.

- **Septicemia:** *Listeria* can be isolated from the blood in adults and neonates who present from the community with nonspecific fever and chills. Bacteremias are more likely in profoundly immunosuppressed hosts but have been seen in alcoholics, diabetics, pregnancy, and normal healthy individuals. The clinical presentation can be indistinguishable from gram-negative sepsis, with high fevers and hypotension (so-called "typhoidal listeremia"). On rare occasion, the diagnosis is suggested by the finding of a monocytosis on the peripheral blood smear, but blood cultures remain the highest yield.

- **Miscellaneous:** Endocarditis, ocular infections, lymphadenitis, osteomyelitis, brain abscess, peritonitis, and other focal infections have been rarely reported.

Diagnosis Except for granulomatosis infantiseptica, the clinical presentations of listeriosis are not unique and microbiological confirmation is necessary. Depending on the clinical site of infection, specimens of blood and body fluids should be sent, as described above. Agglutination studies for antibodies directed against *L. monocytogenes* have little value.

Diagnostic Tests/Procedures
Aerobic Culture, Cerebrospinal Fluid *on page 311*
Blood Culture, Aerobic and Anaerobic *on page 337*
Cerebrospinal Fluid Analysis *on page 354*
Gram's Stain *on page 426*
Lumbar Puncture *on page 477*

Treatment No randomized comparison trials have been performed to determine the drug(s) of choice for listeriosis. *In vitro* data show the organism is susceptible to many antibiotics. The most clinical experience has been limited to penicillin and ampicillin, and they are probably equivalent. Occasionally, penicillin-resistant strains of *Listeria* have been reported, and thus results of susceptibility testing should be followed up on. There is some *in vitro* evidence to suggest the combination of penicillin (or ampicillin) with an aminoglycoside may be synergistic against *Listeria*, and this combination has been used in serious, life-threatening infections. Cephalosporins do not reliably cover this organism and should not be used for cases of *Listeria* meningitis. Consultation with an Infectious Disease specialist is appropriate in complicated cases or in the patient with a penicillin allergy.

Drug Therapy
Recommended
Ampicillin *on page 604*
    or
Ampicillin *on page 604*
    used in combination with
Gentamicin *on page 747*
    or
(Continued)

Listeria monocytogenes (Continued)

Penicillin G, Parenteral, Aqueous on page 860
or
Penicillin G, Parenteral, Aqueous on page 860
used in combination with
Gentamicin on page 747

Alternate

Co-Trimoxazole on page 692

Selected Readings

Armstrong D, "Listeria monocytogenes," Principles and Practice of Infectious Diseases, 4th ed, Mandell GL, Bennett JE, and Dolin R, eds, New York, NY: Churchill Livingstone, 1995, 1880-5.

Gellin BG and Broome CV, "Listeriosis," JAMA, 1989, 261(9):1313-20.

Hof H, Nichterlein T, and Kretschmar M, "Management of Listeriosis," Clin Microbiol Rev, 1997, 10(2):345-57.

Lorber B, "Listeriosis," Clin Infect Dis, 1997, 24(1):1-11.

Lyme Disease Vaccine Guidelines see page 1053

MAC see Mycobacterium avium-intracellulare on page 201

Madura Foot see Dematiaceous Fungi on page 125

MAI see Mycobacterium avium-intracellulare on page 201

Malassezia furfur

Synonyms Pityriasis (Tinea) Versicolor; Pityrosporum orbiculare; Pityrosporum ovale

Microbiology The genus Malassezia contains three species: M. furfur, M. sympodialis, and M. pachydermatis. All are lipophilic yeasts found as indigenous flora of human skin. The distribution of Malessezia correlates with the oily areas of the skin, most notably the scalp, chest, and back. Adolescents have the greatest colonization correlating with the increased activity of the sebaceous glands. The Microbiology Laboratory should be notified if M. furfur is suspected because growth is dependent on the presence of an exogenous source of fatty acids. This is accomplished by overlaying the medium with olive oil. Histopathologic stains reveal filamentous structures; however in culture, Malassezia grows as oval yeast cells measuring up to 6 μm. The colonies are smooth, cream to yellowish brown, and glistening. Optimal growth occurs between 35°C and 37°C.

Epidemiology Although M. furfur is mostly implicated as the etiologic agent of various dermal infections, hematogenous infections especially in debilitated and immunosuppressed patients and neonates occur. Nosocomial outbreaks of both M. furfur and M. pachydermatis bacteremia in neonatal intensive care units attributed to person to person transmission via the hands of medical personnel have been reported. There is a strong correlation of increased risk of Malassezia bacteremia in neonates receiving lipid emulsions through a central venous catheter. The lipids are thought to provide nutrients to the yeasts that have colonized the catheters; however, Malassezia has been reported to cause bacteremias in debilitated adults not receiving any parenteral nutrition.

Clinical Syndromes

- **Cutaneous manifestations:** Folliculitis must be distinguished from other infectious etiologies (eg, bacterial, systemic candidiasis, cryptococcosis, atypical mycobacteria). Biopsy and culture of the skin should be performed. Lesions are usually multiple and distributed over the shoulders, back, and chest. Disseminated candidiasis has a higher predilection for the extremities. Candida folliculitis frequently involves the face. Malassezia folliculitis initially presents as a papulonodular eruption on an erythematous base varying in size from 2-6 mm. Lesions may become pustule or associated with hair follicles. Patients typically complain of intense pruritus.

    Tinea versicolor is a common asymptomatic superficial infection seen in young adults, particularly in warm, humid environments towards the end of summer. It appears as hypo- or hyperpigmented annular lesions of various sizes and shapes. The eruption is asymmetrical occurring on the back, chest, and neck. May go into remission without treatment.

    The role of M. furfur in seborrhoeic dermatitis in HIV-infected individuals is unclear, although some comparative studies have shown efficacy in combined antifungal and steroid therapy. In addition, M. furfur may play a role in atopic dermatitis and seborrhoeic dermatitis in non-HIV infected individuals.

- **Intravenous line sepsis:** Colonization of the central venous catheter occurs prior to *Malassezia* fungemia. Most of the cases of fungemia have been reported in premature infants receiving lipid infusions. Fever is the sole manifestation in approximately 20% of infected infants. May present with apnea, bradycardia or tachycardia, lethargy, cyanosis, tachypnea, and/or hepatosplenomegaly. Plain radiographs of the chest reveal interstitial pneumonitis in 50% to 60% of infants. Leukocytosis and thrombocytopenia occur in 50%. Lipid deposits containing *M. furfur* have been found in the pulmonary arterial walls postmortem. Adults with a history of inflammatory bowel disease or recent abdominal surgery requiring parenteral nutrition are at increased risk of *Malassezia* line sepsis. Most cases are rather indolent with fever being the most common complaint. Peripheral blood cultures are positive in only 25% of cases, which may be due to the low level of fungemia, difficulty in laboratory isolation techniques, adherence to the central venous catheter, or rapid removal of the organism by the pulmonary vasculature.

Diagnosis Gram's stain of the buffy coat should be done in suspected cases of line-associated sepsis. Budding yeast cells can be seen on Gram's, Giemsa, PAS, or silver stains. Suspected cases should be cultured on media overlaid with olive oil. *M. furfur* folliculitis biopsy reveals unipolar budding yeast confined to the epidermis, predominantly near the hair follicles. No pseudohyphae or hyphae are seen. Occasionally, dermal abscess formation in the perifollicular dermis and granulomatous perifolliculitis may be observed. Potassium hydroxide (KOH) preps of skin scrapings of tinea versicolor reveal the characteristic "spaghetti and meatballs" which are strands of filamentous hyphae and yeast cells.

Diagnostic Tests/Procedures
Fungus Culture, Appropriate Site *on page 414*
KOH Preparation *on page 467*

Treatment Treatment of *M. furfur* fungemia requires removal of the central venous catheter with or without systemic antifungal therapy (eg, ketoconazole, itraconazole, fluconazole, or amphotericin B). Folliculitis usually responds to clotrimazole, ketoconazole, or miconazole creams. Diffuse follicular involvement may be treated with any of the systemic azoles. Antipruritics should be prescribed to avoid excoriation and superimposed bacterial infection. Tinea versicolor responds to topical treatment of propylene glycol (50%), selenium sulfide, or azole creams. Systemic azoles are not usually indicated but may be used in refractory cases. Relapse occurs in 60% after 1 year and 80% by 2 years. Seborrhea dermatitis in AIDS may need combination therapy of an azole plus either topical or systemic steroids.

Drug Therapy
Recommended
  Line-Associated:
    Amphotericin B (Conventional) *on page 597*
    Fluconazole *on page 732*
    Itraconazole *on page 785*
    Ketoconazole *on page 791*
  Dermatitides:
    Clotrimazole *on page 688*
    Ketoconazole *on page 791*
    Miconazole *on page 822*
    Selenium Sulfide *on page 917*
    Fluconazole *on page 732*
    Itraconazole *on page 785*

Selected Readings
Marcon MJ and Powell DA, "Human Infections Due to *Malassezia* Species," *Clin Microbiol Rev*, 1992, 5(2):101-19.

Teglia O, Schoch PE, and Cunha BA, "*Malassezia furfur* Infections," *Infect Control Hosp Epidemiol*, 1991, 12(11):676-81.

Welbel SF, McNeil MM, Pramanik A, et al, "Nosocomial *Malassezia pachydermatis* Bloodstream Infections in a Neonatal Intensive Care Unit," *Pediatr Infect Dis J*, 1994, 13(2):104-8.

maltophilia see Stenotrophomonas maltophilia *on page 265*

Measles Virus
Related Information
Recommendations for Measles Vaccination *on page 1044*
(Continued)

Measles Virus (Continued)

Synonyms Rubeola Virus

Microbiology Measles virus is a member of the Paramyxoviridae family (measles virus, mumps virus, parainfluenza virus, canine distemper virus, respiratory syncytial virus, and others). Measles virus is enveloped and contains single-stranded RNA. Measles virus has specific envelope proteins H and F which are responsible for adsorption/hemagglutination and cell penetration/fusion, respectively. Measles virus is extremely labile and is sensitive to light, drying, and naturally occurring enzymes and acids. Measles virus remains extremely infective for several hours as long as it remains moist and in aerosolized droplets. The fact that measles virus is easily spread by inhalation of such droplets and by direct contact with nasal secretions explains why measles virus causes one of the most contagious of all infectious diseases, measles. Measles virus exists in two forms, wild type and vaccine form. The wild type is extremely genetically stable; the same genotype and phenotype exists worldwide.

Epidemiology Measles (archaic term, rubeola) has been observed and recorded for over 2000 years and occurs today in every country. In developing countries, measles affects almost all children younger than 5 years of age and causes 1-2 million deaths per year in children. In the United States, in 1990, there were ca. 27,000 reported cases of measles. More than 80% of the persons who represented these cases had previously received measles vaccine, and approximately 50% of these cases were represented by poor, inner-city preschool children. Humans are the natural reservoir and, for all practical purposes, the only hosts of measles virus.

Clinical Syndromes Measles is an infection of the respiratory tract and central nervous system and can present in at least three syndromes.

- **Conventional measles:** Incubation period, 10-14 days; prodrome of "flu"-like symptoms, conjunctivitis, and other upper respiratory tract symptoms; Koplik spots; typically a 5-day rash which spreads from head to trunk to extremities to palms and soles. Most patients are not contagious after the rash reaches its peak.
- **Mild measles:** Usually observed in infants younger than 1 year of age; similar to conventional measles but is milder and usually is not characterized by all of the typical signs and symptoms of conventional measles.
- **Atypical measles:** More severe and lasts longer than conventional measles; rash usually begins peripherally and progresses toward the trunk; can be confused with chickenpox or Rocky Mountain spotted fever; antibody titers to measles virus often are extremely high.

Diagnosis Measles is usually diagnosed clinically. Measles virus can be isolated in cell culture, but this method is somewhat difficult and usually not practical. The specimens of choice are throat and nasopharyngeal washings. Serology is the diagnostic method of choice. As with most viral serology, diagnosis is made by demonstration of a fourfold rise in measles virus-specific antibody; however, the most widely used tests are immunofluorescence antibody and enzyme immunoassays for measles-specific IgM. A minimal protective IgG antibody level has not been determined. Some laboratories offer direct detection of measles virus-infected cells from nasopharyngeal washings and nasal swabs.

Diagnostic Tests/Procedures

Measles Antibody on page 487

Virus Detection by DFA on page 576

Drug Therapy Comment

No antiviral agents active against measles, but for immune suppressed patients, intravenous immunoglobulins may be indicated.

Drug Therapy

Recommended

Immune Globulin, Intramuscular on page 770

Selected Readings

Gershon AA, "Measles Virus (Rubeola)," *Principles and Practice of Infectious Diseases*, 4th ed, Mandell GL, Bennett JE, and Dolin R, eds, New York, NY: Churchill Livingstone, 1995, 1519-26.

"Measles - United States, First 26 Weeks, 1993," *MMWR Morb Mortal Wkly Rep*, 1993, 42(42):813-6.

Schlenker T, "Measles Resurgent," *Clin Microbiol Newslett*, 1991, 13:156-7.

Siegel CS, "Measles - A Review of the Virological and Serological Methods for Early Detection," *Clin Microbiol Newslett*, 1991, 13:177-9.

Microaerophilic Streptococci see *Streptococcus*-Related Gram-Positive Cocci *on page 278*

Microsporidia

Microbiology Microsporidia are single-cell obligate intracellular parasites which can form spores under extracellular (adverse) environmental conditions. Microsporidia spores are oval to spherical and are 1-20 μm long, depending on the species; however, the spores typically are only 1-5 μm long when found in humans and other mammals. In stained stool preparations, the spores appear as large, fat, gram-negative rods and often have a central and darkly stained band or dot. There are many genera of microsporidia; however, only five genera have been associated with human disease, *Enterocytozoon*, *Encephalitozoon*, *Nosema*, *Pleistophora*, and *Septata*.

Epidemiology Microsporidia are found in many animal species, particularly invertebrates. Microsporidia have been isolated from many human specimens, including stool (by far the most common clinical source), intestine (only the jejunum and duodenum), urine, CSF, liver, skin, sinus/nasal mucosa, cornea, conjunctiva, kidney, and lungs. Microsporidia in the intestines are usually found as complete organisms in the enterocytes and as spores in the stool. Microsporidia, particularly *Enterocytozoon* and *Septata*, probably are pathogens in AIDS patients and probably are responsible for 10% to 20% of the cases of chronic diarrhea in AIDS patients. Less than 20 of the approximately 400 reported cases of microsporidia-associated diarrhea were reported from non-AIDS cases; the remainder were AIDS cases. Most cases have been associated with male homosexuals with AIDS and extremely low CD4 cell counts.

Clinical Syndromes

- **Microsporidia-associated diarrhea:** The most common clinical presentation of microsporidia-associated diarrhea in AIDS patients is gradual onset (eventually chronic) of diarrhea (no blood or mucus), weight loss, nausea, abdominal cramps, and anorexia.

Diagnosis Diagnosis is made by clinical impression and a few laboratory tests. D-xylose and fat malabsorption frequently are present. Histological examination of jejunal and duodenal biopsies can be helpful if pathologists are notified of a suspected case, use appropriate stains, and are familiar with the characteristic morphology of the organism and histological alterations elicited by the organism. The staining characteristics of microsporidia in sections of tissue are variable and unpredictable, and microsporidia often are difficult to recognize in paraffin sections; they are more easily recognized in plastic sections. Microsporidia are easily and reproducibly stained and recognized outside of tissue, specifically in tissue imprint preparations and direct stool smears. Such preparations are best stained by a modified trichrome stain such as that described by Weber (see Selected Readings).

Diagnostic Tests/Procedures

Microsporidia Diagnostic Procedures *on page 489*

Note: Contact laboratory for availability of tests and special instructions.

Treatment Microsporidia-induced diarrhea should be managed with supportive fluid and electrolyte replacement. Although a variety of antiprotazoals have been utilized in the treatment of this infection, success has been limited. Albendazole may have the most clinical success. Metronidazole may also be a useful therapy especially in non-HIV infected patients.

Drug Therapy

Recommended

Metronidazole *on page 817*

Albendazole *on page 585*

Selected Readings

Didier ES, "Microsporidiosis," *Clin Infect Dis*, 1998, 27(1):1-8.

Goodgame RW, "Understanding Intestinal Spore-Forming Protozoa: Cryptospordia, Microsporidia, *Isospora*, and *Clyclospora*," *Ann Intern Med*, 1996, 124(4):429-41.

Lecuit M, Oksenhendler E, and Sarfati C, "Use of Albendazole for Disseminated Microsporidian Infections in a Patient With AIDS," *Clin Infect Dis*, 1994, 19(2):332-3.

Shadduck JA and Greeley E, "Microsporidia and Human Infections," *Clin Microbiol Rev*, 1989, 2(2):158-65.

Sun T, "Microsporidiosis in the Acquired Immunodeficiency Syndrome," *Infect Dis Newslett*, 1993, 12:20-2.

Weber R and Bryan RT, "Microsporidial Infections in Immunodeficient and Immunocompetent Patients," *Clin Infect Dis*, 1994, 19(3):517-21.

(Continued)

Microsporidia *(Continued)*

Weber R, Bryan RT, Owen RL, et al, "Improved Light-Microscopical Detection of Microsporidia Spores in Stool and Duodenal Aspirates. The Enteric Opportunistic Infections Working Group," *N Engl J Med*, 1992, 326(3):161-6.

Weber R, Bryan RT, Schwartz DA, et al, "Human Microsporidial Infections," *Clin Microbiol Rev*, 1994, 7(4):426-61.

Mobiluncus Species

Microbiology *Mobiluncus* species are anaerobic, curved bacteria which are gram-variable (either gram-positive or gram-negative). The organism is highly motile due to its multiple flagella. There are two species, *M. curtisii* and *M. mulieris*. *Mobiluncus* requires enriched media for optimal growth. The organism easily adheres to squamous epithelial cells of the human vagina.

Epidemiology The organism is one of the organisms associated with bacterial vaginosis (see Vaginosis, Bacterial *on page 54*). It has been isolated from the vagina of about 5% of healthy women but in nearly all patients meeting criteria for bacterial vaginosis. The main habitat of *Mobiluncus* is the vagina, but it has been isolated from the urethra of male partners of women with bacterial vaginosis and in rectal cultures of homosexual males.

Clinical Syndromes

- **Bacterial vaginosis:** *Mobiluncus* is one of several organisms associated with bacterial vaginosis. Other purported etiologic agents have included *Gardnerella vaginalis* and the genital *Mycoplasmas*. *Mobiluncus* is usually isolated in culture with other anaerobic organisms. Patients present with vaginal discharge which is typically malodorous and white or gray in appearance. The discharge is homogeneous and coats the vaginal mucosa, with little or no inflammation of the vulva or introitus. There is a fish-like odor to the discharge and the pH of the fluid is usually >4.6. Bacterial vaginosis is associated with "clue cells" which are vaginal epithelial cells coated with mixed organisms, including many gram-negative bacilli.
- **Upper genitourinary infections:** Occasional case reports.
- **Miscellaneous:** Breast abscesses and mastectomy wound infections have been rarely described.

Diagnosis *Mobiluncus* species may be suspected in a woman presenting with bacterial vaginosis, as described in Clinical Syndromes.

Diagnostic Tests/Procedures

Anaerobic Culture *on page 316*
Gram's Stain *on page 426*
(Physician **must** consult the Microbiology Laboratory before any anaerobic vaginal culture is ordered.)

Treatment *Mobiluncus* species are susceptible *in vitro* to a variety of antibiotics, including penicillin. However, most cases of bacterial vaginosis are treated successfully with metronidazole. Formal susceptibility testing is usually not performed.

Drug Therapy

Recommended

Metronidazole *on page 817*

Selected Readings

Spiegel CA, "*Gardnerella vaginalis* and *Mobiluncus* Species," *Principles and Practice of Infectious Diseases*, 4th ed, Mandell GL, Bennett JE, and Dolin R, eds, New York, NY: Churchill Livingstone, 1995, 2050-3.

Moraxella catarrhalis

Synonyms *Branhamella catarrhalis*

Microbiology *Moraxella catarrhalis* (*Branhamella*) is an aerobic, gram-negative diplococcus which resembles *Neisseria* species in its Gram's stain appearance. Although generally considered an organism of low pathogenicity, *M. catarrhalis* has gained increasing attention as a potential pathogen of the upper and lower respiratory tract, particularly in individuals with chronic bronchitis.

In the medical literature this organism has been variously named *Neisseria catarrhalis*, *Branhamella catarrhalis*, and most recently *Moraxella catarrhalis*. *M. catarrhalis* belongs to the family Neisseriaceae. *M. catarrhalis* is a kidney bean shaped coccus 0.6-1.0 μm in diameter, often appearing in pairs or tetrads. During active infection, the organisms can sometimes be seen within the cytoplasm of polymorphonuclear cells, where it is referred to as gram-negative intracellular diplococci. In the laboratory, the organism is readily grown on routine media such as blood agar and can often grow on ordinary media without blood.

Epidemiology *Moraxella catarrhalis* is considered part of the normal flora of the human respiratory tract, particularly in the nasal cavity where it is considered the main natural reservoir for this organism. Thus its isolation in culture does not necessarily imply clinical disease. Less commonly, it has been isolated from the oropharynx of otherwise healthy children and adults, although the prevalence figures vary among different published studies. Higher carriage rates are seen in patients with chronic bronchitis, and there is an established increase in colonization during the winter months.

Clinical Syndromes

- **Exacerbations of chronic obstructive pulmonary disease:** *M. catarrhalis* has been recognized as a potential cause of purulent exacerbations of chronic bronchitis, although still less common than *Streptoccocus pneumoniae* and *Haemophilus influenzae*.
- **Respiratory tract infections in infants and children, particularly in asthmatics.**
- **Acute otitis media.** This organism is the third leading cause of acute otitis media in children, accounting for about 15% of cases, with the highest incidence in the winter months. *M. catarrhalis* can be recovered from specimens of middle ear fluid via tympanocentesis, if clinically indicated.
- **Sinusitis:** *M. catarrhalis* can be a cause of acute sinusitis in both children and adults. It is usually found with other organisms and can be recovered from properly performed sinus aspirates.
- **Acute urethritis:** This organism is occasionally a saprophyte of the genital tract and has been reported to be a rare cause of the urethral syndrome.
- **Other invasive diseases:** Cases of meningitis, endocarditis, septicemia, and peritonitis have been reported, usually in immunosuppressed patients.

Diagnosis The laboratory is easily able to separate it from related *Neisseria* species biochemically. Rapid tests used to speciate *Neisseria* do not react with *Moraxella*. *Moraxella* is frequently recovered from sputum cultures along with a variety of other organisms. Every attempt should be made to obtain a high quality sputum specimen in order to minimize contamination of samples with commensal mouth organisms, which may include *Moraxella*. The finding of many gram-negative diplococci within polymorphonuclear leukocytes on a Gram's stain of expectorated sputum is suggestive of true infection, rather than colonization.

Serologic studies looking for a fourfold rise in antibody titer against *M. catarrhalis* play a limited role for most patients and remain primarily epidemiologic or investigational tools.

Diagnostic Tests/Procedures

Aerobic Culture, Sputum *on page 312*
Blood Culture, Aerobic and Anaerobic *on page 337*
Gram's Stain *on page 426*

Treatment In past years, *Moraxella catarrhalis* was exquisitely sensitive to penicillin. However, in the early 1980s, an increasing number of community isolates were found to produce the enzyme beta-lactamase, which could be either plasmid or chromosomally mediated. It is now estimated that 75% to 85% of strains of *M. catarrhalis* produce beta-lactamase. Such strains generally remain susceptible to oral erythromycin and tetracycline, with only 1% to 2% *in vitro* resistance. Co-trimoxazole is active against most strains of *M. catarrhalis*, which is particularly helpful when empirically treating a patient with an exacerbation of chronic bronchitis. Ampicillin alone is ineffective in treating beta-lactamase producing *M. catarrhalis* and should not be used even if such an organism appears sensitive to ampicillin *in vitro*. The combination of ampicillin or amoxicillin with a beta-lactamase inhibitor such as sulbactam or clavulanate (Augmentin®) is effective against most beta-lactamase positive strains. Finally, the cephalosporins in general appear more stable than penicillins in the presence of *M. catarrhalis* beta-lactamase; however, the results of *in vitro* susceptibility testing remain important in management.

Drug Therapy

Recommended

Co-Trimoxazole *on page 692*

Alternate

Amoxicillin and Clavulanate Potassium *on page 593*

(Continued)

Moraxella catarrhalis (Continued)

Cephalosporins, 2nd Generation *on page 662*

Cephalosporins, 3rd Generation *on page 662*

Clarithromycin *on page 681*

Azithromycin *on page 613*

Fluoroquinolones *on page 736*

Selected Readings

Catlin BW, "*Branhamella catarrhalis*: An Organism Gaining Respect as a Pathogen," *Clin Microbiol Rev*, 1990, 3(4):293-320.

Hager H, Verghese A, Alvarez S, et al, "*Branhamella catarrhalis* Respiratory Infections," *Rev Infect Dis*, 1987, 9(6):1140-9.

Verghese A, Berk SL, "*Branhamella catarrhalis*: A Microbiologic and Clinical Update," *Am J Med*, 1990, 88(Suppl 5A):1S-56S.

Verghese A, Berk SL, "*Moraxella (Branhamella) catarrhalis*," *Infect Dis Clin North Am*, 1991, 5(3):523-38.

MRSA *see Staphylococcus aureus*, Methicillin-Resistant *on page 256*

MRSE *see Staphylococcus epidermidis*, Methicillin-Resistant *on page 261*

MSSA *see Staphylococcus aureus*, Methicillin-Susceptible *on page 258*

MSSE *see Staphylococcus epidermidis*, Methicillin-Susceptible *on page 263*

Mucor Species

Microbiology Mucormycosis refers to opportunistic fungal infections caused by the mold order Mucorales, class Zygomycetes. Contrary to the name, *Mucor* species are rarely implicated in human disease. The most frequent fungi isolated are *Rhizopus*, *Rhizomucor*, and *Absidia*. Mucorales are ubiquitous organisms found worldwide in soil, dust, spoiled fruit, and bread products. They initiate and facilitate decay of organic material.

KOH preparation of infected material reveals sparsely septate mycelia 6-50 µm wide, up to 200 µm long, and rounded sporangia. Growth in culture is rapid at temperatures 25°C to 55°C (optimum temperature 28°C to 30°C) and usually begins as a cottony white mold turning gray to yellow to brown in 3-5 days. Wet mounts reveal sporangiophores arising off clusters of rhizoids (*Mucor* species lack rhizoids). H & E stains typically reveal an abundance of irregular shaped, broad hyphae with right angle branching in the midst of polymorphonuclear infiltrate and round blood vessel walls with or without invasion into the vessel wall.

Epidemiology Mucormycosis is one of the most acute and fulminant fungal infections. It has a distinct predilection for invasion of blood vessel walls with resultant ischemia and necrosis of the adjacent tissue, commonly referred to as "black pus". There are no associations with age, sex, race, or geography. Most frequently seen in poorly controlled diabetics and hematologic malignancies. Infection is secondary to direct inoculation cutaneously or inhalation of spores into the respiratory tract and taken up by alveolar macrophages.

Clinical Syndromes

- **Rhinocerebral:** Generally seen in diabetics, predilection for acidosis. Present with facial pain, headache, and fever. May see black necrotic eschar on palate or nasal mucosa. May involve orbit leading to orbital cellulitis, proptosis, chemosis, cranial nerve involvement, and eventual CNS involvement. Two-thirds develop orbital cellulitis, and 33% develop internal carotid artery thrombosis or cavernous sinus thrombosis. Overall mortality is 80% to 90%.

- **Pulmonary:** Most commonly seen in hematologic malignancies particularly with neutropenia. Present with fever, dyspnea, and chest pain. Typically, no infiltrates seen on chest radiograph secondary to absence of leukocytes. Chest radiograph may reveal necrosis and hemorrhage.

- **Cutaneous:** Usually secondary to direct inoculation from trauma burns. May be secondary to dissemination.

- **Gastrointestinal:** Present with nonspecific signs and symptoms of intra-abdominal abscess. Associated with severe malnutrition, kwashiorkor. Usually diagnosed at autopsy.

- **CNS:** Direct extension from nose or paranasal sinuses. Direct inoculation via intravenous drug abuse. Disseminated disease associated with deferoxamine therapy.

- **Miscellaneous:** Rarely affects bones, kidneys, or mediastinum. Cardiac invasion associated with myocardial infarction, congestive heart failure, valvular incompetence, and pericarditis.

Diagnosis CT scans are useful in delineating extent of rhinocerebral disease. Definitive diagnosis depends on direct examination of infected material revealing characteristic histopathology as cultures of biopsied material frequently do not grow.

Diagnostic Tests/Procedures

Fungus Culture, Biopsy *on page 414*

Fungus Culture, Bronchial Aspirate *on page 416*

KOH Preparation *on page 467*

Treatment Treatment requires extensive surgical debridement, amphotericin B 1-1.5 mg/kg per day and, if possible, correction of the underlying illness. Azoles are still under investigation. Unproven therapies include rifampin, tetracycline, and hyperbaric oxygen.

Drug Therapy

Recommended

Amphotericin B (Conventional) *on page 597*

Selected Readings

Morrison VA and McGlave PB, "Mucormycosis in the BMT Population," *Bone Marrow Transplant*, 1993, 11(5):383-8.

Rinaldi MG, "Zygomycosis," *Infect Dis Clin North Am*, 1989, 3(1):19-41.

Sugar AM, "Mucormycosis," *Clin Infect Dis*, 1992, 14(Suppl 1):S126-9.

Weitzman I, "Emerging Zygomycotic Agents," *Clin Microbiol Newslett*, 1997, 19(11):81-5.

Mumps Virus

Related Information

Immunization Guidelines *on page 1041*

Microbiology Mumps virus is the cause of an acute, nonsuppurative infection of the parotid glands (viral parotitis) which is primarily seen in children and adolescents. Mumps infection can also lead to serious systemic diseases including encephalitis and orchitis.

Mumps virus is an RNA virus of intermediate size (120-200 nm diameter), and belongs to the family Paramyxoviridae. It has two antigens (S and V) which can fix complement. Mumps virus can be grown in cell culture in a diagnostic virology laboratory.

Epidemiology Mumps occurs worldwide and throughout the year, with a peak in the spring (April and May). Humans are the only known reservoir. Epidemics are limited to groups where people live in close quarters, such as military barracks, institutions, or prisons. The incidence of mumps in the United States has declined by 95% since the institution of the mumps vaccine in the late 1960s. However, a significant rise in the number of mumps cases was reported in 1986 and 1987.

The virus has a reputation as being "less contagious" than other childhood illnesses such as measles or chickenpox, but this may not accurately reflect the many mumps infections which are asymptomatic or subclinical. Over 90% of adults are seropositive for mumps, indicating widespread exposure. The infection is rare in children younger than 2 years of age, and peak incidence is between 5 and 9 years of age. Transmission is by direct person-to-person spread of infected salivary secretions. An individual may be infectious for up to 1 week prior to the onset of clinical parotitis, with a peak infectivity 1-2 days before salivary gland swelling. Thus, control of spread is difficult. Mumps has also been isolated from the urine, and this remains a less important but potential route of spread (viruria may persist for weeks). After exposure, the incubation period is 2-4 weeks.

Immunity is life-long. One episode of mumps (even if subclinical) confers protection in almost all cases, and reinfections with mumps have only rarely been reported.

Clinical Syndromes During the several-week incubation period, the virus replicates in the upper respiratory tract and the cervical lymph nodes. Following this period of asymptomatic localized infection, the virus disseminates hematogenously to other organs, including the parotid glands, testes, central nervous system, ovaries, inner ear, and others. Common clinical manifestations include:

- **Acute salivary adenitis:** The salivary glands are thought to be infected during the phase of viremia, although direct extension from the respiratory

(Continued)

Mumps Virus *(Continued)*

tract has also been postulated. Typically, there is an abrupt onset of fever and swelling of the salivary glands. The patient may complain of earache, difficulty chewing, and swallowing. Systemic symptoms (ie, malaise, headache, sore throat, chills) may sometimes precede the acute adenitis, or may follow the onset of parotid swelling. Of the salivary glands, the parotid gland is most commonly involved and is bilateral in two-thirds. The submaxillary and/or the sublingual glands may be infected, alone or in combination with the parotids. In most (but not all) cases, the gland is exquisitely tender to palpation for several days and has a "gelatinous" texture. The ostium of Stensen's duct appears erythematous but frank pus is not expressible, as in bacterial parotitis. Inflammation of the parotid leads to release of salivary amylase, which can be detected in the serum. Most cases resolve in about 1 week without specific intervention.

- **Mumps meningitis:** It is estimated that the mumps virus involves the central nervous system in 50% of cases, although only 10% or less of patients with mumps parotitis develop clinical meningitis. Over 50% of cases of mumps meningitis will have no evidence of parotitis. Patients typically present with an "aseptic meningitis" picture, with headache, photophobia, fever, and stiff neck. Cerebrospinal fluid (CSF) reveals a lymphocytic pleocytosis, sometimes >2000 cells/mm^3, but up to 25% of patients will have a predominance of polymorphonuclear leukocytes, leading to confusion with bacterial meningitis. CSF protein levels are modestly elevated. Hypoglycorrhachia, or a low CSF glucose, is common with mumps meningitis, again potentially causing confusion with bacterial meningitis. Mumps meningitis is self-resolving and benign, and comprises about 1% of aseptic meningitis cases.

- **Mumps encephalitis:** This is a more serious infection than mumps meningitis. Encephalitis may be either "early", occurring at the time of onset of parotitis, or "late", occurring 1-2 weeks later. The "early" cases may be due to direct viral invasion of brain tissue, whereas the "late" cases may be due to an autoimmune, postinfectious demyelinating syndrome (similar to Guillain-Barré). Patients typically present with marked personality changes, decreased sensorium, and high fevers; seizures and aphasia have also been reported. CSF findings are similar to mumps meningitis. Mortality is about 1% to 2%. In the absence of active parotitis, mumps encephalitis is almost impossible to distinguish from herpes simplex encephalitis on clinical grounds. Of all viral encephalitides, mumps is etiologic in only 1% or less due to the success of the mumps vaccine.

- **Epididymoorchitis:** Most cases occur within the first 1-2 weeks following the onset of parotid symptoms, but in some cases, orchitis may occur prior to or without salivary gland involvement. About 25% of mumps cases in postpubertal males are complicated by orchitis. Characteristically, this is part of a biphasic illness, with a dramatic return of systemic symptoms (fever to 40°C, chills, vomiting, headache) accompanied by acute pain and swelling in the testicle. In most cases, there is unilateral testicular pain. Epididymitis is present in the majority of cases. Symptoms usually begin to resolve within 1 week. Sterility is unusual unless there is bilateral testicular involvement complicated by testicular atrophy.

- **Miscellaneous:** Mumps has been reported to cause pancreatitis, oophoritis (5% of postpubertal women), migratory polyarthritis, electrocardiographic abnormalities, myocarditis (rare), and others.

Diagnosis The diagnosis of mumps infection is usually made on clinical grounds, particularly if the characteristic parotid gland inflammation is present. The WBC count is often normal but may show a leukopenia, lymphocytosis, or leukocytosis (with extrasalivary involvement). The serum amylase level stays elevated for several weeks in many cases, even without obvious parotid swelling, and may be useful when mumps encephalitis is suspected.

Laboratory confirmation of the mumps virus is usually not necessary. However, culture or serologic confirmation may be important when mumps encephalitis is a reasonable possibility, extrasalivary mumps is suspected but no parotitis is present, or parotitis is unusually fulminant or prolonged. Laboratory techniques include:

1. Viral culture in cell culture systems. Appropriate specimens include viral swabs of Stensen's duct, saliva, CSF, biopsy material, and sometimes urine.

Blood cultures for mumps virus are low yield. The virus grows well in monkey kidney cells and demonstrates a distinctive cytopathic effect.
2. Serologic studies. Detection of mumps specific IgM antibody is presumptive evidence of recent infection. A fourfold rise in specific IgG titer is also diagnostic.

Diagnostic Tests/Procedures
Mumps Serology *on page 490*
Mumps Virus Culture *on page 491*
Virus Detection by DFA *on page 576*

Treatment There are no antiviral agents proven effective in mumps infection. Mumps immune globulin has been used prophylactically in susceptible individuals during outbreaks but without benefit. A live-attenuated vaccine has been in use in the United States since 1967 and is part of routine pediatric immunizations. The first dose is given around 15 months of age along with the vaccines for measles and rubella, the MMR. The live attenuated vaccine should not be administered to patients with severe immunodeficiencies, including AIDS. An inactivated vaccine is available in such instances.

Drug Therapy Comment
No antiviral agents proven effective.

Selected Readings
Hersh BS, Fine PE, Kent WK, et al, "Mumps Outbreak in a Highly Vaccinated Population," *J Pediatr,* 1991, 119(2):187-93.
Ray CG, "Mumps," *Harrison's Principles of Internal Medicine,* 13th ed, Isselbacher KJ, Braunwald E, Wilson JD, et al, eds, New York, NY: McGraw-Hill, 1994, 830-2.

***Mycobacterium avium* complex** *see Mycobacterium avium-intracellulare on this page*

Mycobacterium avium-intracellulare
Synonyms MAC; MAI; *Mycobacterium avium* complex
Microbiology MAC is an acid-fast bacillus that grows best at 37°C after 10-21 day incubation on selective agar media.

See table in *Mycobacterium tuberculosis* entry *on page 207* for a listing of important and major species of *Mycobacterium* and the pathogenic potential of each species.

Epidemiology Prior to the AIDS epidemic, MAC was extremely rare. Approximately 40% of patients will develop MAC within 2 years of the diagnosis of AIDS if no prophylaxis is given. Median survival was approximately 8-9 months prior to the introduction of potent antiretroviral therapy era. MAC is associated with CD4 counts <50 cells/µL. The incidence of MAC has decreased since the introduction of MAC prophylaxis and potent antiretroviral therapy. MAC disease may start with colonization of the gastrointestinal or respiratory tract and then establish a localized infection with intermittent MAC bacteremia leading to seeding of other organs (primarily to the reticuloendothelial system (RES)). This is followed by an unknown period of proliferation in these extravascular sites until the increasing organism burden results in sustained symptoms and "spillover" sustained bacteremia.

Clinical Syndromes
- **Asymptomatic:** Normal hosts may have colonization in the respiratory or gastrointestinal tracts. Duration of asymptomatic to dissemination in HIV is unknown.
- **Localized:** Focal pneumonia, skin, endophthalmitis, and CNS infections are rare. Localized infection of the GI tract is more common with infection in the duodenum most common. Patients present with nausea, diarrhea, abdominal pain, and, less commonly, biliary obstruction secondary to lymphadenopathy.
- **Disseminated:** Patients present with fever, weight loss, night sweats, anemia, and elevated alkaline phosphatase. Diarrhea (more than three unformed stools daily) is common. Factors associated with MAC include time since diagnosis of AIDS, presence of significant anemia (hemoglobin <8 g/dL), previous opportunistic infection and interruption of antiretroviral therapy. Pathology of infected organs reveal organomegaly, organs which may be yellow secondary to color of organism, histiocytes filled with acid-fast bacilli, and poorly formed granulomas.

Diagnosis Dependent on isolation of MAC from sterile body source. MAC isolated from sputum or GI source may represent colonization, and clinical correlation is recommended. Bone marrow cultures may be more sensitive than
(Continued)

Mycobacterium avium-intracellulare (Continued)

blood cultures due to higher organism burden and earlier infection. Acid-fast bacillus (AFB) stains of the bone marrow may be postive in up to 40% disseminated MAC. Caution should be used when interpreting results of AFB stains as they may represent other mycobacterial disease such as disseminated tuberculosis.

Diagnostic Tests/Procedures

Acid-Fast Stain *on page 305*
Blood Culture, Mycobacteria *on page 342*
Mycobacteria Culture, Biopsy or Body Fluid *on page 493*
Mycobacteria Culture, Sputum *on page 495*

Treatment Disseminated MAC: Macrolide-based therapy is associated with improved survival and decreased relapse rates. Azithromycin 500 mg/day or clarithromycin 500 mg twice daily plus either ethambutol 25 mg/kg/day or rifabutin 300 mg/day. Unknown if initial use of three drugs instead of two drugs is of any benefit. Must remain on therapy for life-long suppression. Initiation of antiretroviral therapy is advised.

Relapse: Should add two drugs not previously used to treat patient. If on macrolide plus ethambutol, add rifabutin and ciprofloxacin. If on macrolide plus rifabutin, add ethambutol and ciprofloxacin. If on macrolide plus ethambutol plus rifabutin, add two of any of the following: ciprofloxacin, clofazimine, or amikacin. Amikacin available in parenteral form only and will require long-term indwelling catheter.

Prophylaxis: Azithromycin 1200 mg orally weekly or clarithromycin 500 mg orally twice weekly or rifabutin 300 mg/day is recommended in all patients with a CD4 nadir <50 cells/μL. Caution should be used when starting macrolide prophylaxis to assure MAC is not present. Initiation of macrolide monotherapy in the setting of MAC infection may result in macrolide resistance. If patient has known colonization with MAC, two-drug prophylaxis is recommended.

Studies are currently in progress to evaluate whether chronic suppressive therapy and prophylaxis can be withdrawn in AIDS patients receiving potent antiretroviral therapy whose CD4 T-cell counts are >100 cells/μL.

Drug Therapy

Recommended

Clarithromycin *on page 681*
used in combination with
Ethambutol *on page 727*
or
Rifabutin(or both) *on page 900*
Azithromycin *on page 613*
used in combination with
Ethambutol *on page 727*
or
Rifabutin(or both) *on page 900*

Alternate

Clofazimine *on page 687*
Amikacin *on page 588*
Ciprofloxacin *on page 678*

Selected Readings

Aberg JA, Yajko DM, and Jacobson MA, "Eradication of AIDS-Related Disseminated *Mycobacterium avium* Complex Infection After 12 Months of Antimycobacterial Therapy Combined With Highly Active Antiretroviral Therapy," *J Infect Dis*, 1998, 178(5):1446-9.

Benson CA and Ellner JJ, "*Mycobacterium avium* Complex Infection and AIDS. Advances in Theory and Practice," *Clin Infect Dis*, 1993, 17(1):7-20.

Falkinham JO 3d, "Epidemiology of Infection by Nontuberculous Mycobacteria," *Clin Microbiol Rev*, 1996, 9(2):177-215.

"Management of *Mycobacterium avium* Complex in Patients With HIV Infection," *Clin Infect Dis*, 1994, 18(Suppl 3):S217-43.

Masur H, "Recommendations on Prophylaxis and Therapy for Disseminated *Mycobacterium avium* Complex Disease in Patients Infected With Human Immunodeficiency Virus," *N Engl J Med*, 1993, 329(12):898-904.

Masur H, Kaplan JE, Holmes KK, et al, "1997 USPHS/IDSA Guidelines for the Prevention of Opportunistic Infections in Persons Infected With Human Immunodeficiency Virus: Disease-Specific Recommendations," *Clin Infect Dis*, 1997, 25(Suppl 3):S313-35.

Nightingale SD, Cameron DW, Gordin FM, et al, "Two Controlled Trials of Rifabutin Prophylaxis Against *Mycobacterium avium* Complex Infections in AIDS," *N Engl J Med*, 1993, 329(12):828-33.

Tartaglione TA, "Therapeutic Options for the Management and Prevention of *Mycobacterium avium* Complex Infection in Patients With the Acquired Immunodeficiency Syndrome," *Pharmacotherapy*, 1996, 16(2):171-82.

Mycobacterium bovis

Synonyms Bacillus, Calmette-Guérin; BCG

Microbiology *Mycobacterium bovis* is an acid-fast bacillus, often shorter and plumper than *M. tuberculosis* (MTB). *M. bovis* grows more slowly than most mycobacterial species and growth can be inhibited by the presence of glycerol in the media. It is biochemically differentiated from MTB by niacin and nitrate reduction tests (*M. bovis* is usually negative for both tests where MTB is generally positive). Unlike MTB, *M. bovis* is microaerophilic, sensitive to thiopin-2-carboxylic acid, and resistant to pyrazinamide. *M. bovis* grows only at 35°C and appears as tiny translucent, smooth, pyramidal colonies. These organisms grow well on most media commonly used for the culture of MTB, including the Lowenstein-Jensen and 7H11. BCG is an attenuated mutant of *M. bovis*.

Epidemiology *Mycobacterium bovis* is known as the agent of bovine tuberculosis. *M. bovis* was a significant cause of "tuberculosis" worldwide in the early 1900s and before. Destruction of animals infected with *M. bovis* and subsequent pasteurization procedures for milk decreased the human infection rate by *M. bovis* dramatically. *M. bovis* was thought to be transmitted not only by ingestion of infected milk but also aerogenously by cow to human transmission. Human to human transmission, which undoubtedly occurs, is quite controversial. The potential for human to cow transmission also may occur through the aerogenous route, as well as through urine of farmers with genitourinary *M. bovis* disease, where feeding areas are contaminated by infectious urine, which is either aerosolized or ingested by cattle. Other animal reservoirs may include pigs, goats, deer, cats, dogs, foxes, badgers, marsupials, rabbits, sheep, and horses.

BCG, which has been used in many parts of the world to immunize individuals against tuberculosis, has also been used to boost immune response and treat carcinoma of the bladder. There are significant numbers of reports of systemic BCG infection developing in these treated or immunized patients. Most cases of serious "BCG" infection are associated with bloodstream absorption of the agent. BCG should not be given to patients until at least 1 week after any surgical manipulation of the bladder or tumor resection.

Clinical Syndromes Unlike tuberculosis, much of the primary disease caused by *M. bovis* occur in the cervical lymph nodes and the GI tract with its related lymphatics; however, *M. bovis* may cause pulmonary disease and cause disease in other extrapulmonary sites in a similar manner to MTB. The most common sites of *M. bovis* infection in children are involvement of the cervical lymph nodes and intra-abdominal organs as reflected in the oral portal of entry. (Incidence is extremely rare since eradication of infected cattle and widespread pasteurization of milk). Disease can occur, however, in any organ system similar to MTB. In adults, extrapulmonary *M. bovis* infection is often a reactivation of disease. The lung is still the most common organ involved when transmission is through bovine contact. *M. bovis* can cause gastric TB, tuberculous meningitis, miliary disease, epidural abscess and spinal tuberculosis, bone and joint infections, and genitourinary infection.

Systemic infection caused by administration of BCG can cause pneumonitis, hepatitis, systemic BCG infection, including life-threatening sepsis, arthritis and arthralgias, skin rash, and genitourinary tract infections. Granulomatous hepatitis may be more of a hypersensitivity reaction than infection. Sepsis following intravesical BCG installation can be lethal. The attenuation of this organism has not rendered it completely harmless. Patients may present with classic symptoms of sepsis including shock, acute respiratory distress, and disseminated intravascular coaguulopathy.

Diagnosis Diagnosis should be based on appropriate history of animal exposure, occupational contact, or receipt of BCG vaccination or chemotherapy. The tuberculin skin test may be useful, except in patients with known exposure to BCG. Appropriate specimen retrieval from suspected infected sites is necessary, with subsequent acid-fast staining and cultures. *M. bovis* will grow in a routine mycobacterial culture.

Diagnostic Tests/Procedures

Acid-Fast Stain *on page 305*

(Continued)

Mycobacterium bovis (Continued)

Mycobacteria Culture, Biopsy or Body Fluid *on page 493*
Mycobacteria Culture, Sputum *on page 495*
Tuberculin Skin Testing, Intracutaneous *on page 557*

Treatment Manifestations of *M. bovis* disease should be treated in a similar manner as tuberculosis, with the exception that all strains are inherently resistant to pyrazinamide. Six month regimens with isoniazid and rifampin (plus ethambutol for the first 2 months) may be adequate. Typical TB treatment courses may be followed. This is also true for disseminated BCG. Organisms are routinely susceptible to all the first and second line antituberculous agents (except pyrazinamide). Susceptibility testing should be performed on all organisms cultured, as mycobacterial infections resistant to one or more drugs have been reported.

Drug Therapy

Recommended

Combinations of 2 or more of the following.

Isoniazid *on page 782*
Rifampin *on page 902*
Ethambutol *on page 727*
Streptomycin *on page 924*

Alternate

If intolerant of a first line antitubercular agent or if multidrug resistance is present, one or more of the alternate antitubercular agents should be substituted:

Antituberculars *on page 611*

Selected Readings

Bass JB Jr, Farer LS, Hopewell PC, et al, "Treatment of Tuberculosis and Tuberculosis Infections in Adults and Children. American Thoracic Society and the Centers for Disease Control and Prevention," *Am J Respir Crit Care Med*, 1994, 149(5):1359-74.

Berlin OG, "Mycobacteria," *Bailey & Scott's Diagnostic Microbiology*, St. Louis, MO: CV Mosby Co, 1990, 597-640.

Dankner WM, Waecker NJ, Essey MA, et al, "*Mycobacterium bovis* Infections in San Diego: A Clinicoepidemiologic Study of 73 Patients and a Historical Review of a Forgotten Pathogen," *Medicine*, 1993, 72(1):11-37.

"Initial Therapy for Tuberculosis in the Era of Multidrug Resistance. Recommendations of the Advisory Council for the Elimination of Tuberculosis," *MMWR Morb Mortal Wkly Rep*, 1993, 42(RR-7):1-8.

Lamm DL, van der Meijden PM, Morales A, et al, "Incidence and Treatment of Complications of Bacillus Calmette-Guérin Intravesical Therapy in Superficial Bladder Cancer," *J Urol*, 1992, 147(3):596-600.

Willett HP, "*Mycobacterium*," *Zinsser Microbiology*, 20th ed, Joklik WK, Willett HP, Amos DB, et al, eds, Norwalk, CT: Appleton & Lange, 1988, 423-48.

Mycobacterium kansasii

Microbiology *Mycobacterium kansasii* is an acid-fast bacillus that is a "nontuberculous" *Mycobacterium*. It is a photochromogen and appears as a long, thick bacillus on clinical specimens. The organism is not well visualized using the Gram's stain and an acid-fast stain is necessary. Similarly, the organism does not grow well on routine bacteriologic media.

See table in *Mycobacterium tuberculosis on page 207* for a listing of important and major species of *Mycobacterium* and the pathogenic potential of each species.

Epidemiology *M. kansasii* has been reported to cause disease worldwide. The highest incidence of disease in the United States has been reported in the southwest and midwest regions. Infection in children is unusual, with most cases reported in the fifth decade of life. Occupational groups at increased risk for *M. kansasii* infection include miners, welders, and painters, among others. There is also an increased incidence of chronic obstructive pulmonary disease in individuals infected with *M. kansasii*. Healthy individuals can be infected by this organism.

Clinical Syndromes

- **Pulmonary infection:** Infection by *M. kansasii* frequently causes a pneumonitis similar to that caused by *Mycobacterium tuberculosis*. Patients present with subacute onset of cough, low grade fevers, and malaise. Routine blood studies are not helpful. A variety of radiographic abnormalities have been reported including cavitary lung disease, pleural effusions, and a miliary pattern. In many cases it is difficult to distinguish the x-ray from tuberculosis.

Some individuals are chronically colonized with this organism, making the clinical interpretation of a positive respiratory culture difficult.

- **Extrapulmonary infection:** *M. kansasii* has been reported to cause cervical lymph node infection, skin lesions (from local inoculation), osteomyelitis, soft tissue infection, renal pelvis obstruction, and dissemination.

Diagnosis Infection with *M. kansasii* mimics tuberculosis both clinically and radiographically. Culture confirmation is essential. Most commonly the diagnosis is established by sending respiratory samples (sputum, bronchoscopy specimens) for acid-fast bacilli (AFB) stain and culture. In cases of extrapulmonary disease, the appropriate body fluid or tissue (urine, lymph node biopsy, etc) should be specified for AFB stain and culture.

Diagnostic Tests/Procedures

Acid-Fast Stain *on page 305*

Mycobacteria Culture, Biopsy or Body Fluid *on page 493*

Treatment In general, *M. kansasii* responds well to antimicrobial therapy. The role on isoniazid has been controversial since this agent has only minimal efficacy against *M. kansasii in vitro.* Current recommendations suggest the combination of isoniazid, rifampin, and ethambutol for initial therapy.

Drug Therapy

Recommended

Isoniazid *on page 782*

Rifampin *on page 902*

Ethambutol *on page 727*

all 3 used in combination

Selected Readings

Bamberger DM, Driks MR, Gupta MR, et al, "*Mycobacterium kansasii* Among Patients Infected With Human Immunodeficiency Virus in Kansas City," *Clin Infect Dis*, 1994, 18(3):395-400.

Mycobacterium Species, Not MTB or MAI

Microbiology Mycobacteria other than *M. tuberculosis* (MTB) and *M. avium-intracellulare* (MAI) (hereafter called "other" mycobacteria) are acid-fast bacilli which have cell walls with high lipid content and are morphologically similar to MTB and MAI. Other mycobacteria are different from MTB and MAI in biochemical reactions, pigmentation, growth rates, natural reservoirs, pathogenesis, manifestations of disease, and susceptibilities to antimicrobial agents. Like MTB, other mycobacteria tend to cause chronic diseases and lesions. There are many species of other mycobacteria, the most commonly isolated are the following: *M. kansasii, M. marinum, M. gordonae, M. ulcerans, M. fortuitum, M. chelonae* subsp *chelonae, M. chelonae* subsp *abscessus,* and *M. scrofulaceum. M. genavense* and *M. haemophilum* are recently recognized other mycobacteria with which most physicians are not familiar. These other mycobacteria are pathogens to humans (usually immunocompromised hosts), grow in blood culture broth but require special growth media for subculture, and can require 4-9 weeks to grow on solid culture media.

See table in *Mycobacterium tuberculosis on page 207* for a listing of important and major species of *Mycobacterium* and the pathogenic potential of each species.

Epidemiology Other mycobacteria are ubiquitous in nature. Natural reservoirs include soil, cattle and other domestic livestock, fish, water, milk and other foods, wild animals, and nonhuman primates. The CDC has reported that other mycobacteria accounted for 35% of non-MTB mycobacteria clinical isolates.

Clinical Syndromes of Mycobacteria

Mycobacterium Infection	Relatively Common Cause
Chronic pulmonary	M. kansasii, M. fortuitum
Cervical lymphadenitis	M. kansasii, M. scrofulaceum
Soft tissue	M. marinum, M. abscessus
Disseminated	M. kansasii
Surgical wound	M. fortuitum, M. chelonae subsp
Skeletal, joint	M. kansasii, M. fortuitum, M. ulcerans
Skin, ulcer, abscess	M. marinum, M. fortuitum, M. abscessus, M. ulcerans, M. chelonae subsp

(Continued)

Mycobacterium Species, Not MTB or MAI *(Continued)*

Humans become infected with other mycobacteria by inhalation of the mycobacteria through the mouth and nose and by direct inoculation into breaks in the skin. Other mycobacteria generally are not transmitted person to person.

Clinical Syndromes Other mycobacteria can cause numerous clinical syndromes, the most common of which are presented in the following table on the previous page.

Mycobacterium fortuitum and *M. chelonei* are two important Runyon group IV "rapid growers", so-named because of their ability to grow in several days when subcultured (initial isolation of the organism may require 1 or more weeks). Both healthy and immunocompromised persons may develop infection with these agents. Skin and soft tissue infections are relatively common manifestations of these organisms and are usually associated with trauma or the presence of a foreign body; this includes infection of postoperative wounds (eg, sternal wounds after cardiac surgery), infections of orthopedic devices such as arthroplasties, breast implant infections, post-traumatic wound infections, and others. Pulmonary infection from inhalation may occur with microabscess formation in the lungs (granuloma formation is less common). Other manifestations include endocarditis, osteomyelitis, and lymphadenitis, but visceral dissemination outside of the lungs is rare. Although disseminated disease has been reported in immunocompromised individuals, a recent review suggests this is an unusual occurrence.

Mycobacterium marinum is the cause of "fishtank granuloma." Infections are characterized by multiple ulcerative skin lesions on an extremity that spread proximally along the lymphatics. The organism grows well in fresh and salt water and is associated with fishtanks, pools, and aquariums. Human disease occurs usually through direct inoculation through a break in the skin. Patients with this clinical syndrome should be asked about exposure to aquarium water or other aquatic activities. Other mycobacteria besides *M. marinum* can cause a similar syndrome, as can infection with *Sporothrix schenckii.*

Mycobacterium scrofulaceum is an important cause of cervical lymphadenitis in children. The disease remains localized, but cure often requires both antimicrobial therapy and surgery.

Mycobacterium ulcerans is pathogenic mainly in tropical countries such as Africa. It characteristically causes a necrotic ulcer on the extremities.

Diagnosis The aforementioned diseases are diagnosed by culture of tissues (**not** swab specimens). Most other mycobacteria will grow in culture in 2-4 weeks. However, growth rates depend on the species and range from 3-60 days. *M. abscessus* soft tissue infections of an extremity can resemble sporotrichosis.

Diagnostic Tests/Procedures

Acid-Fast Stain *on page 305*

Mycobacteria Culture, Biopsy or Body Fluid *on page 493*

Treatment

M. fortuitum: Typically resistant to all common antitubercular agents. Amikacin and cefoxitin can be administered for 2-6 weeks followed by oral therapy with co-trimoxazole or doxycycline for 2-6 months.

M. scrofulaceum: Treatment of choice is usually surgical excision. If necessary, drug therapy regimen should include isoniazid, rifampin, and streptomycin. This organism is also sensitive *in vitro* to the macrolides and cycloserine.

M. marinum: A 6-week (6-month, if deep infection) course of co-trimoxazole or minocycline or rifampin in combination with ethambutol can be used. Surgical excision may also be required.

M. chelonae: Sensitive to amikacin and the macrolides. A 6-month course of clarithromycin may be the regimen of choice.

M. ulcerans: A useful regimen includes a 6-week course of either rifampin in combination with amikacin or ethambutol in combination with co-trimoxazole.

Treatment regimens remain controversial for some of these mycobacterial agents due to a lack of formal clinical trials. Combination therapy is of use with severe infections, but even less data is available concerning the optimal agents to be used. **Antibiotic susceptibility testing is strongly recommended since the drug-susceptibility patterns are not reliably predictable.** Consultation with an Infectious Disease specialist should also be considered.

Selected Readings

Horowitz EA and Sanders WE Jr, "Other *Mycobacterium* Species," *Principles and Practice of Infectious Diseases*, 4th ed, Mandell GL, Bennett JE, and Dolin R, eds, New York, NY: Churchill Livingstone, 1995, 2264-73.

Falkinham JO 3d, "Epidemiology of Infection by Nontuberculous Mycobacteria," *Clin Microbiol Rev*, 1996, 9(2):177-215.

Salfinger M and Wallace RJ, "Susceptibility Testing for Nontuberculosis Mycobacteria: Should It Be Performed?" *Clin Microbiol Newslett*, 1997, 19(9):68-71.

Woods GL and Washington JA 2d, "Mycobacteria Other Than *Mycobacterium tuberculosis*: Review of Microbiologic and Clinical Aspects," *Rev Infect Dis*, 1987, 9(2):275-94.

Mycobacterium tuberculosis

Related Information

HIV Therapeutic Information *on page 1008*

Tuberculosis Guidelines *on page 1114*

Tuberculosis Guidelines *on page 1114*

Synonyms Tubercle Bacillus

Microbiology *Mycobacterium tuberculosis* (MTB) is a fastidious, slowly-growing, aerobic bacterium with a complex cell wall composed of peptidoglycans and many complex, long-chain lipids. The free lipids on the outer layer make *M. tuberculosis* relatively hydrophobic and resistant to many stains used in the laboratory including the Gram's stain and Giemsa stain. It is an acid-fast bacillus, meaning once the organism is stained, it cannot be decolorized by acid solutions.

Mycobacteria can be isolated on solid agar media or in broth cultures (which can be read by automated devices). Growth in broth is usually much more rapid than on agar.

See table for listing of important and major species of *Mycobacterium* and the pathogenic potential of each species.

Clinically Relevant Major Species of *Mycobacterium*

Group	Strict Human Pathogens	Occasional/ Potential Human Pathogens	Usually Environmental/ Rarely Human Pathogens
M. tuberculosis complex	*M. tuberculosis* *M. leprae* *M. africanum* *M. ulcerans*	*M. bovis*	
Photochromogens		*M. kansasii* *M. marinum* *M. simiae* *M. asiaticum*	
Scotochromogens		*M. scrofulaceum* *M. szulgai* *M. xenopi*	*M. gordonae* *M. flavescens*
Nonchromogens	*M. genavense*	*M. avium* *M. intracellulare* *M. hemophilum* *M. malmoense*	
Rapid growers		*M. fortuitum* *M. chelonei*	*M. smegmatis*

Epidemiology Tuberculosis remains one of the most common and deadly diseases throughout the world. It is estimated that 33% of the world's population has been infected with *M. tuberculosis*. There are approximately 30 million active cases of tuberculosis at any time.

In the past 10 years there has been a resurgence of tuberculosis in the United States. In prior years, the number of new cases of tuberculosis had been declining at a rate of about 5% per year, but since the mid 1980s, the case rate began to rise at a rate of about 3% per year; this disturbing reversal has been attributed in large part to the AIDS epidemic. In the United States, over 10 million individuals in the U.S. have been infected with MTB at some point in their lives based on the results of tuberculin skin testing. The majority of active cases of tuberculosis come from this large pool of individuals who have been exposed to MTB in the past and later present with reactivation of latent infection. A smaller number of active cases are attributable to recent exposure of a healthy individual to a person with active tuberculosis.

(Continued)

Mycobacterium tuberculosis *(Continued)*

In the United States, there are many defined groups at high risk for MTB infection:

- individuals with HIV infection
- close contacts (ie, family members and others) of infectious TB cases
- persons with underlying medical conditions which increase the risk of TB (see below)
- persons from foreign countries with a high prevalence of TB
- indigent populations
- alcoholics and persons who use intravenous drugs
- persons residing in nursing homes, prisons, and other long-term care facilities
- healthcare workers

Certain medical conditions predispose a person to the development of active tuberculosis once a person has been infected with the organism:

- HIV infection
- silicosis
- chest x-ray which shows fibrotic lesions, consistent with prior TB
- diabetes
- steroids or other immunosuppressive medications
- lymphomas and other hematologic diseases
- end-stage renal disease, especially those on chronic dialysis
- intestinal bypass
- postgastrectomy
- chronic malabsorption syndromes
- head and neck malignancies
- weight loss of 10% below ideal body weight, from any cause

MTB is transmitted via the respiratory route when an infected individual comes in close contact with a susceptible person. The organism is carried in droplets of respiratory secretions ("airborne droplets") during coughing, sneezing, and speaking; the organism can remain airborne and infectious for a period of time. Person-to-person transmission occurs when a susceptible individual inhales the infectious droplet nuclei. Close household contacts of infected individuals puts others at risk for acquiring infection, although typically several months of exposure may be needed. The degree of contagiousness of a given patient depends on a variety of factors including the number of organisms in the sputum, presence or absence of cavitary lung disease, amount of coughing, length of time on antituberculous therapy, and others.

Clinical Syndromes

- **Primary tuberculosis:** Primary infection, or first exposure to *M. tuberculosis*, often is asymptomatic. Typically, there is a pulmonary infiltrate in the mid or lower lung fields with or without hilar adenopathy. The infiltrates are nonspecific in appearance and are not cavitary. In most cases, the pneumonitis clears without specific therapy and latent infection is established. In some cases, the primary infection progresses and mimics reactivation disease.
- **Latent infection:** Many individuals remain asymptomatic following the primary infection with *M. tuberculosis*. The organism remains latent within macrophages indefinitely. The tuberculin skin test is extremely important in identifying these individuals (see Tuberculin Skin Testing, Intracutaneous *on page 557*). Approximately 1 in 10 persons with infection from *M. tuberculosis* will develop clinical disease at some time in their life unless given preventative therapy.
- **Reactivation tuberculosis:** Patients with reactivation tuberculosis present with weight loss, fever, constitutional symptoms, and a generalized wasting syndrome. Drenching night sweats are common. Often, these individuals are diagnostic dilemmas since pulmonary symptoms may be very mild or absent.
- **Pulmonary tuberculosis:** The majority of cases of active pulmonary tuberculosis are due to reactivation of the latent organism. Reactivation is likely to occur in the upper lobes and the superior segments of the lower lobes due to the oxygen-rich environment. However, disease can involve any area of the lung, especially in diabetics, elderly persons, and persons with AIDS. The absence of apical infiltrates should not be used to exclude tuberculosis; and for practical purposes, TB should be included in the differential diagnosis of

any undiagnosed pneumonia. The extent of disease is also variable, ranging from subtle infiltrates in chest x-ray with minimal cough to the classic cavitary tuberculosis with hemoptysis. If untreated, the pulmonary lesions develop areas of caseation or central necrosis with partial liquefaction.

- **Extrapulmonary tuberculosis:** (See Selected Readings). Tuberculous disease outside the lung parenchyma can be even more difficult to diagnose. Extrapulmonary TB can become clinically apparent during the phase of primary infection, particularly in children. More commonly, extrapulmonary TB represents reactivation of latent infection. It is important to note that a pulmonary lesion of any type will be absent in 50% or more cases of extrapulmonary TB; it is even more uncommon to have a chest x-ray showing active pulmonary infiltrates or cavities. Extrapulmonary TB includes:
  - pleural disease with effusion; the most common form of extrapulmonary TB
  - tuberculous meningitis; often a difficult diagnosis to confirm. Classically, patients present with a chronic meningitis, but a more fulminant variety resembling pyogenic meningitis is well recognized. Because there is often a basilar meningitis, patients frequently develop cranial nerve signs; tuberculous meningitis should be strongly considered in any patient with signs or symptoms of meningitis with cranial nerve deficits. The spinal fluid typically has an elevated protein, low glucose, and a lymphocytic pleocytosis (see Lumbar Puncture *on page 477*), but this pattern can be seen in a number of other disease entities. Often repeated lumbar punctures with high volumes of spinal fluid submitted for mycobacterial culture are required to confirm the diagnosis. However, if the clinical suspicion for tuberculous meningitis is high (ie, positive tuberculin skin test, lymphocytic pleocytosis, etc), antituberculous therapy should be initiated.
  - pericarditis
  - peritonitis
  - tuberculous adenitis or "scrofula" (chronic tuberculous infection of the cervical lymph nodes)
  - osteomyelitis including tuberculosis of the spine (Pott's disease)
  - genitourinary tuberculosis
  - ocular infections including chorioretinitis
  - gastrointestinal tuberculosis
  - cutaneous tuberculosis (lupus vulgaris)
  - miliary tuberculosis; *M. tuberculosis* can disseminate into the lymphohematogenous system either during primary tuberculous infection or during reactivation (more common). This can be a difficult diagnosis to establish, and the chest x-ray can be normal early on.

Diagnosis A high index of suspicion must be maintained for tuberculosis. Laboratory confirmation of suspected cases is essential since the manifestations of MTB are protean. The tuberculin skin test is an important first step in identifying infected patients. Laboratory techniques for identifying *M. tuberculosis* include:

- acid-fast smears and cultures of respiratory secretions
- acid-fast smears and cultures of other potentially infected body fluids or tissues (cerebrospinal fluid, gastric fluid, urine, bone marrow biopsies, joint fluids, and many others)
- rapid methods - amplification of nucleic acid of MTB by the polymerase chain reaction (PCR) and subsequent detection by nucleic acid probes

Diagnostic Tests/Procedures
Acid-Fast Stain *on page 305*
Lumbar Puncture *on page 477*
Mycobacteria Culture, Biopsy or Body Fluid *on page 493*
Mycobacteria Culture, Sputum *on page 495*
Polymerase Chain Reaction *on page 523*
Tuberculin Skin Testing, Intracutaneous *on page 557*

Treatment The treatment of tuberculosis is based on the following principles.

- *M. tuberculosis* becomes resistant to drugs through random, spontaneous genetic mutations. For isoniazid, the proportion of naturally occurring resistant bacteria has been established as 1 in 10^6, and for rifampin, the ratio is 1 bacterium in 10^8.
- A regimen containing multiple drugs to which the organisms are susceptible should be used; susceptibility testing should be done on all isolates.

(Continued)

Mycobacterium tuberculosis (Continued)

- Both isoniazid-resistant MTB and multidrug-resistant MTB are becoming increasing problems (see Selected Readings).
- When patient compliance is poor, directly observed therapy given 3 times per week in an outpatient setting should be strongly considered.
- Failures of therapy are often due to noncompliance with the regimen. The emergence of multidrug therapy is partly due to noncompliance as well.
- Physicians must take into account the immune status of the patient.

The Centers for Disease Control and Prevention has recommended the initial treatment of TB should include four drugs. During the first 2 months, the drug regimen should include isoniazid, rifampin, pyrazinamide, and ethambutol or streptomycin. When drug susceptibility results are available, this regimen should be altered appropriately. In some cases, the four-drug regimen is not necessary but should be based on analysis of the local rate of both isoniazid resistance and multidrug resistance. If the rate of isoniazid resistance in the community is <4%, a two- or three-drug regimen could be used at physician discretion.

Drug Therapy
Recommended
Isoniazid *on page 782*
Rifampin *on page 902*
Rifampin and Isoniazid *on page 905*
Pyrazinamide *on page 884*
Ethambutol *on page 727*
Streptomycin *on page 924*
Note: See Treatment for appropriate regimen.
Alternate
If intolerant of a first-line antitubercular agent or if multidrug resistant and TB is present, one or more of the alternative antitubercular agents should be substituted:
Antituberculars *on page 611*

Selected Readings
Barnes PF and Barrows SA, "Tuberculosis in the 1990s," *Ann Intern Med*, 1993, 119(5):400-10.

Berenguer J, Moreno S, Laguna F, et al, "Tuberculosis Meningitis in Patients Infected With the Human Immunodeficiency Virus," *N Engl J Med*, 1992, 326(10):668-72.

Centers for Disease Control/American Thoracic Society, *Core Curriculum on Tuberculosis*, 2nd ed, Atlanta, GA: U.S. Department of Health and Human Services, Public Health Service, 1991.

Frieden TR, Sterling T, Pablos-Mendez A, et al, "The Emergence of Drug Resistant Tuberculosis in New York City," *N Engl J Med*, 1993, 328(8):521-6.

Goble M, Iseman MD, Madsen LA, et al, "Treatment of 171 Patients With Pulmonary Tuberculosis Resistant to Isoniazid and Rifampin," *N Engl J Med*, 1993, 328(8):527-32.

"Initial Therapy for Tuberculosis in the Era of Multidrug Resistance," *MMWR Morb Mortal Wkly Rep*, 1993, 42(RR-7):1-8.

Snider DE Jr and Roper WL, "A New Tuberculosis," *N Engl J Med*, 1992, 326(10):703-5.

"Treatment of Tuberculosis and Tuberculosis Infection in Adults and Children. American Thoracic Society and the Centers for Disease Control and Prevention," *Am J Respir Crit Care Med*, 1994, 149(5):1359-74.

Mycoplasma hominis and *Mycoplasma genitalium*

Microbiology *Mycoplasma hominis* and *M. genitalium* belong to the organism class called Mollicutes. The class Mollicutes is composed of approximately 160 named species of *Mycoplasma*. The *Mycoplasmas* (including *M. hominis* and *M. genitalium*) are the smallest organisms known to be capable of being free-living and self-replicating, are only 150-250 nm in diameter, do not have cell walls, have deformable membranes, have extremely fastidious growth requirements, and appear as "fried egg" colonies on special growth media.

Epidemiology *Mycoplasmas* are ubiquitous and are commonly found in the mouths, upper respiratory tracts, and lower urogenital tracts of both healthy and diseased humans and animals. In addition, many *Mycoplasmas* are found in plants and insects. *Mycoplasmas* have long been known to cause significant health problems in domestic, commercial, and laboratory animals. Only four of the 13 species of *Mycoplasmas* which have been isolated from humans are associated with human disease: *M. pneumoniae*, *M. hominis*, *M. genitalium*, and *Ureaplasma urealyticum*.

Clinical Syndromes Overwhelming and convincing evidence that *M. hominis* and *M. genitalium* cause disease does not exist. However, evidence does support the idea that *M. hominis* probably causes some cases of pyelonephritis, pelvic inflammatory disease, and postabortion fever; is strongly associated with bacterial vaginosis; causes many cases of postpartum fever; and is associated with various conditions (including arthritis) in immunocompromised persons. The only disease with which *M. genitalium* has been strongly associated is nongonococcal urethritis.

Diagnosis Diseases potentially caused by *M. hominis* and *M. genitalium* are diagnosed clinically and supported by culture results. Consult the clinical laboratory for advice regarding appropriate specimens to collect and appropriate collection procedures and transport medium. **Note:** Special transport medium and conditions are essential for transportation and culture of all *Mycoplasmas*.

Diagnostic Tests/Procedures
Mycoplasma/Ureaplasma Culture *on page 499*

Treatment Although both organisms are in the same genus, their susceptibility patterns are quite different. *Mycoplasma genitalium* mimics *M. pneumoniae*, both of which are susceptible to macrolides, tetracyclines, and fluoroquinolones. *M. hominis* strains resistant to tetracyclines have been appearing more frequently. Susceptibility testing should be performed. Clindamycin can be used in patients with tetracycline-resistant *M. hominis*.

Drug Therapy
Recommended
Mycoplasma hominis:
Clindamycin *on page 684*
Tetracycline *on page 944*
Mycoplasma genitalium:
Macrolides *on page 803*
Tetracycline *on page 944*
Fluoroquinolones *on page 736*

Selected Readings
McCormack WM, "Susceptibility of Mycoplasmas to Antimicrobial Agents: Clinical Implications," *Clin Infect Dis*, 1993, 17(Suppl 1):S200-1.
Shyh-Ching L, "New Understandings of Mycoplasmal Infections and Disease," *Clin Microbiol Newslett*, 1995, 17(22):169-73.
Taylor-Robinson D, "Infections Due to Species of *Mycoplasma* and *Ureaplasma*: An Update," *Clin Infect Dis*, 1996, 23(4):671-82.
Taylor-Robinson D, "*Ureaplasma urealyticum* (T-Strain *Mycoplasma*) and *Mycoplasma hominis*," *Principles and Practice of Infectious Diseases*, 4th ed, Mandell GL, Bennett JE, and Dolin R, eds, New York, NY: Churchill Livingstone, 1995, 1713-8.

Mycoplasma pneumoniae

Synonyms Eaton's Agent

Microbiology *Mycoplasma pneumoniae*, also called Eaton's agent, is the smallest and simplest prokaryote capable of self-replication. Originally, this free-living, strictly aerobic organism was thought to be a virus but later determined to be a bacterium. The diameter of *M. pneumoniae* is 0.2-0.8 μm, and the organism is highly pleomorphic. The organism lacks a cell wall and has only a trilaminar membrane (similar to the structure of the trilaminar membrane which surrounds all bacterial and mammalian cells) enclosing the cell cytoplasm. Although *M. pneumoniae* is classified as a gram-negative bacterium, it retains the Gram's stain poorly and, thus, cannot be reliably seen on routine Gram's stain of clinical specimens such as sputum.

Growth of *M. pneumoniae* in culture requires special laboratory techniques, and a special request for *Mycoplasma* culture must be made. The organism does not grow on routine culture media used for isolating common bacterial respiratory pathogens. *Mycoplasma pneumoniae* requires an exogenous supply of cholesterol and other sterols for membrane synthesis; these nutrients can be supplied by animal sera added to the culture medium, and an exogenous supply of nucleic acids, for synthesis of purines and pyrimidines; this can be supplied by yeast extracts. An artificial, cell-free, selective culture medium is used in many laboratories. This diphasic media is composed of broth (liquid medium) overlying agar. A pH indicator in the agar is used to detect acid produced by *Mycoplasma* as it ferments glucose; a visible color change in the agar is presumptive evidence of *M. pneumoniae*. The colonies of *M. pneumoniae* in culture are 50-100 μm in diameter and have a unique "fried egg" colonial morphology.

Epidemiology *Mycoplasma pneumoniae* infections occur worldwide, with a tendency towards temperate climates. Epidemics of mycoplasmal infections seem to occur every 4-6 years, although outbreaks of epidemic proportions can occur in small communities at any time. Infections with *M. pneumoniae* do not follow a seasonal pattern, unlike many other respiratory pathogens which cause
(Continued)

Mycoplasma pneumoniae (Continued)

bronchitis and/or pneumonia in the winter and spring months (*Streptococcus pneumoniae*, respiratory syncytial virus, influenza A and B, and others). Thus, during summer months, the proportion of respiratory infections due to *Mycoplasma pneumoniae* increases (up to 50% of pneumonia cases), although the actual number of cases stays constant month to month.

One important characteristic of *Mycoplasma* infection is its tendency to spread within a family in a step-wise fashion. Spread within the family is slow (often over weeks), but many, if not all, members become infected. Often the point source for infection in a family can be identified. Clustered cases also occur in military barracks, institutionalized setting, day care centers, and college dormitories but tend to be slower and less complete than spread within families.

The highest rates of infection are in the young; school-aged children and young adults are statistically at highest risk. Although mycoplasmal infections are less common in children younger than 5 years of age, some studies have shown this organism to be a frequent cause of mild, but symptomatic, respiratory infections in this age group. Similarly, the incidence of mycoplasmal infection decreases with advancing age but still remains a sporadic cause of pneumonia in the older adult, which may be overlooked. Transmission of *M. pneumoniae* is via infected respiratory secretions such as nasal discharge. Close contact appears to be necessary for the infection to be spread. The incubation period between exposure to the infection and the first clinical symptoms is about 2-3 weeks.

Clinical Syndromes *Mycoplasma pneumoniae* is pathogenic for the lower respiratory tract and is able to adhere to respiratory epithelium by means of a special protein called P1. This attachment factor is contained in surface projections of the organism which bind to a receptor protein on the surface of the respiratory epithelial cells. Cellular injury takes place probably by several mechanisms including the production of superoxides. In severe cases, there is likely an immunologic component of cellular destruction as well. The organism remains extracellular during infection.

- **Community-acquired pneumonia:** Also known as "walking pneumonia" or "primary atypical pneumonia", this form of *Mycoplasma* infection is seen mainly between 5 and 20 years of age. *Mycoplasma pneumoniae* is the most common cause of pneumonia in this age group. The disease tends to be mild to moderate in severity but is characteristically very slow to resolve. Hospitalization is usually not necessary, and patients remain ambulatory (hence the term "walking pneumonia").

Patients present with prominent constitutional symptoms: persistent headache, malaise, low grade fevers, and muscle aches. Sore throat and ear pain are also present in some cases. The onset of symptoms is gradual and subacute. Respiratory symptoms usually appear after several days of malaise. Patients develop a persistent, nonproductive cough. Purulent sputum, rigors, chest pain, and gross hemoptysis are not prominent features of this infection (although each has been rarely reported). Examination of the lungs may show wheezing, localized rales and/or rhonchi. In some cases, the lungs may be completely clear. Physical findings suggestive of lung consolidation (such as egophony, bronchial breathing, and dullness to percussion) are uncommon and suggestive of other bacterial pathogens. Examination of the head and neck often shows a mild injection of the tympanic membranes, mild pharyngeal erythema, and cervical adenopathy. More severe ear inflammation may be seen in about 15% of cases, with bullous myringitis being classically associated with mycoplasmal pneumonia. However, hemorrhagic bullous myringitis is uncommon, and its absence should not preclude the diagnosis. A nonspecific maculopapular rash is seen in some patients. Chest x-rays typically reveal patchy areas of bronchopneumonia with peribronchial cuffing. Most often the lower lung fields on one side are involved, but multilobar disease can occur. Radiographic findings of lobar consolidation are less common and large pleural effusions are distinctly unusual, both findings suggestive of respiratory pathogens such as *Streptococcus pneumoniae*. The course of atypical pneumonia tends to be protracted, with or without antibiotic treatment. Most patients recover completely, although life-threatening pneumonia with the adult respiratory distress syndrome (ARDS) has been reported.

Complications of *M. pneumoniae* respiratory infection are statistically uncommon. However, unusual and potentially lethal complications have been well-recognized, and the incidence may exceed 10% in hospitalized patients. Respiratory complications include ARDS, pleural effusions, bronchiolitis obliterans, cavitary lung lesions, and bronchiectasis. Nonrespiratory complications include: 1. Mycoplasmal encephalitis, which can be seen when respiratory complaints are minor. Patients present with variable degrees of fever, confusion, and/or personality changes. Mycoplasmal encephalitis is indistinguishable from other forms of infectious encephalitis such as herpes simplex virus encephalitis. This entity should be considered in the differential diagnosis of any patient who presents with encephalitis and a pulmonary infiltrate. Other neurologic complications: transverse myelitis, stroke, postinfectious leukoencephalitis, optic neuritis, polymyositis syndrome, and others. 2. Autoimmune hemolytic anemia, which at times can be quite severe. Such patients have high titers of cold-reacting autoantibodies (cold agglutinins) 3. Erythema multiforme, erythema nodosum. 4. myocarditis, and pericarditis.

- **Tracheobronchitis:** The majority of *M. pneumoniae* infections do not lead to pneumonia. Tracheobronchitis accounts for 70% to 80% of all infections with *M. pneumoniae*, with only about 33% progressing to pneumonia. The clinical presentation of tracheobronchitis is similar to pneumonia, with prominent constitutional symptoms followed by a dry, persistent cough. The chest x-ray in tracheobronchitis remains clear because inflammation is limited primarily to the bronchi. Overall, the disease course is milder than with pneumonia, although the disease course may be equally protracted.

- **Pharyngitis:** *M. pneumoniae* can cause a primary pharyngitis, or mycoplasmal pharyngitis may develop in association with tracheobronchitis or pneumonia. Again, school-aged children and young adults are most commonly involved. Constitutional symptoms are prominent, with fever, headache, and malaise. Patients complain of a severe sore throat and often have difficulty swallowing. On examination, there is tonsillar enlargement, inflammatory exudate, and pharyngeal edema and erythema. Cervical lymphadenopathy is common. The clinical presentation may be confused with streptococcal pharyngitis or primary infectious mononucleosis (from Epstein-Barr virus). Mycoplasmal pharyngitis is probably underdiagnosed.

Diagnosis Diagnosis is made on a clinical basis as described above. A test for cold hemagglutinins can be performed, especially in seriously ill, hospitalized patients. Diagnosis is definitive when the organism is cultured from sputum or throat swab. A rise in antibody titer from acute to convalescent sera is also diagnostic and may occur in up to 80% of patients with pneumonia.

Diagnostic Tests/Procedures
Cold Agglutinin Titer *on page 369*
Mycoplasma Serology *on page 499*
Mycoplasma/Ureaplasma Culture *on page 499*
Polymerase Chain Reaction *on page 523*

Duration of Therapy 2-3 weeks

Treatment The treatment of choice for *M. pneumoniae* infections is erythromycin, although, tetracycline has been shown to be equally effective in clinical trials. Most patients can be treated as outpatients. Patients with severe disease should also receive appropriate supportive care.

Pediatric Drug Therapy
Recommended
Erythromycin *on page 722*

Adult Drug Therapy
Recommended
Erythromycin *on page 722*
Alternate
Tetracycline *on page 944*
Doxycycline *on page 713*
Fluoroquinolones *on page 736*
Azithromycin *on page 613*
Clarithromycin *on page 681*

Selected Readings
Lind K, "Manifestations and Complications of *Mycoplasma pneumoniae* Disease: A Review," *Yale J Biol Med*, 1983, 56(5-6):461-8.
(Continued)

Mycoplasma pneumoniae (Continued)

Mansel JK, Rosenow EC, Smith TF, et al, "*Mycoplasma pneumoniae* Pneumonia," *Chest*, 1989, 95(3):639-46.

Marrie TJ, "*Mycoplasma pneumoniae* Pneumonia Requiring Hospitalization, With Emphasis on Infection in the Elderly," *Arch Intern Med*, 1993, 153(4):488-94.

Murray HW, Masur H, Senterfit LB, et al, "The Protean Manifestations of *Mycoplasma pneumoniae* Infection in Adults," *Am J Med*, 1975, 58(2):229-42.

Waites KB, Bébéar C, Robertson JA, et al, "Laboratory Diagnosis of Mycoplasmal and Ureaplasmal Infections," *Clin Microbiol Newslet*, 1996, 18(14):105-11.

Naegleria fowleri

Microbiology *Naegleria fowleri* is a free-living ameba. It is related to *Acanthamoeba*, another protozoan which is pathogenic for humans. *Naegleria* exists in a trophozoite form (10-30 μm in diameter) and a flagellate form. The trophozoite form can encyst into a smaller spherical cyst (10 μm). The organism is aerobic, and the trophozoite form grows well in a variety of conditions including temperatures up to 45°C which allows it to proliferate in fresh water in temperate climates.

Epidemiology *N. fowleri* is a ubiquitous organism, being isolated in many geographic areas from a variety of environmental sources including fresh water, soil, artificially heated waters, man-made thermal waters, and air. The organism is highly associated with polluted lake or river water, as well as fresh water bodies in warm climates such as Florida. Millions of individuals have been exposed to water contaminated with this ameba, but disease develops only rarely. The immunologic factors that determine disease progression are not known. The major clinical manifestation of *N. fowleri* is primary amebic meningoencephalitis. This disease is seen in otherwise healthy adults and children and is highly associated with swimming in freshwater areas. In the United States, cases have been reported in the southern and central states.

Clinical Syndromes

- **Primary amebic meningoencephalitis:** This rapidly fatal disease usually occurs several days after exposure to freshwater ponds, rivers, or lakes. Patients develop headache, fever, and nuchal rigidity. Severe confusion is common. Death occurs within days. The ameba are likely inhaled through the nose during swimming and penetrate through the olfactory plate into the brain. The grey matter of the brain and the meninges develop extensive hemorrhage and necrosis. The trophozoite forms alone are seen in inflammatory tissue. Myocarditis is also present in many patients at autopsy.

Diagnosis Primary amebic meningoencephalitis should be considered in a young adult who presents with a fulminant encephalitis following fresh water exposure. The diagnosis may be difficult to establish. Head CT scans do not show mass lesions, but there may be contrast enhancement of grey matter and cisterns. Cerebrospinal fluid is usually inflammatory with a variable number of polymorphonuclear leukocytes present and numerous RBCs. Hypoglycorrhachia is usually present, and the CSF protein is elevated. A wet mount of CSF should be performed in addition to the Gram's stain if this disease is even remotely considered because the trophozoites can be disrupted during the Gram's stain. In one series of patients, the *Naegleria* trophozoites were visible on nearly all wet mounts of CSF performed.

Diagnostic Tests/Procedures

Cerebrospinal Fluid Analysis *on page 354*

Computed Transaxial Tomography, Head Studies *on page 374*

Cytology, Body Fluids *on page 386*

Gram's Stain *on page 426*

Treatment Primary amebic encephalitis is rapidly fatal in 95% of cases, although several survivors have been well-described. One patient responded successfully to intravenous and intrathecal amphotericin B, but the optimal regimen is unknown. Immunoglobulin therapy is being investigated as adjunctive therapy due to the poor prognosis of this infection. Consultation with an Infectious Disease specialist is strongly recommended if primary amebic meningoencephalitis is even remotely considered.

Selected Readings

Diedel JS, Harmatz P, Visvesvara GS, et al, "Successful Treatment of Primary Amebic Encephalitis," *N Engl J Med*, 1982, 306:346.

Duma RJ, Rosenblum WI, McGehee RF, et al "Primary Amebic Meningoencephalitis Caused by *Naegleria*. Two New Cases, Responses to Amphotericin B and Review," *Ann Intern Med*, 1971, 74:923-32.

Marciano-Cabral F and Petri WA, "Free-Living Amebae," *Principles and Practice of Infectious Diseases*, 4th ed, Mandell GL, Bennett JE, and Dolin R, eds, New York, NY: Churchill Livingstone, 1995, 2408-15.

Necator americanus see Ancylostoma duodenale on page 66

Neisseria gonorrhoeae

Microbiology *Neisseria gonorrhoeae* is an oxidase- and catalase-positive, gram-negative diplococcus. *N. meningitidis* produces acid from only glucose which differentiates it from the other *Neisseria* species. Typing for different strains of *N. gonorrhoeae* can be performed but are useful only for epidemiologic studies.

The organism readily grows on Thayer-Martin or chocolate media and grows best in the presence of CO_2. Growth is more fastidious than that of *N. meningitidis*.

Epidemiology Humans are the only natural reservoir for *N. gonorrhoeae*. The estimate that 1 million new cases of gonorrhea have occurred each year since the early 1960s is most likely a severe underestimate. Transmission is primarily by sexual contact, with the major reservoir in asymptomatically infected persons. The organism and disease is most commonly found in individuals 20-24 years of age. Fifty percent of women will become infected after a single exposure to an infected male while only 20% of men become infected after a single exposure to an infected female.

Clinical Syndromes In men, gonorrhea is usually limited to burning on urination and a purulent urethral discharge. Ten percent of men will be asymptomatic with 1% or less developing the complications of prostatitis, urethral stricture, or epididymitis. Approximately 50% of women are asymptomatic; when symptoms occur they include dysuria, frequency, vaginal discharge, fever, and abdominal pain. Up to 15% of women with gonorrhea develop pelvic inflammatory disease (PID), with fallopian scarring or subsequent chronic PID, sterility, or ectopic pregnancies. Rectal and pharyngeal colonization and disease may also occur in women and homosexual men.

Disseminated disease may include sepsis, peritonitis, or meningitis, but most commonly causes septic arthritis in patients otherwise asymptomatic. Disseminated disease may be accompanied by petechial or papular lesions. In children, the most common form of gonococcal disease is gonorrhea ophthalmia from contamination through an infected birth canal. This is easily prevented with 1% silver nitrate aqueous drops.

Diagnosis In men with urethral symptoms, Gram's stain of the purulent material is highly sensitive and specific. Gram's stain is less diagnostic in asymptomatic men and clinically useless in diagnosing cervicitis in women because intracellular gram-negative diplococci could be any of the many *Haemophilus* species which are normal vaginal flora. A positive Gram's stain is usually characterized by the presence of gram-negative cocci within or closely associated with polymorphonuclear leukocytes. The Gram's stain of joint fluid can detect organisms in early septic arthritis but is not particularly sensitive for skin lesions or rectal or pharyngeal disease. Specimens from appropriate sites may be inoculated on Thayer-Martin medium when contaminating organisms are present and on chocolate agar if the specimen is from a normally sterile body site. When asymptomatic or cervical disease is expected, the rectum may yield the only positive specimen. Growth is enhanced by CO_2 inoculated media. Blood cultures are positive in early disseminated disease. Infected joint fluid cultures are also usually positive.

Diagnostic Tests/Procedures

Gram's Stain *on page 426*

Neisseria gonorrhoeae Culture *on page 501*

Neisseria gonorrhoeae by Nucleic Acid Probe *on page 500*

Treatment Patients infected with *Neisseria gonorrhoeae* are often coinfected with *C. trachomatis* and should be treated for both.

Uncomplicated gonococcal infections of the cervix, urethra, and rectum: The drugs of choice for these infections include single doses of cefixime 400 mg orally, ceftriaxone 125 mg I.M., ciprofloxacin 500 mg, or ofloxacin 400 mg. Alternative regimens include single doses of spectinomycin I.M., other cephalosporins such as ceftizoxime, cefotaxime, cefotetan, or cefoxitin (probenecid 1 g orally should be added to cefoxitin therapy), enoxacin, lomefloxacin, or norfloxacin.

(Continued)

Neisseria gonorrhoeae (Continued)

Uncomplicated gonococcal infection of the pharynx: The drugs of choice include single doses of ceftriaxone 125 mg I.M., ciprofloxacin 500 mg orally, or ofloxacin 400 mg orally.

If symptoms persist, other organisms should be considered. Also consider reinfection rather than treatment failure, however, culture and sensitivity should be performed. Patients should refer sex partners for evaluation and treatment.

Patients who are intolerant/allergic to cephalosporins or penicillins should be treated with spectinomycin. Pregnant women with cephalosporin intolerance/ allergy should be treated with spectinomycin. Careful follow-up is necessary to assure clinical cure.

Disseminated gonococcal infection: The treatment of choice is ceftriaxone 1 g I.M. or I.V. every 24 hours. Alternative regimens include full courses of cefotaxime, ceftizoxime, ciprofloxacin, ofloxacin, or spectinomycin. Patients can then be switched to oral therapy (cefixime, ciprofloxacin, or ofloxacin) when improvement begins. Patients should be treated for a full week.

Gonococcal conjunctivitis in <u>adults</u>: Ceftriaxone 1 g I.M. one time

Gonococcal meningitis or endocarditis: Ceftriaxone 1-2 g every 12 hours. Meningitis should be treated for 10-14 days; endocarditis for 4 weeks.

Gonococcal infections in infants:

Ophthalmia neonatorum prophylaxis: Instillation of a prophylactic agent into the eyes of all newborns is recommended to prevent gonococcal ophthalmia neonatorum. (Required by law in most states.) Recommended regimens include single application of silver nitrate 1% aqueous, erythromycin 0.5% ophthalmic ointment, or tetracycline 1% ophthalmic ointment.

Ophthalmia neonatorum treatment: Ceftriaxone 25-50 mg/kg I.V. or I.M. in a single dose, not to exceed 125 mg. Topical therapy is inadequate and unnecessary.

Disseminated gonococcal infection and gonococcal scalp abscess in newborns: Conjunctival exudate should be cultured. The drugs of choice include ceftriaxone 25-50 mg/kg/day or cefotaxime 25 mg/kg every 12 hours for 7 days (14 days if meningitis is present).

In children, similar recommendations apply regarding the drugs of choice; doses may vary. Avoid quinolones and tetracyclines.

Pediatric Drug Therapy
Recommended
Ceftriaxone *on page 655*

Adult Drug Therapy
Recommended
Cefixime *on page 636*
Ceftriaxone *on page 655*
Ciprofloxacin *on page 678*
Ofloxacin *on page 847*

Alternate
Spectinomycin *on page 922*
used in combination with
Doxycycline *on page 713*
Ceftizoxime *on page 654*
Cefotaxime *on page 642*
Enoxacin *on page 720*
Norfloxacin *on page 844*

Selected Readings
Baron EJ and Finegold SM, eds, "Aerobic, Gram-Negative Cocci (*Neisseria* and *Branhamella*)," *Bailey & Scott's Diagnostic Microbiology*, St Louis, MO: CV Mosby Co, 1990, 353-62.

Knapp JS, "Antimicrobial Resistance in *Neisseria gonorrhoeae* in the United States," *Clin Microbiol Newslett*, 1999, 21(1):1-7.

Murray PR, Drew WL, Kobayashi GS, et al, eds, "Neisseriaceae," *Medical Microbiology*, St Louis, MO: CV Mosby Co, 1990, 85-97.

"1998 Guidelines for Treatment of Sexually Transmitted Diseases. Centers for Disease Control and Prevention," *MMWR Morb Mortal Wkly Rep*, 1998, 47(RR-1):1-111.

Neisseria meningitidis

Microbiology *Neisseria meningitidis* is an oxidase- and catalase-positive, gram-negative diplococcus. *N. meningitidis* produces acid from glucose and maltose but not from sucrose or lactose, which differentiates it from the other *Neisseria* species. At least nine different serogroups of *N. meningitidis* have been identified on the basis of their polysaccharide capsules. More than 20 serotypes have been identified. Serogroups A, B, C, Y, and W135 are most commonly associated with clinical disease states.

The organism grows on Thayer-Martin or chocolate media and grows best in the presence of CO_2.

Epidemiology *N. meningitidis* is exclusively a human pathogen and causes 3000-4000 cases of meningitis yearly in the United States. *N. meningitidis* is transmitted by droplets among persons with prolonged close contact and who are in direct contact with respiratory secretions. Carriage occurs in 10% to 30% of healthy adults, but disease is rare. Most disease occurs in children 6 months to 5 years of age. Outbreaks occur in other close contact populations such as the military.

Serogroups B and C account for over 75% of cases, and groups W135, Y, and A account for the rest. The last urban epidemic occurred in Brazil in 1971 (serogroups C and A), and the last United States epidemic occurred in 1946 (serogroup A).

Clinical Syndromes *N. meningitidis* causes a wide spectrum of clinical illness which range from a mild nonspecific febrile illness to meningitis and sepsis.

- **Meningitis:** Usually abrupt onset with fever, headache, and meningismus, although the syndrome may be less specific in young children. Mortality is 100% if untreated; 15% if treated appropriately. In meningococcemia, signs and symptoms of sepsis may be seen accompanied by characteristic meningococcal emboli (vasculitic purpura). This syndrome is occasionally preceded by petechial skin lesions. Disseminated intravascular coagulopathy and shock may follow, along with adrenal gland destruction (Waterhouse-Friderichsen syndrome).
- Can also be responsible for urethritis, pneumonias, and arthritis.

Diagnosis Diagnosis is made by Gram's stain and culture of cerebrospinal fluid, blood, etc. Occasionally, the organism can be observed on Gram's stain of the petechial lesions or detected in buffy coat smears. *N. meningitidis* will grow on blood or chocolate agar (best growth with increased CO_2 concentration) or in Thayer-Martin media when multiple organisms are suspected.

Rapid identification can be performed by several laboratory tests, but definitive identification must be made biochemically.

Diagnostic Tests/Procedures
Aerobic Culture, Cerebrospinal Fluid *on page 311*
Bacterial Antigens, Rapid Detection Methods *on page 335*
Gram's Stain *on page 426*
Skin Biopsy *on page 535*

Treatment High dose intravenous penicillin remains the drug of choice for the treatment of meningococcal meningitis. Resistance to penicillin is still exceedingly rare. Chloramphenicol or a third generation cephalosporin are excellent alternatives. Supportive measures are also necessary in patients with meningitis or sepsis.

Prophylaxis for persons with significant exposures to the respiratory secretions of patients with the disease remains controversial. A 2-day regiment of rifampin is recommended (600 mg twice daily for adults, 10 mg/kg twice daily in children, and 5 mg/kg in children younger than 1 month of age). Attempts at eradicating *N. meningitidis* from asymptomatic carriers are impractical and unlikely to be effective.

Drug Therapy
Recommended
Penicillin G, Parenteral, Aqueous *on page 860*
Alternate
Cephalosporins, 3rd Generation *on page 662*
Chloramphenicol *on page 667*

Selected Readings
Baron EJ and Finegold SM, eds, "Aerobic Gram-Negative Cocci (*Neisseria* and *Branhamella*)," *Bailey & Scott's Diagnostic Microbiology*, St Louis, MO: CV Mosby Co, 1990, 353-62.

(Continued)

Neisseria meningitidis (Continued)

Murray PR, Drew WL, Kobayashi GS, et al, eds. "Neisseriaceae," *Medical Microbiology*, St Louis, MO: CV Mosby Co, 1990, 85-97.

Quagliarello V and Scheld WM, "Bacterial Meningitis: Pathogenesis, Pathophysiology, and Progress," *N Engl J Med*, 1992, 327(12):864-72.

Nocardia Species

Microbiology *Nocardia* species are variably acid-fast, "higher order," aerobic bacteria. They belong to the family Nocardiaceae. There are several species of *Nocardia* which are pathogenic for humans, the most common being *Nocardia asteroides* followed by *N. brasiliensis*. Other species occasionally cause human disease such as *N. otitidiscaviarum* (formerly *N. caviae*) and the newly recognized *N. transvalensis*.

Nocardia species have a delicate, branching appearance and may appear fragmented in clinical specimens. The organisms are weakly gram-positive and have a characteristic "beaded" appearance; if present, these characteristics allow rapid preliminary identification. The organisms may be more easily visualized on an acid-fast stain rather than Gram's stain. Most (but not all) strains of *Nocardia* are acid-fast and retain carbol fuchsin when decolorized with a weaker alcohol than the acid alcohol commonly used for staining mycobacterial species. It is important to realize that the acid-fast staining properties of *Nocardia* species differ from those of other acid-fast organisms such as *Mycobacterium tuberculosis*. Laboratories use a **modified** acid-fast stain (eg, a modified Ziehl-Neelsen stain and others) to optimally detect *Nocardia* in direct specimens. In most institutions, the clinician must specifically request a modified acid-fast stain for *Nocardia* if this organism is suspected. In some institutions, a *Nocardia* stain may be part of a routine protocol for processing certain clinical specimens, such as bronchoalveolar lavage fluid from immunocompromised patients.

Nocardia species grow on a variety of standard media employed in microbiology laboratories, including blood agar and Sabouraud's dextrose agar. Growth also occurs on media used for isolation of mycobacteria such as the Lowenstein-Jensen medium. Usually 4-10 days are required before growth of the organism is apparent. When *Nocardia* species are present along with other aerobic bacteria, isolation of *Nocardia* may be delayed for several weeks. *Nocardia* species are most frequently isolated from respiratory specimens; only rarely can they be isolated from standard blood cultures.

Epidemiology *Nocardia* species are distributed worldwide, and there appears to be no geographic clustering of cases. The organisms are ubiquitous in soil and areas of plant decay. Approximately 500-1000 cases are reported in the United States annually. The most common age range is 20-50 years, with several series demonstrating a male predominance. Nocardial infections occur mainly in individuals with defective T-cell immunity (cell-mediated immunity), such as organ transplant recipients, patients with malignancies (lymphoma), those receiving corticosteroids or cytotoxic agents, and persons with AIDS. A 13% incidence was once described in one cardiac transplant center, but other institutions have consistently reported much lower rates. Persons with neutrophil dysfunction also appear at increased risk, and nocardiosis has been well-described in children with chronic granulomatous disease. A large number of other diseases have been associated with nocardiosis including tuberculosis, alcoholism with cirrhosis, inflammatory bowel disease, various forms of vasculitis, pulmonary alveolar proteinosis, sarcoidosis, bronchiectasis, and immunoglobulin deficiencies. Nontuberculous mycobacteria has also been reported as a predisposing condition for nocardial infection. Clinically, significant nocardiosis also may occur in otherwise healthy persons, although the incidence of this has been highly variable.

Although occasional clusters of *Nocardia* infection have been described, most experts feel that the organism is not transmitted person-to-person.

Outside the United States, *Nocardia* species are commonly associated with mycetoma (see Clinical Syndromes). Individuals with frequent contact with soil and other plant matter are at risk for this form of nocardiosis.

Clinical Syndromes Disease usually results from inhalation of the organism leading to colonization in the lung. The organisms may resist local pulmonary defenses including macrophages and immunoglobulins. Infections with *Nocardia* species classically result in abscess formation, with numerous polymorphonuclear leukocytes and only a thin abscess wall.

- **Colonization in healthy persons:** Occasionally immunocompetent persons with no significant lung disease may have positive sputum cultures for *Nocardia*. Clinical evaluation is important in deciding on the role of antibiotics.

- **Respiratory colonization in individuals with chronic obstructive pulmonary disease (COPD):** Several series have reported positive sputum cultures from asymptomatic COPD patients; in most cases, there is no active pneumonia and repeat sputum cultures were negative. Repeated isolation of *Nocardia* in these individuals is more worrisome for active disease, and consultation with an Infectious Disease specialist should be considered.

- **Pneumonia:** Immunosuppressed individuals may develop an isolated pneumonia most commonly from *N. asteroides*. The presentation may be subacute or acute. Symptoms are similar to other bacterial pneumonias with fever, purulent sputum, cough, and dyspnea. Some may have pleuritic chest pain mimicking pneumococcal pneumonia. Since *Nocardia* tends to cause suppurative disease, lung cavitation and empyema are common. Chest x-rays may show a nodular infiltrate, cavities, or a lobar pattern. Direct extension of purulent nocardial infections may occur into the pericardium and other mediastinal structures. Disease outside the lungs may be present in up to 50% of cases.

- **Brain abscess:** *Nocardia* commonly disseminates to the brain in immunosuppressed persons. Multiple brain lesions can occur, and the presentation may be subacute. Nocardial infection should be considered in a patient presenting with pneumonia and brain abscess. Meningitis from *Nocardia* is uncommon.

- **Disseminated nocardial infection:** Approximately 20% of patients with nocardiosis have no apparent lung involvement and instead present with extrapulmonary nocardiosis. The most common presentation is brain abscess. A number of other sites may be involved such as bone, skin, abdomen, and others.

- **Mycetoma:** This is usually seen in persons from tropical or subtropical regions. The pathogenesis of mycetoma is from direct inoculation of the organism into the skin rather than inhalation. The feet and/or hands are the most frequent sites. Chronic nocardial infection may develop with disfiguring skin and soft tissue changes and multiple sinus tracts.

- **Cellulitis and lymphocutaneous nodules:** These forms of direct inoculation are more common in the United States than mycetoma. The cellulitis caused by *Nocardia* species may be difficult to distinguish from other forms of bacterial cellulitis. *Nocardia brasiliensis* may cause subcutaneous nodules that spread on an arm or leg following lymphatic drainage. This may mimic infections caused by *Sporothrix schenckii*.

- **Keratitis:** Occasionally, *Nocardia asteroides* is directly inoculated into the eye following trauma.

Diagnosis *Nocardia* infection should be in the differential diagnosis of any immunocompromised patient presenting with an unexplained pneumonia. The clinical suspicion should be high if there is evidence of extrapulmonary involvement as well, particularly the presence of a central nervous system lesion. Respiratory specimens should be submitted for nocardial stain and culture. The organism may be recovered from induced sputum, but bronchoscopy may be necessary in many cases. It is difficult to isolate *Nocardia* species from blood cultures or cerebrospinal fluid but is readily identified from brain abscesses (if the patient has not received prior antibiotics). Serologic studies for *Nocardia* are not clinically helpful at present.

Diagnostic Tests/Procedures
Acid-Fast Stain, Modified, *Nocardia* Species *on page 307*
Nocardia Culture, All Sites *on page 503*

Treatment The optimal regimen for treating *Nocardia* is still controversial and under study. Sulfonamides have been the cornerstone of therapy and appear to be effective in many cases as monotherapy, even in immunocompromised persons. Sulfisoxazole at high doses (≥6 g/day) has been effective in several studies, as has sulfadiazine. Blood levels may be obtained in serious cases. Cotrimoxazole has also been used with success (given at doses up to 20 mg/kg/day of the trimethoprim component). Some experts have been concerned that (Continued)

Nocardia Species *(Continued)*

the commercially available preparations of co-trimoxazole, such as Bactrim™, may not have enough trimethoprim synergistic activity against *Nocardia*. Other problems with co-trimoxazole include a somewhat higher incidence of drug toxicity than sulfonamides alone, occasional treatment failures, and relapses. However, co-trimoxazole is considered by some to be the treatment of choice.

Minocycline is effective *in vitro* and *in vivo* and can be used if patients develop hypersensitivity to one of the sulfonamides. Other tetracyclines may be less active. A number of other agents have been reported effective in clinical situations including amikacin and imipenem. Many clinicians use combination therapy in life-threatening or refractory cases, although clinical data is very limited. It is still unclear whether combination therapy (eg, sulfisoxazole and amikacin) is superior to a sulfonamide used as monotherapy.

Since *Nocardia* species tend to form abscesses, surgical drainage may be extremely important, particularly with empyema and brain abscess.

Drug Therapy
Recommended
Co-Trimoxazole *on page 692*
Sulfisoxazole *on page 934*
Sulfadiazine *on page 929*
Alternate
Minocycline *on page 823*
Selected Readings
Lerner PI, "Nocardia Species," *Principles and Practice of Infectious Diseases*, 4th ed, Mandell GL, Bennett JE, and Dolin R, eds, New York, NY: Churchill Livingstone, 1995, 2273-80.

Occupational Exposure to Bloodborne Pathogens (Universal Precautions)
see page 1088

Paraflu *see Parainfluenza Virus on this page*

Parainfluenza Virus
Related Information
Immunization Guidelines *on page 1041*
Synonyms Paraflu
Microbiology Parainfluenza viruses (also known as "paraflu") are RNA viruses which frequently cause lower respiratory infections in children and are the most common cause of croup (laryngotracheobronchitis). Parainfluenza viruses are single-stranded RNA viruses with an envelope derived from the host. It belongs to the family Paramyxoviridae and is thus related to the mumps virus and respiratory syncytial virus. Isolates causing human disease have been divided into four serotypes, parainfluenza 1-4. Two glycoproteins are found in the envelope, with hemagglutinin and neuraminidase activity associated with one of the two glycoproteins.

Epidemiology The virus is distributed worldwide. Parainfluenza type 4 is the least common of the serotypes isolated clinically, but this may be due to difficulties in culturing *in vitro*. Parainfluenza viruses are usually considered pathogenic in the pediatric population with antibodies to types 1-3 detectable in almost all children by 8 years of age. Longitudinal studies have shown an interesting pattern; outbreaks of parainfluenza types 1 and 2 tend to occur every other year (usually odd-numbered years) and during fall months, whereas outbreaks of type 3 occur during consecutive years most commonly during the spring. Parainfluenza viruses are a common cause of lower respiratory infections in children, second only to respiratory syncytial virus. Parainfluenza type 3 virus can infect infants in the first month of life. Types 1 and 2 tend to infect children and are important causes of croup. Transmission of the virus is by either direct person-to-person contact or by large droplets (eg, sneezing). The incubation period following exposure is about 3-6 days.

Clinical Syndromes
- **Upper respiratory tract infection:** This occurs particularly in children and is manifested by fever (in >50% of cases), coryza, sore throat, and cough.
- **Croup or laryngotracheobronchitis:** Parainfluenza type 1 is the most common cause of this type of lower respiratory infection. Croup is characterized by a distinctive cough like a "barking seal." In severe cases, the airway may be compromised secondary to subglottal edema, with stridor and respiratory failure. Most cases of croup recover uneventfully within several days.

The differential diagnosis must include epiglottitis from *Haemophilus influenzae* or influenza A.

- **Bronchiolitis or pneumonia:** These forms of lower respiratory infection are characterized by progressive cough with wheezing, dyspnea, and intercostal retractions. The chest radiograph may demonstrate air trapping and interstitial infiltrates.

- **Infection in adults:** Parainfluenza usually causes a mild respiratory infection in adults and is one cause of the common cold. Often adults may experience hoarseness along with the rhinorrhea, sore throat, and cough. Less commonly, tracheobronchitis has been described both in the adult with underlying chronic bronchitis, as well as the otherwise healthy individual. Pneumonia has also been reported in the elderly.

Diagnosis Infection with parainfluenza is suspected when there is a compatible clinical presentation in the appropriate epidemiologic setting, particularly if the "barking seal" cough of croup is recognized. However, the other manifestations of the disease are generally not specific enough to distinguish parainfluenza from other common respiratory viruses, such as respiratory syncytial virus. Microbiologic confirmation is indicated in severe cases (such as bronchiolitis or pneumonia), atypical cases, or if suspected in the adult. In severe cases, it may also be important to rule out respiratory syncytial virus, for which treatment is available. Rapid identification techniques are offered in many virology laboratories, and the identification of the infecting virus may avoid unnecessary antibacterial agents or invasive diagnostic procedures. In mild upper respiratory infections, virologic confirmation is optional.

The best respiratory sample for detecting parainfluenza virus is the nasopharyngeal wash. This is performed at the bedside by gently administering saline into the nares with a standard syringe then aspirating the fluid back into the syringe, capturing saline, mucous, and respiratory epithelial cells. Alternatively, a viral swab may be inserted into the nasopharynx, but fewer respiratory cells are obtained with this technique and the sensitivity is lower. A "respiratory panel" is offered in some microbiology laboratories, whereby a single nasopharyngeal wash (or swab) may be sent for detection of multiple viruses, such as parainfluenza, influenza, respiratory syncytial virus, and others. Laboratory detection methods include:

1. Cell culture, where the clinical specimen is inoculated onto a monolayer of cells. If parainfluenza virus is present, a characteristic change in the appearance of the monolayer is seen, called cytopathic effect (CPE). The turnaround time is variable, and may be over several days, depending on the quality of the specimen and the amount of virus present.
2. Immunofluorescence. This is a rapid technique designed to detect viral presence without culture. Results may be available within hours of sample submission, if necessary.
3. Direct viral antigen detection. This is another early detection method but is still under study.
4. Serologic studies. Specific antibody titers to parainfluenza may be obtained during the acute and convalescent period. Demonstration of a fourfold increase in specific antibody titer is diagnostic of parainfluenza infection. This may be useful if it is important to diagnose a respiratory illness in retrospect (as for an epidemiologic or outbreak study), but contributes little to the immediate management of a new case.

Diagnostic Tests/Procedures

Parainfluenza Virus Antigen by Direct Fluorescent Antibody *on page 512*
Parainfluenza Virus Culture *on page 512*
Parainfluenza Virus Serology *on page 513*

Treatment There are no antiviral agents currently approved for parainfluenza virus, although several are being studied. Bacterial superinfection is always possible and should be considered as a potentially reversible complication in difficult cases. Most cases of croup respond to supportive therapy alone, but severe cases may require intubation.

Drug Therapy Comment

No antiviral agents proven effective.

Selected Readings
Heilman CA, "Respiratory Syncytial and Parainfluenza Viruses," *J Infect Dis*, 1990, 161(3):402-6.
Vainionpää R and Hyypiä T, "Biology of Parainfluenza Viruses," *Clin Microbiol Rev*, 1994, 7(2):265-75.

Parvovirus B19

Microbiology Parvovirus B19 is a small DNA virus which has received increasing attention in recent years. It is the cause of the childhood rash erythema infectiosum ("fifth disease" because it's the "fifth" infectious rash of children) and has been recently linked with a symmetrical adult arthritis, transient aplastic anemia, and chronic anemia in AIDS patients.

Parvovirus B19 is a single-stranded, encapsulated DNA virus which belongs to the family Parvoviridae. There are several other parvoviruses in the same genus as B19, including the common canine parvovirus. However, B19 is a strictly human pathogen and does not cause disease in animals. Infection with B19 is not acquired from dogs (a common misconception); animal parvoviruses have not been shown to cause human disease. The virus predominantly infects erythrocyte precursors in the bone marrow and causes cell lysis. Myeloid precursors in the marrow appear to be spared, although the virus has occasionally been found in peripheral leukocytes. Although parvovirus B19 has been cultured *in vitro* in erythropoietin-stimulated marrow cells, such techniques are not available in clinical virology laboratories. Instead, detection of viral presence is mainly achieved through detection of either specific B19 antibody, viral antigens, or nucleic acid (using polymerase chain reaction).

Epidemiology Infection with parvovirus B19 is common in the United States, beginning in early childhood. Over 50% of the adult population has serologic evidence of prior infection. Many cases are asymptomatic or mild. The primary mode of transmission is most likely respiratory. Outbreaks within families or schools can occur because of a high secondary attack rate which sometimes exceeds 50%. Spread of the virus is facilitated by subclinically infected individuals shedding the virus unknowingly in respiratory secretions. In addition, the individual is infective for several weeks before the characteristic parvovirus rash appears. Based on human volunteer studies, the period of incubation is approximately 1 week (4-14 days).

Clinical Syndromes

- **Erythema infectiosum (slapped cheek):** This is a childhood exanthem caused exclusively by parvovirus B19, also referred to as "fifth disease." Typically, a school-aged child develops a nonspecific febrile illness (low grade fever, malaise, and myalgias), which resolves over several days. Days to weeks later, when the child is feeling well, a brightly erythematous rash develops on the face. This is the characteristic "slapped cheek" rash of erythema infectiosum and is considered benign. Mild constitutional symptoms may accompany the rash (malaise, headache, etc), but the child is usually not infectious at this point. Erythema infectiosum has also been described in the adult and is frequently accompanied by joint symptoms.

- **Adult polyarthropathy:** B19 has recently been associated with a sudden onset, symmetrical polyarthritis syndrome. The great majority of cases have been reported in otherwise healthy women. Patients initially experience a nonspecific viral prodrome, probably corresponding to the period of viremia (B19 nucleic acid has been detected in the serum of some individuals). Several days to weeks later, an acute arthropathy develops, symmetrically involving the small joints of the hands, feet, and knees. Other joints may be involved less commonly (spine, costochondral joints). In addition to these arthralgias, there is often evidence of arthritis and synovitis, with joint stiffness, inflammation, and joint effusions. Arthrocentesis typically shows a mild elevation in WBCs around 3000-6000 cells/mm^3, mostly mononuclear. It is not clear whether B19 arthropathy is due to autoimmune mechanisms or direct viral infection. B19 nucleic acid has been found in the synovial fluid of a single patient (suggesting direct infection) but is generally undetectable in the blood during the arthropathy phase (suggesting an autoimmune etiology). Less than 50% of the cases are accompanied by a rash. When present, the rash appears macular in men and "lace-like" in women. The distribution of the rash is variable but tends to include the arms of legs. In some cases, there is marked involvement of the soles of the feet and the palms (somewhat unusual locations for an exanthem). The typical "slapped cheek" rash of erythema infectiosum is uncommon. The majority of cases of B19 arthropathy resolve completely with observation alone. Occasionally, the polyarthropathy may be persistent or recurrent over a period of years, and recent studies have linked it to a chronic fibromyalgia syndrome. Of

222

note, there are many variations in the presentation of this syndrome, including symmetrical arthritis without a flu-like illness or rash.

- **Transient aplastic crisis:** Parvovirus B19 can cause a severe erythropoietic arrest in patients with a previous underlying blood disorder, especially sickle cell disease, hereditary spherocytosis, thalassemia, hemoglobin SC, and other chronic hemolytic states. (Transient aplastic crisis from B19 usually does not cause anemia in healthy individuals since mature, circulating erythrocytes are spared and continue to circulate for 120 days.) Individuals present with profound fatigue and lethargy, with or without a history of a preceding flu-like illness. Rash and arthralgias are usually not present. Blood counts reveal a severely decreased hemoglobin with absent reticulocytes. Urgent transfusion may be necessary. Examination of the bone marrow shows erythroid hypoplasia with other cell lines usually intact. The finding of giant pronormoblasts in the bone marrow is considered pathognomonic for this infection. B19 viremia has been demonstrated during this time, and patients are potentially still infectious. The aplastic crisis usually resolves within 1-2 weeks.

- **Transient pancytopenia:** Other cells besides the erythrocytes can be involved with an acute parvovirus B19 infection. Potentially life-threatening declines in the neutrophil and/or platelet counts have been reported. In addition, a mild and transient pancytopenia was commonly observed in human volunteers experimentally infected with B19 and likely occurs in natural infections.

- **Chronic anemia in the immunocompromised host:** In these patients, B19 is incompletely cleared after the initial infection and leads to a waxing and waning, persistent infection. Chronic bone marrow suppression may be seen, as the virus causes continued lysis of RBC progenitor cells. Patients may be otherwise asymptomatic despite the chronicity of infection. Cases have been reported in acute leukemia, severe combined immunodeficiency syndrome, bone marrow transplant patients, and HIV-1 infections. The host antibody response to chronic B19 infection is highly variable, and viremia has been seen in patients with a negative parvovirus IgG and IgM. Diagnosis may require demonstration of B19 DNA in the serum by polymerase chain reaction. It is important to recognize this form of chronic anemia because it may respond to immunoglobulin therapy. In 1990, persistent B19 infection was found in a group of HIV-infected patients with red cell aplasia. All patients had giant pronormoblasts in the bone marrow.

- **Perinatal infections:** The developing fetus is at particular risk for complications related to perinatal parvovirus infection. This is due to several factors including the immaturity of the fetal immune system, delayed and incomplete transfer of protective maternal antibody across the placenta, and the need for brisk erythrocyte production in the fetus. Maternal infections with B19 during pregnancy may lead to hydrops fetalis or fetal death. The precise risk of intrauterine transmission to the fetus is unknown, as is the risk of fetal death once transmission has taken place. However, the data available suggest that the majority of pregnant women with acute B19 infections deliver healthy infants. However, fetal demise has been reported following asymptomatic maternal B19 infections. The cause of death in the fetus has been attributed to destruction of erythroid precursors in the liver and bone marrow, followed by edema and congestive heart failure; however, virus has also been identified in tissues such as the heart. Perinatal parvovirus B19 infection has not been associated with congenital abnormalities. Thus, maternal infection is not an indication for an abortion. Although the epidemiology of perinatal parvovirus infections is still evolving, this virus is still an uncommon cause of stillbirths or spontaneous abortions in the general U.S. population (by some estimates, approximately 1% of cases of fetal loss). The Centers for Disease Control has addressed the growing public concern regarding B19 and fetal death by estimating the risks of B19 infection in pregnant women following different exposures to the virus (see Selected Readings). The risk of fetal death in susceptible women exposed to B19 during epidemic outbreaks (school, day care centers) is roughly 1% to 2%.

Diagnosis In the absence of classic erythema infectiosum, parvovirus infection may be difficult to diagnose. The clinician must maintain a high level of suspicion for B19 in patients with unusual skin rashes, arthritis-arthralgia syndromes, aplastic anemia of unknown etiology, and chronic anemia. Laboratory studies are necessary to confirm the diagnosis. These consist of:

(Continued)

Parvovirus B19 *(Continued)*

1. IgG and IgM antibodies specific for parvovirus B19. The presence of IgM antibody in the patient (or in cord blood of the fetus) confirms acute infection. A significant rise in parvovirus IgG during acute and convalescent periods is also diagnostic. A single positive IgG only suggests past infection, and a paired sample is necessary for proper interpretation. Chronic B19 infection in immunosuppressed patients may or may not demonstrate IgG or IgM antibodies and are not completely reliable.

2. Detection of viral antigen is still a research tool and not commercially available as yet.

3. Polymerase chain reaction (PCR), the most sensitive technique, has been employed successfully in many studies, with viral DNA being detected in the serum of individuals with acute viremia as well as a variety of tissues. Contact a large commercial reference laboratory or the Centers for Disease Control and Prevention (Division of Viral Diseases) for inquiries regarding PCR.

4. Electron microscopy for parvovirus-like particles.

5. Histologic specimens, looking for eosinophilic nuclear inclusions (not pathognomonic for B19)

6. Bone marrow aspiration and biopsy. The finding of giant pronormoblasts in Wright-Giemsa stained marrow is characteristic of parvoviral infection.

B19 cannot be detected using the common cell culture systems available in clinical virology laboratories.

Diagnostic Tests/Procedures

Bone Marrow Aspiration and Biopsy *on page 343*
Parvovirus B19 DNA, Qualitative PCR *on page 514*
Parvovirus B19 Serology *on page 514*

Treatment Currently, there is no antiviral agent with significant clinical activity against the B19 virus itself. However, in some cases, the chronic anemia of B19 infection in immunosuppressed patients has been shown to respond dramatically to infusions of intravenous immunoglobulin. This important finding has also been shown in a small cohort of HIV-1 infected individuals with B19-induced anemia.

Drug Therapy Comment

No antiviral agents proven effective.

Selected Readings

Anderson LJ, "Human Parvoviruses," *J Infect Dis*, 1990, 161(4):603-8.

Dollard S, Nasello M, and Menegus M, "Serodiagnosis of Parvovirus Infections: Problems and Pitfalls," *Clin Microbiol Newslett*, 1998, 20(3):21-3.

Faden H, Gary GW Jr, and Anderson LF, "Chronic Parvovirus Infection in a Presumably Immunologically Healthy Woman," *Clin Infect Dis*, 1992, 15(4):595-7.

Frickhofen N, Abkowitz JL, Safford M, et al, "Persistent B19 Parvovirus Infection in Patients Infected With Human Immunodeficiency Virus Type I (HIV-1): A Treatable Cause of Anemia in AIDS," *Ann Intern Med*, 1990, 113(12):926-33.

Kurtzman G, Frickhofen N, Kimball J, et al, "Pure Red-Cell Aplasia of 10 Years' Duration Due to Persistent Parvovirus B19 Infection and Its Cure With Immunoglobulin Therapy," *N Engl J Med*, 1989, 321(8):519-23.

Kurtzman GJ, Cohen B, Meyers P, et al, "Persistent B19 Parvovirus Infection as a Cause of Severe Chronic Anemia in Children With Acute Lymphocytic Leukaemia," *Lancet*, 1988, 2(8621):1159-62.

Woolf AD, Campion GV, Chishick A, et al, "Clinical Manifestations of Human Parvovirus B19 in Adults," *Arch Intern Med*, 1989, 149(5):1153-6.

Pasteurella multocida

Microbiology *Pasteurella multocida* is a gram-negative rod which is primarily a pathogen in wild and domestic animals but is also capable of causing sporadic human diseases such as animal bite infection, osteomyelitis, pneumonia, and sepsis. *P. multocida* is an aerobic, gram-negative coccobacillus which does not form spores. It belongs to the family Pasteurellaceae, and is thus related to *Haemophilus* species. There are six distinct species of *Pasteurella*, but the most common to cause human disease is *Pasteurella multocida*. Special requests for identification for this organism are helpful for the Microbiology Laboratory but are usually not necessary; the organism grows readily on several standard culture media such as blood agar or chocolate agar.

Epidemiology *P. multocida* is a normal commensal of the oropharynx and the gastrointestinal tract of several kinds of animals. However, it is only rarely recovered from the respiratory tract of humans and has been found to be part of the normal oral flora only in individuals with significant animal contact (eg, veterinarians). The frequency of recovery of this organism from a healthy animal depends on the particular animal species, as follows: cats, 50% to 75%; dogs, 10% to 60%; pigs, 50%, and rats, 15%.

Pasteurella has been reported in all age groups. Human infection usually occurs following an animal bite or scratch. One study found that up to 17% of patients being treated in an emergency room for an animal bite ultimately developed a *Pasteurella* infection. Cat scratches or bites cause the majority of *Pasteurella* infections (about 65% of cases). Dog bites are responsible for about 35% of cases. A smaller number of cases of *Pasteurella* infections are due to animal exposures without a clear history of an animal bite or scratch. The patient tends to be frequently exposed to animals (such as a veterinarian, livestock handler, pet shop worker), and the infections are generally in the respiratory tract, although cases of intra-abdominal infection have also been described. A small percentage of patients are infected with *P. multocida* without any significant animal exposure.

Clinical Syndromes

- **Animal bite-wound infections:** Patients who have *Pasteurella* inoculated via a bite wound develop rapid onset of pain, erythema, and edema locally. This may occur within hours of the bite or may be delayed by several days. Common sites include the upper extremities (in particular, hands), legs, and the head and neck region. An important complication is the development of regional lymphadenopathy. Occasionally, *Pasteurella* infection may be the cause of lymph node enlargement of unknown etiology; such patients should be questioned about seemingly minor animal scratches as well. Bite-wound infections are often limited to soft tissue cellulitis or focal abscesses. At times, the course may be complicated by tenosynovitis and osteomyelitis, which can be particularly difficult to treat when involving the hand. Note that the specific entity known as "cat scratch disease" is not caused by *Pasteurella multocida*. The exact cause of this lymphadenopathy syndrome is still being debated.

- **Upper and lower respiratory infections:** This unusual presentation of *Pasteurella* infection may be seen in patients who have had a significant exposure to animals but lack a history of an animal bite. *Pasteurella* has been implicated as a rare cause of bronchitis, sinusitis, and pneumonia in both healthy individuals and those with underlying chronic bronchitis.

- **Infection in the immunocompromised host:** Serious and life-threatening *Pasteurella* infections have been reported in patients with underlying malignancies, organ transplantations, and HIV infection.

- **Miscellaneous infections:** Meningitis, arthritis, peritonitis (particularly patients undergoing peritoneal dialysis), corneal ulcers, ophthalmitis, and urinary tract infections are rarely reported.

Diagnosis *P. multocida* infection should be included in the differential diagnosis of any wound infection following an animal bite or deep scratch. The diagnosis strongly suggested if the onset of local inflammation is within 3-24 hours of the bite and if the animal involved was a cat. Longer periods of incubation are more suggestive of streptococcal or staphylococcal infection, although certainly cases of pasteurellosis may have a delayed onset. The diagnosis is more difficult for nonbite *Pasteurella* infections; the clinician must carefully inquire about unusual or prolonged animal exposures in the workplace and at home.

Diagnostic Tests/Procedures

Blood Culture, Aerobic and Anaerobic *on page 337*
Gram's Stain *on page 426*
Wound Culture *on page 577*

Treatment The drug of choice for pasteurellosis is penicillin. If the infection is minor and limited to soft tissue, a trial of oral penicillin may be attempted (eg, penicillin V, 500 mg orally every 6 hours). If the infection is more serious, parenteral penicillin should be used. This includes deep wound infections of the extremities, osteomyelitis, septic arthritic, tenosynovitis, and pneumonia. Consultation with an Infectious Disease specialist may be useful in complicated cases, where therapy may be prolonged and surgical debridement necessary. Other antimicrobial agents are probably effective but the clinical experience is more limited: tetracycline, ampicillin, possibly ciprofloxacin, and the cephalosporins. Infectious disease consultation may be helpful for therapy with alternative agents.

(Continued)

Pasteurella multocida (Continued)

Drug Therapy
Recommended
Penicillin G, Parenteral, Aqueous *on page 860*
Penicillin V Potassium *on page 865*
Alternate
Amoxicillin and Clavulanate Potassium *on page 593*
Ampicillin and Sulbactam *on page 607*

Selected Readings
Weber DJ, Wolfson JS, Swartz M, et al, "*Pasteurella multocida* Infections. Report of 34 Cases and Review of the Literature," *Medicine (Baltimore)*, 1984, 63(3):133-154.

Pediculus humanus see Lice *on page 188*

Penicillin-Resistant *S. pneumoniae* see Streptococcus pneumoniae, Drug-Resistant *on page 270*

Penicillium marneffei

Microbiology *Penicillium marneffei* is the only dimorphic fungus of the genus *Penicillium*. In the mycelial form on culture, the mold grows relatively fast producing a grayish white and downy or woolly colony in 2-3 days. The underneath of the fungus appears either pink or red due to the production of a soluble red pigment that diffuses into the agar. Over time, the colony becomes more rugose while the aerial mycelia becomes pink. The color of the colony changes from white to light brown to light green after 10 days. Microscopically, it appears as a typical *Penicillium* species characterized by short, branched, septated hyphae with brush-like conidiophores located laterally and terminally. The yeast form grows rapidly appearing as light tan colonies of various textures ranging from smooth to cerebriform. Microscopically, the yeast cells are unicellular 3-6 x 1.5-2 mm in size and vary from round, ellipsoidal, and rectangular shapes. The yeast form may be mixed with hyphal elements. The yeast cells may be distinguished from other yeast by the presence of a white central septum and reproduction by fission, not budding.

Epidemiology The ecological characteristics and geographic distribution are still largely unknown. *P. marneffei* has been isolated from bamboo rats in southeast Asia but is also endemic in the southern part of China. Almost all reported cases have indicated that the infected patients have lived or traveled in southeast Asia particularly Vietnam, Laos, Singapore, Malaysia, Burma, Thailand, Indonesia, Guangxi, or Hong Kong. It occurs more commonly in males. Although the majority of patients who acquire penicilliosis are immunocompromised, there are reports of cases occurring in patients with intact immune systems. *P. marneffei* is the third most common opportunistic infection in patients with AIDS living in northern Thailand following tuberculosis and cryptococcosis. It is classified as an AIDS-defining illness by several southeast Asian countries. There is a 20% mortality in AIDS patients with disseminated disease. Without chronic suppressive therapy, the relapse rate exceeds 50%. The route of transmission is believed to be either from inhalation or ingestion. Autoinoculation in a research laboratory environment has been reported.

Clinical Syndromes
- **Localized disease:** May occur from autoinoculation. Forms a cutaneous lesion and may cause localized lymphadenopathy.
- **Disseminated disease:** Clinically similar to disseminated histoplasmosis and cryptococcosis. Patients present with constitutional symptoms such as fever and weight loss. Various forms of cutaneous lesions are common and are present on the face, upper torso, pinnae, and arms. Patients often have respiratory symptoms including cough and pleuritic pain. Chest radiographs are frequently abnormal revealing infiltrates, nodules, abscesses, or even cavitation. Anemia is commonly seen. Peripheral blood cultures are frequently positive and bone marrow involvement occurs in greater than 25%. Uncommon manifestations include pericarditis, genital ulcers, osteomyelitis, and arthritis.

Diagnosis Diagnosis is dependent on identification of the organism by histopathology and culture. Must be distinguished from *H. capsulatum* as both appear as intracellular organisms; however *H. capsulatum* reproduces by budding whereas *P. marneffei* reproduces by fission. Immunologic assays and PCR remain investigational.

Diagnostic Tests/Procedures
Fungus Culture, Appropriate Site *on page 414*
KOH Preparation *on page 467*
Methenamine Silver Stain *on page 487*

Treatment Non-AIDS: Amphotericin B 0.6 mg/kg/day 1-3 g total dose depending on the severity of the disease

In AIDS: Amphotericin B 0.6 mg/kg/day for 2 weeks followed by itraconazole 200 mg twice daily for 10 weeks followed by itraconazole 200 mg/day for life.

Drug Therapy
Recommended
Non-AIDS:
Amphotericin B (Conventional) *on page 597*
In AIDS:
Amphotericin B (Conventional) *on page 597*
followed by
Itraconazole *on page 785*
Alternate
Itraconazole *on page 785*

Selected Readings
Cooper CR, "From Bamboo Rats to Humans: The Odyssey of *Penicillium marneffei*," *ASM News*, 1998, 64(7):390-7.
Cooper CR Jr and McGinnis MR, "Pathology of *Penicillium marneffei*. An Emerging Acquired Immunodeficiency Syndrome-Related Pathogen," *Arch Pathol Lab Med*, 1997, 121(8):798-804.
Duong TA, "Infection Due to *Penicillium marneffei*, an Emerging Pathogen: Review of 155 Reported Cases," *Clin Infect Dis*, 1996, 23(1):125-30.
Supparatpinyo K, Perriens J, Nelson KE, et al, "A Controlled Trial of Itraconazole to Prevent Relapse of *Penicillium marneffei* Infection in Patients Infected With the Human Immunodeficiency Virus," *N Engl J Med*, 1998, 339(24):1739-43.

Peptostreptococcus see Streptococcus-Related Gram-Positive Cocci *on page 278*

Phaeomycotic Cyst see Dematiaceous Fungi *on page 125*

Phthirus pubis see Lice *on page 188*

Pinworm see Enterobius vermicularis *on page 136*

Pityriasis (Tinea) Versicolor see Malassezia furfur *on page 192*

Pityrosporum orbiculare see Malassezia furfur *on page 192*

Pityrosporum ovale see Malassezia furfur *on page 192*

Plasmodium Species
Related Information
Prevention of Malaria *on page 1057*

Microbiology *Plasmodium* sp are obligate intracellular protozoa related to *Babesia* and *Toxoplasma*. *Plasmodium* sp reproduce sexually in mosquitos. Mosquitos transmit the resulting sporozoites into humans where the organisms reproduce asexually. The sporozoites multiply within the liver; resulting merozoites invade erythrocytes where the merozoites multiply or mature into male and female gametocytes which eventually will be taken up by a mosquito during a blood meal.

Plasmodium sp stain well with Giemsa or Wright-Giemsa and are easily observed in stained peripheral blood smears if parasitemia is heavy enough. There are many species of *Plasmodium*; however, only the following four species infect humans: *P. falciparum*, *P. vivax*, *P. ovale*, and *P. malariae*.

Epidemiology *P. falciparum* is found in tropical areas; *P. vivax* is found throughout many tropical and subtropical parts of the world; *P. ovale* is found in central and west Africa and in some Pacific islands; and *P. malariae* is found sporadically throughout the world. *P. falciparum* and *P. vivax* cause approximately 80% and 15%, respectively, of all cases of malaria. Malaria is the most severe infectious disease of tropical and subtropical areas of the world. One-half of the world's population live in areas where malaria is endemic. Each year approximately 270 million persons become infected with *Plasmodium* sp, approximately 110 million persons develop clinical disease, and 7 million Americans visit areas where malaria is endemic.

Clinical Syndromes After experiencing a prodrome phase of constitutional "flu"-like symptoms, most persons with malaria will experience the hallmark of classic malaria, the paroxysm. A paroxysm is a 3- to 6-hour period of high fever, chills, and rigors. Paroxysms correspond to periodic release of *Plasmodium* merozoites from erythrocytes and the beginning of another life cycle of the organism
(Continued)

Plasmodium Species *(Continued)*

within erythrocytes. Fever patterns are often irregular, but the paroxysm often occurs regularly (eg, every 2 days). Often, patients are asymptomatic between paroxysms. Patients with malaria can experience severe splenomegaly and hepatomegaly. Rupture of the spleen is not uncommon. Anemia is a common complication. Malaria caused by *P. falciparum* is a medically urgent situation and requires immediate diagnosis and medical intervention. Fulminant complications of malaria include renal failure, pulmonary edema, cerebral involvement, and severe reduction of the flow of blood through capillaries.

Diagnosis Smears of peripheral blood must be stained with Giemsa or Wright-Giemsa stains and examined for parasites. Blood should be collected no less than twice per day (preferably, several times a day) until malaria is ruled out or until parasites are observed and identified. The most important and immediate concerns in the management of malaria are to determine if the patient is infected with *Plasmodium* and, if so, to determine if the parasite is *P. falciparum*.

Diagnostic Tests/Procedures

Peripheral Blood Smear, Thick and Thin *on page 519*

Drug Therapy

Recommended

Chloroquine-susceptible:

Chloroquine Phosphate *on page 672*

Quinidine *on page 888*

Chloroquine-resistant:

Mefloquine *on page 809*

Halofantrine *on page 758*

Alternate

Chloroquine-resistant:

Sulfadoxine and Pyrimethamine *on page 931*

Halofantrine *on page 758*

Selected Readings

Garcia LS, "Update on Malaria," *Clin Microbiol Newslett*, 1992, 14:65-9.

Krogstad DJ, "*Plasmodium* Species (Malaria)," *Principles and Practice of Infectious Diseases*, 4th ed, Mandell GL, Bennett JE, and Dolin R, eds, New York, NY: Churchill Livingstone, 1995, 2415-27.

Smith JH, "Malaria: Clinical Laboratory Features," *Clin Microbiol Newslett*, 1995, 17(24):185-8.

Pneumococcus, Drug-Resistant *see Streptococcus pneumoniae*, Drug-Resistant *on page 270*

Pneumocystis carinii

Microbiology *Pneumocystis carinii* has traditionally been classified as a protozoan, although more recent evidence suggests it is more closely related to fungi. Studies using molecular techniques have shown a close homology between *P. carinii* and fungi such as *Saccharomyces* than other protozoans such as *Plasmodium* (the cause of malaria). The organism is unicellular and has three stages: trophozoite, precyst, and cyst. In clinical specimens, the trophozoites are most predominant. The life cycle of *P. carinii* has yet to be fully defined. The organism cannot be cultured reliably in the laboratory, even in research settings. The organism requires special staining to be visible in clinical specimens. Several stains will selectively stain the organism (methenamine-silver, toluidine blue, Wright-Giemsa, and others).

Epidemiology *P. carinii* is distributed worldwide and in animals. Serologic data suggests that infection with this organism is common. Most children show serologic evidence of infection by 4 years of age. Most of these primary infections with *Pneumocystis* in the normal child are insignificant, with either mild or no clinical disease. Individuals with normal immune systems generally are asymptomatic; reactivation or significant reinfection occurs only when the immune system is compromised. Transmission of *P. carinii* is probably by an airborne route. The precise reservoir for the organism in nature is not clear; it is not known if the organism can exist outside of a living host. In humans and animals, the natural reservoir is the lung.

P. carinii causes an opportunistic infection in immunocompromised hosts. Early on, cases of *Pneumocystis carinii* pneumonia (PCP) were described in premature and debilitated infants, institutionalized children, patients with primary immunodeficiency disorders, and adults receiving immunosuppressive medications such as corticosteroids. A defect in the host cell-mediated immunity appeared to be the major risk factor for PCP. More recently, PCP has been and continues to be a common infection in persons with AIDS and is an important AIDS-defining opportunistic infection.

Persons with AIDS are at particularly high risk for PCP. Before the advent of preventative therapy for PCP, about 60% to 80% of AIDS patients developed PCP. Infection with *P. carinii* rarely occurs when the CD4 count is >200 cells/μL, with most cases occurring when the CD4 count is <100 cells/μL.

Clinical Syndromes

- ***Pneumocystis carinii* pneumonia (PCP):** Patients classically present with fever, dyspnea on exertion, and dry cough. AIDS patients often have a very indolent presentation with symptoms present for several weeks. Other symptoms include chills, chest pain, and sputum production. On examination, patients with PCP have tachypnea and tachycardia, but the auscultation of the lungs may be completely normal. Useful laboratory tests include the arterial blood gas, which shows hypoxia, increased alveolar-arterial oxygen gradient, and respiratory alkalosis in most, but not all, patients. The diffusing capacity of the lung (DLCO) at rest or with exercise is decreased in many cases. The chest radiograph usually shows bilateral, symmetrical interstitial pulmonary infiltrates. A variety of unusual chest x-ray findings have been reported including nodules and cavities. In some patients, both the lung examination, arterial blood gas, and chest x-ray are normal.

- **Extrapulmonary pneumocystosis:** Although *P. carinii* most commonly involves the lung, cases of *P. carinii* infection outside the lung have been reported, particularly in AIDS patients receiving aerosolized pentamidine for PCP prophylaxis. These include retinal infection, lymph nodes, liver and spleen, thyroid, ear lesions, skin lesions, and mastoiditis.

Diagnosis The manifestations of *P. carinii* infection in the AIDS patient can be very subtle, and a high index of suspicion must be maintained. Similarly, the non-AIDS patient with PCP may present only with fever and malaise without prominent respiratory symptoms. Laboratory confirmation includes:

- induced sputum for *P. carinii* (usually productive only in immunocompromised patients). Stains for *P. carinii* (toluidine blue, methenamine-silver, Giemsa, immunofluorescence, and calcofluor staining procedures) have been found to be sensitive and convenient.
- bronchoscopy with or without transbronchial biopsy (BAL produces a particularly good specimen)
- open lung biopsy (infrequently required)

Diagnostic Tests/Procedures

Methenamine Silver Stain *on page 487*
Pneumocystis carinii Test *on page 522*

Treatment The mainstays of therapy for *P. carinii* remain co-trimoxazole or intravenous pentamidine. Comparison studies have shown these agents are equally efficacious but fewer adverse reactions have been noted with co-trimoxazole. Thus, co-trimoxazole is considered the agent of choice, usually administered intravenously in serious cases. In mild cases, oral co-trimoxazole may be utilized initially. There is still a high incidence (≥50%) of adverse reactions with co-trimoxazole in AIDS patients with PCP; the incidence is much lower in non-AIDS patients.

Drug Therapy

Recommended

Co-Trimoxazole *on page 692*

Alternate

Pentamidine *on page 866*
Atovaquone *on page 612*
Trimethoprim *on page 957*
    used in combination with
Dapsone *on page 698*

Selected Readings

Caliendo AM, "Enhanced Diagnosis of *Pneumocystis carinii*: Promises and Problems," *Clin Microbiol Newslet*, 1996, 18(15):113-6.

Davey RT Jr, Masur H, "Recent Advances in the Diagnosis, Treatment, and Prevention of *Pneumocystis carinii* Pneumonia," *Antimicrob Agents Chemother*, 1990, 34(4):499-504.

National Institutes of Health - University of California Expert Panel for Corticosteroids as Adjunctive Therapy for *Pneumocystis* Pneumonia, "Consensus Statement on the Use of Corticosteroids as Adjunctive Therapy for *Pneumocystis* Pneumonia in the Acquired Immunodeficiency Syndrome," *N Engl J Med*, 1990, 323(21):1500-4.

(Continued)

Pneumocystis carinii (Continued)

Phair J, Munoz A Detels R, et al, "The Risk of *Pneumocystis carinii* Pneumonia Among Men Infected With Human Immunodeficiency Virus Type 1," *N Engl J Med*, 1990, 322(3):161-5.

"Recommendations for Prophylaxis Against *Pneumocystis carinii* for Adults and Adolescents Infected With Human Immunodeficiency Virus," *MMWR Morb Mortal Wkly Rep*, 1992, 41(No. RR-4):1-11.

Telzak EE, Cote RJ, Gold JW, et al, "Extrapulmonary *Pneumocystis carinii* Infections," *Rev Infect Dis*, 1990, 12(3):380-6.

Wachter RM, Russi MB, Bloch DA, et al, "*Pneumocystis carinii* Pneumonia and Respiratory Failure in AIDS," *Am Rev Respir Dis*, 1991, 143(2):251-6.

Poliovirus

Related Information

Recommended Poliovirus Vaccination Schedule on page 1044

Microbiology Polioviruses are single-stranded RNA viruses which cause poliomyelitis, a central nervous system disease of once epidemic proportions. They belong to the family Picornaviridae (pico-, very small; rna-, ribonucleic acid; -viruses) and the genus Enterovirus. Thus, polioviruses are closely related to such agents as Coxsackieviruses, Enteroviruses, and ECHO viruses. Polioviruses have three distinct serotypes (types 1-3). Infection with one serotype (either natural or vaccine-related) confers serotype-specific immunity; reinfection with a different serotype has been reported.

The virus is tropic for neural tissue. Polioviruses have a narrow tissue tropism in comparison with other Enteroviruses. Polioviruses attach to anterior horn cells of spinal cord gray matter, motor neurons, and dorsal root ganglia by means of a specific receptor (cellular adhesion molecules). The neurovirulence of "wild-type" strains (ie, strains present in the general population) varies enormously. The viral strains used in the polio vaccines are of low neurovirulence and can be distinguished from wild-type strains by means of genomic sequencing and other molecular techniques.

Epidemiology Poliovirus infections were epidemic in the United States in the first half of the twentieth century. In the 1950s, epidemics occurred on a regular basis with an attack rate of 17 cases per 100,000. The introduction of the inactivated polio vaccine (IPV) by Jonas Salk in 1955 was one of the great advances in modern medicine. This introduction was followed soon afterwards by the live-attenuated oral polio vaccine (OPV) developed by Albert Sabin. A striking decline in paralytic and nonparalytic polio cases followed. With the extensive use of the OPV in both North and South America, wild-type strains of polio have nearly disappeared in the Western hemisphere, despite the large number of children who are inadequately immunized. The year 1979 marked the last reported case of endemic, wild-type poliomyelitis in the United States. The most recent case of wild-type paralytic poliomyelitis in either North or South America came from Peru in August 1991. Cases of acute flaccid paralysis continue to be screened by aggressive surveillance programs, but additional wild-type cases have not been recognized through 1992 and the first half of 1993.

Although naturally-occurring cases have been eliminated in this country, rare cases of vaccine-related poliomyelitis still occur. Each of the 5-10 annual cases in the United States can be directly linked to the OPV vaccine. Vaccine-related infections have been reported in recipients of the OPV (usually children), as well as close contacts of vaccine recipients (usually adults). Some experts believe that wild-type polioviruses have essentially been replaced with Sabin vaccine strains; these vaccine strains now circulate widely in the population, presumably causing asymptomatic or mild infections. Poliomyelitis still occurs with some frequency in developing countries outside North and South America. About 120,000 cases were recognized in 1992, mainly in sub-Saharan Africa and the Indian subcontinent. Global eradication of this infection is still possible, although there are multiple factors which account for the persistence of disease. Reintroduction of wild-type polioviruses into the United States from foreign visitors or travelers to endemic areas remains a concern, and justifies continued immunization programs.

Although infection can be induced in experimental animals, humans are believed to be the only natural host of the virus. The infectious cycle begins when the host ingests materials which contain contaminated feces (ie, a fecal-oral route of transmission). Active viral replication takes place in the oropharynx (particularly the tonsils) and in the distal portion of the small bowel (Peyer's patches, intestinal mucosa). This replication is followed by a transient phase of "minor viremia" where virus particles spread hematogenously to various organs and lymph nodes. In the majority of cases, the infection is aborted at this stage by the host immune system; only subclinical or asymptomatic infection results ("abortive poliomyelitis"). Less commonly, viral replication is not controlled by immunologic mechanisms, and virus proliferates in the liver, spleen, marrow, and nodes. This is followed by a "major viremia" in which visceral organs are again seeded hematogenously, including the brain and spinal cord. This "major viremia" corresponds with the prodromal symptoms of poliomyelitis (fever, malaise). The incubation period between exposure and the onset of symptoms has been estimated at 5-35 days.

Clinical Syndromes

- **Asymptomatic illness:** As with other enteroviral infections, the vast majority of infections with poliovirus are asymptomatic, and never go on to develop clinical illness.
- **Aseptic meningitis:** Patients present with fever, headache, and nuchal rigidity. Cerebrospinal fluid characteristically reveals a mild lymphocytic (predominantly polymorphonuclear leukocytes early on, the lymphocytic) with elevated protein in the 40-50 mg/dL range. In some cases the virus may be directly cultured from CSF with cytopathic effect in cell culture in 1 week. There is a rapid clinical recovery within 2-10 days. Poliovirus is a relatively rare cause of the syndrome of aseptic meningitis is indistinguishable from the aseptic meningitis caused by other, more common viruses.
- **Abortive poliomyelitis:** This occurs in less than 10% of polio cases. Patients develop a nonspecific viral syndrome with fever, sore throat, malaise, and abdominal discomfort. Symptoms resolve quickly and there is no progression to paralytic polio.
- **Bulbar poliomyelitis:** In this form of polio, patients initially present with dysphagia and a change in speech due to paralysis of the muscles of the pharynx. Most commonly there is involvement of cranial nerves IX and X, although others may be involved.
- **Polioencephalitis:** Infants are most susceptible to this uncommon manifestation of poliovirus infection. There is alteration in the level of consciousness and seizures are common.
- **Paralytic poliomyelitis:** This is the most feared complication of poliovirus infection and occurs in less than 1 in 1000 cases. Risk factors for this syndrome include prior tonsillectomy, trauma, immunodeficiency, pregnancy, and others. Following an incubation period of 1-5 weeks, patients typically enter a period of "minor illness" (corresponding to viremia), consisting of a flu-like illness with fever, nausea, malaise, headache, sore throat, and vomiting. This nonspecific illness lasts several days then resolves completely. The "major illness" occurs about 1 week later. Patients develop a meningitic syndrome with fever and neck stiffness, along with severe muscle pain often involving the limbs and back. This is followed by the onset of muscle paralysis and weakness. The extent of muscle involvement is highly variable. In mild cases, an isolated muscle group may develop weakness. In severe cases, there may be complete quadriplegia with flaccid paralysis and loss of reflexes. The most common presentation is weakness of one leg or one arm. An important clue to the diagnosis of polio is asymmetric flaccid paralysis. The deficit is purely motor in nearly all cases. Loss of sensation is not part of paralytic poliomyelitis and should bring to mind other diagnoses such as Guillain-Barré syndrome. Following this initial attack, there may be a period of recovery of strength, but this is variable. This is followed by a long period of stability and many persons are able to function at a nearly normal level.
- **Postpolio syndrome:** This syndrome has received much attention in both the medical and lay press. There are roughly 300,000 persons who survived the last epidemic of poliomyelitis in the 1950s, and it appears that all are at risk for the post-polio syndrome. About 30 years after the initial bout of paralytic polio, some individuals have developed fatigue, muscle weakness, and sometimes pain. Most commonly the same muscle group(s) originally involved years ago are once again involved, but in some cases "new" muscle groups also develop weakness. This phenomenon was initially dismissed as being nonorganic, but recent evidence strongly suggests it is a disorder of the motor unit, with objective evidence of ongoing denervation by

(Continued)

Poliovirus *(Continued)*

electromyogram and muscle biopsy even in asymptomatic patients. Although many persons may potentially develop this syndrome, the degree of muscle weakness is not as severe as the original bout of polio and it tends not to progress.

Diagnosis Polioviruses are readily isolated in tissue culture. The highest yield for the virus is from the pharynx early in the illness. Later, virus remains viable in the stool for up to 1 month. The virus is difficult to isolate from cerebrospinal fluid.

Diagnostic Tests/Procedures

Poliovirus Serology *on page 522*
Viral Culture, Central Nervous System Symptoms *on page 570*
Viral Culture, Stool *on page 573*
Viral Culture, Throat *on page 574*

Drug Therapy Comment

No antiviral agents proven effective. Poliovirus vaccine should be administered to all children per routine immunization schedule.

Selected Readings

Colecraft CM, "An Update on Polio," *Clin Microbiol Newslett*, 1998, 20(8):67-72.

Foege WH, "A World Without Polio," *JAMA*, 1993, 270(15):1859-60.

Melnick JL, "Current Status of Poliovirus Infections," *Clin Microbiol Rev*, 1996, 9(3):293-300.

Modlin JF, "Poliovirus," *Principles and Practice of Infectious Diseases*, 4th ed, Mandell GL, Bennett JE, and Dolin R, eds, New York, NY: Churchill Livingstone, 1995, 1613-20.

Munsat TL, "Poliomyelitis - New Problems With an Old Disease," *N Engl J Med*, 1991, 324(17):1206-7.

Postexposure Prophylaxis for Hepatitis B *see page 1054*
Prevention of Malaria *see page 1057*

Proteus Species

Microbiology *Proteus* species are facultative, gram-negative bacilli which belong to the large family Enterobacteriaceae. These organisms are considered "enteric bacilli" because they commonly inhabit the gastrointestinal tract. The two most clinically important *Proteus* species are *Proteus mirabilis* and *Proteus vulgaris*. Biochemically, nearly all strains of *P. mirabilis* are indole-positive; all other clinically relevant *Proteus* species such as *Proteus vulgaris* are indole-negative. *Proteus* species characteristically "swarm" (spread) over the surface of a moist agar plate. The organisms have several features that promote urinary tract infections including fimbriae which facilitate colonization of the organism in the urinary tract and flagella which facilitate motility in the urinary system. In addition, *Proteus* species have the unique ability to produce urease to hydrolyze urea (found in urine of the human host) to ammonium hydroxide which can lead to renal calculi formation and urinary tract infections.

Epidemiology *Proteus* species are found in soil, water, and fecally contaminated materials. They are found in human feces and are considered part of the normal fecal flora. *Proteus* species are some of the most frequently isolated and clinically significant Enterobacteriaceae. In some studies, *Proteus mirabilis* is the second leading cause of community-acquired urinary tract infections, second only to *E. coli*. Aside from urinary tract infections, *Proteus* species rarely cause serious disease in otherwise healthy individuals. However, they are an important cause of hospital-acquired infections in debilitated patients and account for up to 10% to 15% of nosocomial infections in the United States.

Clinical Syndromes

- **Urinary tract infections:** The ability of *P. mirabilis* to hydrolyze urea to ammonia causes a rise in the urine pH. This alkaline urine leads to precipitation of magnesium, calcium, and ammonium and ultimately forms a type of kidney stone called struvite or triple phosphate stones. These stones act as obstructing foreign bodies and can lead to hydronephrosis, chronic and recurrent *Proteus mirabilis* urinary tract infections, pyelonephritis, and renal abscess. As a rule, it is difficult to treat urinary tract infections in the presence of a renal stone; medical therapy with antibiotics alone is often unsuccessful and patients are at risk for urosepsis if the stone is not removed.

- **Pneumonia:** Like other gram-negative bacilli, *Proteus* species can cause serious nosocomial pneumonia particularly in debilitated, ventilator-dependent individuals.

- **Surgical wound infections:** *Proteus* species can cause serious postoperative wound infections, either alone or as part of a polymicrobial infection, particularly in contaminated abdominal wounds.

- **Chronic destructive ear infections:** These organisms have been recovered in patients with a chronic, destructive otitis media similar to necrotizing otitis caused by *Pseudomonas aeruginosa*. This entity can involve the mastoids and central nervous system.
- **Septicemia:** Debilitated hospitalized patients can develop a life-threatening *Proteus* septicemia, most often from a urinary source. Other common origins include biliary tract sepsis (*Proteus* sp are part of the normal fecal flora), abdominal abscesses, catheter-associated bacteremia, and others.

Diagnosis The diagnosis of *P. mirabilis* infection is made by isolation of the organism from appropriate body fluids (urine, sputum, blood, etc). No special culture isolation methods are necessary; *Proteus* species grow readily in standard blood cultures and on solid media. The finding of chronic urinary tract infection in the setting of struvite stones is highly suggestive of *Proteus mirabilis* infection; particularly if there is a consistently high urinary pH.

Diagnostic Tests/Procedures

Aerobic Culture, Appropriate Site *on page 310*
Gram's Stain *on page 426*

Treatment The treatment of *Proteus* infections depends in part on the species involved. *Proteus mirabilis* (indole-negative *Proteus*) was once generally susceptible to most beta-lactams, cephalosporins, and aminoglycosides, but increasing numbers of community-acquired isolates are becoming resistant to these agents. Final antimicrobial selection should be based on antibiotic susceptibility tests. Indole-positive *Proteus* species (including *Proteus vulgaris*) are more commonly hospital-acquired strains and tend to be more antibiotic-resistant than *P. mirabilis*. Multiple beta-lactam resistant *Proteus* strains are becoming more common, as are aminoglycoside-resistant strains; antimicrobial susceptibility testing is crucial in the proper selection of treatment for hospital-acquired *Proteus* infections.

Drug Therapy

Recommended

Cephalosporins, 3rd Generation *on page 662*
Cephalosporins, 1st Generation *on page 661*
Cephalosporins, 2nd Generation *on page 662*

Alternate

Imipenem and Cilastatin *on page 766*
Penicillins, Extended Spectrum *on page 864*
Meropenem *on page 812*
Fluoroquinolones *on page 736*

Selected Readings

Eisenstein BI, "Diseases Caused by Gram-Negative Enteric Bacilli," *Harrison's Principles of Internal Medicine*, 13th ed, Isselbacher KJ, Braunwald E, Wilson JD, et al, eds, New York, NY: McGraw-Hill Inc, 1994, 664.

Prototheca Species

Microbiology *Prototheca* species are unicellular algae which are becoming increasingly recognized as a cause of opportunistic infection. Presently there are three recognized species: *Prototheca wickerhamii*, *P. zopfii*, and *P. stagnora*. These organisms are fungus-like saprophytes which are spherical and about 3-30 μm in size. *Prototheca* lack chlorophyll and reproduce asexually by endosporulation; the presence of endospores helps identify the organism on wet mounts. The organism grows well on Sabaroud-dextrose agar.

Epidemiology *Prototheca* is ubiquitous in the environment (fresh water, soil, trees, and sewage). Human protothecal infections are unusual, with about 60 cases reported in the literature. These cases are distributed worldwide. Approximately half of the reported cases have been in immunocompromised individuals, such as organ transplant recipients, diabetics, and persons with malignancies. Rare cases have been reported in otherwise healthy hosts.

Clinical Syndromes Because of the low incidence of this infection, generalizations about clinical syndromes is difficult. Case reports have included the following.

- **Skin and soft tissue infection:** This appears to be the most common presentation and may be associated with some form of trauma. Patients develop single, usually painless lesion in the skin or subcutaneous tissue which fails to heal spontaneously. Cases of postoperative soft-tissue infection and cutaneous infections in the absence of surgery or other trauma

(Continued)

Prototheca Species *(Continued)*

have been reported. The skin lesion may be indurated, plaque-like, nodular, ulcerated, or even vesicular.

- **Olecranon bursitis:** Some cases reported after trauma.
- **Infection of continuous ambulatory peritoneal dialysis (CAPD) catheters.**
- **Nasopharyngeal ulceration:** Single case report following prolonged endotracheal intubation
- **Meningitis:** Single case report in a patient with AIDS.
- **Disseminated protothecosis:** Two cases have been reported in immunocompetent persons who presented with abdominal pain.

Diagnosis Laboratory confirmation is necessary to make a diagnosis of protothecosis since the clinical syndromes are nonspecific. The organisms may be seen on wet mounts of infected material and can be identified by its characteristic size, morphology, and endospores. Isolation of the organism on fungal media is confirmatory.

Biopsy specimens of infected soft tissue typically show granulomatous inflammation, necrosis, giant cells and chronic inflammation. Microabscesses may also be present. Numerous organisms are typically seen in tissue specimens and stain well with Gomori methenamine silver.

Diagnostic Tests/Procedures

Fungus Culture, Appropriate Site *on page 414*
Methenamine Silver Stain *on page 487*

Treatment The treatment of human protothecosis is controversial, in part due to the limited number of cases. Serious infections have been treated with amphotericin B. Surgical debridement has been used in many of the reported cases of skin and soft tissue infections; adjunctive amphotericin B has been suggested for deeper soft tissue lesions. Bursectomy has been performed in several patients with olecranon bursitis. All patients who developed CAPD catheter infection with prototheca were treated with catheter removal and antifungal agents. *Prototheca* is resistant to flucytosine, and this agent should be avoided. The role of imidazole antifungal agents is not clear. Some cases have responded to fluconazole and ketoconazole, but available data is limited.

Drug Therapy

Recommended

Amphotericin B (Conventional) *on page 597*

Alternate

Fluconazole *on page 732*
Ketoconazole *on page 791*

Selected Readings

Iacoviello VR, De Girolami PC, Lucarini J, et al, "Protothecosis Complicating Prolonged Endotracheal Intubation: Case Report and Literature Review," *Clin Infect Dis*, 1992, 15(6):959-67.

Kaminski ZC, Kapila R, Sharer LR, et al, "Meningitis Due to *Prototheca wickerhamii* in a Patient With AIDS," *Clin Infect Dis*, 1992, 15(4):704-6.

Providencia Species

Microbiology The *Providencia* species are members of the Enterobacteriaceae family. The genus *Providencia* consists of four species, *Providencia rettgeri*, *Providencia alcalifaciens*, *Providencia stuartii*, and *Providencia rustiganii*. These organisms can be differentiated by biochemical and cultural differences. These organisms are considered "enteric bacilli" because they commonly inhabit the gastrointestinal tract. All *Providencia* species are indole-positive, and *P. rettgeri* and some strains of *P. stuartii* are urease-positive. All members of the tribe have O, H, and K antigens. The most important human pathogen species is *P. stuartii*.

Epidemiology Members of the family Enterobacteriaceae can be found as normal colonizers of human and animal intestinal tracts and are commonly found in soil and on plants. *Providencia* species, as well as others in the tribe, are common sources of nosocomial infections, particularly in the urinary tract. Although other members of the family have higher incidences of nosocomial infections and increased antibacterial resistance, *P. stuartii* in particular remains an important and difficult pathogen in this regard.

Clinical Syndromes

- **Urinary tract infections:** Although typically not a cause of community-acquired urinary tract infections, *P. stuartii* is an important pathogen in nosocomial urinary tract infections. Patients particularly at risk are those with catheters, underlying urologic disorders, paraplegia, or advanced age.

- **Pneumonia:** Like other gram-negative bacilli, *Providencia* species can cause serious nosocomial pneumonia, particularly in debilitated, ventilator dependent individuals. Other Enterobacteriaceae cause nosocomial pneumonia more commonly.

- **Septicemia:** Debilitated hospitalized patients can develop life-threatening *Providencia* septicemia, most commonly from a urinary tract source. Other Enterobacteriaceae cause septicemia more often.

- **Gastrointestinal disease:** *P. alcalifaciens* has been associated with outbreaks of gastroenteritis and may have a possible role in the etiology of infectious diarrhea. *P. stuartii* may also be implicated.

Diagnosis The diagnosis of *Providencia* species infections is made by isolation of the organism from the appropriate body fluid (urine, sputum, blood, etc). No special culture isolation methods are necessary; *Providencia* species grow readily in standard blood cultures and on solid media.

Diagnostic Tests/Procedures

Aerobic Culture, Appropriate Site *on page 310*

Blood Culture, Aerobic and Anaerobic *on page 337*

Gram's Stain *on page 426*

Treatment *Providencia* species are typically sensitive to second and third generation cephalosporins, extended spectrum penicillins, carbapenems, quinolones, and aminoglycosides, although increased resistance to all of these drugs has occurred. Gentamicin susceptibility is often variable. Antimicrobial susceptibility testing is crucial in the proper selection of treatment for hospital-acquired *Providencia* infections, with final selection based on susceptibility tests. Co-trimoxazole is also active, particularly in patients with urinary tract infections.

Drug Therapy

Recommended

Cephalosporins, 2nd Generation *on page 662*

Cephalosporins, 3rd Generation *on page 662*

Co-Trimoxazole *on page 692*

Alternate

Imipenem and Cilastatin *on page 766*

Penicillins, Extended Spectrum *on page 864*

Selected Readings

Cornaglia G, Frugoni S, Mazzariol A, et al, "Activities of Oral Antibiotics on *Providencia* Strains Isolated From Institutionalized Elderly Patients With Urinary Tract Infections," *Antimicrob Agents Chemother*, 1995, 39(12):2819-21.

"Enterobacteriaceae," *Bailey & Scott's Diagnostic Microbiology*, Chapter 27, St Louis, MO: CV Mosby Co, 1990, 363-85.

Hawkey BM, "*Providencia stuartii*: A Review of a Multiple Antibiotic Resistant Bacterium," *J Antimicrob Chemother*, 1984, 13:209-26.

Mandell GL, Bennett JE, and Dolin R, *Principles and Practice of Infectious Diseases*, 4th ed, Chapter 196, New York, NY: Churchill Livingstone, 1995.

"Opportunistic Enterobacteriaceae," *Zinsser Microbiology*, 20th ed, Chapter 36, Joklik WK, Willett HP, Amos DB, et al, eds, Norwalk, CT: Appleton & Lange, 1992, 469-70.

Pseudomonas aeruginosa

Microbiology *Pseudomonas aeruginosa* is a lactose-negative, oxidase-positive, nonfermenting, aerobic, gram-negative bacillus with a single flagellum (usually). Strains that produce polysaccharide capsules (glycocalyx) are mucoid in colony appearance, with some strains producing diffusible blue, yellow, or brown pigments (pyocyanin, fluorescein, pyorubin, respectively). *Pseudomonas aeruginosa* can grow on almost all laboratory media at temperatures from 10°C to 40°C. (Optimal growth is at 35°C.)

Epidemiology *Pseudomonas aeruginosa* is ubiquitous; therefore, isolation of the organism on hospital equipment, sinks, etc, is not unexpected and by itself not meaningful. *Pseudomonas aeruginosa* is often considered an opportunistic pathogen because disease occurs most often in patients with neutropenia or neutrophil dysfunction, tissue damage, or other altered host defenses. Presence of *Pseudomonas aeruginosa* in clinical specimens may be contamination or colonization unless accompanied by a correlating clinical scenario.

In the hospital setting, up to 90% of patients staying in intensive care units for more than 7 days may become colonized with *P. aeruginosa*. In some burn

(Continued)

Pseudomonas aeruginosa (Continued)

centers, up to 30% of infections can be attributed to *P. aeruginosa*. *Pseudomonas aeruginosa* is also responsible for approximately 10% of nosocomial infections.

Clinical Syndromes *Pseudomonas aeruginosa* can infect any tissue or organ system including blood, lung, heart, ear, eye, urinary tract, gastrointestinal tract, or musculoskeletal system. Syndromes caused by *Pseudomonas aeruginosa* are usually indistinguishable from those caused by the Enterobacteriaceae with several exceptions. Patients with bacteremia or pneumonia caused by *Pseudomonas aeruginosa* have a higher mortality rate that when caused by the Enterobacteriaceae. *Pseudomonas aeruginosa* is the second most common organism infecting burn patients. Malignant otitis externa is characteristically caused by *P. aeruginosa*.

Diagnosis The only way a diagnosis of *Pseudomonas aeruginosa* infection can be made is by identification of the organism through culture in a patient with a relevant clinical syndrome. No special media or conditions are necessary to grow this organism.

Diagnostic Tests/Procedures

Aerobic Culture, Appropriate Site *on page 310*
Gram's Stain *on page 426*

Treatment Combination of an antipseudomonal penicillin or ceftazidime plus an aminoglycoside is the standard therapy. Combination therapy is necessary for additive or synergistic affects as well as potentially decreasing the emergence of resistant pseudomonal strains. Combination therapy improves outcome in patients with *Pseudomonas aeruginosa* bacteremia. Quinolones and imipenem are active against *Pseudomonas aeruginosa* and should also be used in combination with aminoglycosides in the treatment of serious infection. Quinolones may be used with an antipseudomonal beta-lactam in the treatment of serious *Pseudomonas aeruginosa* infections; in theory, the different mechanisms of action of the two drug classes should be at least additive. Double beta-lactam therapy should be avoided.

Pediatric Drug Therapy

Recommended

Urinary tract infection:
Ceftazidime *on page 651*
Penicillins, Extended Spectrum *on page 864*

Adult Drug Therapy

Recommended

Severe infection:
Ceftazidime *on page 651*
used in combination with
Aminoglycosides *on page 590*
Penicillins, Extended Spectrum *on page 864*
used in combination with
Aminoglycosides *on page 590*

Alternate

Urinary tract infection:
Ceftazidime *on page 651*
Penicillins, Extended Spectrum *on page 864*
Fluoroquinolones *on page 736*
Severe infection:
Imipenem and Cilastatin *on page 766*
or
Meropenem *on page 812*
used in combination with
Aminoglycosides *on page 590*
Ciprofloxacin *on page 678*
used in combination with
Penicillins, Extended Spectrum *on page 864*

Selected Readings

Bisbe J, Gatell JM, Puig J, et al, "*Pseudomonas aeruginosa* Bacteremia: Univariate and Multivariate Analyses of Factors Influencing the Prognosis in 133 Episodes," *Rev Infect Dis*, 1988, 10(3):629-35.

Griffith SJ, Nathan C, Selander RK, et al, "The Epidemiology of *Pseudomonas aeruginosa* in Oncology Patients in a General Hospital," *J Infect Dis*, 1989, 160(6):1030-6.

Hilf M, Yu VL, Sharp J, et al, "Antibiotic Therapy for *Pseudomonas aeruginosa* Bacteremia: Outcome Correlations in a Prospective Study of 200 Patients," *Am J Med*, 1989, 87(5):540-5.

Mendelson MH, Gurtman A, Szabo S, et al, "*Pseudomonas aeruginosa* Bacteremia in Patients With AIDS," *Clin Infect Dis*, 1994, 18(6):886-95.

Murray PR, Drew WL, Kobayashi GS, et al, eds, "Pseudomonadaceae," *Medical Microbiology*, St Louis, MO: CV Mosby Co, 1990, 119-26.

Pollack M, "*Pseudomonas aeruginosa*," *Principles and Practice of Infectious Diseases*, 4th ed, Mandell GL, Bennett JE, and Dolin R, eds, New York, NY: Churchill Livingstone 1995, 1980-2003.

Widmer AF, Wenzel RP, Trilla A, et al, "Outbreak of *Pseudomonas aeruginosa* Infections in a Surgical Intensive Care Unit: Probable Transmission Via Hands of a Health Care Worker," *Clin Infect Dis*, 1993, 16(3):372-6.

Wilson R and Dowling RB, "Lung Infections. 3. *Pseudomonas aeruginosa* and Other Related Species, *Thorax*, 1998, 53(3):213-9.

Zwadyk P, "*Pseudomonas*," *Zinsser Microbiology*, 20th ed, Joklik WK, Willett HP, Amos DB, et al, eds, Norwalk, CT: Appleton & Lange, 1992, 576-83.

Rabies Virus

Related Information

Animal and Human Bites Guidelines *on page 1061*
Immunization Guidelines *on page 1041*

Microbiology Rabies virus is a bullet-shaped single-stranded RNA virus which belongs to the family Rhabdoviridae. A number of important viral proteins have been identified such as viral polymerase, nucleocapsid protein, glycoprotein, and others. Some of these proteins have been used to develop specific diagnostic monoclonal antibodies. Rabies virus can be isolated under the proper conditions in tissue culture. During active rabies infection, the virus can be cultured from a variety of human (and animal) tissues including saliva, brain tissue, respiratory secretions, and urine; the virus is most easily recovered from brain tissue.

The virus is highly neurotropic. When a human is inoculated with rabies virus, the viral glycoprotein attaches to the plasma membrane of cells, possibly the nicotinic acetylcholine receptor. The virus then replicates in skeletal muscle, and when the titer is high enough, it invades nearby sensory and motor nerves and enters the nervous system. It travels along the axon at speeds up to 20 mm/day and eventually reaches the spinal cord. From there, dissemination through the central nervous system occurs rapidly and encephalitis ensues. Other peripheral nerves become involved; the organism can be recovered from the saliva due to infection of nerves in the salivary glands.

Epidemiology Rabies remains primarily a disease of animals, not humans. In many areas of Asia, Africa, and Latin America, canine rabies is poorly controlled, and dogs account for up to 90% of animal rabies cases. In contrast, in Europe and the United States, dogs account for a much lower percentage of cases. In the United States, different species of animals are involved in well-defined geographic areas. For example, raccoons are important in two regions, the eastern seaboard states (New York, New Jersey, Delaware, Virginia) and some southeastern states (Florida, South Carolina, Georgia, Alabama). Skunks predominate in the north central states and California, gray foxes in Texas and Arizona, and coyotes in southern Texas. A total of 10 distinct geographic areas in the United States have been identified; one terrestrial animal predominates and one antigenic variant of the rabies virus predominates. Bats remain an important reservoir of rabies and cause sporadic cases.

Human rabies is distinctly unusual in the United States although it is still problematic in some areas worldwide. In large part, this is due to the control of canine rabies in this country. Between 1980 and 1993, there were 18 reported cases of rabies in the United States with 10 of these acquired outside the country. Of the rabies cases reported since 1960, the great majority involved males younger than 16 years of age or older than 50 years of age. Most cases in the United States are now reported from the following groups:

- U.S. travelers to foreign countries who sustain a dog bite in a rabies-endemic region
- persons bitten by wild animals in the U.S.
- persons with unknown exposure history

A few cases of "nonbite rabies" have been reported. These include:

- laboratory exposure to rabies virus (aerosolized virus)
- rabies contracted from corneal transplant from an infected donor (4 cases)

(Continued)

Rabies Virus *(Continued)*

- inhalation of aerosolized virus in caves with high concentrations of bat secretions (rare)
- contact of virus on mucous membranes, scratches, or eyes (rare)

Clinical Syndromes

- **Clinical rabies:** There is a variable period of incubation before the onset of symptoms (4 days to 19 years), but most cases occur within 1 year of exposure. The initial prodrome of rabies is nonspecific with malaise, fatigue, and fever. In many patients, there may be pain at the initial exposure site. After about 10 days, the patient enters an acute neurologic phase, characterized by bizarre behavior, hyperactivity, and confusion. A small stimulus can elicit short periods of thrashing, biting, and other behaviors. Many patients will display hydrophobia (fear of water); there is often severe laryngospasm and choking when trying to drink water. This will progress to paralysis, which dominates the clinical picture for some days. Patients typically lapse into coma and develop respiratory failure or arrhythmias, leading to death in most cases despite full support in intensive care units. Occasional cases of recovery from rabies have been reported.

Diagnosis Currently, there are no tests available to detect rabies prior to the development of symptoms. The virus is felt to be immunologically "protected" in the muscle cells or nerve cells near the inoculation site, and antibody production occurs late in infection. Rabies encephalitis may be difficult to distinguish from other forms of viral encephalitis. Laboratory tests available include:

- rabies neutralizing antibody
- rabies viral culture of saliva, cerebrospinal fluid, urine, respiratory secretions
- brain biopsy - specimens may be submitted for rabies viral culture; immunofluorescent rabies antibody staining of brain cells; and pathologic examination for Negri bodies, which are cytoplasmic inclusions characteristic of rabies encephalitis seen in 20% to 30% of cases.

Diagnostic Tests/Procedures

Brain Biopsy *on page 352*
Rabies Detection *on page 525*

Treatment There is currently no treatment for rabies once it has become clinically established. Mortality approaches 100%. Thus, the main treatment issues involve rabies prevention, particularly postexposure prophylaxis. The physician deciding whether or not to initiate rabies treatment (rabies vaccine, rabies immunoglobulin) must answer the following questions: Has a significant exposure occurred, and what is the risk that an animal is rabid?

A significant exposure includes the following.

- An animal bite, defined as penetration of the person's skin by teeth with contamination of the wound with saliva
- Contamination of the mucous membranes with saliva or other potentially infectious tissue from an infected animal
- Certain nonbite exposures, including contamination of scratches, scrapes, wounds, or mucous membranes with saliva or other infectious tissues. The risk of rabies after nonbite exposures is extremely rare, although scattered cases have been reported.

Petting a rabid animal or contacting its blood or body fluids is not an exposure. If it appears that a significant exposure has taken place, the physician must determine whether or not the animal was rabid. As outlined by Fishbein and Robinson, this depends on the percentage of animals found to be rabid in the species in the particular geographical area.

Group 1: Rabies is endemic in animal species involved in exposure. This includes:

- bats - anywhere in the United States (3% to 20% positive for rabies)
- terrestrial animals - skunks, raccoons, foxes in areas of United States where rabies is endemic
- dogs in developing countries
- dogs in the United States along the Mexican border.

    For Group 1 exposure, treatment should be initiated for both bite and nonbite exposures.

Group 2: Rabies is not endemic in species involved but is endemic in other wild animals in the area. The risk of rabies is about 10 times lower in these animals compared with the predominant species. These animals include:

- wild carnivores such as wolves, bobcats, bears, and groundhogs. Up to 20% may have rabies. Bite exposures from these should be treated. Nonbite exposures should either be treated or the local health department consulted.
- rodents (squirrels, hamsters, guinea pigs, gerbils, rats, mice) have a low incidence of rabies, 0.01%. Bite exposures should not be treated (or in exceptional cases, the local health department could be consulted). Nonbite exposures should not be treated.
- dogs and cats - in the United States, the risk of rabies in dogs is <1% (except along the Mexican border) in areas where rabies is common in other land animals. In addition, dogs almost always show signs of clinical rabies shortly after the virus is present in saliva. Bite exposure should not be treated if a healthy dog (or cat) is captured; the animal should be observed for 10 days. If the animal develops signs of rabies, treatment in the human should be commenced immediately. If the animal is a stray, it should be sacrificed immediately and the head removed and shipped to an appropriate laboratory. Treatment is delayed pending laboratory testing. The same approach is recommended for nonbite exposures.

Group 3: Rabies is not endemic in the animal species involved in the exposure and is uncommon in other wild animals in the region. This incudes most domestic cats and dogs and wild land animals in Idaho, Washington, Utah, Nevada, and Colorado, where the proportion of rabid animals is very low. For bite or nonbite exposures from Group 3 animals, either consult the local health department or do not treat.

Postexposure treatment consists of:

1. Vigorous wound cleaning - this has been shown to decrease the risk of rabies.
2. Administration or rabies vaccine, either human diploid-cell rabies vaccine or rabies vaccine adsorbed. For persons not previously vaccinated, rabies vaccine should be given 1 mL I.M. on days 0, 3, 7, 14, and 28. Abbreviated regimens have been described. For persons previously vaccinated, the rabies vaccine should be given 1 mL I.M. on days 0 and 3.
3. Administration of rabies immunoglobulin. For persons not previously vaccinated, this should be given at 20 IU/kg of body weight. If possible, one-half the dose should be injected locally near the original wound and the rest given I.M. (using a new needle). For persons previously vaccinated, rabies immunoglobulin is not recommended.

Drug Therapy
Recommended
Rabies Virus Vaccine *on page 893*
Rabies Immune Globulin (Human) *on page 892*

Selected Readings
Fishbein DB and Bernard KW, "Rabies Virus," *Principles and Practice of Infectious Diseases*, 4th ed, Mandell GL, Bennett JE, and Dolin R, eds, New York, NY: Churchill Livingstone, 1995, 1527-43.

Fishbein DB and Robinson LE, "Rabies," *N Engl J Med*, 1993, 329(22):1632-8.

Smith JS, "New Aspects of Rabies With Emphasis on Epidemiology, Diagnosis, and Prevention of the Disease in the United States," *Clin Microbiol Rev*, 1996, 9(2):166-76.

Smith JS, "Rabies," *Clin Microbiol Newslett*, 1999, 21(3):17-23.

Recommendations for Measles Vaccination *see page 1044*
Recommended Poliovirus Vaccination Schedule *see page 1044*

Respiratory Syncytial Virus
Synonyms RSV

Microbiology Respiratory syncytial virus (RSV) is the most common cause of bronchiolitis and pneumonia in infants and children. It is also emerging as a pathogen of the elderly and the immunosuppressed.

RSV is a single-stranded, enveloped RNA virus belonging to the family Paramyxoviridae, and comprises its own genus, *Pneumovirus*. The viral genome codes for at least 10 separate genes. The virus lacks neuraminidase or hemagglutinating activity, which differentiates it from other paramyxoviruses, such as parainfluenza and mumps virus. There are two major subgroups of RSV, group A or B, based on the presence of different surface glycoprotein antigens. The (Continued)

Respiratory Syncytial Virus *(Continued)*

clinical significance of this strain variation is still unknown. RSV is rarely isolated from asymptomatic children and is thus not part of the normal flora.

As with other pathogenic viruses, RSV requires a tissue culture system in the laboratory to support its growth. Clinical specimens can be successfully inoculated onto a variety of cell lines. Of note, live virus from patient secretions can survive for a period of time on environmental surfaces. On a nonporous surface such as a countertop, the virus is still viable up to 7 hours. On a porous surface such as tissue paper or clothing, survival is decreased to about 1 hour.

Epidemiology Infections with RSV are common worldwide, regardless of climate. There is a definite seasonal occurrence to RSV infections, tending to occur almost exclusively in the winter and spring in temperate climates; in temperate climates there is a sharp peak in colder months. In many communities, RSV outbreaks occur every year without fail and often in a very predictable pattern, and at its peak in a season, RSV dominates influenza and other respiratory viruses. Based on studies to determine the prevalence of specific RSV antibody, it appears that nearly all children have been infected with RSV before entering school. Estimates of the attack rates vary according to age. In children younger than 2 years of age, the attack rate for lower respiratory infections was from 9-23 out of 1000, from 2-3 years old it was 7-15 out of 1000, and in the 4-5 year age group, it was 5-8 out of 1000. However, the attack rate for all forms of infection including mild infections is probably much higher based on prospective studies, with some studies estimating 6 per 100. The attack rate is extremely high in day care centers, approaching 100%.

Recurrent infections with RSV are the rule. With each episode of clinical illness, progressively milder forms of infection are seen. Specific neutralizing antibodies develop (IgG, IgM, and secretory IgA) but are not protective. The reason for this is unclear and is not explained by differences in RSV serotypes.

Transmission can be by several routes: self-inoculation of the eyes or nares following contact with contaminated secretions; self-inoculation following contact with contaminated fomites; aerosol spread, when infected individuals are coughing or sneezing (large droplet spread only).

Clinical Syndromes

In children, the major manifestations of RSV include:

- **Upper respiratory infection:** This often mimics the common cold, along with significant fever and profuse rhinorrhea. Typically, lower respiratory infections are preceded by several days of upper tract symptoms.
- **Bronchiolitis:** This is one of the most common manifestations of RSV and is particularly prevalent in infants 2-6 months of age. It is characterized by wheezing, cough, and tachypnea (sometimes 80 breaths per minute) reflecting the hallmark inspiratory and expiratory obstruction of the lower respiratory tract in bronchiolitis. Fever of 38°C to 40°C is common. Chest radiographs may reveal infiltrates, but these are felt to be due to atelectasis and not alveolar consolidation. Most recover spontaneously or with supportive care only, although 1% to 2% may require hospitalization. Bronchiolitis is difficult to separate from pneumonia, and some may have both.
- **Pneumonia:** The presentation of RSV pneumonia is similar to bronchiolitis. Lower respiratory infection in young children is estimated to complicate up to 70% of RSV infections. Chest radiograph abnormalities vary from interstitial infiltrates to consolidation (usually upper and/or middle lobes). Hyperinflation is common. The radiographic findings, however, are not distinctive enough to differentiate RSV pneumonia from other infectious causes of pneumonia, including bacterial pathogens. Fatalities are still uncommon with the notable exception of children with underlying congenital heart disease, pulmonary disease, or compromised immune system.
- **Croup:** RSV is an uncommon cause of croup, accounting for about 5% to 10% of croup cases .
- **Otitis media:** This is quite common in infants. Otitis media may be either primary infection (with symptoms localized to the ear only) or may be secondary to RSV infection elsewhere (usually in the lower respiratory tract).
- **Apnea and the sudden infant death syndrome (SIDS):** Infants with lower respiratory tract infections with RSV have frequent apneic episodes but are self-resolving. Although the cause of SIDS is still unknown, RSV and other

respiratory viruses have been implicated due to the frequent recovery of these pathogens from the lungs of infants with SIDS.

Infections in adults:

- **Upper respiratory tract infections:** In adults, RSV commonly causes an upper respiratory infection somewhat more severe than the common cold. Nasal congestion and cough are prominent, and symptoms may be prolonged, lasting over 1 week. Otalgia is less common in adults. Episodes are self-resolving, but the severity of the URI may cause some to be bedridden for several days.
- **Lower respiratory tract infection:** Tracheobronchitis and pneumonia are relatively uncommon in the otherwise healthy adult. In the elderly patient or the individual with chronic bronchitis, pneumonia can be quite fulminant and clinically mimics the disease as seen in infants. Outbreaks of RSV in the elderly are associated with a high incidence of pneumonia, perhaps up to 50%.
- **Nosocomial infection:** RSV is an important cause of nosocomial viral respiratory infections, both in adults and children. This is particularly problematic in pediatric wards where children are hospitalized during an outbreak of RSV; the virus spreads efficiently to the adult staff with nearly 50% infected.

Diagnosis RSV infection is suspected when there is a compatible clinical presentation, particularly in the setting of a known community outbreak. In the infant and young child, the diagnosis is often made clinically during an outbreak, with microbiologic confirmation reserved for serious or atypical cases. In the adult, RSV infection mimics other viral and bacterial causes of respiratory illness. Routine laboratory studies such as the complete blood count and electrolyte panel are not helpful in making the diagnosis. Microbiological confirmation of RSV is generally unnecessary for mild upper respiratory infections but may be useful in suspected lower respiratory infections or infections in the immunocompromised host. Potentially this may avoid unnecessary antibiotics or invasive diagnostic testing.

There are several laboratory methods available:

1. Viral culture: RSV grows best in continuous cell lines of human origin, such as HEp-2 cells. The virus causes a characteristic cytopathic effect in the cell lines, syncytial formation, from which its name is derived. Culture results may not be available for several days.
2. Direct fluorescent antibody (DFA) detection: This rapid method can detect the presence of RSV in specimens within hours but requires a specimen with cellular material.
3. Enzyme immunoassays (EIA): Another rapid test with results available on the same day.
4. Serologic studies: A fourfold rise in titer of specific antibody to RSV is diagnostic but not useful for immediate diagnosis or treatment.

Diagnostic Tests/Procedures

Respiratory Syncytial Virus Antigen by EIA *on page 527*
Respiratory Syncytial Virus Culture *on page 528*
Respiratory Syncytial Virus Serology *on page 528*

Treatment Treatment is generally supportive, with supplemental oxygen and fluid replacement as needed. Most mild to moderate cases are self-resolving. Severe cases in infants have been treated with the antiviral agent ribavirin, administered as an aerosol. Ribavirin has been shown to improve arterial blood gas values in hypoxic infants, but improvement in mortality or duration of hospitalization has not been demonstrated.

Drug Therapy

Recommended

Ribavirin *on page 899*

Selected Readings

Englund JA, Sullivan CJ, Jordan MC, et al, "Respiratory Syncytial Virus Infection in Immunocompromised Adults," *Ann Intern Med*, 1988, 109(3):203-8.

Smith DW, Frankel LR, Mathers LH, et al, "A Controlled Trial of Aerosolized Ribavirin in Infants Receiving Mechanical Ventilation for Severe Respiratory Syncytial Virus Infection," *N Engl J Med*, 1991, 325(1):24-9.

Rhodococcus equi *see Rhodococcus Species on next page*

Rhodococcus Species

Applies to *Corynebacterium equi; Rhodococcus equi*

Microbiology *Rhodococcus* species are gram-positive, aerobic organisms that may appear as cocci or pleomorphic short or long rods with branching. They are partially acid-fast due to the presence of mycolic acid in their cell walls. There are 16 species of *Rhodococcus* with four species known to be pathogenic in humans. *Rhodococcus equi* is the most common human pathogen and is most typically seen in immunocompromised hosts, particularly in patients with AIDS, lymphoreticular malignancies, and renal transplants. *Rhodococcus* species are members of the informal phylogenetic group actinomycetes.

Although *Rhodococcus* species grows well on routine nonselective media at 35°C, it may be difficult to isolate and identify. They may be misidentified as colonizing diphtheroids, especially in respiratory specimens. It may also be misdiagnosed as a mycobacterial infection given its clinical presentation of cavitary lung lesions with granuloma formation and positive acid-fast stains. They appear on agar as small as 1-3 mm, round, raised, buff to salmon colored colonies. The red-orange pigment that is produced seems to correlate with its ability to produce plasmid-mediated beta-lactamase. *R. equi* is catalase-positive, nonspore-forming, and nonmotile. The various species are differentiated by colonial morphology, biochemical analysis, and DNA analysis.

Epidemiology *Rhodococcus* species are ubiquitous in the environment. *R. equi* can be found widespread in domestic animals and their environment. *R. equi* causes suppurative bronchopneumonia, lymphadenitis, and enteritis in foals less than 6 months of age. The role of animals or soil in transmission is unclear, however, 30% to 50% of infected patients report an exposure to farm animals. It is believed that the primary lesion develops in the lung following inhalation of the soilborne organisms and disseminated hematogenously. Cutaneous inoculation from trauma is the most common mode of transmission in skin, soft tissue, and bone infections.

Clinical Syndromes

- **Pulmonary:** Onset of illness is insidious and the disease progresses slowly. Patients initially present with fever and cough. Chest pain, dyspnea, and weight loss occur over time. Pleural effusions and consolidation may occur but cavitary pneumonia is the most common presentation. Unilobar involvement of one of the lower lobes is most commonly seen on chest radiograph. Associated with cavitary lung lesions in HIV-infected individuals. Pneumonia may be chronic or relapsing. Bacteremia is present in approximately 33%. Mortality is approximately 25%.
- **Skin and soft tissue:** Approximately 50% occurs in immunocompetent hosts. May present as cellulitis, wound infection, subcutaneous nodules, or abscess.
- **CNS:** Has been identified as cause of lymphocytic meningitis in normal host. Meningitis and brain abscess are uncommon manifestations.
- **Endophthalmitis:** Associated with penetrating ocular injuries.
- **Other:** Has been implicated as cause of lymphadenitis, osteomyelitis, paraspinal abscess, pericarditis, peritonitis, pelvic abscesses, and enteritis.

Diagnosis Recovery of organism from sputum may be difficult because the morphology of the organism is similar to that of diphtheroids. Respiratory specimens collected via bronchoscopy, percutaneous drainage, or biopsy may be necessary. Morphological stains including acid-fast are helpful, but isolation and identification of organism is mandatory. Histopathology reveals inflammatory reaction with formation of granulomas which may be caseating. Organisms may be seen intracellular in macrophages. Infected histiocytes are strongly PAS-positive with coarsely granular cytoplasmic inclusions similar to those found in Whipple's disease.

Diagnostic Tests/Procedures

Acid-Fast Stain *on page 305*
Aerobic Culture, Appropriate Site *on page 310*
   (Notify laboratory to look for *Rhodococcus*)
Histopathology *on page 448*
Periodic Acid-Schiff Stain *on page 518*

Treatment The best medical management for *Rhodococcus* species is unknown. Relapses are common; therefore, a prolonged course of antibiotics is recommended. Two to 6 weeks of parenteral antibiotics followed by 4-6 weeks of oral antibiotics that achieve high intracellular concentrations are recommended.

Penicillins, ampicillin, and first-generation cephalosporins are not recommended due to frequently reported resistance that emerges during therapy with these agents. Erythromycin, co-trimoxazole, clarithromycin, and azithromycin all achieve high intracellular concentrations. Clindamycin and chloramphenicol may also be effective. Erythromycin is known to be synergistic with rifampin and are the drugs of choice in veterinary medicine Although vancomycin has poor intracellular penetration, it is very active against *R. equi in vitro*. Imipenem appears to be very effective as well.

Drug Therapy Comment Erythromycin (I.V.) and rifampin (I.V. or oral) can be used initially; rifampin (oral) absorption is excellent in patients with functional GI tract.

Drug Therapy

Recommended

Erythromycin *on page 722*

plus

Rifampin *on page 902*

Alternate

Vancomycin *on page 967*

Imipenem and Cilastatin *on page 766*

Selected Readings

Capdevila JA, Bujan S, Gavaldà J, et al, "*Rhodococcus equi* Pneumonia in Patients Infected With the Human Immunodeficiency Virus. Report of 2 Cases and Review of the Literature," *Scand J Infect Dis*, 1997, 29(6):535-41.

De Marais PL and Kocka FE, "*Rhodococcus* Meningitis in an Immunocompetent Host," *Clin Infect Dis*, 1995, 20(1):167-9.

Frame BC and Petkus AF, "*Rhodococcus equi* Pneumonia: Case Report and Literature Review," *Ann Pharmacother*, 1993, 27(11):1340-2.

Scott MA, Graham BS, Verrall R, et al, "*Rhodococcus equi* - An Increasingly Recognized Opportunistic Pathogen," *Am J Clin Pathol*, 1995, 103(5):649-55.

Rickettsia rickettsii

Microbiology *Rickettsia rickettsii* is the etiologic agent of Rocky Mountain spotted fever (RMSF). The organism is a small coccobacillus measuring 0.2-0.5 μm by 0.3-2.0 μm. It is an obligate intracellular bacteria. The organism can be identified in smears of infected tissue using the Gimenez method, by acridine orange, or by immunofluorescence in tissue sections. The organism does not stain well by Gram's stain. The spotted fever group includes other rickettsial species that are human pathogens, specifically *R. sibirica*, the etiologic agent of North Asian tick typhus, *R. conorii*, the etiologic agent of boutonneuse fever, *R. akari*, the etiologic agent of rickettsialpox, and *R. australis*, the etiologic agent of Queensland tick typhus. The cell walls of these organisms contain lipopolysaccharide and ultrastructurally resemble those of gram-negative rods. They cannot be grown in a cell-free medium but can be isolated in cell culture.

Epidemiology Rocky Mountain spotted fever is transmitted by a tick bite. The tick serves as both vector and main reservoir for the disease. *Dermacentor andersoni* (Rocky Mountain wood tick) and *D. variabilis* (American dog tick) are the main vectors in the United States. The tick transmits *Rickettsia* to humans during feeding. The initial bite may not be symptomatic and is frequently not recommended. Infection may occur as the organisms are released from the ticks salivary gland after 4-6 hours of feeding or when the tick is crushed in an attempt to remove it from the skin. The disease is seen primarily in late spring and summer. In the southeast, most cases are observed in children; while in the western states, adults who work in forestry and related industry have the highest incidence of infection. Incidence is related to tick exposure. There have been few western cases in recent years.

Clinical Syndromes The symptoms of Rocky Mountain spotted fever (RMSF) appear 2-14 days after exposure. There is sudden onset of moderate to high fever, myalgia, severe headache, chills, and conjunctival injection. Abdominal symptoms which may include nausea, pain, vomiting, diarrhea, and tenderness are sometimes present. Young patients may not complain of pain. The hallmark rash is maculopapular, appearing on the extremities by the third day and involving the palms and soles of the feet thereafter. Frequently the rash is generalized. Ultimately more than 90% of patients develop a rash. Late onset or "spotless" fever may delay diagnosis. RMSF without a rash occurs more frequently in blacks and adult patients. The cases are more frequently fatal in blacks than whites, in males, and in adults. Age, glucose-6-phosphate dehydrogenase deficiency, and alcoholism are predispositions to fatal outcome. The (Continued)

Rickettsia rickettsii (Continued)

organisms target the vascular endothelium. The damaged endothelial cells increase vascular permeability with resultant edema, hypovolemia, hypoalbuminemia, and hypotension. The local vascular injuries consume platelets with resultant thrombocytopenia, although clinical DIC is rare. Lung, kidney, CNS, GI tract, pancreas, and skeletal muscle may be symptomatically involved. The case fatality rate is 15% to 20% if specific therapy is not instituted. Overall reported mortality has been about 4% in recent years.

Diagnosis Diagnosis is based on clinical signs and symptoms. Cutaneous biopsy direct immunofluorescence to identify *R. rickettsii* in tissue is available in some institutions. Specific serologic tests confirm the diagnosis. The Weil-Felix test which relies upon cross reaction with the *Proteus* OX-19 and OX-2 antigens is nonspecific and not reliable. Culture is usually not attempted because of technical demands and the extreme infection risk to laboratory workers.

Diagnostic Tests/Procedures

Polymerase Chain Reaction *on page 523*
Rocky Mountain Spotted Fever Serology *on page 529*
Skin Biopsy, Immunofluorescence *on page 538*

Duration of Therapy 7 days or at least 2 days after the patient becomes afebrile

Treatment Patients with severe systemic symptoms should receive supportive therapy. Pulmonary edema caused by extravasation of fluid into the alveolar spaces requires careful management as does overall fluid volume. Doxycycline and tetracycline are considered the drugs of choice. Chloramphenicol is used in pregnant women to avoid the effects of tetracycline on fetal teeth and bones. Chloramphenicol is also favored for children younger than 7 years of age.

The use of erythromycin, β-lactams, aminoglycosides, and co-trimoxazole is not indicated.

Pediatric Drug Therapy
Recommended
    <7 years:
        Chloramphenicol *on page 667*
    >7 years:
        Doxycycline *on page 713*
        Tetracycline *on page 944*
Alternate
    >7 years:
        Chloramphenicol *on page 667*

Adult Drug Therapy
Recommended
    Doxycycline *on page 713*
    Tetracycline *on page 944*
Alternate
    Chloramphenicol *on page 667*
    Ciprofloxacin *on page 678*

Selected Readings

Dumler JS, "Laboratory Diagnosis of Human Rickettsial and Ehrlichial Infections," *Clin Microbiol Newslet*, 1996, 18(8):57-61.

Salgo MP, Telzak EE, Currie B, et al, "A Focus of Rocky Mountain Spotted Fever Within New York City," *N Engl J Med*, 1988, 318(21):1345-8.

Woodward TE, "Rickettsial Diseases," *Harrison's Principles and Practice of Internal Medicine*, 13th ed, Isselbacher KJ, Braunwald E, Wilson JD, et al, eds, New York, NY: McGraw-Hill, 1994, 747-57.

***Rochalimaea* Species** *see Bartonella* Species *on page 76*

Rotavirus

Microbiology Rotavirus is a double-stranded, nonenveloped RNA virus with two icosahedral capsids which make the virus appear as a wheel (Latin: rota) when viewed with an electron microscope. Rotavirus can be cultured but only in special cell cultures and only by special procedures. Therefore, routine culture of rotavirus is not practical. The traditional rotavirus ("typical" rotavirus) occurs worldwide, usually produces disease in young children, has a common group inner capsid antigen (VP6), and is called group A rotavirus. Nongroup A rotaviruses (groups G through F; "atypical" rotavirus) are newly described. Group B rotavirus is clinically important only in China; group C rotavirus in swine.

Epidemiology Rotaviruses are ubiquitous and are found in all parts of the world. Rotaviruses occur year round in tropical climates and mostly in the winter months in temperate climates. Rotaviruses infect humans and most animals. The most common age group affected by rotaviruses is 6 months to 2 years. Most rotaviruses which are clinically important are members of group A. Rotaviruses are spread primarily via the fecal-oral route. The incubation period for rotaviruses is less than 2 days in infants and 2-4 days in adults. Maximum shedding of rotaviruses occurs 2-5 days after the onset of diarrhea. Infant mortality due to rotavirus infection in developing countries is extremely high; in developed countries, mortality is rare. Rotavirus usually does not cause chronic disease.

Clinical Syndromes Rotavirus can cause asymptomatic to fatal disease. The most common form of rotavirus infection is sudden onset of vomiting and diarrhea. Common clinical presentations include vomiting, abdominal pain, diarrhea, and dehydration. Fever is present in ca. 50% of the cases. Rotavirus disease usually lasts 3-9 days, and hospitalization often is required. Nosocomial infections and epidemics are not uncommon.

Diagnosis Rotavirus should be in the differential diagnosis of any newborn or young child with the aforementioned clinical presentations or other form of gastroenteritis. Visualization of rotavirus by electron microscopy is considered by many experts to be the standard method of laboratory diagnosis, but the method is expensive and not widely available. Enzyme immunoassay (EIA) and latex agglutination (LA) are much more widely available and used. Detection of rotavirus antigen by EIA is by far the most practical and cost-efficient method. EIA probably is at least as sensitive as electron microscopy and is a highly recommended method.

Diagnostic Tests/Procedures

Electron Microscopic (EM) Examination for Viruses, Stool *on page 403*
Rotavirus, Direct Detection *on page 529*

Drug Therapy Comment

No antiviral agents proven effective.

Selected Readings

Christensen ML, "Human Viral Gastroenteritis," *Clin Microbiol Rev*, 1989, 2(1):51-89.
Gray LG, "Novel Viruses Associated with Gastroenteritis," *Clin Microbiol Newslett*, 1991, 13:137-40.
Offit PA and Clark HF, "Rotavirus," *Principles and Practice of Infectious Diseases*, 4th ed, Mandell GL, Bennett JE, and Dolin R, eds, New York, NY: Churchill Livingstone, 1995, 1448-55.

RSV *see* Respiratory Syncytial Virus *on page 239*

Rubeola Virus *see* Measles Virus *on page 193*

Salmonella Species

Related Information

Timing of Food Poisoning *on page 1069*

Microbiology *Salmonella* species are gram-negative bacilli which are important causes of bacterial gastroenteritis, septicemia, and a nonspecific febrile illness called typhoid fever. Unfortunately, the classification system for the different *Salmonella* species is complex and confusing to most clinicians. Over 2000 separate serotypes have been identified, and, in the past and currently, each is named as if it was a species. Most experts agree that there are seven distinct subgroups of *Salmonella* (1, 2, 3a, 3b, 4, 5, and 6) each of which contain many serotypes ("species"). The main pathogens in humans are serotypes, *S. choleraesuis*, *S. typhi*, and *S. paratyphi* (all in subgroup 1).

Salmonella is an aerobic gram-negative bacillus in the family Enterobacteriaceae. It is almost always associated with disease when isolated from humans and is not considered part of the normal human flora. As with other members of this family, *Salmonella* carries the endotoxin lipopolysaccharide on its outer membrane, which is released upon cell lysis.

Epidemiology It is estimated that about 3 million new cases of salmonellosis occur each year. *Salmonella* species are found worldwide. Many are easily recovered from animals such as chickens, birds, livestock, rodents, and reptiles (turtles). Some serotypes cause disease almost exclusively in man (*S. typhi*) while others are primarily seen in animals but can cause severe disease when infecting humans (*S. choleraesuis*). Transmission is via ingestion of contaminated materials, particularly raw fruits and vegetables, oysters and other shellfish, and contaminated water. Eggs, poultry, and other dairy products are important sources. Outbreaks have been described in the summer months
(Continued)

Salmonella Species *(Continued)*

where children consume contaminated egg salad. Other outbreaks have been associated with pet turtles, other pets, marijuana, and, rarely, food handlers. The incubation period is about 1-3 weeks. The period of communicability lasts until all *Salmonella* have been eradicated from the stool or urine.

Clinical infection is favored when there is a high inoculum of bacteria in the ingested food, since experimental models suggest that 10^6 bacteria are needed for clinical disease. Contaminated food improperly refrigerated will allow such multiplication. Host factors are important and disease is more likely in immuno-compromised individuals, sickle cell disease, or achlorhydria (gastric acid decreases the viable bacterial inoculum). Although salmonellosis can occur at any age, children are most commonly infected.

Clinical Syndromes The following are the major syndromes associated with salmonellosis. It should be emphasized that these syndromes are often overlapping.

- **Gastroenteritis:** The most common manifestation of *Salmonella* infection. After ingestion of contaminated food, the bacteria are absorbed in the terminal portion of the small intestine. The organisms then penetrate into the lamina propria of the ileocecal area. Following this, there is reticuloendothelial hypertrophy with usually a brisk host immune response. As the organisms multiply in the lymphoid follicles, polymorphonuclear leukocytes attempt to limit the infection. There is release of prostaglandins and other mediators, which stimulates cyclic AMP. This results in intestinal fluid secretion which is nonbloody. Clinically, the patient complains of nausea, vomiting, and diarrhea from several hours to several days after consumption of contaminated food. Other symptoms include fever, malaise, muscle aches, and abdominal pain. Symptoms usually resolve from several days to 1 week, even without antibiotics.

- **Sepsis syndrome:** Patients may present in flora sepsis, indistinguishable from other forms of gram-negative sepsis. Fever, confusion, hypotension, end-organ damage, and poor perfusion may all be seen. *Salmonella* bacteremia may lead to multiple metastatic foci, such as liver abscess, osteomyelitis (particularly with sickle cell disease), septic arthritis, and endocarditis. Mycotic aneurysms may develop following bacteremia, and *Salmonella* is a leading cause of infected aortic aneurysms. Bacteremia is also common in AIDS and repeated relapses with *Salmonella* are common, despite prolonged antibiotics.

- **Typhoid fever:** Also known as enteric fever, this febrile illness is caused classically by *S. typhi.* Following ingestion of the bacteria, the organisms pass into the ileocecal area where intraluminal multiplication occurs. There is a mononuclear host cell response, but the organisms remain viable within the macrophages. The bacteria are carried to the organs of the reticuloendothelial system (spleen, liver, bone marrow) by the macrophages and clinical signs of infection become apparent. Patients complain of insidious onset of fever, myalgias, headache, malaise, and constipation, corresponding to this phase of bacteremia. A pulse-temperature dissociation may be present. A characteristic rash may be seen in about 50% of patients, called "rose spots", which are 2-4 mm pink maculopapular lesions that blanch with pressure, usually on the trunk. Symptoms last for 1 or more weeks. During this time, bacteria multiply in the mesenteric lymphoid tissue, and these areas eventually exhibit necrosis and bleeding. There are microperforations of the abdominal wall. *Salmonella* spreads from the liver through the gallbladder and eventually back into the intestines. This phase of intestinal reinfection is characterized by prominent gastrointestinal symptoms including diarrhea. Overall, fatality with treatment is <2%. A similar, but milder syndrome, can occur with *S. paratyphi,* called paratyphoid fever.

- **Chronic carrier state:** Following infection with *S. typhi,* up to 5% of patients will excrete the bacteria for over 1 year. Such patients are termed chronic carriers and are asymptomatic. Millions of viable bacteria are present in the biliary tree and are shed into the bile and into the feces. Urinary carriage can also occur, particularly in patients who are co-infected with *Schistosoma haematobium.* The chronic carrier state is less important for other *Salmonella* species, where the carriage rate is <1%.

Diagnosis Laboratory confirmation is generally required, since the major syndromes are seldom distinctive enough to be diagnosed solely on clinical criteria. *Salmonella* grows readily on most media under standard aerobic conditions. Cultures from blood, joint aspirations, and cerebrospinal fluid can be plated on routine media. Specimens which are likely to contain other organisms, such as stool or sputum, require selective media, and the laboratory should be appropriately notified. Recovery of *Salmonella* from the stool is the most common means of establishing the diagnosis, and enrichment media are available to maximize the yield. Other laboratory findings may suggest salmonellosis, including a profound leukopenia often seen with typhoid fever.

Recent antimicrobial therapy may render blood and stool cultures negative. In such cases, proctoscopy with biopsy and culture of ulcerations may establish the diagnosis in the enterocolitis syndrome. Serologic tests are not particularly useful in this instance. When typhoid fever is suspected but the patient has already received antimicrobial agents, bone marrow biopsies, as well as skin biopsies of any rose spots, may yield *Salmonella typhi* in culture. Serologic studies are more helpful in diagnosing typhoid fever, but >50% of patients will fail to show the expected rise in agglutinins against the typhoid O antigen.

Diagnostic Tests/Procedures
Blood Culture, Aerobic and Anaerobic *on page 337*
Bone Marrow Culture, Routine *on page 347*
Stool Culture *on page 540*

Treatment Note: *Salmonella* species resistant to multiple antimicrobials are increasing in frequency. *In vitro* susceptibility studies should be performed, particularly in severe cases. Treatment guidelines vary with the type of syndrome, as follows:

Enterocolitis: The majority of cases are self-resolving and do not need antibiotics. Clinical trials have demonstrated that a variety of antibiotics fail to influence the course of mild infections and may prolong excretion of the organisms. For severe cases, or in the immunosuppressed host, a number of antibiotics are usually effective, including ampicillin, chloramphenicol, co-trimoxazole, and third generation cephalosporins.

Typhoid fever: Cases should be treated promptly. Chloramphenicol and ampicillin are effective and have been the most extensively studied. Recent studies show that ciprofloxacin is highly active. Third generation cephalosporins and co-trimoxazole is useful in organisms that are resistant to standard agents.

Bacteremia: Ampicillin, chloramphenicol, co-trimoxazole, and third generation cephalosporins are all effective. However, chloramphenicol should be avoided in endocarditis or mycotic aneurysms. Ciprofloxacin is effective in treating recurrent *Salmonella* bacteremia in AIDS.

Chronic carriage: Ampicillin or amoxicillin for 6 weeks, although elapses are common if there is underlying gallbladder disease cholecystectomy may be an option with repeated relapses. Ciprofloxacin may also be effective.

Drug Therapy
Recommended
Cephalosporins, 3rd Generation *on page 662*
Alternate
Ampicillin *on page 604*
Co-Trimoxazole *on page 692*
Chloramphenicol *on page 667*
Ciprofloxacin *on page 678*

Selected Readings
Levine WC, Buehler JW, Bean NH, et al, "Epidemiology of Nontyphoidal *Salmonella* Bacteremia During the Human Immunodeficiency Virus Epidemic," *J Infect Dis*, 1991, 164(1):81-7.
"Outbreaks of *Salmonella enteritidis* Gastroenteritis - California 1993," *MMWR Morb Mortal Wkly Rep*, 1993, 42(41):793-7.
Rubino JR, "The Economic Impact of Human *Salmonella* Infection," *Clin Microbiol Newslett*, 1997, 19(4):25-9.

Sarcoptes scabiei

Microbiology *Sarcoptes scabiei*, or the human mite, is the causative agent of scabies, a common parasitic infestation of the skin. *Sarcoptes scabiei* is an ectoparasite of humans belonging to the class *Arachnida*. It tends to form skin "burrows" several millimeters wide within the stratum corneum of the epidermis. The fertilized female deposits its eggs in these skin burrows, and the larvae exit after several days to become adults weeks later. The adult is about 0.3 mm long.
(Continued)

Sarcoptes scabiei (Continued)

Epidemiology Scabies is distributed worldwide. The incidence in the United States has been increasing since the 1970s. The reservoir resides in humans, although animal mites can sometimes cause brief human disease. Transmission is person to person by direct contact. Occasionally, transmission may occur when there is contact with heavily contaminated clothing or bedsheets. The incubation period varies from several days to weeks. Infected individuals remain communicable until all the ova and mites are eradicated from the skin.

Clinical Syndromes

- **Human scabies:** Patients present with intense itching, usually in the inter-digital web spaces, along the "belt line," the genital region, the periumbilical area, and also on the wrists, elbows, knees, and feet. Additional areas are common in children, including the hands and face. On physical examination, the characteristic burrows may be seen, appearing linear and several millimeters wide, often in the interdigital spaces. Atypical presentations of scabies may occur, including vesicles and bullae in infants, eczematous eruptions, and urticaria. A variant known as "nodular scabies" has been described in which there are small, brown, intensely pruritic nodules usually on the penis and scrotum. An unusual manifestation of severe scabies called "Norwegian scabies" has been seen in immunocompromised individuals and patients with Down syndrome. The skin is diffusely scaling and thickened as a result of infestation of thousands of mites. Secondary bacterial infections of the skin may occur in all forms of scabies.

- **Animal scabies:** This is due to *Sarcoptes scabiei* var *canis*, carried on some dogs. The clinical presentation is similar to human scabies although burrows are not present.

Diagnosis Infestation with scabies is often suspected when an individual presents with pruritic papules, or an otherwise compatible clinical history. Some patients may present because of a recent history of contact. It should be noted that scabies often imitates other skin lesions, and thus a broad differential diagnosis should be entertained if the linear burrows are not demonstrated. Other diagnostic considerations include impetigo, insect bites, drug eruptions, varicella, eczema, and others.

The linear burrows of the mite can be further demonstrated by applying blue ink over a possible burrow. The ink is drawn into the defect and when excess ink is wiped off with an alcohol pad, the ink within the burrow remains. This and other suspicious areas should covered with oil, the area should be scraped with a sterile blade, the scrapings should be placed into oil on a microscope slide, and the preparation should be examined with a microscope.

Diagnostic Tests/Procedures

Arthropod Identification *on page 334*

Treatment For adults and older children: Lindane 1% lotion or cream is applied to all skin areas from the neck to the toes then washed off after 8-12 hours. During the treatment period, the medication should be reapplied to the hands after routine handwashing; failure to do so may result in treatment failure since the hands are often infected. Lindane is contraindicated in pregnant or lactating women. Of note, lindane has been associated with central nervous system toxicity, particularly when an underlying skin disorder was present to allow greater than normal systemic absorption of drug. The regimen described here is generally safe. The alternative regimen is crotamiton (10%) applied as a thin smear from the neck down and left on for 1 day. A second application is done the following day, then washed off 24 hours later. Crotamiton should be used in individuals with extensive dermatitis.

For children younger than 2 years of age, infants, and pregnant women, crotamiton should be used instead of lindane. Treatment should be administered to sexual partners and close contacts in the same house. Other principles of management include cleaning all potentially contaminated clothes (dry cleaning or machine washing and drying in the hot cycle), prescribing medications for pruritus (Atarax®, diphenhydramine, topical corticosteroids, and others), and treating secondary bacterial infections of the skin with antistaphylococcal antibiotics.

Drug Therapy

Recommended

Lindane *on page 797*

Permethrin *on page 868*
Crotamiton *on page 695*

Schistosoma mansoni

Synonyms Blood Fluke

Microbiology *Schistosoma mansoni* also known as the blood fluke, is a common parasite in South America, the Caribbean, and Africa. The organism causes schistosomiasis (bilharziasis) with diverse clinical manifestations ranging from a mild dermatitis to a fulminant dysentery with bloody stools.

S. mansoni is a parasite classified as a trematode (fluke). As with other trematodes, it appears flat, fleshy, and has a leaf shape. There are two muscular suckers, the oral type being the beginning of an incomplete digestive system and the ventral sucker being an organ of attachment. Unlike other trematodes, *S. mansoni* is not a hermaphrodite and there are separate male and female worms. The intermediate host of *S. mansoni* is the snail, which is necessary for the parasite to complete its life cycle.

The life cycle of the organism begins when the infective forms called cercariae are liberated from the snail. These ciliated, free-swimming organisms travel through fresh water until they reach the human host. The cercariae are able to penetrate intact skin. Following this they enter the circulation and mature in the intrahepatic porta blood. During this developmental period, the parasites coat themselves with a substance that prevents the host from recognizing them immunologically. This remarkable defense explains the mechanism whereby cases of chronic infection have lasted for decades. After 3 weeks of maturation the adult migrates to the mesenteric veins, specifically the small branches of the inferior mesenteric vein near the lower colon. Fertilization occurs in these vessels and eventually eggs are released into the environment, to begin the cycle again.

Epidemiology *S. mansoni* is common in South America (Brazil, Venezuela), the Caribbean (West Indies, Puerto Rico), and Africa. Travelers or immigrants from these areas are the main source for cases seen in the United States. The reservoir for *S. mansoni* is the human, although primates, marsupials, and rodents can also serve as hosts. As noted, transmission occurs when there is skin penetration of the parasite larvae in stool-contaminated waters. The incubation period is 4-6 weeks after skin penetration. There is no defined period of communicability since the parasite is not transmitted person to person. However, ova may be recovered from stools for years.

Clinical Syndromes

- **Asymptomatic infection:** Occurs commonly.
- **Dermatitis:** Following skin penetration by the larvae, a brisk local allergic reaction may be seen, with pruritus, maculopapular lesions, and edema.
- **Cough:** When migrating worms reach the lungs.
- **Mesenteric adenitis:** When the adults begin to lay eggs in the mesenteric vessels, a febrile illness often results. There is abdominal pain, liver tenderness, and malaise. Eventually, the area may become walled off in a foreign-body type reaction, and fibrosis and abscess formation may be seen. Characteristically, there is bloody diarrhea.
- **Chronic infection:** After infection has become established, the patient over time may develop ascites, massive hepatosplenomegaly, lymphadenopathy, white granulomas on the liver called pseudotubercles. Extraintestinal infections may be seen, eggs may be recovered from the spinal cord, lungs, and other areas. Fibrosis is also seen at these other sites. Severe neurologic disease results from the presence of eggs in the spinal cord and brain.

Diagnosis Schistosomiasis is suspected in an individual who resides in an endemic area, or a traveler who has recently returned from such an area who presents with a compatible clinical history. Routine laboratory studies may be helpful, with elevated liver function tests and peripheral blood eosinophilia seen.

The stool examination is critical in confirming the diagnosis. Large eggs 115-175 μm long are seen in established cases. Rectal biopsy may also be considered if serial stool exams are negative but clinical suspicion remains high. The biopsy may reveal the egg tracks laid by the worms in the rectal vessels.

Diagnostic Tests/Procedures

Ova and Parasites, Stool *on page 505*
(Continued)

Schistosoma mansoni (Continued)

Ova and Parasites, Urine or Aspirates *on page 508*

Treatment Asymptomatic cases do not necessarily require treatment. The drugs used have potential toxicities and the situation must be weighed by the physician. The same applies to mild infections; the nature of the patient's immune status must be considered also. Moderate or severe cases respond to praziquantel.

Drug Therapy
Recommended
Praziquantel *on page 880*
Oxamniquine *on page 851*

Selected Readings
Mahmoud AA, "Trematodes (Schistosomiasis) and Other Flukes," *Principles and Practice of Infectious Diseases*, 4th ed, Mandell GL, Bennett JE, and Dolin R, eds, New York, NY: Churchill Livingstone, 1995, 2538-44.

"Schistosomiasis in U.S. Peace Corps Volunteers - Malawi, 1992," *MMWR Morb Mortal Wkly Rep*, 1993, 42(29):565-70.

Scrimgeour EM and Gajdusek DC, "Involvement of the Central Nervous System in *Schistosoma mansoni* and *S. haematobium* Infection: A Review," *Brain*, 1985, 108(Pt 4):1023-38.

Tsang VC and Wilkins PP, "Immunodiagnosis of Schistosomiasis: Screen With FAST-ELISA and Confirm With Immunoblot," *Clin Lab Med*, 1991, 11(4):1029-39.

Serratia Species

Microbiology *Serratia* species are gram-negative rods which are important causes of nosocomial infection and are only rarely associated with community-acquired infections in normal hosts.

Serratia species are moderate-sized aerobic gram-negative bacilli which belong to the large family Enterobacteriaceae. The organisms cannot be identified on the basis of morphologic appearance on Gram's stain alone and are indistinguishable from other Enterobacteriaceae. *Serratia* species are related to such gram-negative bacilli as *Klebsiella*, *Enterobacter*, and *Hafnia* (all belonging to the tribe Klebsielleae). There are several distinct species of *Serratia*, but most human disease is caused by *Serratia marcescens*. Rarely, *Serratia liquefaciens* has been isolated in serious infections. Laboratory identification is generally straightforward. It is unique in that it is the only member of the Enterobacteriaceae to produce extracellular DNase. Special requests for isolation of *Serratia* are not necessary because the organism is not fastidious in its growth requirements. Most clinical isolates will exhibit growth after overnight incubation; the appearance of colonies may be delayed (or completely inhibited) if the patient is receiving antibiotic therapy. *Serratia marcescens* shares several potential virulence factors with other Enterobacteriaceae, including endotoxin, the lipopolysaccharide associated with the outer membrane of the bacteria. When cell lysis occurs (as with antibiotic therapy), the LPS is released into the host and can lead to such inflammatory responses as fever, leukopenia or leukocytosis, hypotension, and disseminated intravascular coagulation. Thus, LPS is regarded as an important mediator of the sepsis syndrome.

Epidemiology In contrast to the other members of the Enterobacteriaceae family, *Serratia* tends to colonize the respiratory and urinary tracts of hospitalized adults more so than the gastrointestinal tract. This colonization probably does not hold true for neonates, in whom the gastrointestinal tract is an important source of the organism. An outbreak of *Serratia marcescens* was reported in a neonatal intensive care unit in 1982; a gastrointestinal reservoir was found to be important. Nosocomial transmission can occur by several routes; the most frequent being hand-to-hand spread via nurses, physicians, and other health-care workers. *Serratia marcescens* has also been associated with hospital outbreaks caused by contaminated respiratory equipment used for inhalational therapy, bronchoscopes, antiseptic fluids, intravenous fluids, scalp-vein needles, peritoneal dialysis catheters, and others. Community-acquired infections with *Serratia* are unusual, and the organism is mainly a nosocomial pathogen. In the 1970s, *Serratia marcescens* was identified as an important cause of endocarditis in intravenous heroin users.

Clinical Syndromes
• **Lower respiratory tract infection:** Nosocomial *Serratia* infections are seen in debilitated, ventilator-dependent patients. *Serratia* and other gram-negative bacilli can asymptomatically colonize the upper respiratory tract of hospitalized patients. Thus, the recovery of *Serratia* from a sputum or

tracheal aspirate culture does not necessarily indicate a significant infection. The diagnosis of a nosocomial pneumonia still rests on standard criteria such as the presence of purulence (many leukocytes) on the Gram's stain of sputum, the presence of a pulmonary infiltrate, and signs of systemic inflammation in the patient. **A positive sputum culture alone is not sufficient justification for initiating antibiotic therapy**.

- **Urinary tract infection:** This infection is also seen in hospitalized patients, often with indwelling Foley catheters. However, *Serratia* may also harmlessly colonize the urine of patients with chronic bladder catheters without causing disease. The decision to initiate antibiotics in such patients should be based on the clinical situation (the presence of pyuria on urinalysis, suprapubic pain, fever, etc). Even the finding of large quantity of *Serratia* in a urine culture (>10^5 colony forming units/mL) by itself does not automatically indicate the need for antibiotic therapy.

- **Hospital-associated bacteremias:** *Serratia* may be recovered from blood cultures in association with a known focus of infection (eg, catheter infection) or may be a "primary bacteremia" with no clear source. Bacteremia may follow instrumentation of the gastrointestinal or urinary tracts.

- **Surgical wound infections**

Diagnosis The clinical presentations of the various nosocomial infections caused by *Serratia marcescens* are not distinctive, and laboratory isolation of the organism is necessary.

Diagnostic Tests/Procedures
Aerobic Culture, Appropriate Site *on page 310*
Gram's Stain *on page 426*

Treatment *Serratia* species present a challenging therapeutic problem. High level drug resistance has been described in some hospital isolates. Preliminary data suggest that the popular third generation cephalosporins may act to select mutants of *Serratia* that are resistant to a wide variety of antibiotics, including both cephalosporins and extended spectrum penicillins. These "stably derepressed mutants" are becoming more common in intensive care units and pose a significant and growing problem. Consultation with an Infectious Disease specialist may be useful in such cases.

Drug Therapy
Recommended
Penicillins, Extended Spectrum *on page 864*
Cephalosporins, 3rd Generation *on page 662*
Alternate
Imipenem and Cilastatin *on page 766*
Aztreonam *on page 615*
Meropenem *on page 812*
Fluoroquinolones *on page 736*

Selected Readings
Campbell JR, Diacovo T, and Baker CJ, "*Serratia marcescens* Meningitis in Neonates," *Pediatr Infect Dis J*, 1992, 11(10):881-6.

Heltberg O, Skov F, Gerner-Smidt P, et al, "Nosocomial Epidemic of *Serratia marcescens* Septicemia Ascribed to Contaminated Blood Transfusion Bags," *Transfusion*, 1993, 33(3):221-7.

Sokalski SJ, Jewell MA, Asmus-Shillington AC, et al, "An Outbreak of *Serratia marcescens* in 14 Adult Cardiac Surgical Patients Associated With 12-Lead Electrocardiogram Bulbs," *Arch Intern Med*, 1992, 152(4):841-4.

Shigella Species
Related Information
Timing of Food Poisoning *on page 1069*

Microbiology *Shigella* species are gram-negative rods which cause a severe diarrheal syndrome, called shigellosis or bacillary dysentery. *Shigella* species belong to the family Enterobacteriaceae and is, for all practical purposes, biochemically and genetically identical to *E. coli*. Four species of *Shigella* have been identified: *S. dysenteriae*, *S. flexneri*, *S. boydii*, and *S. sonnei*. There are approximately 40 serotypes. *Shigella sonnei* is most common in the industrial world and accounts for about 64% of the cases in the United States. *S. flexneri* is seen primarily in underdeveloped countries. Shigellosis can be seen following ingestion of as few as 200 organisms.

Epidemiology Infection with *Shigella* sp is primarily a problem in the pediatric population, with most infections in the 1- to 4-year age group. Outbreaks of epidemic proportions have been described in day care centers and nurseries. The reservoir for the bacteria is in humans. Transmission is by direct or indirect (Continued)

Shigella Species *(Continued)*

fecal-oral transmission from patient or carrier. Hand transmission is important. Less commonly, transmission occurs by consumption of contaminated water, milk, and food. The organism is able to produce outbreaks in areas of poor sanitation, in part due to the low number of organisms required to produce disease. Shigellosis is the most communicable of the bacterial diarrheas.

Clinical Syndromes *Shigella* species invade the intestinal mucosa wherein they multiply and cause local tissue damage. The organisms rarely penetrate beyond the mucosa, and thus the isolation in blood cultures is unusual, even with the toxic patient. Mucosal ulcerations are common. Some strains are known to elaborate a toxin (the shiga-toxin), which contributes to mucosal destruction and probably causes the watery diarrhea seen initially.

- **Dysentery:** Initially, the patient complains of acute onset of fever, abdominal cramping, and large volumes of very watery diarrhea. This phase is entero-toxin-mediated and reflects small bowel involvement. Within 24-48 hours, the fever resolves but the diarrhea turns frankly bloody, with mucous and pus in the stools as well. Fecal urgency and tenesmus are common. This phase reflects direct colonic invasion. This two-phased "descending infection" is suggestive of dysentery. Diarrhea and abdominal pain are almost universally present, but the other symptoms may be absent. Physical examination is variable, and patients may be comfortable or frankly toxic. Rectal examination is often painful due to friable and inflamed rectal mucosa. The course may be complicated from dehydration from diarrhea and vomiting, particularly in the elderly and in infants. Normally, the infection is self limited and resolves within about 1 week even without antibiotics. Complications are unusual and include febrile seizures (particularly in infants), septicemia, and the hemolytic uremic syndrome (usually from the shiga-toxin from *S. dysenteriae* 1).
- **Reactive arthritis:** Following dysentery from *Shigella*, a postinfectious arthropathy resembling Reiter's syndrome has been described, particularly in patients who are HLA-B27 positive.

Diagnosis Dysentery from *Shigella* should be suspected in any patient presenting with fever and bloody diarrhea. A history of a "descending infection" as described above is further suggestive. However, the differential diagnosis of fever with bloody diarrhea is broad and includes salmonellosis, *Campylobacter* enteritis, infection with *E. coli* O157:H7, and inflammatory bowel disease. The WBC count may show either a leukocytosis, leukopenia, or be normal.

There are two important laboratory tests indicated in suspected cases.

1. Stool exam for fecal leukocytes: Numerous white blood cells will be present during the colonic phase of the infection. Note that this is not diagnostic for *Shigella* infections; it indicates that the colonic mucosa is inflamed, from whatever cause. The finding of sheets of fecal leukocytes on smear narrows the differential diagnosis of infectious diarrheas considerably.
2. Stool culture for *Shigella*: Recovery of the organism from stool is more easily performed early in the illness when the concentration in the stool is highest. Samples should be brought to the laboratory as soon as possible to maximize viability, and specific culture for *Shigella* sp should be requested.

Diagnostic Tests/Procedures
Fecal Leukocyte Stain *on page 408*
Stool Culture *on page 540*

Treatment Many cases of *Shigella* dysentery are self-resolving. Some have suggested that antibiotics be reserved for severe cases, but this does not eliminate the reservoir for infection in the community. Antibiotics have been shown to shorten the period of excretion of the organism in the feces, as well as decreasing morbidity. The antibiotic of choice is co-trimoxazole for both children and adults. However, some strains are resistant to co-trimoxazole, particularly in Africa and Southeast Asia, and *in vitro* susceptibility testing should be performed on all isolates. The quinolones have been effective for shigellosis in clinical trials and are useful alternatives. Antimotility agents such as opiates, paregoric, and diphenoxylate (Lomotil®) should be avoided because of the potential for worsening the dysentery and for predisposing to toxic megacolon.

Pediatric Drug Therapy
Recommended
Co-Trimoxazole *on page 692*

Alternate
Ampicillin *on page 604*
Cephalosporins, 3rd Generation *on page 662*

Adult Drug Therapy

Recommended
Ciprofloxacin *on page 678*
Co-Trimoxazole *on page 692*

Alternate
Ampicillin *on page 604*
Cephalosporins, 3rd Generation *on page 662*
Fluoroquinolones *on page 736*

Selected Readings

Ashkenazi S, Amir J, Waisman Y, et al, "A Randomized, Double-Blind Study Comparing Cefixime and Trimethoprim-Sulfamethoxazole in the Treatment of Childhood Shigellosis," *J Pediatr*, 1993, 123(5):817-21.

Baskin DH, Lax JD, and Barenberg D, "*Shigella* Bacteremia in Patients With the Acquired Immune Deficiency Syndrome," *Am J Gastroenterol*, 1987, 82(4):338-41.

Bennish ML, "Potentially Lethal Complications of Shigellosis," *Rev Infect Dis*, 1991, 13(Suppl 4):S319-24.

Halpern Z, Dan M, Giladi M, et al, "Shigellosis in Adults: Epidemiologic, Clinical, and Laboratory Features," *Medicine (Baltimore)*, 1989, 68(4):210-7.

Salam MA and Bennish ML, "Antimicrobial Therapy for Shigellosis," *Rev Infect Dis*, 1991, 13(Suppl 4):S332-41.

Tauxe RV, Puhr ND, Wells JG, et al, "Antimicrobial Resistance of *Shigella* Isolates in the USA: The Importance of International Travelers," *J Infect Dis*, 1990, 162(5):1107-11.

Snuffles *see Bordetella bronchiseptica on page 80*

Sporothrix schenckii

Microbiology *Sporothrix schenckii* is a saprophytic fungus widely dispersed in the soil, on the surface of many plants, and in decaying vegetable matter. The organism is a thermally dimorphic fungus, meaning that it exists in either a yeast or a mold form depending on the temperature. At room temperature, it exists in a mold form, but at warmer temperatures, it grows as a budding yeast. In clinical specimens such as biopsies of skin lesions, *Sporothrix schenckii* appears as a round or oval budding yeast; organisms may be difficult to find in clinical specimens and when present, may have variable size and shape. Thus, culture confirmation of *Sporothrix schenckii* is important. The organism grows relatively well on a variety of fungal media used routinely in microbiology laboratories.

Epidemiology *Sporothrix schenckii* is the causative agent of sporotrichosis or "gardener's disease". Typically, the organism is inoculated directly into the hand or face of a person handling plants or soil containing the organism. *S. schenckii* can be cultured from rose thorns, hay, compost material, mulch, and other decaying plant matter. It is important to obtain a detailed occupational and recreational history in suspected cases of sporotrichosis; individuals at risk include gardeners (particularly those handling roses), florists, landscapers, farmers, loggers, and others. Individuals who are infected with *S. schenckii* generally have a normal immune system. Although zoonotic transmission has been reported, it is much rarer then traumatic implantation of the organism. Several cases have been reported of veterinarians acquiring sporotrichosis from infected cats even without an associated penetrating injury.

The largest documented U.S. outbreak of sporotrichosis occurred in 1988. The outbreak was linked to Wisconsin-grown sphagnum moss used in packing evergreen tree seedlings; 84 individuals from 15 states developed cutaneous sporotrichosis. The attack rate was 17% in New York State, where 13 cases were reported from 109 forestry workers who had handled evergreen seedlings and moss. As expected, the attack rates were highest in those workers spending more time directly exposed to the moss. Although cultures of sphagnum moss from the Wisconsin supplier were negative for *Sporothrix schenckii*, the organism was cultured from multiple samples of the moss obtained from the tree nursery in Pennsylvania thought to be the main source of the outbreak. Several tree-handling procedures at this nursery may have contributed to the outbreak, such as the use of 3-year-old moss to pack seedlings, use of a pond water system to keep the moss wet, use of a polymer gel on the root system of the seedlings, and lengthy storage of moss-packed seedlings prior to shipping. This outbreak emphasized the need for wearing protective gloves and long-sleeved shirts in persons handling evergreens and similar plants.

Clinical Syndromes Sporotrichosis is divided into cutaneous and extracutaneous forms.

(Continued)

Sporothrix schenckii (Continued)

- **Cutaneous sporotrichosis:** This occurs when the organism is inoculated into the subcutaneous tissues following a minor trauma to the extremities or face. The incubation period is variable, from 1 week to several months. Cutaneous sporotrichosis can be classified as either plaque sporotrichosis or lymphocutaneous sporotrichosis. In plaque sporotrichosis, a small red plaque develops on the extremity at the original site of inoculation of the organism. The plaque is nontender and may increase in size but no additional lesions develop. In lymphocutaneous sporotrichosis, the disease begins with a single papular lesion, but in time, multiple similar lesions appear more proximally following the path of lymphatic drainage. These lesions often change from painless papules to ulcers which drain pus or serosanguinous fluid. Interestingly, although new lesions form by lymphangitic spread, axillary (or inguinal) lymph nodes are seldom involved. Both forms of cutaneous sporotrichosis tend to be very chronic if left untreated.

  When examined by light microscopy, the skin lesions in cutaneous sporotrichosis show multinucleated giant cells and epithelioid cells consistent with granulomas; thus, sporotrichosis should be considered in the differential diagnosis of any granulomatous process on an extremity or the face. It is important to note that organisms may not be seen on a single skin biopsy and additional biopsies may be necessary. The finding of an "asteroid body" on histologic section of a skin biopsy is highly suggestive of sporotrichosis but is not reliably present in all biopsies. The asteroid is a fungal organism surrounded by several "rays" that stain with periodic acid-Schiff (PAS). A recent study using electron microscopy suggested that an asteroid body is composed of crystalline products of disintegrated host cells deposited around a central fungal cell.

  A number of clinical entities should be considered in the differential diagnosis of cutaneous sporotrichosis. Some can be eliminated on the basis of epidemiology alone. Diseases to consider include:

  - *Mycobacterium marinum*
  - *Mycobacterium kansasii*
  - pyoderma gangrenosum
  - *Nocardia brasiliensis*
  - *Leishmania* species
  - foreign body granulomas
  - blastomycosis
  - dermatologic diseases (especially with plaque sporotrichosis)

- **Extracutaneous sporotrichosis:** A variety of rare, extracutaneous forms have been described. The most common is osteoarticular sporotrichosis which involves the knee, elbow, wrist, or ankle. There is rarely a history of a plant or thorn injury and typically no skin lesions are present. Patients may present with either single joint involvement or a polyarticular syndrome. The onset is indolent, and the joint develops tenderness, warmth, effusions, and sometimes draining sinuses. Osteoarticular sporotrichosis is a very difficult diagnosis to make; one study reported that it usually took over 2 years to make the correct diagnosis. Other forms of sporotrichosis include:

  - Pulmonary sporotrichosis: Only a few cases have been reported. Patients present with a chronic cavitary pneumonia, usually in an upper lobe. The disease mimics tuberculosis and histoplasmosis. One recent report suggested that the Papanicolaou stain of sputum may be helpful in making this rare diagnosis.

  - Ocular disease: This usually results from penetrating ocular injury to the conjunctiva or surrounding tissues. Eighteen cases of sporotrichoid endophthalmitis have been reported, with only two cases associated with trauma; most have required enucleation.

  - Meningitis: This rare complication has been reported in a few immunocompetent individuals. In one study of meningeal sporotrichosis in 7 patients, the cerebrospinal fluid was frequently negative on both stain and fungal culture initially; repeated lumbar punctures were necessary over a 3- to 11-month period before the organism was cultured.

- Disseminated sporotrichosis: Patients present with multiple skin lesions involving two or more extremities. Blood cultures using the lysis-centrifugation method have been reported positive for *Sporothrix schenckii* in some cases.
- **Sporotrichosis and AIDS:** Systemic sporotrichosis has been reported in patients with advanced HIV infection but remains an infrequent complication. A number of sites of infection have been reported including the lung, liver, spleen, intestine, bone, eye, joints, and disseminated cutaneous lesions. Recently, a case of meningitis was reported in a patient with known cutaneous sporotrichosis and a CD4 cell count of 56/µL. Again, the cerebrospinal fluid was sterile over a 5-month period. The skin lesions responded to a prolonged course of amphotericin B and fluconazole, but the meningeal symptoms worsened on therapy, and on autopsy, *S. schenckii* was found infiltrating into the meninges and brain parenchyma.

Diagnosis The clinical suspicion of sporotrichosis should be confirmed microbiologically because of the number of conditions which can mimic the cutaneous lesions. Cultures of appropriate specimens such as skin biopsies, joint fluid, and bursal fluid will frequently recover the organism. *S. schenckii* is difficult to identify on fungal stains of biopsy specimens or KOH preparations since the organism burden is often low. Cultures of exudates from ulcerative skin lesions are often low-yield. Blood cultures, urine cultures, and sputum are only rarely positive. As noted earlier, cerebrospinal fluid is frequently negative in meningeal sporotrichosis, and multiple samples over time are necessary.

Specific IgG antibodies to *S. schenckii* are available at specialty laboratories but are of limited usefulness. Demonstration of IgG synthesis against the organism in cerebrospinal fluid may be a useful means of diagnosing meningeal sporotrichosis when routine cultures are negative (see Penn et al reference).

Diagnostic Tests/Procedures

Fungus Culture, Body Fluid *on page 415*
Fungus Culture, Cerebrospinal Fluid *on page 416*
Fungus Culture, Skin *on page 417*

Treatment Recently, antifungal susceptibility of *Sporothrix schenckii* to several agents has become available in specialized centers (eg, Dr. Michael Rinaldi, Fungus Testing Laboratory, University Health Science Center, San Antonio, TX). This may be useful in severe or refractory cases. The treatment of choice for cutaneous sporotrichosis is a saturated solution of potassium iodide (SSKI). The mechanism of action of SSKI is obscure. The dose is initiated at 5 drops of SSKI 3 times/day in juice and steadily increased to 40 drops 3 times/day. Toxicity of the medication is common and includes gastrointestinal distress and lacrimation; the dose should be lowered if these symptoms occur. Drug rash is also relatively common, but the medication can usually be continued safely. Local heat is useful in cutaneous disease and can be used either as an adjunctive measure or in patients intolerant of SSKI. The azole antifungal agents may have some activity against *S. schenckii*. Ketoconazole and fluconazole have limited or no activity; itraconazole has *in vitro* activity although the *in vivo* experience is limited.

Extracutaneous sporotrichosis is best treated with amphotericin B. Prolonged courses are usually necessary, and osteoarticular sporotrichosis often requires over 2 g amphotericin. Pulmonary and meningeal sporotrichosis are even more difficult to treat, and a specialist in Infectious Disease should be consulted.

Drug Therapy
Recommended
Cutaneous sporotrichosis:
Potassium Iodide *on page 879*
Extracutaneous sporotrichosis:
Amphotericin B (Conventional) *on page 597*

Selected Readings
Coles FB, Schuchat A, Hibbs JR, et al, "A Multistate Outbreak of Sporotrichosis Associated With Sphagnum Moss," *Am J Epidemiol*, 1992, 136(4):475-87.

Keiser P and Whittle D, "Sporotrichosis in Human Immunodeficiency Virus-Infected Patients: Report of a Case," *Rev Infect Dis*, 1991, 13(5):1027-8.

Penn CC, Goldstein E, and Bartholomew WR, "*Sporothrix schenckii* Meningitis in a Patient With AIDS," *Clin Infect Dis*, 1992, 15(4):741-3.

Rex JH, "*Sporothrix schenckii*," *Principles and Practice of Infectious Diseases*, 4th ed, Mandell GL, Bennett JE, and Dolin R, eds, New York, NY: Churchill Livingstone, 1995, 2321-4.

Roberts GD and Larsh HW, "The Serologic Diagnosis of Extracutaneous Sporotrichosis," *Am J Clin Pathol*, 1971, 56(5):597-600.

SRGPC *see Streptococcus*-Related Gram-Positive Cocci *on page 278*

Staphylococcus aureus, Methicillin-Resistant
Synonyms MRSA
Microbiology Staphylococci derives its name from the Greek word staphyle meaning "bunch of grapes". On Gram's stain, staphylococci are gram-positive cocci, 0.7-1.2 µm, nonspore-forming, occurring singly, in pairs, in short 4-5 cocci chains or clusters. Staphylococci grow rapidly both as an aerobe and anaerobe on blood agar. The colonies are sharply defined, smooth, and 1-4 mm in diameter. Staphylococci are catalase-positive and differ from micrococci by the following: anaerobic acid production from glucose, sensitivity <200 mg/mL lysostaphin, and production of acid from glycerol in the presence of 0.4 mg/mL erythromycin.

Staphylococcus aureus may have a golden pigmentation secondary to carotenoid and produce β-hemolysis on horse, sheep, or human blood agar after an incubation of 24-48 hours. *Staphylococcus epidermidis* and coagulase-negative staph (CNS) are often used interchangeably but recognize that there are over 30 species of CNS of which *S. epidermidis* is the most common. It is important to distinguish three clinically relevant species: *S. aureus*, *S. epidermidis*, and *S. saprophyticus*. See table.

Major Tests for the Differentiation of Human Staphylococci

Test	*Staphylococcus aureus*	*Staphylococcus epidermidis*	*Staphylococcus saprophyticus*
Coagulase	+	–	–
Acid production by mannitol	+	–	+/ –
DNase	+	–	–
Novobiocin resistance	–	–	+
Anaerobic growth	+	+	–
Hemolysis	+	–	–

From Waldvogel FA, "*Staphylococcus aureus* (Including Toxic Shock Syndrome)," *Principals and Practice of Infectious Diseases*, 3rd ed, Mandell GL, Douglas R Jr, and Bennett JE, eds, New York, NY: Churchill Livingstone, 1990, 1490.

Epidemiology Colonization of healthcare workers with MRSA is uncommon. The two major modes of transmission of MRSA is via an infected or colonized patient, or dissemination through an infected or colonized healthcare worker; typically MRSA is transmitted on the hands of a healthcare worker after contact with an infected patient.

MRSA is not a marker for virulence nor spreading, and MRSA has not been shown to spontaneously evolve from MSSA to MRSA during the course of antibiotic therapy. Resistance to methicillin occurs predominantly by intrinsic resistance (penicillin-binding proteins) which is transmitted chromosomally. Five percent to 20% are also resistant to erythromycin, lincomycin, and clindamycin. Rifampin cannot be used alone secondary to a high one-step mutation rate to resistance.

Although universal precautions have been adopted and must be followed by all healthcare personnel, incidence of MRSA continues to rise. The goal of all facilities is ablation of widespread colonization and is difficult to achieve. Contact isolation is recommended.

Clinical Syndromes
- **Localized:** Most common type of infection usually secondary to poor personal hygiene, minor trauma, or diminished skin integrity (ie, eczema, psoriasis)

    Folliculitis - Typically clears with local antiseptic.

    Furuncle - Deep seated infection around a hair follicle beginning as a painful, red nodule then becoming a hot, painful, raised indurated lesion 1-2 cm long, over several days. Predilection for the face, neck, axillae, and buttocks.

    Carbuncle - Deep seated infection of multiple hair follicles that coalesce and spread into the subcutaneous tissue, frequently associated with sinus tracts. Need to exclude septicemia and/or septic thrombophlebitis. If recurrent, should evaluate for underlying phagocytic or metabolic dysfunction.

Impetigo - Typically affects children on exposed areas. Approximately 10% due to *Streptococcus pyogenes* and 10% due to combined staph/strep infections. Begins as a red macule which progresses to a vesicle then to crust. May be confused with HSV and varicella. The bullous form may respond to topical mupirocin or oral antistaphylococcal agents. Nonbullous form usually responds to oral or intramuscular penicillin.

Hydradenitis suppurative - Recurrent pyogenic abscess of apocrine sweat glands, especially axillary, perineal, and genital. Mimics LGV. Usually requires incision and drainage, as well as oral antibiotics.

Mastitis - Occurs in 1% to 3% of nursing mothers. Requires oral antibiotics. Continued nursing is controversial.

Wound infections - Usually occurs 2 days after surgery. May need to explore wound. Requires oral antibiotics 7-10 days. May need I.V. antibiotics 4-6 weeks for underlying prosthesis.

Spreading pyodermas - Surgical intervention needed if necrotizing fasciitis.

- **Pneumonia:** Most frequently occurs a few days after influenza; mortality is 30% to 50%. Acquired via inhalation or hematogenous route. Approximately 33% develop empyemas. Patients present with chest pain, fever, shortness of breath, tachypnea, and a pleural effusion which requires drainage. May be associated with bronchiectasis or obstructive bronchogenic cancer. Hematogenous route usually secondary to right-sided endocarditis, infected intravascular device, or septic phlebitis.
- **Toxic shock syndrome caused by TSST 1 (toxin 1):** Typically occurs in young woman ages 15-25 using tampons. Starts abruptly during menses. Present with fever, profound refractory hypotension, erythroderma with desquamation, multiorgan involvement with profuse diarrhea, mental confusion. Approximately 50% will have elevated creatine kinase, decreased platelets, and leukocytosis. May be seen secondary to surgical wound packages, as well as associated with disseminated staph infections. Mortality is approximately 3%.
- **Staphylococcal scalded skin syndrome (SSSS):** Most commonly occurs in children and neonates; epidemics in neonatal nurseries and day care centers. Usually caused by phage type 2. Starts abruptly with perioral erythema with sunburn-like rash rapidly turning bright red spreading to bullae in 2-3 days and desquamating within 5 days. Positive Nikolsky sign. Recovery in 10 days. Need to exclude toxic epidermal neurolysis and Kawasaki mucocutaneous disease (culture-negative, Nikolsky-negative).
- **Food poisoning:** Usually caused by ingestion of heat stable enterotoxin B. Second most common cause of acute food poisoning. May occur by person-to-person transmission. Incubation 2-6 hours after ingestion of toxin contained in custard filled bakery goods, canned foods, processed meats, potato salads, and ice cream. Patients present with acute salivation, nausea, vomiting progressing to abdominal cramps, and watery, nonbloody diarrhea (risk of dehydration).
- **Musculoskeletal:** Frequent cause of osteomyelitis, septic arthritis, septic bursitis, and, less frequently, pyomyositis. Blood cultures positive in approximately 50% of these cases of osteomyelitis. Need bone biopsy for definitive diagnosis. Typically hematogenous or secondary to local trauma with contiguous infection. Sternoclavicular joint usually follows septic thrombosis of upper limb and often associated with IVDA. Septic arthritis usually secondary to complication of septicemia, rheumatoid arthritis, or prepubertal trauma. (Knee > hip > elbow > shoulder.)
- **Septicemia/endocarditis:** Associated with age extremes, cardiovascular disease, decompensated diabetes, heroin addicts. Mortality remains high (40% to 60%) despite antimicrobial therapy. Thirty-three percent of patients have no focus for infection. Overall incidence of endocarditis with *S. aureus* infection is 10%. *S. aureus* is the second most common cause of native valve endocarditis and continues to rise in incidence in bacteremias thought secondary to IVDA and use of long-term indwelling catheters.

Diagnosis It is not possible to distinguish MRSA from MSSA clinically. Susceptibility testing should be performed on all *S. aureus* isolates. Isolation of *S. aureus* from a patient with suspected toxic shock syndrome (TSS) neither confirms the
(Continued)

Staphylococcus aureus, **Methicillin-Resistant**
(Continued)

diagnosis nor proves that the isolate is the etiological agent of the disease. The isolate must be shown to be capable of producing toxic shock syndrome toxin type 1 (TSST-1). Most isolates of *S. aureus* cultured from patients with clinically proven TSS produce TSST-1. Suspect isolates can be tested for the production of TSST-1 by immunodiffusion, isoelectric focusing, Western blot, and immunoblot techniques. The immunoblot technique is extremely sensitive, specific, rapid, and reliable and is the test of choice. However, the test is not widely available.

Diagnostic Tests/Procedures

Aerobic Culture, Appropriate Site *on page 310*

Gram's Stain *on page 426*

Treatment MRSA is characteristically resistant to penicillins, antistaphylococcal penicillin, erythromycin, lincomycin, clindamycin; somewhat resistant to aminoglycosides and chloramphenicol and sensitive to vancomycin and teicoplanin (not available in U.S.). MRSA will not respond clinically to cephalosporins, even though MRSA often **are susceptible *in vitro***. Both quinolones and teicoplanin have been shown to effective in short-term use, but recent studies show acquired resistance with long-term use. Doxycycline and co-trimoxazole may be used in nonlife-threatening infections if susceptible by *in vitro* testing. Prevention of spread to the other patients is critically important.

Drug Therapy
Recommended

Vancomycin *on page 967*
> or

Vancomycin *on page 967*
> used in combination with

Gentamicin *on page 747*
> or

Vancomycin *on page 967*
> used in combination with

Rifampin *on page 902*

Alternate

The following drug may be used only if susceptible:

Co-Trimoxazole *on page 692*

Doxycycline *on page 713*

Selected Readings

Chambers HF, "Methicillin Resistance in Staphylococci: Molecular and Biochemical Basis and Clinical Implications," *Clin Microbiol Rev*, 1997, 10(4):781-91.

Duckworth GJ, "Diagnosis and Management of Methicillin-Resistant *Staphylococcus aureus* Infection," *BMJ*, 1993, 307(6911):1049-52.

Mounzer KC and diNubile MJ, "Clinical Presentation and Management of Methicillin-Resistant *Staphylococcus aureus* (MRSA) Infections," *Antibiotics for Clinicians*, 1998, 2(Suppl 1):15-20.

Mulligan ME, Murray-Leisure KA, Ribner BS, et al, "Methicillin-Resistant *Staphylococcus aureus*: A Consensus Review of the Microbiology, Pathogenesis, and Epidemiology With Implications for Prevention and Management," *Am J Med*, 1993, 94(3):313-28.

Weckbach LS, Thompson MR, Staneck JL, et al, "Rapid Screening Assay for Toxic Shock Syndrome Toxin Production by *Staphylococcus aureus*," *J Clin Microbiol*, 1984, 20(1):18-22.

Staphylococcus aureus, **Methicillin-Susceptible**

Synonyms MSSA

Microbiology Staphylococci derives its name from the Greek word staphyle meaning "bunch of grapes". On Gram's stain, staphylococci are gram-positive cocci, 0.7-1.2 μm, nonspore-forming, occurring singly, in pairs, in short 4-5 cocci chains or clusters. Staphylococci grow rapidly both as an aerobe and anaerobe on blood agar. The colonies are sharply defined, smooth, and 1-4 mm in diameter. Staphylococci are catalase-positive and differ from micrococci by the following: anaerobic acid production from glucose, sensitivity <200 mg/mL lysostaphin, and production of acid from glycerol in the presence of 0.4 mg/mL erythromycin.

Staphylococcus aureus may have a golden pigmentation secondary to carotenoid and produce β-hemolysis on horse, sheep, or human blood agar after an incubation of 24-48 hours. *Staphylococcus epidermidis* and coagulase-negative staph (CNS) are often used interchangeably but recognize that there are over 30 species of CNS of which *S. epidermidis* is the most common. It is important to distinguish three clinically relevant species: *S. aureus*, *S. epidermidis*, and *S. saprophyticus*. See table in *Staphylococcus aureus*, Methicillin-Resistant *on page 256.*

Epidemiology It is estimated that 20% to 40% of the population are persistent asymptomatic nasal carriers. The carrier state is clinically relevant in that carriers have a higher rate of staphylococci infections as compared to noncarriers. Neonates may be colonized in the perianal area, umbilical stumps, skin, and gastrointestinal tract. Adults are colonized in the anterior nares, skin, and less frequently, vagina. There is an increase carrier rate among hospital personnel, diabetics receiving insulin, hemodialysis patients, and I.V. drug users.

The portal of entry is typically the skin. Patients with chemotaxis defects (ie, Chédiak-Higashi, Wiskott-Aldrich), opsonization defects (ie, complement deficiencies), and staphylocidal defects of polymorphonuclear cells (ie, chronic granulomatous disease) are at increased risk.

Eighty percent to 90% of community-acquired staphylococci are resistant to penicillin. One of the more common forms of resistance is through the production of beta-lactamase, an extracellular enzyme coded for by plasmids that inactivate penicillin by interrupting the β-lactam ring. These organisms are still susceptible to antistaphylococcal penicillins and first generation cephalosporins.

Clinical Syndromes

- **Localized:** Most common type of infection usually secondary to poor personal hygiene, minor trauma, or diminished skin integrity (ie, eczema, psoriasis)

  Folliculitis - Typically clears with local antiseptic.

  Furuncle - Deep seated infection around a hair follicle beginning as a painful, red nodule then becoming a hot, painful, raised indurated lesion 1-2 cm long, over several days. Predilection for the face, neck, axillae, and buttocks.

  Carbuncle - Deep seated infection of multiple hair follicles that coalesce and spread into the subcutaneous tissue, frequently associated with sinus tracts. Need to exclude septicemia and/or septic thrombophlebitis. If recurrent, should evaluate for underlying phagocytic or metabolic dysfunction.

  Impetigo - Typically affects children on exposed areas. Approximately 10% due to *Streptococcus pyogenes* and 10% due to combined staph/strep infections. Begins as a red macule which progresses to a vesicle then to crust. May be confused with HSV and varicella. The bullous form may respond to topical mupirocin or oral antistaphylococcal agents. Nonbullous form usually responds to oral or intramuscular penicillin.

  Hydradenitis suppurative - Recurrent pyogenic abscess of apocrine sweat glands, especially axillary, perineal, and genital. Mimics LGV. Usually requires incision and drainage, as well as oral antibiotics.

  Mastitis - Occurs in 1% to 3% of nursing mothers. Requires oral antibiotics. Continued nursing is controversial.

  Wound infections - Usually occurs 2 days after surgery. May need to explore wound. Requires oral antibiotics 7-10 days. May need I.V. antibiotics 4-6 weeks for underlying prosthesis.

  Spreading pyodermas - Surgical intervention needed if necrotizing fasciitis.

- **Pneumonia:** Most frequently occurs a few days after influenza; mortality is 30% to 50%. Acquired via inhalation or hematogenous route. Approximately 33% develop empyemas. Patients present with chest pain, fever, shortness of breath, tachypnea, and a pleural effusion which requires drainage. May be associated with bronchiectasis or obstructive bronchogenic cancer. Hematogenous route usually secondary to right-sided endocarditis, infected intravascular device, or septic phlebitis.

- **Toxic shock syndrome caused by TSST 1 (toxin 1):** Typically occurs in young woman ages 15-25 using tampons. Starts abruptly during menses. Present with fever, profound refractory hypotension, erythroderma with desquamation, multiorgan involvement with profuse diarrhea, mental confusion. Approximately 50% will have elevated creatine kinase, decreased

(Continued)

Staphylococcus aureus, Methicillin-Susceptible
(Continued)

platelets, and leukocytosis. May be seen secondary to surgical wound packages, as well as associated with disseminated staph infections. Mortality is approximately 3%.

- **Staphylococcal scalded skin syndrome (SSSS):** Most commonly occurs in children and neonates; epidemics in neonatal nurseries and day care centers. Usually caused by phage type 2. Starts abruptly with perioral erythema with sunburn-like rash rapidly turning bright red spreading to bullae in 2-3 days and desquamating within 5 days. Positive Nikolsky sign. Recovery in 10 days. Need to exclude toxic epidermal neurolysis and Kawasaki mucocutaneous disease (culture-negative, Nikolsky-negative).

- **Food poisoning:** Usually caused by ingestion of heat stable enterotoxin B. Second most common cause of acute food poisoning. May occur by person-to-person transmission. Incubation 2-6 hours after ingestion of toxin contained in custard filled bakery goods, canned foods, processed meats, potato salads, and ice cream. Patients present with acute salivation, nausea, vomiting progressing to abdominal cramps, and watery, nonbloody diarrhea (risk of dehydration).

- **Musculoskeletal:** Frequent cause of osteomyelitis, septic arthritis, septic bursitis and less frequently pyomyositis. Blood cultures positive in approximately 50% of these cases of osteomyelitis. Need bone biopsy for definitive diagnosis. Typically hematogenous or secondary to local trauma with contiguous infection. Sternoclavicular joint usually follows septic thrombosis of upper limb and often associated with IVDA. Septic arthritis usually secondary to complication of septicemia, rheumatoid arthritis, or prepubertal trauma. (Knee > hip > elbow > shoulder.)

- **Septicemia/endocarditis:** Associated with age extremes, cardiovascular disease, decompensated diabetes, heroin addicts. Mortality remains high (40% to 60%) despite antimicrobial therapy. Thirty-three percent of patients have no focus for infection. Overall incidence of endocarditis with *S. aureus* infection is 10%. *S. aureus* is the second most common cause of native valve endocarditis and continues to rise in incidence in bacteremias thought secondary to IVDA and use of long-term indwelling catheters.

Diagnosis Diagnosis is made by Gram's stain and culture of appropriate site. Phage typing is a useful epidemiological tool. Antiteichoic antibodies by CIE or RIA are positive in approximately 90% of patients with endocarditis, 20% to 40% positive with bacteremia, and 0% to 60% positive with localized infections. Isolation of *S. aureus* from a patient with suspected toxic shock syndrome (TSS) neither confirms the diagnosis nor proves that the isolate is the etiological agent of the disease. The isolate must be shown to be capable of producing toxic shock syndrome toxin type 1 (TSST-1). Most isolates of *S. aureus* cultured from patients with clinically proven TSS produce TSST-1. Suspect isolates can be tested for the production of TSST-1 by immunodiffusion, isoelectric focusing, Western blot, and immunoblot techniques. The immunoblot technique is extremely sensitive, specific, rapid, and reliable and is the test of choice. However, the test is not widely available.

Diagnostic Tests/Procedures

Aerobic Culture, Appropriate Site *on page 310*
Gram's Stain *on page 426*
Teichoic Acid Antibody *on page 545*

Treatment Topical mupirocin may be useful in eradicating carrier states. Most localized infections will respond to penicillins or antistaphylococcal penicillins or first generation cephalosporins. Deep-seated infections usually require surgical intervention. Penicillin-allergic individuals may be given erythromycin, clindamycin, or tetracycline. Patients with line sepsis without septicemia usually require 5-7 days parenteral antibiotics, whereas therapy is extended 10-14 days with septicemia. Controversy exists as to the removal of the intravascular device, but most authors recommend removing the catheter. Beta-lactam regimens for at least 4-6 weeks plus an aminoglycoside during the first to second week of treatment remains the treatment of choice for left-sided *S. aureus* endocarditis. Patients with β-lactam allergies or failed therapy should be treated with vancomycin plus rifampin. Patients with right-sided endocarditis are typically treated with the same regimens, however, there have been some studies suggesting the efficiency of quinolones. Two-week parenteral regimens are currently being investigated for the treatment of uncomplicated MSSA endocarditis.

Drug Therapy Comment Methicillin-susceptible *Staphylococcus aureus* is sensitive to a wide array of antibiotics including the penicillinase-resistant penicillins, 1st and most 2nd generation cephalosporins (also, *in vitro*, some 3rd generation cephalosporins), macrolides, clindamycin, tetracyclines, sulfonamides, and vancomycin. Although also often susceptible, the quinolones should not be used to treat this organism secondary to the risk of acquired resistance while on therapy. When choosing among these agents for the treatment of serious systemic infections, the penicillinase-resistant penicillins (nafcillin, oxacillin) are the drugs of choice. Organisms typically have higher MICs to vancomycin than to the penicillinase-resistant penicillins. If the organism happens to be penicillin-susceptible, penicillin would be the drug of choice.

Drug Therapy

Recommended

Penicillins, Penicillinase-Resistant *on page 864*

Alternate

Cephalosporins, 1st Generation *on page 661*

Clindamycin *on page 684*

Vancomycin *on page 967*

Selected Readings

Archer GL, "*Staphylococcus aureus*: A Well-Armed Pathogen," *Clin Infect Dis*, 1998, 26(5):1179-81.

Chambers MD, "Short-Course Combination and Oral Therapies of *Staphylococcus aureus* Endocarditis," *Infect Dis Clin North Am*, 1993, 7(1):69-80.

Jensen AG, Espersen F, Skinhoj P, et al "Bacteremic *Staphylococcus aureus* Spondylitis," *Arch Intern Med*, 1998, 158(5):509-17.

Mortara LA and Bayer AS, "*Staphylococcus aureus*, Bacteremia and Endocarditis. New Diagnostic and Therapeutic Concepts," *Infect Dis Clin North Am*, 1993, 7(1):53-68.

Turnidge J and Grayson L, "Optimun Treatment of Staphylococcal Infections," *Drugs*, 1993, 45(3):353-66.

Waldvogel FA, "*Staphylococcus aureus* (Including Toxic Shock Syndrome)," *Principles and Practice of Infectious Diseases*, 4th ed, Mandell GL, Bennett JE, and Dolin R, eds, New York, NY: Churchill Livingstone, 1995, 1754-77.

Weckbach LS, Thompson MR, Staneck JL, et al, "Rapid Screening Assay for Toxic Shock Syndrome Toxin Production by *Staphylococcus aureus*," *J Clin Microbiol*, 1984, 20(1):18-22.

Williams RE and MacKie RM, "The Staphylococci - Importance of Their Control in the Management of Skin Disease," *Dermatol Clin*, 1993, 11(1):201-6.

Staphylococcus epidermidis, Methicillin-Resistant

Synonyms MRSE

Microbiology Staphylococci derives its name from the Greek word staphyle meaning "bunch of grapes". On Gram's stain, staphylococci are gram-positive cocci, 0.7-1.2 μm, nonspore-forming, occurring singly, in pairs, in short 4-5 cocci chains or clusters. Staphylococci grow rapidly both as an aerobe and anaerobe on blood agar. The colonies are sharply defined, smooth, and 1-4 mm in diameter. Staphylococci are catalase-positive and differ from micrococci by the following: anaerobic acid production from glucose, sensitivity <200 mg/mL lysostaphin, and production of acid from glycerol in the presence of 0.4 mg/mL erythromycin.

Staphylococcus aureus may have a golden pigmentation secondary to carotenoid and produce β-hemolysis on horse, sheep, or human blood agar after an incubation of 24-48 hours. *Staphylococcus epidermidis* and coagulase-negative staph (CNS) are often used interchangeably but recognize that there are over 30 species of CNS of which *S. epidermidis* is the most common. It is important to distinguish three clinically relevant species: *S. aureus*, *S. epidermidis*, and *S. saprophyticus*. See table in *Staphylococcus aureus*, Methicillin-Resistant *on page 256*.

Epidemiology Over the past 10 years, MSSE has continued to be the major cause of nosocomial bacteremia and sepsis with a mortality approaching 30%. MSSE is a normal inhabitant of the skin. It synthesizes an extracellular polysaccharide which is associated with persistence of infection, resistance to antibiotics, and a predilection for medical devices. Approximately 24,000 patients annually develop device-related septicemia with the most common being related to insertion site infections.

Thirty percent to 40% of prosthetic valve endocarditis (PVE) is due to CNS compared to 14% due to MSSA. Hickman/Broviac infections are 54% CNS as compared to 20% MSSA. Less than 6% of all pacemaker insertions result in
(Continued)

Staphylococcus epidermidis, Methicillin-Resistant
(Continued)

infections, yet 40% to 50% are due to CNS secondary to contamination at the time of insertion. Similar findings are seen in prosthetic joint infections.

Typically, community-acquired infections are beta-lactam sensitive, whereas most hospital-acquired infections are multiply resistant. Resistance to antistaphylococcal beta-lactams is mediated by the mec gene which confers resistance by encoding a unique penicillin binding protein with low affinity for beta-lactam antibiotics.

Clinical Syndromes

- **Foreign body infections:** Common sites of infection with MSSE include intravascular catheters, pacemakers, prosthetic cardiac valves, vascular grafts, orthopedic appliances, artificial joints, CSF shunts, dialysis catheters, and breast implants.
- **Osteomyelitis:** Most commonly associated with sternal wound infections status post cardiac surgery, although overall frequently rare. Other mode of transmission is via hematogenous spread.
- **Native valve endocarditis:** Less common than PVE; occurs in approximately 5%.
- **Urinary tract infection:** Hospital acquired secondary to manipulation or catheter placement.
- **Endophthalmitis:** Increasing significantly status post intraocular lens placement.

Diagnosis
Diagnosis is made by Gram's stain and culture with sensitivities of appropriate site. Semiquantitative roll technique by Dennis Maki in which catheter is rolled over surface of blood agar plate is useful in suggesting a true intravascular catheter sepsis when both blood culture grows MSSE and count >15 colonies on blood agar plate.

Diagnostic Tests/Procedures
Aerobic Culture, Appropriate Site *on page 310*
Gram's Stain *on page 426*

Treatment
Vancomycin remains the drug of choice for MRSE. More than 50% of all isolates are resistant to tetracycline, chloramphenicol, clindamycin, and erythromycin. MRSE is usually sensitive to rifampin and gentamicin, but resistance develops quickly and neither drug can be used as a sole agent. Although not available in the U.S., teicoplanin may be of benefit. Antimicrobial therapy for PVE should consist of vancomycin, rifampin, and/or gentamicin for 4-6 weeks. UTIs secondary to MRSE may be treated with co-trimoxazole if susceptible.

Drug Therapy
Recommended
Vancomycin *on page 967*
  or
Vancomycin *on page 967*
  used in combination with
Gentamicin *on page 747*
  or
Vancomycin *on page 967*
  used in combination with
Rifampin *on page 902*

Alternate
The following drug may be used only if susceptible:
Co-Trimoxazole *on page 692*

Selected Readings
Christensen GD, "The 'Sticky' Problem of *Staphylococcus epidermidis* Sepsis," *Hosp Pract (Off Ed)*, 1993, 28(9A):27-36, 38.

Hachem RY and Raad I, "Clinical Presentation and Management of Methicillin-Resistant *Staphylococcus epidermidis* (MRSE) Bloodstream Infections," *Antibiotics for Clinicians*, 1998, 2(Suppl 1):21-4.

Lai KK and Fontecchio SA, "Infections Associated With Implantable Cardioverter Defibrillators Placed Transvenously and Via Thoracotomies: Epidemiology, Infection Control, and Management," *Clin Infect Dis*, 1998, 27(2):265-9.

Rupp ME and Archer GL, "Coagulase-Negative Staphylococci: Pathogens Associated With Medical Progress," *Clin Infect Dis*, 1994, 19(2):231-43.

Whitener C, Caputo GM, Weitekamp MR, et al, "Endocarditis Due to Coagulase-Negative Staphylococci," *Infect Dis Clin North Am*, 1993, 7(1):81-96.

Staphylococcus epidermidis, Methicillin-Susceptible

Synonyms MSSE

Microbiology Staphylococci derives its name from the Greek word staphyle meaning "bunch of grapes". On Gram's stain, staphylococci are gram-positive cocci, 0.7-1.2 μm, nonspore-forming, occurring singly, in pairs, in short 4-5 cocci chains or clusters. Staphylococci grow rapidly both as an aerobe and anaerobe on blood agar. The colonies are sharply defined, smooth, and 1-4 mm in diameter. Staphylococci are catalase-positive and differ from micrococci by the following: anaerobic acid production from glucose, sensitivity <200 mg/mL lysostaphin; and production of acid from glycerol in the presence of 0.4 mg/mL erythromycin.

Staphylococcus aureus may have a golden pigmentation secondary to carotenoid and produce β-hemolysis on horse, sheep, or human blood agar after an incubation of 24-48 hours. *Staphylococcus epidermidis* and coagulase-negative staph (CNS) are often used interchangeably but recognize that there are over 30 species of CNS of which *S. epidermidis* is the most common. It is important to distinguish three clinically relevant species: *S. aureus*, *S. epidermidis*, and *S. saprophyticus*. See table in *Staphylococcus aureus*, Methicillin-Resistant *on page 256*.

Epidemiology Over the past 10 years, MSSE has continued to be the major cause of nosocomial bacteremia and sepsis with a mortality approaching 30%. MSSE is a normal inhabitant of the skin. It synthesizes an extracellular polysaccharide which is associated with persistence of infection, resistance to antibiotics, and a predilection for medical devices. Approximately 24,000 patients annually develop device-related septicemia with the most common being related to insertion site infections.

Thirty percent to 40% of prosthetic valve endocarditis (PVE) is due to CNS compared to 14% due to MSSA. Hickman/Broviac infections are 54% CNS as compared to 20% MSSA. Less than 6% of all pacemaker insertions result in infections, yet 40% to 50% are due to CNS secondary to contamination at the time of insertion. Similar findings are seen in prosthetic joint infections.

Typically, community-acquired infections are beta-lactam sensitive, whereas most hospital-acquired infections are multiply resistant. Resistance to antistaphylococcal beta-lactams is mediated by the mec gene which confers resistance by encoding a unique penicillin binding protein with low affinity for beta-lactam antibiotics.

Clinical Syndromes
- **Foreign body infections:** Common sites of infection with MSSE include intravascular catheters, pacemakers, prosthetic cardiac valves, vascular grafts, orthopedic appliances, artificial joints, CSF shunts, dialysis catheters, and breast implants.
- **Osteomyelitis:** Most commonly associated with sternal wound infections status post cardiac surgery, although overall frequently rare. Other mode of transmission is via hematogenous spread.
- **Native valve endocarditis:** Less common than PVE; occurs in approximately 5%.
- **Urinary tract infection:** Hospital acquired secondary to manipulation or catheter placement.
- **Endophthalmitis:** Increasing significantly status post intraocular lens placement.

Diagnosis Diagnosis is made by Gram's stain and culture with sensitivities of appropriate site. Semiquantitation roll technique by Dennis Maki in which catheter is rolled over surface of blood agar plate is useful in suggesting a true intravascular catheter sepsis when both blood culture grows MSSE and count >15 colonies on a blood agar plate.

Diagnostic Tests/Procedures

Aerobic Culture, Appropriate Site *on page 310*

Gram's Stain *on page 426*

Treatment First choice antibiotic in MSSE infections are penicillins or antistaphylococcal penicillins (penicillinase-resistant). For most medical device infections, the medical device must be removed. Current recommendations for pacemaker infection is to remove the pacer during the second week of parenteral antibiotics before reimplantation. Sixty-seven percent of prosthetic joint infection occur during the first 2 years. If the joint is not loose, 6 weeks of (Continued)

Staphylococcus epidermidis, Methicillin-Susceptible (Continued)

parenteral antibiotics are recommended. If the joint is loose, then removal of the joint plus parenteral antibiotics for 6 weeks is recommended. For nonlife-threatening infections with MSSE, a first generation cephalosporin may be used. For penicillin allergic individuals, clindamycin, vancomycin, doxycycline or co-trimoxazole based on susceptibility testing may be used.

Drug Therapy

Recommended

Penicillins, Penicillinase-Resistant *on page 864*

Alternate

Cephalosporins, 1st Generation *on page 661*

Clindamycin *on page 684*

Vancomycin *on page 967*

Selected Readings

Christensen GD, "The 'Sticky' Problem of *Staphylococcus epidermidis* Sepsis," *Hosp Pract (Off Ed),* 1993, 28(9A):27-36, 38.

Lai KK and Fontecchio SA, "Infections Associated With Implantable Cardioverter Defibrillators Placed Transvenously and Via Thoracotomies: Epidemiology, Infection Control, and Management," *Clin Infect Dis,* 1998, 27(2):265-9.

Raad I, Alrahwan A, and Rolston K, "*Staphylococcus epidermidis*: Emerging Resistance and Need for Alternative Agents," *Clin Infect Dis,* 1998, 26(5):1182-7.

Rupp ME and Archer GL, "Coagulase-Negative Staphylococci: Pathogens Associated With Medical Progress," *Clin Infect Dis,* 1994, 19(2):231-43.

Whitener C, Caputo GM, Weitekamp MR, et al, "Endocarditis Due to Coagulase-Negative Staphylococci," *Infect Dis Clin North Am,* 1993, 7(1):81-96.

Staphylococcus saprophyticus

Microbiology Staphylococci derives its name from the Greek word staphyle meaning "bunch of grapes". On Gram's stain, staphylococci are gram-positive cocci, 0.7-1.2 μm, nonspore-forming, occurring singly, in pairs, in short 4-5 cocci chains or clusters. Staphylococci grow rapidly both as an aerobe and anaerobe on blood agar. The colonies are sharply defined, smooth, and 1-4 mm in diameter. Staphylococci are catalase-positive and differ from micrococci by the following: anaerobic acid production from glucose, sensitivity <200 mg/mL lysostaphin, and production of acid from glycerol in the presence of 0.4 mg/mL erythromycin.

Staphylococcus aureus may have a golden pigmentation secondary to carotenoid and produce β-hemolysis on horse, sheep, or human blood agar after an incubation of 24-48 hours. *Staphylococcus epidermidis* and coagulase-negative staph (CNS) are often used interchangeably but recognize that there are over 30 species of CNS of which *S. epidermidis* is the most common. It is important to distinguish three clinically relevant species: *S. aureus, S. epidermidis,* and *S. saprophyticus.* See table in *Staphylococcus aureus*, Methicillin-Resistant *on page 256.*

Epidemiology *Staphylococcus saprophyticus* is a common cause of urinary tract infections (UTIs) in sexually active young women, elderly men, and children. The use of spermicide-coated condoms has been associated with an increase risk of UTI in young women. Highest frequency occurs during late summer and early autumn; reasons unclear.

Clinical Syndromes

- **Urinary tract infection (UTI):** Present with acute dysuria, back or flank pain, and temperature <38.5°C. Hematuria and pyuria are usually present.

Diagnosis Diagnosis depends on isolation of organism from urine. Counts as low as 10^2 CFU/mL in young women with symptoms is considered significant.

Diagnostic Tests/Procedures

Urine Culture, Clean Catch *on page 565*

Treatment First choice therapy is co-trimoxazole. Controversy exists whether single dose, 3-day, 7-day, or 10-day course are equally effective. Studies suggest that for women, a 3-day course is equally effective to a 7-day course. Alternative therapies include nitrofurantoin, ampicillin, first generation cephalosporin, or quinolone based on susceptibility testing.

Drug Therapy

Recommended

Co-Trimoxazole *on page 692*

Alternate
Nitrofurantoin *on page 842*
Ampicillin *on page 604*
Cephalosporins, 1st Generation *on page 661*
Fluoroquinolones *on page 736*

Selected Readings
Abrahamsson K, Hansson S, Jodal U, et al, "*Staphylococcus saprophyticus* Urinary Tract Infections in Children," *Eur J Pediatr*, 1993, 152(1):69-71.

Elder NC, "Acute Urinary Tract Infection in Women. What Kind of Antibiotic Therapy Is Optimal?" *Postgrad Med*, 1992, 92(6):159-62, 165-6, 172.

Fihn SD, Boyko EJ, Chen CL, et al, "Use of Spermicide-Coated Condoms and Other Risk Factors for Urinary Tract Infection Caused by *Staphylococcus saprophyticus*," *Arch Intern Med*, 1998, 158(3):281-7.

Stenotrophomonas maltophilia

Synonyms *maltophilia*; *Xanthomonas maltophilia*

Microbiology *Stenotrophomonas maltophilia* is a lactose-negative, oxidase-negative, nonfermenting, aerobic, gram-negative bacillus with polar flagella. *S. maltophilia* is an obligate aerobe with optimal growth at 35°C. The organism grows well on common laboratory media as smooth, glistening, gray/light yellow, nonhemolytic colonies.

Epidemiology *Stenotrophomonas maltophilia* is ubiquitous and is considered an opportunistic pathogen. It can be isolated from natural water sources, sewage, soil, and a variety of plant environments. It can also be found in human feces and a wide range of nosocomial sources including fomites. The increasing presence of this organism is most likely due to antimicrobial selective pressure and the increase in debilitated patients. Virulence factors for *Stenotrophomonas maltophilia* have not been extensively investigated.

Clinical Syndromes *Stenotrophomonas maltophilia* can infect any tissue or organ system including blood, lung, heart, skin, soft tissue, bone and joint, ophthalmologic, gastrointestinal tract, urinary tract, or musculoskeletal system. Syndromes caused by *Stenotrophomonas maltophilia* are usually indistinguishable from those caused by the Enterobacteriaceae. Organisms are often grown as part of mixed cultures; therefore, distinguishing colonization from true infection is often difficult. Risk factors associated with *S. maltophilia* infections include prior antibiotic therapy, central lines, immunosuppression, prolonged hospitalization, intensive care admissions, mechanical ventilation, and others.

Diagnosis The only way a diagnosis of *Stenotrophomonas maltophilia* infection can be made is by identification of the organism through culture in a patient with a relevant clinical syndrome. No special media or conditions are necessary to grow this organism.

Diagnostic Tests/Procedures
Aerobic Culture, Appropriate Site *on page 310*
Blood Culture, Aerobic and Anaerobic *on page 337*
Gram's Stain *on page 426*

Treatment *Stenotrophomonas maltophilia* is resistant to a wide variety of antimicrobial agents. The organism is almost always resistant to imipenem, and often resistant to extended spectrum penicillins, cephalosporins and the fluoroquinolones. *Stenotrophomonas maltophilia* is typically susceptible to co-trimoxazole with alternative therapies dependent on susceptibility testing. Synergy may exist with co-trimoxazole and Timentin® and co-trimoxazole and minocycline.

Drug Therapy
Recommended
Co-Trimoxazole *on page 692*
Alternate
Consider alternate agents only if susceptible.
Fluoroquinolones *on page 736*
Ticarcillin and Clavulanate Potassium *on page 950*
Ceftazidime *on page 651*
Doxycycline *on page 713*
Minocycline *on page 823*

Selected Readings
Denton M and Kerr KG, "Microbiological and Clinical Aspects of Infection Associated With *Stenotrophomonas maltophilia*," *Clin Microbiol Rev*, 1998, 11(1):57-80.

Elting LS and Bodey GP, "Septicemia Due to *Xanthomonas* Species and Non-Aeruginosa *Pseudomonas* Species: Increasing Incidence of Catheter-Related Infections," *Medicine (Baltimore)*, 1990, 69(5):296-306.

Marshall WF, Keating MR, Anhalt JP, et al, "*Xanthomonas maltophilia*: An Emerging Nosocomial Pathogen," *Mayo Clin Proc*, 1989, 64(9):1097-104.

(Continued)

Stenotrophomonas maltophilia (Continued)

Murray PR, Drew WL, Kobayashi GS, et al, eds, "Pseudomonadaceae," *Medical Microbiology*, St Louis, MO: CV Mosby Co, 1990, 119-26.

Penzak SR and Abate BJ, "*Stenotrophomonas (Xanthomonas) maltophilia*: A Multidrug-Resistant Nosocomial Pathogen," *Pharmacotherapy*, 1997, 17(2):293-301.

Streptococcus agalactiae

Synonyms Group B *Streptococcus*

Microbiology *Streptococcus agalactiae* is a β-hemolytic *Streptococcus* first recognized in 1938 as a cause of puerperal sepsis ("childbed fever"). By the Lancefield serogroup classification of β-hemolytic streptococci, *S. agalactiae* is also known as Group B *Streptococcus*. Like other streptococci, *S. agalactiae* are gram-positive cocci that appear to form chains when grown in broth. When the organism is growing on a blood agar plate, there is an area of complete hemolysis surrounding the colony, a finding called β-hemolysis. Several streptococci are β-hemolytic including Group A streptococci (*Streptococcus pyogenes*), and Groups B, C, and G streptococci. *S. agalactiae* does not require special media for growth and is readily isolated from clinical specimens.

Epidemiology The spectrum of Group B streptococcal infections has been changing over the past years. In the 1970s, this organism was a leading cause of neonatal meningitis and sepsis and was an important cause of maternal peripartum infections, such as postpartum endometritis and bacteremia. More recently, surveillance studies in the 1990s have shown an incidence of 3-4 cases of invasive *S. agalactiae* infections per 100,000 adults. The majority of these infections have appeared in nonpregnant adults. A recent report in 1993 suggested an increasing incidence of invasive Group B infections in nonpregnant adults, but the reasons for this increase were unclear.

Adult groups at risk for serious Group B disease include persons with AIDS, diabetes mellitus, and cancer. Newborns are also at high risk for infection, although the presence of maternal IgG antibodies to the organism correlates with protection from serious infection in the neonate. Serious *S. agalactiae* infections are uncommon in infants older than 3 months of age, even though specific antibodies usually are not present.

Clinical Syndromes

- **Asymptomatic carriage in pregnant females:** It is estimated that 15% to 25% of women are asymptomatic carriers of Group B streptococci. Many such women who are carriers of Group B streptococci during pregnancy can be identified by culture of the rectum and/or vagina at approximately 26 weeks of gestation. However, the presence of Group B *Streptococcus* at this time (26 weeks) does **not** predict the presence of Group B *Streptococcus* at **birth**, the time when detection of the bacterium is most clinically significant. Of this group, those women who have risk factors for infant infection are candidates for preventative therapy during delivery (see Treatment). These risk factors include premature labor, fever, premature or prolonged rupture of membranes, multiple gestations, or a history of prior Group B infection in a previous neonate. Prevention of Group B neonatal infections in this manner is recommended by the American College of Obstetricians and Gynecologists, and the American Academy of Pediatrics.

- **Invasive infections in neonates:** Infection is acquired during passage through a colonized birth canal. "Early onset" infections occur within 1 week and often less than 1 day. Approximately 50% of infants born to mothers with vaginal and rectal carriage of Group B streptococci will themselves become colonized; however, only a small percentage will develop symptomatic infection. In general, neonates are bacteremic with this organism, and many develop pneumonia with a respiratory distress syndrome. "Late-onset" infections occur between 1 week and 3 months, and meningitis is most frequently seen.

- **Invasive infections in the adult:** Pregnancy-related *S. agalactiae* infections include peripartum fever, endometritis, chorioamnionitis, often with bacteremia. In nonpregnant adults, common infections include cellulitis, diabetic ulcer infections, urinary tract infections, septic arthritis, and pneumonias. A variety of serious complications have been seen including endocarditis, pelvic abscesses, meningitis, and others.

Diagnostic Tests/Procedures

Aerobic Culture, Appropriate Site *on page 310*

Group B *Streptococcus* Antigen Test *on page 429*

Treatment Group B streptococci are susceptible to penicillins, although they exhibit less *in vitro* sensitivity than Group A streptococci. Adults with invasive, localized infections such as pyelonephritis or infected joint spaces should be treated with relatively high doses of penicillin G, approximately 12 million units daily. Patients with life-threatening infections such as endocarditis should receive 18 (or more) million units of penicillin G daily.

Neonates with Group B bloodstream infections should also receive penicillin G. Some limited data suggest *in vitro* synergy between penicillin and gentamicin, and many pediatricians will use this combination. Therapy is usually continued 10-14 days or more due to the risk of relapse in such conditions as meningitis.

As described above, pregnant women who are found to be carriers of Group B streptococci in the vagina or rectum **at the time of birth** may be candidates for antibiotic prophylaxis if an additional risk factor to the infant is identified. Prophylactic administration of ampicillin to the mother at the time of delivery has been shown to decrease the rate of infection of the newborn. Indiscriminate prophylaxis of all pregnant women who are carriers of Group B streptococci is not recommended.

Drug Therapy
Recommended
Penicillin G, Parenteral, Aqueous *on page 860*
Amoxicillin *on page 592*
Ampicillin *on page 604*
Alternate
Cephalosporins, 1st Generation *on page 661*
Erythromycin *on page 722*
Vancomycin *on page 967*

Selected Readings
Gallagher PG and Watanakunakorn C, "Group B Streptococcal Bacteremia in a Community Teaching Hospital," *Am J Med*, 1985, 78(5):795-800.

Schwartz B, Schuchat A, Oxtoby MJ, et al, "Invasive Group B Streptococcal Disease in Adults," *JAMA*, 1991, 266(8):1112-4.

Verghese A, Mireault K, and Arbeit RD, "Group B Streptococcal Bacteremia in Men," *Rev Infect Dis*, 1986, 8(6):912-7.

***Streptococcus*, Anaerobic** see *Streptococcus*-Related Gram-Positive Cocci *on page 278*

Streptococcus anginosus see *Streptococcus*, Viridans Group *on page 279*

Streptococcus bovis
Synonyms Group D *Streptococcus*
Applies to *Streptococcus equinus*
Microbiology *Streptococcus bovis* and *Streptococcus equinus* possess the Group D lipoteichoic acid antigen in their cell walls. Since 1984, the enterococci have been classified in a separate genus (*Enterococcus*). *S. bovis* is associated with human infections while *S. equinus* is found predominantly in the alimentary tract of horses. These organisms are gram-positive cocci which appear in chains. They are β-hemolytic on rabbit blood, α-hemolytic or nonhemolytic on sheep blood. The ability to cause hemolysis on laboratory media does not correlate with clinical virulence.
Epidemiology *Streptococcus bovis* is a minor part of the normal flora of man where it is found in the genital and intestinal tracts. In sheep and cows, it inhabits the intestinal tract. Infection with *Streptococcus bovis* is correlated with colon and rectal carcinoma and hepatic dysfunction. These organisms have low intrinsic virulence.
Clinical Syndromes *Streptococcus bovis* is a cause of endocarditis and bacteremia primarily in the elderly. Eighty percent of cases occur in patients 60 years of age or older. The association with colon carcinoma is attributed to production by the tumor of transferrin-like chelators that facilitate bacterial growth. One-third of patients with *S. bovis* endocarditis are found to have an adenocarcinoma, villous adenoma, or colonic polyp. The association with liver disease may be the result of altered hepatic secretion of bile salts or immunoglobulins and compromise of the hepatic reticuloendothelial system. Bacteremia associated with *S. bovis* is polymicrobial in approximately 20% of cases.
Diagnosis The diagnosis of *S. bovis* endocarditis is established by positive blood culture in a patient with mild fever and malaise. The disease onset is usually
(Continued)

Streptococcus bovis (Continued)

gradual. Low grade fever, arthralgia and cardiac murmurs, splenomegaly, splinter hemorrhages, Roth spots, Osler nodes, and embolic phenomenon may also be presenting features. If *S. bovis* is recovered, a thorough search for adenocarcinoma of the colon or rectum should be undertaken.

Diagnostic Tests/Procedures

Aerobic Culture, Appropriate Site *on page 310*
Blood Culture, Aerobic and Anaerobic *on page 337*

Duration of Therapy Endocarditis: 4 weeks; nonendocarditis: 7-10 days

Treatment Differentiation between nonenterococcal Group D streptococci (primarily *S. bovis*) and enterococci (now classified in separate genus *Enterococcus* including *E. faecalis*, *E. faecium*, and *E. durans*) is important in regard to antimicrobial susceptibility. *S. bovis* is sensitive to penicillin (90% have penicillin MIC <0.2 µg/mL), ampicillin, cephalothin, and clindamycin. Endocarditis due to *S. bovis* is frequently treated with parenteral penicillin G as monotherapy. *Enterococcus* species generally have much higher MICs, usually 2-4 µg/mL and are resistant to achievable levels of cephalosporins and clindamycin. Therapy for enterococci requires use of a penicillin or vancomycin in combination with an aminoglycoside. See also *Enterococcus* Species *on page 137* and *Streptococcus* Viridans Group *on page 279*.

Penicillin G, 10-20 million units/day I.V. in divided doses every 4 hours for 4 weeks for organism with an MIC ≤0.1 µg/mL. Addition of gentamicin or streptomycin may result in more rapid cure. Streptomycin dosage 7.5 mg/kg I.M. every 12 hours or gentamicin 1 mg/kg I.V. every 8 hours for the first 2 weeks of therapy with penicillin being continued for the full 4 weeks. An additional alternative in cefazolin 1-2 g I.V. or I.M. every 6-8 hours for 4 weeks.

Vancomycin, 15 µg/kg I.V. every 12 hours for 4 weeks.

Drug Therapy

Recommended

Penicillin G, Parenteral, Aqueous *on page 860*

Alternate

Vancomycin *on page 967*

Selected Readings

Zarkin BA, Lillemoe KD, Cameron JL, et al, "The Triad of *Streptococcus bovis* Bacteremia, Colonic Pathology, and Liver Disease," *Ann Surg*, 1990, 211(6):786-92.

Streptococcus equinus *see Streptococcus bovis on previous page*

Streptococcus intermedius *see Streptococcus, Viridans Group on page 279*

Streptococcus milleri Group *see Streptococcus, Viridans Group on page 279*

Streptococcus mitis *see Streptococcus, Viridans Group on page 279*

Streptococcus morbillorum *see Streptococcus, Viridans Group on page 279*

Streptococcus mutans *see Streptococcus, Viridans Group on page 279*

Streptococcus pneumoniae

Microbiology *Streptococcus pneumoniae* was called "the captain of the men of death" by Sir William Osler because of its lethality. It remains a leading cause of acute lobar pneumonia, otitis media, and meningitis. *Streptococcus pneumoniae* is an encapsulated gram-positive coccus. Classically, the organism appears lancet-shaped and commonly in pairs or short chains. Colonies appear circular, dimpled or mucoid, and dome-shaped. They cause α-hemolysis when grown aerobically on blood agar. There are several determinants of pathogenicity:

- the polysaccharide capsule, which protects the organism from phagocytosis
- adherence, which allows colonization of epithelial cells
- enzymes, such as neuraminidase (which allows growth in mucous secretions) and proteases (which degrade IgA and facilitate colonization)
- toxins, such as pneumolysis O, which directly inhibits phagocytic activity

Epidemiology *S. pneumoniae* is a common colonizer of the nasopharynx of healthy individuals. Estimates of this carriage state range from 5% to >70% and appears more common in children. Carriage seems highest in the winter and spring months, which is also the most common period for true infection. New serotypes of *Streptococcus pneumoniae* are acquired throughout the year. When true infection occurs, it is often with a new serotype rather than the serotype associated with years of carriage. Patients with chronic bronchitis are frequently colonized in the nasopharynx and respiratory tree with pneumococcus, and purulent exacerbations of bronchitis are often associated with this organism.

Clinical Syndromes

- **Pneumonia:** Typically, pneumococcal pneumonia begins abruptly with sudden fever and shaking chills, which resolves. Pleuritic pain may be quite severe. The patient often develops a cough productive of "rusty" mucopurulent sputum. Complications include parapneumonic effusion, empyema, bacteremia, and meningitis. *Streptoccocus pneumoniae* is still the most common cause of community-acquired pneumonia in adults.

- **Otitis media:** *S. pneumoniae* is a leading cause, accounting for 35% to 50% of the cases.

- **Meningitis:** *S. pneumoniae* is the most common etiology for community-acquired meningitis in adults. Often, this is preceded by pulmonary infection or a mild upper respiratory infection. Predisposing factors include alcoholism, sickle cell disease, multiple myeloma, and general debility.

- **Bacteremia:** This may occur in 25% or more of patients with pneumococcal pneumonia and >80% of patients with meningitis. Endocarditis has also been described.

Diagnosis The finding of lancet-shaped gram-positive cocci in ordinarily sterile body fluids such as cerebrospinal fluid, blood, sinus aspirates, or pleural fluid is diagnostic of *S. pneumoniae* infection. However, such a finding is not necessarily diagnostic when found in expectorated sputum since respiratory colonization is common (particularly in chronic bronchitics). With respiratory secretions, it is important to note the presence of both polymorphonuclear leukocytes, as well as numerous pneumococci on Gram's stain; this combination is suggestive of true infection, but physician judgment is critical.

Antigen detection techniques are widely available for identifying the soluble pneumococcal capsular polysaccharide. Latex agglutination may be used to identify *S. pneumoniae* antigens from sterile body fluids such as cerebrospinal fluid. It may be useful (but only occasionally) in patients with suspected pneumococcal meningitis who have recently been treated with antibiotics which could interfere with recovery of the organism. However, Gram's stain and cultures are much more preferred to latex agglutination.

Diagnostic Tests/Procedures

Aerobic Culture, Appropriate Site *on page 310*
Bacterial Antigens, Rapid Detection Methods *on page 335*
Gram's Stain *on page 426*

Treatment Penicillin is the drug of choice for *Streptoccocus pneumoniae*. Recently, strains of *S. pneumoniae* resistant to penicillin have been reported, particularly in Western Europe. The incidence of penicillin-resistance is still quite low in the United States but is a worrisome trend. Some authors have suggested using vancomycin for empiric therapy of pneumococcal meningitis until antibiotic susceptibility patterns of the specific isolate are known.

Drug Therapy

Recommended

Meningitis:
> Penicillin G, Parenteral, Aqueous *on page 860*
Nonmeningitis:
> Penicillin G, Parenteral, Aqueous *on page 860*

Alternate

Meningitis:
> Vancomycin *on page 967*
> Chloramphenicol *on page 667*
Nonmeningitis:
> Macrolides *on page 803*
> Erythromycin *on page 722*
> Vancomycin *on page 967*
> Cephalosporins, 1st Generation *on page 661*

Selected Readings

Kronenberger CB, Hoffman RE, Lezotte DC, et al, "Invasive Penicillin-Resistant Pneumococcal Infections: A Prevalence and Historical Cohort Study," *Emerg Infect Dis*, 1996, 2(2):121-4.

Musher DM, "Infections Caused by *Streptococcus pneumoniae*: Clinical Spectrum, Pathogenesis, Immunity, and Treatment," *Clin Infect Dis*, 1992, 14(4):801-7.

Musher DM, Watson DA, and Dominguez EA, "Pneumococcal Vaccination: Work to Date and Future Prospects," *Am J Med Sci*, 1990, 300(1):45-52.

(Continued)

Streptococcus pneumoniae (Continued)

Pallares R, Gudiol F, Linares J, et al, "Risk Factors and Response to Antibiotic Therapy in Adults With Bacteremic Pneumonia Caused by Penicillin-Resistant Pneumococci," *N Engl J Med*, 1987, 317(1):18-22.

Streptococcus pneumoniae, Drug-Resistant

Synonyms DRSP; Penicillin-Resistant *S. pneumoniae*; Pneumococcus, Drug-Resistant

Microbiology *Streptococcus pneumoniae* is a gram-positive coccus which has a lancet-shaped appearance. Nearly all clinical isolates have a polysaccharide capsule in addition to the pneumococcal cell wall. The pneumococcal cell wall consists of mainly teichoic acid and peptidoglycan. β-lactam antibiotics such as penicillin act at the level of the cell wall by covalently binding to key enzymes in the cell wall which mediate cell wall integrity and synthesis. Enzymes such as endo-, trans- and carboxypeptidases cross-link the many peptide side chains of the cell wall and are called "penicillin-binding proteins (PBPs)." The importance of PBPs has come to the forefront recently due to the emergence of penicillin-resistant strains of pneumococci which result from alterations in these enzymes.

In the past 20 years, the number of drug-resistant *S. pneumoniae* (DRSP) isolates has increased from a scattered case reports from Australia and Africa to a global problem involving all countries including the United States. DRSP results from stepwise mutations of the bacterial genes which encode for PBPs. These genes are considered "mosaic genes" in that the coding region includes segments of genetic material derived from other related streptococcal species. It is postulated that the DNA sequences encoding these altered PBPs originally came from other streptococcal species which already exhibited varying degrees of penicillin resistance (eg, viridans streptococci). Multiple alterations in PBPs decrease the binding affinity of penicillin and other β-lactam antibiotics for these proteins, decreasing their efficacy. These mutations are chromosomally mediated and do not appear to alter the virulence of the organism; that is, penicillin-resistant pneumococci are neither more or less virulent than penicillin-sensitive isolates.

The altered PBP genes appear to spread readily to other strains of *S. pneumoniae* in a horizontal fashion, and these mutations appear to be stable. Of the 90 known serotypes of *S. pneumoniae*, the majority of penicillin-resistant isolates belong to serotypes 6, 9, 14, 19, and 23. As with penicillin-susceptible strains of *S. pneumoniae*, the organism is spread via a respiratory route from person to person such that some individuals become colonized in the nasopharynx. This state of colonization generally lasts from weeks to months. Nasopharyngeal colonization is felt to precede more invasive disease such as pneumonia or meningitis. The proportion of persons colonized with DRSP who develop invasive disease is currently under study. Clones of DRSP have been documented to spread horizontally, and this tendency has certainly contributed to the rapid dissemination of resistant isolates across the world.

Resistance of *S. pneumoniae* to other β-lactam antibiotics such as the cephalosporins is also mediated by PBPs. The *in vitro* susceptibility of penicillin-resistant *S. pneumoniae* to the various cephalosporins is variable, with the third-generation cephalosporins being more predictably active (see Treatment). *S. pneumoniae* can also be resistant to antibiotics other than the β-lactam antibiotics, through mechanisms other than alterations in PBPs. Resistance can be acquired through conjugation with other related streptococci such that there is a change in the antimicrobial target, as with the macrolides (eg, erythromycin), fluoroquinolones (eg, ciprofloxacin), trimethoprim, and others. This phenomenon of multidrug resistance in *S. pneumoniae* (resistance to two or more antibiotics) is seen more commonly in isolates which are resistant to penicillin. It is unusual to see resistance to non-β-lactam antibiotics in penicillin-sensitive *S. pneumoniae*.

Epidemiology Until recently, nearly all clinical isolates of *S. pneumoniae* were exquisitely susceptible to penicillin. Testing for resistance was not necessary and serious pneumococcal infections could be treated confidently with penicillin without awaiting antibiotic susceptibility testing. The first report of a penicillin-resistant isolate causing disease came from Australia in 1967. Since then reports from countries such as New Guinea, Australia, and South Africa have shown an increase in DRSP from 12% in the 1970s to over 30% in the 1980.

DRSP is now reported globally and in some regions over one-half of pneumococcal isolates have either intermediate or high level penicillin resistance. This rapid spread of DRSP is due to at least two factors, horizontal spread of resistant clones and emergence of new clones of DRSP due to heavy use of antibiotics.

In the United States, several recent epidemiologic studies have shown that about 25% to 30% of pneumococcal isolates are now resistant to penicillin (either intermediate or high-level resistance). This increase has mainly taken place over the last decade. However, not all communities have this high a rate; penicillin-resistance appears quite variable across the United States, with some regions having <5% DRSP (usually rural) compared with rates >30% in some urban areas. Surveillance studies have shown that rates of DRSP can vary markedly within the same community, from hospital to hospital, and from adults to children. One problem regarding accurate surveillance of resistance trends is that DRSP is not a mandatory reportable illness. To address this, the Centers for Disease Control has launched an initiative to track resistant isolates nationwide.

Several risk factors have been identified for the development of DRSP:

- age younger than 6 years of age
- recent treatment with antibiotics
- multiple comorbid diseases
- child attending day care (and family members of same)
- the elderly
- HIV infection and other immunodeficiency states
- recent hospitalization
- residence in a nursing home or prison

Much of the development and spread of DRSP is due to the heavy use of antimicrobial agents for children in day care centers. Common conditions such as acute otitis media and other upper respiratory infections in these populations have led to the empiric and often inappropriate use of antimicrobial agents in children with the emergence of new DRSP clones.

Clinical Syndromes

- **Meningitis caused by DRSP**: A number of case series have described *S. pneumoniae* meningitis caused by strains that were either intermediate or highly resistant to penicillin. The clinical features of meningitis due to DRSP are the same as with penicillin-susceptible pneumococci, a finding consistent with the fact that drug-resistant isolates are not more virulent. The therapy of meningitis caused by DRSP is complex although a general consensus has been reached (see Treatment).
- **Pneumonia caused by DRSP**: Only a limited amount of information is available concerning the clinical course and outcomes of pneumonia caused by DRSP. In one study of children in South Africa with pneumococcal pneumonia, the clinical presentation of children with penicillin-resistant and penicillin-susceptible strains were equivalent. A similar finding was noted in a large U.S. pediatric multicenter pneumococcal surveillance study. Interestingly, a number of cases of pneumonia caused by DRSP have been treated successfully with penicillin, in contrast with the treatment of meningitis (see Treatment).
- **Others**: Bacteremia, acute otitis media, and sinusitis have all been reported to be caused by DRSP. Only a limited amount of information is available for clinical presentations and outcomes of these conditions.

Diagnosis Infections caused by penicillin-resistant *S. pneumoniae* are indistinguishable at the bedside from those caused by penicillin-susceptible isolates, and laboratory determination of drug resistance is essential. However, although infection with *S. pneumoniae* may be suspected early on because of a Gram's stain of a clinical specimen (lancet-shaped diplococci), or on the basis of the clinical presentation alone, results of *in vitro* susceptibility testing is not generally available for 24 hours or more. Rapid assays to detect DRSP in 6 hours or less are being developed at this time but remain research tools.

The National Committee for Clinical Laboratory Standards (NCCLS) has recommended that all isolates of *S. pneumoniae* obtained from usually sterile sites undergo testing for penicillin resistance. This is accomplished by screening isolates using a 1 mcg oxacillin disk. If the oxacillin disk results in a zone of

(Continued)

Streptococcus pneumoniae, Drug-Resistant
(Continued)

inhibition of bacterial growth ≥20 mm, the isolate is considered penicillin-suscep-tible, and further laboratory testing is not necessary. If the oxacillin zone diam-eter is ≤19 mm, then penicillin resistance is considered probable. Screening with the oxacillin disk is 99% sensitive and fairly specific (80% to 90%) and should detect almost all isolates resistant to penicillin and extended-spectrum cephalosporins (eg, ceftriaxone or cefotaxime). Those isolates that appear nonsusceptible by oxacillin disk should then undergo further testing using stan-dard quantitative minimal inhibitory concentration (MIC) tests against penicillin, extended-spectrum cephalosporin(s), chloramphenicol, vancomycin, and other drugs. MIC testing should be performed by established methods such as the broth microdilution procedure (using Mueller-Hinton broth with 3% lysed horse blood), agar dilution, disk diffusion, or antimicrobial gradient strips (eg, E-test), but not by automated methods.

The NCCLS has defined the following MIC breakpoints for interpreting the susceptibility of *S. pneumoniae* to penicillin:

susceptible: MIC of penicillin ≤0.06 µg/mL

intermediate: MIC of penicillin 0.1-1.0 µg/mL

resistant: MIC of penicillin ≥2.0 µg/mL

These breakpoints of susceptible, intermediate, and resistant are based on several factors including available data on clinical response to antibiotic therapy and on achievable levels of penicillin in blood. The NCCLS has defined interpre-tive standards for *S. pneumoniae* MIC breakpoints for a number of other antibi-otics, including non-β-lactam antibiotics.

Diagnostic Tests/Procedures

Aerobic Culture, Appropriate Site *on page 310*

Bacterial Antigens, Rapid Detection Methods *on page 335*

Gram's Stain *on page 426*

Treatment It is important to note that recommendations for treatment of penicillin-intermediate and penicillin-resistant *S. pneumoniae* are evolving, and in many situations a consensus has not been reached. Only a limited amount of informa-tion is available to correlate clinical failure with the interpretive MIC breakpoints (ie, to determine if an isolate of *S. pneumoniae* that is penicillin-resistant *in vitro* actually fails to respond to therapy with penicillin). To complicate matters, it is likely that the significance of penicillin resistance is not the same for meningitis, pneumonia, bacteremia, and upper respiratory infections, given varying concen-trations of the drug at each site. The following recommendations are based on current data, which is likely to change. An infectious disease consultation should be considered in difficult cases.

Meningitis due to DRSP: More information is available for treatment of acute meningitis caused by penicillin-intermediate and penicillin-resistant *S. pneumo-niae* isolates than other infections caused by pneumococci. Clinical failures have been reported when penicillin has been used to treat intermediate and high level resistant strains. Extended spectrum cephalosporins are useful for treating inter-mediately resistant strains as long as the MIC was <2.0 µg/mL, since treatment failures have been reported with use of the cephalosporins above this level. For high level resistant strains of *S. pneumoniae* to penicillin and cephalosporins, treatment with vancomycin and an extended spectrum cephalosporin is indi-cated due to some animal data suggesting the combination is synergistic in this setting. Some authors recommend adding vancomycin to an extended spectrum cephalosporin even when the isolate is only intermediately resistant to cephalosporins (ie, MIC for ceftriaxone = 1 µg/mL), but other authors do not. No vancomycin-resistant isolates of *S. pneumoniae* have been described to date, but the liberal use of vancomycin is not advised due to concerns about potential resistance developing in the future. Rifampin may have some potential role for highly penicillin- and cephalosporin-resistant isolates, but little clinical data is available. Recommendations are as follows.

Recommended Treatment for Meningitis Due to DRSP

Penicillin MIC	Ceftriaxone or Cefotaxime MIC	Recommended Therapy
<0.1 µg/mL	≤0.5 µg/mL	Penicillin I.V. (high dose)
0.1-1.0 µg/mL	≤0.5 µg/mL	Ceftriaxone or cefuroxime
	1.0 µg/mL	Ceftriaxone or cefuroxime, +/- vancomycin
	≥2.0 µg/mL	Ceftriaxone + vancomycin
≥2.0 µg/mL	any MIC value	Ceftriaxone + vancomycin, +/- rifampin

Pneumonia due to DRSP: Only a limited amount of information is available concerning the clinical significance of DRSP in pneumonia, and a variety of regimens have been proposed in recent years. Several large clinical studies suggest that *in vitro* penicillin resistance is not as significant with pneumococcal pneumonia when compared with meningitis, and some authorities feel that penicillin can still be used when the isolate is intermediately resistant to penicillin, up to and including an MIC of 2 µg/mL. In part this has been justified by the significantly higher concentrations of drug in respiratory tissue than in cerebrospinal fluid, along with other immunologic and host defense factors which influence clinical outcome. Some authors have modified the MIC breakpoints set forth by the NCCLS for defining intermediate and resistant isolates when applied to pneumococcal pneumonia, since the original breakpoints were based on data available for meningitis. Little information is available concerning the newer quinolones such as trovafloxacin in this setting. Recommendations are as follows:

Recommended Treatment for Pneumonia Due to DRSP

Penicillin MIC	Ceftriaxone MIC	Recommended Therapy
<0.1 µg/mL	<8.0 µg/mL	For outpatient therapy (clinically mild disease), oral β-lactam antibiotics (amoxicillin, cefuroxime axetil, and others) with or without a single dose of ceftriaxone
		For inpatient therapy, I.V. penicillin or cefuroxime. Alternative, third generation cephalosporin.*
>2.0 µg/mL	<8.0 µg/mL	Ceftriaxone or cefotaxime*
>2.0 µg/mL	≥8.0 µg/mL	Vancomycin

* Some authors feel that a third generation cephalosporin such as ceftriaxone is not justified in this situation due to the likelihood of success with penicillin or cefuroxime

Drug Therapy
Recommended
Meningitis:
  Ceftriaxone *on page 655*
    in combination with
  Vancomycin *on page 967*
    with or without
  Rifampin *on page 902*

Pneumonia:
  Vancomycin *on page 967*
Alternate
Pneumonia:
  Levofloxacin *on page 795*
  Sparfloxacin *on page 921*
  Grepafloxacin *on page 752*

Selected Readings
Campbell GD and Silberman R, "Drug-Resistant *Streptococcus pneumoniae*," *Clin Infect Dis*, 1998, 26(5):1188-95.

"Defining the Public Health Impact of Drug-Resistant *Streptococcus pneumoniae*: Report of a Working Group," *MMWR Morb Mortal Wkly Rep*, 1996, 45(RR-1):1-20.

Kaplan SL, "*Streptococcus pneumoniae*: Impact of Antibiotic Resistance in Pediatrics," *Curr Probl Pediatr*, 1997, 27(5):187-95.

Klugman KP and Feldman C, "The Clinical Relevance of Antibiotic Resistance in the Management of Pneumococcal Pneumonia," *Infect Dis Clin Pract*, 1998, 7:180-4.

Tomasz A, "Antibiotic Resistance in *Streptococcus pneumoniae*," *Clin Infect Dis*, 1997, 24(Suppl 1):S85-8.

Streptococcus pyogenes

Synonyms GABHS; Group A β-Hemolytic *Streptococcus*; Group A *Strepto-coccus*

Microbiology *Streptococcus pyogenes* are gram-positive, spherical cocci, which frequently appear in chains. Group A refers to a specific carbohydrate (Lancefield) antigen which is part of the cell wall and is used for serogrouping streptococcal species. The M-protein, of which there are more than 100 sero-types, is associated with resistance to phagocytosis by polymorphonuclear leukocytes. M-protein acts by decreasing alternative complement pathway acti-vation and thereby limiting deposition of C3 on the surface of the bacteria. Immunity results from the development of type specific antibodies to the M-protein. Serum antibodies are thought to be protective against invasive infection but do not prevent the carrier state. Lipoteichoic acid on the surface of group A streptococci is responsible for binding the bacteria to the epithelial cell membranes of the oropharynx initiating colonization which is the first stage in infection. The hyaluronic acid capsule also is an additional virulence factor. Extracellular products produced by group A streptococci include streptolysin O, deoxyribonuclease B (DNase B), and hyaluronidase. These antigens evoke the formation of antibodies which (when detected in serum) confirm recent strepto-coccal infection in cases of acute glomerulonephritis or acute rheumatic fever. In addition, DNases A, C, and D; streptolysin S; proteinase; nicotinamide adenine deaminase; streptokinase; and the pyrogenic exotoxins A, B, C, and D are produced. These exotoxins cause the rash of scarlet fever, alter the blood-brain barrier, damage organs and may cause shock, block the reticuloendothelial system, and alter T-cell function. The effects of these toxins are thought to be mediated by hypersensitivity of the host to the toxins, as well as the direct toxic effect. In culture at 35°C, *Streptococcus pyogenes* is β-hemolytic on blood agar. Streptococci are catalase-negative. Presumptive diagnosis can be made by bacitracin susceptibility followed by confirmation using agglutination or coagglu-tination or other rapid antigen-antibody specific tests.

Epidemiology Infections due to *Streptococcus pyogenes* are ubiquitous in temperate and semitropical areas. They are less common in the tropics. Inap-parent infections are as frequent as clinical infections. Serotypes associated with acute glomerulonephritis include 1, 3, 4, 12, and 25 in association with throat infections and 2, 4, 9, 55, 57, 58, 59, and 60 in association with skin infections. M types associated with rheumatic fever include 1, 3, 5, 6,14, 18, 19, and 24. The lists are not comprehensive.

Rheumatic fever remains a major public health concern in developing countries. Strep throat occurs with a peak incidence in late winter and spring. Children and adolescents are most often affected. Outbreaks occur in school and military recruit populations. Foodborne epidemics may occur during any season. The outbreaks are most frequently associated with milk, milk products, deviled eggs, and egg salad. The reservoir for *Streptococcus pyogenes* is man; transmission is by direct or intimate contact. Transmission by hand contact or objects is rare. Nasal carriers are particularly prone to transmit the disease. Eradication of the carrier state may require several courses of antimicrobials and is difficult.

Clinical Syndromes *Streptococcus pyogenes* is a frequently encountered and ubiquitous pathogen. Acute pharyngitis ("strep throat") and impetigo or pyoderma are the most common clinical presentations. Other manifestations include septicemia, otitis, sinusitis, cellulitis, peritonsillar and retropharyngeal abscess, pneumonia, lymphangitis, gangrene, myositis, vaginitis, peripheral sepsis, perianal cellulitis, and scarlet fever. Group A streptococcal infections are associated with important nonsuppurative sequelae specifically acute glomerulo-nephritis, acute rheumatic fever, and rarely toxic shock-like syndrome.

Patients with streptococcal sore throat may have minimal symptoms or may develop fever, painful sore throat, exudative tonsillitis and/or pharyngitis, and anterior cervical adenopathy. The pharynx, tonsillar pillars, and soft palate may exhibit petechiae against a background of edema and erythema. Otitis media and peritonsillar abscess often complicate severe cases. Acute glomerulone-phritis may follow with a mean time of 10 days. Acute rheumatic fever may follow in 7-35 days with a mean of 19 days.

Scarlet fever is characterized by a fine erythematosus rash which blanches on pressure. It has a sandpaper-like touch and is commonly seen over the neck, chest, folds of the axilla, groin, elbow, and inner thigh. It is the result of infection by a strain-producing erythrogenic toxin to which the patient is sensitive but not immune. Acute glomerulonephritis and rheumatic fever can follow.

The American Heart Association (AHA) guidelines for the diagnosis of initial attack of rheumatic fever (Jones Criteria, 1992 Update). See table.

Guidelines for the Diagnosis of Initial Attack of Rheumatic Fever (Jones Criteria, 1992 Update)*

Major Manifestations†
Carditis
Polyarthritis
Chorea
Erythema marginatum
Subcutaneous nodules
Minor Manifestations‡
Clinical findings
Arthralgia
Fever
Laboratory findings
Elevated acute phase reactants
Erythrocyte sedimentation rate
C-reactive protein
Prolonged PR interval
Supporting Evidence of Antecedent Group A Streptococcal Infection§
Positive throat culture or rapid streptococcal antigen test
Elevated or rising streptococcal antibody titer

*If supported by evidence of preceding group A streptococcal infection, the presence of two major manifestations or of one major and two minor manifestations indicates a high probability of acute rheumatic fever.

From Diagnosis of Rheumatic Fever – Special Writing Group, "Guidelines for the Diagnosis of Rheumatic Fever," *JAMA*, 1992, 268(15):2069-73.

A case definition has been developed for Group A streptococcal toxic shock syndrome (TSS) which should facilitate diagnosis and may lead to the evolution of prevention strategies and more effective therapy. See Tables 1 and 2 on the next page.

Diagnosis Clinical diagnosis of "strep throat" is only 30% to 60% sensitive. Throat culture is the gold standard for the diagnosis of streptococcal pharyngitis. Culture obtained during an active infection in an untreated patient is almost always positive. The culture does not distinguish between acute streptococcal infection and streptococcal carriers with viral infections. The vast majority of symptomatic sore throat patients have viral sore throat. Rapid tests for the detection of Group A streptococcal antigen are specific (~95%), but sensitivity varies widely from 60% to 90%. Their sensitivity is less than that of throat culture. **A negative antigen test should be confirmed by a culture**. The organism is readily recovered by routine aerobic culture from other sites.

Diagnostic Tests/Procedures
Aerobic Culture, Appropriate Site *on page 310*
Antideoxyribonuclease-B Titer, Serum *on page 322*
Antistreptolysin O Titer, Serum *on page 330*
Gram's Stain *on page 426*
Group A *Streptococcus* Antigen Test *on page 428*
Streptozyme *on page 544*
Throat Culture for Group A Beta-Hemolytic *Streptococcus on page 550*

Treatment Patients who have had rheumatic fever are at high risk of suffering recurrent attacks if they develop streptococcal upper respiratory infections. Even asymptomatic infections can cause recurrence, and recurrence can occur in optimally treated symptomatic infections. Thus, continuous prophylaxis with antimicrobials is recommended. This therapy should be continued into the patient's early 20s and for at least 5 years after the last recurrence. Patients who

(Continued)

Streptococcus pyogenes (Continued)

Table 1. Proposed Case Definition for the Streptococcal Toxic Shock Syndrome*

I. Isolation of group A streptococci (*Streptococcus pyogenes*)

A. From a normally sterile site (eg, blood, cerebrospinal, pleural, or peritoneal fluid, tissue biopsy, surgical wound, etc)

B. From a nonsterile site (eg, throat, sputum, vagina, superficial skin lesion, etc)

II. Clinical signs of severity

A. Hypotension: Systolic blood pressure ≤90 mm Hg in adults or <5th percentile for age in children **and**

B. Two or more of the following signs:

- Renal impairment: Creatinine ≥177 μmol/L (≥2 mg/dL) for adults or greater than or equal to twice the upper limit of normal for age. In patients with pre-existing renal disease, a twofold or greater elevation over the baseline level

- Coagulopathy: Platelets ≤100 x 10⁹/L (≤100,000/mm³) or disseminated intravascular coagulation defined by prolonged clotting times, low fibrinogen level, and the presence of fibrin degradation products

- Liver involvement: Alanine aminotransferase (ALT), aspartate aminotransferase (AST), or total bilirubin levels greater than or equal to twice the upper limit of normal for age. In patients with pre-existing liver disease, a twofold or greater elevation over the baseline level

- Adult respiratory distress syndrome defined by acute onset of diffuse pulmonary infiltrates and hypoxemia in the absence of cardiac failure, or evidence of diffuse capillary leak manifested by acute onset of generalized edema, or pleural or peritoneal effusions with hypoalbuminemia

- A generalized erythematous macular rash that may desquamate

- Soft-tissue necrosis, including necrotizing fasciitis or myositis, or gangrene

*An illness fulfilling criteria IA and II (A and B) can be defined as a **definite** case. An illness fulfilling criteria IB and II (A and B) can be defined as a **probable** case if no other etiology for the illness is identified.

Table 2. Classification of Group A Streptococcal Infection*

I. **Streptococcal toxic shock syndrome (streptococcal TSS):** Defined by criteria in Table 1

II. **Other invasive infections:** Defined by isolation of group A streptococci from a **normally sterile site** in patients not meeting criteria for streptococcal TSS

A. Bacteremia with no identified focus

B. Focal infections with or without bacteremia. Includes meningitis, pneumonia, peritonitis, puerperal sepsis, osteomyelitis, septic arthritis, necrotizing fasciitis, surgical wound infections, erysipeas, and cellulitis

III. **Scarlet fever:** Defined by a scarlatina rash with evidence of group A streptococcal infection, most commonly pharyngotonsillitis

IV. **Noninvasive infections:** Defined by the isolation of group A streptococci from a nonsterile site

A. Mucous membrane: Includes pharyngitis, tonsillitis, otitis media, sinusitis, vaginitis

B. Cutaneous: Includes impetigo

V. **Nonsuppurative sequelae:** Defined by specific clinical findings with evidence of a recent group A streptococcal infection

A. Acute rheumatic fever

B. Acute glomerulonephritis

*Examples of conditions in each category are not inclusive.

From Streptococcal Toxic Shock Syndrome Case Definition Working Group, "Defining the Group A Streptococcal Toxic Shock Syndrome," *JAMA*, 1993, 269(3):390-1.

have had carditis are at relatively high risk for recurrences of carditis. Discontinuance of prophylaxis should not be undertaken without consideration of the epidemiological risk factors for the particular patient (ie, likelihood of exposure to school children, day care, military recruit, college student, etc). The American Heart Association (AHA) has recommended the following therapy.

Primary Prevention of Rheumatic Fever
(Treatment of Streptococcal Tonsillopharyngitis)

Agent	Dose	Mode	Duration
Benzathine penicillin G	600,000 units for patients <60 lb 1,200,000 units for patients >60 lb	I.M.	Once
	or		
Penicillin V (phenoxymethyl penicillin)	250 mg 3 times/day	P.O.	10 days
For individuals allergic to penicillin:			
Erythromycin estolate	20-40 mg/kg/day 2-4 times/day (maximum: 1 g/day)	P.O.	10 days
	or		
Erythromycin ethylsuccinate	40 mg/kg/day 2-4 times/day (maximum: 1 g/day)	P.O.	10 days

The following agents are acceptable but usually not recommended: amoxicillin, dicloxacillin, oral cephalosporins, and clindamycin.

The following are not acceptable: sulfonamides, trimethoprim, tetracyclines, and chloramphenicol.

From Dajani AS, Bisno AL, and Chung KJ, "Prevention of Rheumatic Fever," *Circulation,* American Heart Association, 1988, 78:1082-6.

Secondary Prevention of Rheumatic Fever
(Prevention of Recurrent Attacks)

Agent	Dose	Mode
Benzathine penicillin G	1,200,000 units	I.M., every 4 weeks*
	or	
Penicillin V	250 mg twice daily	P.O.
	or	
Sulfadiazine	0.5 g once daily for patients <60 lb 1 g once daily for patients >60 lb	P.O.
For individuals allergic to penicillin and sulfadiazine:		
Erythromycin	250 mg twice daily	P.O.

*In high-risk situations, administration every 3 weeks is advised.

From Dajani AS, Bisno AL, and Chung KJ, "Prevention of Rheumatic Fever," *Circulation,* 1988, 78:1082-6.

Drug Therapy
Recommended
Penicillin G, Parenteral, Aqueous *on page 860*
Alternate
Erythromycin *on page 722*
Vancomycin *on page 967*
Cephalosporins, 1st Generation *on page 661*
Selected Readings
Bisno AL, "Group A Streptococcal Infections and Acute Rheumatic Fever," *N Engl J Med,* 1991, 325(11):783-93.

Bisno AL, Gerber MA, Gwaltney JM, et al, "Diagnosis and Management of Group A Streptococcal Pharyngitis: A Practice Guideline. Infectious Diseases Society of America," *Clin Infect Dis,* 1997, 25(3):574-83.

Campos JM, "Laboratory Diagnosis of Group A Streptococcal Pharyngitis," *Infect Dis Clin Prac,* 1993, 2:303-7.

(Continued)

Streptococcus pyogenes (Continued)

Denny FW Jr, "Group A Streptococcal Infections - 1993," *Curr Probl Pediatr*, 1993, 23(5):179-85.

Fiorentino M, "The Return of Rheumatic Fever: A Segue to the Understanding of Group A *Strepto-coccus*," *Clin Microbiol Newslet*, 1996, 18(4):25-9.

Hoge CW, Schwartz B, Talkington DF, et al, "The Changing Epidemiology of Invasive Group A Streptococcal Infections and the Emergence of Streptococcal Toxic-Shock Like Syndrome," *JAMA*, 1993, 269(3):384-9.

"Invasive Group A Streptococcal Infections - United Kingdom, 1994," *MMWR Morb Mortal Wkly Rep*, 1994, 43(21):401-2.

Musher DM, Hamill RJ, Wright CE, et al, "Trends in Bacteremic Infection Due to *Streptococcus pyogenes* (Group A *Streptococcus*), 1986-1995," *Emerg Infect Dis*, 1996, 2(1):54-6.

Schwartz B, Facklam RR, and Breiman RF, "Changing Epidemiology of Group A Streptococcal Infection in the USA," *Lancet*, 1990, 336(8724):1167-71.

Stevens DL, "Streptococcal Toxic-Shock Syndrome: Spectrum of Disease, Pathogenesis, and New Concepts in Treatment," *Emerg Infect Dis*, 1995, 1(3):69-78.

Streptococcus-Related Gram-Positive Cocci

Synonyms Anaerobic *Streptococcus*; SRGPC; *Streptococcus*, Anaerobic

Applies to Microaerophilic Streptococci; *Peptostreptococcus*

Microbiology *Streptococcus*-related gram-positive cocci (SRGPC) which are clinically important include species of the genera *Peptostreptococcus*, *Streptococcus*, and *Gemella*. SRGPC which rarely cause clinical infections include species of the genera *Peptococcus*, *Coprococcus*, *Ruminococcus*, *Sarcina*, and *Staphylococcus saccharolyticus*. *Peptostreptococcus* is the most significant pathogen and is recovered almost as frequently (~25%) as *Bacteroides fragilis* from clinical specimens. *Peptostreptococcus* and *Bacteroides* species are frequently recovered together and in combination with aerobic bacteria in abscess cavities throughout the body. The *Peptostreptococcus* species most frequently recovered include *P. magnus*, *P. asaccharolyticus*, *P. prevotii*, and *P. anaerobius*. SRGPC are speciated by biochemical and chromatographic methods in the laboratory. Reclassification of these species utilizing modern DNA, ribosomal RNA, and cell wall polysaccharide content analyses will continue.

Epidemiology SRGPC comprise a large portion of the normal flora of the mouth, intestinal tract, and vagina. Infections in humans are often the result of contamination from normal flora sites or contiguous extension of infection from colonized sites onto adjacent tissues.

Clinical Syndromes SRGPC are often recovered from abscesses, frequently in polymicrobial infections, at virtually any site in the body. More often than not, SRGPC are contaminants if isolated with other bacteria, and clinical interpretation of their presence is often difficult. Head and neck infections include infection of paranasal sinuses, brain abscess, dental abscess, lateral (pharyngomaxillary) and retropharyngeal space infections, and in Ludwig's angina (bilateral submandibular and sublingual cellulitis often, 50% to 90%, of dental origin). Thoracic infections include lung abscess and empyema. Abdominal infections include liver abscess, visceral abscess, and pelvic and perirectal abscesses. Skin and subcutaneous tissue infections often involve devitalized or necrotic skin, muscle, and subcutaneous tissue. Specific examples include anaerobic streptococcal myositis, a fulminant disease characterized by pain, marked edema, crepitant myositis, and a purulent or seropurulent exudate that on Gram's stain reveals gram-positive cocci in chains. Progressive synergistic gangrene is caused by polymicrobic infection with *Staphylococcus aureus* and microaerophilic or anaerobic streptococci. The infection occurs around surgical incisions as an ulcerated lesion with surrounding gangrenous tissue. Chronic burrowing ulcer is an infection of deep soft tissue. It erodes (burrows) through subcutaneous tissue to erupt as an ulcer at a distant site.

Diagnosis Documentation of the diagnosis of infection with SRGPC requires that potentially contaminating normal flora be excluded from the cultures. Needle aspiration of loculated pus by the percutaneous route is a frequently good approach. Often Gram's stain yields more information than culture because of the fastidious nature of the organisms (difficult to recover by usual laboratory methods) and the frequent polymicrobial nature of the infections.

Diagnostic Tests/Procedures

Anaerobic Culture *on page 316*

Gram's Stain *on page 426*

Duration of Therapy 7-10 days

Treatment Successful therapy for anaerobic and microaerophilic streptococcal infections usually involves debridement or drainage of involved area or abscess and intravenous antimicrobial therapy usually with intravenous penicillin.

Drug Therapy

Recommended

Penicillin G, Parenteral, Aqueous *on page 860*

Alternate

Cephalosporins, 1st Generation *on page 661*

Clindamycin *on page 684*

Vancomycin *on page 967*

Streptococcus salivarius see *Streptococcus*, Viridans Group *on page 279*

***Streptococcus sanguis* I** see *Streptococcus*, Viridans Group *on page 279*

***Streptococcus sanguis* II** see *Streptococcus*, Viridans Group *on page 279*

Streptococcus Species

Refer to

Streptococcus agalactiae on page 266

Streptococcus bovis on page 267

Streptococcus pneumoniae on page 268

Streptococcus pyogenes on page 274

Streptococcus-Related Gram-Positive Cocci *on page 278*

Streptococcus, Viridans Group *on page 279*

Streptococcus, Viridans Group

Synonyms Viridans Streptococci

Applies to *Gemella morbillorum; Streptococcus anginosus; Streptococcus intermedius; Streptococcus milleri* Group; *Streptococcus mitis; Streptococcus morbillorum; Streptococcus mutans; Streptococcus salivarius; Streptococcus sanguis* I; *Streptococcus sanguis* II

Microbiology Historically "viridans" or green streptococci were separated from other "β-hemolytic" strains of streptococci by their ability to produce α-hemolysis ("greening") on blood agar, although many strains produce γ-hemolysis (nonhemolytic). More recently, antigenic, physiological, biochemical, and DNA homology techniques have resulted in more precise characterization of these organisms. The Lancefield serogroup (eg, A, B, C, D, etc) cross species lines. New species are being described and many reclassifications have been made. *S. bovis* and *S. pneumoniae* are α-hemolytic. Upon isolation of α, β, or nonhemolytic streptococci on blood agar, presumptive identification of nongroup A, B, or D can be made be resistance to bacitracin, negative hippurate or CAMP test, negative or weakly reactive bile esculin hydrolysis, negative PYR test, negative pyruvate, and failure to grow in 6.5% NaCl.

Some of these organisms are nutritionally fastidious and can require complex supplemented media. CO_2 may enhance growth. There is no correlation between serogroup and biochemical speciation. Speciation can be accomplished by biochemical testing. *S. morbillorum* has been transferred to the genus *Gemella*.

Clinical Syndromes Clinically, viridans streptococci are associated primarily with endocarditis, although infection of all tissues have been reported. *S. sanguis* I, *S. sanguis* II, and *S. mitis* are most frequently implicated in endocarditis, while *S. intermedius* is associated with noncardiac suppurative infections. *S. anginosus* and *S. constellatus* are closely related and are sometimes classified together with *S. intermedius* and *Streptococcus* MG as *Streptococcus milleri* or *S. milleri* group.

Viridans streptococci often pose a problem as they may be detected in blood culture as the result of transient insignificant bacteremia or may represent insignificant contaminants. Fifty percent of all bacterial endocarditis is due to viridans streptococci which is often diagnosed in patients with valvular heart disease. The course is subacute with cure rates in excess of 90%. Transient seeding of the blood by viridans streptococci is regarded as a commonplace occurrence. The organism has low intrinsic virulence. See table on next page.

Diagnosis Diagnosis is usually accomplished by repeated positive blood culture or recovery of the organism in cultures from the affected site.

(Continued)

Streptococcus Viridans Group

Species	Alternate Nomenclature	Lancefield Groups	Normal Human Habitat	Normal Veterinary Habitat	Human Disease	Veterinary Disease
S. acidominimus		NG, E, F	Oropharynx, teeth surface, skin, intestinal tract	Milk, genital and intestinal tracts	Rare	—
S. anginosus, S. constellatus, S. intermedius	S. milleri	NG, A, C, F, G, K	Oropharynx, teeth surface, skin, intestinal tract		Endocarditis, suppurative infections, abcesses, bacteremia	—
S. bovis		D	Genital and intestinal tracts	Bovine and sheep – intestinal tracts	Endocarditis, bacteremia	Endocarditis
S. cremoris		N	Oropharynx	Milk	Rare	Mastitis
S. dysgalactiae	S. equisimilis	C, G, L	Upper respiratory tract, skin, vagina	Bovine and sheep	—	Mastitis
S. lactis		N	Oropharynx	Milk	Rare	Mastitis
S. mitis S. sanguis II	S. mitior	NG, A, C, F, G, H, K, M, O	Oropharynx, intestinal tract		Endocarditis, caries	—
S. morbillorum	Gemella morbillorum	NG	Intestinal and urogenital tracts		Endocarditis, suppurative infections	—
S. mutans		NG, E, F, K	Teeth surface, intestinal tract		Endocarditis, caries	—
S. pneumoniae		—	Upper respiratory tract		Common	—
S. salivarius		NG, F, H, K	Oropharynx, intestinal tract		Endocarditis	—
S. sanguis I	S. mitior	NG, C, F, H, K	Teeth surface, intestinal tract		Endocarditis, caries	—
S. suis		D (R, S, T)		Swine	Rare	Bacteremia, bone and joint infections
S. uberis		NG, E, F, K		Milk, oropharynx, skin, intestinal tract	Rare	Mastitis

NG = nongroupable.

Adapted from Gallis HA, "Viridans and β-Hemolytic (Non-Group A, B, and D) Streptococci," *Principles and Practice of Infectious Diseases*, Mandell GL, Douglas RG Jr, and Bennett JE, eds, New York, NY: Churchill Livingstone, 1990; 1563-72, with permission.

Diagnostic Tests/Procedures
Aerobic Culture, Appropriate Site *on page 310*
Blood Culture, Aerobic and Anaerobic *on page 337*
Gram's Stain *on page 426*
Duration of Therapy Endocarditis: 4 weeks; nonendocarditis: 7-10 days
Treatment Susceptibility testing has not been standardized for fastidious CO_2-requiring *Streptococcus* species. Most isolates are reported to be susceptible to penicillin with MICs <0.06 µg/mL. Rare isolates have penicillin MICs >1.0 µg/mL. Other effective agents include cephalosporins (first and second generation), cefotaxime, clindamycin, erythromycin, and vancomycin. *In vitro* resistance to aminoglycosides is observed; however, synergy is observed *in vitro* with cell wall active agents.

Penicillin G, 10-20 million units/day I.V. in divided doses every 4 hours for 4 weeks for organisms with an MIC ≤0.1 µg/mL. Addition of gentamicin or streptomycin may result in more rapid cure. Streptomycin dosage 7.5 mg/kg I.M. every 12 hours or gentamicin 1 mg/kg I.V. every 8 hours for the first 2 weeks of therapy with penicillin being continued for the full 4 weeks. An additional alternative in cefazolin 1-2 g I.V. or I.M. every 6-8 hours for 4 weeks.

Vancomycin, 15 µg/kg I.V. every 12 hours for 4 weeks.

Drug Therapy
Recommended
Endocarditis:
Penicillin G, Parenteral, Aqueous *on page 860*
  or
Penicillin G, Parenteral, Aqueous *on page 860*
  used in combination with
Gentamicin *on page 747*
Nonendocarditis:
Penicillin G, Parenteral, Aqueous *on page 860*
Alternate
Endocarditis:
Vancomycin *on page 967*
  or
Vancomycin *on page 967*
  used in combination with
Gentamicin *on page 747*
Nonendocarditis:
Cephalosporins, 1st Generation *on page 661*
Vancomycin *on page 967*
Selected Readings
Bochud PY, Eggiman P, Calandra T, et al, "Bacteremia Due to Viridans *Streptococcus* in Neutropenic Patients With Cancer: Clinical Spectrum and Risk Factors," *Clin Infect Dis*, 1994, 18(1):25-31.
Burden AD, Oppenheim BA, Crowther D, et al, "Viridans Streptococcal Bacteremia in Patients With Haematological and Solid Malignancies," *Eur J Cancer*, 1991, 27(4):409-11.
Elting LS, Bodey GP, and Keefe BH, "Septicemia and Shock Syndrome Due to Viridans Streptococci: A Case-Control Study of Predisposing Factors," *Clin Infect Dis*, 1992, 14(6):1201-7.

Strongyloides stercoralis
Microbiology *Strongyloides stercoralis* is a small roundworm (nematode) which can cause human disease in several ways. The "direct" cycle of infection begins when the human comes in contact with soil containing the worm in its infective (filariform) larval stage. *Strongyloides* penetrates the skin and enters the circulation of the host. When the worms reach the alveolar capillaries, a pulmonary phase begins in which the parasites enter the alveoli and ascend the respiratory tract. Once in the pharynx, the organisms are swallowed. Maturation and reproduction occur in the small intestine. The fertilized adult female burrows into the mucosa of the upper small intestine and begins to lay eggs. The larvae which hatch are in a noninfectious (rhabditiform) stage; they eventually bore through the intestinal epithelium to reach the bowel lumen and are passed in the feces. The rhabditiform larvae can transform to infective filariform larvae in soil, thus completing the cycle.

In addition to this direct cycle, *Strongyloides* can also reproduce without a human host. In this "indirect cycle," larvae are passed into the soil, as described above. If proper environmental conditions are present, larvae mature into adult helminths capable of reproduction. After copulation, large numbers of new larvae are produced, potentially infectious to humans.
(Continued)

Strongyloides stercoralis (Continued)

A less common but clinically important aspect of *Strongyloides* is its "**autoinfection cycle.**" Instead of being passed in the stool, noninfectious larvae transform into infectious larvae in the lumen of the intestine. They can then reenter the host circulation either by boring through the intestinal wall or penetrating the perianal skin. This "autoinfection" can cause repeated infections over the years and at times can be life-threatening because of the associated heavy worm burden ("hyperinfection syndrome").

Epidemiology *Strongyloides* infections occur worldwide. Infections are common in the tropics where the prevalence may approach 50% in some areas. In the United States, the disease is much less common, even in the southern states where the most number of cases are reported (prevalence <4%). In addition to the direct penetration of the skin, *Strongyloides* can be sexually transmitted.

Clinical Syndromes

- **Asymptomatic infection:** About 33% of infected individuals have no symptoms.

- **Abdominal pain and diarrhea (sometimes bloody):** This usually occurs as the larvae hatch in the intestinal mucosa and are passed through the lumen. Complications include ileus, weight loss, and malabsorption syndromes. Important clues to the diagnosis are concomitant peripheral eosinophilia and an urticarial skin rash.

- **Eosinophilic pneumonitis, a Löffler's-type syndrome:** This is similar to other hookworm infections which have a prominent pulmonary phase. Patients present with fever, cough, and wheezing as the larvae migrate through the pulmonary circulation and alveoli. A pruritic rash may be seen.

- **Autoinfection** (see Microbiology): Chronic and recurrent *Strongyloides* infections can occur over months or years because of the organism's ability to autoinfect the host. These patients can present with a wide variety of symptoms, either gastrointestinal (nausea, vomiting, abdominal pain, explosive diarrhea) and/or pulmonary (wheezing, cough) depending on the phase of the parasite's life cycle. Immunocompromised individuals are at risk for life-threatening, disseminated hyperinfections with massive worm burdens. The majority of cases have been reported in organ transplant recipients and in patients with lymphoma or leukemia; in some cases, hyperinfection occurs in otherwise healthy individuals. An overwhelming pneumonitis is characteristically seen with cough, dyspnea, bronchospasm, and sputum production. Peripheral eosinophilia is common but may be absent. Other complications include bacterial sepsis, respiratory failure, bacterial meningitis, and death. The hyperinfection syndrome is an uncommon manifestation of strongyloidiasis.

- ***Strongyloides* in AIDS:** In the past, disseminated *Strongyloides* has been regarded as an AIDS-defining condition in people who are seropositive for HIV. However, it has proven a relatively uncommon occurrence even in patients from endemic areas.

Diagnosis Strongyloidiasis should be suspected in travelers or immigrants from an endemic area and presenting with diarrhea and eosinophilia. It should also be considered in the differential diagnosis of eosinophilic pneumonia (Löffler's-type syndrome) or unexplained diarrhea in an immunocompromised patient. Peripheral eosinophilia, while important, may be absent. In all cases, laboratory confirmation is essential and includes:

- Stool examination to identify the characteristic larval forms (rather than the eggs, which are rarely found). A single negative fecal exam does not rule out strongyloidiasis.

- Duodenal aspiration to identify the organism in the upper intestinal tract. This can be done as part of an upper endoscopic procedure.

Diagnostic Tests/Procedures

Ova and Parasites, Stool *on page 505*

Ova and Parasites, Urine or Aspirates *on page 508*

Treatment The drug of choice for strongyloidiasis is thiabendazole. However, it is well known that treatment failures occur with the standard drug doses for unclear reasons. A recent report has suggested that ivermectin may also be effective in people with AIDS.

Since disseminated *Strongyloides* is seen in organ transplant recipients, individuals from endemic areas awaiting transplantation should be carefully screened and treated if positive.

Drug Therapy
Recommended
Thiabendazole *on page 947*
Ivermectin *on page 787*

Selected Readings
Gompels MM, Todd J, Peters BS, et al, "Disseminated Strongyloidiasis in AIDS: Uncommon but Important," *AIDS,* 1991, 5(3):329-32.

Longworth DL and Weller PF, "Hyperinfection Syndrome With Strongyloidiasis," *Curr Clin Top Infect Dis,* 1986, 10:1-26.

Torres JR, Isturiz R, Murillo J, et al, "Efficacy of Ivermectin in the Treatment of Strongyloidiasis Complicating AIDS," *Clin Infect Dis,* 1993, 17(5):900-2.

Tapeworms see Cestodes *on page 94*

Timing of Food Poisoning see page 1069

Tinea Nigra *see* Dematiaceous Fungi *on page 125*

T-*Mycoplasma* *see* Ureaplasma urealyticum *on page 292*

Toxo *see Toxoplasma gondii on this page*

Toxoplasma gondii

Synonyms Toxo

Microbiology *Toxoplasma gondii* is a sporozoan of the order Coccidia and suborder *Eimeria.* The three forms of *T. gondii* are trophozoites (previously referred as tachyzoites), tissue cysts, and oocysts. The trophozoite is crescent to oval shape, 4 x 8 µm in size, and stains with both Wright and Giemsa stains. The trophozoite invades all nucleated cells, resides in vacuoles, and reproduces to form cysts. Tissue cysts measure 10-200 µm and may contain up to 3000 organisms. These cysts may remain dormant for years and can become reactivated. The organisms stain PAS positive, but the cyst wall itself stains very weakly positive. The oocysts measure 10-12 µm and are produced only in cats. All three forms are pathogenic to humans.

Epidemiology *Toxoplasma* infects nearly all animals and birds. It is the most widely distributed of all intracellular parasites. Prior to the AIDS epidemic, the majority of cases were benign and self-limited. There are still approximately 3000 cases of congenital toxoplasmosis reported per year with an average of 0.6 cases per 1000 pregnancies in the United States. Toxoplasmosis is the most common focal CNS infection in AIDS. It is estimated that 5% to 10% of AIDS patients have toxoplasmosis although 25% to 50% of AIDS patients will have positive IgG titers indicating previous exposure suggesting that reactivation plays an important role. In heart, but not renal or liver, transplantation, 50% of the seronegative recipients who receive seropositive donor hearts develop toxoplasmosis with a mortality rate exceeding 75%. Bone marrow transplant patients appear to be at increased risk of reactivation.

Humans become infected by ingesting the cysts either through contamination with cat feces or undercooked meat, especially pork and lamb, or through direct inoculation via blood transfusions, laboratory accidents, or congenital transmission. After ingestion of the cysts, digestive enzymes disrupt the cyst wall and release viable organisms that invade the mucosa and disseminate.

Clinical Syndromes
- **Asymptomatic lymphadenitis:** Eighty percent to 90% of patients present with asymptomatic cervical lymphadenitis.
- **Mononucleosis syndrome:** Some patients may present with fever, malaise, myalgias, sore throat, maculopapular rash, and hepatosplenomegaly which is self-limited and often confused with viral illnesses such as EBV. Rarely, patients develop myocarditis or pneumonitis.
- **Congenital:** Pregnant women who acquire toxoplasmosis during the first trimester have a 25% risk of fetal transmission resulting in spontaneous abortions, stillborns, or severe disease. Sixty-five percent of infants born to women infected during the third trimester have subclinical infection with ultimately 85% developing chorioretinitis or neurological sequelae. The number of congenital cases continues to decline probably because of increased awareness of food and cat hygiene during pregnancy.
- **Ocular:** Vast majority of chorioretinitis is due to congenital toxoplasmosis. Patients in their second or third decade of life present with blurred vision, scotoma, eye pain, and photophobia. Fundoscopic examination reveals characteristic exudative retinal lesions. Typically bilateral in congenital toxoplasmosis and unilateral in acquired infection.

(Continued)

Toxoplasma gondii (Continued)

- **Pulmonary:** Second most common site after the brain in AIDS patients with CD4 T-cell counts <50 cells/μL. Present with fever, nonproductive cough, and dyspnea. Chest x-ray usually reveals bilateral interstitial infiltrates.
- **Encephalitis:** Increased incidence in homosexual AIDS patients. Patients present with headache, seizures, disorientation, fever, and focal neurological deficits depending on size, location, and number of lesions. MRI is more sensitive than CT. *Toxoplasma* typically appears as multiple small lesions with predilection for corticomedullary junction and basal ganglia, whereas lymphoma usually presents with a large solitary lesion with subependymal spread or ventricular encasement. Differential diagnosis of CNS mass lesions in AIDS is toxoplasmosis 50% to 70%, primary CNS lymphoma 20% to 30%, progressive multifocal leukoencephalopathy 10% to 20%, and, less frequently, Kaposi sarcoma, tuberculosis, fungal, or herpes. Serological test may be of limited value given 3% false-negative and increased seropositivity in AIDS.

Diagnosis Diagnosis depends on serological tests and biopsy. Ocular *Toxoplasma* is diagnosed by clinical examination. Biopsy material reveals trophozoites.

Diagnostic Tests/Procedures

Brain Biopsy *on page 352*

Lymph Node Biopsy *on page 482*

Muscle Biopsy *on page 491*

Polymerase Chain Reaction *on page 523*

Toxoplasma Antigen by ELISA *on page 552*

Toxoplasma Serology *on page 552*

Treatment

Acute infection: Treatment should consist of sulfadiazine 1-1.5 g every 6 hours plus pyrimethamine 50-100 mg everyday plus leucovorin. Co-trimoxazole (based on TMP 10 mg/kg/day) every 12 hours may be as efficacious as sulfadiazine/pyrimethamine. If intolerant of sulfa, may substitute sulfadiazine with clindamycin 450-600 mg every 6 hours. In patients intolerant of either sulfadiazine or clindamycin, the following may be substituted: azithromycin 1200 mg orally daily, clarithromycin 1 g orally twice daily or atovaquone 750 mg orally 4 times/day plus pyrimethamine and folinic acid. Induction therapy should be given for at least 6 weeks until the lesions have resolved or stabilized at a reduced size. Ninety percent of patients will show clinical or radiographic improvement within 10-14 days of therapy. Patients without either clinical or radiographic improvement should have brain biopsy to confirm diagnosis.

A commonly employed presumptive diagnostic method is to empirically treat all AIDS patients with mass lesions for 2 weeks with antitoxoplasmosis agents and then re-evaluate clinically and radiographically. However, in patients with a negative toxoplasmosis IgG and the absence of the characteristic toxoplasmosis lesions on MRI or presence of lesions suggestive of lymphoma, the likelihood of toxoplasmosis is significantly less than 1%, and it is recommended that the patient undergo an immediate brain biopsy for definitive diagnosis and prompt appropriate intervention.

Maintenance (chronic suppression): Patients must be continued on suppressive therapy to avoid reactivation. Sulfadiazine 500-1000 mg orally every 6 hours plus pyrimethamine 25-75 mg orally daily plus folinic acid 10 mg orally daily (A 3 times/week regimen of sulfadiazine 1 g twice daily plus pyrimethamine 50 mg plus folinic acid 10 mg revealed similar efficacy in a small study.) or co-trimoxazole (based on 5 mg/kg TMP) orally every 12 hours. Alternate: Clindamycin 300-450 mg orally every 6 hours plus pyrimethamine 25-75 mg orally daily and folinic acid 10 mg orally daily.

In patients intolerant of either sulfadiazine or clindamycin, the following may be substituted (unknown efficacy): atovaquone, azithromycin, clarithromycin, or dapsone. Dapsone should not be used for acute infection as it has no effect on tissue cysts but may be used as an alternate for chronic suppressive therapy.

Prophylaxis: Preventive measures include avoidance of cat feces and freezing at -20°C, thawing, and heating to >60°C to destroy cysts in contaminated meats.

Chemoprophylaxis should be initiated if a patient has a CD4 count <100 cells/µL and is seropositive for IgG antibody to *T. gondii* and is not already receiving a regimen for PCP prophylaxis that is also effective for toxoplasmosis.

Current recommended prophylaxis: Co-trimoxazole DS orally daily; dapsone 50-100 mg orally daily plus pyrimethamine 50 mg and leucovorin 25 mg/week; or dapsone 200 mg plus pyrimethamine 75 mg and leucovorin 25 mg/week. Efficacy of clindamycin/pyrimethamine, macrolides, or atovaquone for prophylaxis is unknown.

Drug Therapy
Recommended
Pyrimethamine *on page 886*
  used in combination with
Sulfadiazine *on page 929*
Co-Trimoxazole *on page 692*

Alternate
Clindamycin *on page 684*
  used in combination with
Pyrimethamine *on page 886*

Selected Readings
Campagna AC, "Pulmonary Toxoplasmosis," *Semin Respir Infect*, 1997, 12(2):98-105.

Franzen C, Altfeld M, Hegener P, et al, "Limited Value of PCR for Detection of *Toxoplasma gondii* in Blood From Human Immunodeficiency Virus-Infected Patients," *J Clin Microbiol*, 1997, 35(10):2639-41.

Joiner KA and Dubremetz JF, "*Toxoplasma gondii*: A Protozoan for the Nineties," *Infect Immun*, 1993, 61(4):1169-72.

McCabe R and Chirurgi V, "Issues in Toxoplasmosis," *Infect Dis Clin North Am*, 1993, 7(3):587-604.

Torre D, Casari S, Speranza F, et al, "Randomized Trial of Trimethoprim-Sulfamethoxazole Versus Pyrimethamine-Sulfadiazine for Therapy of Toxoplasmic Encephalitis in Patients with AIDS. Italian Collaborative Study Group," *Antimicrob Agents Chemother*, 1998, 42(6):1346-9.

Torres RA, Weinberg W, Stansell J, et al, "Atovaquone for Salvage Treatment and Suppression of Toxoplasmic Encephalitis in Patients With AIDS. Atovaquone/Toxoplasmic Encephalitis Study Group," *Clin Infect Dis*, 1997, 24(3):422-9.

Wong SY and Remington JS, "Toxoplasmosis in Pregnancy," *Clin Infect Dis*, 1994, 18(6):853-61.

Treponema pallidum
Related Information
HIV Therapeutic Information *on page 1008*

Microbiology *Treponema pallidum* (subspecies *pallidum*) is a thin, gram-negative bacterium which belongs to the order Spirochaetales. It is one of the clinically important spirochetes and is thus related to such agents as *Borrelia burgdorferi* (the cause of Lyme disease) and *Leptospira* (the cause of leptospirosis). *T. pallidum* is the etiologic agent of syphilis. The organism is thin, long, helical, and coiled and is difficult to see by light microscopy. Visualization of the organism in clinical specimens requires special techniques other than the Gram's stain or Giemsa stain. There are no clinically available culture systems for *T. pallidum*, and microbiologic identification of the organism depends on such techniques as darkfield microscopy, direct fluorescent antibody stains, silver stains, and serologic tests.

Epidemiology Syphilis occurs exclusively in humans. The vast majority of cases are acquired via sexual contact with an infected person. Other modes of acquisition include congenital transmission to the newborn and blood transfusion, but these are much less common.

Despite public health measures, the incidence of syphilis has continued to increase to epidemic proportions. In the United States, the number of syphilis cases increased dramatically in the late 1980s, with a near doubling of total reported cases. In 1992, there were over 120,000 reported cases of syphilis (at all stages), but this number grossly underestimates the true number of infections since many cases are undiagnosed. In many urban areas in the U.S., the number of syphilis cases has increased dramatically despite a lower incidence in the homosexual community, the population previously at highest risk. In large part, this change in the at-risk population is due to the increased use of crack cocaine and the exchange of sex for drugs. Sex partners are almost impossible to locate in some urban areas and a substantial number of crack users have undiagnosed syphilis. Currently, the groups at highest risk for syphilis are black, heterosexual men and black, heterosexual women. There has also been an increase in the number of cases of congenital syphilis corresponding roughly to the increase in primary and secondary syphilis in heterosexual women.

(Continued)

Treponema pallidum (Continued)

Sexual partner notification remains an important part of infection control measures. About 50% of partners named by an actively infected individual will also have syphilis; many partners will either be actively infected themselves or will have incubating syphilis.

Clinical Syndromes Syphilis commonly presents in one of several stages: primary, secondary, latent (early latent and late latent), or tertiary syphilis. However, it should be remembered that syphilis has been called "the great mimic" in medical literature because of its protean manifestations and tendency to mimic other diseases.

- **Primary syphilis:** This is an important cause of the common clinical syndrome of "genital ulceration with regional lymphadenopathy". This syndrome is caused by syphilis, primary herpes simplex virus infection, lymphogranuloma venereum, donovanosis, and chancroid. It may be difficult for the clinician to diagnose this on the basis of clinical findings alone. The hallmark of primary syphilis is the genital chancre. The syphilitic chancre is typically a single, painless ulcer with raised and indurated borders. The base of the ulcer is clean, usually without purulence. Up to 33% of syphilitic ulcers, however, may be mildly painful. The chancre can be found on the penis, rectum, anal verge, mouth, labia, or cervix. In the absence of treatment, chancres persist for up to 6 weeks. In addition, inguinal lymphadenopathy is present in the majority of cases of primary syphilis (about 80%). The onset of adenopathy usually occurs at the same time as the genital lesion. Characteristically, the adenopathy is painless (like the chancre), and the nodes are firm. In 70% of cases, the adenopathy is bilateral. Constitutional symptoms are usually absent in primary syphilis. In some individuals, primary syphilis goes unnoticed, especially if the chancre is small and painless. The chancre is teeming with live and active organisms and is an excellent source of material (serum and lymphatic fluid) for a darkfield examination.

- **Secondary syphilis:** In the absence of specific therapy for primary syphilis, further clinical manifestations may develop. Secondary syphilis may occur up to 2 years after initial infection. In secondary syphilis, there is evidence of a systemic illness and often the diagnosis may be difficult to make. The manifestations of secondary syphilis are protean. The most common finding is a skin rash, which is present in about 90% of cases. This rash may be macular, papular, papulosquamous, pustular, or nonspecific. The rash of secondary syphilis is somewhat unique in that it often involves the palms of the hands and soles of the feet; only a limited number of infectious and noninfectious conditions cause a rash in this distribution. In secondary syphilis, mouth or throat lesions are present in about 33% of cases, and the original genital chancre may still be present in some (15% to 20%). Hair loss can be an important clue to the diagnosis; involvement of the hair follicles (follicular syphilides) causes areas of alopecia. Condylomata lata are large fleshy papular lesions that may form in the perianal and genital areas and are characteristic of secondary syphilis. Constitutional symptoms such as fevers, myalgias, and weight loss are also common. There may be evidence of central nervous system involvement in a number of cases; about 1% to 2% met present with acute meningitis, both clinically and by cerebrospinal fluid analysis. A larger number (up to 40%) may have asymptomatic abnormalities in the spinal fluid. The Centers for Disease Control have stated that a routine lumbar puncture in secondary lues is not indicated. However, if there is evidence of auditory, cranial nerve, meningeal, or ocular manifestations of syphilis, a lumbar puncture and careful ophthalmologic exam (including slit-lamp) should be performed.

  A variety of unusual manifestations of secondary syphilis have been well-described including nephropathy, hepatitis, arthritis, colitis, and others.

- **Latent syphilis:** The natural history of untreated secondary syphilis is that the illness resolves spontaneously after 3-12 weeks, although viable organisms persist. In the absence of specific treatment, patients enter a stage of "latency". These patients have no symptoms related to syphilis, and the only clue for the diagnosis of latent infection is a positive serologic test for syphilis. It is important for the physician to perform a careful history and physical examination looking for signs and symptoms of tertiary syphilis;

only then should patients be classified as truly "latent". Patients are classified as having "early latent" disease if they are asymptomatic and have acquired infection within the past year. Those with no symptoms and infection of longer than 1-year duration are said to have "late latent" syphilis. In the asymptomatic patient with a positive serology, it may sometimes be difficult to distinguish early from late latent disease.

The role of lumbar puncture in latent syphilis has recently been addressed by the Centers for Disease Control. The yield of spinal fluid analysis in detecting unsuspected tertiary syphilis in a patient who appears to have only latent syphilis is low. Lumbar puncture should be considered in the following situations:
- patients with neurologic abnormalities
- evidence of other syphilitic disease, such as aortitis, gummas, iritis
- treatment failure
- concomitant HIV infection
- RPR or VDRL titer >1:32, unless infected <1 year
- if treatment with antibiotics other than penicillin is anticipated
• **Tertiary syphilis:** This includes the following:
- asymptomatic neurosyphilis
- symptomatic neurosyphilis, or tabes dorsalis
- cardiovascular syphilis
- syphilitic uveitis
- late benign syphilis (gummas)
• **Syphilis and AIDS:** Syphilis in the HIV-infected individual can be highly aggressive. Patients progress from primary to tertiary syphilis over several years, as opposed to several decades in the non-HIV infected individual. When the clinical findings suggest syphilis (at any stage) but the standard serologic tests are negative, the diagnosis should be pursued with a biopsy, darkfield exam, or DFA antibody staining. Treatment of syphilis in the AIDS patient is no different; penicillin should be used if at all possible. A lumbar puncture should be considered in any patient with HIV and syphilis. A VDRL or RPR should be obtained at 1, 2, 3, 6, 9, and 12 months. If the titers fail to decrease fourfold, retreat with penicillin and perform a lumbar puncture.

Diagnosis The definitive methods for diagnosing early syphilis are darkfield examination (of active lesions) and direct fluorescent antibody tests on active lesions or tissue biopsies. Serologic tests for syphilis, while commonly used, are not diagnostic. A presumptive diagnosis of active syphilis can be made using one of various serologic tests, which are classified as follows:

   Nontreponemal tests: Venereal Disease Research Laboratory (VDRL), rapid plasma reagin (RPR)
   Treponemal: Fluorescent treponemal antibody absorbed test (FTA-ABS), microhemagglutination assay for antibody to *Treponema pallidum* (MHA-TP), and *Treponema pallidum* immobilization test (TPI)

Both a treponemal and nontreponemal test are generally necessary to presumptively diagnose primary syphilis. As a rule, the treponemal tests stay positive for life following the initial infection, whether or not appropriate therapy has been administered. Since treponemal tests do not correlate with disease activity, they are usually reported as either positive or negative. In contrast, nontreponemal tests do correlate with the activity of disease, reaching high titers with primary infection or recent reinfection and falling over time following appropriate therapy. Nontreponemal tests are reported as quantitative titers. The adequacy of therapy can be determined using serial RPR (or VDRL) tests; ideally the same test in the same laboratory should be followed sequentially.

In primary syphilis, the VDRL is positive in about 70% of cases (treated or untreated), and the RPR is positive in about 80% of cases. Thus, it is important to realize that a substantial number of patients with a typical syphilitic chancre may have a negative nontreponemal test. In contrast, the VDRL and RPR are positive in nearly 100% of individuals with secondary syphilis, treated or untreated.

The treponemal tests may also be falsely negative in primary syphilis. The percent positive for the FTA-ABS is 85%, for the MHA-TP is 65%, and the TPI is 50%.

The sensitivity of the specific diagnostic tests for syphilis are summarized in the following table.
(Continued)

Treponema pallidum (Continued)

Diagnostic Tests in Syphilis

Test	Primary*	Secondary*	Late†
Nontreponemal			
VDRL	70	99-100	1
RPR	80	99-100	0
Treponemal			
FTA-ABS	85	100	98
TPHA or MHA-TP	65	100	95

*Treated or untreated

†Treated

Diagnostic Tests/Procedures

Darkfield Examination, Syphilis *on page 394*
FTA-ABS, Cerebrospinal Fluid *on page 409*
FTA-ABS, Serum *on page 410*
MHA-TP *on page 488*
RPR *on page 530*
VDRL, Cerebrospinal Fluid *on page 570*

Treatment The proper treatment of syphilis depends on the stage of infection. Primary, secondary, and early latent syphilis (defined as syphilis of <1-year duration) are treated with benzathine penicillin G, 2.4 million units I.M. (one dose). For the penicillin-allergic patient, the alternative is doxycycline, 100 mg orally twice daily for 2 weeks.

The recommended therapy for the respective stages of syphilis are summarized in the table.

Syphilis Therapy

Stage	Recommended	Alternative
Primary	Benzathine penicillin G I.M.: 2.4 million units x 1	Doxycycline P.O.: 100 mg twice daily for 2 weeks*
Secondary		
Early latent <1 year		
Latent >1 year	Benzathine penicillin G I.M.: 2.4 million units every week x 3	Doxycycline P.O.: 100 mg twice daily for 4 weeks*
Gummas		
Cardiovascular		
Neurosyphilis	Aqueous penicillin G I.V.: 12-24 million units/day for 14 days	Procaine penicillin I.M.: 2-4 million units/day and probenecid 500 mg 4 times/day for 10-14 days

*Avoid tetracyclines during pregnancy.

From U.S. Public Health Service Recommendations, "1993 Sexually Transmitted Diseases Treatment Guidelines," *MMWR Morbid Mortal Wkly Rep*, 1993, 42:1-102.

Drug Therapy

Recommended

Primary, secondary, latent syphilis:
Penicillin G Benzathine, Parenteral *on page 859*
Neurosyphilis:
Penicillin G, Parenteral, Aqueous *on page 860*

Alternate

Primary, secondary, latent syphilis:
Doxycycline *on page 713*
Neurosyphilis:
Penicillin G Procaine *on page 862*

Selected Readings

Hook EW 3d, "Diagnosing Neurosyphilis," *Clin Infect Dis*, 1994, 18(3):295-7.

Hook EW 3d and Marra CM, "Acquired Syphilis in Adults," *N Engl J Med*, 1992, 326(16):1060-9.

Lukehart SA and Holmes KK, "Syphilis," *Harrison's Principles of Internal Medicine*, 13th ed, Isselbacher KJ, Braunwald E, Wilson JD, et al, eds, New York, NY: McGraw-Hill, 1994, 726-36.

Musher DM "Syphilis," *Infect Dis Clin North Am*, 1987, 1(1):83-95.

Musher DM, Hamill RJ, and Baughn RE, "Effect of Human Immunodeficiency Virus (HIV) Infection on the Course of Syphilis and on the Response to Treatment," *Ann Intern Med*, 1990, 113(11):872-81.

"1998 Guidelines for Treatment of Sexually Transmitted Diseases. Centers for Disease Control and Prevention," *MMWR Morb Mortal Wkly Rep*, 1998, 47(RR-1):1-111.

Trichinella spiralis

Microbiology *Trichinella spiralis*, a nematode, is the infectious agent of human trichinosis. The adult male worm measures 1.5 mm in length and the adult female measures 2-4 mm. The average lifespan is 4 months. Identification is made by demonstration of the characteristic encapsulated larvae in biopsy specimens of infected muscles. The cyst wall is derived from the host cell muscle. The larva may incite an inflammatory reaction characterized by surrounding lymphocytes and eosinophils and eventual larval calcification.

Epidemiology *Trichinella* is found worldwide except Australia and several Pacific islands. Trichinosis results from consumption of undercooked pork, unsanitary cooking practices, and contaminated meats. Its reservoirs include pigs, horses, bears, and Arctic mammals. The three subspecies reflect three sylvatic cycles - arctic, temperate, and tropical.

The incidence in the United States continues to decline probably because of increased public awareness, commercial freezing, and legislature prohibiting feeding of raw garbage to swine. From 1982-1986, approximately 57 cases per year were reported with three associated deaths. From 1987-1990, 206 cases were reported to the CDC. Most of the cases reported in the U.S. are associated with improperly cooked game animals and travel to Mexico, Asia, and other endemic areas.

Trichinosis results from ingestion of encysted larvae in the contaminated meat. The acid-pepsin environment in the stomach digest the cyst wall, releasing the infectious larvae which burrow and attach to the mucosa at the base of the villi. Over a 6-10 day period, the larvae molt four times to become sexually mature adult worms which attach to the duodenal and jejunal mucosa producing between 200-1500 larvae over the next 2 weeks. The newborn or first stage larvae penetrate the gut mucosa into the lamina propria. An immunologic reaction partially mediated by IgE-mast cell system results in release of vasoactive substances that promote intestinal motility and secretion (diarrhea). The larvae then migrate into the draining lymphatics and blood vessels and have a high predilection to invade muscles of increased use and blood flow (ie, diaphragm, extraocular muscles, masseters, tongue, deltoids, and gastrocnemius). Once penetrated into the skeletal muscle, the larvae elicit a host inflammatory response which surrounds the larvae and creates granulomas and calcifications. Only larvae that encyst mature. Larvae may remain viable and infective for many years even in calcified cysts.

The severity of the symptoms is directly related to the larvae load. Patients usually remain asymptomatic with 1-10 larvae per gram muscle and systemic illness occurs with 50-100 larvae per gram.

Clinical Syndromes

- **Asymptomatic:** Ninety percent to 95% infections are asymptomatic.
- **Self-limited:** 1-2 weeks after ingestion, patients experience enteric phase associated with nonbloody diarrhea and abdominal cramps. Approximately 2-4 weeks later, patients experience fever, intense myalgia especially extraocular and masseters, periorbital edema, conjunctivitis, headache, and/or subconjunctival and subungual petechia. Ninety percent will have peripheral eosinophilia which peaks at 3-4 weeks. Absence of eosinophilia is a poor prognostic sign. Approximately 50% will have elevated CK and LDH enzymes.
- **Arctic trichinosis:** Described in northern Canada and Alaska in which patients have eaten contaminated walruses or seals. Associated with diarrhea lasting up to 14 weeks, mild and transitory myalgia without fever, peripheral eosinophilia, and no pathogens isolated in stools to explain etiology.
- **Myocarditis:** Incidence of approximately 5% of symptomatic patients. Typically occurs 3 weeks after larvae migration and presents with tachycardia and chest pain mimicking infarction. Patients have myocardium invasion without encystment. EKG reveals benign, reversible nonspecific EKG changes. May develop nonspecific inflammatory myocarditis predominantly eosinophilic and sometimes associated with pericarditis. Fewer than 0.1% patients die from cardiac complications (ie, congestive heart failure).

(Continued)

Trichinella spiralis (Continued)

- **Pulmonary:** Up to 6% symptomatic patients may develop cough and dyspnea on exertion presumed secondary to larvae migration associated with infiltrates, hemorrhage, and allergic granulomatous reactions.
- **CNS:** Prevalence of 10% to 24% in symptomatic patients. In the first 2 weeks when larvae migration is maximal, CNS invasion can occur which appears as meningoencephalitis with delirium and confusion. Larvae encystment may result in focal neurological deficits, anal/urinary sphincter dysfunction, cranial nerve palsies especially VI and VII, seizures, vertigo, anisocoria, tinnitus, diminished auditory acuity, or ataxia. Papilledema, hemianopia, aphasia, and paresis have been reported. CNS and peripheral nerve deficits generally resolve in 4-6 months but may persist up to 10 years. May also cause eosinophilic meningitis. CT scan is usually normal but may see multiple nodular or ring enhancing lesions 3-8 mm and calcification. EEG reveals nonspecific abnormalities consistent with diffuse encephalopathy.

Diagnosis CDC case definition must fit one of two criteria:

1. Positive muscle biopsy or positive serology titer in a patient with clinical symptoms compatible with trichinosis including eosinophilia, fever, myalgias, or periorbital edema.
2. In an outbreak (at least one person must fit above criteria), must have either a positive serology titer or clinical symptoms compatible with trichinosis in a person who shared the implicated meat source.

IgM and IgE serology tests are helpful in distinguishing active from previous infection.

Diagnostic Tests/Procedures
Ova and Parasites, Stool *on page 505*
Trichinella Serology *on page 555*

Treatment Majority of symptomatic patients need supportive care only as infection is self-limited. Benzimidazole carbonates may be given. Mebendazole 200-400 mg three times/day for 3 days followed by 400-500 mg three times/day for 10 days is active against both invasive and encystment stages. Mebendazole does not cross the blood-brain barrier. Thiabendazole 25 mg/kg twice daily for 7 days is indicated to eliminate gut-dwelling adult worms. It is not effective against larval stages in tissue. Not well tolerated secondary to increased gastrointestinal side effects. Albendazole is still under investigation. Steroids (prednisone 40-60 mg daily) may reduce inflammation and is recommended in serious infections.

Overall prognosis is related to severity and intensity of initial infection as well as effectiveness of antiparasitic agents, anti-inflammatory agents, patients immune status, and whether any end-organ damage was rendered. Mortality related to pulmonary, cardiac, and CNS involvement.

All patients traveling outside the United States should receive pre-travel counseling. Smoking, microwaving, and freezing contaminated meats are not reliable means of eliminating trichinosis.

Drug Therapy Comment
Steroids used in combination with mebendazole in serious infections.

Drug Therapy
Recommended
Mebendazole *on page 808*
Alternate
Thiabendazole *on page 947*

Selected Readings
Capó V and Despommier DD, "Clinical Aspects of Infection With *Trichinella* spp," *Clin Microbiol Rev*, 1996, 9(1):47-54.

McAuley JB, Michelson MK, and Schantz PM, "*Trichinella* Infection in Travelers," *J Infect Dis*, 1991, 164(5):1013-6.

Trichomonas vaginalis

Microbiology *Trichomonas vaginalis* is the causative agent of trichomoniasis, a sexually transmitted vaginal infection. *Trichomonas vaginalis* is a flagellated protozoan which exists only in the trophozoite stage. It is easily visualized on wet mount slides under low power and high dry (40x).

Epidemiology The organism is transmitted by sexual intercourse, and the only known reservoir is humans. Occasional transmission can be indirect via contact with contaminated articles. The incubation period is 4-20 days. The period of communicability lasts the duration of the infection. Asymptomatic infections are common.

Clinical Syndromes

- **Vaginitis:** Trichomonas is a common cause of vaginitis and must be distinguished from other causes of vaginitis, such as Candida and Gardnerella vaginalis (the cause of bacterial vaginosis). Typically, there is a vaginal discharge accompanied by vulvar pruritus, dyspareunia, and dysuria. The vaginal discharge is often profuse, thin, frothy, and gray to yellow in color. On pelvic exam, there may be mild erythema of the vaginal walls and endocervix. In severe cases, there are vaginal erosions and petechiae, and occasionally a "strawberry cervix" may be seen where the endocervix is erythematous, granular, and friable. Addition of 10% KOH to the vaginal discharge liberates a fishy odor, as with bacterial vaginosis. On wet prep or Gram's stain, there are many polymorphonuclear cells seen, reflecting the inflammatory nature of this form of vaginitis (as opposed to bacterial vaginosis). On wet prep, the motile trichomonads can be seen under low power and high dry, establishing the diagnosis. Asymptomatic infection is very common, and it is estimated that 50% of women carrying Trichomonas are asymptomatic.

- **Urethritis in males:** Infection with Trichomonas accounts for about 5% of cases of nongonococcal urethritis in males. This is characterized by persistent dysuria with a nonpurulent urethral discharge and may be suspected in patients who have failed the usual tetracycline regimens.

- **Prostatitis:** Trichomonas is a rare but reported cause of prostatitis in males.

Diagnosis The symptoms of vaginitis are not specific enough to distinguish infection with Trichomonas from other causes. In addition, patients may present following exposure to a sexual partner with Trichomonas and have no symptoms. Pelvic examination is mandatory in the female, as is a wet prep of any vaginal discharge. The finding of motile trichomonads is diagnostic. Negative wet mounts may be seen in asymptomatic women or in women who have recently douched. Gram-stained smears are useful in diagnosing bacterial vaginosis but add little to the yield for Trichomonas detection. Occasionally, forms resembling Trichomonas are incidentally found on Papanicolaou smears of the cervix. Since the cytologic smear is not the ideal procedure for identifying this organism, the patient should be promptly re-examined and a fresh wet mount obtained to confirm the presence of the protozoan. Culture techniques for Trichomonas are available in some specialized laboratories but is not usually necessary.

Prostatic and urethral secretions may similarly be examined for motile trichomonads. This may be a reasonable procedure in symptomatic males with persistent symptoms of urethritis where gonorrhea and Chlamydia have been excluded. Occasionally, the organism can be visualized in spun urine sediment.

Diagnostic Tests/Procedures

Trichomonas Preparation on page 555

Treatment Both symptomatic and asymptomatic individuals should be treated, the latter to decrease the incidence of reinfection from a sexual partner. The recommended regimen is metronidazole 2 g orally as a single dose. Alternatively, metronidazole can be given as 500 mg orally twice daily for 7 days. If failure occurs on the single dose regimen, the patient should be given the full 7-day regimen. In refractory cases, a patient may be given up to 2 g orally daily for 3-5 consecutive days. Such cases warrant consultation with an Infectious Disease specialist and in vitro testing of the isolate in culture for metronidazole resistance.

The sexual partners should be treated with either the 2 g single dose regimen or the 500 mg twice daily regimen for 7 days. During pregnancy, metronidazole is contraindicated based on data suggesting the drug is mutagenic in rodents. No other agent is reliable, although some authors have suggested clotrimazole intravaginally if necessary in the first trimester. During the second or third trimester of pregnancy, severe cases may be treated with a single 2 g dose at the discretion of the physician.

Drug Therapy Comment

Treat sexual partners as well.

Drug Therapy
Recommended

Metronidazole on page 817

(Continued)

Trichomonas vaginalis (Continued)

Selected Readings

"1998 Guidelines for Treatment of Sexually Transmitted Diseases. Centers for Disease Control and Prevention," *MMWR Morb Mortal Wkly Rep*, 1998, 47(RR-1):1-111.

Krieger JN, Tam MR, Stevens CE, et al, "Diagnosis of Trichomoniasis. Comparison of Conventional Wet-Mount Examination With Cytologic Studies, Cultures, and Monoclonal Antibody Staining of Direct Specimens," *JAMA*, 1988, 259(8):1223-7.

Lossick JG, "The Diagnosis of Trichomoniasis," *JAMA*, 1988, 259(8):1230.

Lossick JG and Kent HL, "Trichomoniasis: Trends in Diagnosis and Management," *Am J Obstet Gynecol*, 1991, 165(4):1217-22.

Sears SD and O'Hare J, "*In Vitro* Susceptibility of *Trichomonas vaginalis* to 50 Antimicrobial Agents," *Antimicrob Agents Chemother*, 1988, 32(1):144-6.

Sugarman B and Mummaw N, "Effects of Antimicrobial Agents on Growth and Chemotaxis of *Trichomonas vaginalis*," *Antimicrob Agents Chemother*, 1988, 32(9):1323-6.

Wolner-Hanssen P, Krieger JN, Stevens CE, et al, "Clinical Manifestations of Vaginal Trichomoniasis," *JAMA*, 1989, 261(4):571-6.

Tubercle Bacillus *see Mycobacterium tuberculosis on page 207*

Tuberculosis Guidelines *see page 1114*

TWAR *see Chlamydia pneumoniae on page 95*

Ureaplasma urealyticum

Synonyms T-*Mycoplasma*

Microbiology *Ureaplasma urealyticum* is a potential human pathogen formerly known as T-*Mycoplasma* (the "T" standing for tiny). The organism belongs to the *Mycoplasma* group (class: Mollicutes; order: Mycoplasmatales, family: Mycoplasmataceae, genus: *Ureaplasma*). As with other *Mycoplasmas*, *Ureaplasma* is one of the smallest free-living organisms in existence, intermediate in size between viruses and bacteria. Important points regarding its microbiology include the organism is very difficult to see using standard light microscopy, the organism picks up the Gram's stain poorly, the lack of a cell wall makes the organism resistant to beta-lactam antibiotics, and *Ureaplasma* demonstrates complex nutritional requirements necessitating special medium for optimal growth in culture.

Because of the fastidious nature of *Ureaplasma*, it is important to consult with the Microbiology Laboratory prior to obtaining cultures, particularly if important body fluids are sent (such as blood cultures, cerebrospinal fluid, synovial fluid, etc). Specimen collection is important; both the proper transport media (eg, 2 SP, Sp-4) and proper swabs (eg, calcium alginate, wire loops, and others) must be used. The organism can occasionally grow in routine blood culture media and blood agar plates, but the yield is low.

Epidemiology Infants: *Ureaplasma* is a common colonizer of the urogenital tract in infants. The organism can be cultured from the genital tract of roughly 33% of female infants. In most cases, the organism is acquired from the mother as the newborn passes through an infected birth canal. Male infants are colonized less frequently. After 2 years, the rate of colonization for both sexes decreases significantly, but some children have persistently positive genital tract cultures. Colonization rates are higher in sexually abused children.

Adults: Colonization of the adult urogenital tract is also quite common, but the pathogenesis is usually from sexual contact. Studies have shown that *Ureaplasma* can be cultured from the cervix and vagina in 40% to 80% of sexually active women, nearly all being asymptomatic. Risk factors for colonization include multiple sexual partners, lower socioeconomic status, and perhaps black race. Adults who are sexually inexperienced have low rates of colonization. Thus, the finding of a positive urogenital culture for *Ureaplasma* must be interpreted cautiously since in many cases the organism is a harmless commensal.

Clinical Syndromes *Ureaplasma* has been associated with a variety of diseases, but many of these associations are supported only at the case report level and remain controversial. The evidence for causality can be divided as follows:

Good evidence supporting the role of *Ureaplasma urealyticum*:

- **Nongonococcal urethritis (NGU) in the adult male:** The etiologic role of *Ureaplasma* in this common syndrome is supported by evidence from animal models and human volunteer studies. In addition, a small number of placebo-controlled antibiotic trials in males with urethritis has demonstrated improvement in urethral symptoms in the group receiving tetracyclines. The number of NGU cases caused by *Ureaplasma* is unknown.

- **Postpartum bacteremia:** *Ureaplasma* has been isolated from blood cultures in case reports of women with postpartum fever following vaginal delivery. Bloodstream infections with *Ureaplasma* have also been reported following abortions. The role of this organism in postpartum or postabortal fever is still unclear since blood cultures for *Ureaplasma* are rarely obtained.

- **Urethroprostatitis:** *Ureaplasma* appears to be a cause of acute urethroprostatitis in rare cases. There is no evidence to date proving *Ureaplasma* as a cause of chronic urethroprostatitis.

- **Epididymitis:** A single case report has shown *Ureaplasma* to be a likely causative pathogen in an acute case of epididymitis.

- **Septic arthritis:** An unusual septic arthritis due to *Ureaplasma urealyticum* has been described in patients with underlying hypogammaglobulinemia. Joint aspirations have yielded the organism in pure culture. Other clinical features that have accompanied the septic arthritis include subcutaneous abscesses and chronic cystitis. Septic arthritis due to *Ureaplasma* has also been reported in renal transplant patients. Important clinical clues to this syndrome include an immunocompromised host, synovial fluid on arthrocentesis that is "culture-negative" on routine testing, evidence of joint destruction without macroscopic purulence in the joint, and lack of improvement on conventional antibiotic therapy.

- **Chorioamnionitis:** Women who carry *Ureaplasma* in the urogenital tract chronically may potentially develop colonization of the endometrium during pregnancy. Cases have been described where *U. urealyticum* has been repeatedly isolated from amniotic fluid containing inflammatory cells. Symptoms may or may not be present. A low-grade chronic amnionitis has been described and may be associated with premature spontaneous labor and delivery.

- **Respiratory infection in newborns:** Increasing evidence has shown that *Ureaplasma* is a potential cause of congenital pneumonia, probably from acquisition *in utero*. Premature, low-birth weight infants appear to be at risk. The clinical spectrum of respiratory infection has ranged from asymptomatic colonization of the airways to overwhelming pneumonia with acute respiratory distress syndrome. In some cases, endotracheal aspirates, lung biopsies, and lung tissue at autopsy have all yielded pure cultures of *Ureaplasma* with histologic evidence of pneumonia. Blood cultures and cerebrospinal fluid may also be positive for *Ureaplasma*. However, it is important to note that *Ureaplasma* is frequently a harmless colonizer of the airways, and the diagnosis of ureaplasmal pneumonia must be made cautiously.

- **Chronic respiratory disease in neonates:** *Ureaplasma* has been implicated as a risk factor for bronchopulmonary dysplasia, based on limited evidence.

- **Newborn meningitis:** Several studies suggest that *Ureaplasma* may be an important but under-recognized cause of meningitis in premature infants. A fulminant meningitis with intraventricular hemorrhage has been described, but there may also be a more chronic and indolent form. This remains a controversial topic.

Limited evidence supporting the role of *Ureaplasma urealyticum*:
- **Pelvic inflammatory disease**
- **Renal calculi**
- **Reiter's syndrome**
- **Infertility**
- **Repeated spontaneous abortions**
- **Pyelonephritis**

Diagnosis Isolation of the organism from the appropriate site or body fluid is essential for confirming the diagnosis, since the clinical syndromes described above are not specific for *Ureaplasma*. The main errors in diagnosis are failure to consider this organism in the differential diagnosis of a disease syndrome, improper specimen collection, and failure to ask the laboratory to specifically culture for *Ureaplasma* (or *Mycoplasma*). Routine culturing techniques can occasionally yield the organism, but this is not recommended. Serologic testing has limited usefulness. The polymerase chain reaction using the 16S rRNA gene sequence has been described but is currently only a research tool.
(Continued)

Ureaplasma urealyticum (Continued)

Another potential error is confusing colonization of *Ureaplasma* at a body site with true disease. Several of the clinical syndromes described above are only loosely associated with the particular disease entity. There is a risk for overdiagnosis and overtreatment.

Diagnostic Tests/Procedures

Genital Culture for *Ureaplasma urealyticum* on page 424

Treatment Because *Ureaplasma* has no cell wall, it is resistant to penicillins, cephalosporins, sulfonamides, and other cell wall-active antibiotics. The organism is often resistant *in vitro* to aminoglycosides, clindamycin, and chloramphenicol. About 90% of *Ureaplasma* strains are sensitive to the tetracyclines, and these are the drugs of choice. Tetracycline resistance has been described and is likely to increase; most strains of tetracycline-resistant *Ureaplasma* remain sensitive to erythromycin. Recent *in vitro* studies have shown a potential role for the quinolones (particularly sparfloxacin), but little clinical data is available yet.

A difficult situation arises when there is life-threatening *Ureaplasma* infection in the newborn. Tetracyclines are generally contraindicated in this age group, but some have reported the use of intravenous doxycycline in severe neonatal meningitis. Erythromycin is the drug of choice in patients younger than 8 years of age, but the penetration into the spinal fluid is poor. Consultation with an Infectious Disease specialist may be warranted in these cases.

Pediatric Drug Therapy

Recommended

Erythromycin on page 722

Alternate

>7 years:

Tetracycline on page 944

Adult Drug Therapy

Recommended

Erythromycin on page 722
Tetracycline on page 944
Doxycycline on page 713

Alternate

Clarithromycin on page 681
Azithromycin on page 613

Selected Readings

Cassell GH, Waites KB, Watson HL, et al, "*Ureaplasma urealyticum* Intrauterine Infection: Role in Prematurity and Disease in Newborns," *Clin Microbiol Rev*, 1993, 6(1):69-87.

Forgacs P, Kundsin RB, Margles SW, et al, "A Case of *Ureaplasma urealyticum* Septic Arthritis in a Patient With Hypogammaglobulinemia," *Clin Infect Dis*, 1993, 16(2):293-4.

Taylor-Robinson D, "*Ureaplasma urealyticum* (T-strain *Mycoplasma*) and *Mycoplasma hominis*," *Principles and Practice of Infectious Diseases*, 4th ed, Mandell GL, Bennett JE, and Dolin R, eds, New York, NY: Churchill Livingstone, 1995, 1713-8.

Valencia GB, Banzon F, Cummings M, et al, "*Mycoplasma hominis* and *Ureaplasma urealyticum* in Neonates With Suspected Infection," *Pediatr Infect Dis J*, 1993, 12(7):571-3.

Waites KB, Bébéar C, Robertson JA, et al, "Laboratory Diagnosis of Mycoplasmal and Ureaplasmal Infections," *Clin Microbiol Newslet*, 1996, 18(14):105-11.

Waites KB, Crouse DT, and Cassell GH, "Antibiotic Susceptibilities and Therapeutic Options for *Ureaplasma urealyticum* Infections in Neonates," *Pediatr Infect Dis J*, 1992, 11(1):23-9.

Varicella-Zoster Virus

Related Information

Immunization Guidelines on page 1041

Synonyms Herpes Zoster; VZV

Microbiology VZV is the cause of two different clinical entities, chickenpox (also called varicella) and shingles (also called zoster or herpes zoster).

Epidemiology Chickenpox (varicella): Approximately 3 million cases of primary chickenpox occur annually, leading to over 500,000 physician visits. Most cases occur in the late winter and spring. Humans are the only known reservoir for VZV. Transmission is probably via respiratory secretions, although this point has been difficult to substantiate. Intimate contact between a susceptible host (who is seronegative) and an individual actively shedding virus is necessary for transmission. Chickenpox still remains predominantly a pediatric disease, with >90% of all cases reported in children younger than 3 years of age. Household contacts of infected children are at high risk for varicella. The estimated secondary attack rate in susceptible family members is about 90%; the secondary attack rate in susceptible school mates approaches 40%. The incubation period between exposure and clinical disease is about 14 days, with a range of 10-20 days. Patients can be infectious and spread virus to others for about 2 days prior to the appearance of any skin rash. Patients remain infectious until all skin vesicles have crusted over (5 days or more).

Shingles (zoster): This is also a common disorder, with nearly 10% of the general population afflicted at some time. Almost 1.5 million physician office visits are for management of shingles. Shingles is predominantly a disease of the elderly, although immunocompromised patients are accounting for an increasing fraction. Cases appear sporadically in the population rather than in clusters, due to the pathogenesis of the disease. Herpes zoster results from reactivation of VZV which has remained latent in dorsal root ganglia of peripheral or cranial nerves since the original episode of chickenpox. The factors that govern both latency and reactivation are still under study, but clearly host immune competency is important. Shingles is not spread from one individual to another in the same manner as chickenpox, although the lesions of herpes zoster do contain active VZV and can potentially infect susceptible individuals.

Clinical Syndromes

- **Chickenpox in the normal child:** In the otherwise healthy child, chickenpox is generally a benign, self-limited infection. Typically, the child presents with fever, malaise, and a new generalized skin eruption. The skin rash is distinctive and consists of hundreds of discrete circular lesions. An individual lesion will pass through several stages over time: lesions first appear as vesicles with clear fluid ("dew drops"), then vesicles containing purulent fluid (pustules), then ruptured pustules, and then hard scabs. New vesicles continue to emerge for several days as older ones reach the scab stage. Thus, the rash of chickenpox characteristically has lesions in all stages of evolution at any single point in time. Patients complain of fatigue, pruritus, and anorexia. Lesions can be found in nearly all areas of the skin, and in some cases, the mucous membranes as well. The disease remains active for about 5 days. Complications are unusual in healthy children. Secondary bacterial infection of excoriated skin lesions is the most common complication in children. A variety of unusual neurologic syndromes has been reported in association with chickenpox including cerebellar ataxia (characterized by vertigo, abnormal gait, fever, and vomiting; usually resolves over weeks without treatment), encephalitis (characterized by confusion, personality changes, and seizures; a particularly worrisome complication, with up to 20% of cases resulting in death), cerebral angiitis, meningitis, and Reye's syndrome (particularly if aspirin is given). In clinical trials, acyclovir has demonstrated a statistically significant benefit in normal children (2-12 years of age) with chickenpox. This benefit, however, is small. New lesion formation was decreased from 2.5 days to 2 days, and the number of lesions was decreased from 350 to 300. Acyclovir did not alter the rate of serious complications or spread of infection within the family. The U.S. Food and Drug Administration has supported the use of acyclovir in this setting. The cost-benefit ratio of routine acyclovir use in normal children is likely to be low, since the disease is usually benign. Supportive care remains the mainstay of treatment.

- **Chickenpox in the healthy adult:** About 10% of adults do not acquire VZV infection in childhood and thus remain susceptible to primary infection later in life. Infection in the adult is more severe than in childhood, with varicella pneumonitis a significant concern. Data derived from studies of military recruits suggest that varicella pneumonia may be underdiagnosed. Pulmonary infiltrates were found on chest x-ray in 16% of all recruits with primary varicella, most of whom had no respiratory complaints.

   Perinatal varicella can occur when a pregnant woman develops chickenpox. This is unusual because most adult females are seropositive and immune. Maternal varicella can result in transmission to the fetus, especially if maternal infection occurs several days before delivery. The fetus may be born with visceral VZV dissemination, central nervous system abnormalities, skin scarring and other defects collectively called the congenital varicella syndrome. Potentially infected neonates are candidates for varicella zoster immune globulin (with or without antiviral drugs).

(Continued)

Varicella-Zoster Virus *(Continued)*

Clinical trials examining chickenpox in normal adolescents and adults have shown acyclovir to be effective when administered within 24 hours of symptoms. The treatment effect demonstrated in this older age group is greater than similar studies in children. The U.S. FDA has also approved the use of oral acyclovir for chickenpox in healthy adults and teenagers. Pregnant women who contract varicella pneumonia are frequently given intravenous acyclovir because of the high mortality of this complication in pregnancy. Newborns with perinatal varicella probably benefit from acyclovir, although formal data to support this practice are limited.

- **Chickenpox in the immunocompromised host:** Morbidity and mortality are high in this population, with >50% of children suffering visceral complications. Mortality approaches 20% overall. Most reported cases of life-threatening varicella have been described in leukemic children. Other risk groups include patients with solid tumors, lymphoproliferative malignancies, and organ transplant recipients. The skin rash tends to be more severe, with delayed time to crusting of lesions. Pneumonitis, hepatitis, and encephalitis are common.

HIV-infected children who develop chickenpox are also at risk for serious disease. In addition to the visceral complications as noted above, these children are at risk for an unusual, chronic form of the infection, where recurrent vesicular eruptions take place. Several clinical trials have been performed to examine the efficacy of antiviral agents in this setting. Acyclovir decreased the incidence of varicella pneumonia but did not alter the natural history of skin lesions. Intravenous acyclovir has been recommended for both adults and children who are immunosuppressed.

- **Shingles in the normal host:** Most cases of shingles occur in normal individuals 60-90 years of age, although cases have been reported in all age groups including children. Reactivation of VZV is heralded by localized pain along a dermatomal distribution, the phase of "acute neuritis". After 2-3 days of pain, the skin erupts with papules and vesicles along the same unilateral dermatomal distribution. As with primary varicella, the skin lesions evolve from fluid-filled vesicles into pustules and later scabs. The number of skin lesions is variable. Pain can be quite severe and may require narcotics. New lesions continue to form over 3-5 days. The disease stays active for about 1 week, but complete healing requires several additional weeks, particularly in the elderly.

Selective involvement of the ophthalmic branch of the trigeminal nerve (cranial nerve V) is called herpes zoster ophthalmicus. Keratitis, uveitis, and other ocular complications may result in visual loss if untreated. Involvement of the geniculate ganglion results in the Ramsay Hunt syndrome - vesicles in the external auditory canal, facial palsy, and loss of taste in the anterior two-thirds of the tongue. Other serious complications of herpes zoster in the normal host include cutaneous dissemination and aseptic meningitis. Unlike chickenpox, visceral complications such as pneumonitis and hepatitis are rare. The most common complication of herpes zoster is postherpetic neuralgia, particularly problematic in the elderly. The incidence of this is unclear. Pain persists in the involved dermatome for months after the skin eruption has resolved. Narcotics are only partially helpful, and patients may be quite disabled from the pain; nerve blocks have been attempted with variable success.

Several clinical trials have been conducted to evaluate the efficacy of acyclovir in herpes zoster in the normal adult. Acyclovir improved the healing time of skin lesions (only by 24 hours) but had a variable and often negligible effect on postherpetic neuralgia. This is an important limitation because postherpetic neuralgia is the most commonly encountered complication and a particularly frustrating problem for physicians. The U.S. FDA has recommended licensure of acyclovir in this setting, but other experts believe the benefit of acyclovir to be small and decisions regarding treatment should by made on a case-by-case basis. Certainly herpes zoster ophthalmicus and other complications warrant prompt treatment.

- **Herpes zoster in the immunocompromised host:** Severe herpes zoster has been described in patients with lymphoma, leukemia, organ transplant recipients, solid malignancies, and those receiving chemotherapy or chronic corticosteroids. Skin lesions frequently extend beyond the original dermatomal distribution. The period of new lesion formation may continue for weeks, and healing is delayed. Generalized skin dissemination has been observed in nearly 25% of patients. Fifty percent of those patients with cutaneous dissemination will progress to visceral dissemination. In HIV-infected individuals, herpes zoster is also severe and potentially life-threatening. Often multiple dermatomes are involved, and recurrences are common. A chronic form of herpes zoster has been described in patients with advanced AIDS.

Acyclovir has been shown to clearly benefit the immunocompromised host. It is generally given intravenously for 7 days or more. Chronic suppressive doses of oral acyclovir have been given to HIV-infected patients with recurrent herpes zoster. Acyclovir-resistant VZV has been isolated from some individuals on chronic therapy, but this appears to still be uncommon.

Diagnostic Tests/Procedures

Herpes Cytology *on page 444*
Polymerase Chain Reaction *on page 523*
Skin Biopsy *on page 535*
Varicella-Zoster Virus Culture *on page 568*
Varicella-Zoster Virus Serology *on page 569*
Virus Detection by DFA *on page 576*

Drug Therapy

Recommended

Treatment:
Acyclovir *on page 581*
Valacyclovir *on page 965*
Famciclovir *on page 729*
Prophylaxis:
Varicella Virus Vaccine *on page 970*

Selected Readings

Arvin AM, "Varicella-Zoster Virus," *Clin Microbiol Rev*, 1996, 9(3):361-81.
Brunell PA, "Varicella in Pregnancy, the Fetus, and the Newborn: Problems in Management," *J Infect Dis*, 1992, 166(Suppl 1):S42-7.
Dunkle LM, Arvin AM, Whitley RJ, et al, "A Controlled Trial of Acyclovir for Chickenpox in Normal Children," *N Engl J Med*, 1991, 325(22):1539-44.
Straus SE, Ostrove JM, Inchauspé G, "Varicella-Zoster Virus Infections. Biology, Natural History, Treatment, and Prevention," *Ann Intern Med*, 1988, 108(2):221-37.
Wallace MR, Bowler WA, Murray NB, et al, "Treatment of Adult Varicella with Oral Acyclovir. A Randomized, Placebo-Controlled Trial," *Ann Intern Med*, 1992, 117(5):358-63.
Watson PN and Evans RJ, "Postherpetic Neuralgia: A Review," *Arch Neurol*, 1986, 43(8):836-40.
Whitley RJ, "Varicella-Zoster Virus," *Principles and Practice of Infectious Diseases*, 4th ed, Mandell GL, Bennett JE, and Dolin R, eds, New York, NY: Churchill Livingstone, 1995, 1345-51.
Wood MJ, Johnson RW, McKendrick MW, et al, "A Randomized Trial of Acyclovir for 7 Days or 21 Days With and Without Prednisolone for Treatment of Acute Herpes Zoster," *N Engl J Med*, 1994, 330(13):896-900.

Vibrio cholerae

Related Information

Timing of Food Poisoning *on page 1069*

Microbiology *Vibrio cholerae* is an oxidase-positive, fermentative, gram-negative rod that can have a comma-shaped appearance on initial isolation. *V. cholerae* can be subdivided by the production of endotoxin and agglutination in 0-1 antisera with the nomenclature of *V. cholerae* 0-1, atypical or nontoxigenic 0-1, or non-0-1. The serogroup 0-1 can further be subdivided into the El Tor and Classic cholera biotypes which can be further subdivided into a variety of serotypes. The major virulence factor of *V. cholerae* is the extracellular enterotoxin produced by the 0-1 strain, although nontoxin-producing organisms have been implicated in some outbreaks.

V. cholerae is a facultative anaerobe which grows best at a pH of 7.0 and at a wide temperature range (18°C to 37°C). *Vibrio* species can be differentiated from other gram-negative bacilli by their sensitivity to 0129 and may be speciated by a variety of biochemical tests.

Epidemiology Cholera is usually spread by contamination of water and food by infected feces, with fecal contamination of water being the principal vehicle of transmission. Person-to-person transmission is less common due to the large organism load necessary for infection. Asymptomatic carriers play a minor role in cholera outbreaks. Outbreaks may be seasonally dependent based on either (Continued)

Vibrio cholerae (Continued)

temperature or rainfall. Transmission by food can be eliminated by thorough cooking. Adequate sanitation is the best means of cholera prevention.

There have been several pandemics of cholera reported since 1817, originating in Bengal and subsequently spreading to a variety of geographic locations, responsible for hundreds of thousands of deaths. The latest pandemic originated in Indonesia in 1961 and moved to the Western hemisphere. In 1991, a cholera outbreak in Peru and 20 other countries in the Western hemisphere accounted for over 600,000 cases with 5000 deaths caused by El Tor 0-1.

Clinical Syndromes After a 2- to 5-day incubation period, classic cholera is characterized by an abrupt onset of vomiting and profuse watery diarrhea with flecks of mucus (rice water stool). Fluid losses can be significant (up to 20 L/ day). Hypovolemic shock and metabolic acidosis can cause death within a few hours of onset, especially in children. Mortality, in untreated cases, is as high as 60%. Milder forms of the disease also occur, especially with the non-0-1 cholera.

Diagnosis Organisms can be identified by darkfield microscopy showing large numbers of comma-shaped organisms with significant motility. However, this test is relatively insensitive and is nonspecific. Thiosulfate-citrate-bile salt-sucrose agar (TCBS) or alkaline peptone broth are used to facilitate growth and identification. Positive identification depends on serologic and biochemical testing.

Diagnostic Tests/Procedures
Fecal Leukocyte Stain on page 408
Stool Culture, Uncommon Organisms on page 543

Treatment Early and rapid replacement of fluid and electrolytes can decrease the mortality to <1%. Oral rehydration is usually successful, but in severe cases, intravenous replacement is required. When fluid and electrolyte imbalances are corrected, cholera is a short, self-limiting disease lasting a few days. According to the MMWR, doxycycline, tetracycline, co-trimoxazole, erythromycin, and fura-zolidone have all demonstrated effectiveness in decreasing the diarrhea and bacterial shedding in this disease. The usual recommendation is doxycycline 300 mg as a single dose for adults, and co-trimoxazole 5 mg/kg, twice daily for 3 days.

Pediatric Drug Therapy
Recommended
<7 years:
Co-Trimoxazole on page 692
>7 years:
Tetracycline on page 944
Doxycycline on page 713
Alternate
>7 years:
Co-Trimoxazole on page 692

Adult Drug Therapy
Recommended
Doxycycline on page 713
Tetracycline on page 944
Alternate
Co-Trimoxazole on page 692

Selected Readings
"Cholera Associated With International Travel, 1992," MMWR Morb Mortal Wkly Rep, 1992, 41(36):664-7.

Falkow S and Mekalanos J, "The Enteric Bacilli and Vibrios," Microbiology, 4th ed, Davis BD, Dulbecco R, Eisen HN, et al, eds, Philadelphia, PA: JB Lippincott Co, 1990, 561-87.

Johnston JM, Becker SF, McFarland LM, "Vibrio vulnificus: Man and the Sea," JAMA , 1985, 253(19):2850-3.

Levine WC and Griffin PM, "Vibrio Infections on the Gulf Coast: The Results of a First Year of Regional Surveillance. Gulf Coast Vibrio Working Group," J Infect Dis, 1993, 167(2):479-83.

Rabbani GH, "Cholera," J Clin Gastroenterol, 1986, 15(3):507-28.

Tacket CO, Brenner F, Blake PA, "Clinical Features and an Epidemiological Study of Vibrio vulni-ficus Infections," J Infect Dis, 1984, 149(4):558-61.

"Update: Cholera -- Western Hemisphere, and Recommendations for Treatment of Cholera," MMWR Morb Mortal Wkly Rep, 1991, 40(32):562-5.

"Vibrio vulnificus Infections Associated With Raw Oyster Consumption - Florida, 1981-1992," MMWR Morb Mortal Wkly Rep, 1993, 42(21):405-7.

Zwadyk P, "Vibrionaceae," Zinsser Microbiology, 20th ed, Joklik WK, Willett HP, Amos DB, et al, eds, Norwalk, CT: Appleton & Lange, 1992, 566-76.

Viridans Streptococci *see Streptococcus,* Viridans Group *on page 279*

VZV *see* Varicella-Zoster Virus *on page 294*

Xanthomonas maltophilia *see Stenotrophomonas maltophilia on page 265*

Yersinia enterocolitica

Microbiology *Yersinia enterocolitica* is a gram-negative bacillus named in honor of the French bacteriologist Alexander Yersin, who discovered *Yersinia pestis* (the cause of plague) in 1894. *Y. enterocolitica* is an unusual cause of enterocolitis, terminal ileitis mimicking acute appendicitis, and septicemia. The organism is an aerobic gram-negative rod, nonlactose fermenting, which is motile at 25°C. It is unusual in that it grows better at somewhat cooler temperatures than do other pathogenic gram-negative rods (25°C to 32°C). It also is able to grow well at 4°C, which is the basis for CEM.

Epidemiology *Yersinia enterocolitica* is endemic in many animals which serve as reservoirs: cattle, pigs, dogs, cats, and others. The usual route of human infection is via ingestion of contaminated food, milk, and water. There have been three major foodborne epidemics in the United States: June 1982 - outbreak in several states linked to consumption of milk pasteurized at a plant in Memphis, Tennessee; 172 positive cultures from cases in Tennessee, Arkansas, and Mississippi, where patients presented with diarrhea, fever, abdominal pain. It also included 24 cases of extraintestinal infections including throat, blood, urinary tract, central nervous system, and wounds; 1976 - contaminated chocolate milk in New York State; 1982 - contaminated tofu in Washington state.

Clinical Syndromes

- **Enterocolitis:** *Yersinia enterocolitica* is a rare cause of enterocolitis. The severity of symptoms can be quite variable and can range from mild fever, diarrhea and abdominal pain, to fulminant colitis with spiking fevers and rectal bleeding.

- **Mesenteric adenopathy with or without terminal ileitis:** This form of *Yersinia* infection is known to mimic acute appendicitis. Patients present with right lower quadrant pain, fever, and leukocytosis. Upon laparotomy the appendix is normal but enlarged mesenteric lymph nodes are palpable and when cultured will yield the organism. This has been described primarily in adolescents, although cases have been reported in adults.

- **Polyarthritis:** This has been described as the sole manifestation of *Yersinia enterocolitica* infection or as a secondary manifestation of gastrointestinal infection. Well documented cases have been described in Scandinavia, where up to 30% of cases develop erythema nodosum, and 10% to 30% develop polyarthritis (especially associated with HLA-B27 haplotype). *Yersinia* antigens have recently been found in synovial fluid cells from patients suffering from reactive arthritis following *Yersinia* infection.

- **Liver abscess:** *Yersinia* is a rare but reported cause of liver abscess in the absence of typical enterocolitis symptoms.

- **Ascending infection of an extremity:** Recently, cases of infections of the hand and upper extremity due to *Yersinia enterocolitica* have been described. These infections occurred in adults preparing contaminated chitterlings (pig intestines) with local inoculation into the hand via small cuts.

- **Septicemia:** *Yersinia* is an unusual cause of community-acquired septicemia but may occur following ingestion of heavily contaminated food. Risk factors for septicemia are cirrhosis, malignancy, diabetes mellitus, and patients with iron overload syndromes (such as hemachromatosis, frequent blood transfusions). Typically, there is fever, myalgias, confusion, and possibly hypotension. Symptoms of enterocolitis, such as diarrhea and abdominal pain, may be completely absent, adding to the diagnostic confusion. Elevated liver enzymes and muscle enzymes may occur. Blood cultures are often positive for the organism.

- **Miscellaneous:** Other manifestations of *Yersinia* infection include osteomyelitis, meningitis, pharyngitis (without enterocolitis), and intra-abdominal abscess.

Diagnosis In the absence of an outbreak, the diagnosis of enterocolitis due to *Yersinia* is difficult to make on clinical grounds alone. Thus, laboratory confirmation is important in most cases. Appropriate specimens for culture include stool, blood, lymph node, pharyngeal exudates, ascites fluid, and cerebrospinal fluid. Joint aspiration fluid may be sent for *Yersinia* culture in the appropriate clinical setting (ie, reactive polyarthritis following a diarrheal illness), but the yield is extremely low. The laboratory should be notified if a stool specimen is being

(Continued)

Yersinia enterocolitica (Continued)

examined for *Yersinia*. Serologic tests for specific antibody production to *Yersinia enterocolitica* are available in some laboratories.

Diagnostic Tests/Procedures

Aerobic Culture, Appropriate Site *on page 310*
Stool Culture, Uncommon Organisms *on page 543*

Treatment Many cases of enterocolitis and mesenteric adenitis secondary to *Yersinia* are self-resolving, and the role of antibiotics is unclear. Patients with *Yersinia* septicemia, however, definitely require antibiotic therapy since the mortality approaches 50%. The organism is susceptible *in vitro* to a number of agents, including third generation cephalosporins, piperacillin, co-trimoxazole, and aminoglycosides. Most isolates are resistant to penicillin, ampicillin, and first generation cephalosporins. The optimal drug regimen *in vivo* has not been defined in the literature. For serious infections, it seems reasonable to treat initially with a combination (eg, third generation cephalosporin and aminoglycoside) until the patient has stabilized.

Adult Drug Therapy

Recommended

Severe infection:

Cephalosporins, 3rd Generation *on page 662*
used in combination with
Aminoglycosides *on page 590*

Selected Readings

Bottone E and Sheehan DJ, "*Yersinia enterocolitica*: Guidelines for Serologic Diagnosis of Human Infections," *Rev Infect Dis*, 1983, 5(5):898-906.

Bottone EJ, "*Yersinia enterocolitica*: The Charisma Continues," *Clin Microbiol Rev*, 1997, 10(2):257-76.

Centers for Disease Control, "*Yersinia enterocolitica* Bacteremia and Endotoxin Shock Associated With Red Blood Cell Transfusions - United States, 1991," *JAMA*, 1991, 256(17):2174-5.

Cover TL and Aber RC, "*Yersinia enterocolitica*," *N Engl J Med*, 1989, 321(1):16-24.

Gayraud M, Mollaret HH, et al, "Antibiotic Treatment of *Yersinia enterocolitica* Septicemia: A Retrospective Review of 43 Cases," *Clin Infect Dis*, 1993, 17(3):405-10.

Naqvi SH, Swierkosz EM, and Gerard J, "Presentation of *Yersinia enterocolitica* Enteritis in Children," *Pediatr Infect Dis J*, 1993, 12(5):386-9.

Yersinia pestis

Microbiology *Yersinia pestis* is the etiological agent of plague. All of the 11 species of *Yersinia* are aerobic, gram-negative rods, are well established members of the family Enterobacteriaceae, and have been isolated from human clinical specimens. At least three species of *Yersinia* are unequivocal human pathogens: *Y. pestis*, *Y. enterocolitica*, and *Y. pseudotuberculosis*.

Epidemiology *Yersinia pestis* infections are rare in the United States. From 1970 to 1991, 295 cases were reported to the Center for Disease Control and Prevention. Plague occurs worldwide; most cases occur in Asia and Africa. In the United States, plague occurs (rarely) in New Mexico, Arizona, California, Utah, and Colorado. Yersinioses are zoonotic infections that usually affect rodents, small animals, and birds. Rats are the natural reservoir of *Y. pestis* in areas of urban ("city") plague; small animals such as ground squirrels, wood rats, rabbits, and cats are the natural reservoirs of *Y. pestis* in areas of sylvatic ("country") plague. Humans are accidental hosts of *Yersinia* species. Humans become infected with the bacterium after being bitten by fleas of the aforementioned animals, or, much less commonly, by handling infected animals or inhaling aerosolized *Y. pestis* generated by a person with pulmonary plague.

Clinical Syndromes Plague: Plague presents in many different and protean clinical forms: bubonic, septicemic, pneumonic, cutaneous, and meningitic. After an incubation period of 2-8 days, most patients with **bubonic plague**, the most common form, experience fever, chills, headache, aches, extreme exhaustion, and lymphadenitis. At the same time, extremely painful bubos develop in the groin, axilla, or neck. These patients have overwhelming numbers of bacteria in their blood. Patients with **septicemic plague** also have tremendous numbers of bacteria in their blood; however, these patients have a more septic presentation, and bubos usually are not present. **Pneumonic plague** is a complication of bubonic plague and is characterized by cough, chest pain, difficulty breathing, and hemoptysis; bubos might or might not be present. Pneumonic plague, if not treated immediately, has a very high mortality rate and can be rapidly fatal within 1 day. The natural progression of plague is from the bubonic, to the septicemic, to the pneumonic forms. The overall mortality rate for untreated cases of plague is 50% to 60%.

Diagnosis Diagnosis of plague is mainly a clinical diagnosis. Laboratories must be notified if *Y. pestis* is suspected as an etiological agent because many laboratories do not routinely suspect *Y. pestis* or culture clinical specimens for *Y. pestis* because special media and techniques easily can be used to enhance isolation of the bacterium and because the colonial morphology of *Y. pestis* is not typical of many other gram-negative rods. Culture is the most productive test for the laboratory diagnosis of plague. *Yersinia pestis* is not fastidious and grows well on blood agar media and many enteric media. Many commercial bacterial identification systems do not include *Y. pestis* in their databases. The most appropriate clinical specimens for culture include blood, biopsy or aspirate of bubo, sputum, cerebrospinal fluid, and cutaneous biopsy.

Diagnostic Tests/Procedures
Aerobic Culture, Appropriate Site *on page 310*
Blood Culture, Aerobic and Anaerobic *on page 337*

Treatment Supportive care is essential. The antibiotic of choice is streptomycin. Gentamicin, tetracyclines, and chloramphenicol are all effective alternatives. Timely treatment can potentially reduce mortality from plague to 10%.

Travelers to endemic areas are generally at low risk for developing infection. The CDC does, however, recommend the following precautions: avoid rat-infested areas; generous use of insect repellents and insecticides including body, clothing, and bedding application; avoid handling sick or dead animals. The CDC also recommends the use of prophylactic antibiotics if the risk of exposure is high. Tetracycline or doxycycline should be used in adults, and sulfonamides used for children younger than 8 years of age. Plague vaccine requires multiple dosing over several months for protection and is therefore not recommended for immediate protection during outbreaks.

Drug Therapy
Recommended
Streptomycin *on page 924*
Alternate
Gentamicin *on page 747*
Tetracycline *on page 944*
Doxycycline *on page 713*
Chloramphenicol *on page 667*

Selected Readings
Butler T, "*Yersinia* Infections: Centennial of the Discovery of the Plague Bacillus," *Clin Infect Dis*, 1994, 19(4):655-63.

Butler TB, "*Yersinia* Species (Including Plague)," *Principles and Practice of Infectious Diseases*, 4th ed, Mandell GL, Bennett JE, and Dolin R, eds, New York, NY: Churchill Livingstone, 1995, 2070-8.

Craven RB, Maupin GO, Beard ML, et al, "Reported Cases of Human Plague Infections in the United States, 1970-1991," *J Med Entomol*, 1993, 30(4):758-61.

Crook LD and Tempest B, "Plague. A Review of 27 Cases," *Arch Intern Med*, 1992, 152(6):1253-6.

"Human Plague - United States, 1993-1994," *MMWR Morb Mortal Wkly Rep*, 1994, 43(13):242-6.

Perry RD and Fetherston JD, "*Yersinia pestis* - Etiologic Agent of Plague," *Clin Microbiol Rev*, 1997, 10(1):35-66.

Reisner B, "Plague - Past and Present," *Clin Microbiol Newslett*, 1996, 18(20):153-6.

DIAGNOSTIC TESTS/PROCEDURES

LIVERPOOL
JOHN MOORES UNIVERSITY
AVRIL ROBARTS LRC
TEL. 0151 231 4022

Abdomen, CT *see* Computed Transaxial Tomography, Abdomen Studies *on page 373*

Abdomen Ultrasound *see* Ultrasound, Abdomen *on page 560*

Abdominal Paracentesis *see* Paracentesis *on page 509*

Abscess Aerobic and Anaerobic Culture

Related Information

Antimicrobial Susceptibility Testing, Aerobic and Facultatively Anaerobic Organisms *on page 323*
Antimicrobial Susceptibility Testing, Anaerobic Bacteria *on page 327*
Genital Culture *on page 423*
Wound Culture *on page 577*

Applies to Aerobic Culture, Abscess; Anaerobic Culture, Abscess

Test Includes Culture for aerobic and facultative anaerobic organisms. Culture for anaerobic organisms usually must be specifically requested and may require a separate specimen.

Patient Preparation Aseptic preparation of the aspiration site. The overlying and adjacent areas must be carefully decontaminated to eliminate isolation of potentially contaminating anaerobes which colonize the skin surface.

Special Instructions The laboratory should be informed of the specific site of specimen, age of patient, current antibiotic therapy, clinical diagnosis, and time of collection.

Clinical Observations Suggestive of Anaerobic Infection

Foul-smelling discharge
Location of infection in proximity to a mucosal surface
Necrotic tissue, gangrene, pseudomembrane formation
Gas in tissues or discharges
Endocarditis with negative routine blood cultures
Infection associated with malignancy or other process producing tissue destruction
Infection related to the use of aminoglycosides (oral, parenteral, or topical)
Septic thrombophlebitis
Bacteremic picture with jaundice
Infection resulting from human or other bites
Black discoloration of blood-containing exudates (may fluoresce red under ultraviolet light in *B. melaninogenicus* infections)
Presence of "sulfur granules" in discharges (actinomycosis)
Classical clinical features of gas gangrene
Clinical setting suggestive for anaerobic infection (septic abortion, infection after gastrointestinal surgery, genitourinary surgery, etc)

From Bartlett JG," Anaerobic Bacterial Infections of the Lung," *Chest,* 1987, 91:901-9, with permission.

Specimen Fluid, pus, abscess wall tissue, or other material properly obtained from an abscess for optimal yield. Specimens for anaerobic culture should be accompanied by a specimen for aerobic culture from the same site. Aspirated fluid is acceptable for anaerobic culture if it is submitted in a properly capped syringe or an approved anaerobic transport device.

Container Anaerobic transport container swab with anaerobic transport medium and aerobic transport media or swab may be used if aspirated fluid is not available. However, swabs always provide inferior specimens.

Collection Specimens are to be collected from a prepared site using sterile technique. Contamination with normal flora from skin, rectum, vaginal tract, all mucus membranes, or other body surfaces must be avoided. Some anaerobes will be killed by contact with oxygen for only a few seconds. Ideally, pus obtained by needle aspiration through an intact surface, which has been aseptically prepared, is put directly into an anaerobic transport device or transported directly to the laboratory in the original syringe. Sampling of open lesions is enhanced by deep aspiration using a sterile needle and syringe. Curettings of the base of an open lesion may also provide a good yield. If irrigation is necessary, nonbacteriostatic sterile normal saline may be used. Pulmonary samples may be obtained by transtracheal percutaneous needle aspiration by physicians trained in this procedure or by use of a special sheathed catheter. If swabs must be used, two should be collected; one for culture and one for Gram's stain. Specimens collected and transported in syringes should be transported to the laboratory within 30 minutes of collection.

Storage Instructions If syringe is used to transport specimen to the laboratory, all air should be expelled, and the needle removed.

Causes for Rejection Specimens which have been exposed to air, refrigerated, or delayed in transit have a less-than-optimal yield. Specimens from sites which have anaerobic bacteria as normal flora (eg, throat, feces, colostomy stoma, rectal swabs, bronchial washes, cervical-vaginal mucosal swabs, sputums, skin and superficial wounds, voided or catheterized urine) **are not** acceptable for anaerobic culture because of contamination by the normal flora.

Turnaround Time Cultures showing no bacterial growth can generally be reported after 2-3 days. However, initial growth may not appear for up to 7 days. Complete reports of cultures with anaerobic bacteria may take as long as 2 weeks after receipt of culture, depending upon the nature and number of the organisms isolated.

Reference Range No growth of anaerobic bacteria

Use Determine microbial etiology of the abscess and provide a guide for therapy

Limitations The only sources for specimens with established validity for meaningful anaerobic culture in patients with pleuropulmonary infections are blood, pleural fluid, transtracheal aspirates, transthoracic pulmonary aspirates, specimens obtained at thoracotomy, and fiberoptic bronchoscopic aspirates using the protected brush or sheathed catheter. Aspirated pleural fluid is preferred for patients with empyema. Blood cultures yield positive results in less than 5% of cases of anaerobic pulmonary infection.

Mycobacterium sp or *Nocardia* sp which may cause abscesses will **not** be recovered even if present, since extended incubation periods, aerobic incubation, and special media are necessary for their isolation. Cultures for these organisms should be specifically requested.

Contraindications Bronchoscopically obtained specimens are extremely poor specimens because the instrument becomes contaminated by organisms normally contaminating the oropharynx during insertion. Culture of specimens from sites harboring endogenous anaerobic organisms or contaminated by endogenous organisms (usually sites at or contiguous with any mucus membrane) usually will be misleading with regard to etiology and selection of appropriate therapy.

Additional Information In open wounds, anaerobic organisms may play an etiologic role, whereas aerobes may represent superficial contamination. Serious anaerobic infections are often due to mixed flora which are pathologic synergists. Anaerobes frequently recovered from closed postoperative wound infections include *Bacteroides fragilis*, approximately 50%; *Bacteroides* sp, approximately 25%; *Peptostreptococcus* sp, approximately 15%; and *Fusobacterium* sp, approximately 25%. Anaerobes are seldom recovered in pure culture (10% to 15% of cultures). Aerobes and facultative anaerobes when present are frequently found in lesser numbers than the anaerobes. Anaerobic infection is most commonly associated with operations involving opening or manipulating the bowel, mucus membranes, or a hollow viscus (eg, appendectomy, cholecystectomy, colectomy, gastrectomy, bile duct exploration, etc). The ratio of anaerobes to facultative anaerobes is normally about 10:1 in the mouth, vagina, and sebaceous glands and at least 1000:1 in the colon.

Selected Readings

Brook I, "A 12 Year Study of Aerobic and Anaerobic Bacteria in Intra-abdominal and Postsurgical Abdominal Wound Infections," *Surg Gynecol Obstet*, 1989, 169(5):387-92.

Finegold SM, Jousimies-Somer HR, and Wexler HM, "Current Perspectives on Anaerobic Infections: Diagnostic Approaches," *Infect Dis Clin North Am*, 1993, 7(2):257-75.

Styrt B and Gorbach SL, "Recent Developments in the Understanding of the Pathogenesis and Treatment of Anaerobic Infections," *N Engl J Med*, 1989, 321(4):240-6.

Swenson RM, "Rationale for the Identification and Susceptibility Testing of Anaerobic Bacteria," *Rev Infect Dis*, 1986, 8(5):809-13.

Acid-Fast Stain

Related Information

Mycobacteria Culture, Cerebrospinal Fluid *on page 494*
Mycobacteria Culture, Sputum *on page 495*

Synonyms AFB Smear; Atypical *Mycobacterium* Smear; Kinyoun Stain; *Mycobacterium* Smear; TB Smear; Ziehl-Neelsen Stain

(Continued)

Acid-Fast Stain *(Continued)*

Applies to Auramine-Rhodamine Stain; Fluorochrome Stain

Test Includes Acid-fast stain. For diagnosis, acid-fast stain and culture are usually ordered together. For monitoring therapy, stain alone may be sufficient.

Abstract Acid-fast bacilli are so called because they are surrounded by a waxy envelope that is resistant to destaining by acid-alcohol. Either heat (classic Ziehl-Neelsen) or a detergent (Tergitol Kinyoun method) is required to allow the stain to penetrate the cell wall. Once stained, acid-fast bacteria resist decolorization, whereas other bacteria are destained with acid-alcohol.

Patient Preparation Same as for mycobacteria culture of given site

Special Instructions The laboratory should be informed of the source of the specimen. Specimens may be divided for fungus culture and stain (KOH) preparation, mycobacteria culture and acid-fast smear, and routine bacterial culture and Gram's stain only if the specimen is accompanied by appropriate requests for these procedures and if the specimen is of adequate volume for all tests requested.

Specimen The appropriate specimen for an acid-fast smear is the same as for culture. See specific site mycobacteria culture listings for details.

Container Same as for culture of specific site

Collection See specific mycobacteria culture listings for specific site.

Causes for Rejection Insufficient specimen volume, specimen received on a swab

Turnaround Time Routine: 24-48 hours; stat (if available): 2 hours

Reference Range No mycobacteria identified. Positive smears usually are reported in a quantitative manner such as a number of bacilli per field or entire smear.

Use Determine the presence of mycobacteria, monitor the course of antimycobacterial therapy; establish the diagnosis of mycobacterial infection in undiagnosed granulomatous disease, fever of unknown origin (FUO), and in patients suspected of having a defect in cellular immunity (eg, AIDS, lymphoma, etc)

Limitations Cultures are more sensitive than smears; therefore, the smear may be negative when culture is positive. Fluorochrome stains (auramine-rhodamine) are more sensitive than carbol-fuchsin stains. Nonpathogenic acid-fast bacilli can be present as normal flora. Culture is necessary to determine the specific species of *Mycobacterium* present, however a presumptive determination of whether *Mycobacterium tuberculosis* or mycobacteria other than *M. tuberculosis* (formerly called "atypical mycobacteria") are present can be made. DNA probes, which are more sensitive and specific than smears for the diagnosis of mycobacterial infection are now in use in some laboratories.

Methodology Acid-fast stain of concentrated or unconcentrated specimen

Additional Information A stat acid-fast smear can be performed by some laboratories upon special request. However, concentration procedures are not usually performed on a stat basis. Very active infection is required to produce a positive without concentration. In extrapulmonary tuberculosis, the acid-fast stain can be useful in yielding a rapid diagnosis. Routine acid-fast staining and culturing of CSF for AFB is rarely, if ever, productive. However, positive smears have been reported from CSF in 67% of cases of culture-proven tuberculous meningitis, lymph nodes biopsy in 80% of miliary tuberculosis cases, 75% peritoneal biopsies in peritonitis, and urine in 80% of the cases of renal tuberculosis.

Acid-fast stains performed on gastric aspirates and urine when positive are reliable indicators of true mycobacterial disease. However, tap water can contain *M. gordonae* and can be responsible for false-positive results. Klotz and Penn have reported the sensitivity, compared to culture, as approximately 30% for gastric aspirates and approximately 50% for urine. False-positives were negligible, <1%.

The sensitivity and specificity of acid-fast staining for the diagnosis of pulmonary mycobacteria tuberculosis infection in a large prospective study was 53.1% and 99.8%, respectively, and 81.5% and 98.4%, respectively, for culture.

Selected Readings
Gordin F and Slutkin G, "The Validity of Acid-Fast Smears in the Diagnosis of Pulmonary Tuberculosis," *Arch Pathol Lab Med*, 1990, 114(10):1025-7.

Klotz SA and Penn RL, "Acid-Fast Staining of Urine and Gastric Contents is an Excellent Indicator of Mycobacterial Disease," *Am Rev Respir Dis*, 1987, 136(5):1197-8.

Levy H, Feldman C, Sacho H, et al, "A Re-evaluation of Sputum Microscopy and Culture in the Diagnosis of Pulmonary Tuberculosis," *Chest*, 1989, 95(6):1193-7.

Morris A, Reller LB, Salfinger M, et al, "Mycobacteria in Stool Specimens: The Nonvalue of Smears for Predicting Culture Results," *J Clin Microbiol*, 1993, 31(5):1385-7.

Murray PR, Elmore C, and Krogstad DJ, "The Acid-Fast Stain: A Specific and Predictive Test for Mycobacterial Disease," *Ann Intern Med*, 1980, 92(4):512-3.

Acid-Fast Stain, Modified, *Cryptosporidium* *see* Cryptosporidium Diagnostic Procedures, Stool *on page 381*

Acid-Fast Stain, Modified, *Nocardia* Species

Related Information

Actinomyces Culture, All Sites *on next page*
Gram's Stain *on page 426*
Methenamine Silver Stain *on page 487*
Nocardia Culture, All Sites *on page 503*
Periodic Acid-Schiff Stain *on page 518*

Synonyms Hank's Stain; *Nocardia* Species Modified Acid-Fast Stain

Test Includes Modified acid-fast stain. Culture generally must be ordered specifically as such. The recovery of *Nocardia* sp usually requires special culture techniques.

Abstract Infections with *Nocardia* sp may resemble many other more common diseases. Because therapy differs, it is important to establish a definitive diagnosis, preferably by culture. The diagnosis of nocardiosis should be considered in unexplained cavitary lung disease, granulomatous lung disease of established cause not responsive to appropriate therapy, brain abscess particularly in the presence of cavitary lung disease, alveolar proteinosis, with mycetoma, and in any patient in whom a disseminated granulomatous disease is considered.

Specimen Appropriate preparation, specimen and container for smear is the same as for culture

Causes for Rejection Insufficient specimen volume, specimen received on a dry swab

Reference Range No acid-fast organisms seen

Use Determine the presence or absence of *Nocardia* sp which are usually, but not invariably, acid-fast when stained by the modified acid-fast stain. *Actinomyces* and *Streptomyces* sp which may be microscopically similar to *Nocardia* on Gram's stain, are negative with the modified acid-fast stain. Establish the etiology of maduromycosis and of fever of unknown origin in patients with suspected defects of cellular immunity (eg, AIDS, Hodgkin's disease, lymphoma, and so forth).

Limitations *Nocardia* sp do not always stain acid-fast by this method; consequently, the presence of branching, gram-positive bacilli on Gram's stain suggests that Gram's stain might have greater sensitivity. *Nocardia* sp, however, cannot be distinguished from *Actinomyces* sp and other closely related organisms by Gram's stain. Organisms from clinical material are more likely to be "modified acid-fast" than those from culture.

Methodology Kinyoun stain followed by relatively less severe decolorization with 3% acid alcohol (940 mL of 95% ethanol and 60 mL of concentrated HCl). If clumps or granules are observed, they should be crushed between two glass slides and examined microscopically.

Additional Information Nocardiosis has also been reported with lupus, rheumatoid arthritis, and liver disease. Aggressive diagnostic procedures are often necessary to obtain appropriate specimen for definitive diagnosis. Organisms consistent with *Nocardia* sp can be identified presumptively on Gram's stain and modified acid-fast stain pending more definitive diagnosis by culture. Examination of sputum with *Nocardia* may show thin, crooked, weakly to strongly gram-positive, modified acid-fast positive, irregularly staining or beaded filaments. Opaque or pigmented sulfur granules may occasionally be present in direct smear of pus. Colonization without apparent infection may occur.

Selected Readings

Beaman BL and Beaman L, "*Nocardia* Species: Host-Parasite Relationships," *Clin Microbiol Rev*, 1994, 7(2):213-64.

Javaly K, Horowitz HW, and Wormser GP, "Nocardiosis in Patients With Human Immunodeficiency Virus Infection. Report of 2 Cases and Review of the Literature," *Medicine (Baltimore)*, 1992, 71(3):128-38.

Koneman EW, Allen SD, Janda WM, et al, *Color Atlas and Textbook of Diagnostic Microbiology*, 4th ed, Philadelphia, PA: JB Lippincott Co, 1992, 505.

McNeil MM and Brown JM, "The Medically Important Aerobic Actinomycetes: Epidemiology and Microbiology," *Clin Microbiol Rev*, 1994, 7(3):357-417.

(Continued)

Acid-Fast Stain, Modified, *Nocardia* Species
(Continued)

Osoagbaka OU and Njoku-Obi AN, "Presumptive Diagnosis of Pulmonary Nocardiosis: Value of Sputum Microscopy," *J Appl Bacteriol*, 1987, 63(1):27-38.

Wilson JP, Turner HR, Kirchner KA, et al, "Nocardial Infections in Renal Transplant Recipients," *Medicine (Baltimore)*, 1989, 68(1):38-57.

Acromioclavicular Joint, Left or Right, X-ray *see* Bone Films *on page 343*

Actinomyces Culture, All Sites

Related Information

Acid-Fast Stain, Modified, *Nocardia* Species *on previous page*
Gram's Stain *on page 426*
Nocardia Culture, All Sites *on page 503*

Applies to Intrauterine Device Culture; IUD Culture; Sulfur Granule, Culture

Test Includes Anaerobic culture for *Actinomyces* sp and direct microscopic examination of Gram's stain for sulfur granules and gram-positive branching bacilli

Abstract Actinomycosis is a chronic progressive suppurative disease characterized by the formation of multiple abscesses, draining sinuses, and dense fibrosis. The classic presentations include cervicofacial, thoracic, abdominal, and pelvic infections.

Patient Preparation Cleanse the skin around the opening of a draining sinus with an alcohol swab, allow to dry, and obtain the specimen from as deep within the sinus as possible. Submit aspirated material or tissue. Do not submit a swab specimen.

Special Instructions In tissues, *Actinomyces* sp produce chronic suppuration with formation of multiple draining sinuses. Examination of material from such sinuses often reveals tangled masses of filamentous elements and granules called sulfur granules. The presence of sulfur granules is highly suggestive of *Actinomyces* infection. If actinomycosis is suspected clinically, the laboratory should be informed. The specific site of specimen, current antibiotic therapy, and clinical diagnosis should be provided.

Specimen Exudate, material from draining sinus

Container Anaerobic specimen transport medium

Collection *Actinomyces* sp are fastidious anaerobic organisms. It is, therefore, essential that the specimen be placed into the appropriate anaerobic transport tube and delivered to the laboratory as quickly as possible. If a syringe is used, expel all air before transferring into the tube. Swabs invariably collect poor specimens, but if used, should be transported in anaerobic transport medium. With a draining sinus, obtain the specimen by aspirating as far into the sinus as possible.

Storage Instructions Specimens should be transported immediately to the laboratory and processed as soon as possible.

Causes for Rejection Specimens exposed to air, specimens which have been refrigerated or have an excessive delay in transit, have a less than optimal yield. Specimens from sites which have anaerobic bacteria as normal flora (eg, throat, feces, colostomy stoma, rectal swabs, bronchial washes, cervical-vaginal mucosal swabs, sputums, skin and superficial wounds, voided or catheterized urine), may **not** be acceptable for anaerobic culture because of contamination by the normal flora.

Turnaround Time Preliminary reports are usually available after 7 days. Cultures with no growth may be reported after 14 days.

Reference Range No *Actinomyces* isolated. *A. israelii* is a normal inhabitant of the mouth, oropharynx, and gastrointestinal tract.

Use Detect infections due to *Actinomyces* sp; establish the etiology of granulomatous disease, chronic draining sinus, and fever of unknown origin (FUO) particularly in immunocompromised patients

Limitations Inform the laboratory that actinomycosis is clinically suspected, to ensure that cultures will be incubated long enough to permit recovery of *Actinomyces* sp; *Actinomyces* sp are relatively slow growing and will often fail to grow in the period in which most laboratories incubate routine cultures. Additionally, even when incubated appropriately, recovery of *Actinomyces* sp may be hindered by overgrowth with obligate and facultative anaerobic bacteria.

Methodology Anaerobic culture including thioglycolate broth media

Additional Information If granules are detected on the gauze pad covering a draining sinus, submit the granules to the laboratory. A Gram's stain and culture should be performed on such granules. On smear branching gram-positive rods may be found. They may be similar in appearance to other actinomycetes including species of *Nocardia*, *Streptomyces*, and also *Mycobacterium*. Actinomycetes are not stained by the modified acid-fast stain used for *Nocardia* sp. Several species of *Actinomyces* are responsible for human infection. *Actinomyces israelii* is the most significant. *A. naeslundii*, *A. odontolyticus*, *A. viscosus*, and *Arachnia propionica* also have been reported as human pathogens. Pelvic and perirectal infections have been associated with intrauterine devices (IUDs). A classic presentation of actinomycosis is as a painless lump in the jaw. *Actinomyces* may be found in rare instances of recurrent ventral hernia following appendectomy for appendicitis. The diagnosis of actinomycosis in many settings requires consideration of the possibility followed by persistence on the part of laboratory personnel.

Selected Readings
Bellingan GJ, "Disseminated Actinomycosis," *BMJ*, 1990, 301(6764):1323-4.

Feder HM Jr, "Actinomycosis Manifesting as an Acute Painless Lump of the Jaw," *Pediatrics*, 1990, 85(5):858-64.

Holtz HA, Lavery DP, and Kapila R, "Actinomycetales Infection in the Acquired Immunodeficiency Syndrome," *Ann Intern Med*, 1985, 102:203-5.

Levine LA and Doyle CJ, "Retroperitoneal Actinomycosis: A Case Report and Review of the Literature," *J Urol*, 1988, 140(2):367-9.

Nahass RG, Scholz P, Mackenzie JW, et al, "Chronic Constrictive Pericarditis, A Case Report and Review of the Literature," *Arch Intern Med*, 1989, 149(5):1202-3.

Persson E, "Genital Actinomycosis and *Actinomyces israelii* in the Female Genital Tract," *Adv Contracept*, 1987, 3:115-23, (review).

Acute Phase Reactant *see* C-Reactive Protein *on page 378*

Adenovirus Antibody Titer
Related Information
Adenovirus Culture *on this page*

Special Instructions Acute and convalescent sera should be tested simultaneously.

Specimen Serum

Container Red top tube or serum separator tube

Sampling Time Acute and convalescent sera drawn 12-21 days apart

Reference Range A fourfold increase in titer of paired sera is indicative of a virus infection. Titers suggestive of no previous exposure are usually ≤1:16.

Use Establish the diagnosis of adenovirus infection; can be useful in differential diagnosis of respiratory ailments, hemorrhagic cystitis, and keratoconjunctivitis

Limitations The specific adenovirus serotype responsible for infection and the distinction between IgG and IgM titers cannot be determined by complement fixation test. Complement fixation tests are of low sensitivity, particularly in children.

Methodology Complement fixation (CF), hemagglutination inhibition (HAI), enzyme-linked immunosorbent assay (ELISA), serum neutralization, indirect immunofluorescent assay (IFA)

Additional Information There are 41 different types of adenovirus, and many infections are both asymptomatic and persistent. Thus, serologic evidence of adenovirus, and even isolation of an adenovirus from a patient, may be coincidental rather than the cause of the patient's present complaints.

Selected Readings
Bryan JA, "The Serologic Diagnosis of Viral Infections," *Arch Pathol Lab Med*, 1987, 111(11):1015-23.

Hierholzer JC, "Adenoviruses," *Manual of Clinical Laboratory Immunology*, 4th ed, Rose NR, de Macario EC, Fahey JL, et al, eds, Washington, DC: American Society for Microbiology, 1992, 590-5.

Adenovirus Culture
Related Information
Adenovirus Antibody Titer *on this page*
Viral Culture, Throat *on page 574*

Test Includes Culture for adenovirus only; adenovirus usually is detected in a routine/general virus culture

Specimen Midstream urine, stool, nasopharyngeal secretions, eye exudates, throat swab or tissue

(Continued)

Adenovirus Culture *(Continued)*

Container Sterile container. Swabs should be placed into cold viral transport medium.

Storage Instructions Keep specimens cold and moist. Adenoviruses are more stabile than are most other viruses; however, specimens should not be stored or refrigerated for long periods of time. Specimens should be delivered immediately to the clinical laboratory.

Causes for Rejection Dry specimen, specimen not in proper viral transport medium, specimen not refrigerated during transport, specimen fixed in formalin

Turnaround Time Variable (1-14 days) and depends on culture method used and amount of virus in the specimen

Reference Range No virus isolated

Use Aid in the diagnosis of disease caused by adenovirus (eg, conjunctivitis, cystitis, pneumonia, and pharyngoconjunctivitis)

Limitations Rule out or identify adenovirus **only**

Methodology Inoculation of specimen into cell cultures, incubation of cell cultures, observation of characteristic cytopathic effect, and identification by fluorescent monoclonal antibody

Additional Information Adenoviruses can be the etiologic agent of respiratory infections in children up to 6 years of age and of ocular infections in both children and adults. Adenovirus respiratory infections can mimic pertussis.

Serology to detect adenovirus antibodies is often helpful in establishing a diagnosis.

Selected Readings

Hierholzer JC, "Adenoviruses," *Manual of Clinical Microbiology*, 5th ed, Balows A, Hausler WJ Jr, Herrmann KL, et al, eds, Washington, DC: American Society for Microbiology, 1991, 896-903.

Hierholzer JC, "Adenoviruses - A Spectrum of Human Diseases," *Clin Microbiol Newslett*, 1992, 14(15):113-20.

Hierholzer JC, "Adenoviruses in the Immunocompromised Host," *Clin Microbiol Rev*, 1992, 5(3):262-74.

Adenovirus Culture, Stool *see* Viral Culture, Stool *on page 573*

ADNase-B *see* Antideoxyribonuclease-B Titer, Serum *on page 322*

Aerobic Blood Culture *see* Blood Culture, Aerobic and Anaerobic *on page 337*

Aerobic Bone Marrow Culture *see* Bone Marrow Culture, Routine *on page 347*

Aerobic Culture, Abscess *see* Abscess Aerobic and Anaerobic Culture *on page 304*

Aerobic Culture, Appropriate Site

Refer to

Aerobic Culture, Body Fluid *on page 310*

Aerobic Culture, Cerebrospinal Fluid *on page 311*

Aerobic Culture, Sputum *on page 312*

Aerobic Culture, Body Fluid

Related Information

Anaerobic Culture *on page 316*

Histopathology *on page 448*

Synonyms Body Fluid Culture, Routine

Applies to Ascitic Fluid Culture; Bone Marrow Culture; Culture, Biopsy; Joint Fluid Culture; Pericardial Fluid Culture; Peritoneal Fluid Culture; Pleural Fluid Culture; Surgical Specimen Culture; Synovial Fluid Culture

Test Includes Aerobic culture of biopsy or body fluid specimens

Patient Preparation Aseptic preparation of biopsy site

Special Instructions The laboratory should be informed of the specific source of the specimen, age of patient, current antibiotic therapy, and clinical diagnosis. Specimens may be divided for fungus culture and stain, mycobacteria culture and acid-fast stain, and routine bacterial culture and Gram's stain only if the specimen is of adequate volume for all tests requested.

Specimen Surgical tissue, bone marrow, biopsy material from normally sterile site or aseptically aspirated body fluid

Container Sterile container with lid, no preservative. Bone marrow aspirates and body fluids may be directly inoculated into blood culture media. Contact the laboratory and obtain approval before inoculating fluids into blood culture media.

Collection Do **not** submit fluid collected with a swab. This type of specimen is rarely productive. The portion of the fluid specimen submitted for culture should be separated (utilizing sterile technique) from the portion submitted for histopathology.

Storage Instructions The specimen should be transported immediately to the laboratory.

Causes for Rejection Specimens in fixative, specimens collected on swabs, specimens having an excess transit time to the laboratory. Specimens which have been refrigerated have a less than optimal yield.

Turnaround Time Preliminary reports are available at 24 hours. Cultures with no growth are reported after 48 hours. Reports on specimens from which pathogens are isolated require a minimum of 48 hours for completion.

Reference Range No growth

Use Isolate and identify aerobic organisms causing infections in tissue

Limitations If anaerobes are suspected submit a properly collected specimen. See listings Anaerobic Culture *on page 316* and Abscess Aerobic and Anaerobic Culture *on page 304*. If mycobacteria or fungi are suspected see Mycobacteria Culture, Biopsy or Body Fluid *on page 493*, or Fungus Culture, Body Fluid *on page 415* for detailed instructions.

Methodology Aerobic culture

Additional Information The specimen should be obtained before empiric antimicrobial therapy is started.

Selected Readings
Gorbach SL, "Treatment of Intra-abdominal Infection," *Am J Med*, 1984, 76(5A):107-10.

Aerobic Culture, Cerebrospinal Fluid

Related Information
Cerebrospinal Fluid Analysis *on page 354*

Synonyms Cerebrospinal Fluid Aerobic Culture

Applies to Ventricular Fluid Culture

Test Includes Aerobic culture and Gram's stain (stat) if requested. Gram's stain, cell count, differential, glucose, and protein levels are usually requested. Additional fluid if available may be used for additional cultures and other diagnostic tests such as those for bacterial or cryptococcal antigen and/or for acid-fast stain.

Abstract The major tests to be performed on the CSF for meningitis are the Gram's stain and the bacteriologic culture. The "gold standard" for the diagnosis of bacterial meningitis is the isolation of a bacterium from the cerebrospinal fluid. Diagnosis of meningitis is made by blood culture and examination and culture of CSF.

Patient Preparation Aseptic preparation of the aspiration site

Special Instructions The laboratory should be informed of the specific source of specimen, age of patient, current antibiotic therapy, clinical diagnosis, and time of collection.

Specimen Cerebrospinal fluid

Container Sterile CSF tube

Collection Tubes should be numbered 1, 2, 3 with tube #1 representing the first portion of the sample collected. Contamination with normal flora from skin or other body surfaces must be avoided. The second or third tube collected during lumbar puncture is most suitable for culture, as skin contaminants from the puncture usually are washed out with fluid collected in the first two tubes. Since blood cultures are often positive in subjects with bacterial meningitis, blood cultures should be requested as well. Peripheral blood white cell count and differential are usually abnormal in patients with meningitis and represent an important part of the clinical investigation.

Storage Instructions The specimen should be transported immediately to the laboratory. If the specimen cannot be processed immediately, it should be kept at room temperature or placed in an incubator. Refrigeration inhibits viability of certain anaerobic organisms and may prevent the recovery of the common aerobic pathogens *Streptococcus pneumoniae*, *Neisseria meningitidis*, and *Haemophilus influenzae*.

Turnaround Time Preliminary reports are usually available at 24 hours. Cultures with no growth can be reported after 72 hours. Reports of cultures from which pathogens are isolated require a minimum of 48 hours for completion.

Reference Range No growth
(Continued)

Aerobic Culture, Cerebrospinal Fluid *(Continued)*

Use Isolate and identify pathogenic organisms causing meningitis, shunt infection, brain abscess, subdural empyema, cerebral or spinal epidural abscess, bacterial endocarditis with embolism. The time honored Gram's stain and aerobic CSF cultures in suspected bacterial meningitis are fundamental to appropriate diagnosis and treatment.

Limitations Cultures may be negative in partially treated cases of meningitis. Gram's stain is the single most useful laboratory test to diagnose bacterial meningitis. However, Gram's stains should be interpreted with care. Gram-positive organisms may decolorize (ie, stain gram-negative in partially treated cases). Acridine orange stain (AO) may have better sensitivity than Gram's stain in detecting the presence of organisms in partially treated cases of meningitis but it is not at all widely used.

Methodology Aerobic culture

Additional Information See table in Cerebrospinal Fluid Analysis *on page 354* for laboratory values of components of CSF from healthy persons and from persons with meningitis. *Haemophilus influenzae, Neisseria meningitidis,* and *Streptococcus pneumoniae,* the most commonly isolated pathogens, can be serotyped if requested. Infections of cerebrospinal fluid shunts pose a difficult clinical problem. Organisms cultured include coagulase-negative staphylococci, *S. aureus, Streptococcus,* viridans group, enterococci, and *H. influenzae.* Culture of CSF or shunt fluid is diagnostic. Simultaneous blood cultures are rarely positive. Removal of the catheter and later replacement are frequently required to eradicate the infection. Susceptibility testing will be performed if indicated.

Selected Readings

Feigin RD, McCracken GH Jr, and Klein JO, "Diagnosis and Management of Meningitis," *Pediatr Infect Dis J,* 1992, 11(9):785-814.

Gray LD and Fedorko DP, "Laboratory Diagnosis of Bacterial Meningitis," *Clin Microbiol Rev,* 1992, 5(2):130-45.

Greenlee JE, "Approach to Diagnosis of Meningitis - Cerebrospinal Fluid Evaluation," *Infect Dis Clin North Am,* 1990, 4(4):583-98.

Wenger JD, Hightower AW, Facklam RR, et al, "Bacterial Meningitis in the United States, 1986: Report of a Multistate Surveillance Study," *J Infect Dis,* 1990, 162(6):1316-23.

Aerobic Culture, Sputum

Related Information

Anaerobic Culture *on page 316*
Legionella pneumophila Culture *on page 469*
Mycoplasma pneumoniae Diagnostic Procedures *on page 497*

Synonyms Sputum Culture, Aerobic

Applies to Bronchial Washings Culture; Bronchoscopy Culture; Percutaneous Transtracheal Culture Routine; Tracheal Aspirate Culture; Transtracheal Aspirate Culture

Test Includes Culture of aerobic organisms and usually Gram's stain

Patient Preparation The patient should be instructed to remove dentures, rinse mouth, and gargle with water. The patient should then be instructed to cough deeply and expectorate sputum into proper container.

Special Instructions The laboratory should be informed of the specific site of specimen, the age of patient, current antibiotic therapy, clinical diagnosis, and time of collection.

Specimen Sputum, first morning specimen preferred; tracheal aspiration, bronchoscopy specimen, or transtracheal aspirate

Container Sputum container, sputum trap, sterile tracheal aspirate, or bronchoscopy aspirate tube

Collection Specimen collected, at time of bronchoscopy, by aspiration or by transtracheal aspiration by a physician skilled in the procedure. The specimen should be transported to laboratory within 1 hour of collection for processing.

Storage Instructions Refrigerate if the specimen cannot be promptly processed.

Causes for Rejection Specimens spilled or leaking onto the outside of the container pose excessive risk to laboratory personnel and may not be acceptable to the laboratory.

Turnaround Time Preliminary reports are usually available at 24 hours. Cultures with no growth or normal flora are usually reported after 48 hours. Reports on specimens from which pathogens are isolated require at least 48 hours for completion.

Reference Range Normal upper respiratory flora. Tracheal aspirate and bronchoscopy specimens usually are contaminated with normal oral flora. Transtracheal aspiration: no growth.

Use Isolate and identify potentially pathogenic organisms present in the lower respiratory tract. Presence or absence of normal upper respiratory flora is often reported.

Limitations An adequate sputum specimen should contain many neutrophils and few to no squamous epithelial cells, which are indicative of contamination with saliva. Results obtained by culture without evaluation for contamination may be noncontributory or misleading. A carefully collected and Gram's-stained specimen with neutrophils and gram-positive lancet-shaped diplococci can provide strong support for a clinical diagnosis of pneumococcal pneumonia.

In bronchoscopy and aspirated specimens reduction of contamination may be accomplished by a head-down position to reduce gravitational flow of saliva, when combined with quantitative culture techniques. Oral contamination may successfully be reduced by using a protected brush (PBC) catheter. The use of the PBC and bronchoalveolar lavage increases the overall diagnostic yield. Quantitation aids interpretation. Qualitatively, a bronchial washing is no better than sputum. If anaerobic bacteria are suspected in a transtracheal aspiration, a properly collected specimen for anaerobic culture should be submitted.

Methodology Aerobic culture following appropriate specimen selection. The most important step in the evaluation of a specimen is to be certain that the secretions that are examined are the product of the inflammatory process in the bronchi and not oropharyngeal material. All laboratories should perform this step.

Additional Information Potential pathogens recovered by usual sputum culture methods include: *Staphylococcus aureus*, *Haemophilus influenzae*, *Streptococcus pneumoniae*, *Neisseria meningitidis*, *Haemophilus parainfluenzae*, *Pseudomonas aeruginosa*, *Escherichia coli*, *Proteus* sp, *Moraxella catarrhalis*, *Bacteroides fragilis*, and rarely many other organisms. *Haemophilus* sp and *Neisseria* sp may not be isolated and identified by routine procedures. Thus, if their presence is clinically suspected, specific isolation procedures should be requested. See table.

Bacterial Species Recovered From Sputa in 103 Acute Bronchitic Exacerbations

	Number	Percent of All Types Cultured	Percent of Sputa Cultured
H. influenzae	41	24.0	39.8
H. parainfluenzae	29	17.0	28.2
S. pneumoniae	34	19.9	33.0
M. catarrhalis	19	11.1	18.4
N. meningitidis	5	2.9	4.9
K. pneumoniae	8	4.7	7.8
P. aeruginosa	4	2.3	3.9
Other possible pathogens	14	8.2	13.6
Unlikely pathogens	17	9.9	16.5

From Chodosh S, "Acute Bacterial Exacerbations in Bronchitis and Asthma," *Am J Med*, 1987, 82(Suppl 4A):154-63, with permission.

Organisms such as *Bordetella pertussis*, *Chlamydia pneumoniae Corynebacterium diphtheriae*, *Legionella pneumophila*, *Mycoplasma pneumoniae*, and *Mycobacterium tuberculosis* require special laboratory tests for isolation. Clinical suspicion of involvement by these agents should be communicated to the laboratory. See also listings for the specific agents.

The critical criteria for the diagnosis of acute bacterial infection of the bronchi are obtained from examination and culture of the sputum. The presence of bacteria in numbers greater than when the patient's condition is stable and a significant increase (ie, doubling) in the numbers of neutrophils present are essential laboratory criteria for the diagnosis of an acute bronchitic exacerbation. Gram's stain results more closely reflect the clinical outcome and along with the criterion of (Continued)

Aerobic Culture, Sputum *(Continued)*

the number of neutrophils in the sputum should be laboratory basis for determining success. Other commonly recognized agents causing pneumonia are listed in the following tables.

Spectrum of Frequent Etiologic Agents in Pneumonia

Aerobic Bacteria	Anaerobes	Fungi
Gram-positive aerobes	Bacteroides melaninogenicus	Aspergillus
Streptococcus pneumoniae	Fusobacterium	Coccidioides immitis
Staphylococcus aureus	Peptostreptococcus	Histoplasma capsulatum
Streptococcus pyogenes	Bacteroides fragilis	Blastomyces dermatitidis
Gram-negative aerobes	Actinomyces israelii	Cryptococcus neoformans
Haemophilus influenzae		Zygomycetes
Legionella pneumophila		
Escherichia coli		
Klebsiella pneumoniae		
Pseudomonas aeruginosa		
Viruses	**Parasites**	**Other**
Respiratory syncytial virus	Pneumocystis carinii	Mycoplasma pneumoniae
Parainfluenza virus	Ascaris lumbricoides	Chlamydia trachomatis
Influenza virus	Toxocara canis and catis	Chlamydia psittaci
Adenovirus	Filaria	Mycobacterium tuberculosis
Enterovirus	Strongyloides stercoralis	Chlamydia TWAR strains
Rhinovirus	Hookworms	Nocardia
Measles virus	Paragonimus	
Varicella-zoster virus	Echinococcus	
Rickettsia	Schistosomes	
Coxiella burnetii		
Cytomegalovirus		
Hantavirus		

From Cohen GJ, "Management of Infections of the Lower Respiratory Tract in Children," *Pediatr Infect Dis*, 1987, 6:317-23, with permission.

Community-Acquired Bacterial Pneumonias: Frequency of Various Pathogens	%
Streptococcus pneumoniae	40-60
Haemophilus influenzae	2.5-20
Gram-negative bacilli	6-37
Staphylococcus aureus	2-10
Anaerobic infections	5-10
Legionella	0-22.5
Mycoplasma pneumoniae	5-15
Nosocomial Pneumonias: Frequency of Various Pathogens	**%**
Klebsiella	13
Pseudomonas aeruginosa	10-12
Staphylococcus aureus	3-10.6
Escherichia coli	4-7.2
Enterobacter	6.2
Group D Streptococcus	1.3
Proteus and Providencia	6
Serratia	3.5
Pneumococcus	10-20
Aspiration pneumonia anaerobic pneumonia*	5-25
Legionella*	0-15

*The specific incidence of pneumonias caused by *Mycoplasma*, *Legionella*, and anaerobes is difficult to document because of the technical problems in isolating the organisms.

From Verghese A and Berk SL, "Bacterial Pneumonia in the Elderly Medicine," 1983, 62:271-85, with permission.

Selected Readings

Bartlett JG, Brewer NS, and Ryan KJ, "Laboratory Diagnosis of Lower Respiratory Tract Infections," *Cumitech 7*, Washington, DC: American Society for Microbiology, 1978.

Boerner DF and Zwadyk P, "The Value of the Sputum Gram's Stain in Community-Acquired Pneumonia," *JAMA*, 1982, 247(5):642-5.

Stratton CW, "Bacterial Pneumonias - An Overview With Emphasis on Pathogenesis, Diagnosis, and Treatment," *Heart Lung*, 1986, 15(3):226-44.

Aerobic Culture, Tissue *see* Biopsy Culture, Routine *on page 337*

AFB Culture, Biopsy *see* Mycobacteria Culture, Biopsy or Body Fluid *on page 493*

AFB Culture, Bronchial Aspirate *see* Mycobacteria Culture, Sputum *on page 495*

AFB Culture, Gastric Aspirate *see* Mycobacteria Culture, Sputum *on page 495*

AFB Culture, Sputum *see* Mycobacteria Culture, Sputum *on page 495*

AFB Smear *see* Acid-Fast Stain *on page 305*

AIDS Antigen *see* p24 Antigen *on page 509*

AIDS Blood Culture *see* Blood Culture, Mycobacteria *on page 342*

AIDS Virus Culture *see* Human Immunodeficiency Virus Culture *on page 459*

Amebiasis Serological Test *see* Entamoeba histolytica Serology *on page 404*

Amikacin Level

Related Information

Antibiotic Level, Serum *on page 321*

Synonyms Amikin® Level, Blood

Applies to Kanamycin (Kantrex®) Level

Abstract Aminoglycoside antibiotics, including amikacin, are used primarily to treat infections caused by aerobic gram-negative bacilli. Amikacin has a narrow therapeutic window. Its use in life-threatening infections makes it mandatory that effective levels be achieved without overdosing.

Specimen Serum

Container Red top tube or serum separator tube

Collection Not more than 30 minutes before the next dose for trough level; for peak level draw 15-30 minutes after completion of infusion or 45-75 minutes following intramuscular injection. Specify dosage, time of dosage, and all other coadministered antimicrobials. For send outs, ship specimen frozen in plastic vial on dry ice.

Storage Instructions Separate serum within 1 hour of collection, refrigerate or freeze until assayed.

Reference Range Therapeutic: peak: 15-25 µg/mL (SI: 26-43 µmol/L) (depends in part on the minimal inhibitory concentration of the drug against the organism being treated); trough: <10 µg/mL (SI: <17 µmol/L).

Critical Values Toxic: peak: >35 µg/mL (SI: >60 µmol/L); trough: >10 µg/mL (SI: >17 µmol/L)

Use Peak levels are necessary to assure adequate therapeutic levels for organism being treated. Trough levels are necessary to reduce the likelihood of nephrotoxicity.

Limitations High peak levels may not have strong correlation with toxicity.

Methodology High performance liquid chromatography (HPLC), fluorescence polarization immunoassay (FPIA), enzyme immunoassay (EIA)

Additional Information Amikacin is cleared by the kidney and accumulates in renal tubular cells. **Nephrotoxicity** is most closely related to the length of time that trough levels exceed 10 µg/mL (SI: >17 µmol/L). Creatinine levels should be monitored every 2-3 days as an indicator of impending renal toxicity. The initial toxic result is nonoliguric renal failure that is usually reversible if the drug is discontinued. Continued administration of amikacin may produce oliguric renal failure. Nephrotoxicity may occur in as many as 10% to 25% of patients receiving aminoglycosides; most of this toxicity can be avoided by monitoring levels and adjusting dosing schedules accordingly.

Aminoglycosides may also cause irreversible **ototoxicity** that manifests itself clinically as hearing loss. Aminoglycoside ototoxicity is relatively uncommon and (Continued)

Amikacin Level (Continued)

clinical trials in which levels were carefully monitored and dosing adjusted failed to show a correlation between auditory toxicity and plasma aminoglycoside levels. In situations where dosing is not adjusted, however, sustained high levels may be associated with ototoxicity. This association is far from clear cut, and new once-daily dosing regimens (and associated high peak serum concentrations) that fail to enhance toxicity further complicate the understanding of this issue.

Selected Readings

Edson RS and Terrell CL, "The Aminoglycosides," Mayo Clin Proc, 1991, 66(11):1158-64.
Porter WH, "Therapeutic Drug Monitoring," Clin Chem, Taylor EH, ed, New York, NY: John Wiley and Sons, 1989, 217-48.

Amikin® Level, Blood see Amikacin Level on previous page

Amphotericin B Level

Synonyms Fungizone® Level, Blood

Abstract Amphotericin B is a clinically useful but highly toxic antifungal agent. Newer, less toxic agents are available. However, for many serious fungal infections, amphotericin B is still used despite its toxicity.

Specimen Serum

Container Red top tube or serum separator tube

Reference Range Therapeutic range: 1.0-2.0 µg/mL (SI: 1.0-2.2 µmol/L)

Use Monitor serum levels for potential toxicity and correlation with in vitro susceptibility data

Limitations Assays for amphotericin B are performed only in a few reference laboratories. In routine clinical use it is probably more prudent to follow creatinine, potassium, bicarbonate, and magnesium concentrations and the CBC, than to perform amphotericin B assays.

Methodology High performance liquid chromatography (HPLC), bioassay

Additional Information Amphotericin B therapy frequently induces fever, chills, nausea, and reversible bone marrow suppression.

Additionally, approximately 80% of patients develop increased creatinine concentrations, and occasional patients show an acute deterioration in **renal function**; when creatinine levels exceed 3.0 µg/mL it is advisable to withhold amphotericin B for several days and resume therapy at a lower dose.

Because the pharmacokinetics and biodistribution of the drug are not clearly defined, it may be useful to correlate serum levels with desired concentrations determined by in vitro susceptibility testing. Susceptibility testing, however, is not widely available, is not well standardized, and may not accurately predict clinical response. Amphotericin B can increase digitalis toxicity and decrease the anti-Candida effect of miconazole, and its toxicities are additive with those of aminoglycosides.

Selected Readings

Bodey GP, "Topical and Systemic Antifungal Agents," Med Clin North Am, 1988, 72(3):637-59.
Drutz DJ, "Newer Antifungal Agents and Their Use, Including an Update on Amphotericin B and Flucytosine," Curr Clin Top Infect Dis, Remington JS and Swartz MN, eds, New York, NY: McGraw-Hill Book Co, 1982, 3:97-135.
Terrell CL and Hughes CE, "Antifungal Agents Used for Deep-Seated Mycotic Infections," Mayo Clin Proc, 1992, 67(1):69-91.

Amplicor™ HCV Monitor see Hepatitis C Viral RNA, Quantitative PCR on page 441

Anaerobic Bacterial Susceptibility see Antimicrobial Susceptibility Testing, Anaerobic Bacteria on page 327

Anaerobic Blood Culture see Blood Culture, Aerobic and Anaerobic on page 337

Anaerobic Culture

Related Information

Aerobic Culture, Body Fluid on page 310
Aerobic Culture, Sputum on page 312
Biopsy Culture, Routine on page 337

Applies to Biopsy Culture, Anaerobic; Body Fluid Anaerobic Culture; Bronchial Aspirate Anaerobic Culture; Cerebrospinal Fluid Anaerobic Culture; Cyst Culture, Anaerobic; Surgical Specimen Anaerobic Culture; Tissue Anaerobic Culture; Transtracheal Aspirate Anaerobic Culture

Test Includes Isolation and identification of anaerobic organisms; susceptibility testing may be performed if clinically warranted.

Patient Preparation Sterile preparation of the site

Special Instructions The following information will assist the laboratory in the proper processing of the specimen: specific site of specimen, current antibiotic therapy, age and sex of patient, collection time and date, and clinical diagnosis.

Specimen Surgical tissue, biopsy material from normally sterile site, aspirated fluids, etc. Specimen for anaerobic culture should be accompanied by a specimen for aerobic culture from the same site.

Container Fluids: anaerobic transport container or original syringe; tissue: sterile container, no preservative

Collection Specimens are to be collected from a prepared site using sterile technique. Contamination with normal flora from skin, rectum, vagina, or other body surfaces **must** be avoided.

Storage Instructions Transport specimen to the laboratory within 30 minutes. Do not refrigerate. Refrigeration inhibits viability of certain anaerobic organisms and also the common important aerobic pathogens *Neisseria meningitidis*, *Streptococcus pneumoniae*, and *Haemophilus influenzae*.

Causes for Rejection Specimen not received in appropriate transport container or sterile container, specimen in fixative. Specimens delayed in transport to the laboratory and specimens which have been refrigerated have a less than optimal yield. Specimens from unacceptable sites (see above) may not be acceptable for anaerobic culture because of contamination by the normal flora.

Turnaround Time Cultures showing no bacterial growth will be reported after 2 days. Complete reports of cultures with anaerobic bacteria may take as long as 2 weeks after receipt of culture depending upon the nature and number of the organisms isolated.

Reference Range No growth of anaerobic bacteria

Use Anaerobic cultures are indicated particularly when suspected infections are related to mucus membranes, gastrointestinal tract, pelvic organs, associated with malignancy, related to use of aminoglycosides, or occur in a setting where the diagnosis of gas gangrene or actinomycosis is considered. Anaerobic culture is especially indicated when an exudate has a foul odor or if the exudate has a grayish discoloration and is hemorrhagic. Frequently, more than one organism is recovered from an anaerobic infection.

Limitations Specimens received in anaerobic transport containers are less-than-optimal for aerobic or fungal cultures.

Contraindications Specimens absolutely contraindicated for anaerobic culture include the following: oral, GI, skin, urogenital, throat, sputum, bronchial wash, bowel contents, void urine, vaginal, cervical, material adjacent to a mucus membrane from a wound or decubitus.

Additional Information Biopsy culture is particularly useful in establishing the diagnosis of anaerobic osteomyelitis, clostridial myonecrosis, intracranial actinomycosis and pleuropulmonary infections. In cases of osteomyelitis, biopsy is mandatory. Anaerobic infections of soft tissue include the following: anaerobic cellulitis, necrotizing fasciitis, clostridial myonecrosis (gas gangrene), anaerobic streptococcal myositis or myonecrosis, synergistic nonclostridial anaerobic myonecrosis, and infected vascular gangrene. These infections, particularly clostridial myonecrosis, necrotizing fasciitis, and nonclostridial anaerobic myonecrosis, may be fulminant and are frequently characterized by the presence of gas and foul smelling necrotic tissue. Empiric therapy based on likely pathogens should be instituted as soon as appropriate cultures are collected.

Oral contamination of bronchial aspirates can be minimized by using a telescoping double catheter with a plug to protect the brush. Even by this method, many anaerobes might not survive transit to the laboratory because of aeration of specimens and transport to the laboratory in an inappropriate transport device. Because of difficulty in interpretation, the usefulness of bronchial aspirate anaerobic cultures collected in the usual manner by routine bronchoscopy (ie, contaminated with oral flora), has been questioned. Pleuropulmonary infections caused by anaerobic organisms are most often secondary to aspiration of oropharyngeal contents. They may also be caused by septic emboli or from intra-abdominal infections (ie, subphrenic abscess, diverticulitis, appendicitis, etc). Community-acquired aspiration pneumonia, necrotizing pneumonia with multiple small abscesses, frank lung abscess, and pulmonary empyema yield significant anaerobes, 60% to 95% of cases, if appropriate culture technique is (Continued)

Anaerobic Culture *(Continued)*

employed. The characteristic foul smelling odor of an anaerobic infection may not be present early in the course.

Selected Readings

Allen SD and Siders JA, "An Approach to the Diagnosis of Anaerobic Pleuropulmonary Infection," *Clin Lab Med*, 1982, 2(2):285-303.

Bartlett JG, Alexander J, Mayhew J, et al, "Should Fiberoptic Bronchoscopy Aspirates be Cultured?" *Am Rev Respir Dis*, 1976, 114(1):73-8.

Finegold SM, "Anaerobic Bacteria: General Concepts," *Principles and Practice of Infectious Diseases*, 4th ed, Mandell GL, Bennett JE and Dolin R, eds, New York, NY: Churchill Livingstone, 1995, 2156-73.

Finegold SM, "Anaerobic Infections," *Surg Clin North Am*, 1980, 60(1):49-64.

Willis AR, "Anaerobic Bacterial Diseases Now and Then. Where Do We Go From Here?" *Rev Infect Dis*, 1984, 6(Suppl 1):S293-9.

Anaerobic Culture, Abscess *see* Abscess Aerobic and Anaerobic Culture *on page 304*

Ancobon® Level *see* Flucytosine Level *on page 408*

Anergy Control Panel *see* Anergy Skin Test Battery *on this page*

Anergy Skin Test Battery

Related Information

Fungal Skin Testing *on page 411*

Tuberculin Skin Testing, Intracutaneous *on page 557*

Synonyms Anergy Control Panel; Anergy Skin Testing; Delayed Reaction Intracutaneous Tests; Skin Test Battery

Test Includes Injection of several common antigenic substances into the skin, such as *Candida*, *Trichophyton*, and mumps antigens. Anergy skin testing is an *in vivo* means of evaluating the cell-mediated immune system. Skin injection sites are examined at 24, 48, and 72 hours. The development of local erythema and induration indicates an adequate delayed hypersensitivity response, and implies competent T-cell function. Failure to respond to any skin test antigen is termed cutaneous anergy, and is seen in a variety of systemic disorders.

Patient Preparation Procedure and risks are explained to the patient. No specific skin preparation is necessary. However, those patients with generalized skin disease, such as psoriasis, should be examined beforehand to ensure that there are suitable areas of normal appearing skin. Although testing need not be performed by a physician, one should be immediately available in the event of a systemic reaction.

Aftercare If no adverse reaction has occurred within 30 minutes, patient may be discharged from the testing center. Test sites should be kept reasonably clean for 72 hours. No restrictions on bathing are necessary. Patient should contact physician if severe local reactions develop, extensive erythema beyond the test site occurs, or if fever, dyspnea, or lightheadedness develops.

Special Instructions Requisition should include a list of all current medications, with attention to corticosteroids or other immunosuppressive agents.

Complications Anergy skin testing is generally quite safe. However, as with other forms of skin testing, immediate local reactions to antigens are distinctly unusual but possible. These reactions are usually IgE-mediated and lead to an immediate wheal and flare reaction. Rarely, serious local reactions have been reported to various antigens commonly included in the test battery; these include vesiculation, skin necrosis, and extensive erythema. Systemic reactions have been reported only on an individual case basis.

Equipment Antigens used for anergy testing are commercially prepared liquid extracts of a variety of foreign substances. These antigens are chosen because ubiquitous exposure to these substances is expected in the general population. Thus, in any randomly selected subgroup, a high rate of delayed hypersensitivity skin reactions would be anticipated. Commonly used bacterial antigens include streptococcal antigen (derived from *Streptococcus* group CH 46A), *Proteus* antigen (often from *Proteus mirabilis* IM 2104 strain), and in some centers, tuberculin is also included. Fungal antigens frequently employed include *Candida* antigen (derived from *Candida albicans* strain 2111), *Trichophyton* antigen (from *Trichophyton mentagrophytes*), and frequently histoplasmin is used (from *Histoplasma capsulatum*). Toxoids are also included in the test battery, usually tetanus toxoid (from *Clostridium tetani*, Harvard strain 401) and diphtheria toxoid (from *Corynebacterium diphtheriae*). Mumps skin test antigen is a viral antigen derived from inactivated mumps virus cultured in chick embryo.

The choice of antigens and total number employed has yet to be standardized. Most test centers use less than five antigens in their routine battery, but considerable variation exists, with the total number ranging from 1-11. In studies, 90% of 750 hospitalized patients reacted to one or more of the following: mumps, *Candida*, *Trichophyton*, and tuberculin. Increasing the total number of antigens improved the rate of skin reactions by only 1%. With respect to the individual selection of antigens, a representative battery might therefore include mumps, *Candida*, and *Trichophyton*; this combination is commonly seen in practice. However, in one literature review, more than thirty different antigens were found to be in routine use at major centers. Disposable plastic or glass tuberculin syringes, 0.5-1 mL are also required, along with 26- or 27-gauge short ($^1/_4$" to $^1/_2$") beveled needles, some alcohol pads, and gauze. An alternative anergy testing technique has been developed in recent years to address the aforementioned lack of standardization in antigen selection and number. Termed the Multitest® CMI system, seven standardized antigens and one control are simultaneously injected by means of a multiple puncture device. Antigens used in the system are tetanus toxoid, diphtheria toxoid, streptococcal antigen, *Proteus*, tuberculin, *Candida*, and *Trichophyton*. This device obviates the need for separate syringes, needles, and antigens.

Technique Traditional method: Antigens are injected separately. Antigens are individually drawn up into tuberculin syringes immediately prior to testing. The volar aspects of the arms or forearms are the preferred test sites. Only normal appearing skin should be used. Sites are prepared with alcohol swabs. Using a 26- or 27-gauge needle, each antigen is injected intradermally at a 45° angle, bevel down. A small bleb approximately 2-3 mm in diameter should be raised; usually an injected volume of 0.05 mL is sufficient. Care should be taken to avoid deeper subcutaneous injections. Each antigen is separately planted in this fashion with adequate spacing between injection sites (>2 cm).

Multipuncture method: Antigens are placed simultaneously by means of the Multitest® CMI device. Seven antigens and one glycerol control are standardized with respect to selection and concentration and are preloaded onto this disposable plastic device. A different antigen coats each of seven multiple puncture heads, which are spaced approximately 2 cm apart, in two parallel rows of four. The skin over the forearm is held taut. The device is then oriented per manufacturer's instructions ("T" bar towards the head) and applied to the skin with a rocking motion. Each head must sufficiently puncture the skin.

Regardless of technique, all tests sites should be examined immediately and at 24, 48, and 72 hours. Date and time of injection must be recorded. The precise location, identity, and concentration of each antigen should be recorded, most often in a pictorial format or standardized table. It may be helpful to circle and label each antigen with a waterproof pen directly onto the skin, but this must not replace formal notations in the medical chart.

Data Acquired The transverse diameter of induration at each test site should be carefully measured by both inspection and palpation. Results are recorded in millimeters at the appropriate 24-hour intervals. Areas of erythema are also measured but play a minor role in most grading schemes.

Reference Range Normal individuals should demonstrate a positive skin reaction to one or more test antigens.

Critical Values A positive skin test is usually defined as the presence of induration and accompanying erythema ≥5 mm in transverse diameter at an injection site at 24, 48, or 72 hours. Immediate skin reactions (ie, within minutes) are due to mechanisms other than cellular immunity and do not define a positive test. When the Multitest® CMI system is used, induration ≥2 mm in transverse diameter is considered significant. This disparity in definition between the intradermal and multiple puncture technique results from a variety of technical factors including volume of antigen introduced, depth of skin penetration, etc. A state of anergy is defined as an inability to mount an appropriate delayed hypersensitivity response. In clinical practice this is manifested as a complete absence of reactivity to a skin test battery of at least four to five antigens. Some authorities require repetition of the test battery at least once before labeling a patient "anergic". Normal individuals are expected to develop a positive skin test in response to at least one antigen, barring technical error. Anergy may be present (Continued)

Anergy Skin Test Battery *(Continued)*

as a generalized defect in T-cell function, as in sarcoidosis, AIDS, or tuberculosis, or as a specific defect in cellular immunity, as in mucocutaneous candidiasis where T-cell response to *Candida* is selectively deficient. There are numerous causes of anergy and may be categorized as follows:

- infections: bacterial, tuberculosis, disseminated fungal infections, viral (influenza, mumps, mononucleosis, hepatitis, and others), parasitic
- congenital: cell-mediated deficiency (DiGeorge syndrome), combined cellular and humoral deficiency (Nezelof's, Wiskott-Aldrich syndrome, etc)
- acquired/iatrogenic: neoplasms (solid tumors, lymphomas, leukemias), medications (corticosteroids, antineoplastic agents, methotrexate, and others), AIDS
- rheumatic diseases: rheumatoid arthritis, lupus, Behçet's disease
- miscellaneous: uremia, diabetes mellitus, inflammatory bowel disease, sarcoidosis, extremes of age, malnutrition

However, anergy skin testing by itself does not distinguish amongst these conditions from a diagnostic viewpoint. Clinically, anergy testing is most useful in evaluating the patient who presents with chronic or recurrent infections, or infection with unusual organisms. In such cases, formal evaluation of the immune system may be warranted. This may include assessment of all four major components of the immune system: cell-mediated (T-cell) immunity, antibody-mediated (B-cell) immunity, phagocytic system (polymorphonuclear leukocytes, macrophages), and complement. Often a careful history and physical, with attention to infectious diseases, will identify the particular component deficiency. Anergy testing is an appropriate and recommended screening procedure for suspected deficiencies in cell-mediated immunity, often characterized by fungal, mycobacterial, or disseminated viral infections (eg, varicella-zoster, cytomegalovirus, herpes simplex virus). Among the many laboratory tests available to evaluate host defense, anergy testing is rightfully obtained soon after the history and physical (along with a complete blood count with differential) but prior to more elaborate *in vitro* investigation of T-cell function. These latter tests include T-cell surface marker studies, T-cell subsets, and response to mitogens (such as pokeweed mitogen, phytohemagglutinin, concanavalin A). Some individuals demonstrate partial or inconclusive responses to skin testing. This is seen as a "borderline" skin induration diameter (ie, 1-4 mm) or as a poor reactivity rate when a large antigen battery is employed (ie, one positive reaction out of ten tested). These patients have sometimes been called "hypoergic," which implies a partially impaired delayed hypersensitivity response. The clinical significance of this phenomenon is unclear at present.

Use

- Objectively demonstrate cutaneous anergy in cases of suspected cellular immune system deficiency (T-cell dysfunction); often this procedure is performed as part of an initial immune system assessment, but may also be repeated in a serial fashion in cases of protracted or chronic illness
- Serve as a "control" skin test accompanying the tuberculin skin test (or other specific antigen tests); this allows more accurate interpretation of a negative tuberculin test; patients with generalized cutaneous anergy predictably fail to react to injected tuberculin despite prior exposure to *M. tuberculosis*
- Establish the presence of cutaneous anergy prior to more extensive *in vitro* evaluation of lymphocyte and monocyte function
- Less commonly, to help predict postoperative morbidity and mortality, especially in the patient with sepsis
- Occasionally, to provide general prognostic information in patients with cancer

Limitations "Traditional" skin test battery limitations, mentioned previously, include variation in selection and total number of antigens used as well as a lack of standardization of antigen potency. However, some practitioners consider the inability to select and interchange antigens in the Multitest® CMI system a major drawback. False-positive reactions may occur:

- when an immediate wheal and flare is interpreted as delayed hypersensitivity
- when intradermal bleeding is interpreted as erythema
- when dermographism is present

False-negative reactions may be caused by:

- lack of antigen potency

- subcutaneous injection
- inadequate dose or concentration
- incomplete skin puncture by the Multitest® device
- attenuated skin response, as in atopic dermatitis

Contraindications

- Prior systemic reaction to any antigen included in the skin test battery; alternate antigens may be substituted in most cases
- Known hypersensitivity to a stabilizer or diluent used in commercial antigen preparations; for example, mumps skin test antigen is derived from virus incubated in chicken embryo and preserved in thimerosal. Patients should therefore be questioned regarding feather and egg allergy as well as sensitivity to thimerosal prior to administering mumps antigen. Depending on the particular antigens selected, published manufacturer's warnings should be reviewed and potential hypersensitivity reactions avoided.

Selected Readings

Gordin FM, Hartigan PM, Klimas NG, et al, "Delayed-Type Hypersensitivity Skin Tests Are an Independent Predictor of Human Immunodeficiency Virus Disease Progression," *J Infect Dis*, 1994, 169(4):893-7.

Kniker WT, Anderson CT, McBryde JL, et al, "Multitest CMI for Standardized Measurement of Delayed Cutaneous Hypersensitivity and Cell-Mediated Immunity. Normal Values and Proposed Scoring System for Healthy Adults in the U.S.A.," *Ann Allergy*, 1984, 52(2):75-82.

Anergy Skin Testing *see* Anergy Skin Test Battery *on page 318*

Animal and Human Bites Guidelines *see page 1061*

Ankle Arthrogram *see* Arthrogram *on page 334*

Ankle, Left or Right, X-ray *see* Bone Films *on page 343*

Anti-B19 Parvovirus IgG Antibodies *see* Parvovirus B19 Serology *on page 514*

Anti-B19 Parvovirus IgM Antibodies *see* Parvovirus B19 Serology *on page 514*

Antibacterial Activity, Serum *see* Serum Bactericidal Test *on page 533*

Antibiotic-Associated Colitis Toxin Test *see* Clostridium difficile Toxin Assay *on page 367*

Antibiotic Level, Serum

Related Information

Amikacin Level *on page 315*
Chloramphenicol Serum Level *on page 367*
Flucytosine Level *on page 408*
Gentamicin Level *on page 425*
Tobramycin Level *on page 551*
Vancomycin Level *on page 568*

Synonyms Antimicrobial Assay

Abstract Assays for antimicrobial agents in serum are performed for two primary reasons: 1. to ensure therapeutic levels, and 2. to monitor for potentially toxic levels. In most situations, it is not necessary to monitor antimicrobial levels because serum levels are relatively predictable based on dosing; *in vitro* susceptibility testing uses those predictable levels to determine clinical efficacy. Similarly, toxicity is not always related to serum levels. It may be more appropriate to monitor for toxicity by following determinants of hematologic, renal, or hepatic function. In certain situations however (eg, aminoglycoside antibiotics which have a narrow therapeutic range and a high potential for toxicity), it is essential to follow serum levels.

Specimen Serum

Container Red top tube or serum separator tube

Sampling Time Peak: 30 minutes after 30 minute I.V. infusion; 1 hour after I.M. dose. Trough: immediately prior to next dose.

Collection Keep frozen if not assayed immediately.

Causes for Rejection Incomplete clinical information (eg, specific antimicrobial, dosage and schedule, other concurrent antimicrobials)

Reference Range Therapeutic range depends on agent being tested for, and minimal inhibitory concentration of drug against organism. Selected ranges in µg/mL are presented as a guide only. See table on next page.

Possible Panic Range See entries on aminoglycoside drugs.

Use Evaluate adequacy of serum antibiotic level; detection of toxic levels

(Continued)

Antibiotic Level, Serum *(Continued)*

Antibiotic Level, Serum

Drug	Peak		Trough	
	µg/mL	SI: µmol/L	µg/mL	SI: µmol/L
Amikacin	15-25	26-43	<10	<17
Chloramphenicol	25	77		
Flucytosine	100	775		
Gentamicin	4-10	8-21	<2	<4
Netilmicin	4-8	8.0-17.0	1-2	0.7-1.4
Streptomycin	5-20	9-34	<5	<9
Tobramycin	4-10	8-21	<2	<4
Vancomycin	20-40	13.6-27.2	5-10	3.4-6.8

Selected ranges in µg/mL are presented as a guide only.

Limitations May not be technically possible in a patient taking more than one antibiotic

Methodology Bioassay: cephalosporins, clindamycin, erythromycin, metronidazole, penicillins, polymyxin, tetracycline, trimethoprim. High performance liquid chromatography: chloramphenicol, flucytosine, mezlocillin. Fluorescence polarization immunoassay (FPIA): amikacin, gentamicin, tobramycin, kanamycin, streptomycin, vancomycin, neomycin, netilmicin.

Additional Information With the increasing availability of *in vitro* sensitivity testing expressed as the minimal inhibitory or bactericidal concentration of an antibiotic, measurement of serum levels of these drugs has taken on practical clinical importance. This is especially true for agents with narrow therapeutic ranges and significant toxicity. It should be remembered, however, that in most patients, cure of infection depends on numerous host factors as well as on antibiotics. Therefore, antibiotic levels should not be relied on as the sole guide to therapy.

Selected Readings

Donowitz GR and Mandell GL, "Drug Therapy. Beta-Lactam Antibiotics," *N Engl J Med*, 1988, 318(8):490-500.

Rosenblatt JE, "Laboratory Tests Used to Guide Antimicrobial Therapy," *Mayo Clin Proc*, 1991, 66(9):942-8.

Smith AL and Opheim E, "Comparison of Methods for Clinical Quantitation of Antibiotics," *Curr Clin Top Infect Dis*, Remington JS and Swartz MN, eds, New York, NY: McGraw-Hill Book Co, 1983, 4:333-57.

Antideoxyribonuclease-B Titer, Serum

Related Information

Antistreptolysin O Titer, Serum *on page 330*
Streptozyme *on page 544*

Synonyms ADNase-B; Anti-DNase-B Titer; Antistreptococcal DNase-B Titer; Streptodornase

Specimen Serum

Container Red top tube or serum separator tube

Causes for Rejection Excessive hemolysis, chylous serum

Reference Range Preschool: ≤60 units; school: ≤170 units; adult: ≤85 units; A rise in titer of two or more dilution increments between acute and convalescent sera is significant.

Use Document recent streptococcal infection

Limitations Normal ranges may vary in different populations

Contraindications Not valid in patients with hemorrhagic pancreatitis

Methodology Colorimetry based on hydrolysis of DNA

Additional Information Presence of antibodies to streptococcal DNase is an indicator of recent infection, especially if a rise in titer can be documented. This test has both theoretical and technical advantages over the ASO test: it is more sensitive to streptococcal pyoderma, it is not so subject to false-positives due to liver disease, and one need not worry about test invalidation due to oxidation of reagents.

Anti-DNase-B Titer *see* Antideoxyribonuclease-B Titer, Serum *on this page*

Antifungal Susceptibility Testing

Related Information

Periodic Acid-Schiff Stain *on page 518*

Synonyms Fungi, Susceptibility Testing; Susceptibility Testing, Fungi

Test Includes Broth dilution, agar dilution and disc diffusion testing of antifungal agents. Results may be quantitative or qualitative.

Special Instructions Consult the laboratory to determine availability and choice of methods.

Specimen Pure isolate of the organism

Causes for Rejection Organism disposed of prior to request for testing.

Reference Range See table on next page.

Use Determine susceptibility of isolated fungi to available therapeutic agents, predict probable clinical response, explain observed or suspected therapeutic failures, determine if primary or secondary resistance is present

Limitations This test procedure is usually available only from specialized laboratories. Methods for fungal susceptibility testing are not as yet as standardized as for bacteria. Stability and solubility of some of the agents cause technical difficulty.

Methodology Standardized methods are evolving for the susceptibility of yeasts. The availability of a choice of therapeutic agents will continue to cause laboratories to attempt to provide susceptibility data with a useful predictive value for clinicians.

Additional Information Interpretation of *in vitro* susceptibility data for antifungal drugs is hindered by the absence of standardized test criteria. Thus, it is extremely difficult to identify a clear relation between minimal inhibitory concentrations and clinical outcome. The situation appears more readily resolvable for yeast-like fungi than for filamentous fungi since the former are more easily quantified by standardized microbiologic techniques.

Selected Readings

Bennett JE, "Antifungal Agents," *Principles and Practice of Infectious Diseases*, New York, NY: John Wiley & Sons, 1985, 263-70.

Espinel-Ingroff A, "Antifungal Susceptibility Testing," *Clin Microbiol Newslett*, 1996, 18(21):161-7.

Fromtling RA, "Overview of Medically Important Antifungal Azole Derivatives," *Clin Microbiol Rev*, 1988, 1(2):187-217.

Shadomy S and Pfaller MA, "Laboratory Studies With Antifungal Agents: Susceptibility Tests and Quantitation in Body Fluids," *Manual of Clinical Microbiology*, 5th ed, Balows A, Hausler WJ Jr, Herrmann KL, et al, eds, Washington, DC: American Society for Microbiology, 1991, 1173-83.

Anti-HCV (IgM) *see* Hepatitis C Serology *on page 437*

Anti-Hepatitis E Virus *see* Hepatitis E Serology *on page 443*

Anti-HEV *see* Hepatitis E Serology *on page 443*

Antimicrobial Assay *see* Antibiotic Level, Serum *on page 321*

Antimicrobial Removal Device (ARD) Blood Culture *see* Blood Culture, Aerobic and Anaerobic *on page 337*

Antimicrobial Susceptibility Testing, Aerobic and Facultatively Anaerobic Organisms

Related Information

Abscess Aerobic and Anaerobic Culture *on page 304*

Penicillinase Test *on page 517*

Serum Bactericidal Test *on page 533*

Synonyms Kirby-Bauer Susceptibility Test; MIC; Minimum Inhibitory Concentration Susceptibility Test; Susceptibility Testing, Aerobic and Facultatively Anaerobic Organisms

Test Includes Qualitative or quantitative determination of antimicrobial susceptibility of an isolated organism

Abstract The purpose of antimicrobial susceptibility testing is to determine the degree of activity of antimicrobial agents against specific pathogens.

Specimen Viable pure culture of aerobic or facultatively anaerobic rapidly growing organism

Turnaround Time Usually 1 day after isolation of a pure culture

Reference Range As of December, 1993, the National Committee for Clinical Laboratory Standards revised interpretations of antimicrobial susceptibility testing results. The interpretation "moderately susceptible" has been eliminated. The current interpretations of results are "susceptible," "intermediate," and "resistant."

(Continued)

In vitro Antifungal Activities of Four Antifungal Agents Against Pathogenic Fungi*

Organism	Amphotericin B		Flucytosine (5-FC)		Miconazole		Ketoconazole
	MIC (µg/mL)	MFC (µg/mL)	MIC (µg/mL)	MFC (µg/mL)	MIC (µg/mL)	MFC (µg/mL)	MIC (µg/mL)
Pathogenic yeasts							
Cryptococcus neoformans	0.05-0.78†	0.1-12.5	0.10-100#	0.39->100	0.05-3.13	0.05-25	0.1-32
Candida albicans	0.2-0.78•	0.39-0.78	0.05-12.5#	0.10->100	0.1-2.0•	0.1-10	<0.1-128
Candida sp not C. albicans	0.2-1.56•	0.39-6.25	0.10-50#	0.20->100	<0.1-2.0	0.1->10	<0.1-64
Torulopsis glabrata	0.1-0.4	0.2-0.78	0.05-1.56	0.4->100	0.5-10	2-10	1-64
Trichosporon sp	0.78-3.13	1.56-3.13	25-100	>100	0.2-25	0.2->100	
Geotrichum sp	0.4-1.56	0.78-3.13	1.56-12.5	25->100	0.1-2	0.5->10	
Filamentous fungi							
Pseudallescheria (Petriellidium) boydii	1.56->100#	>100	Resistant		0.5§	0.05	0.1-4#
Aspergillus sp including A. fumigatus	0.05-8	6.25->100	0.2-1.56#	>100	0.4->100	0.8->100	0.1-100
Blastomyces dermatitidis	0.05-0.2	0.1-0.4	Resistant		≤0.25	ND	0.1-2
Xylohypha bautiano	3.13->100	3.13->100	3.13-12.5#	12.5->100	0.5->64	ND	0.1-64
Coccidioides immitis	0.1-0.78	0.70-1.56	Resistant		0.25-1.0	ND	0.1-0.8

In vitro Antifungal Activities of Four Antifungal Agents Against Pathogenic Fungi*Continued

Organism	Amphotericin B		Flucytosine (5-FC)		Miconazole			Ketoconazole
	MIC (µg/mL)	MFC (µg/mL)	MIC (µg/mL)	MFC (µg/mL)	MIC (µg/mL)	MFC (µg/mL)		MIC (µg/mL)
Histoplasma capsulatum	0.05–1.0	0.05–0.2	Resistant		≤0.25	ND		0.1–0.5
Phialophora sp and other dematiaceous fungi	0.05–>128	6.25–>128	Variable susceptibility	Resistant	0.05–32	ND		0.1–64
Sporothrix schenckii	1.56–12.5	3.13–>100	Resistant		1–2	ND		0.1–16
Zygomycetes	0.78–1.56	1.56–>100	Variable susceptibility	Resistant				
Control organisms								
S. cerevisiae ATCC 36375, etc	0.1	0.2	0.05	0.10	0.20	0.39		0.20
C. pseudotropicalis ATCC 28838			0.05	0.10	0.10	0.20		0.05

*Based upon both data obtained at the Medical College of Virginia, Virginia Commonwealth University, Richmond, and a review of the literature. In vitro data for nystatin is not included because of the narrow clinical spectrum of this agent; however, most isolates of Candida species and Torulopsis species should be clinically susceptible (MIC ≤10 µg/mL) to nystatin. MFC, minimal fungicidal concentration; ND, not determined.

†Expected ranges of MICs and MFCs.

#Resistance not uncommon.

•Resistance reported but rare.

§Only limited data available.

‡ In vitro susceptibility of Aspergillus sp to ketoconazole is highly species dependent.

From Shadomy S and Pfaller MA, "Laboratory Studies With Antifungal Agents: Susceptibility Tests and Quantitation in Body Fluids," Manual of Clinical Microbiology, 5th ed, Washington, DC, American Society for Microbiology, 1991, 1173–83, with permission.

Antimicrobial Susceptibility Testing, Aerobic and Facultatively Anaerobic Organisms *(Continued)*

Use Determine the antimicrobial susceptibility of organisms involved in infectious processes when the susceptibility of the organism cannot be predicted from its identity

Methodology Disc diffusion, broth dilution, agar dilution, or microbroth dilution.

Additional Information Effective antimicrobial therapy is usually selected with the intent of achieving peak level 2-4 times the MIC at the site of infection. An antimicrobial level 10 times the MIC is usually sought in urinary tract infections. The "breakpoints" indicate clinically achievable levels and relate to MICs above which organisms are resistant and would not be expected to respond to readily achievable levels of antimicrobial therapy.

Susceptible: This category implies that an infection due to the strain may be appropriately treated with the dosage of antimicrobial agent recommended for that type of infection and infecting species, unless otherwise contraindicated.

Intermediate: This interpretation implies clinical applicability in body sites where the agent is physiologically concentrated (eg, in urine) or when a high dose of agent can be administered (eg, penicillins). In some cases "intermediate" applies to an MIC literally between a "susceptible" MIC and a "resistant" MIC. Such MICs are due to small uncontrollable technical errors/factors.

Resistant: Strains falling in this category are not inhibited by the usually achievable systemic concentrations of the agent with normal dosage schedules and/or fall in the range where specific microbial resistance mechanisms are likely (eg, beta-lactamases), and clinical efficacy has not been reliable in treatment studies. See table.

Major Mechanisms of Bacterial Antimicrobial Resistance

Enzymatic inactivation or modification of drug

- β-lactamase hydrolysis of β-lactam ring with subsequent inactivation of β-lactam antibiotics
- Modification of aminoglycosides by acetylating, adenylating, or phosphorylating enzymes
- Modification of chloramphenicol by chloramphenicol acetyltransferase

Decreased drug uptake or accumulation

- Intrinsic or acquired lack of outer membrane permeability
- Faulty or lacking antibiotic uptake and transport system
- Antibiotic efflux system (eg, tetracycline resistance)

Altered or lacking antimicrobial target

- Altered penicillin-binding proteins (β-lactam resistance)
- Altered ribosomal target (eg, aminoglycoside, macrolide, and lincomycin resistance)
- Altered enzymatic target (eg, sulfonamide, trimethoprim, rifampin, and quinolone resistance)

Circumvention of drug action consequences

- Hyperproduction of drug targets or competitive substrates (eg, sulfonamide and trimethoprim resistance)

Uncoupling of antibiotic attack and cell death

- Bacterial tolerance and survival in presence of usually bactericidal drugs (eg, β-lactams and vancomycin)

Selected Readings

Gill VJ, Witebsky FG, and MacLowry JD, "Multicategory Interpretive Reporting of Susceptibility Testing With Selected Antimicrobial Concentrations. Ten Years of Laboratory and Clinical Experience," *Clin Lab Med*, 1989, 9(2):221-38.

Hindler JA and Thrupp LD, "Interpretive Guidelines for Antimicrobial Susceptibility Test Results: What Do They Mean?" *Clin Microbiol Newslett*, 1989, 17:129-36.

"Methods for Dilution Antimicrobial Susceptibility Tests for Bacteria Which Grow Aerobically - Third Edition; Approved Standard. Document M7-A3," Vol 13, Villanova, PA: National Committee for Laboratory Standards, 1993.

"Performance Standards for Antimicrobial Disk Susceptibility Tests -Fifth Edition; Approved Standard. Document M2-A5," Vol 13, Villanova, PA: National Committee for Laboratory Standards, 1993.

Rosenblatt JE, "Laboratory Tests Used to Guide Antimicrobial Therapy," *Mayo Clin Proc*, 1991, 66(9):942-8.

Antimicrobial Susceptibility Testing, Anaerobic Bacteria

Related Information

Abscess Aerobic and Anaerobic Culture *on page 304*

Penicillinase Test *on page 517*

Synonyms Anaerobic Bacterial Susceptibility; MIC, Anaerobic Bacteria; Susceptibility Testing, Antimicrobial, Anaerobic Bacteria

Special Instructions The laboratory should be consulted regarding appropriateness and scope of anaerobic susceptibility testing in a particular clinical setting.

Specimen Viable pure culture of anaerobic organism

Turnaround Time 2-5 days from time organism is isolated and identified

Reference Range See table on next page.

Use Susceptibility test results are usually reported on anaerobic bacterial isolates only on special request to the laboratory. Susceptibility testing of anaerobes is not usually performed. It may be indicated for individual patient isolates when the selection of therapeutic agents is critical. This situation may occur because of failure of empiric therapy or because of lack of response to empiric therapy. Difficulty in making empiric decisions due to lack of precedent, specific infections which may be appropriate for the determination of anaerobic susceptibility include brain abscess, endocarditis, osteomyelitis, joint infection, infection of prosthetic devices or vascular grafts.

Limitations Breakpoints are not well defined or universally accepted for categorization of susceptible and resistant. Methods are still being developed to standardize testing, reporting, and interpretation of anaerobic susceptibility tests for the broth disc elution and microdilution methods. Anaerobic infections are frequently mixed involving aerobic and anaerobic flora, thus, the predictive value of an anaerobic susceptibility test for a successful clinical outcome may be limited by the complexity of the clinical infection.

Contraindications Anaerobe isolate from patient is not available or fails to give adequate growth for susceptibility testing.

Methodology Broth disc elution, broth microdilution, and agar dilution technique; beta-lactamase testing

Additional Information At present, routine susceptibility testing of anaerobic isolates is not recommended. Infections involving anaerobes frequently contain mixed flora and appropriate drainage rather than antimicrobial therapy seems to be the most crucial factor in the successful treatment of these infections.

Indications for anaerobic susceptibility testing include:

- determination of susceptibility of anaerobes to new antimicrobial agents
- monitoring susceptibility patterns by geographic area
- monitoring susceptibility patterns in local hospitals
- assisting in the management of selected individual patients.

Many anaerobes grow so slowly that by the time isolation and susceptibility testing is completed (6-14 days), the results are of little clinical value. Most anaerobes have very predictable *in vitro* susceptibility patterns that appear to have changed little over the years. For these reasons, many laboratories perform anaerobic susceptibility testing only on anaerobic isolates from blood, pleural fluid, peritoneal fluid, and CSF. In cases of chronic anaerobic infections (septic arthritis, osteomyelitis, etc), susceptibility testing may be done by special request. The physician should contact the laboratory regarding the specific antibiotic(s) to be tested and the testing method (broth disk, MICs, etc) available.

Organisms that are recognized as virulent (ie, *Bacteroides fragilis* group, pigmented *Bacteroides* sp, *Bacteroides gracilis*, certain *Fusobacterium*, *Clostridium perfringens*, and *Clostridium ramosus*) may also be considered for testing.

Selected Readings

Finegold SM, "Susceptibility Testing of Anaerobic Bacteria," *J Clin Microbiol*, 1988, 26(7):1253-6.

Rosenblatt JE, "Susceptibility Testing of Anaerobic Bacteria," *Clin Lab Med*, 1989, 9(2):239-54, (review).

Styrt B and Gorbach SL, "Recent Developments in the Understanding of the Pathogenesis and Treatment of Anaerobic Infections," *N Engl J Med*, 1989, Part I, 321(4):240-6 and Part II, 321(5):298-302.

Zebransky RJ, "Revisiting Anaerobe Susceptibility Testing," *Clin Microbiol Newslett*, 1989, 11:185-92.

Typical Sensitivities of Important Anaerobic Pathogens to Major Classes of Antibiotics

Antibiotic	B. fragilis Group	B. melaninogenicus Group	Fusobacterium	Clostridium	Propionibacterium	Actinomyces	Peptostreptococcus
Penicillin G	− to +	− to +++	++	+ to ++	+++	+++	+++
Antipseudomonal penicillins	++ to +++	+ to +++	+++	+++	+++	+++	+++
Cefoxitin	++	+++	++ to +++	− to ++	+++	+++	+++
Imipenem-cilastatin	+++	+++	++	+++	+++	+++	+++
Combinations of beta-lactam and beta-lactamase inhibitor	+++	+++	+++	+++	+++	+++	+++
Clindamycin	++ to +++	+++	+++	++	+++	+++	+++
Chloramphenicol	+++	+++	+++	+++	+++	+++	+++
Metronidazole	+++	+++	+++	+++	−	−	++ to +++

− denotes that <50% of the strains were susceptible.

+ denotes that 50% to 70% of the strains were susceptible.

++ denotes that 70% to 90% of the strains were susceptible.

+++ denotes that >90% of the strains were susceptible.

From Styrt B and Gorbach SL, "Recent Developments in the Understanding of the Pathogenesis and Treatment of Anaerobic Infections," *N Engl J Med*, 1989. Part I, 321:240-6 and Part II, 321:298-302 (review), with permission.

Antimycobacterial Susceptibility Testing

Related Information
Mycobacteria Culture, Biopsy or Body Fluid *on page 493*

Synonyms Mycobacteria, Susceptibility Testing; Susceptibility Testing, Mycobacteria

Test Includes Panel of antimycobacterial agents tested against isolates at appropriate concentrations

Specimen Pure isolate of an organism

Causes for Rejection Specimen not available for testing.

Turnaround Time 4-6 weeks after organism is isolated

Use Determine the susceptibility of the isolated organism to a panel of antimycobacterial agents

Limitations Susceptibilities cannot be reported if the organism fails to grow on test media.

Methodology Agar dilution. Some laboratories use the Bactec® broth system to determine susceptibility to some antimycobacterial agents. The CDC recommends this broth method. See table.

Antimicrobials Commonly Used for Mycobacterial Susceptibility Testing

Antituberculosis Drugs	
Primary	**Secondary**
Ethambutol	Capreomycin
Isoniazid	Ciprofloxacin
Pyrazinamide	Cycloserine
Rifampin	Ethionamide
Streptomycin	Kanamycin
Other Mycobacterial Isolates*	
Primary	**Secondary**
Amikacin	Azithromycin
Ciprofloxacin	Clarithromycin
Ethambutol	Clofazimine
Isoniazid	Doxycycline
Rifampin	
Streptomycin	
Sulfonamides	
Tobramycin	

*Drug regimens will depend on the mycobacterial species identified.

From Wolinsky E, "Mycobacterial Diseases Other Then Tuberculosis," *Clin Infect Dis*, 1992, 15:1-12, with permission.

Additional Information Susceptibilities are performed on the first organism isolated from a patient, and at 3- to 6-month intervals if that organism continues to be isolated while the patient is on therapy. Susceptibility tests should be performed in patients with recurrent tuberculosis as resistant strains are common in recurrent infection. Failure to take all drugs in a multidrug regimen can lead to a shift toward resistant organisms and treatment failure. Atypical or environmental mycobacteria, particularly stains of the *M. avium* complex, have variable susceptibility within species. Frequently, they are resistant to oral therapy.

Selected Readings
Heifets L, "Qualitative and Quantitative Drug Susceptibility Tests in Mycobacteriology," *Am Rev Respir Dis*, 1988, 137(5):1217-22.
Swenson JM, Wallace RJ Jr, Silcox VA, et al, "Antimicrobial Susceptibility of Five Subgroups of *Mycobacterium fortuitum* and *Mycobacterium chelonae*," *Antimicrob Agents Chemother*, 1985, 28(6):807-11.
Van Scoy RE and Wilkowske CJ, "Antituberculous Agents," *Mayo Clin Proc*, 1992, 67(2):179-87.
Wallace RJ Jr, Swenson JM, Silcox VA, et al, "Treatment of Nonpulmonary Infections Due to *Mycobacterium fortuitum* and *Mycobacterium chelonei* Based on In Vitro Susceptibilities," *J Infect Dis*, 1985, 152(3):500-14.

Antistreptococcal DNase-B Titer *see* Antideoxyribonuclease-B Titer, Serum *on page 322*

Antistreptolysin O Titer, Serum

Related Information

Antideoxyribonuclease-B Titer, Serum *on page 322*

Streptozyme *on page 544*

Synonyms ASO

Specimen Serum

Container Red top tube or serum separator tube

Causes for Rejection Excessive hemolysis

Reference Range Less than 2 years of age: usually <50 Todd units; 2-5 years: <100 Todd units; 5-19 years: <166 Todd units; adults: <125 Todd units. A rise in titer of four or more dilution increments from acute to convalescent specimens is considered to be significant regardless of the magnitude of the titer. For a single specimen, ASO titers ≤166 Todd units are considered normal, but higher titers may be "normal" in demographic groups, or may be associated with chronic pharyngeal carriage.

Use Document streptococcal infection. A marked rise in titer or a persistently elevated titer indicates that a *Streptococcus* infection or poststreptococcal sequelae are present. Elevated titers are seen in 80% to 85% of patients with acute rheumatic fever and in 95% of patients with acute glomerulonephritis.

Limitations False-positive ASO titers can be caused by increased levels of serum betalipoprotein produced in liver disease and by contamination of the serum with *Bacillus cereus* and *Pseudomonas* sp. ASO is usually not formed as a result of streptococcal pyoderma. Test is subject to technical false-positives due to oxidation of reagents.

Methodology Hemolysis inhibition, latex agglutination (LA)

Additional Information Streptolysin is a cytolysin produced by group A streptococci. In an infected individual streptolysin O acts as a protein antigen, and the patient mounts an antibody response. A rise in titer begins about 1 week after infection and peaks 2-4 weeks later. In the absence of complications or reinfection, the ASO titer will usually fall to preinfection levels within 6-12 months. Both clinical and laboratory findings should be correlated in reaching a diagnosis.

Selected Readings

Ayoub EM and Harden E, "Immune Response to Streptococcal Antigens: Diagnostic Methods," *Manual of Clinical Laboratory Immunology*, 4th ed, Rose NR, de Macario EC, Fahey JL, et al, eds, Washington, DC: American Society for Microbiology, 1992, 427-34.

Escobar MR, "Hemolytic Assays: Complement Fixation and Antistreptolysin O," *Manual of Clinical Microbiology*, 5th ed, Balows A, Hausler WJ Jr, Herrmann KL, et al, eds, Washington, DC: American Society for Microbiology, 1991, 73-8.

Keren DF and Warren JS, *Diagnostic Immunology*, Baltimore, MD: Williams & Wilkins, 1992, 168-70.

Arbovirus Serology *see* Encephalitis Viral Serology *on page 404*

ARD, Blood Culture *see* Blood Culture, Aerobic and Anaerobic *on page 337*

Arterial Line Culture *see* Intravenous Line Culture *on page 464*

Arthritis Series, X-ray *see* Bone Films *on page 343*

Arthrocentesis

Synonyms Closed Joint Aspiration; Joint Tap

Test Includes Passing a needle into a joint space and aspirating synovial fluid for diagnostic analysis

Patient Preparation Procedure and risks are explained and consent is obtained. No intravenous pain medications or sedatives are required.

Aftercare Determined by results of procedure, as outlined by physician. May range from joint immobilization with passive range of motion, as in septic arthritis, to full weight bearing, as in effusions secondary to osteoarthritis. No specific joint positioning postprocedure has been demonstrated to reduce complications.

Complications Arthrocentesis is usually a safe procedure, especially when performed on an easily accessible joint such as the knee. Potential complications include:

- iatrogenic joint space infection (if properly performed, incidence has been estimated at 1 in 15,000 cases)
- hemorrhage or hematoma formation (usually when alternative approaches are used and blood vessels are ruptured on the flexor surface of the joint)

- local pain caused by needle trauma to the periosteum
- injury to cartilage, particularly problematic due to slow repair rate
- tendon rupture
- nerve palsies

Equipment Alcohol swabs, povidone-iodine prep solution, sterile gloves and towels, gauze, and forceps. Local anesthesia with ethyl chloride vinyl spray and/or lidocaine 1% with appropriate syringes and subcutaneous needles. If the joint to be aspirated is large, use 18- or 20-gauge 1.5" needle on a 20 mL syringe (additional syringes should be available). If joint is small or effusion minimal, use 20- or 22-gauge 1.5" needle on 3 mL syringe. In this latter case, additional tubes for fluid collection will not be needed. Otherwise, use three sterile tubes for collection, the first one with either EDTA additive or a small amount of heparin. If gonococcal arthritis is suspected, obtain chocolate (Thayer-Martin) media. Glass slides and polarized microscope are necessary if crystalline arthropathy is suspected.

Technique The following description details the technique of knee arthrocentesis, a joint commonly aspirated by the generalist. Patient is instructed to lie supine and remain relaxed. Physician selects the type of approach: suprapatellar, para-patellar, or infrapatellar. The parapatellar approach is popular and effective with tense effusions. Here, the knee is placed in 20° flexion to relax the quadriceps. The preferred entry site is the midportion of the patella (approximately 2 cm superior to the inferior portion of the patella), preferably the medial aspect. This site is marked by indenting the skin with the retracted end of a ballpoint pen. The skin is prepped with alcohol first then povidone-iodine. Some clinicians prefer strict aseptic technique (5-minute scrub, masks, gowns, and drapes) whereas others do not use even sterile gloves or drapes. We prefer a middle-ground approach, using sterile gloves and drapes but foregoing masks and gowns. The use of local anesthesia also varies amongst practitioners. If the joint is tense, and anatomical landmarks easily palpable, we prefer cutaneous anesthesia with only a spray of ethyl chloride solution. Alternatively, a subcutaneous wheal of lidocaine may be raised in the usual fashion. Injection of lidocaine into deeper structures is not usually required (where it may potentially interfere with culture results because of bacteriostatic properties). Following this, the needle-on-syringe is passed through the marked skin site and advanced slowly while aspirating. A "pop" may be felt as the needle penetrates the capsule. The needle should be directed parallel to the plane of the synovial capsule if the parapatellar approach is used. Once fluid is returned, the needle should not be advanced further in order to avoid cartilage damage. Only mild suction should be used to aspirate so that trauma and hemorrhage do not occur. In general, joint effusions should be drained completely. A blind "search" with the needle (often with vigorous aspiration) is hazardous and should not be attempted. Forceps may be used to stabilize the needle if several syringe changes are required. Once completed, withdraw the needle, apply pressure, and place adhesive tape over puncture site. If persistent pain is encountered during the procedure, trauma to cartilage or periosteum is likely. Do not reflexly anesthetize these deeper tissues with lidocaine; instead, withdraw the needle and redirect it along a new plane. Correct placement of the needle in the joint space is normally painless. In the case of a "dry tap," folds of synovium may be acting as a valve obstructing the needle lumen. Reposition the needle slightly, or if there is fluid in the syringe, inject a small amount to clear the needle bevel. This problem can be avoided by using the infrapatellar approach. The technique for suprapatellar and infrapatellar aspiration has been detailed elsewhere. The suprapatellar approach is most useful in tense effusions where the suprapatellar bursa (usually in communication with the joint space) is visibly distended. While easily performed, there is a potential for sinus tract formation especially if the entry site is directly over the bursa, rather than several centimeters away. The infrapatellar approach has a low risk of cartilage damage compared with the parapatellar approach and is useful for patients with marked flexion contractures of the knee. However, clinicians may not be familiar with the technical details of this approach. Similar principles apply to aspiration of joints other than the knee.

Data Acquired A wide array of tests on synovial fluid is available. Routine tests on effusions of unknown etiology include: cell count, glucose, Gram's stain and routine culture, and microscopic examination for crystals (urate, calcium, pyrophosphate dihydrate). Optional tests include: viscosity, mucin clot test, uric acid level, and culture for *Neisseria gonorrhoeae*, tuberculosis, fungi, *Mycoplasma*

(Continued)

Arthrocentesis *(Continued)*

pneumoniae, nontuberculous, acid-fast bacteria, etc. Occasionally, ordered tests include: synovial fluid protein, LDH, cytology, rheumatoid factor, complement.

Specimen Synovial fluid

Container For small fluid volumes, send capped syringe without needle to laboratory; otherwise, fluid may be carefully transferred to sterile tubes.

Collection Tube 1: Gram's stain and culture; tube 2: mucin clot, if ordered (no heparin); tube 3: (add heparin or EDTA) cell count, chemistries, crystals, additional studies. If gonococcal arthritis is suspected, chocolate (Thayer-Martin) agar should be available either at the bedside or during specimen processing in the microbiology laboratory.

Storage Instructions Specimen should be hand carried to the laboratory. Delay in processing may cause spuriously low synovial fluid glucose levels or false-negative results.

Normal Findings In the absence of disease, synovial fluid usually cannot be aspirated. Normal synovial fluid is clear and viscous. A drop placed between the thumb and forefinger (or two microscope slides) can form a string >2 cm long as the fingers are separated, indicating high viscosity. Similarly, the mucin clot test is performed by adding 1 mL of synovial fluid to a 5% solution of acetic acid. Normally, a firm clot forms. Both tests reflect high viscosity of synovial fluid caused by leukocyte hyaluronic acid. Cell count and differential normally reveal <200 WBCs/mm^3 with <25% neutrophils. Chemistries show protein <2 g/dL, uric acid <8 mg/dL, synovial glucose nearly equal to serum glucose, and synovial LDH less than serum LDH. Gram's stain and cultures are negative (acellular).

Critical Values Abnormal synovial fluid can be divided into four diagnostic categories. Considerable overlap exists among these categories and correlation with the clinical presentation is required.

Group I synovial fluids are seen commonly in degenerative joint disease (osteo-arthritis) and trauma. Fluid is clear or yellow tinged, viscous and mucin clot firm. WBC count is <200/mm^3 with <25% neutrophils (often mononuclears >50%). Chemistries including glucose are normal and microbiologic cultures are negative. This is considered a "noninflammatory" effusion. Some inflammatory conditions may at times cause a group I fluid, such as acute rheumatic fever and systemic lupus erythematosus.

Group II fluids are "inflammatory" in nature. Diseases leading to this category include: crystal-induced arthropathies (gout, CPPD or "pseudogout"), rheumatoid arthritis, connective tissue diseases (SLE, polymyositis, etc), ankylosing spondylitis and other seronegative spondyloarthropathies (Reiter's syndrome, psoriatic arthritis), and acute rheumatic fever. Synovial fluid appears opaque and turbid from cellular fragmentation. Viscosity is similar to water and the "string test" yields only short strings. Mucin clot testing results in a friable gel rather than a tight, rope-like clot. WBC counts are elevated, 5000-75,000/mm^3 with >50% neutrophils. Synovial glucose tends to be lower than serum glucose, especially if synovial WBCs are elevated (neutrophils consume glucose). Gram's stain and cultures are negative.

Group III effusions are characteristic of septic arthritis. Fluid appears grossly turbid and may be frankly purulent. WBC count as a rule is >50,000/mm^3 and may be >1,000,000/mm^3. Differential shows preponderance of neutrophils (>90%), with the exception of tuberculous arthritis where lymphocytes may comprise 50% of leukocytes. Synovial glucose is characteristically <50% of simultaneous serum glucose and this finding strongly suggests septic arthritis. Glucose values <10 mg/dL have been reported and support classification into group III (rather than group II) in cases where WBC count is moderately elevated. However, sensitivity of low glucose levels in the septic joint is approximately 50%. Gram's stain yield in group III effusions varies with the bacteria isolated. In patients with staphylococcal septic arthritis, the Gram's stain is diagnostic in 75% of cases in patients with gram-negative arthritis, 50% of Gram's stains are diagnostic, but with gonococcal arthritis, only 25% of Gram's stains are positive. In nongonococcal septic arthritis, the bacterial culture is more helpful than the Gram's stain, the former being positive in 85% to 95% of cases (provided no recent antibiotic use). However, with gonococcal arthritis, the culture is less sensitive, with only a 25% positive yield.

Group IV synovial effusions are grossly hemorrhagic. Etiologies include: systemic abnormalities (eg, excessive heparin anticoagulation, severe thrombocytopenia) and local joint pathology (eg, femur fracture, neuropathic joint).

As mentioned earlier, diagnostic groups are not mutually exclusive. Certain disease entities may fall into more than one diagnostic category. For example, synovial fluid in acute rheumatic fever may appear as either a group I or a group II effusion; neuropathic arthropathy may appear as group I or IV, and lupus-associated effusions as group I or II. In addition, an individual patient may suffer from more than one pathologic process over the course of time. For example, a joint effusion from rheumatoid arthritis (group II effusion) maybe a predisposing factor to the later development of bacterial arthritis (group III) and both may be present in the same patient. Finally, some diseases may change from one diagnostic category to another over a short time period. For example, septic arthritis in an early stage may present with a low synovial WBC count and normal glucose (group I) and only later on progress to a typical septic arthritis (group III) picture on subsequent arthrocentesis.

Use Diagnostic indications include:
- joint effusions of unknown etiology
- arthritis of unclear etiology
- all cases of suspected infectious arthritis (bacterial, fungal, tuberculous)
- confirmation of a diagnosis strongly suspected on clinical grounds, such as suspected gout in patients with podagra
- monitoring synovial fluid response to antibiotic therapy in established cases of septic arthritis

Therapeutic indications include:
- decompression of a tense, painful joint effusion
- evacuation of pus in bacterial arthritis (repeated closed drainage)
- removal of inflammatory cells and crystals in selected cases of gout or pseudogout
- intra-articular injection of corticosteroids

Contraindications
- local infection along the proposed needle entrance tract (eg, overlying cellulitis, periarticular infection)
- uncooperative patient, especially if unable to keep the joint immobile throughout procedure
- difficulty identifying boney landmarks
- a poorly accessible joint space, as in hip aspiration in the obese patient
- inability to demonstrate a joint effusion on physical examination, except when septic arthritis is strongly suspected (and effusions may be barely detectable)

In addition, some authors consider bacteremia (documented or suspected) a contraindication to arthrocentesis based on the theoretical concern of seeding a sterile joint when the entering needle ruptures surrounding capillaries. No data is available to support or refute this and clinical judgment must be individualized in each case. If infectious arthritis is suspected, arthrocentesis should be promptly performed even with documented bacteremia. However, more elective indications for the procedure, such as corticosteroid injection, should be deferred, at physician's discretion.

Additional Information Arthrocentesis is indispensable for the accurate diagnosis (or exclusion) of septic arthritis and crystal-induced arthropathy and therein lies its greatest utility. Despite the difficulties with the classification scheme described above, synovial fluid findings in both these treatable conditions is often pathognomonic. Practically, the procedure carries a low risk of complications and can be performed in minutes when an accessible joint is involved. The general physician often handles aspirations of the knee, elbow, and first metatarsal phalangeal joint. When septic arthritis is suspected in a less accessible area, such as the sacroiliac joint, aspiration should not be delayed due to a lack of familiarity. Rheumatologic or orthopedic consultation should be obtained.

Selected Readings
Gatter RA, "Arthrocentesis Technique and Intrasynovial Therapy," *Arthritis and Allied Conditions: A Textbook of Rheumatology*, 11th ed, Chapter 39, McCarty DJ, ed, Philadelphia, PA: Lea & Febiger, 1989.

Rodnan GP and Schumacher HR, "Examination of Synovial Fluid," *Primer on the Rheumatic Diseases*, 8th ed, Chapter 90, Atlanta, GA: Arthritis Foundation, 1983.

(Continued)

Arthrocentesis *(Continued)*

Simon RR and Brenner BE, "Orthopedic Procedures," *Emergency Medicine Procedures and Techniques*, 2nd ed, Chapter 7, Baltimore, MD: Williams & Wilkins, 1987, 192-243.

Arthrogram

Synonyms Joint Study

Applies to Ankle Arthrogram; Elbow Arthrogram; Hip Arthrogram; Knee Arthrogram; Shoulder Arthrogram; Temporomandibular Joint Arthrogram; Wrist Arthrogram

Patient Preparation Informed consent is obtained

Aftercare No strenuous activity involving the joint of interest for 24 hours.

Equipment 22-gauge needle, contrast medium, and fluoroscopic and x-ray equipment

Technique Local anesthesia is instilled at the appropriate site. A small gauge needle is inserted into the joint space. Any fluid within the joint space is aspirated and sent for appropriate chemical or bacteriologic analysis. Contrast medium and air are then inserted into the joint space under fluoroscopic guidance. Radiographs and occasionally tomograms are then obtained in multiple projections.

Data Acquired Visualization of the components of the joint space including the cartilage, ligaments, menisci, and connecting bursa

Normal Findings The joint space should not contain fluid. The cartilaginous surfaces and menisci should be smooth without evidence for erosions, tears, or disintegration.

Use Evaluate damage to the cartilage, ligaments, and bony structures composing the joint

Limitations Large joint effusions can be difficult to aspirate completely, thus resulting in dilution of the contrast material and poor visualization of the joint space structures.

Contraindications Bleeding abnormalities

Selected Readings

Resnick D, "Arthrography, Tenography and Bursography," *Diagnosis of Bone and Joint Disorders*, 2nd ed, Resnick D and Niwayama G, eds, Philadelphia, PA: WB Saunders Co, 1988, 302-444.

Arthropod Identification

Synonyms Ectoparasite Identification; Insect Identification

Applies to Bed Bugs Identification; Body Lice Identification; *Cimex* Identification; Crab Lice Identification; Deer Tick Identification; Flea Identification; Head Lice Identification; *Ixodes dammini* Identification; Lice Identification; Mite Identification; Nits Identification; *Pediculus humanus* Identification; *Phthirus pubis* Identification; Pubic Lice Identification; *Sarcoptes scabiei* Skin Scrapings Identification; Skin Scrapings for *Sarcoptes scabiei* Identification; Tick Identification

Specimen Gross arthropod, skin scrapings

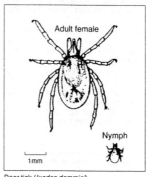

Deer tick (*Ixodes dammini*)

Container Screw cap tube or screw cap jar

Collection Arthropods (gross) are to be submitted in alcohol (70%) or formalde-hyde in tube or container with secure closure. To establish the diagnosis of scabies, skin scrapings may be collected with a scalpel and a drop of mineral oil. The liquid may be examined directly or alternatively the organism may be teased away from its burrow or papule with a needle or scalpel.

Storage Instructions Room temperature, fill the container with preservative as completely as possible to avoid damage to the specimen by air bubbles in the container

Turnaround Time 1-2 hours; if referral to a state or federal laboratory is required, 2-4 weeks

Reference Range No arthropod identified

Use Identify arthropods affecting humans; establish the presence of ectoparasite infestation

Methodology Macroscopic evaluation

Selected Readings

Hobbs GD and Harrell RE Jr, "Brown Recluse Spider Bites: A Common Cause of Necrotic Arach-nidism," *Am J Emerg Med*, 1989, 7(3):309-12.

Nelson JA and Bouseman JK, "Human Tick-Borne Illnesses: United States," *Clin Microbiol Newslett*, 1992, 14(14):105-12.

Pratt HD and Smith JW, "Arthropods of Medical Importance," *Manual of Clinical Microbiology*, 5th ed, Balows A, Hausler WJ Jr, Herrmann KL, et al, eds, Washington, DC: American Society for Microbiology, 1991, 796-810.

Ascites Fluid Tap *see* Paracentesis *on page 509*

Ascitic Fluid Culture *see* Aerobic Culture, Body Fluid *on page 310*

Ascitic Fluid Cytology *see* Cytology, Body Fluids *on page 386*

Ascitic Fluid Fungus Culture *see* Fungus Culture, Body Fluid *on page 415*

ASO *see* Antistreptolysin O Titer, Serum *on page 330*

***Aspergillus* Immunodiffusion** *see* Fungal Serology *on page 410*

Aspirates for Ova and Parasites *see* Ova and Parasites, Urine or Aspirates *on page 508*

Atypical *Mycobacterium* Smear *see* Acid-Fast Stain *on page 305*

Auramine-Rhodamine Stain *see* Acid-Fast Stain *on page 305*

B19 DNA *see* Parvovirus B19 DNA, Qualitative PCR *on page 514*

Bacterial Antigens by Coagglutination *replaced by* Bacterial Antigens, Rapid Detection Methods *on page 335*

Bacterial Antigens by Counterimmunoelectrophoresis *replaced by* Bacterial Antigens, Rapid Detection Methods *on page 335*

Bacterial Antigens, Rapid Detection Methods

Related Information

Group A *Streptococcus* Antigen Test *on page 428*

Group B *Streptococcus* Antigen Test *on page 429*

Synonyms Cerebrospinal Fluid Latex Agglutination for Bacterial Antigens; Latex Agglutination, Bacterial Antigens, Cerebrospinal Fluid

Replaces Bacterial Antigens by Coagglutination; Bacterial Antigens by Counter-immunoelectrophoresis

Test Includes Qualitative determination of the presence of antigens of *H. influ-enzae*, *S. pneumoniae*, *N. meningitidis*. Test may also identify subgroups of above organisms and may include testing for group B *Streptococcus* and *E. coli* K1 antigen in neonates. Gram's stain and culture are preferable to bacterial antigen testing, and results of Gram's stain must be coordinated with antigen testing by knowledgeable laboratory workers.

Abstract Rapid adjunctive tests include latex agglutination, which is more sensi-tive than coagglutination. False-negative results occur. *Clinical Microbiology Procedures Handbook* (Isenberg HD, ed) indicates that **these latex agglutina-tion tests are not intended as a substitute for bacterial culture. Confirma-tory diagnosis of bacterial meningitis infection is possible only with appropriate culture procedures.** Similar observations are published by others as well. Concentration of antigen depends on variables including the number of bacteria, the duration of infection, and the presence or absence of specific antibodies which may prevent antigen detection. Several publications recognize these tests' shortcomings and describe the rapid diagnostic tests as not essen-tial but note that they may be helpful in establishing an etiologic diagnosis rapidly.

Patient Preparation Usual aseptic aspiration

(Continued)

Bacterial Antigens, Rapid Detection Methods
(Continued)

Specimen Cerebrospinal fluid, serum, urine

Container Sterile CSF tube, red top tube, sterile urine container

Storage Instructions Keep refrigerated

Reference Range Negative

Use Detect bacterial antigens in CSF for the rapid diagnosis of meningitis. The method may be applied to other body fluids, blood culture supernatants, and urine (depending on the body fluid tested and the test used).

Limitations May be negative in early meningitis. **Does not replace Gram's stain and culture.** Group B *Streptococcus* and the *E. coli* K1 antigen are frequently not tested on infants over 6 months of age. The sensitivity of the tests vary from 55% to 100% depending on the specificity of the antibody and the concentration of antigen in the specimen. Nonspecific cross reactions occur. False-positive reactions and nonspecific agglutination occur. Antigenic cross-over (cross reactions) are seen (eg, *E. coli* K1 and *N. meningitidis* group B). The sensitivity of commercial antigen detection kits remains imperfect, the sensitivity differing substantially with various organisms and in various clinical series. False-negative results occur, especially those taken early in the disease, with low antigen load. Pneumococcal and *Haemophilus* strains not possessing capsular antigens may not be detected by immunological techniques. Pneumococcal antigen is not detected in urine.

Many authors have stated that these tests are expensive and have, usually, no impact on patient care. Physicians are urged to order only Gram's stain and culture. These tests can be used later if stain and culture results are negative. Counterimmunoelectrophoresis is no longer in common clinical use.

Methodology Latex agglutination and coagglutination

Additional Information Antigen detection methods should never be substituted for culture and Gram's stain. Culture and Gram's stain must always have priority when only very limited quantities of CSF are available.

The rapid diagnosis of group A and group B *Streptococcus* infection is discussed specifically in Group A *Streptococcus* Screen and Group B *Streptococcus* Screen test listings.

Selected Readings

Gray LD and Fedorko DP, "Laboratory Diagnosis of Bacterial Meningitis," *Clin Microbiol Rev*, 1992, 5(2):130-45.

Greenlee JE, "Approach to Diagnosis of Meningitis - Cerebrospinal Fluid Evaluation," *Infect Dis Clin North Am*, 1990, 4(4):583-98.

Isenberg HD, "Bacterial Antigen Detection by Latex Agglutination," *Clinical Microbiology Procedures Handbook*, Washington DC: American Society for Microbiology, 1992, 2:9.2.-9.2.4.

Rodewald LE, Woodin KA, Szilágyi PG, et al, "Relevance of Common Tests of Cerebrospinal Fluid in Screening for Bacterial Meningitis," *J Pediatr*, 1991, 119(3):363-9.

Smith AL, "Bacterial Meningitis," *Pediatr Rev*, 1993, 14(1):11-8.

Bacterial Inhibitory Level, Serum *see* Serum Bactericidal Test *on page 533*

Bacterial Smear *see* Gram's Stain *on page 426*

Bacteria Screen, Urine *see* Leukocyte Esterase, Urine *on page 473*

Bacteria Screen, Urine *see* Nitrite, Urine *on page 503*

Basement Membrane Antibodies *see* Skin Biopsy, Immunofluorescence *on page 538*

bDNA Testing for HIV *see* HIV-1 RNA, Quantitative bDNA, 3rd Generation *on page 451*

Bed Bugs Identification *see* Arthropod Identification *on page 334*

Beta-Hemolytic Strep Culture, Throat *see* Throat Culture for Group A Beta-Hemolytic *Streptococcus* on page 550

Beta-Lactamase Production Test *see* Penicillinase Test *on page 517*

Beta-Lactam Ring *see* Penicillinase Test *on page 517*

Biopsy *see* Histopathology *on page 448*

Biopsy Culture, Aerobic *see* Biopsy Culture, Routine *on next page*

Biopsy Culture, Anaerobic *see* Anaerobic Culture *on page 316*

Biopsy Culture, Fungus *see* Fungus Culture, Biopsy *on page 414*

Biopsy Culture, Routine

Related Information

Anaerobic Culture *on page 316*

Histopathology *on page 448*

Applies to Aerobic Culture, Tissue; Biopsy Culture, Aerobic; *Brucella* Culture, Tissue; Culture, Biopsy; Cyst Culture, Aerobic; Surgical Specimen Culture, Routine; Tissue Culture, *Brucella*; Tissue Culture, Routine

Patient Preparation Aseptic preparation of biopsy site

Special Instructions The following information must be provided to the laboratory and will assist the laboratory in the proper processing of the specimen; specific site of specimen, current antibiotic therapy, age and sex of patient, collection time and date, and clinical diagnosis.

Specimen Surgical tissue, bone marrow, biopsy material from normally sterile site or aseptically aspirated body fluid

Container Sterile container with lid, no preservative. Bone marrow aspirates and body fluids may be directly inoculated into blood culture media.

Collection The portion of the biopsy specimen submitted for culture should be separated from the portion submitted for histopathology by the surgeon or pathologist utilizing sterile technique.

Storage Instructions Transport specimen to the laboratory immediately.

Causes for Rejection Specimen not received in appropriate sterile container, specimen received in preservative, excessive delay in transport. If an unacceptable specimen is received the nursing station will be notified and another specimen will be requested before disposal of the original specimen.

Turnaround Time Preliminary reports are available at 24 hours. Cultures with no growth will be reported after 48 hours. Reports on specimens from which pathogens are isolated require a minimum of 48 hours for completion.

Reference Range No growth

Use Isolate and identify organisms causing infections in tissue

Limitations If anaerobes are suspected submit a properly collected specimen.

Additional Information The specimen should be obtained before empiric antimicrobial therapy is started.

Biopsy *Legionella* Culture *see Legionella pneumophila Culture on page 469*

Biopsy of Lung (Transbronchial) for *Pneumocystis* *see Pneumocystis carinii Test on page 522*

Blastomycosis Immunodiffusion *see Fungal Serology on page 410*

Blind Liver Biopsy *see Liver Biopsy on page 474*

Blood Cell Profile *see Complete Blood Count on page 369*

Blood Count *see Complete Blood Count on page 369*

Blood Culture, Aerobic and Anaerobic

Related Information

Blood Culture, Fungus *on page 341*

Blood Culture, Mycobacteria *on page 342*

Synonyms Aerobic Blood Culture; Anaerobic Blood Culture; Culture, Blood

Applies to Antimicrobial Removal Device (ARD) Blood Culture; ARD, Blood Culture; Blood Culture, Lysis Centrifugation; Blood Culture With Antimicrobial Removal Device (ARD)

Test Includes Isolation of both aerobic and anaerobic bacteria and susceptibility testing on all significant isolates

Patient Preparation The major difficulty in interpretation of blood cultures is contamination by skin flora. This difficulty can be markedly reduced by careful attention to the details of skin preparation and antisepsis prior to collection of the specimen.

After location of the vein by palpation, the venipuncture site should be vigorously scrubbed and cleansed with 70% alcohol (isopropyl or ethyl) and then swabbed in a circular motion concentrically from the center outward using tincture of iodine or a povidone iodine solution. **The iodine should be allowed to dry before the venipuncture is undertaken.** If palpation is required during the venipuncture, the glove covering the palpating finger tip should be disinfected.

In iodine sensitive patients, a double alcohol, green soap, or acetone alcohol preparation may be substituted.

(Continued)

Blood Culture, Aerobic and Anaerobic *(Continued)*

Aftercare Iodine used in the skin preparation should be carefully removed from the skin after venipuncture.

Special Instructions The requisition should state current antibiotic therapy and clinical diagnosis.

Specimen Blood. The yield of positives is not increased by culturing arterial blood even in endocarditis.

Container Bottles of trypticase soy broth or other standard medium, one vented (for aerobes), one unvented (for anaerobes)

Collection A single blood culture is rarely indicated and to be discouraged unless medically necessary. More than four cultures in 24 hours is also not indicated (not necessary). Ideally, 2-3 cultures (1 hour apart) taken over 24 hours is adequate to recover bacteria causing septicemia.

Blood cultures should be drawn prior to initiation of antimicrobial therapy. If more than one culture is ordered at the same time (such should be ordered only in medically urgent situations), the specimens should be drawn from separately prepared sites. A syringe and needle, transfer set or pre-evacuated set of tubes containing culture media may be used to collect blood. Collection tubes should be held below the level of the venipuncture to avoid reflux. A sample volume of 10-20 mL (more is always better) in adults, 1-5 mL in pediatric patients is usually collected for each set.

If a syringe and needle or transfer set is used, the top of the blood culture bottles should also be aseptically prepared with alcohol only. See table.

Blood Culture Collection

Clinical Disease Suspected	Culture Recommendation	Rational
Sepsis, meningitis osteomyelitis, septic arthritis, bacterial pneumonia	Two sets of cultures - one from each of two prepared sites, the second drawn after a brief time interval, then begin therapy.	Assure sufficient sampling in cases of intermittent or low level bacteremia. Minimize the confusion caused by a positive culture resulting from transient bacteremia or skin contamination.
Fever of unknown origin (eg, occult abscess, empyema, typhoid fever, etc)	Two sets of cultures - one from each of two prepared sites, the second drawn after a brief time interval (30 minutes). If cultures are negative after 24-48 hours obtain two more sets, preferably prior to an anticipated temperature rise.	The yield after four sets of cultures is minimal. A maximum of three sets per patient per day for 3 consecutive days is recommended.
Endocarditis:		
Acute	Obtain three blood culture sets within 2 hours, then begin therapy.	95% to 99% of acute endocarditis patients (untreated) will yield a positive in one of the first three cultures.
Subacute	Obtain three blood culture sets on day 1, repeat if negative after 24 hours. If still negative or if the patient had prior antibiotic therapy, repeat again.	Adequate sample volume despite low level bacteremia or previous therapy should result in a positive yield.
Immunocompromised host (eg, AIDS):		
Septicemia, fungemia mycobacteremia	Obtain two sets of cultures from each of two prepared sites; consider lysis concentration technique to enhance recovery for fungi and mycobacteria.	Low levels of fungemia and mycobacteremia frequently encountered.
Previous antimicrobial therapy:		
Septicemia, bacteremia; monitor effect of antimicrobial therapy	Obtain two sets of cultures from each of two prepared sites; consider use of antimicrobial removal device (ARD) or increased volume >10 mL/set.	Recovery of organisms is enhanced by dilution, increased sample volume, and removal of inhibiting antimicrobials.

Transient bacteremia caused by brushing teeth, bowel movements, etc or by local irritations caused by scratching of the skin, may cause positive blood cultures as can contamination by skin flora at the time of collection. Interpretation of results can be enhanced by collecting blood cultures separated by time intervals (1 hour is acceptable and useful). Cultures should be taken as early as possible in the course of a febrile episode.

Storage Instructions Specimens collected in tubes with SPS (sodium polyanetholesulfonate) should be processed without delay. The specimen should be transferred to appropriate blood culture media **immediately** to avoid any possible decrease in yield due to storage or prolonged contact with SPS.

Causes for Rejection Unlabeled bottles are not acceptable.

Turnaround Time Common laboratory procedure is to issue a final culture report after 5-7 days. A preliminary culture report based upon Gram's stain and primary subculture is usually available at 24 hours. Positive blood cultures must be reported immediately by telephone and followed with a written report.

Reference Range Negative

Interpretation of Positive Blood Cultures

Virtually **any** organism, including normal flora, **can** cause bacteremia.
A negative culture result does not necessarily rule out bacteremia; false-negative results occur when pathogens fail to grow.
A positive culture result does not necessarily indicate bacteremia; false-positive results occur when contaminants grow.
Gram-negative bacilli, anaerobes, and fungi should be considered pathogens until proven otherwise.
The most difficult interpretation problem is to determine whether an organism that is usually considered normal skin flora is a true pathogen.

From Flournoy DJ and Adkins L, "Understanding the Blood Culture Report," *Am J Infect Control*, 1986,14:41-6, with permission.

Use Isolate and identify potentially pathogenic organisms causing bacteremia, septicemia, meningitis, and other microbiologic states

Limitations Three negative sets of blood cultures in the absence of antimicrobial therapy are usually sufficient to exclude the presence of bacteremia. One set is seldom, if ever, sufficient. Prior antibiotic therapy may cause negative blood cultures or delayed growth. Blood cultures from patients suspected of having *Brucella* or *Leptospira* must be requested as special cultures. Consultation with the laboratory for special culture procedures for the recovery of these organisms prior to collecting the specimen is recommended. See the listings *Leptospira* Culture *on page 472*, and Blood Culture, *Brucella on page 340* for the proper method of collection of these specimens. Yeast often are isolated from routine blood cultures. However, if yeast or other fungi are specifically suspected, a separate fungal blood culture should be drawn along with each of the routine blood culture specimens. See separate listing for proper collection of blood fungus culture. *Mycobacterium avium-intracellulare* (MAI) is frequently recovered from blood of immunocompromised patients particularly those with acquired immunodeficiency syndrome, AIDS. Special procedures are required for the recovery of these organisms, ie, lysis filtration concentration or use of a special mycobacteria blood culture medium. Radiometric methods facilitate the recovery of mycobacteria from blood.

Contraindications Use of a 2% iodine preparation is contraindicated in the preparation of patients sensitive to iodine. Green soap may be substituted for the iodine or alcohol acetone alone may be used.

Methodology Early subculture of aerobic bottle; visual, radiometric, or infrared monitoring. Aerobic and anaerobic culture in broth media usually with subculture to blood agar and chocolate agar. In the lysis centrifugation procedure, blood is lysed and centrifuged using a Du Pont Isolator™ tube or similar method. The sediment is divided to media appropriate for growing aerobic and anaerobic bacteria, fungi, and mycobacteria.

Additional Information Sequential blood cultures in nonendocarditis patients and using a 20 mL sample results in an 80% positive yield after the first set, a 90% yield after the second set, and a 99% yield after the third set. **Volume of blood** cultured seems to be more important than the specific culture technique being employed by the laboratory. The isolation of coagulase-negative *Staphylococcus* (CNS) poses a critical and difficult clinical dilemma. Although CNS is the most commonly isolated organism from blood cultures, only a few (6.3%) of the isolates represent "true" clinically significant bacteremia. Conversely, CNS is (Continued)

Blood Culture, Aerobic and Anaerobic *(Continued)*

well recognized as a cause of infections involving prosthetic devices, cardiac valves, CSF shunts, dialysis catheters, and indwelling vascular catheters. Ultimately the physician is responsible for determining whether an organism is a contaminant or a pathogen. The decision is based on both laboratory and clinical data. Frequently this determination includes patient data (ie, patient history), physical examination, body temperatures, clinical course, and laboratory data (ie, culture results, white blood cell count, and differential). Clinical experience and judgment may play a significant role in resolving this clinical dilemma.

The use of a lysis centrifugation system or specific fungal blood culture media have been reported to increase the recovery rate and decrease the time of fungal recovery compared to traditional or biphasic blood culture systems. Recovery of mycobacteria and *Legionella* may also be enhanced by lysis filtration. In patients who have received antimicrobial drugs, four to six blood cultures may be necessary. Any organism isolated from the blood is usually tested for susceptibility. It is not recommended to culture blood while antimicrobials are present unless verification of an agent's efficacy is needed. This is confirmed with a single culture.

The use of antimicrobial removal devices (ARD) or resin bottles to attempt to increase the yield of blood cultures drawn from patients on antimicrobial therapy is controversial. Some microorganisms are occasionally not recovered with the use of ARD blood cultures. It is therefore advised that at least one culture in a series of three be requested without the use of the ARD bottles. ARD blood cultures are substantially more expensive than routine blood cultures. There is no consensus as to the effectiveness of the ARD cultures in enhancing recovery of organisms.

The diagnosis of bacterial meningitis is accomplished by blood culture, as well as culture and examination of the cerebrospinal fluid. Most children with bacterial meningitis are initially bacteremic.

Selected Readings

Aronson MD and Bor DH, "Blood Cultures," *Ann Intern Med*, 1987, 106(2):246-53.
MacLowry JD, "Clinical Microbiology of Bacteremia an Overview," *Am J Med*, 1983, 75(1B):2-6.
Reller BL, Murray PR, and MacLowry JD, "Blood Cultures II," *Cumitech 1A*, Washington, DC: American Society for Microbiology, 1982, (review).

Blood Culture, AIDS *see* Blood Culture, Mycobacteria *on page 342*

Blood Culture, *Brucella*

Synonyms *Brucella* Blood Culture; Undulant Fever, Culture

Patient Preparation See preparation procedures under listing for Blood Culture, Aerobic and Anaerobic *on page 337*.

Special Instructions The laboratory must be informed of the request for *Brucella* **blood culture.** Collection time, date, age of patient, current antibiotic therapy, clinical diagnosis, and relevant history.

Specimen Blood

Container Castañeda bottle; *Brucella* broth and agar; conventional trypticase soy broth (TSB)

Collection Should be drawn prior to administration of antibiotics, and before an expected temperature rise. Follow collection procedure in Blood Culture, Aerobic and Anaerobic.

Causes for Rejection Specimens not received in appropriate bottles will have less than optimal yield.

Turnaround Time 6 weeks

Reference Range No growth

Use Establish the diagnosis of brucellosis

Limitations Blood cultures for *Brucella* are primarily useful in the early acute phase of the disease. Recovery of *Brucella* is limited by the relatively low level of bacteremia and the fastidious nature of the organism. Yield may be increased by culturing larger volumes of blood in a conventional trypticase soy broth or use of a lysis centrifugation concentration technique.

Methodology *Brucella* broth and agar, held at least 21 days with or without lysis concentration. Trypticase soy broth (TSB) cultures yield acceptable results (93% of possible isolates). Blood clot cultures utilizing a variety of methods provide no advantage over more conventional TSB cultures for the isolation of *Brucella melitensis*. The use of a lysis concentration procedure was found to be superior to the use of the Castañeda procedure (biphasic medium) for the recovery of *Brucella* from clinical specimens. *Brucella* may be recovered using the Roche Septi-Chek® system with growth observed on the chocolate section of the paddle. The organism appears as a small slow-growing white colony. It is a gram-negative coccobacillus. **The handling of cultures and specimens as well as the inhalation of dust-containing *Brucella* organisms is dangerous to laboratory workers**. A biologic safety cabinet should be used for all suspected isolates.

Additional Information Bone marrow culture and serologic testing of acute and convalescent specimens for *Brucella* antibodies may be useful when cultures of peripheral blood are negative. In animals, brucellosis has a bacteremic phase followed by localization in the reproductive tract and reticuloendothelial system. The disease is common worldwide, particularly in the countries of the former Soviet Union, Mediterranean, Latin America, and Spain. One hundred and six cases were reported in the U.S. in 1986. Most brucellosis in the U.S. occurs in abattoir workers, farmers and rarely veterinarians. Symptoms may be subclinical, subacute, acute relapsing and chronic. Undulant fever is most typical of *B. melitensis*. Symptoms may include abdominal pain and may mimic appendicitis or cholecystitis. Unpasteurized milk may be a source of infection. Risk factors raising an index of suspicion include travel, food, and occupation. Serologic confirmation of the diagnosis may be helpful.

Selected Readings
Etemadi H, Raissadt A, Pickett MJ, et al, "Isolation of *Brucella* spp. From Clinical Specimens," *J Clin Microbiol*, 1984, 20(3):586.

Finegold SM and Baron EJ, *Bailey and Scott's Diagnostic Microbiology*, 7th ed, St Louis, MO: CV Mosby Co, 1986, 440-3.

Moyer NP, Holcomb LA, and Hausler WJ Jr, "*Brucella*," *Manual of Clinical Microbiology*, 5th ed, Balows A, Hausler WJ Jr, Herrmann KL, et al, eds, Washington, DC: American Society for Microbiology, 1991, 457-62.

Blood Culture for CMV *see* Cytomegalovirus Culture, Blood *on page 389*

Blood Culture, Fungus

Related Information
Blood Culture, Aerobic and Anaerobic *on page 337*

Synonyms Fungus Blood Culture; Fungus Culture, Blood

Test Includes Routine blood culture and inoculation of specific fungal media at time of collection; identification of any fungi isolated

Patient Preparation See Blood Culture, Aerobic and Anaerobic *on page 337*.

Special Instructions Inform the laboratory of the specific request for fungus blood culture. The following information will assist the laboratory in the proper processing of the specimen: specific site of specimen, current antibiotic therapy, age and sex of patient, collection time and date, and clinical diagnosis.

Specimen Blood

Container Routine and special fungal blood culture media

Collection Standard blood culture collection procedures.

Storage Instructions Transport specimen to the laboratory immediately.

Turnaround Time Preliminary reports are usually available in one to two days. Negative cultures are commonly reported at 4-6 weeks.

Reference Range No fungi grown

Use Isolate and identify fungi; establish the diagnosis of fungemia, fungal endocarditis, and disseminated mycosis in immunocompromised patients, oncology patients, transplant patients, patients with leukemia and lymphoma, and patients with the acquired immunodeficiency syndrome (AIDS)

Limitations A single negative culture does not rule out the presence of fungal infection. Fungal blood cultures are most effective in isolating *Candida albicans* and *Candida glabrata* (*Torulopsis glabrata*). If other fungal species are suspected, a biopsy or bone marrow fungus culture should be considered. *Blastomyces dermatitidis* usually is not recovered from blood.

Additional Information Fungemia may complicate therapy with steroids, antineoplastic drugs, radiation therapy, broad spectrum antibiotic therapy, venous or arterial catheterization, hyperalimentation, and the acquired immunodeficiency syndrome (AIDS). Intravenous drug abusers are prone to *Candida* endocarditis. Although many fungal species including *Histoplasma capsulatum*, *Coccidioides immitis*, *Cryptococcus neoformans*, and many other unusual isolates are recoverable from blood cultures, the most common cause of fungemia is *Candida albicans* followed by other *Candida* sp including *Candida glabrata* (*Torulopsis* (Continued)

Blood Culture, Fungus *(Continued)*

glabrata). In most cases fungemia represents a failure of the host defense system. Fungemia may be caused by contamination of an indwelling catheter or, in the critically ill and immunocompromised patient, contamination of the gastro-intestinal and less frequently the urinary tract.

Blood Culture, *Leptospira* *see Leptospira Culture on page 472*

Blood Culture, Lysis Centrifugation *see Blood Culture, Aerobic and Anaerobic on page 337*

Blood Culture, Mycobacteria

Related Information
Blood Culture, Aerobic and Anaerobic *on page 337*

Applies to AIDS Blood Culture; Blood Culture, AIDS

Patient Preparation Usual sterile preparation

Special Instructions Request test specifically. Not part of routine blood culture. Contact the laboratory prior to collecting blood.

Specimen Blood

Container Aerobic blood culture bottle

Storage Instructions Incubate if unable to deliver to the laboratory on the day of collection.

Causes for Rejection Other bacteria present

Use Isolate mycobacteria, especially *M. avium-intracellulare*

Additional Information Mycobacterial usually are identified to genus and species, and susceptibility tests will be done usually without special request. Contact the laboratory for details and special collection instructions.

Blood Culture With Antimicrobial Removal Device (ARD) *see Blood Culture, Aerobic and Anaerobic on page 337*

Blood Smear for Malarial Parasites *see Peripheral Blood Smear, Thick and Thin on page 519*

Blood Smear for Trypanosomal/Filarial Parasites *see Microfilariae, Peripheral Blood Preparation on page 489*

Body Cavity Fluid Cytology *see Cytology, Body Fluids on page 386*

Body Fluid Anaerobic Culture *see Anaerobic Culture on page 316*

Body Fluid Culture, Routine *see Aerobic Culture, Body Fluid on page 310*

Body Fluid Fungus Culture *see Fungus Culture, Body Fluid on page 415*

Body Lice Identification *see Arthropod Identification on page 334*

Body Surface Areas of Adults and Children *see page 991*

Bone Biopsy

Applies to Percutaneous Biopsy of Musculoskeletal Lesions and Synovial Membranes

Test Includes This procedure involves the passage of a needle, either under fluoroscopic or computed tomographic guidance, into an area of bony abnormality to facilitate precise histologic and/or bacteriologic diagnosis. In many clinical situations, this procedure can establish definitive diagnosis without the disadvantages of surgery making it a useful alternative to open biopsy. In selected cases of arthritis, examination of the synovium may provide precise diagnostic clues or useful information about the nature of the arthritic process. A biopsy of the synovium can be performed through an open arthrotomy, percutaneous biopsy, or as part of an arthroscopic procedure during which the synovium can be visualized.

Patient Preparation Biopsies are performed in the Radiology Department. Skeletal biopsies are usually done under local anesthesia, with the exception of children and restless patients who are placed under general anesthesia or heavy sedation. Local anesthesia facilitates communication between the patient and the physician performing the procedure. Should the patient complain of radiating pain, the needle can be repositioned. Spinal biopsies necessitate a 24-hour hospitalization. Other anatomic areas may be biopsied on an outpatient basis. The patient should not eat on the morning of the examination. An intravenous catheter is generally placed for I.V. access and the patient is usually administered both a sedative and a medication for pain.

Specimen There are a wide variety of commercially available needles for these procedures. A needle aspiration biopsy consists of aspiration of fluid for cytologic and/or bacteriologic analysis. A core biopsy, however, requires a larger needle and allows retrieval of a core of tissue for histopathologic interpretation.

Use When there is a need for a tissue or bacteriologic diagnosis in situations where it is desirable to forego open biopsy

Selected Readings
Bard M and Laredo JD, *Interventional Radiology in Bone and Joint*, New York, NY: Springer-Verlag Wien, 1988.

Bone Films

Applies to Acromioclavicular Joint, Left or Right, X-ray; Ankle, Left or Right, X-ray; Arthritis Series, X-ray; Calcaneus (heel), Left or Right, X-ray; Clavicle, Left or Right, X-ray; Elbow, Left or Right, X-ray; Femur, Left or Right, X-ray; Finger, Left or Right Hand, X-ray; Foot, Left or Right, X-ray; Forearm, Left or Right, X-ray; Hand, Left or Right, X-ray; Hands and Wrist Arthritis, X-ray; Hip, Left or Right, and Pelvis, X-ray; Hip, Left or Right, X-ray; Hips Arthritis, X-ray; Humerus, Left or Right, X-ray; Knee, Left or Right, X-ray; Knees Arthritis, X-ray; Patella of Knee, Left or Right, X-ray; Pelvis AP, X-ray; Pelvis Stereo, X-ray; Postreduction Films, X-ray; Scanogram, X-ray; Scapula, Left or Right, X-ray; Shoulder, Left or Right, X-ray; Shoulder Stereo, Left or Right, X-ray; Shoulder to Include Axial View, Left or Right, X-ray; Shoulders Arthritis, X-ray; Sternoclavicular Joint, Left or Right, X-ray; Thumb, Left or Right, X-ray; Tibia and Fibula, Left or Right, X-ray; Toes of Foot, Left or Right, X-ray; Wrist, Left or Right, X-ray

Test Includes Upper extremity and shoulder girdle: fingers, thumb, hands, wrists, wrists for carpal tunnel, wrists for navicular views, PA hands and wrists for arthritis, forearm, elbow, humerus, scapula, shoulder for trauma, shoulder for inflammatory process, shoulder to include axial view, clavicle, nonweight bearing and weight bearing views of acromioclavicular joints, bilateral comparison sternoclavicular joints, and postreduction films.

Lower extremity and pelvis: AP pelvis, stereo pelvis, pelvis and hips, hips for congenital deformity, hips for arthritis, femur, knee, weight bearing, knees for arthritis, knees with patellar views, knees with tunnel views, tibia-fibula, ankles, ankles with stress views, calcaneus, feet, toes.

Bony thorax: ribs, unilateral or bilateral, sternum.

Patient Preparation The parts under scrutiny should bear the lightest possible dressing. Patient must wear x-ray gown to department.

Special Instructions Requisition must state: if safe for patient to sit, stand, and move extremities. If questions of liability or compensation are known to exist in the case. If there is a question of fracture, how long ago injury occurred, and any previous fractures. In case of foreign bodies, state their nature since many are not visible on x-ray examination. If dressings, bivalved casts, and splints may be removed. If "wet reading" is desired. By appointment, call appropriate number. Send completed and signed requisition to Radiology. Comparison views on request. Specify right or left.

Use Evaluate bones for the presence of metastatic and primary neoplasms, trauma, infectious disease, degenerative and reactive processes

Limitations Metal appliances, casts and dressings containing aluminum paste, lead water, or Epsom salts obscure or obliterate all detail

Methodology The affected body part will be moved, if possible, into two or three different positions so films can be obtained.

Bone Marrow *see* Bone Marrow Aspiration and Biopsy *on this page*

Bone Marrow Aspiration and Biopsy

Applies to Bone Marrow; Bone Marrow Iron Stain; Bone Marrow Sampling; Bone Marrow Trephine Biopsy; Iron Stain

Test Includes Aspiration and/or biopsy of bone marrow (BM) for microscopic analysis. Both procedures are carried out under local anesthesia at the patient's bedside. For aspiration, a specialized hollow needle is advanced into the intramedullary cavity (usually iliac crest). Approximately 0.4 mL liquid marrow and bone fragments are aspirated into a syringe, then smeared onto a slide. Frequently, a bone marrow biopsy is performed as a complementary, but separate, procedure (different equipment and site). A specialized biopsy needle (eg, Jamshidi needle) is used to obtain a core of solid cortical bone. This technique (Continued)

Bone Marrow Aspiration and Biopsy *(Continued)*

preserves the normal marrow architecture of the biopsy sample and allows for formal histologic analysis.

Patient Preparation Technique and risks of the procedure are explained to the patient and consent is obtained. Considerable patient apprehension often accompanies this procedure and requires thorough, step-by-step explanation beforehand. If coagulopathy is known or suspected, a recent CBC and PT/PTT should be drawn. Requisition must state in advance any special studies to be performed on specimen, such as AFB stain, Congo red stain for amyloid, cytogenetics studies, etc. Contact referring physician if any questions arise or contact appropriate laboratories directly. Patients are commonly premedicated with a short-acting benzodiazepine or analgesic such as meperidine.

Aftercare Needle puncture site(s) are covered with a dry sterile dressing. If the bone marrow biopsy is performed from the posterior iliac crest, patient must lie on back for a full 30 minutes before being discharged. In the presence of a low-grade coagulopathy or mild thrombocytopenia, direct pressure should be applied by operator (not patient) to puncture sites until local bleeding ceases. Instruct patient to keep dressings dry. Ideally, puncture sites should be examined approximately 24 hours later by nurse or physician, but this is not always feasible.

Special Instructions This procedure requires at least two operators. The first obtains the aspiration and/or biopsy specimen in a sterile fashion (usually a physician or specialized nurse clinician) and the second immediately examines and prepares the specimen (usually a nurse or technologist from the Hematology Laboratory).

Complications Bone marrow sampling is considered a relatively safe but invasive procedure. Minor complications include local bleeding, hematoma, and discomfort at the needle puncture site. Local infection is rarely seen if proper aftercare is followed. Major complications have been reported with sternal biopsy (Bahir 1963), including fatal puncture of mediastinal structures. Historical reports of fistula formation, osteomyelitis, and profuse bleeding were associated with biopsy of what are now considered nonstandard sites, such as the tibia. Minimal complications are associated with sampling of the iliac crest, the preferred site.

Equipment Commercially assembled trays for aspiration and biopsy are widely available. These prepackaged kits typically contain a bone marrow biopsy needle (usually Jamshidi needle), aspiration needle (usually Illinois needle), various syringes (5 mL, 10 mL, 20 mL), assorted needles (18-gauge, 25-gauge), and 1% lidocaine with epinephrine for local anesthesia. Also included are gauze, sterile gloves, drapes and towels, No 11 scalpel blade, and alcohol and iodine prep. The Jamshidi needle is a large-bore (usually 11-gauge), hollow needle with a tapered tip, thin metal stylet, and wide plastic grip to allow easy needle rotation. The Illinois needle is somewhat smaller, but likewise comes with a stylet and plastic sheath for improved grip. Smaller gauge needles are available for use in the pediatric population.

Technique The procedure is performed by experienced operators only. May be carried out at the bedside if adequate lighting is available, otherwise done in a procedure room.

Aspiration: Preferred site is the posterior superior iliac spine (PSIS), alternatively the sternum. Patient is placed on his side or lies prone. Landmarks are identified by palpation - the PSIS primarily, but the anterior superior iliac spine also. A wide circular area (approximately 5" in diameter) overlying the PSIS is prepped with povidone-iodine in the usual sterile fashion. Using the 25-gauge needle and lidocaine, the skin directly over the PSIS is anesthetized. Following this, deeper structures are liberally anesthetized with the 18-gauge needle, including a several centimeter area of the periosteum. A 4 mm long skin incision is made over the PSIS by means of the No 11 scalpel blade, then extended deeper through fatty tissues down to the anesthetized periosteum. The Illinois aspiration needle (with stylet in place) is advanced through this soft tissue incision and firmly into the cortex of the PSIS, using a constant rotary motion of the needle ("drilling"). Once the needle has penetrated approximately 1 cm into the marrow cavity, the stylet is removed and a 10 mL syringe is attached to the open (distal) end of the aspiration needle. At least 4-5 mL marrow is aspirated using firm suction. This volume is adequate for most routine hematologic studies, but larger volumes are usually needed for fungal or tuberculous cultures, cytogenetics, cell markers, etc. This step often causes the most patient discomfort. After aspiration, the syringe is detached and immediately handed over to the technologist in order to prevent the specimen from clotting (aspiration needle is still in the PSIS). The technologist examines the specimen grossly for marrow particles, which may be visible to the naked eye. If present, this signifies that an adequate marrow specimen has likely been obtained; if absent, the aspiration needle is redirected slightly and the previous listed steps repeated. After completion, the needle is removed and direct pressure applied.

Biopsy: May be carried out immediately following aspiration, while patient is still under local anesthesia. Preferred site is again the PSIS; however, unlike bone marrow aspiration, biopsy is never obtained from the sternum. A Jamshidi biopsy needle is passed through the same skin and soft tissue incision used for aspiration (alternatively, a completely new site may be used). However, a separate hole in the PSIS must be made. Once into the cortical bone, the needle is advanced using a pronounced clockwise/counterclockwise rotary motion. The needle is oriented along an imaginary line connecting the PSIS and the anterior superior iliac spine, forcing a slight angle of the needle with respect to the skin. The needle should **not** be advanced perpendicular to the skin; this results in poor quality biopsies (often with mostly cartilage). The stylet is then removed. The "drilling" is continued until the needle is at least 2 cm deep into the cortex. This may be estimated by periodically replacing the stylet into the needle and noting the distance the stylet protrudes. The biopsy core is subsequently "sheared off" by the following maneuvers:

- needle is rotated a full 10 turns clockwise then 10 turns counterclockwise
- needle is withdrawn slightly and redirected at a different angle
- needle is readvanced
- steps 1-3 are repeated (until the core is sheared off). The needle is withdrawn, again using rotary motions so as not to lose the core. The blunt obturator or "push wire" is passed through the sharp tip of the Jamshidi needle and the specimen pushed gently out of the needle base and onto a sterile gauze. The technologist immediately makes imprints of the core then places the specimen in fixative.

The techniques for aspiration and biopsy outlined are generally agreed upon in major textbooks. However, some clinicians strongly believe that bone marrow biopsy should always **precede** aspiration, despite the "textbook" recommendations. They argue that artifacts in the core biopsy may be induced by aspiration.

Specimen The bone marrow aspirate is immediately examined for visible bone spicules. The presence of these small spicules suggests an adequate specimen. Direct smears of the aspirate fluid are prepared by the technologist at the bedside. These smears consist of marrow particles and free marrow cells spread onto coverslips. This technique helps to preserve the cytologic appearance of individual blood cells. Bone marrow biopsy samples are handled differently. In many institutions, touch preparations are made first, before specimen fixation. The marrow specimen is touched gently to a clean glass slide in several places, without smearing. These "touch preps" are allowed to air-dry and subsequently undergo routine staining. This technique also helps preserve cytologic detail. Once the touch preparations are completed, the remainder of the specimen is placed in a fixative such as formalin or Zenker's solution. The specimen is then processed according to individual laboratory protocol (for example, overnight fixation, decalcification, wash steps, dehydration, and serial sectioning). Routine stains are performed on processed specimens. These include hematoxylin and eosin (H & E), Wright-Giemsa stain, and iron stain. Optional studies may be obtained at physician request such as cytogenetic analysis, flow cytometry, electron microscopy, and amyloid stains. The Hematology Laboratory must be notified in advance for these studies. Bone marrow specimens may also be submitted for microbiological analysis. Cultures may be obtained for aerobic and anaerobic bacteria, fungi (eg, *Histoplasma capsulatum*), acid-fast bacilli (eg, *Mycobacterium tuberculosis* or *Mycobacterium avium-intracellulare*), and viruses (cytomegalovirus). Fixatives should **not** be added to specimens submitted for culture. Again, it is important to notify the Microbiology Laboratory in advance for these cultures.

Reference Range The bone marrow aspirate and biopsy are reviewed by a staff pathologist or hematologist. The preliminary report on the bone marrow aspirate may often be available several hours after the procedure, on request. Normal values for bone marrow cell lines in the adult are as follows:
(Continued)

Bone Marrow Aspiration and Biopsy *(Continued)*

Granulocytes
- blasts: 0% to 1 %
- promyelocytes: 1% to 5%
- neutrophil myelocytes and metamyelocytes: 7% to 25%
- neutrophil bands and segs: 20% to 60%
- eosinophils: 0% to 3%
- basophils: 0% to 1%
- monocytes: 0% to 2%
- lymphocytes: 5% to 15%
- plasma cells: 0% to 2%

Erythrocytes
- proerythrocytes: 0% to 1%
- early erythrocytes: 1% to 4%
- late erythrocytes: 10% to 20%
- normoblasts: 5% to 10%

The above bone marrow differential cell counts are calculated from the bone marrow aspirate specimen. Other useful data provided by the bone marrow aspirate include:
- myeloid/erythroid ratio (normal ratio 3-4:1)
- total cells counted
- overall cellularity
- erythropoiesis
- granulopoiesis

The bone marrow biopsy provides additional information on marrow architecture (which cannot be obtained from the aspirate). When examining the biopsy specimen, the pathologist may comment on:
- gross description including size of sample
- overall cellularity
- presence of granulomas
- infiltrative marrow processes such as lymphoma, carcinoma, granulomas
- iron stores
- results of special stains

Use Bone marrow sampling is indicated in the evaluation of a wide variety of hematologic disorders, usually noted first on the CBC or peripheral smear. It is also useful in the diagnosis of systemic diseases which may potentially involve the marrow, such as infectious or granulomatous processes. Bone marrow aspiration and biopsy should be considered separate procedures, although indications often overlap. Indications for bone marrow **aspiration** include:
- evaluation of severe anemia, especially when etiology is in doubt and reticulocyte count is low
- evaluation of macrocytic anemia, to confirm the presence of megaloblastic anemia or to exclude sideroblastic anemia and normoblastic erythropoiesis
- leukopenia and/or thrombocytopenia, to differentiate excessive consumption from decreased production
- persistent leukocytosis of unknown etiology
- suspected myelodysplastic syndrome
- suspected leukemia, to confirm diagnosis and to classify subtype (FAB categorization)
- suspected immunoglobulin disorders, such as multiple myeloma, for diagnosis and staging
- evaluation of lipid storage diseases
- evaluation of suspected iron storage abnormalities
- acquisition of marrow for chromosomal analysis
- acquisition of tissue for microbiological culture (fungi, bacteria, mycobacteria, parasites)
- evaluation of response to therapy for hematologic malignancies

Bone marrow biopsy preserves the marrow architecture and is useful in evaluating systemic diseases secondarily involving the marrow. Bone marrow **biopsy** indications include:
- evaluation of pancytopenia
- evaluation of possible myelophthisic anemia (bone marrow infiltrated with leukemic cells, metastatic tumor, lymphoma, granulomas, etc)
- diagnosis and staging of solid tumors or lymphoma

- evaluation of selected cases of fever of unknown origin
- diagnosis of systemic amyloidosis when other methods have failed
- suspected cases of myelofibrosis
- evaluation of myeloproliferative syndromes (polycythemia vera, essential thrombocythemia, etc)
- failed bone marrow aspiration attempts (the so-called "dry tap")

Authorities differ on the exact indications for both bone marrow aspiration and biopsy. Some believe that most hematologic abnormalities are adequately evaluated by bone marrow aspiration alone (without biopsy). Bone marrow biopsy should not be routinely performed with aspiration, it is argued, due to the following reasons:

- diagnosis can often be made by aspiration
- significant patient discomfort accompanies biopsy
- there is needless expense and patient risk

Thus, bone marrow biopsy should only be performed if specific indications are present (as listed).

Other experts routinely include a biopsy whenever aspiration is performed. The following reasons are cited.

- Bone marrow biopsy may be diagnostic in cases where aspiration is negative or equivocal.
- It is nearly impossible to predict in advance which aspiration attempts will be technically difficult.
- Bone marrow biopsy actually causes less discomfort than aspiration in some cases.
- Cost-benefit analysis may favor the combined approach. The cost to physician, technologist, and patient may be doubled if patient is forced to undergo a separate bone marrow biopsy at a later date.

Contraindications

- uncooperative patient
- cellulitis, osteomyelitis, or radiation therapy involving the proposed site of needle entry
- severe, noncorrectable coagulopathy
- thoracic aortic aneurysm if a sternal approach is used
- Paget's disease involving the iliac bone represents a high risk situation, due to excessive bleeding at trephine biopsy site (but not necessarily a contraindication)

Selected Readings

Batjer JP, "Preparation of Optimal Bone Marrow Samples," Lab Med, 1979, 10:101-6.

Beckstead JH, "The Bone Marrow Biopsy: A Diagnostic Strategy," Arch Pathol Lab Med, 1986, 110(3):175-9.

Brynes RK, McKenna RW, and Sundberg RD, "Bone Marrow Aspiration and Trephine Biopsy: An Approach to a Thorough Study," Am J Clin Pathol, 1978, 70(5):753-9.

Williams WJ and Nelson DA, "Examination of the Marrow," Hematology, 4th ed, Chapter 3, WJ Williams, E Beutler, AJ Erslev, et al, eds, New York, NY: McGraw-Hill, 1990, 24-31.

Bone Marrow Culture see Aerobic Culture, Body Fluid on page 310

Bone Marrow Culture, Routine

Synonyms Aerobic Bone Marrow Culture; Routine Bone Marrow Culture

Test Includes Culture and Gram's stain if requested. Properly collected specimens must also be cultured for anaerobes.

Patient Preparation Usual sterile preparation of aspiration site.

Special Instructions Add 0.1-0.2 mL heparin 10,000 units/mL to sterile tube or Anaport vial

Specimen Bone marrow

Container Sterile tube or Anaport vial containing 0.1-0.2 mL heparin 10,000 units/mL

Collection The specimen will be divided for aerobic, fungus, anaerobic, mycobacteria cultures and smears, volume permitting if accompanied by appropriate requisitions

Storage Instructions Transport specimen to the laboratory immediately. Do not refrigerate.

Causes for Rejection Clots, inadequate volume for studies requested. Specimen will not be discarded without consultation with the attending physician. (Continued)

Bone Marrow Culture, Routine *(Continued)*

Turnaround Time Stat Gram's stain: 1 hour. Physician will be notified of all positive smears or cultures. Preliminary results are reported at 24 hours with broth held for 5-7 days.

Reference Range No growth

Use Isolate and identify etiologic agent

Bone Marrow Iron Stain *see* Bone Marrow Aspiration and Biopsy *on page 343*

Bone Marrow Mycobacteria Culture *see* Mycobacteria Culture, Biopsy or Body Fluid *on page 493*

Bone Marrow Sampling *see* Bone Marrow Aspiration and Biopsy *on page 343*

Bone Marrow Trephine Biopsy *see* Bone Marrow Aspiration and Biopsy *on page 343*

Bone Scan

Synonyms Bone Scintigraphy; Radionuclide Bone Scan; Whole Body Bone Scan

Applies to Bone Scan With Flow; Three-Phase Bone Scan

Test Includes The patient receives an intravenous injection of a technetium-99m (^{99m}Tc) phosphonate radiopharmaceutical which localizes in bone with intensity proportional to the degree of metabolic activity present. Three hours after the injection, whole body and appropriate regional skeletal images are acquired. An initial dynamic flow study and/or early images may also be acquired if osteomyelitis, osteonecrosis, Legg-Calvé-Perthes disease, septic arthritis, or other inflammatory disease is suspected (three-phase technique).

Patient Preparation Patient should have all RIA blood work performed, or at least drawn, prior to injection of any radioactive material. The patient does not need to be fasting or NPO for this procedure. Patient should be encouraged to drink fluids during the waiting period before scanning and will be asked to void just before scanning begins.

Special Instructions Requisition must state the current patient diagnosis in order to select the most appropriate radiopharmaceutical and/or imaging technique. When ordering liver and bone scans for the same patient, schedule liver scan at least 1 day before the bone scan. **DURATION OF PROCEDURE:** 3-4.5 hours. This includes a 2-3 hour delay after tracer injection to allow adequate localization in bone. **RADIOPHARMACEUTICAL:** ^{99m}Tc phosphonate compound.

Technique The application of single-photon emission tomography (SPECT) techniques may contribute significantly to the diagnostic accuracy of this imaging study.

Causes for Rejection Other recent Nuclear Medicine procedure may interfere. If uncertain, call the Nuclear Medicine Department.

Turnaround Time A written report will be sent to the patient's chart and/or to the referring physician.

Normal Findings Homogeneous and symmetric distribution of activity throughout all skeletal structures

Use Bone imaging is extremely sensitive for the detection of infection or malignancy involving any part of the skeleton. It is the most appropriate screening test for these conditions, since scan abnormalities are present long before structural defects develop radiographically. Bone scans are also accurate for localizing lesions for biopsy, excision, or debridement. Stress fractures can be diagnosed by bone scan when radiographs are completely normal.

Limitations In postoperative orthopedic patients and diabetics, additional imaging with gallium or indium-labeled white blood cells may help to confirm the presence of active infection and serve as a baseline for later comparison

Selected Readings

Datz FL, "Radionuclide Imaging of Joint Inflammation in the 90s," *J Nucl Med*, 1990, 31(5):684-7.

Gupta NC and Prezio JA, "Radionuclide Imaging in Osteomyelitis," *Semin Nucl Med*, 1988, 18(4):287-99.

Jacobson AF, Cronin EB, Stomper PC, et al, "Bone Scans With One or Two Abnormalities in Cancer Patients With No Known Metastases: Frequency and Serial Scintigraphic Behavior of Benign and Malignant Lesions," *Radiology*, 1990, 175(1):229-32.

Lusins JO, Danielski EF, and Goldsmith SJ, "Bone SPECT in Patients With Persistent Back Pain After Lumbar Spine Surgery," *J Nucl Med*, 1989, 30(4):490-6.

Matin P, "Basic Principles of Nuclear Medicine Techniques for Detection and Evaluation of Trauma and Sports Medicine Injuries," *Semin Nucl Med*, 1988, 18(2):90-112.

McDougall IR and Keeling CA, "Complications of Fractures and Their Healing," *Semin Nucl Med*, 1988, 18(2):113-25.

McNeil BJ, "Value of Bone Scanning in Neoplastic Disease," *Semin Nucl Med*, 1985, 14(4):277-86.

Palmer E, Henrikson B, McKusick K, et al, "Pain as an Indicator of Bone Metastasis," *Acta Radiol*, 1988, 29(4):445-9.

Bone Scan With Flow *see* Bone Scan *on previous page*

Bone Scintigraphy *see* Bone Scan *on previous page*

***Bordetella pertussis* Antibodies** *see Bordetella pertussis* Serology *on page 351*

Bordetella pertussis Direct Fluorescent Antibody

Related Information

Bordetella pertussis Nasopharyngeal Culture *on this page*

Bordetella pertussis Serology *on page 351*

Synonyms *Bordetella pertussis* Smear; Nasopharyngeal Smear for *Bordetella pertussis*

Replaces Cough Plate Culture for Pertussis

Test Includes Fluorescent antibody stain to detect *Bordetella pertussis* on smear

Patient Preparation Patient must not be on antimicrobial therapy.

Special Instructions Laboratory supervisor should be notified 24 hours before collection of specimen so that a special isolation medium can be prepared.

Specimen Nasopharyngeal swab

Container Nasopharyngeal swab, sterile saline

Collection Swab is passed through nose gently and into nasopharynx. Stay near septum and floor of nose. Rotate and remove. Specimen must be hand transported to the laboratory immediately following collection.

Storage Instructions Do not refrigerate. Transport to the laboratory immediately.

Causes for Rejection Specimen not received in appropriate sterile container or on appropriate isolation medium, specimen more than 2 hours old. Cough plates are unacceptable.

Reference Range No *B. pertussis* detected

Use Detect and identify *B. pertussis* and *B. parapertussis*, establish diagnosis of whooping cough

Limitations Direct detection assays are always limited by the adequacy of the sample. Bacteria may be difficult to detect if there are few bacteria present in the specimen or too much mucoid material.

Contraindications Lack of clinical symptoms of pertussis; previous antibiotic therapy

Methodology Direct fluorescent antibody (DFA)

Additional Information The procedure enables early presumptive identification of *Bordetella pertussis*, the agent of whooping cough. Definitive cultural identification should be completed. There is also available a test for serum agglutinating antibodies, which if present may be titered over time to indicate exposure.

Bordetella pertussis Nasopharyngeal Culture

Related Information

Bordetella pertussis Direct Fluorescent Antibody *on this page*

Bordetella pertussis Serology *on page 351*

Synonyms Nasopharyngeal Culture for *Bordetella pertussis*; Pertussis Culture; Whooping Cough Culture

Replaces Cough Plate Culture for Pertussis; Throat Culture for *Bordetella pertussis*

Test Includes Specific culture and identification of *Bordetella pertussis* and *Bordetella parapertussis*

Patient Preparation Patient should not be on antimicrobial therapy prior to the collection of the specimen.

Special Instructions Consult the laboratory prior to collection of the specimen so that the special isolation medium can be obtained. The laboratory should be made aware of the specific request to screen for *Bordetella pertussis* with information relevant to current antibiotic therapy and current diagnosis.

Specimen Nasopharyngeal swab

Container Flexible calcium alginate swab (Calgiswab®) and Bordet-Gengou plate. Transport medium composed of half strength Oxoid charcoal agar CM19 supplemented with 40 µg/mL cephalexin and 10% hemolyzed defibrinated horse blood may be used.

(Continued)

Bordetella pertussis Nasopharyngeal Culture
(Continued)

Collection Shape the flexible swab into the contour of the nares. Pass the swab gently through the nose. Leave swab in place near septum and floor of nose for 15-30 seconds. Rotate and remove. The recovery of the organism depends on collecting an adequate specimen. Inoculate the plate or transport medium directly at the bedside.

The following procedure optimizes the laboratory diagnosis of pertussis.

- Collect nasopharyngeal specimens in the early stage of illness. Providing specimen collection kits facilitates the appropriate specimen collection and transportation.
- For swab collected specimens, use a transport medium consisting of half strength Oxoid charcoal agar supplemented with 10% hemolyzed, defibrinated horse blood, and 40 µg/mL cephalexin.
- Inoculate a selective primary plating medium composed of Oxoid charcoal agar, 10% defibrinated horse blood, and 40 µg/mL cephalexin. A nonselective medium without cephalexin may be used in addition to the selective medium.
- Perform direct fluorescent antibody (DFA) tests on appropriately collected nasopharyngeal secretions with *B. pertussis*- and *B. parapertussis*-conjugated antisera to facilitate an earlier diagnosis.
- After inoculating primary plating media, retain swabs in the original transport medium at room temperature. If cultures become overgrown with indigenous bacterial flora or fungi, use swabs to inoculate additional media.
- Identify suspicious isolates with appropriate cultural and biochemical tests. The DFA test performed on growth from isolated colonies is an excellent procedure for confirmatory or definitive identification.

Storage Instructions The specimen should not be refrigerated. It should be transported to the laboratory as soon as possible after collection.

Causes for Rejection Specimen not received on appropriate isolation medium. Excessive delay in transit to the laboratory results in less than optimal yield.

Turnaround Time Preliminary reports are generally available at 24 hours if pathogens other than *B. pertussis* are isolated. Growth of *Bordetella pertussis* takes at least 72 hours to be detected. Cultures with no growth are usually reported after 1 week. Reports on specimens from which *B. pertussis* has been isolated generally require at least 1 week for completion.

Reference Range No *B. pertussis* or *B. parapertussis* isolated

Use Isolate and identify *B. pertussis*, and *B. parapertussis*; establish the diagnosis of whooping cough

Limitations Cough plates are less reliable than nasopharyngeal specimens.

Contraindications Lack of clinical symptoms of pertussis; previous antibiotic therapy; history of vaccination is a relative contraindication

Methodology Culture on selective medium (selective chocolate agar with 10% defibrinated horse blood and 40 µg/mL cephalexin), presumptive confirmation by direct fluorescent antibody (DFA). Culture after enrichment in transport medium for 48 hours increases yield.

Additional Information Direct fluorescent antibody (DFA) procedures provide more rapid results and have been increasingly used in the diagnosis of *B. pertussis* infection. The DFA procedures are most useful in the first 2-3 weeks of the illness. DFA test detected 42 of 164 (26%) of patients who proved culture positive for *B. pertussis* and 8 of 38 (21%) of patients who proved culture positive for *B. parapertussis*. False-negatives may be caused by inadequate specimens having little cellular material (leukocytes and brush border epithelial cells).

Selected Readings

Friedman RL, "Pertussis: The Disease and New Diagnostic Methods," *Clin Microbiol Rev*, 1988, 1(4):365-76.

Halperin SA, "Interpretation of Pertussis Serologic Tests," *Pediatr Infect Dis J*, 1991, 10(10):791-2.

Halperin SA, Bortolussi R, and Wort AJ, "Evaluation of Culture, Immunofluorescence, and Serology for the Diagnosis of Pertussis," *J Clin Microbiol*, 1989, 27(4):752-7.

Herwaldt LA, "Pertussis in Adults: What Physicians Need to Know," *Arch Intern Med*, 1991, 151(8):1510-2.

Marchant CD, Loughlin AM, Lett SM, et al, "Pertussis in Massachusetts, 1981-1991: Incidence, Serologic Diagnosis, and Vaccine Effectiveness," *J Infect Dis*, 1994, 169(6):1297-305.

Young SA, Anderson GL, and Mitchell PD, "Laboratory Observations During an Outbreak of Pertussis," *Clin Microbiol Newslett*, 1987, 9:22, 176-9.

Bordetella pertussis Serology

Related Information

Bordetella pertussis Direct Fluorescent Antibody *on page 349*

Bordetella pertussis Nasopharyngeal Culture *on page 349*

Synonyms *Bordetella pertussis* Antibodies; *Bordetella pertussis* Titer; Pertussis Serology

Test Includes Enzyme-linked immunosorbent assay to detect antibodies to *Bordetella pertussis* and/or pertussis toxin

Specimen Serum

Container Red top tube

Storage Instructions Refrigerate serum at 4°C.

Reference Range Absent IgM antibody; less than fourfold rise in titer in paired sera

Use Evaluate acute infection with or immunity following vaccination for *Bordetella pertussis*

Methodology Microhemagglutination, enzyme-linked immunosorbent assay (ELISA)

Additional Information Patients with acute infection develop IgG, IgM, and IgA antibodies to febrile agglutinogens; and IgM and IgA antibodies are probably diagnostic. Following vaccination, IgG and IgM antibodies can be demonstrated, except in infants. IgA antibodies do not develop.

Selected Readings

Manclark CR, Meade BD, and Burstyn DG, "Serologic Response to *Bordetella pertussis*," *Manual of Clinical Laboratory Immunology*, 4th ed, Vol 2, Rose NR, Conway de Macario E, Fahey JL, et al, eds, Washington, DC: American Society for Microbiology, 1986, 388-94.

Mertsola J, Ruuskanen O, Kuronen T, et al, "Serologic Diagnosis of Pertussis: Evaluation of Pertussis Toxin and Other Antigens in Enzyme-Linked Immunosorbent Assay," *J Infect Dis*, 1990, 161(5):966-71.

Tomoda T, Ogura H, and Kurashige T, "Immune Responses to *Bordetella pertussis* Infection and Vaccination," *J Infect Dis*, 1991, 163(3):559-63.

***Bordetella pertussis* Smear** *see Bordetella pertussis Direct Fluorescent Antibody on page 349*

***Bordetella pertussis* Titer** *see Bordetella pertussis Serology on this page*

Borreliosis Serology *see Lyme Disease Serology on page 481*

Borreliosis Serology *see Lyme Disease Serology by Western Blot on page 482*

Botulism, Diagnostic Procedure

Synonyms *Clostridium botulinum* Toxin Identification Procedure; Infant Botulism, Toxin Identification; Sudden Death Syndrome

Abstract A neurotoxin, botulin, may be produced by *C. botulinum* in foods which have been improperly preserved. Characteristics of this type of food poisoning include vomiting and abdominal pain, disturbances of vision, motor function and secretion, mydriasis, ptosis, dry mouth, and cough.

Special Instructions The laboratory must be notified prior to obtaining specimen in order to prepare for transport of the specimen to the State Health Laboratory or Center for Disease Control.

Specimen Vomitus, serum, stool, gastric washings, cerebrospinal fluid or autopsy tissue; food samples

Container Sterile wide-mouth, leakproof, screw-cap jar; red top tube

Storage Instructions Keep refrigerated at 4°C except for unopened food samples.

Turnaround Time 3-7 days

Reference Range No toxin identified, no *Clostridium botulinum* isolated

Use Diagnose infant botulism, sudden death syndrome, floppy baby syndrome, classic botulism in adults

Limitations The toxin from *C. botulinum* binds almost irreversibly to individual nerve terminals; thus, serum and cerebrospinal fluid specimens may yield false-negative results.

Contraindications Due to the difficulty in performance of the diagnostic test and because of the extensive epidemiological studies initiated upon receipt of the specimen, State Department of Health Laboratories require specific clinical symptomatology for infant botulism. Therefore, they should be consulted early to optimize handling of the suspect case.

Methodology Toxin neutralization test in mice, isolation of *Clostridium botulinum* from feces

(Continued)

Botulism, Diagnostic Procedure *(Continued)*

Additional Information The classic presentation of **infant botulism** is hypotonia (floppy baby syndrome), constipation, difficulty in feeding, and a weak cry. Some cases of sudden death syndrome have been traced to ingesting honey containing *C. botulinum*. Both *C. botulinum* and *C. butyricum* have been identified as species capable of toxin production. Autointoxication may occur from toxin production during organism growth in tissue, the intestinal tract in both adults and infants, and in wounds. Botulism has been reported with cocaine-associated sinusitis.

Selected Readings

Hatheway CL, "Toxigenic Clostridia," *Clin Microbiol Rev*, 1990, 3(1):66-98.

Schmidt RD and Schmidt TW, "Infant Botulism: A Case Series and Review of the Literature," *J Emerg Med*, 1992, 10(6):713-8.

Wigginton JM and Thill P, "Infant Botulism. A Review of the Literature," *Clin Pediatr (Phila)*, 1993, 32(11):669-74.

Brain Biopsy

Related Information

Rabies Detection *on page 525*

Test Includes Routine histopathologic diagnosis. Special tests are requested by physician.

Special Instructions Submit specimen in formalin for routine histology. Requisition must state operative diagnosis and source of specimen.

Specimen Brain tissue biopsy

Container Test tube

Collection For needle biopsies of brain, an open-end rather than side-opening needle should be used. All types of brain biopsies are best placed on saline-moistened Gelfoam®. Do not place on gauze or immerse in saline. Arrange for specimen to be in hands of neuropathologist in shortest possible time, otherwise store in refrigerator. Do not freeze.

Storage Instructions Any necessary storage should be done in formaldehyde in a closed container.

Causes for Rejection Unlabeled specimen container, insufficient material, improper fixative

Turnaround Time 24 hours to 3 weeks, depending on nature of clinical problem

Reference Range Results interpreted by neuropathologist

Use Morphologic evaluation of brain disease

Limitations The size of the tissue sample is often a limiting factor. Brain biopsy does not offer an answer in most obscure neurological diseases.

Additional Information The most commonly sought pathogens in brain biopsies are herpesvirus and *Toxoplasma*, especially in immunocompromised hosts. Special arrangements must be made for electron microscopy or immunoperoxidase studies.

Brain, CT *see* Computed Transaxial Tomography, Head Studies *on page 374*

Bronchial Aspirate Anaerobic Culture *see* Anaerobic Culture *on page 316*

Bronchial Aspirate Fungus Culture *see* Fungus Culture, Bronchial Aspirate *on page 416*

Bronchial Aspiration for *Pneumocystis* *see* Pneumocystis carinii Test *on page 522*

Bronchial Biopsy *see* Histopathology *on page 448*

Bronchial Washings Culture *see* Aerobic Culture, Sputum *on page 312*

Bronchoalveolar Lavage (BAL) *see* Fungus Culture, Bronchial Aspirate *on page 416*

Bronchopulmonary Lavage for *Pneumocystis* *see* Pneumocystis carinii Test *on page 522*

Bronchoscopic *Legionella* Culture *see* Legionella pneumophila Culture *on page 469*

Bronchoscopy Culture *see* Aerobic Culture, Sputum *on page 312*

Bronchoscopy, Fiberoptic

Synonyms Flexible Bronchoscopy

Test Includes Direct visual examination of upper airway, vocal cords, and tracheobronchial tree out to the fourth to sixth division bronchi. Other procedures such as washings, brush biopsy bronchoalveolar lavage, endobronchial and transbronchial biopsy are also included depending on the clinical indications.

Patient Preparation NPO after midnight for a morning bronchoscopy and NPO after light breakfast for afternoon procedures. Routine medications (especially antiasthmatic drugs) may be taken at any time with a small amount of water. Routine lab work including clotting times, BUN, CBC, and platelet count is essential to exclude a coagulopathy - especially if a biopsy is to be performed. Some measure of pulmonary function is useful (spirometry, blood gases) to assess pulmonary reserve and document bronchospasm. Premedication with a narcotic (meperidine 25-75 mg) or minor tranquilizer (diazepam 10 mg) is given parenterally 15-30 minutes before the procedure. Atropine 0.4 mg I.M. is given as a vagolytic agent at the same time unless contraindicated by the presence of arrhythmia, narrow angle glaucoma, or urinary retention.

Aftercare NPO for 2 hours or longer after the procedure until the gag reflex is fully recovered. Because of the premedication, outpatients are not allowed to drive until the following day. Transient fever and mild hemoptysis may be noted for the next 24 hours.

Equipment A fiberoptic bronchoscope and halogen or xenon light source are necessary for this airway exam. The bronchoscope is equipped with a thumb lever which allows angulation of the distal end of the instrument. A 2-2.6 mm hollow channel runs the length of the scope and allows injection of medication and aspiration of secretions for airway clearance and obtaining bronchial washings and lavage. It is also utilized for the passage of instruments, such as bronchial brushes and forceps.

Technique Procedure may be performed with the patient in supine or sitting position. Patient gargles with 2% lidocaine solution or alternatively tetracaine 2% aerosolized spray (Cetacaine®) is used to anesthetize the pharynx. The bronchoscope tip is lubricated with Xylocaine® jelly and introduced transnasally or transorally with the use of a bite block. Lidocaine 2% solution is then injected through the bronchoscopic channel in 2 mL aliquots for anesthesia of the vocal cords and entire tracheobronchial tree. Lidocaine has definite toxicity (seizures and respiratory arrest) and the total dosage should generally not exceed 400 mg. The duration of action generally lasts 20-30 minutes. Once adequate anesthesia has been obtained, a detailed visual examination is performed. Subsequently other procedures such as biopsies, washings, and brushings can be carried out.

Data Acquired This examination provides information regarding the patency and normality of the central airways. It is used as a vehicle for sampling the airways and lung parenchyma itself via brushing and biopsy techniques.

Specimen Bronchial washings, brushings, biopsy, or lavage

Container Formalin jars, mucous specimen containers, slides in 95% alcohol

Turnaround Time Reports: Written in chart at time of procedure.

Normal Findings Normal endobronchial examination.

Use The major utility is in the assessment of malignant disease, early diagnosis of carcinoma, assessment of operability, transbronchial or endobronchial lung biopsy, hemoptysis (not massive), persistent chronic cough, removal of foreign bodies (minor role), and diagnosis of lung infections especially in immunocompromised hosts. Other uses include difficult endotracheal intubation.

Limitations Limited usefulness in retrieving foreign bodies and the management of massive hemoptysis.

Contraindications Asthma, severe hypoxemia, serious arrhythmia unstable angina pectoris, recent myocardial infarction, and poor patient cooperation. All of these are only relative contraindications and vary depending on the clinical situation and experience of the bronchoscopist. When bronchoscopy involves biopsy procedures, coagulopathies or bleeding tendencies are contraindications.

Additional Information The procedure is markedly safe. Large reviews have shown that approximately 50% of the life-threatening complications are associated with premedication or topical anesthesia. The risk seems highest in patients with underlying cardiac disease and the elderly. Patients with underlying bronchospastic disease are particularly prone to bronchospasm and laryngospasm and thus should be under optimal treatment before undertaking bronchoscopy. A drop in pO_2 of approximately 20 mm Hg occurs, and therefore supplemental oxygen administration is indicated. Transient fever and pneumonia occur in a small number of patients. Bleeding can occur from the nose or

(Continued)

Bronchoscopy, Fiberoptic (Continued)

tracheobronchial tree although this complication is mainly associated with transbronchial biopsy.

Selected Readings

Ackart RS, Foreman DR, and Klayton RJ, "Fiberoptic Bronchoscopy in Outpatient Facilities, 1982," Arch Intern Med, 1983, 143(1):30-1.

Fulkerson WJ, "Current Concepts. Fiberoptic Bronchoscopy," N Engl J Med, 1984, 311(8):511-15.

Ikeda S, Atlas of Flexible Bronchofiberoscopy, Baltimore, MD: University Park Press, 1974.

Lukomsky GI, Ovchinnikov AA, and Bilal A, "Complications of Bronchoscopy: Comparison of Rigid Bronchoscopy Under General Anesthesia in Flexible Bronchoscopy Under Topical Anesthesia," Chest, 1981, 79(3):316-21.

Marini JJ, Pierson DJ, and Hudson LD, "Acute Lobar Atelectasis: A Prospective Comparison of Fiberoptic Bronchoscopy and Respiratory Therapy," Am Rev Respir Dis, 1979, 119(6):971-8.

Mitchell DM, Emerson CJ, and Collyer J, "Fiberoptic Bronchoscopy: Ten Years On," Br Med J, 1980, 281(6236):360-3.

Pereira W, Kovnat DM, Khan MA, et al, "Fever and Pneumonia After Flexible Fiberoptic Bronchoscopy," Am Rev Respir Dis, 1975, 112(1):59-64.

Perry LB, "Topical Anesthesia for Bronchoscopy," Chest, 1978, 73(Suppl 5):691-3.

Sackner MA, "Bronchofiberoscopy," Am Rev Respir Dis, 1975, 111(1):62-88.

Schnapf BM, "Oxygen Desaturation During Fiberoptic Bronchoscopy in Pediatric Patients," Chest, 1991, 99(3):591-4.

Sen RP and Walsh TE, "Fiberoptic Bronchoscopy for Refractory Cough," Chest, 1991, 99(1):33-5.

Trouillet JL, Guiguet M, Gibert C, et al, "Fiberoptic Bronchoscopy in Ventilated Patients. Evaluation of Cardiopulmonary Risk Under Midazolam Sedation," Chest, 1990, 97(4):927-33.

Bronchoscopy Fungus Culture see Fungus Culture, Sputum on page 419

Bronchoscopy Mycobacteria Culture see Mycobacteria Culture, Sputum on page 495

Brucella Blood Culture see Blood Culture, Brucella on page 340

Brucella Culture, Tissue see Biopsy Culture, Routine on page 337

Buffy Coat Culture for CMV see Cytomegalovirus Culture, Blood on page 389

Buffy Coat Viral Culture see Cytomegalovirus Culture, Blood on page 389

Bullous Pemphigoid Antibodies see Skin Biopsy, Immunofluorescence on page 538

C 100-3 see Hepatitis C Serology on page 437

Calcaneus (heel), Left or Right, X-ray see Bone Films on page 343

Campylobacter pylori, Gastric Biopsy Culture see Helicobacter pylori Culture, Gastric Biopsy on page 433

Campylobacter pylori Serology see Helicobacter pylori Serology on page 433

Campylobacter pylori Urease Test and Culture see Helicobacter pylori Culture and Urease Test on page 432

Casts, Urine see Urinalysis on page 562

Catheter Culture, Intravenous see Intravenous Line Culture on page 464

Catheter Tip Culture see Intravenous Line Culture on page 464

CBC see Complete Blood Count on page 369

Cefinase (Nitrocefin) Testing see Penicillinase Test on page 517

Cell Sorting Fluorescence Activation see Lymph Node Biopsy on page 482

Cephalosporinase Production Testing see Penicillinase Test on page 517

Cerebrospinal Fluid Aerobic Culture see Aerobic Culture, Cerebrospinal Fluid on page 311

Cerebrospinal Fluid Anaerobic Culture see Anaerobic Culture on page 316

Cerebrospinal Fluid Analysis

Related Information

Aerobic Culture, Cerebrospinal Fluid on page 311
Fungus Culture, Cerebrospinal Fluid on page 416
VDRL, Cerebrospinal Fluid on page 570
Viral Culture, Central Nervous System Symptoms on page 570

Synonyms CSF Analysis; Lumbar Puncture Analysis; Spinal Fluid Analysis; Spinal Tap

Test Includes Color of supernatant, turbidity, WBC/mm^3, polys/mm^3, lymphs/mm^3, RBC/mm^3, percent of crenated RBC, protein, sugar, and sometimes VDRL.

Abstract Examination of cerebrospinal fluid (CSF) contributes to diagnosis and sometimes management of infections of the central nervous system, meningitis, encephalitis, instances of vasculitis, demyelinating diseases, tumors, paraneo-plastic entities, polyneuritis, instances of cerebrovascular disease, and cases of seizure disorders and confusional states.

Patient Preparation Aseptic preparation for aspiration

Special Instructions Specimen should be delivered to the laboratory **promptly**.

When a diagnosis of meningitis is considered, culture of other materials as well as culture of CSF may be helpful. Most children with bacterial meningitis are initially bacteremic, and blood cultures are of value. In neonates and small children, urine culture may be positive. Cultures and Gram's stains of petechiae may provide immediate diagnosis.

Specimen Cerebrospinal fluid

Container Sterile test tubes from lumbar puncture tray

Collection Specimens of spinal fluid and blood, for culture, should be obtained prior to initiation of antibiotic treatment of meningitis. Tubes must be labeled with patient's name, date, and labeled with number indicating sequence in which tubes were obtained.

Storage Instructions Do **not** store; specimen should be processed as soon as possible.

Causes for Rejection Unlabeled tubes, insufficient specimen, clotted or refrigerated specimen, improper dispensation of specimen

Reference Range Adults: 0-5 cells/mm^3, all lymphocytes and monocytes; 0 red blood cells; protein: lumbar 15-50 mg/dL, cisternal 15-25 mg/dL, ventricular 6-15 mg/dL; glucose 50-80 mg/dL. Younger than 1 month: <32 cells/mm^3, 1 month to 1 year: <10 cells/mm^3, 1-4 years: <8 cells/mm^3, 5 years to puberty: <5 cells/mm^3; in the premature neonate: <29 cells/mm^3

Laboratory Values of Components of CSF From Healthy Persons and From Patients With Meningitis*

Source	CSF Laboratory Value			
	Protein (mg/dL)	Glucose (mg/dL)†	Leukocytes (/μL)	Predominant Cell Type (%)
Healthy persons newborns	15-170	34-119	0-30	
adults	15-50	40-80	0-10	Lymphocytes (63-99) Monocytes (3-37) PMN (0-15)
Adult patients with: bacterial meningitis	>100	<40	>1000	PMN (>50)
fungal meningitis	Increased	<30	Increased	Lymphocytes
viral or aseptic meningitis	<100	Normal‡	<500	PMN (early) and lymphocytes (late)

*Data are commonly observed values. Notable exceptions to these values and overlap of values elicited by different etiological agents are not uncommon. PMN = polymorphonuclear leukocytes.

†CSF glucose/serum glucose ratio usually is 0.6 (adults) or 0.74-0.96 (neonates and preterm babies). In patients with bacterial meningitis, the ratios usually are <0.5 (adults) and <0.6 (neonates and preterm babies).

‡Lower than normal glucose concentrations have been observed during some non-infectious disease processes and in some patients with viral meningoencephalitis due to herpesviruses, varicella-zoster virus, mumps virus, lymphocytic choriomeningitis virus, and enteroviruses.

From Gray LD and Fedorko DP, "Laboratory Diagnosis of Bacterial Meningitis," *Clin Microbiol Rev*, 1992, 5(2):133.

Possible Panic Range Increased number of cells

Use Evaluate bacterial or viral encephalitis, meningitis, meningoencephalitis, mycobacterial or fungal infection, parasitic infestations, primary or secondary malignancy, leukemia/malignant lymphoma of CNS, trauma, vascular occlusive disease, vasculitis, heredofamilial and/or degenerative processes. The tables outline findings, including those with subdural empyema, brain abscess, ventricular empyema, cerebral epidural, abscess, spinal epidural abscess, tuberculosis, syphilis, sarcoidosis, and other entities.

The nucleated blood cell count in the cerebrospinal fluid is described as superior to any combination of the other CSF tests for bacterial meningitis. In patients who have not received antimicrobial agents, the ultimate diagnosis of bacterial meningitis is based on results of culture. The cell count and differential (Continued)

Cerebrospinal Fluid Analysis (Continued)

count are mandatory, and a Gram's stain must be examined promptly in work up of possible meningitis. The CSF must be cultured; glucose and protein are necessary, as well, in the work-up for possible meningitis. **Viral infection,** as well as **bacterial meningitis,** can elicit neutrophil leukocytosis in blood and CSF. Seasonal curves for viral and bacterial infection go in opposite directions; although viral meningitis is a disease of midsummer, bacterial meningitis is relatively more common in the winter.

Signals of possible meningeal infection in the newborn: leukocyte count >30 cells/mm^3 with >60% PMNs, CSF protein >100 mg/dL, and/or CSF glucose <40% than that in blood are found with bacterial meningitis. CSF WBC counts >10 cells/mm^3 in very young infants, and >5 cells/mm^3 in older infants, and children with >1 PMN/mm^3 are abnormal. See table on next page.

Limitations A traumatic (bloody) tap may make interpretation difficult. Normal CSF may be found early in meningitis.

Additional Information See table on next page for laboratory values of components of CSF from healthy persons and from patients with meningitis.

More extensive testing: cytology, conventional cultures and cultures for myco-bacteria, fungi, and viruses, additional chemistry and serologic determinations must usually be ordered separately.

Correction for traumatic tap: If cell counts and protein determinations are performed on CSF and blood obtained at the same time, correction for "bloody tap" can be calculated. All CSF measurements should be made from the same tube. The ratio of RBC count CSF to RBC count blood provides a factor which when multiplied by the blood WBC count or blood protein level indicates the expected level of contribution of these parameters from the blood to the spinal fluid. These contributed WBC or protein values can then be subtracted from the respective values measured in the spinal fluid. For example:
1. RBCs (CSF)/RBCs (blood) x WBCs (blood) or x protein (blood).
2. WBCs (CSF) or protein (CSF) - product calculated in 1 = true CSF WBC or true CSF protein.

If the peripheral blood is normal and traumatic tap had occurred, about 1 WBC is added to the CSF for each 700 RBCs that have been transferred into the CSF. RBC contamination from a traumatic tap does not adversely affect the laboratory diagnosis of bacterial meningitis.

Antigen detection methods cannot replace culture and Gram's stain. Gram's stain and culture must always have priority over antigen detection testing. A bacterial culture is the major test to be performed on cerebrospinal fluid for meningitis. It is the "gold standard" for diagnosis. A requirement for 50 or more leukocytes per μL of CSF has been proposed as justification for bacterial antigen testing. Another group found a CSF nucleated blood cell count <6/mm^3 provided a criterion for an abbreviated CSF evaluation. There is substantial mortality and morbidity in subjects with bacterial meningitis. Neurologic sequelae are found in as many as 33% of all survivors, especially newborns and children. Especially when bacterial meningitis follows an insidious pattern, diagnostic delay may be unavoidable. Eight of 21 survivors of neonatal meningitis were normal, 8 had mild and 5 had moderate to severe sequelae in a culture-proven series.

White cell pleocytosis is found in only 33% of patients with multiple sclerosis (MS). The white count rarely exceeds 20 cells/mm^3. Most patients with MS (66%) have normal total proteins. In contrast, patients with the demyelinating disease Guillain-Barré syndrome usually have no excess white cells but show elevated CSF protein of 100-500 mg/dL.

Selected Readings

Bonadio WA, Smith DS, Goddard S, et al, "Distinguishing Cerebrospinal Fluid Abnormalities in Children With Bacterial Meningitis and Traumatic Lumbar Puncture," *J Infect Dis,* 1990, 162(1):251-4.

Felgin RD and Cherry JD, *Textbook of Pediatric Infectious Diseases,* Philadelphia, PA: WB Saunders Co, 1987, 488.

Feigin RD, McCracken GH Jr, and Klein JO, "Diagnosis and Management of Meningitis," *Pediatr Infect Dis J,* 1992, 11(9):785-814.

Gray LD and Fedorko DP, "Laboratory Diagnosis of Bacterial Meningitis," *Clin Microbiol Rev,* 1992, 5(2):130-45.

Cerebrospinal Fluid Cryptococcal Latex Agglutination see Cryptococcal Antigen Serology, Serum or Cerebrospinal Fluid on page 379

Initial Cerebrospinal Fluid Findings in Suppurative Diseases of the Central Nervous System and Meninges

Condition	Pressure (mm H₂O)	Leukocytes/mm³	Protein (mg/dL)	Glucose (mg/dL)	Specific Findings
Acute bacterial meningitis	Usually elevated; average, 300	Several hundred to >60,000; usually a few thousand; occasionally <100 (especially meningococcal or early in disease); PMNs* predominate	Usually 100-500, occasionally >1000	<40 in >50% of cases	Organism usually seen on smear or culture in >90% of cases
Subdural empyema	Usually elevated; average, 300	<100 to a few thousand; PMNs predominate	Usually 100-500	Normal	No organisms seen on smear or culture unless concurrent meningitis
Brain abscess	Usually elevated	Usually 10-200; fluid is rarely acellular; lymphocytes predominate	Usually 75-400	Normal	No organisms seen on smear or culture
Ventricular empyema (rupture of brain abscess)	Considerably elevated	Several thousand to 100,000; usually >90% PMNs	Usually several hundred	Usually <40	Organism may be seen on smear or culture
Cerebral epidural abscess	Slightly to modestly elevated	Few to several hundred or more cells; lymphocytes predominate	Usually 50-200	Normal	No organisms seen on smear or culture
Spinal epidural abscess	Usually reduced with spinal block	Usually 10-100; lymphocytes predominate	Usually several hundred	Normal	No organisms seen on smear or culture
Thrombophlebitis (often associated with subdural empyema)	Often elevated	Few to several hundred; PMNs and lymphocytes	Slightly to moderately elevated	Normal	No organisms seen on smear or culture

357

Initial Cerebrospinal Fluid Findings in Suppurative Diseases of the Central Nervous System and Meninges *(Continued)*

Condition	Pressure (mm H_2O)	Leukocytes/mm³	Protein (mg/dL)	Glucose (mg/dL)	Specific Findings
Bacterial endocarditis (with embolism)	Normal or slightly elevated	Few to <100; lymphocytes and PMNs	Slightly elevated	Normal	No organisms seen on smear or culture
Acute hemorrhagic encephalitis	Usually elevated	Few to >1000; PMNs predominate	Moderately elevated	Normal	No organisms seen on smear or culture
Tuberculous infection	Usually elevated; may be low with dynamic block in advanced stages	Usually 25-100, rarely >500; lymphocytes predominate, except in early stages when PMNs may account for 80% of the cells	Nearly always elevated, usually 100-200; may be much higher if dynamic block	Usually reduced; <50 in 75% of cases	Acid-fast organisms may be seen on smear of protein coagulum (pellicle) or recovered from inoculated guinea pig or by culture
Cryptococcal infection	Usually elevated; average, 225	Average, 50 (0-800); lymphocytes predominate	Average, 100; usually 20-500	Reduced in >50% the cases; average 30; often higher in patients with concomitant diabetes mellitus	Organisms may be seen in India ink preparation and on culture (Sabouraud's medium); will usually grow on blood agar; may produce alcohol in cerebrospinal fluid from fermentation of glucose
Syphilis (acute)	Usually elevated	Average, 500; usually lymphocytes; rare PMNs	Average, 100; globulin often high, with abnormal colloidal gold curve	Normal (rarely reduced)	Positive results of reagin test for syphilis; spirochetes not demonstrable by usual techniques of smear or culture
Sarcoidosis	Normal to considerably elevated	0 to <100 mononuclear cells	Slight to moderate elevation	Normal	No specific findings

*Polymorphonuclear leukocytes

From Feigin RD and Cherry JD, eds, *Textbook of Pediatric Infectious Diseases*, Vol 1, Philadelphia, PA: WB Saunders, 1992, 410, with permission.

Cerebrospinal Fluid Fungus Culture *see* Fungus Culture, Cerebrospinal Fluid *on page 416*

Cerebrospinal Fluid India Ink Preparation *see* India Ink Preparation *on page 460*

Cerebrospinal Fluid Latex Agglutination for Bacterial Antigens *see* Bacterial Antigens, Rapid Detection Methods *on page 335*

Cerebrospinal Fluid Tap *see* Lumbar Puncture *on page 477*

Cerebrospinal Fluid VDRL *see* VDRL, Cerebrospinal Fluid *on page 570*

Cervical *Chlamydia* Culture *see* Chlamydia Culture *on this page*

Cervical Culture *see* Genital Culture *on page 423*

Cervical Culture for T-Strain *Mycoplasma* *see* Genital Culture for *Ureaplasma urealyticum on page 424*

Cervical Culture for *Ureaplasma urealyticum* *see* Genital Culture for *Ureaplasma urealyticum on page 424*

Cervical *Trichomonas* Smear *see* Trichomonas Preparation *on page 555*

Cervix Culture *Neisseria gonorrhoeae* *see* Neisseria gonorrhoeae Culture *on page 501*

Cervix, *Mycoplasma* Culture *see* Mycoplasma/Ureaplasma Culture *on page 499*

Chest Films

Synonyms CXR; PA; PA and Lateral CXR

Test Includes PA and lateral exposures of the chest. Sagel and his colleagues published an article in 1974 questioning the efficacy of screening examinations of the chest and whether or not lateral views should be obtained. Both medical and economic factors were considered. The study was based on a review of PA and lateral views of the chest in 10,597 examinations and reached the following conclusions.

- Routine screening for hospital admission or for surgery was not warranted for patients younger than 20 years of age.
- Lateral projection could be eliminated in routine screening of patients 20-39 years of age.
- Lateral projection should be obtained at any age when disease of the chest is suspected.
- Lateral projection should be obtained in screening examinations of patients older than 40 years of age.

Patient Preparation Remove medals, lockets, and other jewelry from neck. Arrange hair, when long, high on head so that no locks hang over chest or shoulders.

Special Instructions The chest x-ray can be modified in various ways to answer specific questions. For example, while the standard PA view of the chest is obtained in full inspiration, a pneumothorax will be more readily appreciated when the film is exposed in expiration. Decubitus films are helpful in differentiating mobile fluid in the pleural space from fluid loculations or pleural thickening. A lordotic view of the chest may be helpful in evaluating the apices. Oblique views of the chest done with 45° angulation in the right anterior oblique projection and 60° angulation in the left anterior oblique projection with barium opacifying the esophagus at the time of exposure are helpful in evaluating the size of the various cardiac chambers. A standard radiographic examination of the chest in addition to the modifications mentioned may be scheduled by calling the Radiology Department.

Use Evaluate lungs and thoracic bones for presence of metastatic and primary neoplasm, infectious disease, degenerative and reactive processes, trauma, and surgical change; evaluate the heart and great vessels

Selected Readings
Sagel SS, Evens RG, Forrest JV, et al, "Efficacy of Routine Screening and Lateral Chest Radiographs in a Hospital-Based Population," *N Engl J Med*, 1974, 291(19):1001-4.

Chickenpox Culture *see* Varicella-Zoster Virus Culture *on page 568*

Chickenpox Titer *see* Varicella-Zoster Virus Serology *on page 569*

Chlamydia Culture

Related Information
Chlamydia pneumoniae Serology *on page 361*
Chlamydia psittaci Serology *on page 362*
Chlamydia Species Serology *on page 362*
(Continued)

Chlamydia Culture *(Continued)*

Chlamydia trachomatis by DFA *on page 363*
Chlamydia trachomatis by DNA Probe *on page 364*
Genital Culture *on page 423*

Synonyms TRIC Agent Culture

Applies to Cervical *Chlamydia* Culture; Eye Swab *Chlamydia* Culture; Lympho-granuloma Venereum Culture; Urethral *Chlamydia* Culture

Test Includes Cell culture to detect *Chlamydia*

Special Instructions Availability and specific specimen collection requirements for *Chlamydia* cultures vary. Consult the laboratory for specific instructions, swabs, and transport materials prior to collection of the specimen.

Specimen *Chlamydia* is an intracellular organism; therefore, infected cells must be obtained by swabbing the urethra, cervix, rectum, conjunctiva, posterior nasopharynx, or throat.

Container Culturette® (Dacron) swabs should be used. Use specific *Chlamydia* transport medium.

Collection

Urethra: Remove mucous/pus by using a separate swab; discard this swab. The swab should be inserted 2-4 cm into the urethra. Use firm pressure to scrape cells from the mucosal surface. If possible repeat with second swab. Patient should not urinate within 1 hour prior to specimen collection.

Cervix: Remove mucous/pus with a Culturette® and discard this swab. Use a new swab (Culturette®) and use firm and rotating pressure to obtain specimen. May be combined with a urethral swab into same transport medium. This two-swab method is highly recommended.

Rectum: Sample anal crypts with a Culturette®.

Conjunctiva: Remove mucous and exudate with a separate swab; discard this swab. Use a Culturette® and firm pressure to scrape away epithelial cells from upper and lower lids.

Posterior nasopharynx or throat: Collect epithelial cells by using a Culturette®.

Storage Instructions Deliver inoculated transport medium **immediately** to laboratory. Specimens must be **refrigerated** during storage and transportation or frozen at -70°C if stored more than 2 days.

Turnaround Time Cultures with no growth usually will be reported after 4-7 days. Rapid culture methods for detection of *Chlamydia* require a minimum of 48 hours.

Reference Range No *Chlamydia* isolated

Use Aid in the diagnosis of infections caused by *Chlamydia* (eg, cervicitis, trachoma, conjunctivitis, pelvic inflammatory disease, pneumonia, urethritis, nongonococcal urethritis, pneumonitis, and sexually transmitted diseases).

Limitations Culture may be negative in presence of *Chlamydia* infection. Culture is probably not the gold standard for the detection of *C. trachomatis*. The sensitivity of culture probably is only 70% to 90% because *C. trachomatis* does not always survive transit to the laboratory and because sampling is often inadequate even with (multiple) swabs.

Methodology Inoculation of specimen onto McCoy cell culture and subsequent detection of *Chlamydia*-infected cells by immunofluorescence and monoclonal antibody

Additional Information This organism infects the endocervical columnar epithelial cells and will not be found in the inflammatory cells. In obtaining the specimen, clean the area of inflammatory cells and then attempt to scrape epithelial cells for culturing by using a new, separate swab. The results of cytological diagnosis of chlamydial infection of the female genital tract have been disappointing. Papanicolaou-stained cervical smears are not reliable enough to help establish or exclude the presence of *Chlamydia*. In patients with vaginal discharge or other genital tract symptomatology of unknown etiology, cervical cytology can be useful in identifying patients who should be cultured for *Chlamydia*. Direct immunofluorescence techniques and enzyme immunoassays are available to detect *Chlamydia* in clinical specimens. These methods usually provide reliable results in high-prevalence populations and detect both viable and nonviable organisms. Selection of the most efficient method for recovery of

Chlamydia depends upon the incidence in the patient population and the local availability of the various methods. Urine culture for *Chlamydia* is not a sensitive procedure and generally should not be done. The incidence of cervical infection with *Chlamydia trachomatis* is two to three times that of gonorrhea: 4% to 9% in private office settings, 6% to 23% in family planning clinics, and 20% to 30% in sexually transmitted diseases clinics.

Culture should be the test-of-choice (i) in cases of child abuse, ascending pelvic infections, and rectal and throat infections, and (ii) when a test-for-cure is desired.

Chlamydia is a single genus and consists of the following:
- *C. trachomatis* (serotypes A-K): inclusion conjunctivitis, trachoma, and genital infections
- *C. trachomatis* (serotypes L1-L3): lymphogranuloma venereum
- *C. psittaci*: psittacosis
- *C. pneumoniae* (TWAR): respiratory infections

Serology to detect antibodies to each of the three species of *Chlamydia* is available.

Laboratory diagnosis of *C. pneumoniae* infections is not widely available; commercial tests for *C. pneumoniae* are not available. *C. pneumoniae* is responsible for approximately 10% of community-acquired pneumonias. The cells (McCoy) usually used to culture *C. trachomatis* will not reliably support the growth of *C. pneumoniae*. Recent studies have shown that other cell lines (H 292 and HEp-2) are more appropriate. However, culture using these cells is not generally available. An alternate, widely used method for the laboratory diagnosis of *C. pneumoniae* infection is serology by microimmunofluorescence. Currently, this serological test is the most sensitive and specific laboratory test for *C. pneumoniae*.

Selected Readings

Grayston JT, "*Chlamydia pneumoniae*, Strain TWAR," *Chest*, 1989, 95(3):664-9.

Grayston JT, Campbell LA, Kuo CC, et al, "A New Respiratory Tract Pathogen: *Chlamydia pneumoniae* Strain TWAR," *J Infect Dis*, 1990, 161(4):618-25.

Hipp SS and Coles FB, "The Virtues of *Chlamydia* Culture," *Clin Microbiol Newslett*, 1994, 16(5):37-9.

Le Scolea LJ Jr, "The Value of Nonculture Chlamydial Diagnostic Tests," *Clin Microbiol Newslett*, 1991, 13(3):21-4.

Lombardo JM and Gadol CL, "*Chlamydia trachomatis*: A Perfect Test?" *Clin Microbiol Newslett*, 1990, 12(13):100-2.

Schachter J, "Laboratory Aspects of Chlamydial Infections," *Adv Exp Med Biol*, 1987, 224:73-7.

Chlamydia pneumoniae Serology

Related Information

Chlamydia Culture *on page 359*
Chlamydia psittaci Serology *on next page*
Chlamydia Species Serology *on next page*
Chlamydia trachomatis by DFA *on page 363*
Chlamydia trachomatis by DNA Probe *on page 364*

Synonyms *Chlamydia*, TWAR Strain; TWAR Strain *Chlamydia*

Test Includes Pan-reactive for trachoma, psittacosis, LGV, and TWAR

Specimen Serum

Container Red top tube or serum separator tube

Storage Instructions Separate serum and refrigerate.

Causes for Rejection Excessive hemolysis, chylous serum, inadequate labeling

Reference Range Negative. Titers <1:64 suggest no current or previous infection. A fourfold or greater increase in antibody titer in paired specimens usually provides unequivocal evidence of recent infection.

Use Evaluate possible chlamydial infection

Limitations The antigen (lipopolysaccharide) used in the test is group specific and not species specific. A very high "background" of immunity in the general population makes interpretation of results difficult.

Methodology Indirect fluorescent antibody (IFA)

Additional Information A new *Chlamydia* species, *C. pneumoniae* (TWAR strain), is a frequent cause of acute respiratory disease. *C. pneumoniae* antibody has been found in 25% to 60% of adults. The determination of species or type specific antibodies to *C. psittaci*, *C. trachomatis*, and *C. pneumoniae* strain is complicated by cross reactive antigens or nonspecific stimulation of
(Continued)

Chlamydia pneumoniae Serology (Continued)

antichlamydial antibodies. Thus, a panel of *Chlamydia* must be tested to determine specific titers and establish the strongest reactions. The panel to differentiate *C. pneumoniae*, *C. psittaci*, and *C. trachomatis* may be requested from a microbiology reference laboratory.

Selected Readings

Grayston JT, "*Chlamydia pneumoniae*, Strain TWAR Pneumonia," *Annu Rev Med*, 1992, 43:317-23.

Hammerschlag MR, "*Chlamydia pneumoniae*: A New Respiratory Pathogen," *Infect Dis Newslett* 1992, 11(1):1-4.

***Chlamydia psittaci* Antibody** see *Chlamydia psittaci* Serology *on this page*

Chlamydia psittaci Serology

Related Information

Chlamydia Culture *on page 359*
Chlamydia pneumoniae Serology *on previous page*
Chlamydia Species Serology *on this page*
Chlamydia trachomatis by DFA *on next page*
Chlamydia trachomatis by DNA Probe *on page 364*

Synonyms *Chlamydia psittaci* Antibody

Special Instructions Acute and convalescent samples are recommended.

Specimen Serum

Container Red top tube or serum separator tube

Reference Range Less than a fourfold increase in titer in paired sera

Use Diagnose psittacosis

Limitations Antibody response may be suppressed if patient has been treated with antibiotics

Methodology Complement fixation (CF), microimmunofluorescence

Additional Information Most patients with psittacosis develop high titers of complement fixing antibody and in some with the proper clinical setting a single very high titer may be strongly supportive of the diagnosis. Specific IgM antibody can sometimes be demonstrated.

To detect psittacosis antibody, an antigen specific for *C. psittaci* must be included in the test system. There may be significant antibody titers in veterinarians and patients with Reiter's syndrome.

Selected Readings

Schachter J, "*Chlamydia*," *Manual of Clinical Laboratory Immunology*, 3rd ed, Rose NR, Friedman H, and Fahey JL, eds, Washington, DC: American Society for Microbiology, 1986, 587-92.

***Chlamydia* Smear** see Ocular Cytology *on page 505*

Chlamydia Species Serology

Related Information

Chlamydia Culture *on page 359*
Chlamydia pneumoniae Serology *on previous page*
Chlamydia psittaci Serology *on this page*
Chlamydia trachomatis by DFA *on next page*
Chlamydia trachomatis by DNA Probe *on page 364*

Test Includes Detection of antibody titer to *Chlamydia* species

Specimen Serum

Container Red top tube

Collection Collect acute phase blood as soon as possible after onset (no later than 1 week). Convalescent blood should be drawn 1-2 weeks after acute (no less than 2 weeks after onset).

Reference Range Negative. A fourfold increase in titer in paired sera is usually indicative of chlamydial infection. Determination of IgM antibody may be helpful in differentiating acute infection from prior exposure.

Use Evaluate possible chlamydial infection

Limitations The antigen (lipopolysaccharide) used in the test is group specific and not species specific. In cases of conjunctivitis, nongonococcal urethritis, and pneumonia of the newborn, there is usually **not** an antibody response detectable by complement fixation. A very high "background" of immunity in the general population makes interpretation of results difficult.

Methodology Complement fixation (CF), indirect fluorescence antibody (IFA), enzyme immunoassay (EIA)

Additional Information Because of the high prevalence of antibodies to *Chlamydia*, especially in patients being evaluated for urethritis or possible venereal disease, results of serologic tests must be interpreted with caution. Very high titers, rising titers, or IgM specific antibody should be sought. In a patient being evaluated for chlamydial disease of the genitourinary tract, culture as well as serology should be obtained, as well as a serologic test for syphilis and a culture for *Neisseria gonorrhoeae*.

Selected Readings

Ehret JM and Judson FN, "Genital *Chlamydia* Infections," *Clin Lab Med*, 1989, 9(3):481-500.

Miettinen A, Heinonen PK, Teisala K, et al, "Antigen-Specific Serum Antibody Response to *Chlamydia trachomatis* in Patients With Pelvic Inflammatory Disease," *J Clin Pathol*, 1990, 43(9):758-61.

Schachter J, "Chlamydiae," *Manual of Clinical Laboratory Immunology*, 4th ed, Rose NR, de Macario EC, Fahey JL, et al, eds, Washington, DC: American Society for Microbiology, 1992, 661-6.

Chlamydia trachomatis by DFA

Related Information

Chlamydia Culture *on page 359*
Chlamydia pneumoniae Serology *on page 361*
Chlamydia psittaci Serology *on previous page*
Chlamydia Species Serology *on previous page*
Chlamydia trachomatis by DNA Probe *on next page*

Synonyms MicroTrak®

Test Includes Examination of specimen, specifically for *Chlamydia trachomatis*

Patient Preparation For urogenital specimens, patient should not urinate 1 hour prior to collection.

Special Instructions Specify specimen origin. Include all pertinent information, label slide and collection pack.

Specimen Direct smear

Container Single well (8 mm) glass slide, Dacron swabs (one large, one small), one cytobrush, methanol fixative (0.5 mL vial). These items are contained in a commonly used direct detection kit (collection pack) known as MicroTrak®.

Collection **Endocervical with cytology brush:** Nonpregnant women. Use large swab to remove exudate or mucous from exocervix. Insert cytobrush into cervical os past the squamocolumnar junction. Rest 2-3 seconds, rotate brush 360 degrees to gather columnar cells and withdraw brush. Do not touch vaginal walls with brush, and prepare slides immediately by rotating and twisting brush back and forth across center of slide well.

Endocervical with swab: Pregnant women. Use large swab to remove exudate or mucous from exocervix. Insert another large Dacron swab until tip is no longer visible, rotate swab 5-10 seconds, and withdraw swab. Do not touch vaginal walls and prepare slides immediately. Firmly roll one side of swab over top half of well. Turn swab over and roll other side over bottom half of slide well.

Urethral: Males. Patient should not urinate 1 hour before sampling. Remove pus or exudate with separate swab, insert small swab with wire shaft 2-4 cm into penis. Gently rotate swab to dislodge cells, rest swab 2 seconds, withdraw swab, and prepare slide immediately as above.

Rectal: Symptomatic patients only. Use large swab. Insert approximately 3 cm into anal canal. Move swab from side to side to sample crypts. If fecal contamination occurs, discard swab and obtain another specimen. Prepare slide immediately as above.

Conjunctival: Neonates, symptomatic only. Use large separate swab to gently remove pus or discharge and discard. If both eyes are sampled, swab less affected eye first. Swab inside of lower, then upper lid, and prepare slide immediately as above.

Nasopharyngeal: Neonates, symptomatic only. Use small swab or nasal aspirator. Collect specimen from posterior nasopharynx using standard collection method. If swab was used, prepare slide immediately. If nasal aspirate was collected, deliver to laboratory technician immediately for slide preparation.

All specimens: Write patient name and date on slip and outside of collection pack. Allow specimen to air dry. Lay slide flat and flood with methanol fixative. Let entire quantity evaporate. Refold pack without touching fixed specimen. (Continued)

Chlamydia trachomatis by DFA *(Continued)*

Storage Instructions Refrigerate slides at 2°C to 8°C or at room temperature (20°C to 30°C) until taken to the laboratory. Slides must be stained within 7 days of collection.

Causes for Rejection Specimen not labeled, slide received broken, less than 10 columnar or cuboidal epithelial cells on slide, slide more than 7 days old

Turnaround Time The time required to stain and examine the specimen is generally less than 1 hour. Turnaround time depends on staffing within the laboratory.

Reference Range Unsatisfactory specimen; negative or positive for *Chlamydia*

Use Aid in the diagnosis of disease caused by *Chlamydia* (eg, pneumonitis, sexually transmitted disease, inclusion conjunctivitis, trachoma, and pneumonia)

Limitations The direct detection of *C. trachomatis* is a useful tool in screening high-risk populations and in clinical situations where rapid positive results may be useful. However, the direct fluorescent antibody procedure is no more sensitive than the cell culture procedure. The number of cells on the slide can be too low for diagnosis.

Methodology Direct fluorescent antibody (DFA)

Additional Information The *Chlamydia trachomatis* direct test uses fluorescein-conjugated monoclonal antibodies (reactive with all 15 known serotypes of *C. trachomatis*) to detect elementary bodies in clinical smears. This test detects only *Chlamydia trachomatis* major outer membrane protein (MOMP); the test does not distinguish between living and dead organisms. Therefore, the test does not necessarily serve as a test-of-cure.

Chlamydia trachomatis, primarily a human pathogen, has been implicated in neonatal/infantile conjunctivitis and afebrile pneumonia. Thirty-three percent to 50% of babies born vaginally to mothers with chlamydial infection of the cervix will be infected; the majority of these neonates will develop inclusion conjunctivitis and/or a respiratory tract infection that can lead to the distinctive (afebrile) pneumonia syndrome.

Conjunctivitis: Conjunctivitis in infected neonates usually occurs between the 5th and 12th day after birth. In neonates born to mothers with premature rupture of the membranes, *C. trachomatis* has been detected, in rare cases, as early as the first day following birth.

Afebrile pneumonia: Many neonatal chlamydial infections also involve the respiratory tract. Respiratory infections usually occur secondarily to inclusion conjunctivitis. Rhinitis is often a prodrome for severe lower respiratory tract involvement. Signs of chlamydial pneumonia include cough, tachypnea, inspiratory rales, and, in more severe cases, vomiting and periods of apnea.

Selected Readings

Barnes RC, "Laboratory Diagnosis of Human Chlamydial Infections," *Clin Microbiol Rev*, 1989, 2(2):119-36.

Chlamydia trachomatis by DNA Probe

Related Information

Chlamydia Culture *on page 359*
Chlamydia pneumoniae Serology *on page 361*
Chlamydia psittaci Serology *on page 362*
Chlamydia Species Serology *on page 362*
Chlamydia trachomatis by DFA *on previous page*

Synonyms *Chlamydia trachomatis* DNA Detection Test; DNA Hybridization Test for *Chlamydia trachomatis*; DNA Test for *Chlamydia trachomatis*; PACE2®

Test Includes Direct detection of *Chlamydia trachomatis* nucleic acid in swab specimens.

Patient Preparation When taking urethral specimens the patient should not have urinated for 1 hour prior to collection.

Specimen Swab specimen collected from the genitourinary tract of a male or female patient

Container Special DNA transport medium is provided by the laboratory and should not be substituted. A kit containing a swab and special transport medium is made by Gen-Probe, Inc, and is required for this test.

Collection Currently the DNA test for *Chlamydia trachomatis* is FDA-approved only for urethral, cervical, and conjunctival specimens.

For a male the urethra is swabbed by rotating the swab 2-3 cm into the urethra. This should provide enough epithelial cells from the infected site to detect *C. trachomatis*. The swab is then placed in the transport tube for shipping to the laboratory.

For females, the Gen-Probe® kit provides two swabs. The cervix or endocervix should be swabbed and with one swab first to clean the area and the second swab is used to collect the specimen. The swab is inserted 2-3 cm into the endocervix and then rotated to collect the epithelial cells from the infected site. The swab is then put immediately into the transport tube and shipped to the laboratory.

For conjunctival specimens, use a "male" collection kit, clean away exudate with a separate swab and discard the swab, thoroughly swab the lower and upper conjunctiva each two to three times. Place the swab immediately into the transport tube with medium for transport to the laboratory.

Storage Instructions The specimens should be kept at room temperature or refrigerated. Do not freeze.

Causes for Rejection Contamination with urine; specimen frozen (which lyses the cells collected); gross blood in specimen

Turnaround Time Usually results are available within 24 hours of receipt of the specimen.

Reference Range The results of a normal test should be negative for *Chlamydia trachomatis* DNA. A sexually active, asymptomatic individual may harbor *C. trachomatis* in rates ranging from 0% to 7%.

Use Rapid detection of *C. trachomatis* in clinical specimens

Limitations DNA detection test cannot be done in child abuse cases. Cell culture is the only approved test in these cases. However, this test can be used to confirm positive culture results.

Methodology This test detects *C. trachomatis* ribosomal RNA directly from swab specimens. This requires denaturation of the RNA in the specimens by heating, hybridization with a specific DNA probe and detection of bound probe after several washing steps. Detection is done by using a probe labeled with an acridinium ester which releases a burst of light when in the presence of H_2O_2.

Additional Information Approximately 4 million cases of *C. trachomatis* occur annually in the United States, and it is considered a serious sexually transmitted disease problem. The detection of *C. trachomatis* RNA provides a diagnostic test that has several advantages over the traditional culture method. The turnaround time is shorter, it is less labor intensive, and it provides an objective result that makes interpretation easier. The RNA detection test for *C. trachomatis* has been proven to have an equivalent sensitivity to the antibody-based test (EIA and fluorescent antibody detection methods) and to have a greater specificity than these tests. However, at the present time this test cannot be done exclusively if a child abuse case is involved. These cases must be detected with a cell culture test.

Selected Readings
Barnes RC, "Laboratory Diagnosis of Human Chlamydial Infections," *Clin Microbiol Rev*, 1989, 2(2):119-36.

Ehret JM and Judson FN, "Genital *Chlamydia* Infections," *Clin Lab Med*, 1989, 9(3):481-500.

Peterson EM, Oda R, Alexander R, et al, "Molecular Techniques for the Detection of *Chlamydia trachomatis*," *J Clin Microbiol*, 1989, 27(10):2359-63.

Chlamydia trachomatis DNA by LCR

Synonyms *C. trachomatis* LCx®

Specimen Urine, urethral or endocervical swab

Container Preservative-free, sterile plastic container for urine; LCx® STD swab specimen collection and transport kit

Collection Wait at least 1 hour after the previous urination before collecting the specimen. Collect the first 20 mL of voided urine into a sterile container. Follow directions in LCx® kit for swab specimens. Avoid contamination with spermicidal agents, feminine powder sprays, blood, or large amounts of mucous.

Storage Instructions Refrigerate urine specimen. Follow directions in LCx® kit for swab specimens.

Reference Range Not detected

Use Diagnose *Chlamydia trachomatis* infection in women and men; screen asymptomatic individuals for *Chlamydia trachomatis* infection

(Continued)

Chlamydia trachomatis DNA by LCR (Continued)

Testing performed on:
- Symptomatic individuals
- Sexual partners of infected individuals (symptomatic and asymptomatic)
- Individuals in high-risk populations:
  - women and teens attending STD clinics, family-planning clinics, or prenatal clinics
  - women undergoing elective abortion
  - women residing in detention facilities
  - sexually active women younger than 20 years of age
  - women 20-24 years of age who either have inconsistent use of barrier contraception **or** new or multiple sexual partners during the last 3 months
  - women older than 24 years of age who have inconsistent use of barrier contraception **and** new or multiple sexual partners during the last 3 months
  - women being evaluated for infertility

Methodology Ligase chain reaction (LCR) amplification and microparticle enzyme immunoassay (MEIA), hybridization of C. trachomatis DNA to four C. trachomatis cryptic plasmid-specific oligonucleotide probes

Sensitivity: 1-5 organisms/assay

Additional Information Chlamydia trachomatis account for more than 4 million sexually transmitted infections each year, often spread unknowingly by asymptomatic individuals. The asymptomatic nature of the disease frequently precludes diagnosis and simple, yet effective, treatment. Without treatment, the infection may result in nongonococcal urethritis, epididymitis, and infertility in men; pelvic inflammatory disease (PID), ectopic pregnancy, and infertility in women; and nasopharyngeal infection, inclusion conjunctivitis, and pneumonia in neonates.

The diagnostic gold standard, until recently, has been culture of organisms from urethral or endocervical swab specimens; however, specimen collection is uncomfortable for the patient and sensitivity is only 70% to 85%. Antibody tests are also available, as is antigen detection by direct immunofluorescence, enzyme immunoassay (EIA), DNA probe (without amplification), polymerase chain reaction (PCR), or ligase chain reaction (LCR). Diagnostic sensitivity and specificity are greatest in nucleic acid amplification methods (PCR and LCR). The LCR method may be performed on a urine specimen, eliminating the need for discomfort associated with swab specimen collection and enabling detection of the 5% to 30% of infected women with urethra-only infections which cannot be detected with endocervical swab specimens.

Diagnostic sensitivity is 95% for urine specimens and 97% for urethral and endocervical swab specimens; specificity is 99% for both urine and swab specimens. When assessing treatment success or failure, test results are reliable only if the specimen was collected 3 or more weeks post therapy. Earlier specimen collection may result in a false-positive result due to the persistence of nucleic acids following therapy. Spermicidal agents, feminine powder sprays, blood, or large amounts of mucus may interfere with test results.

This test is not recommended for medicolegal cases.

Selected Readings
Chernesky MA, Jang D, Lee H, et al, "Diagnosis of Chlamydia trachomatis Infections in Men and Women by Testing First-Void Urine by Ligase Chain Reaction," J Clin Microbiol, 1994, 32(11):2682-5.

Chernesky MA, Lee H, Schachter J, et al, "Diagnosis of Chlamydia trachomatis Urethral Infection in Symptomatic and Asymptomatic Men by Testing First-Void Urine in a Ligase Chain Reaction Assay," J Infect Dis, 1994, 170(5):1308-11.

Lee HH, Chernesky MA, Schachter J, et al, "Diagnosis of Chlamydia trachomatis Genitourinary Infection in Women by Ligase Chain Reaction Assay of Urine," Lancet, 1995, 345(8944):213-6.

Rumpianesi F, Donati M, Negosanti M, et al, "Detection of Chlamydia trachomatis by a Ligase Chain Reaction Amplification Method," Sex Transm Dis, 1996, 23(3):177-80.

Schachter J, Stamm WE, Quinn TC, et al, "Ligase Chain Reaction to Detect Chlamydia trachomatis Infection of the Cervix," J Clin Microbiol, 1994, 32(10):2540-3.

Stary A, Tomazic-Allen S, Choueiri B, et al, "Comparison of DNA Amplification Methods for the Detection of Chlamydia trachomatis in First-Void Urine From Asymptomatic Military Recruits," Sex Transm Dis, 1006, 23(2):97-102.

Chlamydia trachomatis DNA Detection Test see Chlamydia trachomatis by DNA Probe on page 364

Chlamydia, TWAR Strain see Chlamydia pneumoniae Serology on page 361

Chloramphenicol Serum Level

Related Information

Antibiotic Level, Serum *on page 321*

Synonyms Chloromycetin®; Mychel-S®

Abstract Chloramphenicol is an antimicrobial agent whose use has been greatly reduced in recent years because of the introduction of a wide variety of less toxic alternative agents. It is still appropriately used to treat certain rickettsial infections or penicillin-allergic patients with bacterial meningitis. Life-threatening bone marrow toxicity is not closely associated with high serum levels.

Specimen Serum

Container Red top tube or serum separator tube

Sampling Time Collect for trough level immediately before next dose; for peak level about 2 hours after oral dose, 30 minutes after I.V. dose (time to peak can be variable)

Storage Instructions Freeze processed specimen

Reference Range Therapeutic range: 10-25 µg/mL (SI: 31-77 µmol/L), trough <5 µg/mL (SI: <15 µmol/L)

Critical Values Toxic range: >25 µg/mL (SI: >77 µmol/L)

Use Monitor drug therapy; monitor for potential toxicity

Limitations Reversible dose related bone marrow depression may occur when serum/plasma concentration >25 µg/mL (SI: >77 µmol/L). Idiosyncratic bone marrow aplasia is a rare event that usually occurs weeks to months after completing therapy, but approximately 25% occur during the course of therapy. Hematologic studies should be performed before and during therapy.

Methodology High performance liquid chromatography (HPLC), gas-liquid chromatography (GLC), immunoassay

Additional Information Chloramphenicol is an extremely effective antibacterial agent which unfortunately has both idiosyncratic and dose-related toxicities. Half-life is 1.6-3.3 hours longer in infants and patients with hepatic and renal disease. The dose related toxicity is, in adults, bone marrow suppression. "Gray syndrome," a type of circulatory collapse, occurs primarily in infants whose livers are unable to metabolize chloramphenicol effectively. Idiosyncratic aplastic anemia occurs in between 1 in 20,000 and 1 in 40,000 exposures. There are a number of chloramphenicol drug interactions since chloramphenicol can inhibit hepatic microsomal metabolism, increasing the serum concentration of phenytoin, tolbutamide, and dicumarol. Phenobarbital may be elevated in the presence of chloramphenicol.

Selected Readings

Baselt RC, *Analytical Procedures for Therapeutic Drug Monitoring and Emergency Toxicology*, Davis, CA: Biomedical Publications, 1980, 71-5.

de Louvois J, Mulhall A, and Hurley R, "Comparison of Methods Available for Assay of Chloramphenicol in Clinical Specimens," *J Clin Pathol*, 1980, 33(6):575-80.

Smilack JD, Wilson WR, and Cockerill FR 3d, "Tetracyclines, Chloramphenicol, Erythromycin, Clindamycin, and Metronidazole," *Mayo Clin Proc*, 1991, 66(12):1270-80.

Chloromycetin® *see* Chloramphenicol Serum Level *on this page*

CIE for Group B Streptococcal Antigen *see* Group B *Streptococcus* Antigen Test *on page 429*

Cimex Identification *see* Arthropod Identification *on page 334*

Clavicle, Left or Right, X-ray *see* Bone Films *on page 343*

Closed Joint Aspiration *see* Arthrocentesis *on page 330*

Clostridium botulinum Toxin Identification Procedure *see* Botulism, Diagnostic Procedure *on page 351*

Clostridium difficile Toxin Assay

Related Information

Fecal Leukocyte Stain *on page 408*

Synonyms Antibiotic-Associated Colitis Toxin Test; Pseudomembranous Colitis Toxin Assay; Toxin Assay, *Clostridium difficile*

Test Includes Toxin detection

Special Instructions When antibiotic-associated colitis is suspected a toxin assay rather than a *C. difficile* culture should be ordered on the stool.

Specimen Stool or proctoscopic specimen

Container Stool container with lids (swabs are inadequate because of small volume)

(Continued)

Clostridium difficile Toxin Assay *(Continued)*

Collection Keep specimen **cold** and transport immediately to prevent deterioration of toxin. Specimens can be frozen if transportation will be delayed.

Storage Instructions If the specimen cannot be processed immediately, it should be stored under refrigeration.

Turnaround Time 1-2 days depending on the availability and on the protocol of laboratory

Reference Range Presence of toxin is indicative of disease. Isolation of organism (*C. difficile*) may occur in a small percentage of normal adults (5% to 21%) and in normal newborns. Isolation of the organism without demonstration of toxin production is a nonspecific finding because only certain isolates are toxigenic.

Use Determine the presence or absence of antibiotic-related colitis caused by *C. difficile* toxin

Limitations Results given as titers are not significant as such because size/amounts of original specimens are usually not standardized. Results should be given as positive or negative, and any titer result should be interpreted as simply positive.

The latex agglutination test is simple and rapid, but it does not detect (is not specific for) toxin A, the protein thought to be primarily responsible for pseudomembranous colitis.

Methodology Latex agglutination test to detect toxin, toxin neutralization test in tissue culture (toxin), selective anaerobic culture (organism)

Additional Information Antibiotic-associated pseudomembranous colitis has been shown to result from the action of toxins produced by the organism, *C. difficile*. The disease has been associated with clindamycin but now it is recognized that pseudomembranous colitis can follow administration of virtually any antibiotic. More than 70% of cases in a large study were associated with cephalosporin therapy. The clinical spectrum of antibiotic-induced syndromes caused by *C. difficile* includes patients with symptoms of acute abdomen with little or no diarrhea, as well as cases with fulminant life-threatening diarrhea. Nosocomial transmission and reinfection with different strains occurs as do spontaneous cases without prior antimicrobial therapy. In cases where cessation of antibiotic therapy does not produce a response, specific therapy with oral vancomycin, metronidazole or oral bacitracin may be effective. The detection of the toxin (rather than culture of the organism or detection of the organism by latex agglutination) is essential in determining the etiology of this potentially fatal disease. In a recent report of 40 patients with *C. difficile*-associated diarrhea, 70% were positive in the cytotoxin assay, 78% positive in the LA test, and 90% culture positive. Fifty-three control patients had a 2%, 8%, and 4% positive rate respectively (ie, a small percentage of false-positives). A reasonable strategy might be to screen with the LA test and perform the toxin assay in cases which are positive. The routine use of culture is not appropriate because of the costs and the high rate of recovery of strains which do not produce toxin. Cytotoxin results are slightly more predictive of *C. difficile* disease than latex-positive results. Neither method alone is able either to predict or rule out all cases accurately. The organism is known to produce an enterotoxin, toxin A and a cytotoxin, toxin B. The exact role of each of these toxins, in clinical disease, remains unclear.

Selected Readings
Fekety R, and Shah AB, "Diagnosis and Treatment of *Clostridium difficile* Colitis," *JAMA*, 1993, 269(1):71-5.

Gerding DN, Olson MM, Peterson LR, et al, "*Clostridium difficile*-Associated Diarrhea and Colitis in Adults," *Arch Intern Med*, 1986, 146(1):95-100.

Kelly MT, Champagne SG, Sherlock CH, et al, "Commercial Latex Agglutination Test for Detection of *Clostridium difficile*-Associated Diarrhea," *J Clin Microbiol*, 1987, 25(7):1244-7.

Knoop FC, Owens M, and Crocker IC, "*Clostridium difficile*: Clinical Disease and Diagnosis," *Clin Microbiol Rev*, 1993, 6(3):251-65.

Lyerly DM, "Epidemiology of *Clostridium difficile* Disease," *Clin Microbiol Newslett*, 1993, 15(7):49-56.

Lyerly DM, Krivan HC, and Wilkins TD, "*Clostridium difficile*: It's Disease and Toxins," *Clin Microbiol Rev*, 1988, 1(1):1-18.

Wexler H, "Diagnosis of Antibiotic-Associated Disease Caused by *Clostridium difficile*," *Clin Microbiol Newslett*, 1989, 11:25-32.

CLO™ Test *see* Helicobacter pylori Culture and Urease Test *on page 432*

CMG *see* Cystometrogram, Simple *on page 382*

CMV Antigenemia *see* Cytomegalovirus Antigenemia *on page 386*

CMV Antigen Test *see* Cytomegalovirus Antigenemia *on page 386*

CMV Culture *see* Cytomegalovirus Culture *on page 388*

CMV Culture *see* Cytomegalovirus Culture, Blood *on page 389*

CMV DNA Hybrid Capture *see* Cytomegalovirus DNA Hybrid Capture *on page 390*

CMV Early Antigen FA Method *see* Cytomegalovirus Isolation, Rapid *on page 392*

CMV-IFA *see* Cytomegalovirus Serology *on page 392*

CMV-IFA, IgG *see* Cytomegalovirus Serology *on page 392*

CMV-IFA, IgM *see* Cytomegalovirus Serology *on page 392*

CMVS, Culture *see* Urine Culture, Clean Catch *on page 565*

CMV Shell Vial Method *see* Cytomegalovirus Isolation, Rapid *on page 392*

CMV Titer *see* Cytomegalovirus Serology *on page 392*

CMV-Vue™ Assay *see* Cytomegalovirus Antigenemia *on page 386*

Coagglutination Test for Group A Streptococci *see* Group A *Streptococcus* Antigen Test *on page 428*

***Coccidioides* Immunodiffusion** *see* Fungal Serology *on page 410*

Cold Agglutinin Titer

Test Includes Titer of patient's serum against type O blood cells at 2°C to 8°C

Special Instructions Transport blood immediately to laboratory.

Specimen Serum

Container Red top tube or serum separator tube

Storage Instructions After clotting at 37°C, separate serum from cells if specimen is to be stored overnight in refrigerator.

Causes for Rejection Refrigeration of the specimen before separating serum from cells; specimen not allowed to clot at 37°C

Reference Range Screen: negative; titer: <1:32

Use Occasionally, the cold agglutination titer is useful in supporting the diagnosis of primary atypical pneumonia (infection with *Mycoplasma pneumoniae*). Because it is nonspecific, the test generally is not recommended. Tests for specific antibodies to *Mycoplasma pneumoniae* are much more useful and specific than are tests for cold agglutinins.

Limitations False-negatives may occur if serum is refrigerated on the clot; only half of patients with *M. pneumoniae* infection will have positive test; many positive results are associated with a wide variety of nonspecific conditions

Additional Information The i and I RBC antigens appear to be ceramide heptasaccharides and decasaccharides. The fetal i RBCs change after birth so that by 18 months red cells carry largely I. The i substance has been found in saliva, milk, amniotic fluid, ovarian cyst fluid, and serum.

The most common cause of elevated cold agglutinin in high titers is an infection with *Mycoplasma pneumoniae*. *M. pneumoniae* has I-like antigen specificity. Fifty-five percent of patients with disease have rising titers. In primary atypical *Mycoplasma pneumoniae* pneumonia, cold agglutinins appear approximately 1 week after onset; the titer increases in 8-10 days, peaks at 12-25 days, and rapidly falls after day 30. Antibiotic therapy may interfere with antibody formation. Ninety percent of those who are severely affected or have prolonged illness will have a positive cold agglutination titer.

Cold agglutinins are usually IgM autoantibodies directed against the Ii antigens of human RBCs. These antibodies may be found in patients with cold agglutinin disease or may occur transiently following a number of acute infectious illnesses. Cold agglutinins of cold agglutinin disease are usually monoclonal IgM kappa. Cold antibodies of IgG, IgA, or IgM type directed against Ii antigens may be found in infectious mononucleosis. Antibodies reacting near physiologic temperatures are more likely to be clinically important. Detection of cold agglutinins may be useful in patients where cold blood is to be used such as in a blood cardioplegia unit.

Complete Blood Count

Synonyms Blood Cell Profile; Blood Count; CBC; Hemogram

Test Includes WBC, Hct, Hgb, differential count, RBC, WBC and RBC morphology, RBC indices, platelet estimate, platelet count, RDW, and histograms. Although RBC, WBC, and platelet histograms are not available on patient charts, they are helpful to the technologist in detecting problems with
(Continued)

Complete Blood Count *(Continued)*

patients and quality control. Even though the histograms are not on the chart, they can be viewed in the laboratory along with the blood smear. New analyzers also provide automated 5-part white cell differentials: granulocytes, monocytes, lymphocytes, eosinophils, and basophils.

Abstract The standard automated test for evaluation of RBC, WBC, and platelets

Specimen Whole blood

Container Lavender top (EDTA) tube

Collection Mix specimen 10 times by gentle inversion. If specimen is not brought to the laboratory immediately refrigeration is required. If the anticipated delay in arrival is more than 4 hours, two blood smears should be prepared immediately after the venipuncture and submitted with the blood specimen.

Causes for Rejection Improper tube, clotted specimen, hemolyzed specimen, dilution of blood with I.V. fluid

Reference Range Accompanying tables summarize differences in red cell parameter normal ranges, note especially important age and sex variances. Refer to tables.

Critical Values Hematocrit: <18% or >54%; hemoglobin: <6.0 g/dL or >18.0 g/dL; WBC on admission: <2500/mm^3 or >30,000/mm^3

Use Evaluate anemia, leukemia, reaction to inflammation and infections, peripheral blood cellular characteristics, state of hydration and dehydration, polycythemia, hemolytic disease of the newborn; manage chemotherapy decisions

Limitations Hemoglobin may be falsely high if the plasma is lipemic or if the white count is >50,000 cells/mm^3. "Spun" (manual centrifuged) microhematocrits are approximately 3% higher (due to plasma trapping) compared to automated hematocrit levels. The increase is especially pronounced in cases of polycythemia (increased Hct levels) and when the cells are hypochromic and microcytic. The spun Hct level (as compared to Coulter S) may be 12% higher at Hct levels of 70% and MCV of 48 fL with decrease in change to 3% higher at Hct levels of 70% with MCV of 100 fL. Cold agglutinins (high titer) may cause

Mean Hematologic Values for Low-Birth-Weight Infants*

Weight and Gestational Age at Birth	Age at Testing	Hemoglobin (g/dL)	Hematocrit (%)	Reticulocytes (%)
	3 d	17.5±1.5	54±5	8.0±3.5
	1 wk	15.5±1.5	48±5	3.0±1.0
	2 wk	13.5±1.1	42±4	3.0±1.0
<1500 g, 28-32 wk	3 wk	11.5±1.0	35±4	—
	4 wk	10.0±0.9	30±3	6.0±2.0
	6 wk	8.5±0.5	25±2	11.0±3.5
	8 wk	8.5±0.5	25±2	8.5±3.5
	10 wk	9.0±0.5	28±3	7.0±3.0
	3 d	19.0±2.0	59±6	6.0±2.0
	1 wk	16.5±1.5	51±5	3.0±1.0
	2 wk	14.5±1.1	44±5	2.5±1.0
1500-2000 g, 32-36 wk	3 wk	13.0±1.1	39±4	—
	4 wk	12.0±1.0	36±4	3.0±1.0
	6 wk	9.5±0.8	28±3	6.0±2.0
	8 wk	9.5±0.5	28±3	5.0±1.5
	10 wk	9.5±0.5	29±3	4.5±1.5
	3 d	19.0±2.0	59±6	4.0±1.0
	1 wk	16.5±1.5	51±5	3.0±1.0
	2 wk	15.0±1.5	45±5	2.5±1.0
2000-2500 g, 36-40 wk	3 wk	14.0±1.1	43±4	—
	4 wk	12.5±1.0	37±4	2.0±1.0
	6 wk	10.5±0.9	31±3	3.0±1.0
	8 wk	10.5±0.9	31±3	3.0±1.0
	10 wk	11.0±1.0	33±3	3.0±1.0

*Mean ±1 SD.

From Johnson TR, "How Growing Up Can Alter Lab Values in Pediatric Laboratory Medicine," *Diag Med* (special issue), 1982, 5:13-8, with permission.

Red Cell Values on First Postnatal Day*

Gestational Age (wk)	24-25	26-27	28-29	30-31	32-33	34-35	36-37	Term
RBC (x 10^6/mm³)	4.65 ±0.43	4.73 ±0.45	4.62 ±0.75	4.79 ±0.74	5.0 ±0.76	5.09 ±0.5	5.27 ±0.68	5.14 ±0.7
Hgb (g/dL)	19.4 ±1.5	19.0 ±2.5	19.3 ±1.8	19.1 ±2.2	18.5 ±2.0	19.6 ±2.1	19.2 ±1.7	19.3 ±2.2
Hct (%)	63 ±4	62 ±8	60 ±7	60 ±8	60 ±8	61 ±7	64 ±7	61 ±7.4
MCV (fL)	135 ±0.2	132 ±14.4	131 ±13.5	127 ±12.7	123 ±15.7	122 ±10.0	121 ±12.5	119 ±9.4
Retic (%)	6.0 ±0.5	9.6 ±3.2	7.5 ±2.5	5.8 ±2.0	5.0 ±1.9	3.9 ±1.6	4.2 ±1.8	3.2 ±1.4

*Mean values ±1 SD.

From Zaizov R and Matoth Y, "Red Cell Values on the First Postnatal Day During the Last 16 Weeks of Gestation," *Amer J Hematol*, 1976, 1:2, 275-8, with permission.

Mean Hematologic Values for Full-Term Infants, Children, and Adults*

Age	Hgb (g/dL)	Hct (%)	RBC (x 10^6/mm³)	MCV (fL)	MCH (pg)	MCHC (g/dL)
Birth (cord blood)	17.1±1.8	52.0±5	4.64±0.5	113±6	37±2	33±1
1 d	19.4±2.1	58.0±7	5.30±0.5	110±6	37±2	33±1
2-6 d	19.8±2.4	66.0±8	5.40±0.7	122±14	37±4	30±3
14-23 d	15.7±1.5	52.0±5	4.92±0.6	106±11	32±3	30±2
24-37 d	14.1±1.9	45.0±7	4.35±0.6	104±11	32±3	31±3
40-50 d	12.8±1.9	42.0±6	4.10±0.5	103±11	31±3	30±2
2-2.5 mo	11.4±1.1	38.0±4	3.75±0.5	101±10	30±3	30±2
3-3.5 mo	11.2±0.8	37.0±3	3.88±0.4	95±9	29±3	30±2
5-7 mo	11.5±0.7	38.0±3	4.21±0.5	91±9	27±3	30±2
8-10 mo	11.7±0.6	39.0±2	4.35±0.4	90±8	27±3	30±1
11-13.5 mo	11.9±0.6	39.0±2	4.44±0.4	88±7	27±2	30±1
1.5-3 y	11.8±0.5	39.0±2	4.45±0.4	87±7	27±2	30±2
5 y	12.7±1.0	37.0±3	4.65±0.5	80±4	27±2	34±1
10 y	13.2±1.2	39.0±3	4.80±0.5	81±6	28±3	34±1
Male	15.5±1.1	46.0±3.1	5.11±0.38	90.1±4.8	30.2±1.8	33.7±1.1
Female	13.7±1.0	40.9±3	4.51±0.36	90.1±4.8	30.2±1.8	33.7±1.1

*Mean ±1 SD.

From Johnson TR, "How Growing Up Can Alter Lab Values in Pediatric Laboratory Medicine," *Diag Med* (special issue), 1982, 5:13-8, with permission.

spurious macrocytosis and low RBC count. This results when RBC couplets are "seen" and processed as single cells by the detection circuitry. Keeping the blood warm and warming the diluent prior to and during counting can correct this problem.

Methodology Varies considerably between institutions. Most laboratories have high capacity multichannel instruments in place (available from multiple commercial sources). The majority measure RBC and WBC parameters on the basis of changes in electrical impedance as cells and platelets are pulled through a tiny aperture. These are highly automated devices with extensive computer processing of the electrical signals after analog/digital conversion. Accuracy (with proper standardization) and precision (usually in the 0.5% to 2% range) is significantly improved over older manual and semiautomated methods. Some instruments count light impulses that are generated as cells flow across a laser beam.

Additional Information Presence of one or more of the following may be indications for further investigation: hemoglobin <10 g/dL, hemoglobin >18 g/dL, MCV >100 fL, MCV <80 fL, MCHC >37%, WBC >20,000/mm³, WBC <2000/mm³, presence of sickle cells, significant spherocytosis, basophilic stippling, stomatocytes,significant schistocytosis, oval macrocytes, tear drop red blood cells, eosinophilia (>10%) monocytosis (>15%), nucleated red blood cells in (Continued)

Proposed Classification of Anemic Disorders Based on Red Cell Mean (MCV) and Heterogeneity (RDW)

MCV Low RDW Normal (microcytic homogeneous)	MCV Low RDW High (microcytic heterogeneous)	MCV Normal RDW Normal (normocytic homogeneous)	MCV Normal RDW High (normocytic heterogeneous)	MCV High RDW Normal (macrocytic homogeneous)	MCV High RDW High (macrocytic heterogeneous)
Heterozygous thalassemia*	Iron deficiency*	Normal	Mixed deficiency*	Aplastic anemia	Folate deficiency*
Chronic disease*	S/β-thalassemia	Chronic disease* chronic liver disease††	Early iron or folate deficiency*	Preleukemia†	Vitamin B_{12} deficiency
	Hemoglobin H	Nonanemic hemoglobinopathy (eg, AS, AC)	Anemic hemoglobinopathy (eg, SS, SC)*		Immune hemolytic anemia
	Red cell fragmentation	Transfusion†	Myelofibrosis		Cold agglutinins
		Chemotherapy	Sideroblastic*		Chronic lymphocytic leukemia, high count
		Chronic lymphocytic leukemia			
		Chronic myelocytic leukemia†			
		Hemorrhage			
		Hereditary spherocytosis			

*MCV alone <90% sensitive.

†RDW alone <30% sensitive.

From Bessman JD Jr, Gilmer PR, Gardner FH, "Improved Classification of Anemias by MCV and RDW," *Am J Clin Pathol,* 1983, 80:324, with permission. The data for sensitivity of RDW and MCV in each disease category can be obtained from the authors.

other than the newborn, malarial organisms or the possibility of malarial organisms, hypersegmented (five or more nuclear segments) PMNs, agranular PMNs, Pelger-Huët anomaly, Auer rods, Döhle bodies, marked toxic granulation, mononuclears in which apparent nucleoli are prominent (blast type cells), presence of metamyelocytes, myelocytes, promyelocytes, neutropenia, presence of plasma cells, peculiar atypical lymphocytes, significant increase or decrease in platelets. Some quantitative elements of the CBC are related to each other, normally, such that examination of the results of any individual analysis allow for the application of a simple but effective case individualized quality control maneuver. The RBC count, hemoglobin, and hematocrit may be analyzed by applying a "rule of three." If red cells are normochromic/normocytic, the RBC count times 3 should approximately equal the hemoglobin and the hemoglobin multiplied by 3 should approximate the hematocrit. If there is significant deviation from this relation, one should check for supporting abnormalities in RBC indices and peripheral smear. The indices themselves offer a quick quality control check of the CBC. If patient transfusion can be excluded, then RBC indices should vary little consecutively from day to day. Anemias have been classified on the basis of their MCV and RDW (RBC heterogeneity). This classification has been especially helpful in the separation of iron deficiency from thalassemia. Heterozygous thalassemia has a normal RDW while RDW is high with iron deficiency.

In iron deficiency, the RDW is usually increased before the MCV decreases. Although this is somewhat controversial, it serves as an inexpensive screen for common iron deficiency anemia. See table on previous page.

Selected Readings

Beautyman W and Bills T, "Osmotic Error in Erythrocyte Volume Determinations," *Am J Hematol*, 1982, 12(4):383-9.

England JM, Walford DM, Waters DA, et al, "Re-assessment of the Reliability of the Haematocrit," *Br J Haematol*, 1972, 23(2):247-56.

Fraser CG, Wilkinson SP, Neville RG, et al, "Biologic Variation of Common Hematologic Laboratory Quantities in the Elderly," *Am J Clin Pathol*, 1989, 92(4):465-70.

Computed Transaxial Tomography, Abdomen Studies

Synonyms Abdomen, CT; CT, Lower Abdomen; CT, Total Abdomen; CT, Upper Abdomen

Test Includes CT scan of liver, spleen, kidneys, pancreas, aorta, retroperitoneum, gastrointestinal tract, pelvis. **Note:** In some departments, a request for a CT study of the abdomen will yield a study extending inferiorly to the pubic symphysis. In others, the study will extend only to the pelvic brim.

Patient Preparation Patient's oral intake restricted to fluid only for 4 hours prior to the examination. Medication schedule should not be interrupted. Should the patient have recently undergone a barium examination of the gastrointestinal tract, a digital radiograph obtained with the scanner prior to commencement of the procedure may be helpful in excluding the presence of barium within the bowel. The latter may produce significant artifact and thus render the study nondiagnostic. Where possible, all CT scan studies of the abdomen should be performed prior to normal GI barium studies. A recent serum creatinine is requested on all patients 60 years of age and older, patients with known significant atherosclerotic disease, diabetes mellitus, or with pre-existing renal disease. Intravenous contrast material is routinely administered for this examination. Physician may opt to omit intravenous contrast. Patients undergoing a CT study of the abdomen are requested to drink approximately 450 mL of a dilute barium solution (approximately 1% barium) commencing 1 hour prior to the examination. Inclusion of the pelvis in this examination requires further patient preparation.

Special Instructions CT scan of the abdomen may be requested by a practicing physician. The abdominal area of interest should be specified along with pertinent clinical history. This will allow the diagnostic radiologist to tailor the examination for maximum diagnostic yield. For example, studies being performed for detection of renal calculi should be performed without contrast material, as the contrast, when excreted from the kidney, will mask the presence of small calculi within the collecting system. Adequate evaluation of small structures within the abdomen may require modification of technique such as thin slices or overlapping slices. A further example would be in the evaluation of the liver for primary or metastatic tumor. Maximum yield in the demonstration of such abnormalities requires examination both with and without contrast material.
(Continued)

Computed Transaxial Tomography, Abdomen Studies
(Continued)

Equipment This examination may be performed on any one of many commercially available computerized tomography scanners.

Technique Standard examination of the abdomen consists of 1 cm contiguous slices obtained from the dome of the diaphragm to the pelvic brim or pubic symphysis depending upon whether one groups the pelvis with the abdomen or treats it separately.

Causes for Rejection Patients with residual barium within the GI tract from a prior conventional barium study - this nondilute barium produces considerable artifact rendering the examination suboptimal and often nondiagnostic, uncooperative patients who are not candidates for sedation/anesthesia

Turnaround Time A verbal telephone report of the scan will be given to the referring physician if specified. A written report will be available.

Use Diagnose and/or evaluate cysts, tumors, masses, aneurysm, metastases, abscesses, and trauma. The modality is also often used for staging of known tumors.

Contraindications Patient cooperation is of the utmost importance as the examination requires the patient to remain motionless for the duration of the study. The time of the study will vary from 20-40 minutes depending on the equipment being used. Children and uncooperative adults may require sedation.

Additional Information Patients should be informed that the examination may take 45 minutes to 1 hour and that oral contrast and intravenous contrast are commonly required. If the pelvis is included with the abdominal CT study, rectal contrast material and placement of a vaginal tampon in the case of females may also be required. The patient's medical record should accompany the patient. This will furnish the radiologist with sufficient information to tailor the examination as he/she deems appropriate. For example, patients suspected of an adrenal adenoma may require thin (2 mm) slices through the adrenal glands for the detection of such an abnormality.

Selected Readings

Halvorsen RA Jr and Thompson WM, "Computed Tomographic Staging of Gastrointestinal Tract Malignancies, Part I. Esophagus and Stomach," *Invest Radiol*, 1987, 22(1):2-16.

Thompson WM and Halvorsen RA Jr, "Computed Tomographic Staging of Gastrointestinal Tract Malignancies, Part II," *Invest Radiol*, 1987, 22(2):96-105.

Computed Transaxial Tomography, Appropriate Site
Refer to

Computed Transaxial Tomography, Abdomen Studies *on page 373*
Computed Transaxial Tomography, Head Studies *on page 374*
Computed Transaxial Tomography, Thorax *on page 376*

Computed Transaxial Tomography, Head Studies
Synonyms Brain, CT; Head Studies, CT

Test Includes CT scan of the brain

Patient Preparation The examination should be ordered and a requisition with information pertaining to the reason for the request and the clinical history should be completed by the referring physician. If there is the slightest possibility that intravenous contrast material will be administered, the patient's oral intake should be limited to liquids for at least 4 hours prior to the examination. Care must be taken to ensure the patient does not become dehydrated and medications should not be interrupted. A recent serum creatinine is requested on patients with pre-existing renal disease, diabetes mellitus, significant atherosclerotic disease, and advancing age (60 years and older). Agitated patients and children may require sedation prior to the examination. In these cases, an order for the appropriate sedative and dose should be recently recorded within the patient's chart. Sedatives should be administered by a physician within the Radiology Department.

Equipment Any commercially available computed tomographic scanner

Technique CT scans of the head are usually obtained at 15° angulation to the orbitomeatal line, a line connecting the lateral canthus of the eye with the external auditory canal. Contiguous slices 8 or 10 mm in thickness are obtained from the vertex of the skull to the foramen magnum. The orbital roof should be included. The patient is positioned supine for the examination. The head is placed securely in a head holder. The chin is flexed comfortably towards the chest. The appropriate 15° angulation can be obtained by angulation of the gantry if necessary.

Use Evaluate known or suspected primary or secondary neoplasm, cystic lesions, hydrocephalus, head trauma, seizure disorder, multiple sclerosis, atrophy, Alzheimer's disease, normal pressure hydrocephalus, Parkinson's disease, dementia, depression, organic brain syndrome, etc

Contraindications Assuming a cooperative or quiescent patient, there are no absolute contraindications to a CT scan of the head. A decision must be taken, however, as to whether the study is to be done with or without intravenous contrast material. While each case must be assessed individually, the following broad guidelines may be helpful. Those studies indicated by virtue of a recent infarct, cerebrovascular accident or stroke, or those being done for assessment of atrophy, Alzheimer's disease, normal pressure hydrocephalus, Parkinson's disease, hydrocephalus, evaluation of an intraventricular shunt, assessment of ventricular size, subdural hematoma, or suspected dementia are examined without contrast material. Patients for whom the indication is headache, psychiatric condition (such as anorexia or bulimia), tumor follow-up, rule out tumor, rule out metastasis, multiple sclerosis, seizure disorders, depression, and organic brain syndrome are generally studied with contrast material. Patients in whom the indication is one of infection, abscess, meningitis, transient ischemic attack, arteriovenous malformation, remote subdural hematoma, or who have recently undergone a craniotomy and are being studied for postoperative evaluation are best studied with and without contrast material. Patients with a known diagnosis of plasmacytoma or multiple myeloma should not receive intravenous contrast material. Patients with compromised renal function may or may not benefit from intravenous contrast material. A recent serum creatinine and BUN will be helpful in deciding whether or not the latter group of patients receive contrast material.

Computed Transaxial Tomography, Paranasal Sinuses

Synonyms Paranasal Sinuses, CT; Sinuses, CT

Test Includes The examination is composed of contiguous 3-5 mm slices obtained from the inferior portion of the maxillary sinuses, cephalad to the superior extent of the frontal sinuses.

Patient Preparation Patients oral intake should be restricted to fluid for 4 hours prior to the examination. Medication schedule should not be interrupted. Administration of intravenous contrast material is at the discretion of the diagnostic radiologist. If a patient is being evaluated for trauma or inflammatory disease of the paranasal sinuses, no intravenous contrast material is usually administered. If a mass is identified in the course of the examination, or if a patient is known to have a tumor, then intravenous contrast material is usually given. Because of this, a recent serum creatinine is requested in all patients 60 years of age and older and those patients with known significant atherosclerotic disease, diabetes mellitus, or pre-existing renal disease. Children and uncooperative adults may require sedation.

Special Instructions If the nasopharynx is to be included in the examination, the study should be extended inferiorly to the hard palate or slightly below. The oral pharynx may be included by continuing to the base of the tongue. If there is a question of tumor invasion of the orbit from a sinus then coronal sections are very helpful.

Technique This examination may be performed in any one of many commercially available computerized tomographic scanners. Standard examination of the paranasal sinuses consist of 3-5 mm contiguous slices as previously described.

Turnaround Time Verbal telephone report of the scan will be given to the referring physician if specified. A written report will be available.

Use Diagnose and/or evaluate tumors, masses, metastases, inflammatory conditions, and traumatic involvement. The modality is commonly used for staging of tumors.

Contraindications Patients who are not candidates for sedation/anesthesia, uncooperative patient; patient cooperation is of the utmost importance as the examination requires the patient to remain motionless for the duration of the study.

Additional Information Some departments offer a limited CT study of the paranasal sinuses which is competitive with plain film radiographs of the sinus in terms of pricing. This consists of 5 or 6 transaxial images through the sinus obtained parallel to Reid's baseline. The examination is achieved by obtaining a
(Continued)

Computed Transaxial Tomography, Paranasal Sinuses
(Continued)

lateral digital image of the skull. From this the distance between the hard palate and the superior aspect of the frontal sinuses is measured. The distance is then divided by 5 or 6 to get the interslice distance. The slice thickness is 3-5 mm.

Selected Readings

Harnsberger HR, Osborn AG, and Smoker RK, "CT in the Evaluation of the Normal and Diseased Paranasal Sinuses," *Seminars in the Ultrasound, CT and MR,* 1986, 7:68-90.

Computed Transaxial Tomography, Thorax

Test Includes CT study of the chest extending from the lung apices to the posterior costophrenic sulci. The study may extend inferiorly to image the adrenal glands because they are a relatively frequent site of metastasis from primary lung carcinoma.

Patient Preparation The patients should be limited to a liquid diet for at least 4 hours prior to the CT examination. Medication schedules should be maintained. The use of intravenous contrast material may be required at the discretion of the diagnostic radiologist. Because of this, a recent serum creatinine is requested in all patients 60 years of age and older, and those patients with known significant atherosclerotic disease, diabetes mellitus, or pre-existing renal disease. In the case of children who need sedation, a recent (within 30 days) recording of the child's weight and a written order by the child's physician must be in the patient's medical record. All children should be accompanied by a responsible adult. Opacification of the esophagus with thick barium paste may be of value in some cases and administration should be at the discretion of the diagnostic radiologist.

Special Instructions The exam may be requested by a practicing physician. The area of interest must be specified along with pertinent clinical history and reason for the CT scan. The test should be complete in 10-30 minutes. Intravenous contrast material may be administered.

Equipment The examination may be performed on any number of commercially available CT scanners.

Technique A routine CT study of the chest consists of sequential 1 cm slices obtained from the apices through the posterior costophrenic sulci. The study may be extended to include the adrenal glands if a diagnosis of primary bronchogenic carcinoma is known or suspected. The technique may vary depending upon the indications for the study. The examination may be tailored by the diagnostic radiologist to answer specific questions. For example, the questionably abnormal pulmonary hilum on conventional films may require 5 mm contiguous sections subsequent to the intravenous administration of contrast material. The latter will facilitate enhancement of major vascular structures thus highlighting normal and abnormal anatomy. Similarly, densitometric evaluation of a solitary pulmonary nodule will require contiguous 2 mm slices throughout the nodule without intravenous contrast material. This maneuver will facilitate evaluation of the nodule for the presence and distribution of calcium within it. All modifications of the conventional contiguous 1 cm slice protocol throughout the chest are made at the discretion of the radiologist. The patient's medical record should accompany the patient to the department in order to ensure that the radiologist is furnished with sufficient information to tailor the examination appropriately.

Causes for Rejection Inability of the patient to cooperate is the major problem. Should the uncooperative patient not be a candidate for sedation and/or anesthesia, the study cannot be performed.

Turnaround Time A verbal telephone report of the scan will be given to the referring physician if specified. A written report will be available.

Use The examination facilitates evaluation of abnormalities of the lungs, mediastinum, pleura, and chest wall. Conventional PA and lateral views of the chest represent the basic screening tool in the identification of abnormalities involving the thorax. The axial anatomic display and superior density discrimination of computed tomography provides information pertaining to the extent of disease and more precise characterization of abnormalities initially noted on physical examination, chest films or on the barium swallow.

Contraindications Patient cooperation is of utmost importance as the examination requires the patient to remain motionless for the duration of the study. The time of the study will vary from 10-30 minutes depending on the equipment being used. Children and uncooperative adults may require sedation.

Selected Readings
Naidich DP, Zerhouni EA, Hutchins GM, et al, "Computed Tomography of the Pulmonary Parenchyma, Part 1: Distal Air-space Disease," *J Thorac Imaging*, 1985, 1(1):39-53.

Zerhouni EA, Naidich DP, Stitik FP, et al, "Computed Tomography of the Pulmonary Parenchyma, Part 2: Interstitial Disease," *J Thorac Imaging*, 1985, 1(1):54-64.

Conjunctival Smear *see* Ocular Cytology *on page 505*

Corneal Smear *see* Ocular Cytology *on page 505*

***Corynebacterium diphtheriae* Culture, Throat** *see* Throat Culture for *Corynebacterium diphtheriae on page 549*

Cough Plate Culture for Pertussis *replaced by Bordetella pertussis* Direct Fluorescent Antibody *on page 349*

Cough Plate Culture for Pertussis *replaced by Bordetella pertussis* Nasopharyngeal Culture *on page 349*

Counterimmunoelectrophoresis for Group B Streptococcal Antigen *see* Group B *Streptococcus* Antigen Test *on page 429*

***Coxiella burnetii* Titer** *see* Q Fever Serology *on page 525*

Coxsackie A Virus Culture *see* Enterovirus Culture *on page 405*

Coxsackie A Virus Serology

Related Information
Enterovirus Culture *on page 405*

Specimen Serum

Container Red top tube or serum separator tube

Sampling Time Acute and convalescent sera drawn at least 14 days apart are required

Reference Range Less than a fourfold increase in titer in paired sera. Most healthy people do not have titers >1:8. Titers ≥1:32 are especially diagnostic. Titers ≤1:8 could represent cross reactions with other enteroviruses.

Use Establish the diagnosis of Coxsackie A virus infection (eg, in viral myocarditis)

Limitations Neutralizing antibodies develop quickly and persist for many years after infection, making demonstration of a rise in titer difficult. There are at least 24 types/serotypes of Coxsackie A virus. Therefore, serotypes detected will depend on particular reagents used in a particular test. Consult the laboratory for serotypes detected.

Methodology Viral neutralization, complement fixation (CF)

Additional Information Coxsackie A virus produces a wide spectrum of disease including aseptic meningitis, myositis, encephalitis, respiratory illnesses, herpangina, hand-foot-and-mouth disease, rash, and generalized systemic infection. Documentation of infection by serology is difficult and diagnosis may depend on culture.

Selected Readings
Melnick JL, "Enteroviruses," *Manual of Clinical Laboratory Immunology*, 4th ed, Rose NR, de Macario EC, Fahey JL, et al, eds, Washington, DC: American Society for Microbiology, 1992, 631-3.

Coxsackie B Virus Culture *see* Enterovirus Culture *on page 405*

Coxsackie B Virus Serology

Related Information
Enterovirus Culture *on page 405*

Test Includes Coxsackie B_1, B_2, B_3, B_4, B_5, B_6 virus titers

Specimen Serum

Container Red top tube or serum separator tube

Sampling Time Acute and convalescent sera drawn 10-14 days apart are required.

Reference Range Less than a fourfold increase in titer in paired sera

Use Establish the diagnosis of Coxsackie B virus infection

Limitations Neutralizing antibodies arise quickly, last for years, and may make the demonstration of a rising titer difficult. Tests for complement fixing antibodies are insensitive and nonspecific. There are six types/serotypes of Coxsackie B virus. Consult the laboratory to determine if test detects some or all six types.

Methodology Complement fixation (CF), viral neutralization

Additional Information Coxsackie B virus causes a wide variety of clinical illness, including pleurodynia (Bornholm's disease), aseptic meningitis, carditis/myocarditis, rash, pulmonary infection, a generalized systemic infection, and (Continued)

Coxsackie B Virus Serology *(Continued)*

several neonatal diseases and syndromes. Approximately 50% of clinical myocarditis and pericarditis is caused by Coxsackie B. Since culture is frequently unrewarding, diagnosis may depend on serologic studies.

Recently there has been interest in various viral assays for postviral fatigue syndrome. Antibody to Coxsackie B virus is not helpful in this assessment.

Selected Readings

Melnick JL, "Enteroviruses," *Manual of Clinical Laboratory Immunology*, 4th ed, Rose NR, de Macario EC, Fahey JL, et al, eds, Washington, DC: American Society for Microbiology, 1992, 631-3.

Miller NA, Carmichael HA, Calder BD, et al, "Antibody to Coxsackie B Virus in Diagnosing Postviral Fatigue Syndrome," *BMJ*, 1991, 302(6769):140-3.

Coxsackie Virus Culture, Stool *see* Viral Culture, Stool *on page 573*

Crab Lice Identification *see* Arthropod Identification *on page 334*

C-Reactive Protein

Related Information

Sedimentation Rate, Erythrocyte *on page 532*
Serum Bactericidal Test *on page 533*

Synonyms Acute Phase Reactant; CRP

Specimen Serum

Container Red top tube or serum separator tube

Causes for Rejection Excessive hemolysis, chylous serum

Reference Range <8 μg/mL

Use Used similarly to erythrocyte sedimentation rate. CRP is a nonspecific acute phase reactant protein used as an indicator of infectious disease and inflammatory states, including active rheumatic fever and rheumatoid arthritis. Progressive increases correlate with increases of inflammation/injury. CRP is a more sensitive, rapidly responding indicator than is ESR. CRP may be used to detect early postoperative wound infection and to follow therapeutic response to anti-inflammatory agents.

Limitations Frozen specimens may give false-positive results; oral contraceptives may affect results

Methodology Agglutination, nephelometry, radioimmunoassay (RIA)

Additional Information CRP is a pentameric globulin with mobility near the gamma zone. It is an acute phase reactant which rises rapidly, but nonspecifically, in response to tissue injury and inflammation. It is particularly useful in detecting occult infections, acute appendicitis, particularly in leukemia and in postoperative patients. In uncomplicated postoperative recovery, CRP peaks on the third postop day, and returns to preop levels by day 7. It may also be helpful in evaluating extension or reinfarction after myocardial infarction, and in following response to therapy in rheumatic disorders. It may help to differentiate Crohn's disease (high CRP) from ulcerative colitis (low CRP), and rheumatoid arthritis (high CRP) from uncomplicated lupus (low CRP). When used to evaluate patients with arthritis, serum is the preferred specimen. There is no advantage to examining synovial fluid for CRP.

Selected Readings

Dowton SR and Colten HR, "Acute Phase Reactants in Inflammation and Infection," *Semin Hematol*, 1988, 25(2):84-90.

Van Lente F, "The Diagnostic Utility of C-Reactive Protein," *Hum Pathol*, 1982, 13(12):1061-3.

Creatinine Clearance

Related Information

Body Surface Areas of Adults and Children *on page 991*
Creatinine Clearance Estimating Methods in Patients With Stable Renal Function *on page 993*

Applies to GFR; Glomerular Filtration Rate

Replaces Urea Clearance; Urea Nitrogen Clearance

Test Includes Serum creatinine, urine creatinine

Patient Preparation Avoid cephalosporins. If possible, drugs should be stopped beforehand. Have patient drink water before the clearance is begun, and continue good hydration throughout the clearance.

Special Instructions Blood creatinine should be ordered at the same time. Requisition should state date and time collection started, date and time collection finished, patient's age, height, and weight.

Specimen 24-hour urine and serum; test can be done for shorter periods

Container Plastic urine container and red top tube

Collection Instruct the patient to void at 8 AM and discard the specimen. Then collect all urine including the final specimen voided at the end of the 24-hour collection period (ie, 8 AM the next morning). Keep specimen on ice during collection. Bottle must be labeled with patient's name, date and time for a 24-hour collection.

Especially for creatinine clearance, accuracy and precision of collection are important. Complete, carefully timed (usually 24-hour) collection is needed; 4-hour and 12-hour collections are acceptable.

Storage Instructions Refrigerate

Causes for Rejection No blood creatinine ordered, urine specimen not timed

Reference Range Children: 70-140 mL/min/1.73 m^2 (SI: 1.17-2.33 mL/s/1.73 m^2); adult male: 85-125 mL/min/1.73 m^2 (SI: 1.42-2.08 mL/s/1.73 m^2); adult female: 75-115 mL/min/1.73 m^2 (SI: 1.25-1.92 mL/s/1.73 m^2)

Use Renal function test to estimate glomerular filtration rate (GFR); evaluate renal function in small or wasted subjects; follow possible progression of renal disease; adjust dosages of medications in which renal excretion is pivotal (eg, aminoglycosides, methotrexate, cisplatin)

Limitations Exercise may cause increased creatinine clearance. The glomerular filtration rate is substantially increased in pregnancy. Ascorbic acid, ketone bodies (acetoacetate), hydantoin, numerous cephalosporins and glucose may influence creatinine determinations. Trimethoprim, cimetidine, quinine, quinidine, procainamide reduce creatinine excretion. Icteric samples, lipemia, and hemolysis may interfere with determination of creatinine.

Since tubular secretion of creatinine is fractionally more important in progressing renal failure, the creatinine clearance overestimates GFR with high serum creatinine levels.

While ingestion of meats may cause some increase in creatinine excretion, in practice this seems to make little difference. Intraindividual variation in creatinine clearance is about 15%. Males excrete more creatinine and have slightly higher clearance than females.

Methodology Jaffé reaction (alkaline picrate). The calculation for corrected creatinine clearance in mL/minute: = [(urine volume per minute x urine creatinine)/serum creatinine] x (1.73/surface area of body in square meters). Body surface area is obtained from nomograms which require age, height, and weight. See Appendix table Body Surface Area of Adults and Children *on page 991*.

Additional Information Glomerular filtration rate declines about 10% per decade after age 50. Some patients with significant impairment of glomerular filtration rate have only slightly elevated serum creatinine.

Creatinine clearance is calculated on the basis of the surface area of the patient. The estimated error of determining creatinine clearance utilizing serum and 24-hour urine collection has been found to be in the range of 10% to 15%.

Any test requiring a 24-hour urine collection may also be run on this specimen, eg, protein, quantitative, 24-hour urine.

Selected Readings

Levey AS, Perrone RD, and Madias NE, "Serum Creatinine and Renal Function," *Annu Rev Med*, 1988, 39:465-90.

Luke DR, Halstenson CE, Opsahl JA, et al, "Validity of Creatinine Clearance Estimates in the Assessment of Renal Function," *Clin Pharmacol Ther*, 1990, 48(5):503-8.

Van Lente F and Suit P, "Assessment of Renal Function by Serum Creatinine and Creatinine Clearance: Glomerular Filtration Rate Estimated by Four Procedures," *Clin Chem*, 1989, 35(12):2326-30.

Creatinine Clearance Estimating Methods in Patients With Stable Renal Function *see page 993*

CRP *see C-Reactive Protein on previous page*

Cryptococcal Antigen Serology, Serum or Cerebrospinal Fluid

Related Information

Cryptococcus Serology *on next page*

Fungus Culture, Cerebrospinal Fluid *on page 416*

India Ink Preparation *on page 460*

Methenamine Silver Stain *on page 487*

(Continued)

Cryptococcal Antigen Serology, Serum or Cerebrospinal Fluid (Continued)

Periodic Acid-Schiff Stain on page 518

Synonyms Cerebrospinal Fluid Cryptococcal Latex Agglutination; *Cryptococcus* Antigen, Blood; *Cryptococcus* Latex Antigen Agglutination; Spinal Fluid Cryptococcal Latex Agglutination

Test Includes Testing patient's serum or CSF for the presence of cryptococcal antigen (with rheumatoid factor/nonspecific control)

Abstract Cryptococcal antigen testing is the single most useful diagnostic test for cryptococcal meningitis.

Specimen Serum or cerebrospinal fluid

Container Red top tube, sterile CSF tube

Reference Range Negative

Use Establish the diagnosis of *Cryptococcus neoformans* infection

Limitations False-positive results can occur in patients with rheumatoid arthritis, but test controls usually eliminate this possibility. The test is less frequently positive in serum than in CSF. Disseminated cryptococcal infections usually result in a positive serum test. False-negatives occur.

Methodology Latex agglutination with rheumatoid factor/nonspecific control and in some laboratories pronase pretreatment.

Additional Information Presence of cryptococcal capsular polysaccharide is indicative of cryptococcosis. Samples should either be treated to remove rheumatoid factor and other interfering factors or tested to distinguish between positivity due to cryptococcal antigen and that due to interfering factors. If this distinction cannot be made the test cannot be interpreted. Pretreatment of the specimen with pronase reduces false-positives and increases the likelihood of positivity of the method.

The cryptococcal antigen test is positive in about 85% to 90% of cases of cryptococcal meningitis, while the India ink test is positive in ≤50%. The cryptococcal antigen test has been reported to be able to detect antigen in 95% of AIDS patients with cryptococcal disease. Culture of cerebrospinal fluid for fungus should be performed in patients who are suspected of having cryptococcosis.

Selected Readings

Gray LD and Roberts GD, "Experience With the Use of Pronase to Eliminate Interference Factors in the Latex Agglutination Test for Cryptococcal Antigen," *J Clin Microbiol,* 1988, 26(11):2450-1.

Greenlee JE, "Approach to Diagnosis of Meningitis - Cerebrospinal Fluid Evaluation," *Infect Dis Clin North Am,* 1990, 4(4):583-98.

Kaufman L and Reiss E, "Serodiagnosis of Fungal Diseases," *Manual of Clinical Laboratory Immunology,* 4th ed, Rose NR, de Macario EC, Fahey JL, et al, eds, Washington, DC: American Society for Microbiology, 1992, 506-28.

Cryptococcosis, IFA see *Cryptococcus* Serology on this page

Cryptococcosis, Indirect Fluorescent Antibody Titer see *Cryptococcus* Serology on this page

Cryptococcus Antigen, Blood see Cryptococcal Antigen Serology, Serum or Cerebrospinal Fluid on previous page

Cryptococcus Latex Antigen Agglutination see Cryptococcal Antigen Serology, Serum or Cerebrospinal Fluid on previous page

Cryptococcus Preparation see India Ink Preparation on page 460

Cryptococcus Serology

Related Information

Cryptococcal Antigen Serology, Serum or Cerebrospinal Fluid on previous page
Periodic Acid-Schiff Stain on page 518

Synonyms Cryptococcosis, IFA; Cryptococcosis, Indirect Fluorescent Antibody Titer

Special Instructions Sequential assays may be desirable

Specimen Serum

Container Red top tube or serum separator tube

Reference Range Negative

Use Diagnosis and prognosis of cryptococcal infections

Limitations A negative test result does not rule out infection because an antibody response may be reduced by circulating antigen bound to antibody. Cross reactions of the IFA test have been reported with blastomycosis, histoplasmosis, and some other fungal infections.

Methodology Tube agglutination, indirect fluorescent antibody

Additional Information Antibody titers ≥1:2 are suggestive of infection with *Cryptococcus neoformans*. Antibody can be detected early in the course of the disease, but if the disease progresses, excess antigen may be produced and render antibodies undetectable. With effective chemotherapy, the antigen titer declines and antibody may once again be demonstrated. Antibodies may persist for long periods even after cessation of chemotherapy.

Selected Readings

Heyworth MF, "Immunology of *Giardia* and *Cryptosporidium* Infections," *J Infect Dis*, 1992, 166(3):465-72.

Kaufman L and Reiss E, "Serodiagnosis of Fungal Diseases," *Manual of Clinical Laboratory Immunology*, 4th ed, Rose NR, de Macario EC, Fahey JL, et al, eds, Washington, DC: American Society for Microbiology, 1992, 506-28.

***Cryptococcus* Stain** *see* India Ink Preparation *on page 460*

Cryptosporidium Diagnostic Procedures, Stool

Related Information

Fecal Leukocyte Stain *on page 408*
Periodic Acid-Schiff Stain *on page 518*

Synonyms Acid-Fast Stain, Modified, *Cryptosporidium*

Test Includes Examination of stool for the presence of *Cryptosporidium*

Special Instructions Procedures for the detection of *Cryptosporidium* in humans have recently become available in most clinical laboratories. Consult the laboratory regarding availability of the procedure and specific specimen collection instructions before collecting the specimen.

Specimen Fresh stool; stool preserved with 10% formalin or sodium acetate-acetic acid formalin preservative

Container Stool container with lid

Collection Transport fresh specimen to laboratory promptly following collection. Specimen on outside of container poses excessive risk of contamination to laboratory personnel.

Reference Range Negative

Use A part of the differential work-up of diarrhea, particularly in immunocompromised hosts and suspected AIDS patients; establish the diagnosis of cryptosporidiosis by demonstration of the oocysts

Limitations The organisms are most readily demonstrated in diarrheal stools. Forms of *Blastocystis hominis* may cause confusion if Giemsa stain is used. Most recommended procedures cannot be performed on polyvinyl alcohol (PVA) preserved specimens.

Methodology Phase contrast microscopy after floatation concentration technique (Sheather's method) is not particularly sensitive; modified acid-fast stain on air-dried smears. Auramine and carbol-fuchsin stain is used by some laboratories for screening. An immunofluorescence test is also available.

Additional Information *Cryptosporidium* is a coccidian parasite of the intestines and respiratory tract of many animals including mice, sheep, snakes, turkeys, chickens, monkeys, and domestic cats. It is a cause of severe and chronic diarrhea in patients with hypogammaglobulinemia and the acquired immune deficiency syndrome. The organism is widely recognized as a disease of the immunocompromised patient, however it can also cause disease in immunocompetent patients. Animal contact, travel to an endemic area, living in a rural environment, and day care attendance by toddlers have been recognized as risk factors for the development of cryptosporidiosis. Perinatal infection has been reported. Children are more prone to develop infection than are adults. In children, the disease is a self-limited gastroenteritis; in immunocompromised patients a profound enteropathy results. There is a seasonal variation in incidence with the highest frequency reported in summer and autumn. The organism can be demonstrated in biopsies of small bowel and colon, adherent to surface of the epithelial cells (Giemsa stain). Most therapeutic regimens for cryptosporidiosis are not successful unless immunosuppression is reversed.

Selected Readings

Baron EJ, Schenone C, and Tanenbaum B, "Comparison of Three Methods for Detection of *Cryptosporidium* Oocysts in a Low-Prevalence Population," *J Clin Microbiol*, 1989, 27(1):223-4.

(Continued)

Cryptosporidium Diagnostic Procedures, Stool (Continued)

Current WL, "The Biology of *Cryptosporidium*," *Am Soc Microbiol News*, 1988, 54:605-11, (review).

Current WL and Garcia LS, "Cryptosporidiosis," *Clin Microbiol Rev*, 1991, 4(3):325-58.

Petersen C, "Cryptosporidiosis in Patients Infected With the Human Immunodeficiency Virus," *Clin Infect Dis*, 1992, 15(6):903-9.

Soave R and Armstrong D, "*Cryptosporidium* and Cryptosporidiosis," *Rev Infect Dis*, 1986, 8(6):1012-23.

Crystals, Urine *see* Urinalysis *on page 562*

CSF Analysis *see* Cerebrospinal Fluid Analysis *on page 354*

CSF Fungus Culture *see* Fungus Culture, Cerebrospinal Fluid *on page 416*

CSF Mycobacteria Culture *see* Mycobacteria Culture, Cerebrospinal Fluid *on page 494*

CSF VDRL *see* VDRL, Cerebrospinal Fluid *on page 570*

CT, Lower Abdomen *see* Computed Transaxial Tomography, Abdomen Studies *on page 373*

C. trachomatis LCx® *see* Chlamydia trachomatis DNA by LCR *on page 365*

CT, Total Abdomen *see* Computed Transaxial Tomography, Abdomen Studies *on page 373*

CT, Upper Abdomen *see* Computed Transaxial Tomography, Abdomen Studies *on page 373*

Culdocentesis *see* Cytology, Body Fluids *on page 386*

Culture, Biopsy *see* Aerobic Culture, Body Fluid *on page 310*

Culture, Biopsy *see* Biopsy Culture, Routine *on page 337*

Culture, Blood *see* Blood Culture, Aerobic and Anaerobic *on page 337*

Culture for *Leptospira* *see* Leptospira Culture *on page 472*

Culture, HSV Only *see* Herpes Simplex Virus Isolation, Rapid *on page 447*

Culture, *Legionella pneumophila* *see* Legionella pneumophila Culture *on page 469*

CXR *see* Chest Films *on page 359*

Cyst Culture, Aerobic *see* Biopsy Culture, Routine *on page 337*

Cyst Culture, Anaerobic *see* Anaerobic Culture *on page 316*

Cyst Culture, Fungus *see* Fungus Culture, Biopsy *on page 414*

Cystometrogram, Simple

Synonyms CMG; Cystometry; Filling Cystometrogram; Simple CMG; Urodynamic Testing of Bladder Function

Test Includes Bedside evaluation of urinary bladder function in selected patients with urinary incontinence or retention. The bladder is passively filled with sterile water through a transurethral Foley catheter. Intravesical pressures are measured with an open manometer as bladder volume increases. Information regarding bladder sensation, capacity, and contractility is obtained.

Patient Preparation Technique and risks of the procedure are explained to the patient and consent is obtained. Ideally, patient should be off sedatives, cholinergics, or anticholinergics prior to testing. Indwelling Foley catheters should be removed well in advance so that residual volume may be measured. No pain medications or anxiolytics are routinely necessary. Patient is asked to void, if possible, immediately prior to procedure.

Aftercare No specific postprocedure restrictions are required and previous activity level may be resumed. At physician discretion, a urinalysis (and possibly urine culture) may be ordered on follow-up, 48-72 hours later.

Special Instructions Simple cystometry may be easily performed by a trained nurse or physician assistant and in most cases does not require direct physician supervision. This is a considerable advantage over complex cystometry which is usually performed in the Urodynamics Laboratory.

Complications This procedure is considered relatively safe. The vast majority of patients tolerate simple cystometry with minimal problems. Reported complications are similar to those seen with straight catheterization, such as local urethral discomfort, hematuria, and urinary tract infection. The precise complication rate is not known, but in one study involving 171 incontinent geriatric patients, <8% developed new urinary symptoms consistent with infection and <2% required antibiotic therapy.

Equipment Standard Foley catheter or 14F red rubber catheter required. Alternatively, a 3-channel Foley catheter (often used for bladder irrigation) may be used. Also needed are a urinary catheterization tray (drapes, lubricant, iodine, gloves, syringes, etc), Y-connector, 50 mL syringe, sterile water in graduated container, sterile tubing, nonsterile measuring basin. An open manometer, such as a spinal manometer, is commonly used.

Technique Numerous minor variations in technique have been described with the choice depending on physician preference and patient logistics. In its simplest form, a manometer is not used. After voiding, patient is placed in supine position and a Foley catheter (or 14F red rubber straight catheter) is inserted transurethrally into the bladder. Residual urine volume is measured and the catheter is left in place. With the bladder empty, the patient is requested to relax completely and avoid all bladder or abdominal contractions for the remainder of the procedure. The inner piston of a 50 mL syringe is removed and the syringe tip inserted into the distal (open) end of the catheter. Using the syringe as a funnel, room temperature sterile water is infused through the syringe and catheter in 50 mL increments. The syringe is elevated so the highest level of the fluid column is always 15 cm above the symphysis pubis. Thus, fluid enters the bladder by gravity drainage and not forcibly by syringe pressure. After each 50 mL water, the height of the water column is observed. Patient subjectively reports first perceptible sensation of bladder fullness and first strong urge to void. When patient notes a strong voiding urge, additional volume is added in 25 mL increments until discomfort is reported or an involuntary bladder contraction occurs. A bladder contraction appears as a sharp and sustained rise in the water column despite attempted voluntary bladder relaxation (and may be seen at any time during the procedure). The procedure is terminated at this stage. This brief sequence of maneuvers has been described in several formal studies comparing simple and complex multichannel cystometry. A common and time-honored variation of this procedure requires the use of a spinal manometer. Initial steps are identical. After residual volume is measured, a Y-connector is attached to the distal end of the Foley. Through one arm of the Y-connector, sterile water in a calibrated reservoir is instilled by gravity drainage. The other arm is connected to an open spinal manometer via sterile connecting tubing. An anaeroid manometer (Lewis cystometer) may also be used. Pressure within the tubing system is "bled off" into the manometer port. As water incrementally fills the bladder, increasing intravesicular pressure is transmitted back through the tubing and is crudely estimated by the height of the water column in the manometer. A plot of bladder pressure versus volume may be constructed in this manner. Alternatively, a 3-channel Foley may be used. Again, fluid is introduced through 1-catheter channel, but in this technique the spinal manometer is connected to a physically separate channel. This allows more accurate intravesical pressure estimations. When bladder pressure is measured in the fluid in the flow channel (as in the Y-connector arrangement), several confounding variables are introduced, such as the internal resistance to fluid in the catheter. Some of these variables are eliminated by this simple maneuver.

Data Acquired
- residual volume (mL)
- threshold for sensation of bladder fullness (mL) - the volume at which patient reports first sensation of fullness
- maximum cystometric capacity (mL) - the volume at which patient describes a strong urge to void, or the volume just prior to an involuntary contraction
- bladder contractility (presence and number of involuntary bladder contractions, as defined)

If a manometer is used, additional data includes:
- pressure-volume characteristics of the bladder during filling, this is termed the cystometrogram - bladder pressure (ordinate) plotted against volume (abscissa)
- bladder compliance, defined as $\Delta V/\Delta P$ and is derived from the cystometrogram

Normal Findings Approximated as follows:
- residual volume - usually minimal or no urine obtained
- threshold for sensation of bladder fullness, 100-200 mL
- maximum capacity, 400-500 mL
- bladder contractility, no involuntary contractions noted
- cystometrogram, normally divided into the following four phases: (see figure on next page)
- compliance - normally very high in phase two of the cystometrogram (approaching infinity)

(Continued)

Cystometrogram, Simple *(Continued)*

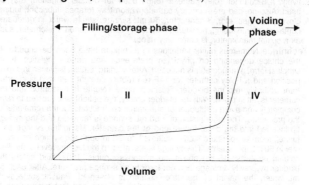

Phase 1: Initial pressure rise, stabilizes at the initial filling pressure or "resting pressure," normally approximately 10 cm H_2O.

Phase 2: The tonus limb, where compliance is high; pressure normally is low and remains constant as volume increases.

Phase 3: The limit of bladder elastic properties; increasing volume causes marked pressure increases. Patient normally can still voluntarily control micturition, even through maximum bladder capacity has almost been reached.

Phase 4: Voluntary voiding (not tested with simple cystometry).

Idealized cystometrogram. Note that the voiding phase is only assessed with complex cystometry. Reproduced with permission from Wein AJ, et al, *Urol Clin North Am,* 1988, 15(4):613.

Critical Values Residual volume: Significant postvoid residual may result from sensory neuropathy, lower motor neuron (LMN) disease, or bladder outlet resistance (functional or mechanical).

Threshold of sensation: Decreased sensation (ie, threshold >200 mL) is seen with sensory neuropathies such as diabetes mellitus, tabes dorsalis, cauda equina syndrome, or normal variant.

Maximum capacity: Decreased in a variety of disorders including upper motor neuron (UMN) disease, fibrotic bladder (eg, tuberculous interstitial cystitis), dysfunctionalized bladder, etc. Increased capacity (>500 mL) is seen with sensory neuropathy, LMN disease, chronic obstruction, bladder "training".

Contractility: Involuntary contractions at volumes less than capacity are abnormal. This condition has been called "detrusor hyper-reflexia" and "uninhibited" or "unstable" bladder. Increased contractility is found in various stroke syndromes, UMN lesions, hypertrophic bladder. Contractility is absent or weak in LMN lesions, sensory neuropathies, or voluntary inhibition.

Cystometrogram: Both the pattern of the tracing (pressure vs volume) and the absolute values should be compared against a standard normal curve. Some cystometrogram patterns may be diagnostic but tracings generated from simple cystometry are crude and may be difficult to interpret.

Compliance: A noncompliant bladder may result from a variety of disorders, including bladder wall fibrosis, bladder contraction, idiopathic male enuresis.

Use The exact indications for simple cystometry are controversial. Even amongst urologists, considerable debate exists in the medical/surgical literature considering the optimal role of this procedure. Simple cystometry is useful in the patient with persistent urinary incontinence or retention felt to be secondary to impaired bladder filling or storage. Common clinical indications for this test include:
- suspected "neurogenic bladder"

- suspected detrusor motor instability, the hyper-reflexive bladder
- suspected abnormalities in bladder sensation, capacity, or contractility
- the geriatric patient with persistent urinary incontinence of unclear etiology (controversial)

Simple cystometry is less useful in evaluating the following conditions:
- suspected stress urinary incontinence in the female
- suspected psychogenic urinary incontinence in the male
- suspected urinary obstruction in the male

Limitations Procedure has questionable utility in the diagnosis of voiding disorders due to structural abnormalities, such as stress urinary incontinence or prostatic hypertrophy with retention, or complex voiding disorders. By nature, passive filling of the bladder is nonphysiologic and may potentially alter measured variables (eg, bladder capacity) in yet-to-be-understood ways. Only urologic function related to the bladder is assessed. Urine flow, force, urethral function, and myoneural coordination are not tested. Numerous technical factors may lead to false-positive or false-negative results. As previously mentioned, intravesical pressure is only crudely estimated by spinal manometry and is limited by confounding factors, such as inflow tubing resistance. Phase 4 of the standard cystometrogram is not evaluated (ie, the voiding phase of micturition). Complex cystometry is required for this. Increases in intra-abdominal pressure will alter pressure readings. This is not controlled for adequately in this procedure. Increases in manometric pressure readings may be due to increased intravesical pressure, increased abdominal wall pressure, or both. Thus, any abdominal muscle contraction may be misinterpreted as a bladder contraction. Although the examiner may simply observe the patient's abdomen for signs of muscle contraction, this is imprecise. With complex cystometry this is avoided by simultaneously recording intravesical and anorectal pressures (which estimate intra-abdominal pressure). The cystometrogram generated by manometer readings is discontinuous and crude. Provocative measures (position changes, medications, etc) are not routinely performed. These are usually reserved for complex cystometry.

Contraindications
- patient refusal
- the demented patient with severe cognitive impairment; this procedure requires the patient to accurately report sensations of bladder filling
- inability to pass transurethral Foley catheter
- active urinary tract infection

Additional Information The main advantage of simple cystometry is its convenience and low cost in comparison with more complex urodynamic testing. It may be performed by a trained nurse in less than minutes and need not be done in a hospital setting. Thus, it has been advocated for the evaluation of the nursing home patient or the elderly clinic patient. Several studies have compared simple and complex cystometry directly. Sutherst and Brown (1984) found that simple cystometry achieved a sensitivity of 100% for bladder instability with 89% specificity (when compared with complex cystometry as a gold standard). Ouslander (1988) also showed a high degree of correlation between the two tests in terms of bladder capacity and stability. However, the role of cystometry has not been clearly defined. Some authorities believe that only a small percentage of patients with voiding disorders need to undergo cystometry. This subpopulation may be identified using statistically derived algorithms based primarily on historical and physical examination findings. Others feel that the urologic history is misleading often enough (or inaccurate in the demented geriatric patient) to justify frequent use of simple cystometry. In many cases, it is argued, management of a voiding disorder will be influenced by the objective results from cystometry. In all cases, test results must be interpreted in conjunction with the clinical suspicion.

Selected Readings
Hilton P and Stanton SL, "Algorithmic Method for Assessing Urinary Incontinence in Elderly Women," *Br Med J [Clin Res]*, 1981, 282(6268):940-2.

Hinman F Jr, "Office Evaluation of Urodynamic Problems," *Urol Clin North Am*, 1979, 6(1):149-54.

Ouslander J, Leach G, Abelson S, et al, "Simple Versus Multichannel Cystometry in the Evaluation of Bladder Function in an Incontinent Geriatric Population," *J Urol*, 1988, 140(6):1482-6.

Sutherst JR and Brown MC, "Comparison of Single and Multichannel Cystometry in Diagnosing Bladder Instability," *Br Med J [Clin Res]*, 1984, 288(6432):1720-2.

Tanagho EA, "Urodynamic Studies," *Smith's General Urology*, Tanagho EA and McAninch JW, eds, 12th ed, Chapter 21, Norwalk, CT: Appleton and Lange, 1988, 452-72.

(Continued)

Cystometrogram, Simple *(Continued)*

Wein AJ, English WS, and Whitmore KE, "Office Urodynamics," *Urol Clin North Am*, 1988, 15(4):609-23.

Cystometry *see* Cystometrogram, Simple *on page 382*

Cytology, Body Fluids

Synonyms Body Cavity Fluid Cytology; Effusion, Cytology; Fluids, Cytology

Applies to Ascitic Fluid Cytology; Culdocentesis; Paracentesis Fluid Cytology; Pericardial Fluid Cytology; Peritoneal Fluid Cytology; Pleural Fluid Cytology; Synovial Fluid Cytology; Thoracentesis Fluid Cytology

Test Includes Cytologic evaluation of smears, cytocentrifuge preparations, filters, and cell block when indicated

Patient Preparation Patient should sign informed consent prior to procedure. Puncture site should be carefully cleaned and prepped as for any tap.

Special Instructions Add 1 mL of heparin per 100 mL of fluid anticipated (each mL of heparin contains 1000 units). Include pertinent clinical information on requisition - previous malignancy, drugs, radiation therapy, history of alcohol abuse, or infection suspected.

Specimen Fresh body fluid

Container 150 mL vacuum heparinized bottle

Collection Gently agitate the flask as fluid is collected to mix the heparin with the fluid

Storage Instructions After hours place in the refrigerator

Causes for Rejection Fixation of any type, improper labeling or requisition, gross contamination due to spillage, prolonged period (over 24 hours) at room temperature

Use Establish the presence of primary or metastatic neoplasms; aid in the diagnosis of rheumatoid pleuritis, systemic lupus erythematosus, myeloproliferative and lymphoproliferative disorders, fungal and parasitic infestation of serous cavities, and fistulas involving serous cavities. Examination of synovial fluid from a joint effusion may aid in the diagnosis of metabolic arthritis (gout or pseudogout), rheumatoid arthritis, or traumatic arthritis. Examination of effusion is more sensitive and specific than blind pleural biopsy in the diagnosis of malignant pleural disease.

Limitations Allowing fluid to stand for prolonged period before processing may cause deterioration and artifact. Cells in fluids of long duration may be degenerated on first tap and a second tap may be required after reaccumulation for best cytologic detail. Clots may contain diagnostic cells which are unavailable for sampling.

Contraindications Documented bleeding diathesis is a relative contraindication

Additional Information Fluids should be submitted **fresh, unfixed**, and **heparinized** to provide well-preserved, representative, diagnostic material. Exfoliated cells deteriorate rapidly in the effusion, both in and out of the body. The amount of heparin recommended is minimal but adequate to prevent clotting of body cavity fluids and act as a preservative, though excess amounts will not alter cytologic detail. Cytologic evaluation may include the type of neoplasm and suggest its site of origin. The more clinical information provided, especially prior malignancy, prior radiation or chemotherapy, and relevant clinical findings, the better the diagnostic yield.

Selected Readings

Dekker A and Bupp PA, "Cytology of Serous Effusions. An Investigation Into the Usefulness of Cell Blocks Versus Smears," *Am J Clin Pathol*, 1978, 70(6):855-60.

Frist B, Kahan AV, and Koss LG, "Comparison of the Diagnostic Values of Biopsies of the Pleura and Cytologic Evaluation of Pleural Fluids," *Am J Clin Pathol*, 1979, 72(1):48-51.

O'Hara MF, Cousar JB, Glick AD, et al, "Multiparameter Approach to the Diagnosis of Hematopoietic-Lymphoid Neoplasms in Body Fluids," *Diagn Cytopathol*, 1985, 1(1):33-8.

Spieler P and Gloor F, "Identification of Types and Primary Sites of Malignant Tumors by Examination of Exfoliated Tumor Cells in Serous Fluids," *Acta Cytol*, 1985, 29(5):753-67.

Wahl RW, "Curschmann's Spirals in Pleural and Peritoneal Fluids," *Acta Cytol*, 1986, 30(2):147-51.

Cytomegalovirus Antigenemia

Related Information

Cytomegalovirus Culture *on page 388*
Cytomegalovirus Culture, Blood *on page 389*
Cytomegalovirus DNA Hybrid Capture *on page 390*
Cytomegalovirus Isolation, Rapid *on page 392*

Cytomegalovirus Serology *on page 392*

Synonyms CMV Antigenemia; CMV Antigen Test; CMV-Vue™ Assay; pp65 Antigenemia

Test Includes Rapid detection of CMV in polymorphonuclear leukocytes (PMNs) from venous blood. The antigenemia assay detects the lower matrix protein pp65 of CMV (the UL83 gene product) in CMV-infected leukocytes. The pp65 protein is a specific marker for active CMV infection and is present early in infection. The assay is performed by preparing a direct smear of PMNs on a slide, adding a monoclonal antibody specific for pp65, immunostaining (either immunofluorescence or immunoperoxidase), and counting the number of CMV-infected cells. The assay has also been used to quantify the presence of CMV in the blood (ie, to determine the CMV "viral load").

Special Instructions Larger volumes of blood from patients with severe neutropenia may be necessary in order to increase the number of leukocytes available for staining. One study suggested that patients should have an absolute neutrophil count (ANC) of 0.2 x 10^3/mm³ for the assay to be accurate.

Specimen Blood; some investigators have modified the assay successfully to identify CMV-infected cells from other body fluids such as bronchoalveolar lavage fluid and cerebrospinal fluid, but this application remains mainly a research tool.

Container Lavender top (EDTA) tube; green top (heparin) tube or blue top (sodium citrate) tube also acceptable

Collection Clinical specimen must be transported to the laboratory as soon as possible, since the optimal time from collection to the preparation of PMN smears is <6 hours. Some laboratories may have an early cutoff time for accepting specimens due to the complex and manual nature of the assay and may perform the test only once during the day using fresh blood. Other laboratories may accept specimens throughout the day; late specimens are partially processed (slides of PMNs prepared), and the remainder of the assay performed the next morning. The laboratory should be contacted regarding optimal timing of specimen collection especially during evenings and weekends.

Storage Instructions Maximum time from collection to slide preparation is 6 hours. Longer storage may result in excessive loss of leukocytes and may significantly decrease identification and quantification of the virus.

Turnaround Time Same day or the following day

Reference Range Laboratories differ in reporting protocols. Some laboratories may report only a qualitative result for the detection of CMV (ie, yes or no). Others will issue a quantitative result (ie, the number of PMNs antigen positive per slide).

Use The CMV antigenemia test is one of several assays for CMV that have become popular for identifying patients at highest risk for serious CMV disease. The assay is the key element of a "pre-emptive approach" for management of CMV infection in many transplant centers. This therapeutic strategy is based on the identification of early subclinical disease by the use of a reliable laboratory test which can identify a subgroup of patients at the highest risk for clinical disease. CMV dissemination in the blood is now understood to be an important early step in the pathogenesis of CMV disease, and the early detection of circulating antigen-positive PMNs hopefully can identify infection before the development of disease. Pre-emptive therapy differs from prophylactic therapy in that pre-emptive therapy is based on a specific marker for disease (usually a positive laboratory test) which has sufficient predictive power to justify starting antimicrobial therapy. In contrast, prophylactic therapy is started before there is evidence of infection and involves treating larger numbers of people than the pre-emptive approach. CMV antigenemia was one of the first assays used for pre-emptive therapy.

Methodology Some laboratory variation in performing the assay persists, despite efforts to standardize the methodology. One commercially-available kit (CMV-vue™ kit, Incstar Corp) is performed as follows: PMNs are isolated from fresh EDTA-treated blood using 0.5 mL 5% dextran. Contaminating erythrocytes are lyzed using lysing medium. The PMNs are washed and suspended in phosphate-buffered saline and adjusted to make a 2 x 10^6 cells/mL suspension. A 25 µL specimen sample is applied to test wells on the microscope slide. Specimens are fixed in acetone. Slides are stained by an indirect immunoperoxidase technique using mouse monoclonal antibodies directed against the pp65 early structural protein of CMV. This is followed by a horseradish peroxidase labeled
(Continued)

Cytomegalovirus Antigenemia *(Continued)*

anti-mouse antibody. Positively stained cells are viewed by light microscopy. Results are expressed as the number of positive cells relative to the total number of cells per slide.

Additional Information In several studies, CMV antigenemia has proven more sensitive than traditional CMV cell culture techniques and equal to or less sensitive than CMV polymerase chain reaction (PCR). A number of studies have looked at the ability of the antigenemia test to quantify the CMV viral load. The ability of the antigenemia test to predict significant clinical disease later has been variable and appears to depend in part on the type of organ transplant. In general, the higher the degree of CMV antigenemia (ie, the higher the CMV viral load), the better the positive predictive value for the development of clinical disease. For example, one study of allogeneic marrow transplant recipients showed the positive predictive value >1 antigen-positive cell per slide of 75% and the negative predictive value of 72%. In one study of kidney transplant recipients, more than 100 antigen-positive cells per 50,000 cells gave a positive predictive value of 75% and a negative predictive value of 88%. Studies have also attempted to define a CMV-antigenemia threshold over which antiviral therapy should be started. For example, one study suggested that ganciclovir should be started if the assay showed >100 positive cells/slide for heart transplant recipients. Other studies have suggested the threshold is >10 positive cells/slide for kidney transplant recipients, and >2 positive cells/slide for allogeneic bone marrow transplant recipients. (For an in-depth review of CMV antigenemia quantification see the review by Boeckh and Boivin). Although this assay has a reasonable predictive power in transplant recipients, it is clear from several studies that patients with CMV disease may still have a negative antigenemia test, and not all patients with a positive test will go on to develop disease.

The antigenemia assay has also been used to predict the development of CMV disease in persons with AIDS. Several studies have shown that a >50 positive cells/2×10^5 cells in a person with AIDS is correlated with CMV-related symptoms. Three studies have shown that a positive antigenemia test (one or more positive cells/slide) had a positive predictive value for CMV disease of about 45%. Less data is available regarding the utility of antigenemia assay in AIDS than in transplant recipients. Recent studies have instead focused on the use of CMV PCR as a better predictor of CMV disease in AIDS.

CMV antigenemia is a rapid means of CMV detection with results available the same day or the following day. Since it does not require cell culture systems, the assay does not require expensive laboratory equipment. However, the assay is still relatively complex to perform and requires a significant amount of "hands-on" time by trained technicians. One significant limitation is the requirement for rapid specimen processing (within 6 hours). Samples are difficult to batch, and thus, the assay is not well suited for high-volume virology laboratories. Despite these limitations, the assay has proven to be a sensitive and reasonably accurate test for guiding pre-emptive therapy.

Selected Readings

Boeckh M and Boivin G, "Quantitation of Cytomegalovirus: Methodologic Aspects and Clinical Applications," *Clin Microbiol Rev,* 1998, 11(3):533-54.

Erice A, Holm MA, Gill PC, et al, "Cytomegalovirus (CMV) Antigenemia Assay Is More Sensitive Than Shell Vial Cultures for Rapid Detection of CMV in Polymorphonuclear Blood Leukocytes," *J Clin Microbiol,* 1992, 30(11):2822-5.

Erice A, Holm MA, Sanjuan MV, et al, "Evaluation of CMV-vue™ antigenemia Assay for Rapid Detection of Cytomegalovirus in Mixed-Leukocyte Blood Fractions," *J Clin Microbiol,* 1995, 33(4):1014-5.

Landry ML and Ferguson D, "Comparison of Quantitative Cytomegalovirus Antigenemia Assay With Culture Methods and Correlation With Clinical Disease," *J Clin Microbiol,* 1993, 31(11):2851-6.

Cytomegalovirus Culture

Related Information

Cytomegalovirus Antigenemia *on page 386*
Cytomegalovirus Culture, Blood *on next page*
Cytomegalovirus DNA Hybrid Capture *on page 390*
Cytomegalovirus Isolation, Rapid *on page 392*
Cytomegalovirus Serology *on page 392*

Synonyms CMV Culture; Viral Culture, Cytomegalovirus

Test Includes Culture for CMV only; CMV also is usually detected in a routine/general virus culture

Special Instructions Obtain viral transport medium from the laboratory prior to collecting the specimen.

Specimen Urine, throat, bronchoalveolar lavage, bronchial washings, lung biopsy

Container Sterile container; cold viral transport medium for swabs

Collection

Urine: A first morning clean catch urine should be submitted in a sterile screw cap container.

Throat: Rotate swab in both tonsillar crypts and against posterior oropharynx. Place swab in tube of viral transport medium, break off end of swab and tighten cap. This specimen is not particularly productive.

Storage Instructions Do not freeze specimens. Keep specimens cold and moist. Specimens should be delivered to the laboratory and handed to a technologist within 30 minutes of collection. If freezing is absolutely necessary, add an equal amount of 0.4 M sucrose-phosphate to the specimen before freezing.

Causes for Rejection Dry specimen, specimen not refrigerated during transport, specimen fixed in formalin, unlabeled specimen

Turnaround Time Variable (1-14 days) and depends on culture method used and amount of virus in the specimen

Reference Range No virus isolated

Use Aid in the diagnosis of disease caused by CMV (eg, viral infections, pneumonia, and organ transplant-related disease)

Methodology Inoculation of specimen into cell cultures, incubation of cultures, observation of characteristic cytopathic effect, and identification by fluorescent monoclonal antibody

Additional Information CMV infections are very common and are usually asymptomatic. CMV infections are frequently severe and life-threatening in immunocompromised patients including organ recipients and AIDS patients.

CMV is the most frequent cause of congenital viral infections in humans and occurs in about 1% of all newborns. Approximately 90% have no clinical symptoms at birth. Ten percent to 20% of these infants will develop complications before school age. Congenital infection may occur as a result of either primary or recurrent maternal infection.

Serology for the detection of cytomegalovirus is available, but the results are often of limited value unless a fourfold rise in titer can be documented.

Selected Readings
Chou S, "Newer Methods for Diagnosis of Cytomegalovirus Infection," *Rev Infect Dis*, 1990, 12(Suppl 7):S727-36.

Griffiths PD and Grundy JE, "The Status of CMV as a Human Pathogen," *Epidemiol Infect*, 1988, 100(1):1-15.

Landini MP, "New Approaches and Perspectives in Cytomegalovirus Diagnosis," *Prog Med Virol*, 1993, 40:157-77.

Cytomegalovirus Culture, Blood

Related Information
Cytomegalovirus Antigenemia *on page 386*
Cytomegalovirus Culture *on previous page*
Cytomegalovirus DNA Hybrid Capture *on next page*
Cytomegalovirus Isolation, Rapid *on page 392*
Cytomegalovirus Serology *on page 392*

Synonyms Blood Culture for CMV; Buffy Coat Culture for CMV; Buffy Coat Viral Culture; CMV Culture

Test Includes Culture of buffy coat for cytomegalovirus

Specimen Blood

Container Heparinized syringe or green top (heparin) tube

Collection Heparinize a 2 mL syringe with sterile preservative-free heparin. Invert the syringe several times after the blood is drawn to mix the blood thoroughly with the heparin. As an alternative, two 10 mL heparinized tubes may be used if transport of a syringe is difficult.

Storage Instructions Do not store specimen. Transport to the laboratory immediately in sealed plastic bag with request form.

Causes for Rejection Excessive hemolysis, delay in transport, leaking syringes

Turnaround Time Positive cultures will be reported when identification is made. Negative cultures will be reported after 28 days.

Reference Range No virus isolated

(Continued)

Cytomegalovirus Culture, Blood *(Continued)*

Use Detect cytomegaloviremia

Limitations Yield of CMV from this specimen may be high in patients with the acquired immunodeficiency syndrome (AIDS), but significantly lower in non-AIDS patients.

Methodology Cell culture for isolation and identification by indirect fluorescent antibody (IFA)

Cytomegalovirus DNA Hybrid Capture

Related Information

Cytomegalovirus Antigenemia *on page 386*

Cytomegalovirus Culture *on page 388*

Cytomegalovirus Culture, Blood *on previous page*

Cytomegalovirus Isolation, Rapid *on page 392*

Cytomegalovirus Serology *on page 392*

Synonyms CMV DNA Hybrid Capture; Digene CMV Hybrid Capture DNA; DNA Hybrid Capture, CMV; Murex CMV DNA Hybrid Capture Assay

Test Includes CMV hybrid capture (HC) is a new molecular hybridization assay designed for the direct detection of CMV nucleic acid in white blood cells. This assay differs from polymerase chain reaction (PCR) assays since there are no viral amplification steps with HC. In the United States, the assay is commercially available as the Digene CMV Hybrid Capture System™ (Digene Corp, Silver Spring, MD).

HC is relatively simple to perform, rapid (6 hours), and does not require tissue culture techniques or molecular amplification steps. HC technology uses a CMV RNA probe which is capable of binding to a 40,000 base pair segment of the CMV genome. When the probe binds with the target CMV DNA, a "hybrid" of RNA-DNA is formed. The hybrids are then "captured" or immobilized within a special tube coated with antibodies specifically directed against the hybrids. A signal-amplified sandwich capture technique is used, and the hybrids are detected with chemiluminescent substrate. Light emitted is measured as relative light units. The intensity of light is proportional to the amount of target CMV DNA present in the specimen. The assay has been approved for qualitative determinations of CMV (virus absent or present) but can be easily set up for quantitative measurements (eg, copies/mL whole blood).

There are two versions of HC reported in the literature. Version 1 has a lower limit of detection of about 5000 copies of CMV per mL whole blood. Version 2 has a lower limit of about 700 copies per mL whole blood; only Version 2 is available commercially.

Specimen Whole blood

Container Lavender top (EDTA) tube

Storage Instructions Whole blood may be stored for up to 6 days at 4°C without a significant change in results. The ability to store the original specimen for several days is an important advantage for the HC assay and allows for flexible specimen collection on nights and weekends, and shipping specimens to reference laboratories is simplified. This is in contrast to the CMV antigenemia assay which requires prompt processing of fresh specimens within 6 hours.

For research purposes, a cell pellet can be extracted in several simple steps and frozen at -20°C for testing at a later date.

Turnaround Time Results available the same day or the following day, depending on the laboratory protocol.

Reference Range Laboratories may differ in how results are reported. Some laboratories may provide only a qualitative result for the detection of CMV (ie, yes/no); others will issue a quantitative result (eg, the number of CMV copies/mL whole blood).

Use

- Determine if the cause of a mononucleosis-like syndrome is from CMV (fever, myalgias, leukopenia, reactive lymphocytosis, pharyngitis, spleno-megaly). CMV may cause a syndrome similar to infectious mononucleosis from Epstein-Barr virus in both immunocompetent and immunocompro-mised hosts.

- Determine if CMV infection is the cause of fever in an immunocompromised host who has no identifiable focus of infection (ie, the "CMV syndrome"). Laboratory testing in this setting must be interpreted cautiously since some patients may asymptomatically shed CMV in the blood during febrile episodes.

- Determine if CMV may be the cause of disease in a patient with an identified source of infection (ie, the transplant patient with a new pulmonary infiltrate of unknown etiology). Again, a positive DNA result must be interpreted carefully.

- Identify high-risk patients early in the course of CMV infection (ie, "pre-emptive therapy") (see Additional Information).

Limitations CMV hybrid capture is currently performed in a limited number of laboratories. In addition, some laboratories may require a specific request in advance for quantitative rather than qualitative HC results, since several control standards must be included in each test run to calculate a quantitative result.

Methodology A minimum of 3.5 mL whole blood is incubated for 15 minutes in a RBC-lysing solution. WBCs are spun down, washed, and resuspended. The sample is denatured with base which lyses the cells and separates the strands of DNA. A target-specific, single-stranded RNA probe to CMV DNA is added, creating an RNA:DNA hybrid. The RNA probe is large, containing approximately 38 kb of sequences. Hybridization takes place over 2 hours at 70°C. The captured hybrid is detected with a second set of RNA:DNA antibodies conjugated to alkaline phosphatase. Each 38 kb RNA:DNA hybrid binds approximately 1000 antibody conjugate molecules, and each is bound to three alkaline phosphatase molecules. Because each captured hybrid binds up to 3000 alkaline phosphatase molecules, the resulting signal is amplified at least 3000-fold. Substrate is then added. Upon cleavage by the alkaline phosphatase, the substrate produces light that is measured on a luminometer in relative light units. The intensity of the light emitted denotes the presence or absence of target DNA in the specimen.

Additional Information CMV hybrid capture is one of several assays for CMV that have been used to identify patients at highest risk for serious CMV disease. Because HC is a relatively new assay, most of the studies have compared HC to CMV cell culture and to CMV pp65 antigenemia (see separate listings). It is hoped that the HC assay will prove to be equivalent to the pp65 antigenemia as part of a "pre-emptive approach" for management of CMV infection in many transplant centers. This therapeutic strategy is based on the identification of early subclinical disease by the use of a reliable laboratory test which can identify a subgroup of patients at the highest risk for clinical disease. CMV dissemination in the blood is now understood to be an important early step in the pathogenesis of CMV disease, and the early detection of CMV DNA ("DNA-emia") hopefully can identify infection before the development of disease. Pre-emptive therapy differs from prophylactic therapy in that pre-emptive therapy is based on a specific marker for disease (usually a positive laboratory test) which has sufficient predictive power to justify starting antimicrobial therapy. In contrast, prophylactic therapy is started before there is evidence of infection and involves treating larger numbers of people than the pre-emptive approach.

CMV antigenemia was one of the first assays used for pre-emptive therapy. HC and pp65 antigenemia appear to have comparable sensitivity and specificity based on the results of several comparison trials. How well the HC and pp65 antigenemia assays correlate in terms of quantitation of CMV is unknown. Larger studies are underway to study the quantitative aspects of HC. Several questions remain to be answered: (1) is there a "threshold" CMV DNA level as determined by HC that is associated with clinical disease, (2) what are the positive and negative predictive values of HC in predicting end-organ disease, (3) how does HC compare with other methods for CMV quantitation including pp65 antigenemia and quantitative PCR, and (4) how useful is HC in monitoring response to therapy?

HC has several advantages over existing assays for CMV. Because there are no target amplification steps, HC avoids the problem of contamination seen with PCR. In addition the problems with enzymatic inhibitors reported with PCR have not been noted with HC. HC also has several advantages over pp65 antigenemia, including the ease of specimen preparation, the stability of the original specimen for several days prior to laboratory processing, ability to batch specimens for large runs, and an objective, semiautomated means of viral quantification.

(Continued)

LIVERPOOL JOHN MOORES UNIVERSITY
LEARNING SERVICES

Cytomegalovirus DNA Hybrid Capture *(Continued)*

Selected Readings

Barrett-Muir WY, Aitken C, Templeton K, et al, "Evaluation of the Murex Hybrid Capture Cytomegalovirus DNA Assay Versus Plasma PCR and Shell Vial Assay for Diagnosis of Human Cytomegalovirus Viremia in Immunocompromised Patients," *J Clin Microbiol*, 1998, 36(9):2554-6.

Boeckh M and Boivin G, "Quantitation of Cytomegalovirus: Methodologic Aspects and Clinical Applications," *Clin Microbiol Rev*, 1998, 11(3):533-54.

Bossart W, Bienz K, and Wunderli W, "Surveillance of Cytomegalovirus After Solid-Organ Transplantation: Comparison of pp65 Antigenemia Assay With a Quantitative DNA Hybridization Assay," *J Clin Microbiol*, 1997, 35(12):3303-4.

Mazzulli T, Wood S, Chua R, et al, "Evaluation of the Digene Hybrid Capture System for Detection and Quantitation of Human Cytomegalovirus Viremia in Human Immunodeficiency Virus-Infected Patients," *J Clin Microbiol*, 1996, 34(12):2959-62.

Veal N, Payan C, Fray D, et al, "Novel DNA Assay for Cytomegalovirus Detection: Comparison With Conventional Culture and pp65 Antigenemia Assay," *J Clin Microbiol*, 1996, 34(12):3097-100.

Cytomegalovirus Isolation, Rapid

Related Information

Cytomegalovirus Antigenemia *on page 386*
Cytomegalovirus Culture *on page 388*
Cytomegalovirus Culture, Blood *on page 389*
Cytomegalovirus DNA Hybrid Capture *on page 390*
Cytomegalovirus Serology *on this page*

Synonyms CMV Early Antigen FA Method; CMV Shell Vial Method

Test Includes Inoculation of cell cultures in shell vials, 16-hour incubation, and immunofluorescence staining of CMV early nuclear antigen with monoclonal antibodies; conventional cell culture inoculation

Specimen Urine, bronchoalveolar lavage, blood, tracheal aspirates, appropriate autopsy and biopsy specimens

Container Sterile container; cold viral transport medium for swabs

Collection

Urine: A first morning clean catch urine should be submitted in a sterile screw cap container.

Throat: Rotate swab in both tonsillar crypts and against posterior oropharynx. Place swab in tube of viral transport medium, break off end of swab and tighten cap. This specimen is not particularly productive.

Turnaround Time Overnight to 2 days depending on method and capability of laboratory

Reference Range No CMV detected

Use Aid in the diagnosis of disease caused by CMV (eg, viral infections, pneumonia, and organ transplant-related disease)

Limitations The rapid shell vial method for the detection of CMV has been reported to be more sensitive than conventional cell culture.

Methodology Specimens are centrifuged onto cell cultures grown on coverslips in the bottoms of 1-dram shell vials. Centrifugation greatly accelerates virus attachment and penetration. After incubation, fluorescein-labeled monoclonal antibodies are applied to the infected cells to detect viral antigens that are expressed in the membranes of the cells. Characteristic fluorescent foci indicate the presence of virus.

Selected Readings

Gleaves CA, Smith TF, Shuster EA, et al, "Comparison of Standard Tube and Shell Vial Cell Culture Techniques for the Detection of Cytomegalovirus in Clinical Specimens," *J Clin Microbiol*, 1985, 21(2):217-21.

Smith TF, "Rapid Methods for the Diagnosis of Viral Infections," *Lab Med*, 1987, 18:16-20.

Cytomegalovirus Serology

Related Information

Cytomegalovirus Antigenemia *on page 386*
Cytomegalovirus Culture *on page 388*
Cytomegalovirus Culture, Blood *on page 389*
Cytomegalovirus DNA Hybrid Capture *on page 390*
Cytomegalovirus Isolation, Rapid *on this page*

Synonyms CMV-IFA; CMV Titer

Applies to CMV-IFA, IgG; CMV-IFA, IgM

Test Includes IgG and IgM testing of acute sera in neonates, patients suspected of post-transfusion CMV infection, immunosuppressed patients, and maternity cases; IgG testing of acute and convalescent sera

Specimen Serum

Container Red top tube or serum separator tube

Sampling Time Acute and convalescent sera drawn 10-14 days apart are required

Storage Instructions Store at 4°C or freeze.

Reference Range IgM <1:8 and IgG <1:16 is considered nondiagnostic. A four-fold increase in titer in paired sera drawn 10-14 days apart is usually indicative of acute infection.

Use Support the diagnosis of cytomegalovirus infection

Limitations Heterophil antibodies and presence of rheumatoid factor may cause false-positive IgM results. Fetal IgM antibody to maternal IgG may also cause false-positive results. Because of high levels of "background" antibody in adult populations, a single antibody determination is not useful. For rapid confirmation of new CMV infection, rapid shell vial culture for CMV is superior to serology.

Methodology Indirect fluorescent antibody (IFA), enzyme immunoassay (EIA)

Additional Information A single titer is rarely significant if past history is unknown. A fourfold or greater rise in CMV titer between acute and convalescent specimens is evidence of infection. A single IgM specific titer >1:8 is also excellent evidence of acute infection. CMV causes an infectious mononucleosis syndrome clinically indistinguishable from heterophil positive mononucleosis, a very common disease. Significant CMV titers are found almost universally in patients with AIDS, and CMV genome has been demonstrated in the cells of Kaposi's sarcoma. CMV is a significant cause of postcardiotomy, post-transplant and postpump hepatitis syndromes.

Although serology is a useful method to detect CMV infections, the newer shell vial culture can more reliably identify symptomatic CMV infections in immuno-compromised patients.

Several new EIA tests agree well with the IFA serology and provide a more objective measure of infection status than the subjective IFA test.

Selected Readings

Bryan JA, "The Serologic Diagnosis of Viral Infections," *Arch Pathol Lab Med*, 1987, 111(11):1015-23.

Marsano L, Perrillo RP, Flye MW, et al, "Comparison of Culture and Serology for the Diagnosis of Cytomegalovirus Infection in Kidney and Liver Transplant Recipients," *J Infect Dis*, 1990, 161(3):454-61.

Van Enk RA, James KK, and Thompson KD, "Evaluation of Three Commercial Enzyme Immunoassays for *Toxoplasma* and Cytomegalovirus Antibodies," *Am J Clin Pathol*, 1991, 95(3):428-34.

Waner JL and Stewart JA, "Cytomegalovirus," *Manual of Clinical Laboratory Immunology*, 4th ed, Rose NR, de Macario EC, Fahey JL, et al, eds, Washington, DC: American Society for Microbiology, 1992, 563-7.

Darkfield Examination, Leptospirosis

Related Information

Leptospira Culture *on page 472*

Leptospira Serology *on page 472*

Mycoplasma pneumoniae Diagnostic Procedures *on page 497*

Synonyms Darkfield Microscopy, *Leptospira*; Leptospirosis, Darkfield Examination

Test Includes Examination of serum, urine, or CSF for organisms

Specimen Urine, serum, cerebrospinal fluid

Container Sterile plastic urine container, red top tube, or sterile CSF tube

Causes for Rejection Specimen dried out

Use Evaluate the presence of *Leptospira* to establish the diagnosis of leptospirosis. The failure to detect leptospires does not rule out their presence.

Limitations Culture for *Leptospira* is a more valuable and sensitive test. The concentration of leptospires in blood and CSF is low. Therefore, concentration by centrifugation with sodium oxalate or heparin can be useful. The incidence of false-positives is increased because fibrils and cellular extrusions can be mistaken for organisms. Extreme technical expertise is required.

Methodology A very small drop of fluid is distributed in a thin layer between a glass coverslip and slide. Positives should be confirmed by serologic or cultural methods. The typical morphology helicoidal, flexible organisms 6-20 μm long and 0.1 μm in diameter usually with semicircular hooked ends should be observed before a presumptive diagnosis is made. Artifacts are common. (Continued)

Darkfield Examination, Leptospirosis *(Continued)*

Additional Information *Leptospira* are present in blood early in course of the disease (first week only). After 10-14 days they may be found in the urine. Urine must be neutral or alkaline. Culture has much greater value for diagnosis.

Darkfield microscopy is best used to demonstrate leptospires in specimens in which a high concentration of organisms is present, ie, tissue from animals (guinea pig or hamster), inoculation including blood, peritoneal fluid, or liver suspensions. Urine or kidney suspensions from swine, dogs, and domestic animals may also yield positive darkfield examination.

Selected Readings
Alexander AD, "*Leptospira,*" *Manual of Clinical Microbiology,* 5th ed, Balows A, Hausler WJ Jr, Herrmann KL, et al, eds, Washington, DC: American Society for Microbiology, 1991, 554-9.

Darkfield Examination, Syphilis

Related Information
FTA-ABS, Serum *on page 410*
RPR *on page 530*
VDRL, Cerebrospinal Fluid *on page 570*

Synonyms Darkfield Microscopy, Syphilis; Syphilis, Darkfield Examination; *Treponema pallidum* Darkfield Examination

Test Includes Cleansing of chancre, procurement of specimen, and darkfield examination

Patient Preparation The surface of the chancre is cleansed and roughened by the physician with a swab or gauze moistened with saline. This removes exudate and excess bacteria contamination. Serum is then collected from the surface of the chancre using a small pipette. The serum is placed on a slide or coverslip. Alternatively, the specimen can be collected by directly touching the slide to the lesion. The object is to obtain clear serum exudate from the subsurface of the lesion. It is then examined by darkfield microscopy.

Specimen Moist serum from the base of a cleansed unhealed chancre. The youngest lesion available is best. The chance of identification of treponemes decreases with the age of the lesion as it dries and heals.

Causes for Rejection Healed chancre, previous treatment, ointment, dried up specimen

Reference Range *Treponema pallidum* has a rapid and purposeful motion as it travels across the microscopic field. The organisms appear as a tight corkscrew. The organisms are 1.0 to 1.5 times the diameter of an RBC in length.

Use Determine the presence of characteristic spirochetes in lesions suspected of being syphilis

Limitations Darkfield examination is of limited value in oral and rectal lesions because of the normal presence of other nonpathogenic spirochetes. Dry or bloody specimens render this examination worthless. The specimen should be examined within 15 minutes of collection because the organisms lose motility with decrease in temperature.

Contraindications Antibiotic therapy prior to the darkfield examination. The organisms are rapidly cleared following therapy.

Methodology Darkfield microscopy. Motile organisms are observed to rotate around their long axis and to bend, snap, and flex along their length. A smooth translational back and forth directed movement is also apparent.

Additional Information *Treponema* can be found in skin lesions and lymph nodes in secondary syphilis but are more plentiful in primary chancres. They cannot be grown in culture.

Selected Readings
Fitzgerald TJ, "*Treponema,*" *Manual of Clinical Microbiology,* 5th ed, Balows A, Hausler WJ Jr, Herrmann KL, et al, eds, Washington, DC: American Society for Microbiology, 1991, 567-71.
Larsen SA, "Syphilis," *Clin Lab Med,* 1989, 9(3):545-57.

Darkfield Microscopy, *Leptospira* see Darkfield Examination, Leptospirosis *on previous page*

Darkfield Microscopy, Syphilis see Darkfield Examination, Syphilis *on this page*

Davidsohn Differential *replaced by* Infectious Mononucleosis Serology *on page 462*

Deer Tick Identification *see* Arthropod Identification *on page 334*

Delayed Hypersensitivity Fungal Skin Tests *see* Fungal Skin Testing *on page 411*

Delayed Reaction Intracutaneous Tests *see* Anergy Skin Test Battery *on page 318*

Delta Agent Serology *see* Hepatitis D Serology *on page 442*

Delta Hepatitis Serology *see* Hepatitis D Serology *on page 442*

Dermatitis Herpetiformis Antibodies *see* Skin Biopsy, Immunofluorescence *on page 538*

Dermatophyte Fungus Culture *see* Fungus Culture, Skin *on page 417*

Digene CMV Hybrid Capture DNA *see* Cytomegalovirus DNA Hybrid Capture *on page 390*

Diphtheria Culture *see* Throat Culture for *Corynebacterium diphtheriae on page 549*

Direct Detection of Virus *see* Virus Detection by DFA *on page 576*

Direct Fluorescent Antibody Smear for *Legionella pneumophila* *see* Legionella *pneumophila* Smear *on page 470*

Direct Fluorescent Antibody Test for Virus *see* Virus Detection by DFA *on page 576*

Direct Immunofluorescent Studies, Biopsy *see* Immunofluorescent Studies, Biopsy *on page 460*

DNA Hybrid Capture, CMV *see* Cytomegalovirus DNA Hybrid Capture *on page 390*

DNA Hybridization Test for *Chlamydia trachomatis* *see* Chlamydia trachomatis by DNA Probe *on page 364*

DNA Hybridization Test for *Neisseria gonorrhoeae* *see* Neisseria gonorrhoeae by Nucleic Acid Probe *on page 500*

DNA Probe for *Legionella* *see* Legionella DNA Probe *on page 469*

DNA Probe for Mycobacteria *see* Mycobacteria Culture, Sputum *on page 495*

DNA Test for *Chlamydia trachomatis* *see* Chlamydia trachomatis by DNA Probe *on page 364*

DNA Test for *Neisseria gonorrhoeae* *see* Neisseria gonorrhoeae by Nucleic Acid Probe *on page 500*

Eaton Agent Titer *see* Mycoplasma Serology *on page 499*

EB Nuclear Antigens *see* Epstein-Barr Virus Serology *on page 406*

EBV Culture *see* Epstein-Barr Virus Culture *on page 406*

EB Virus Titer *see* Epstein-Barr Virus Serology *on page 406*

EBV Titer *see* Epstein-Barr Virus Serology *on page 406*

Echocardiography, M-Mode

Synonyms M-Mode Echo; Unidimensional Echo

Test Includes M-mode echocardiography, the first form of cardiac ultrasound used in clinical practice, takes its name from the motion of the cardiac structures that was possible to visualize when this diagnostic method was introduced. M-mode echocardiography provides an "ice pick" view of the heart with a very high temporal and unidimensional space resolution, so that it provides an excellent method to measure chamber dimensions and to time cardiac events.

Patient Preparation No special patient preparation is required. Fasting is not necessary. The procedure can be done at any time. In scheduling patients that will have multiple cardiac diagnostic procedures it will be best to order the echocardiogram before Holter monitoring since the multiple electrodes placed on the chest for this procedure may interfere with the performance of the echocardiogram. Also, if a patient is to have a stress test on the same day, enough time (2-3 hours) should be allowed after the exercise test to perform the echocardiogram under basal conditions.

Special Instructions In most cases the M-mode echocardiogram is performed as part of a more complete cardiac ultrasound study that includes either 2-D echocardiography and/or Doppler echocardiography. The test that provides the most information should be requested, although sometimes this decision is left to the personnel in the Echo Laboratory. A complete cardiac ultrasound study takes anywhere from 60-90 minutes, the "M-mode" part of it takes approximately 30 minutes. To optimize the diagnostic yield of the echocardiogram a note relating the reason for the request should be made in the patient's chart or in a requisition form. Other useful information to be presented includes patient's age, weight, and height.

Technique A patient arriving at the Echo Laboratory is greeted by the laboratory personnel. He/she is asked about any previous experience with the procedure (Continued)

Echocardiography, M-Mode (Continued)

and is given a brief description of the test. Patient is asked to undress from the waist up and is given a gown with the opening in the front. Three electrodes for EKG monitorization are placed on the chest and the patient is asked to lie in a left lateral decubitus position. Currently, most M-mode echocardiograms are obtained by using a 2-D echocardiographic probe and selecting M-mode information from it. Briefly, the transducer is placed at the left parasternal border, the long axis view is selected, and the M-mode line is moved from the left ventricle to the mitral valve and finally to the aorta and left atrium. Recordings at these levels are registered in a strip chart recorder, a video recorder, or a page printer. These recordings become part of the report and of the Echo Laboratory file.

Normal Findings Adequate interpretation of M-mode echocardiography requires knowledge of the normal values of the dimension of the cardiac chambers and great arteries (see table), and an understanding of the normal motion of the valves and different walls of the cardiac system. Distinct abnormalities can be characterized by M-mode echocardiography for many cardiovascular disorders.

Normal M-Mode Echocardiographic Values

	Mean (cm)	Range (cm)
RVD	1.7	0.9-2.6
LVIDD	4.7	3.5-5.7
PLVWT	0.9	0.6-1.1
IVSWT	0.9	0.6-1.1
LA	2.9	1.9-4.0
AO	2.7	2.0-3.7
FS	36%	34%-44%

RVD = Right ventricular dimension

LVIDD = Left ventricular internal dimension in diastole

PLVWT = Posterior left ventricular wall thickness

IVSWT = Interventricular wall thickness

LA = Left atrium

AO = Aorta

FS = Fractional shortening

From Feigenbaum H, *Echocardiography*, 4th ed, Philadelphia, PA: Lea & Febiger, 1986, with permission.

Use The most common indications for this test include:
- wall thickness measurement of interventricular septum, posterior left ventricular wall and right ventricular free wall
- measurement of end-diastolic and end-systolic left ventricular internal dimensions
- percent of fractional shortening (difference between end-diastolic and end-systolic dimensions divided by end-diastolic dimension)
- measurement of right ventricular dimension; measurement of the anteroposterior diameter of the ascending aorta and left atrium.

M-mode echocardiography is **most useful** in:
- diagnosis of pericardial effusion
- left ventricular hypertrophy
- generalized left ventricular dysfunction
- hypertrophic obstructive cardiomyopathy
- mitral valve prolapse
- mitral stenosis
- left atrial myxoma

Contraindications There are no contraindications for M-mode echocardiography but patients with chronic obstructive lung disease or marked obesity will usually have tests of poor diagnostic quality.

Selected Readings

Sahn DJ, DeMaria A, Kisslo J, et al, "Recommendations Regarding Quantitation in M-Mode Echocardiography: Results of a Survey of Echocardiographic Measurements," *Circulation*, 1978, 58(6):1072-83.

Echovirus Culture see Enterovirus Culture on page 405

Echovirus Culture, Stool *see* Viral Culture, Stool *on page 573*
Ectoparasite Identification *see* Arthropod Identification *on page 334*
EEG *see* Electroencephalography *on this page*
Effusion, Cytology *see* Cytology, Body Fluids *on page 386*

Ehrlichia Serology
Related Information
Rocky Mountain Spotted Fever Serology *on page 529*
Test Includes Antibody to *Ehrlichia canis*
Specimen Serum
Container Red top tube or serum separator tube
Sampling Time Acute and convalescent serum 14-21 days apart are recommended.
Storage Instructions Separate serum and refrigerate.
Causes for Rejection Inadequate labeling, excessive hemolysis, chylous serum
Use Establish the diagnosis of ehrlichiosis
Methodology Indirect fluorescent antibody (IFA)
Additional Information Newly recognized human ehrlichiosis is a disease caused by a Rickettsiaceae (*Ehrlichia*) family member which is well known for causing disease in animals. Human infection with an *Ehrlichia canis*-like organism was first described in the United States in 1986. Preliminary data suggest that human ehrlichiosis is tickborne, and that most human cases present with symptoms suggestive of RMSF without the rash or as "spotless" RMSF. *E. canis* is found in white blood cells, in particular, polymorphonuclear leukocytes and mononuclear cells. During acute illness, intracellular inclusions (in monocytes) of *E. canis* can be observed on peripheral blood smears. IgG titers of 1:16-1:32 are considered equivocal while IgG titers ≥1:64 are indicative of *E. canis* infection. Titers which show a fourfold or greater increase in IgG or the presence of IgM against *E. canis* is indicative of recent or current infection. Serological testing for *E. canis* is performed only in research and specialty reference laboratories.
Selected Readings
Goldman DP, Artenstein AW, and Bolan CD, "Human Ehrlichiosis: A Newly Recognized Tick-Borne Disease," *Am Fam Physician*, 1992, 46(1):199-208.
McDade JE, "Ehrlichiosis - A Disease of Animals and Humans," *J Infect Dis*, 1990, 161(4):609-17.
Rikihisa Y, "The Tribe Ehrlichieae and Ehrlichial Diseases," *Clin Microbiol Rev*, 1991, 4(3):286-308.

Elbow Arthrogram *see* Arthrogram *on page 334*
Elbow, Left or Right, X-ray *see* Bone Films *on page 343*
Electrodiagnostic Study *see* Electromyography *on page 399*
Electroencephalogram *see* Electroencephalography *on this page*

Electroencephalography
Synonyms EEG; Electroencephalogram
Applies to Somatosensory Evoked Potentials
Test Includes Analysis of the electrical activity of the brain using scalp electrodes. This procedure is based on the principle that neurons within the cerebral cortex will normally generate low-amplitude electrical potentials. Electrodes positioned over specific regions of the cortex are able to detect these signals. Brain rhythms are then amplified and transmitted to a multichannel polygraph which records waveforms with automatic ink pens on moving paper. This written document, often more than 100 pages, is called the electroencephalogram. It is a continuous plot of voltage (vertical axis) versus time (horizontal axis). Abnormalities in the EEG brain wave pattern may be diagnostic of specific neurologic diseases. EEG is an indispensable means of evaluating gray matter disease and it is the only electrophysiologic measure of ongoing cortical function.
Patient Preparation Details of the procedure are discussed with the patient. When possible, sedative medications should be discontinued well in advance. This includes benzodiazepines, barbiturates, ethanol, etc. Fasting prior to EEG is not necessary, in fact, relative hypoglycemia has been reported to alter the EEG. The patient should also be reasonably rested beforehand since sleep deprivation has been known to cause alpha-rhythm abnormalities. If the patient has already been receiving anticonvulsant agents (eg, phenytoin (Dilantin®), carbamazepine) the management is more complex. The decision to withdraw or continue anticonvulsants prior to EEG testing should be handled by the physician. When approaching the patient with a new-onset seizure disorder (witnessed or suspected), many clinicians will obtain the initial EEG while the
(Continued)

Electroencephalography *(Continued)*

patient is still on an anticonvulsant agent. If results are negative, the EEG may be repeated later after discontinuing anticonvulsants for 1-2 days. Although this approach is admittedly cautious, it reduces the chance of seizure "breakthrough". Patient should wash hair the night before the test. Hair cream, oils, spray, and lacquer should not be applied after washing.

Aftercare If an overnight sleep study has been performed, patient is not permitted to drive home afterwards. Otherwise, if a routine (wake) EEG is performed no specific postprocedure restrictions are necessary. If anticonvulsant medications were discontinued specifically for the EEG, the patient is instructed to restart medications until notified by physician.

Special Instructions Requisition for EEG from the ordering physician should state patient's age, brief clinical history, overall impression, and reason for EEG. Special requests can be made for overnight study, sleep study, nasopharyngeal leads, activation procedures, evoked response testing, etc.

Complications EEG is considered a safe procedure and is well tolerated. The following "activation" techniques may be successful in inducing a seizure, but this is a desired "complication".

Technique At the start of the procedure, surface electrodes are placed on the scalp over designated areas. From 8-20 electrodes may be used, each approximately 0.5 cm in diameter. The patient is asked to rest comfortably on the examining table, first with eyes open, then closed. The underlying electrical activity of the cerebral cortex is measured (deeper structures are more difficult to measure). The signals are amplified, filtered, and transmitted to a polygraph. The electrical signals detected at each electrode move a separate ink writing pen on the polygraph. Thus, activity within anatomically different areas of the brain (temporal lobe, occipital, frontal, etc) are recorded on separate "channels". A continuous graph is produced on moving paper plotting voltage (vertical axis) versus time (horizontal axis). The written record may be several hundred pages long. Testing requires approximately 1 hour. Several "activation" measures may be attempted in order to induce a seizure under controlled laboratory conditions. These include:

- hyperventilation (leads to acute respiratory alkalosis and cerebral vasoconstriction)
- stroboscopic stimulation
- sleep EEG (for suspected temporal lobe epilepsy)

Use Common indications for EEG in general practice include:

- evaluation of the patient with a suspected seizure disorder; EEG is unique in its ability to objectively document the presence of seizure activity. In addition, EEG is crucial in localizing the site of a seizure focus and classifying the nature of epileptiform discharges. EEG is nearly always abnormal during an acute generalized seizure (eg, grand mal, petit mal), and frequently abnormal during an acute focal seizure (eg, Jacksonian). The EEG may also have diagnostic utility during the interictal period with abnormal discharges seen in 80% of patients with petit mal and 60% of patients with grand mal seizures.
- assessment of coma and other impairments in mental status; the EEG is abnormal in nearly every case of metabolic encephalopathy or ischemic encephalopathy, but is normal in most psychiatric conditions. In some instances, EEG may reveal important etiologic data not suspected clinically. For example, when coma is caused by hepatic encephalopathy, barbiturate overdose, or subclinical status epilepticus, distinctive and diagnostic EEG waveforms may be seen.
- diagnosis of certain infections of the central nervous system (CNS); characteristic EEG patterns may be seen in herpes simplex encephalitis, Creutzfeldt-Jakob disease, and subacute sclerosing panencephalitis.

Additional roles for EEG include:

- diagnosis of intracranial mass lesions; EEG is capable of diagnosing and localizing lesions such as brain tumors, abscesses, meningiomas, etc. However, this test cannot reliably distinguish between these entities. In recent years, the CT scan and MRI scan have supplanted the EEG in the evaluation of space occupying lesions.
- evaluation of cerebrovascular disease; in a patient who has suffered a recent cortical stroke, EEG can demonstrate regional electrical abnormalities in the distribution of the thrombosed vessel. In the patient who has suffered a

subcortical stroke ("lacunar stroke"), the EEG is usually normal even though the patient is hemiplegic. Thus, EEG may play a role in distinguishing cortical from subcortical stroke syndromes. In addition, EEG has been used in the past to diagnose and localize subarachnoid hemorrhage. However, CT scan or MRI scan have become the diagnostic tests of choice for stroke and subarachnoid hemorrhage.

- assessment of head injury; following a cerebral concussion, EEG is usually normal, but after a cerebral contusion, EEG is usually abnormal (although nonspecific). EEG has also been used to predict the subset of patients with head trauma who will go on to develop a seizure disorder.
- evaluation of persistent sleep disorders; overnight EEG recording is included as part of the polysomnogram (along with other monitoring techniques).
- intraoperative monitoring of cerebral activity; EEG may be used during certain neurosurgical procedures, carotid endarterectomies, and some non-neurologic surgeries as well (eg, cardiothoracic surgery). It is also useful in assessing depth of anesthesia.
- evaluation of suspected pseudoseizures; the EEG is normal despite generalized clonic movements
- EEG is characteristically **normal** in the following: multiple sclerosis (in severe cases some nonspecific changes may be seen); delirium tremens; Wernicke-Korsakoff's syndrome; Alzheimer's disease; cryptococcal meningitis; cerebral concussion; psychiatric disturbances, including bipolar disorder; tension headache; pseudoseizures.

Contraindications No absolute contraindications exist for EEG.

Selected Readings

Adams RD and Victor M, *Principles of Neurology*, 4th ed, New York, NY: McGraw-Hill Book Co, 1989, 19-31.

Aminoff MJ, *Electrodiagnosis in Clinical Neurology*, 2nd ed, New York, NY: Churchill-Livingstone, 1986.

Chusid JG, *Correlative Neuroanatomy and Functional Neurology*, 18th ed, Los Altos, CA: Lange Medical Publications, 1982, 223-44.

Davis TL and Freemon FR, "Electroencephalography Should Not Be Routine in the Evaluation of Syncope in Adults," *Arch Intern Med*, 1990, 150(10):2027-9.

Kiloh LG, McComas AJ, and Osselton JW, *Clin Electroencephalography*, 4th ed, London, England: Butterworth's Publishers, 1981.

Niedermeyer E and DaSilva FL, *Electroencephalography*, 2nd ed, Baltimore, MD: Urban and Schwarzenberg, 1987.

Spehlmann R, *EEG Primer*, Elsevier, North Holland: Biomedical Press, 1981.

Wee AS, "Is Electroencephalography Necessary in the Evaluation of Syncope?" *Arch Intern Med*, 1990, 150(10):2007-8.

Electromyography

Synonyms Electrodiagnostic Study; EMG

Test Includes Insertion of a needle electrode into skeletal muscle to measure electrical activity and assess physiologic function. In this procedure, percutaneous, extracellular needle electrodes are placed into a selected muscle group. Muscle action potentials (AP) are detected by these electrodes, amplified, and displayed on a cathode ray oscilloscope. In addition, fluctuations in voltage are heard as "crackles" over a loudspeaker, permitting both auditory and visual analysis of the muscle APs. Testing is performed with the muscle at rest, with a mild voluntary contraction, and with maximal muscle contraction (where recruitment pattern and interference are noted). Unlike nerve conduction studies, EMG does not involve external electrical stimulation. Muscle APs (normal or abnormal) are physiologically generated. In various diseases of the motor system, typical electrical abnormalities may be present: increased insertional activity, abnormal motor unit potentials, fibrillations, fasciculations, positive sharp waves, decreased recruitment pattern, and others. EMG assesses the integrity of upper motor neurons, lower motor neurons, the neuromuscular junction, and the muscle itself. However, EMG is seldom diagnostic of a particular disease entity. Its major use lies in differentiating between the following disease classes: primary myopathy, peripheral motor neuron disease, and disease of the neuromuscular junction. As with nerve conduction velocity studies (with which EMG is usually paired), EMG should be considered an extension of the history and physical examination.

Patient Preparation Details of procedure are reviewed with the patient. Considerable patient apprehension often accompanies "needle tests" and calm reassurance from the medical team will go far in allaying such anxieties. Aspirin products should be discontinued 5-7 days beforehand. Nonsteroidal agents (Continued)

Electromyography *(Continued)*

should also be stopped several days in advance. Routine medications may be taken on the morning of the examination. If coagulopathy is suspected, appropriate hematologic tests should be ordered (PT/PTT, CBC, bleeding time, etc). If a primary muscle disease is suspected, creatine phosphokinase (CPK) level should be drawn prior to needle examination. Routine EMG testing may cause minor elevations in CPK up to one and one-half times baseline. However, striking elevations in CPK, as seen with polymyositis or muscular dystrophy, are not associated with EMG testing.

Aftercare No specific activity restrictions are necessary. Patient may resume previous activity level.

Special Instructions Requisition from ordering physician should include brief clinical history, tentative neurologic diagnosis, and the specific limb(s) or muscle group(s) in question. Physician should also state whether nerve conduction studies are desired, although in some centers these may be added at the neurologist's discretion.

Complications Local discomfort at the site of needle insertion is common. This is often mild in severity and has no significant sequelae. Pneumothorax has been rarely documented in the literature. This was associated with needle examination of paraspinal muscles. Transient bacteremia has been reported, but routine antibiotic prophylaxis for patients with high-risk cardiac lesions is not generally recommended.

Equipment EMG is performed in a specially equipped procedure room, usually reserved for electrodiagnostic studies. Basic instrumentation includes:

- needle electrodes; these may be monopolar (sharpened, coated steel wires), coaxial, or bipolar (two wires within a needle). These needles record electrical activity from muscle fibers directly contacting the tip, as well as fibers within a several millimeter radius.
- amplifier with filters
- cathode ray oscilloscope with the vertical axis measuring voltage, the horizontal axis measuring time. This device usually has an audio amplifier and loudspeaker, which converts APs to sound energy.
- data storage apparatus (eg, magnetic tape recorder)

Technique A brief neurologic examination is performed prior to the start of the procedure. For EMG of the extremities, patient lies recumbent on the examination table. When paraspinal muscles are tested, the patient adopts a prone position. No intravenous sedatives or pain medications are used. Local anesthesia is also not required despite the generous number of needle insertions. The skin is cleansed thoroughly with alcohol pads, as necessary. Patient is instructed to relax as much as possible. The following steps are carried out.

- Recording needle electrode is inserted percutaneously into the muscle under consideration. The initial electrical activity of the muscle, as seen on the oscilloscope screen and heard over the loudspeaker, is termed the **insertional activity**.
- Next, the needle is held stationary and the muscle action potentials during voluntary relaxation are recorded.
- Patient performs a mild, submaximal contraction of the test muscle. The summed muscle action potentials - the motor unit potential - are observed on the oscilloscope.
- Finally, a maximal muscle contraction is carried out. The compound action potentials generated during this maneuver are studied for **interference** and **recruitment pattern**.

Needle examination is, by nature, a slow and labor-intensive process. Numerous muscles must be tested individually including both symptomatic and clinically asymptomatic muscles. Within a specific muscle, several independent sites may need to be examined, particularly when the muscle has a large surface area. A number of myopathic processes are focal and sampling errors even within an individual muscle are possible (ie, disease process may effect proximal portion of a muscle, sparing distal fibers).

Normal Findings Results are interpreted by neurologist or physiatrist with preliminary impression written in chart immediately. A formal, typed report is completed several days later. The fundamental principles underlying test interpretation are as follows.

- Insertional activity: Immediately upon needle insertion, there is a brief burst of electrical activity lasting <300 msec. This "insertional activity" is heard over the loudspeaker and may be increased or decreased in various disease states.

- Electrical activity at rest: Muscle tissue is normally silent at rest. No action potentials are seen on the oscilloscope.

- Minimal muscle contraction: When a minimal contraction is performed, several motor unit potentials (MUPs) are activated. Several individual APs are normally visible on the oscilloscope at a rate of 4-5/second. The idealized configuration of a single MUP is depicted in the following figure (see normal column).

- Full voluntary contraction: As the strength of the muscle contraction increases, further muscle units are "recruited". On the oscilloscope the APs appear more disorganized and individual APs can no longer be recognized. At the peak of a contraction the "complete recruitment pattern" is seen, which represents a compilation of motor unit potentials firing asynchronously. The normal interference pattern is considered "full," that is, the amplitude of APs is high (≤5 mV) and firing rate is fast (40/second).

EMG FINDINGS

LESION / EMG Steps	NORMAL	NEUTOGENIC LESION		MYOGENIC LESION		
		Lower Motor	Upper Motor	Myopathy	Myotonia	Polymyositis
1 Insertional Activity	Normal	Increased	Normal	Normal	Myotonic Discharge	Increased
2 Spontaneous Activity	—	Fibrillation / Positive Wave	—	—	—	Fibrillation / Positive Wave
3 Motor Unit Potential	0.5-1.0 mV / 5-10 ms	Large Unit / Limited Recruitment	Normal	Small Unit / Early Recruitment	Myotonic Discharge	Small Unit / Early Recruitment
4 Interference Pattern	Full	Reduced / Fast Firing Rate	Reduced / Slow Firing Rate	Full / Low Amplitude	Full / Low Amplitude	Full / Low Amplitude

Idealized EMG findings, normal, neurogenic lesions, and myogenic lesions. Reproduced with permission from Kimura J, Chapter 13, "Types of Abnormality," *Electrodiagnosis in Diseases of Nerve and Muscle: Principles and Practice*, 2nd ed, Philadelphia, PA: FA Davis, 1989, 263.

Critical Values Abnormalities in one or more of the previously stated parameters may be seen.

Insertional activity: Increased in both neurogenic disorders (eg, lower motor nerve disease) and myogenic disorders (eg, polymyositis), and thus is considered nonspecific. Decreased insertional activity is less common, but may be associated with far advanced denervation or myopathy, especially when muscle is replaced by fat or collagen. A distinctive insertional pattern is seen with myotonia, an unusual neurologic disorder, and is termed "myotonic discharge".

Abnormal activity at rest: Instead of the electrical silence which characterizes the muscle at rest, spontaneous action potentials in single muscle fibers ("fibrillation potentials") may be observed in several disease states.

Fibrillations are seen 1-3 weeks after destruction of a lower motor neuron. Denervated muscle fibers develop heightened chemosensitivity and individual muscle fibers contract spontaneously. The phenomenon of "positive sharp waves" may also be seen. Fibrillations may also occur with severe polymyositis when extensive areas of necrosis interrupt nerve innervation. The naked eye is unable to perceive fibrillations.

Fasciculations represent random contractions of a full motor unit, often visible through the skin. (A motor unit is comprised of an anterior horn cell, axon, neuromuscular junction, and the numerous muscle fibers supplied by the axon.) Fasciculations may be benign, with no other EMG abnormalities observed. They may also be associated with amyotrophic lateral sclerosis, other anterior horn cell diseases, nerve root compression, herniated nucleus pulposus syndrome, acute polyneuropathy, and others.

(Continued)

Electromyography *(Continued)*

Abnormalities in the motor unit potential (MUP): Individual motor unit potentials are distinguishable during a submaximal muscle contraction. Abnormalities in amplitude, shape (number of phases, serrations, configuration), and duration are possible. Increased MUP amplitude is seen in lower motor neuron disease but is normal in upper motor neuron disease. Decreased MUP amplitude is characteristic of polymyositis and other myopathies and duration of the MUP is also decreased.

Abnormalities in interference pattern: The normal "full recruitment" pattern seen during maximal muscle contraction is often compromised in disease states. In myogenic lesions, such as polymyositis and myotonia, the amplitude of the MUPs is significantly decreased but the recruitment pattern is normal (ie, the number of activated motor units is normal but the number of muscle fibers per motor unit is diminished). In LMN lesions, the number of motor units recruited is decreased. In severe cases of neuropathy, the maximum interference pattern resembles that of a single MUP, with individual potentials visible. Amplitude of MUPs may be normal. These findings are summarized in the previous figure.

Use In the neurologic literature, EMG has been performed in a wide variety of clinical situations, many of which are experimental or highly specialized in nature. Common indications for EMG in general practice include the following.

Evaluation of the patient with clinical features of primary muscle disease (symmetric and proximal weakness, muscle atrophy, intact sensory system, etc). Examples include:

- muscular dystrophy
- glycogen storage disease
- myotonia
- inflammatory myopathies (systemic lupus, sarcoidosis, infectious myopathies)
- polydermatomyositis
- alcoholic myopathy
- endocrine myopathies, and others

Evaluation of the patient with lower motor neuron disease, including:

- suspected peripheral nerve lesions, such as diffuse peripheral neuropathies, spinal root lesions, and trauma
- suspected disease of the anterior horn cells (characterized by asymmetric weakness, muscle atrophy, fasciculations), as in amyotrophic lateral sclerosis or poliomyelitis

Assessment of the patient with suspected upper motor neuron disease, when prior imaging studies are inconclusive. This includes occult lesions of the corticospinal tract (syringomyelia, tumor) and, less commonly, lesions of the cerebral tract (tumor, CVA). Evaluation of the patient with suspected neuromuscular junction disease (NMJ). This includes myasthenia gravis and the paraneoplastic Eaton-Lambert syndrome. Conventional EMG, as described here, is not the diagnostic test of choice for myasthenia gravis. However, other forms of EMG such as single fiber EMG and repetitive stimulation tests are highly specific for NMJ disease. Assessment of the patient with severe and persistent muscle cramps. Serial documentation of response to therapy for known cases of myopathy or neuropathy. Identification of significantly diseased muscle groups to help guide muscle biopsy (if clinical examination is not inconclusive). EMG is less useful in:

- the restless legs syndrome
- transient, self-resolving muscle cramps
- uncomplicated cases of polymyalgia rheumatica unless the diagnosis is in doubt or underlying myositis is suspected
- routine cases of fibrositis/fibromyalgia (EMG abnormalities have recently been documented in the medical literature but needle examination is not routinely indicated)

Contraindications The following situations represent relative contraindications:

- severe coagulopathy, including hemophilia and marked thrombocytopenia. It should be noted that EMG has been performed safely with platelet counts as low as 20,000/mm^3, but this is not recommended.
- systemic anticoagulation (eg, intravenous heparin, oral Coumadin®)
- patients with an unusual susceptibility to systemic infections (EMG has been known to cause transient bacteremia)

- patients undergoing a muscle biopsy after EMG require special consideration. It is well known that needle insertion and manipulation during EMG may cause local microscopic tissue damage on a traumatic basis. Histologically, this damage may be confused with a focal myopathy. Thus, some experts avoid detailed needle examinations of the specific muscle group which will be biopsied (although EMG testing of surrounding muscle groups is frequently performed).

Selected Readings

Adams RD and Victor M, *Principles of Neurology*, 4th ed, New York, NY: McGraw-Hill Book Co, 1989, 1009-27.

Aminoff MJ, *Electromyography in Clinical Practice*, 2nd ed, New York, NY: Churchill-Livingstone, 1987.

Goodgold J and Eberstein A, *Electrodiagnosis of Neuromuscular Diseases*, 3rd ed, Baltimore, MD: Williams & Wilkins, 1983.

Griggs RC, Bradley WG, and Shahani B, "Approach to the Patient With Neuromuscular Disease," *Harrison's Principles of Internal Medicine*, 12th ed, Wilson JD, Braunwald E, Isselbacher KJ, et al, eds, New York, NY: McGraw-Hill Book Co, 1991, 2088-96.

Johnson EW and Wiechers D, "Electrodiagnosis," *Krusen's Handbook of Physical Medicine and Rehabilitation*, 3rd ed, Kottke FJ, Stillwell GK, and Lehmann JF, eds, Philadelphia, PA: WB Saunders Co, 1982, 56-85.

Kimura J, *Electrodiagnosis in Diseases of Nerve and Muscle: Principles and Practice*, 2nd ed, Philadelphia, PA: FA Davis Co, 1989.

Electron Microscopic (EM) Examination for Viruses, Stool

Related Information

Histopathology *on page 448*

Skin Biopsy *on page 535*

Synonyms EM Examination for Viruses; EM of Enteric Viruses; Enteric Viruses by EM; Gastrointestinal Viruses by EM

Applies to Rotavirus Detection by EM

Test Includes Direct visualization of virions

Special Instructions Laboratory must be notified prior to requesting examination of any specimen by EM.

Specimen Stool from the acute, diarrheal phase of disease

Container Sterile vial, tube, Petri dish, or stool carton

Sampling Time As soon as possible after the onset of disease

Turnaround Time Less than 1 day

Use Demonstration of viral particles (eg, rotavirus, Norwalk virus, calcivirus, astrovirus, and coronavirus) in stool specimens from patients with suspected viral gastroenteritis

Limitations Generally, EM visualization of virus particles is not as sensitive as is cell culture, except for detecting nonculturable viruses such as rotavirus. EM can detect viruses if they are present in quantities of 10^6 to 10^7 particles/mL. This sensitivity is appropriate for agents causing diarrhea but is not sufficiently sensitive for the detection of other potential pathogens.

It is often difficult to differentiate (by EM) the aforementioned viruses.

Methodology Diluted stool (either with or without being mixed with patient serum) is mixed with an electron-opaque heavy metal solution such as phosphotungstic acid. The stool solution is placed onto an electron-lucent grid support and examined by electron microscopy. Virions or virions agglutinated by specific antibodies (if present in serum) appear as a negative image against a black surrounding background.

Additional Information Very few clinical Microbiology/Virology Laboratories have access to electron microscopes.

Selected Readings

Christensen ML, "Human Viral Gastroenteritis," *Clin Microbiol Rev*, 1989, 2(1):51-89.

Drew WL, "Diagnostic Virology," *Clin Lab Med*, 1987, 7(4):721-40.

Gray LD, "Novel Viruses Associated With Gastroenteritis," *Clin Microbiol Newslett*, 1991, 13(18):137-44.

Miller SE, "Diagnostic Virology by Electron Microscopy," *Am Soc Microbiol News*, 1988, 54:475-81.

EM Examination for Viruses *see* Electron Microscopic (EM) Examination for Viruses, Stool *on this page*

EMG *see* Electromyography *on page 399*

EM of Enteric Viruses *see* Electron Microscopic (EM) Examination for Viruses, Stool *on this page*

Encephalitis Viral Serology

Synonyms Arbovirus Serology

Abstract Encephalitogenic arboviruses commonly seen in North America (ie, California encephalitis (LaCrosse), Western equine encephalitis, Eastern equine encephalitis, and St Louis encephalitis viruses). Arboviruses (arthropod-borne viruses) are a taxonomically heterogeneous group of viruses grouped together because they are all transmitted to humans via an arthropod vector.

Specimen Serum

Container Red top tube

Collection Acute and convalescent sera drawn 10-14 days apart

Reference Range Less than a fourfold titer increase in paired sera. CSF IgM: negative; hemagglutination inhibition: ≤1:80; complement fixation: ≤1:32; immunofluorescence: ≤1:128.

Use Support the diagnosis of infection with encephalitis viruses

Limitations Cross-reacting antibodies from previous infections or from immunization for yellow fever may produce false-positive results, particularly when assays are performed on unpaired sera.

Additional Information Central nervous system infection by California encephalitis (LaCrosse), Western equine encephalitis, Eastern equine encephalitis, or St Louis encephalitis viruses may manifest as aseptic meningitis, encephalitis, or meningoencephalitis. There is a seasonal distribution for these infections that reflects their mode of transmission to humans by mosquitos. In the United States, the incidence of arboviral infection is low as is the prevalence of antibodies to these agents in the general population. Consequently, a positive result in an unpaired specimen is **presumptive** evidence for a recent infection. A fourfold increase in titer or a positive CSF IgM test is confirmatory. Antibody detection is the diagnostic test of choice as these viruses are essentially nonculturable in routine diagnostic virology laboratories.

Selected Readings

Bale JF Jr, "Viral Encephalitis," *Med Clin North Am*, 1993, 77(1):25-42.

Calisher CH, "Medically Important Arboviruses of the United States and Canada," *Clin Microbiol Rev*, 1994, 7(1):89-116.

Tsai TF, "Arboviruses," *Manual of Clinical Laboratory Immunology*, 4th ed, Chapter 91, Rose NR, Conway de Macario E, Fahey JL, et al, eds, Washington, DC: American Society for Microbiology, 1992, 606-18.

Endocervical Culture see Genital Culture *on page 423*

Endoscopic Biopsy see Histopathology *on page 448*

Entamoeba histolytica Serology

Synonyms Amebiasis Serological Test

Patient Preparation Fasting blood sample required

Specimen Serum

Container Red top tube or serum separator tube

Reference Range IHA titer: <1:128; CF titer: <1:8; immunodiffusion test: negative

Use Diagnose systemic amebiasis

Limitations Sensitivity is highest in extraintestinal amebiasis, lower in amebic dysentery, and lowest in asymptomatic carriers. Some false-positives occur in patients with ulcerative colitis. Recently a serine-rich recombinant *Entamoeba histolytica* protein has proven to be a useful antigen to assist in the serodiagnosis of *Entamoeba* which has disseminated.

Methodology Complement fixation (CF), indirect hemagglutination (IHA), immunodiffusion (ID), indirect fluorescent antibody (IFA), enzyme immunoassay (EIA)

Additional Information Indirect hemagglutination is positive in 87% to 100% of patients with liver abscesses and more than 85% of patients with acute amebic dysentery. Fewer than 6% of uninfected individuals react in the test. Amebic serology when negative is strong evidence against amebic liver abscess. IHA titers of 1:128 or greater are considered to be clinically significant, and a fourfold rise in titer is diagnostic evidence. Although titers will decrease over time, serology may remain positive for as long as 2 years, even after curative therapy.

Selected Readings

Bruckner DA, "Amebiasis," *Clin Microbiol Rev*, 1992, 5(4):356-69.

Kagan IG and Maddison SE, "Serodiagnosis of Parasitic Diseases," *Manual of Clinical Laboratory Immunology*, 4th ed, Rose NR, de Macario EC, Fahey JL, et al, eds, Washington, DC: American Society for Microbiology, 1992, 529-43.

Maddison SE, "Serodiagnosis of Parasitic Diseases," *Clin Microbiol Rev*, 1991, 4(4):457-69.

Reed SL, "Amebiasis: An Update," *Clin Infect Dis*, 1992, 14(2):385-93.
Stanley SL Jr, Jackson TF, Reed SL, et al, "Serodiagnosis of Invasive Amebiasis Using a Recombinant *Entamoeba histolytica* Protein," *JAMA*, 1991, 266(14):1984-6.

Enteric Pathogens Culture, Routine *see* Stool Culture *on page 540*

Enteric Viruses by EM *see* Electron Microscopic (EM) Examination for Viruses, Stool *on page 403*

Enterobiasis Test *see* Pinworm Preparation *on page 520*

***Enterobius vermicularis* Preparation** *see* Pinworm Preparation *on page 520*

Enterohemorrhagic *E. coli*, Stool Culture *see* Stool Culture, Diarrheagenic *E. coli on page 542*

Enteroinvasive *E. coli*, Stool Culture *see* Stool Culture, Diarrheagenic *E. coli on page 542*

Enteropathogenic *E. coli*, Stool Culture *see* Stool Culture, Diarrheagenic *E. coli on page 542*

Enterotoxigenic *E. coli*, Stool Culture *see* Stool Culture, Diarrheagenic *E. coli on page 542*

Enterovirus Culture

Related Information
Coxsackie A Virus Serology *on page 377*
Coxsackie B Virus Serology *on page 377*

Applies to Coxsackie A Virus Culture; Coxsackie B Virus Culture; Echovirus Culture; Poliovirus Culture

Test Includes Culture for Coxsackie A virus, Coxsackie B virus, echovirus, and poliovirus

Specimen Stool (best specimen), rectal swab, cerebrospinal fluid, upper and lower respiratory tract specimens, blood, throat swab (good specimen), various organs and tissues

Container Sterile container

Sampling Time It is important to obtain specimens very early in the disease; however, virus is shed in the stool for weeks.

Storage Instructions Enteroviruses are rather hardy; however, specimens should be refrigerated or placed into cold virus transport medium and delivered immediately to the clinical laboratory.

Causes for Rejection Dry specimen, specimen not in proper viral transport medium, specimen not refrigerated during transport, specimen fixed in formalin, unlabeled specimen

Turnaround Time Variable (1-4 days) and depends on culture method used and amount of virus in specimen

Reference Range No virus isolated

Use Aid in the diagnosis of disease caused by enteroviruses (eg, polio, congenital viral infections, and meningitis (aseptic))

Limitations Cell culture generally does not support the growth of Coxsackie A enteroviruses. Inoculation of suckling mice is the preferred method to isolate Coxsackie A virus.

Methodology Inoculation of specimens into cell culture, incubation, and observation of characteristic cytopathic effect. Specimens suspected of containing Coxsackie A virus are inoculated into suckling mice which are then observed for flaccid paralysis without encephalitis.

Some (usually reference) laboratories can identify specific enteroviruses by using a battery of specific enterovirus-neutralizing antibodies. These antibodies are useful in identifying and typing Coxsackie A, Coxsackie B, echovirus, and poliovirus.

Additional Information Infrequently, aseptic meningitis is caused by Coxsackie A virus types which require animal inoculation for isolation.

Selected Readings
Dowsett EG, "Human Enteroviral Infections," *J Hosp Infect*, 1988, 11(2):103-15.
Menegus MA, "Enteroviruses," *Manual of Clinical Microbiology*, 5th ed, Balows A, Hausler WJ Jr, Herrmann KL, et al, eds, Washington, DC: American Society for Microbiology, 1991, 943-7.
Modlin JF and Kinney JS, "Perinatal Enterovirus Infections," *Adv Pediatr Infect Dis*, 1987, 2:57-78.
Moore M and Morens DM, "Enteroviruses, Including Polioviruses," *Textbook of Human Virology*, Belshe RB, ed, Littleton, MA: PSG Publishing Co, 1984, 407-83.

Enterovirus Culture, Stool *see* Viral Culture, Stool *on page 573*

Enzyme Immunoassay for Group A *Streptococcus* Antigen *see* Group A *Streptococcus* Antigen Test *on page 428*

EPEC, Stool Culture see Stool Culture, Diarrheagenic *E. coli* on page 542

Epstein-Barr Early Antigens see Epstein-Barr Virus Serology on this page

Epstein-Barr Viral Capsid Antigen see Epstein-Barr Virus Serology on this page

Epstein-Barr Virus Culture

Related Information

Epstein-Barr Virus Serology on this page

Synonyms EBV Culture

Applies to Lymph Node Culture; Lymphocyte Culture; Spleen Cell Culture

Test Includes Culture for EBV only

Special Instructions The laboratory must be notified prior to receipt of specimen.

Specimen Blood, lymph node, spleen, tumor biopsies, throat garglings (for isolation of excreted virus)

Container Green top (heparin) tube; sterile container

Storage Instructions Blood specimen can be maintained at room temperature but should be immediately transported to the laboratory. Biopsy specimen should be sent to the Virology Laboratory immediately after collection.

Causes for Rejection Dry specimen, specimen not in proper viral transport medium, specimen not refrigerated during transport, specimen fixed in formalin, unlabeled specimen, specimen not received in sterile container, excessive delay in transit to laboratory

Turnaround Time 4-6 weeks

Reference Range No growth of lymphocyte culture

Use Aid in the diagnosis of disease caused by EBV (eg, infectious mononucleosis, chronic fatigue syndrome, and Burkitt's lymphoma)

Limitations Cell culture for EBV is not diagnostically practical because it proliferates only in B lymphocytes. Cell culture requires at least 4 weeks, and the virus is ubiquitous in humans.

Methodology Virus is given opportunity to grow for 4 weeks in a lymphocyte culture. Virus-infected cells will proliferate; if virus is not present, lymphocytes will die.

Additional Information Viral serology (usually immunofluorescence) is the preferred diagnostic method. EBV persists regularly in the lymphoreticular system of EBV-infected individuals. EBV-positive lymphoblast lines can be established frequently from peripheral leukocytes and lymph node cells from those individuals.

Selected Readings

Lennette ET, "Epstein-Barr Virus," *Manual of Clinical Microbiology*, 5th ed, Balows A, Hausler WJ Jr, Herrmann KL, et al, eds, Washington, DC: American Society for Microbiology, 1991, 847-52.

Okano M, Thiele GM, Davis JR, et al, "Epstein-Barr Virus and Human Diseases: Recent Advances in Diagnosis," *Clin Microbiol Rev*, 1988, 1(3):300-12.

Epstein-Barr Virus Serology

Related Information

Epstein-Barr Virus Culture on this page

Infectious Mononucleosis Serology on page 462

Synonyms EB Virus Titer; EBV Titer

Applies to EB Nuclear Antigens; Epstein-Barr Early Antigens; Epstein-Barr Viral Capsid Antigen; VCA Titer

Test Includes Serology for several EBV antigens

Specimen Serum

Container Red top tube or serum separator tube

Reference Range

- Patients with no history of infectious mononucleosis: IgG anti-VCA: <1:10; IgM anti-VCA: <1:10; anti-EBNA: <1:5; early antigen: <1:10.
- Patients with previous infectious mononucleosis by history: IgG anti-VCA: ≥1:10; IgM anti-VCA: ≤1:10; anti-EBNA: ≥1:50; early antigen: <1:10.
- Patients with current or active infection: Many combinations of results are possible. Consult the laboratory for interpretation of specific results.

Use Diagnose Epstein-Barr virus infection, heterophil-negative mononucleosis, hereditary sex-linked lymphadenopathy

Limitations Despite much publicity, these tests are neither sensitive nor specific for chronic fatigue syndrome

Contraindications The Epstein-Barr viral test need not be done on patients who have heterophil antibodies, symptoms, physical findings, and lymphocyte morphology consistent with infectious mononucleosis. Typically, this test is performed on the ~15% of patients who are heterophil-negative and are still suspected of having infectious mononucleosis.

Methodology Indirect fluorescent antibody (IFA), enzyme-linked immunosorbent assay (ELISA)

Additional Information Epstein-Barr virus is a herpes group virus which is almost ubiquitous. It is the cause of classic infectious mononucleosis, and is causally implicated in the pathogenesis of Burkitt's lymphoma, some nasopharyngeal carcinomas, and rare hereditary lymphoproliferative disorders. The serologic response to EB virus includes antibody to early antigen, which is usually short lived, IgM and IgG antibodies to viral capsid antigen (VCA), and antibodies to nuclear antigen (EBNA).

Although most cases of infectious mononucleosis can be diagnosed on the basis of clinical findings, blood count and morphology, and a positive test for heterophil antibody, as many as 20% may be heterophil-negative, at least at presentation (heterophil may become positive when repeated in a few days). In some of these cases, a test for Epstein-Barr virus antibodies may be useful.

Of the numerous antibodies that may be assayed, viral capsid antibody is the most useful. A high presenting titer is good evidence for EB virus infection. Since titers are generally high by the time a patient is symptomatic, it may not be possible to demonstrate the fourfold rise in titer usually recommended. Even a very high titer may be due to past infection, so IgA and IgM titers should be measured to establish acute infection. Persistent absence of antibody to viral capsid is good evidence against EB virus infection.

Antibody to EB virus nuclear antigen (EBNA) usually develops 4-6 weeks after infection, so its presence early during an acute illness should lead one to consider diagnosis other than EB virus infectious mononucleosis.

Patients with nonkeratinizing squamous carcinoma of the nasopharynx may have elevated levels of IgG antibody to EB early antigen, but the rarity of this condition and the 10% to 20% false-positive rate vitiate its usefulness for screening. Such patients may also have IgA antibodies to VCA.

The most controversial use of EBV serology is in chronic fatigue syndrome, a complaint predominantly but not exclusively of young to middle-aged women, characterized by long persistent debilitating fatigue and a panoply of usually mild somatic complaints. In the initial reports of this illness, chronic infection with EBV was suggested as the cause, and EBV serology suggested as a diagnostic tool. In the past several years, although the legitimacy of a chronic fatigue syndrome seems to have been established, the inappropriateness of EBV serology for diagnosis has been realized. The high levels of EBV antibodies in the general population, their long persistence, and the poor correlation of antibody titers with symptoms combine to make EBV serology useless in diagnosing, following, or ruling out chronic fatigue syndrome.

IgG antibody to early antigen occurs in patients with Hodgkin's disease in higher titer than expected. This observation suggests the possibility that EB virus activation plays a pathogenetic role in Hodgkin's disease.

Selected Readings

Erlich KS, "Laboratory Diagnosis of Herpesvirus Infections," *Clin Lab Med*, 1987, 7(4):759-76.

Merlin T, "Chronic Mononucleosis: Pitfalls in the Laboratory Diagnosis," *Hum Pathol*, 1986, 17(1):2-8.

Sumaya CV and Jenson HB, "Epstein-Barr Virus," *Manual of Clinical Laboratory Immunology*, 4th ed, Rose NR, de Macario EC, Fahey JL, et al, eds, Washington, DC: American Society for Microbiology, 1992, 568-75.

Thiele GM and Okano M, "Diagnosis of Epstein-Barr Virus Infections in the Clinical Laboratory," *Clin Microbiol Newslett*, 1993, 15(6):41-8.

Esophageal Echo *see* Transesophageal Echocardiography *on page 553*

Esterase, Leukocyte, Urine *see* Leukocyte Esterase, Urine *on page 473*

Eye Smear for Cytology *see* Ocular Cytology *on page 505*

Eye Swab *Chlamydia* Culture *see* Chlamydia Culture *on page 359*

FA Smear for *Legionella pneumophila* *see* Legionella pneumophila Smear *on page 470*

5-FC Level *see* Flucytosine Level *on next page*

Fecal Leukocyte Stain

Related Information

Clostridium difficile Toxin Assay *on page 367*
Cryptosporidium Diagnostic Procedures, Stool *on page 381*
Stool Culture *on page 540*
Stool Culture, Diarrheagenic *E. coli on page 542*

Test Includes Methylene blue, Gram's, or Wright's stain of stool smear

Patient Preparation Collect specimen prior to barium procedures if possible.

Specimen Fresh random stool, rectal swab

Container Culturette®, sealed plastic stool container

Collection Transport specimen to laboratory as soon as possible after collection, significant deterioration of the specimen occurs with prolonged storage.

Storage Instructions Refrigerate

Causes for Rejection Insufficient specimen volume. Specimens which are delayed in transit are less than optimal.

Turnaround Time 1 hour

Reference Range Few, if any, leukocytes

Use Assist in the differential diagnosis of diarrheal disease

Limitations Ten percent to 15% of stools which yield an invasive bacterial pathogen have an absence of fecal leukocytes. Many bacterial intestinal pathogens do not elicit a leukocyte response in stool. Fecal leukocytes are present in idiopathic inflammatory bowel disease.

Methodology Smear of stool (preferably mucus) with one drop methylene blue (or other stain), coverslip, and observe the presence of leukocytes.

Additional Information Conditions associated with varying degrees of fecal leukocytes, blood and/or mucus include diffuse antibiotic associated colitis, ulcerative colitis, shigellosis, *Campylobacter*, *Yersinia*, amebiasis, and some diarrheagenic *E. coli* infection. Conditions associated with an absence of fecal leukocytes include toxigenic bacterial infection, giardiasis, and viral infections. In a review the methylene blue stain for polymorpholeukocytes had a high sensitivity (85%) and specificity (88%) for bacterial diarrhea (*Shigella*, *Salmonella*, *Campylobacter*). Positive predictive value was poor (59%). Negative predicative value was 97%. In the presence of a history of abrupt onset, greater than four stools per day and no vomiting before the onset of diarrhea, the methylene blue stain for fecal polymorphonuclear leukocytes was a very effective presumptive diagnostic test for bacterial diarrhea. A positive occult blood test may also be suggestive of acute bacterial diarrhea. Neither method is sufficiently sensitive or specific to pre-empt the use of culture. Similar findings including a sensitivity of 81% and specificity 74% were observed when both tests were positive.

Selected Readings

Bishop WP and Ulshen MH, "Bacterial Gastroenteritis," *Pediatr Clin North Am*, 1988, 35(1):69-87.
Harris JC, Dupont HL, and Hornick RB, "Fecal Leukocytes in Diarrheal Illness," *Ann Intern Med*, 1972, 76(5):697-703.
Siegel D, Cohen PT, Neighbor M, et al, "Predictive Value of Stool Examination in Acute Diarrhea," *Arch Pathol Lab Med*, 1987, 111(8):715-8.

Femur, Left or Right, X-ray *see* Bone Films *on page 343*

Filarial Infestation *see* Microfilariae, Peripheral Blood Preparation *on page 489*

Filariasis Peripheral Blood Preparation *see* Microfilariae, Peripheral Blood Preparation *on page 489*

Filling Cystometrogram *see* Cystometrogram, Simple *on page 382*

Finger, Left or Right Hand, X-ray *see* Bone Films *on page 343*

Flea Identification *see* Arthropod Identification *on page 334*

Flexible Bronchoscopy *see* Bronchoscopy, Fiberoptic *on page 352*

Flucytosine Level

Related Information

Antibiotic Level, Serum *on page 321*

Synonyms Ancobon® Level; 5-FC Level; 5-Fluorocytosine Level

Abstract Flucytosine is an antifungal agent often used in conjunction with amphotericin B for treatment of fungal meningitis and endocarditis. Bone marrow toxicity and hepatotoxicity are occasionally seen in patients being treated with flucytosine.

Specimen Serum

Container Red top tube

Sampling Time Peak serum levels are reached 4-6 hours after a single oral dose. During ongoing therapy, peak levels are reached 1-2 hours after successive doses.

Reference Range Therapeutic: 50-100 µg/mL (SI: 390-775 µmol/L)

Possible Panic Range 100-125 µg/mL (SI: 775-970 µmol/L)

Use Monitor for bone marrow toxicity; evaluate weekly if patient has normal renal function, more often if renal function is abnormal.

Limitations Serum levels do not correlate well with clinical toxicity. The hypothesis of serum level associated adverse effects has been inferred from case reports but has not been definitively studied.

Methodology High performance liquid chromatography (HPLC), gas chromatography/mass spectrometry (GC/MS)

Additional Information Clinical use of flucytosine is associated with significant frequency of life-threatening bone marrow suppression which occurs most often when blood levels are >100 µg/mL (SI: >775 µmol/L) for 2 or more weeks. The bone marrow suppression is usually reversible. It is most likely to occur in patients with underlying hematologic disorders or in patients undergoing myelosuppressive therapy.

Selected Readings

Bodey GP, "Topical and Systemic Antifungal Agents," *Med Clin North Am*, 1988, 72:637-59.

Gerson B, "Flucytosine," *Clin Lab Med*, 1987, 7(3):541-4.

Terrell CL and Hughes CE, "Antifungal Agents Used for Deep-Seated Mycotic Infections," *Mayo Clin Proc*, 1992, 67(1):69-91.

Fluids, Cytology see Cytology, Body Fluids on page 386

Fluorescent Rabies Antibody Test see Rabies Detection on page 525

Fluorescent Treponemal Antibody Adsorption see FTA-ABS, Serum on next page

Fluorochrome Stain see Acid-Fast Stain on page 305

5-Fluorocytosine Level see Flucytosine Level on previous page

Follow-up Ultrasound Abdomen see Ultrasound, Abdomen on page 560

Follow-up Ultrasound Retroperitoneal see Ultrasound, Abdomen on page 560

Foot, Left or Right, X-ray see Bone Films on page 343

Forearm, Left or Right, X-ray see Bone Films on page 343

***Francisella tularensis* Antibodies** see Tularemia Serology on page 559

FRA Test see Rabies Detection on page 525

FTA-ABS, Cerebrospinal Fluid

Related Information

VDRL, Cerebrospinal Fluid on page 570

Synonyms *Treponema pallidum* Antibodies, CSF

Test Includes CSF specimens are adsorbed (FTA - ABS) with nonpathogenic *Treponema* sp and tested.

Specimen Cerebrospinal fluid

Container Clean, sterile CSF tube

Causes for Rejection Bloody specimen

Reference Range Nonreactive

Use Test for the presence of *Treponema pallidum* antibodies; VDRL is preferred over the FTA when examining CSF.

Limitations The interpretation of FTA results when performed on CSF is not clearly defined. False-positive results may occur particularly if the specimen is not adsorbed prior to testing. VDRL on cerebrospinal fluid is recommended by the Center for Disease Control to help establish the diagnosis of neurosyphilis. However, while a positive CSF VDRL is strong evidence for active neurosyphilis, a negative does not rule it out. An FTA-ABS on CSF can be positive in cases of neurosyphilis when CSF VDRL is negative, but this combination of results is not common. Unfortunately, the CSF FTA-ABS test is less specific than CSF VDRL for distinguishing currently active neurosyphilis from past syphilis infection. Therefore, a correlation of the clinical facts with the serologic findings is essential for each case. One useful guide when screening for neurosyphilis is to first detect a serum FTA-ABS and/or a VDRL or RPR.

Methodology Indirect immunofluorescence of killed *Treponema* after serum adsorption of antibodies to nonpathogenic *Treponema* sp

(Continued)

FTA-ABS, Cerebrospinal Fluid *(Continued)*

Selected Readings

Davis LE and Schmitt JW, "Clinical Significance of Cerebrospinal Fluid Tests for Neurosyphilis," *Ann Neurol,* 1989, 25(1):50-5.

Larsen SA, Pope V, and Quan TJ, "Immunologic Methods for the Diagnosis of Spirochetal Diseases," *Manual of Clinical Laboratory Immunology,* 4th ed, Rose NR, de Macario EC, Fahey JL, et al, eds. Washington, DC: American Society for Microbiology, 1992, 467-81.

Young H, Moyes A, McMillan A, et al, "Enzyme Immunoassay for Anti-Treponemal IgG: Screening or Confirmatory Test?," *J Clin Pathol,* 1992, 45(1):37-41.

FTA-ABS, Serum

Related Information

Darkfield Examination, Syphilis *on page 394*

RPR *on page 530*

VDRL, Cerebrospinal Fluid *on page 570*

Synonyms Fluorescent Treponemal Antibody Adsorption

Applies to Serologic Test for Syphilis

Patient Preparation Patient should be fasting if possible

Specimen Serum

Container Red top tube or serum separator tube

Reference Range Nonreactive

Use Confirm the presence of *Treponema pallidum* antibodies; establish the diagnosis of syphilis

Limitations FTA-ABS test for syphilis usually is positive in the treponemal diseases pinta, yaws and bejel, and falsely positive in patients with numerous diseases associated with increased or abnormal globulins, antinuclear antibodies, lupus erythematosus (beaded pattern), old age, pregnancy, and drug addiction (although drug addicts are likely to have true positives as well). As many as 2% of the general population may have a false-positive. Borderline results are inconclusive and cannot be interpreted; they may indicate a very low level of treponemal antibody or may be due to nonspecific factors. Further follow-up and serological confirmation with the treponemal immobilization test may be helpful.

Methodology Indirect immunofluorescence of killed *Treponema* after serum adsorption of antibodies to nonpathogenic *Treponema* sp

Additional Information FTA-ABS is the most sensitive test in all stages of syphilis, and is the best confirmatory test for a serum reactive to a screening test such as RPR. Occasionally, patients with ocular (uveitis) syphilis or otosyphilis will have a negative VDRL while their FTA-ABS is positive. FTA-ABS cannot be used to follow disease activity or response to treatment, because it will remain high for life. A modification of the test can detect IgM-specific antibodies, which may distinguish true congenital syphilis from placental transfer of maternal antibodies. However, tests for anti-*Treponema* IgM are not widely available. When a positive serum FTA-ABS is required before performing CSF VDRL examination, the specificity of the CSF test is markedly improved.

Although not officially recommended for testing cerebrospinal fluid, the FTA test, unabsorbed, can be performed on some spinal fluids with excellent specificity. At present this application of the test should be restricted to reference laboratories.

Selected Readings

Albright RE Jr, Christenson RH, Emlet JL, et al, "Issues in Cerebrospinal Fluid Management. CSF Venereal Disease Research Laboratory Testing," *Am J Clin Pathol,* 1991, 95(3):397-401.

Davis LE and Schmitt JW, "Clinical Significance of Cerebrospinal Fluid Tests for Neurosyphilis," *Ann Neurol,* 1989, 25(1):50-5.

Farnes SW and Setness PA, "Serologic Tests for Syphilis," *Postgrad Med,* 1990, 87(3):37-41, 45-6.

Larsen SA, Pope V, and Quan TJ, "Immunologic Methods for the Diagnosis of Spirochetal Diseases," *Manual of Clinical Laboratory Immunology,* 4th ed, Rose NR, de Macario EC, Fahey JL, et al, eds, Washington, DC: American Society for Microbiology, 1992, 467-81.

Fungal Immunodiffusion *see Fungal Serology on this page*

Fungal Precipitin Test *see Fungal Serology on this page*

Fungal Serology

Synonyms Fungal Immunodiffusion; Fungal Precipitin Test

Applies to *Aspergillus* Immunodiffusion; Blastomycosis Immunodiffusion; *Coccidioides* Immunodiffusion; Histoplasmosis Immunodiffusion

Specimen Serum

Container Red top tube or serum separator tube

Reference Range Negative or no bands identified

Use Confirm and aid in the differential diagnosis of aspergillosis, blastomycosis, histoplasmosis, and coccidioidomycosis

Limitations Results reported as positive or negative; no titer is given

Contraindications Prior skin test may give a single precipitin band ("M") with histoplasmin

Methodology Immunodiffusion (ID), enzyme-linked immunosorbent assay (ELISA)

Additional Information

Blastomycosis: A band of identity with the "A" reference antibody from an infected human indicates active infection or recent past infection. This detects about 80% of cases. A negative test has little value and in no way excludes the existence of blastomycosis. Cross reacting antibodies producing lines of partial identity are seen in patients with histoplasmosis and coccidioidomycosis.

Aspergillosis: Sera can be tested against a polyvalent antigen mixture, or a series of species preparations. The greater the number of bands, the greater the likelihood of either a fungus ball or invasive aspergillosis. A negative test does not rule out aspergillosis. Nonidentity bands could be due to presence of CRP. Cross reactions occur in cases of histoplasmosis, coccidioidomycosis and blastomycosis, or may indicate antibody to an *Aspergillus* species other than *Aspergillus fumigatus*. Bands due to reaction with C-reactive protein can be removed by sodium citrate.

Coccidioidomycosis: A band of identity with coccidioidin indicates infection but may be negative early. Some individuals continue to produce detectable antibodies up to 1 year after clinical recovery from active disease. A negative test does not exclude coccidioidomycosis.

Histoplasmosis: "H" and "M" precipitin bands are of diagnostic significance and if both are present indicate active infection. "H" identity bands alone are rarely seen; they are always associated with active infection. "M" identity bands alone indicate active infection, recent past infection (within the past year), or recent positive histoplasmin skin test (within past 2 months). The absence of precipitin antibodies does not rule out histoplasmosis.

Unfortunately, because of poorly standardized reagents and inherent biologic cross-reactivity, and interference from complement, the general clinical utility of measuring or detecting fungal antibodies is low. Only the detection of CSF antibodies to *Coccidioides* is truly diagnostic. For this reason, much effort is now devoted to tests for detecting fungal antigens, of which the most useful presently is the latex agglutination test for cryptococcal antigen.

Selected Readings

Drutz DJ, "Antigen Detection in Fungal Infections," *N Engl J Med*, 1986, 314(2):115-7.

Kaufman L and Reiss E, "Serodiagnosis of Fungal Diseases," *Manual of Clinical Laboratory Immunology*, 4th ed, Rose NR, de Macario EC, Fahey JL, et al, eds, Washington, DC: American Society for Microbiology, 1992, 506-28.

Tang CM and Cohen J, "Diagnosing Fungal Infections in Immunocompromised Hosts," *J Clin Pathol*, 1992, 45(1):1-5.

Fungal Skin Testing

Related Information

Anergy Skin Test Battery *on page 318*
Tuberculin Skin Testing, Intracutaneous *on page 557*

Synonyms Delayed Hypersensitivity Fungal Skin Tests; Skin Tests for Histoplasmosis, Blastomycosis, Coccidioidomycosis

Test Includes Intradermal injection of fungal antigen(s) to determine if a delayed hypersensitivity reaction is present to a given fungus. Skin test sites are examined at 24, 48, and 72 hours for induration which, if present, implies prior infection with the tested fungus.

Patient Preparation Procedure and risks are explained to the patient. No specific skin preparation is necessary. However, those patients with generalized skin disorders such as extensive psoriasis should be examined beforehand for suitable areas of normal appearing skin. If immediate hypersensitivity to the fungal antigen is even remotely suspected, physician should be in attendance.

Aftercare Fifteen to 30 minutes after injections, sites should be examined for adverse reactions ranging from the IgE wheal and flare response to systemic (Continued)

Fungal Skin Testing *(Continued)*

reactions; otherwise, close observation postprocedure is generally not necessary and patients should be instructed to keep test sites clean for 72 hours. No restrictions on bathing or cleaning injection sites are necessary.

Special Instructions Requisition should state the specific fungal antigens to be planted, as well as whether a simultaneous skin anergy panel is desired. Current medications should also be included in the requisition, with attention to corticosteroids or other immunosuppressive agents.

Complications As with other forms of skin testing, immediate IgE-mediated local reactions are possible, although unusual. Erythema, vesiculation, and skin necrosis may be seen, at times involving large areas. Systemic reactions, including anaphylaxis, have rarely been reported. Patients with infection with *Coccidioides immitis* who manifest erythema nodosum may be at an increased risk of a major systemic reaction after skin testing. However, in the vast majority of cases, fungal skin testing is safe.

Equipment Skin test materials are derived from cultures of the appropriate fungi and most are available commercially in standardized concentrations. Common fungal antigens tested include *Histoplasma capsulatum*, *Coccidioides immitis*, *Blastomyces dermatitidis* (not available commercially), *Candida*, and *Trichophyton*. Disposable plastic or glass tuberculin syringes are required along with 26- or 27-gauge short ($1/4$" to $1/2$") beveled needles.

Technique The volar aspect of the forearm is prepped with alcohol swabs. Skin test material(s) are injected intradermally so that discrete wheals are raised. Generally, 0.1 mL skin test antigen is injected, but more dilute solutions may be used if a severe reaction is anticipated. Subcutaneous injections should be avoided. Multiple fungal antigens may be injected at separate sites using this method. Test sites should be examined at 24, 48, and 72 hours. Date and time of injection should be recorded along with the location of each fungal antigen.

Data Acquired The transverse diameter of induration should be carefully measured by inspection and palpation and results recorded (in millimeters) at 24-hour intervals. Areas of erythema, however, are not as important as induration and are excluded in most grading schemes unless extensive (>10 mm).

Normal Findings No induration or erythema

Critical Values A positive skin test is defined by many authorities as a diameter of induration ≥5 mm. Induration of 0-4 mm is considered negative. Alternatively, a standardized grading scale, which is popular with general delayed-type hypersensitivity skin testing, may be used:

- 0: no reaction
- 1+: erythema >10 mm and/or induration 1-5 mm
- 2+: induration 6-10 mm
- 3+: induration 11-20 mm
- 4+: induration >20 mm

The interpretation of a positive (or negative) skin test is so problematic that the clinical utility of fungal skin testing is significantly limited. A positive reaction indicates only that exposure to the relevant fungus has occurred at some time in the past, whether recent or remote. In addition, fungal infections are endemic in many areas of the United States, where >90% of the local population may be skin test positive following asymptomatic or subclinical infections (eg, histoplasmosis in the Ohio River Valley). Thus, in the individual patient with suspected active fungal infection, a positive skin test adds little new diagnostic information and fails to establish the fungus as the infecting agent. This becomes especially relevant if the patient has ever lived in a known endemic area. In the patient with pulmonary nodules, the importance of a positive test is also unclear. Some authorities consider a positive histoplasmin test in an area of low prevalence as strong evidence for histoplasmosis. Others argue that lung nodules may still be due to bronchogenic carcinoma despite a positive histoplasmin test, and skin testing adds little to clinical decision making. Similarly, a negative skin test presents major problems in interpretation. Lack of reactivity may be seen in the following situations:

- no previous fungal infection
- previous fungal infection in an immunocompromised patient
- acute systemic fungal infection, where skin test positivity is often delayed for 2-4 weeks
- waning skin test reactivity to a given fungus, as occurs in the elderly
- technical errors in antigen placement

Even the documentation of skin test conversion (ie, negative test converting to positive or serial testing) is regarded as only indirect evidence of fungal exposure in the interim and does not necessarily imply active infection. Regarding the specific fungal antigens, the derivative of *Histoplasma capsulatum* is termed histoplasmin. An older preparation of histoplasmin cross reacted frequently with *Blastomyces* and *Coccidioides* and caused a rise in complement fixation titers to *Histoplasma*. A newer histoplasmin preparation ameliorates, but does not entirely eliminate, these problems. The histoplasmin skin test may cause a spurious increase in *Histoplasma* complement fixation titers. Since the CF serologic test is clinically more useful than the histoplasmin skin test, serologies should be drawn first in suspected cases. Coccidioidomycosis skin testing shares many of the same interpretive difficulties as histoplasmosis testing, such as waning reactivity over time, delay in test positivity during acute fungal infection, and areas of high prevalence. Two preparations of *Coccidioides* antigen are available, the older coccidioidin (derived from the mycelia phase) and Spherulin® (derived from lysed spherules). Spherulin® may have superior sensitivity and has been found to be positive in 30% more cases than coccidioidin. Although testing is not useful in the individual with suspected *Coccidioides* pneumonia, it may provide prognostic information in culture proven cases. In a classic study, patients with disseminated coccidioidomycosis had a higher survival rate if their skin test was positive (75%) compared with those who tested negative (15%). Patients with limited coccidioidomycosis almost always develop a positive test; failure to do so may predict impending disseminated disease. Use of the coccidioidin preparation may cause false-positive histoplasmosis serologic tests, but neither Spherulin® nor coccidioidin interferes with serologic tests for coccidioidomycosis. Coccidioidal skin tests are generally positive before coccidioidal serologic tests; some clinicians use this fact to justify skin testing in acute cases (despite its limited diagnostic utility). Skin tests for blastomycosis are presently of questionable value due to poor sensitivity and specificity, even in the study of epidemics. Fungal antigens derived from *Candida albicans* and *Trichophyton* are primarily used only for anergy testing because of high prevalence of positive skin tests in the general population.

Use Fungal skin testing has been applied for the following reasons:

- as an epidemiologic tool for defining geographic regions of endemic fungal infection

- as a diagnostic aid in individual cases of suspected primary fungal infection (limited usefulness)

- as a prognostic indicator in culture-proven cases of fungal infection (particularly coccidioidomycosis)

- as a component of a comprehensive cutaneous anergy panel, used to assess the integrity of a patient's cell-mediated immune system (T-cell function); this standardized panel is usually comprised of *Candida*, mumps, and *Trichophyton* antigens

Contraindications Prior systemic reaction to fungal skin testing; known immediate hypersensitivity (IgE-mediated) to the specific fungus to be tested; known immediate hypersensitivity to mercury, which is contained in some commercial preparations of *Coccidioides* antigen; the presence of erythema nodosum (high risk for adverse reaction - see following information).

Additional Information Fungal skin testing is a form of delayed hypersensitivity skin testing and as such is an assessment of cell-mediated immunity. Delayed hypersensitivity is a clinical phenomenon based on the reaction of the skin to intradermal injection of an antigen. It is a common form of immune protection against a wide range of infectious agents, including fungi. Following initial exposure to a fungus, a population of transformed T-lymphocytes is created, the so-called memory cells. When fungal antigen is introduced intradermally at a later date, these sensitized T cells are activated and initiate a cascade involving lymphokines, neutrophils, and macrophages. Clinically, this is manifested by the delayed formation of significant skin induration. Delayed hypersensitivity fungal skin testing should be differentiated from immediate hypersensitivity skin testing. The former is primarily T-cell mediated and the latter is mediated by IgE mechanisms. Skin testing for common allergies to molds or fungi is carried out using the percutaneous allergy testing method and is IgE-mediated. Similarly, skin tests for immediate hypersensitivity to *Aspergillus fumigatus* also use this method. This is commonly obtained in the evaluation of patients with suspected allergic bronchopulmonary aspergillosis.

Fungi, Susceptibility Testing *see* Antifungal Susceptibility Testing *on page 323*

Fungizone™ Level, Blood *see* Amphotericin B Level *on page 316*

Fungus Blood Culture *see* Blood Culture, Fungus *on page 341*

Fungus Culture, Appropriate Site

Refer to

Fungus Culture, Biopsy *on page 414*

Fungus Culture, Body Fluid *on page 415*

Fungus Culture, Bronchial Aspirate *on page 416*

Fungus Culture, Cerebrospinal Fluid *on page 416*

Fungus Culture, Skin *on page 417*

Fungus Culture, Sputum *on page 419*

Fungus Culture, Urine *on page 421*

Fungus Culture, Biopsy

Related Information

Histopathology *on page 448*

Methenamine Silver Stain *on page 487*

Periodic Acid-Schiff Stain *on page 518*

Sporotrichosis Serology *on page 540*

Synonyms Biopsy Culture, Fungus; Fungus Culture, Tissue

Applies to Cyst Culture, Fungus; Fungus Culture, Surgical Specimen

Patient Preparation Usual sterile preparation of biopsy site

Special Instructions The following information will assist the laboratory in the proper processing of the specimen: specific site of specimen, current antibiotic therapy, age and sex of patient, collection time and date, and clinical diagnosis.

Specimen Surgical specimen. **Swab specimens are not acceptable. Tissue must be submitted.**

Container Sterile test tube or container

Collection The portion of the biopsy submitted for culture should be separated from the portion submitted for histopathology by the surgeon or pathologist utilizing sterile technique. The laboratory should be informed of the fungal species suspected. Every effort should be made to collect the specimen early in the day so that it may be processed promptly, assuring optimal yield.

Storage Instructions Transport specimen to the laboratory immediately. Do not store or refrigerate.

Causes for Rejection Specimen in fixative solution, specimen not received in a sterile container.

Turnaround Time Physician will be notified of positive cultures. Negatives are reported after 4 weeks.

Reference Range No growth

Use Isolate and identify fungi; establish the diagnosis of fungemia, fungal endocarditis, and disseminated mycosis in immunocompromised patients, oncology patients, transplant patients, patients with leukemia and lymphoma, and patients with the acquired immunodeficiency syndrome (AIDS)

Limitations A single negative culture does not rule out the presence of fungal infection

Additional Information Optimal isolation of fungi from tissue is accomplished by processing **as much tissue as possible**. Swabs should be submitted only when adequate tissue is not available. Depending upon the geographic area *Histoplasma capsulatum, Blastomyces dermatitidis,* and *Coccidioides immitis,* among the deep pathogenic fungi, are most frequently isolated. Immunocompromised patients, transplant patients, and patients with acquired immunodeficiency syndrome (AIDS), are susceptible to opportunistic mycoses. The most frequently encountered are *Candida albicans, Cryptococcus neoformans,* and *Aspergillus* sp. The recovery of a recognized fungal pathogen from a wound culture or draining sinus is significant. Isolates such as *Candida* sp and *Aspergillus* sp are often environmental in origin and must be interpreted in the clinical context.

Selected Readings

Gray LD and Roberts GD, "Laboratory Diagnosis of Systemic Fungal Diseases," *Infect Dis Clin North Am,* 1988, 2(4):779-803.

Musial CE, Cockerill FR 3d, and Roberts GD, "Fungal Infections of the Immunocompromised Host: Clinical and Laboratory Aspects," *Clin Microbiol Rev,* 1988, 1(4):349-64.

Fungus Culture, Blood *see* Blood Culture, Fungus *on page 341*

Fungus Culture, Body Fluid

Related Information

Histopathology *on page 448*
Methenamine Silver Stain *on page 487*
Periodic Acid-Schiff Stain *on page 518*
Sporotrichosis Serology *on page 540*

Synonyms Body Fluid Fungus Culture

Applies to Ascitic Fluid Fungus Culture; Fungus Culture, Bone Marrow; Fungus Culture, Surgical Specimen; Fungus Culture, Tissue; Joint Fluid Fungus Culture; Pericardial Fluid Fungus Culture; Peritoneal Fluid Fungus Culture; Pleural Fluid Fungus Culture; Surgical Specimen Fungus Culture; Synovial Fluid Fungus Culture; Thoracentesis Fluid Fungus Culture Bone Marrow Fungus Culture; Tissue Fungus Culture; Wound Fungus Culture

Patient Preparation Aseptic preparation of biopsy site or site of body fluid aspiration

Special Instructions The laboratory should be informed of the specific source of specimen. Specimens may be divided for fungus culture, mycobacteria culture and acid-fast smear, and routine bacterial culture and Gram's stain only if the specimen is of adequate volume for all tests requested.

Specimen Body fluid, blood, bone marrow

Container Sterile container with lid

Collection The portion of the fluid specimen submitted for culture should be separated from the portion submitted for cytology by the surgeon or pathologist utilizing sterile technique. The laboratory should be informed of the fungal species suspected. Every effort should be made to collect the specimen early in the day so as it may be processed promptly, assuring optimal yield. Multiple daily fungal blood cultures are not necessary. Single daily cultures for 2-3 days are sufficient.

Storage Instructions Specimens should not be stored or refrigerated. The specimen should be transported to the laboratory as soon as possible after collection.

Causes for Rejection Specimen in fixative

Turnaround Time Negatives are reported after 4 weeks

Reference Range No growth

Use Isolate and identify fungi; establish the diagnosis of fungemia, fungal endocarditis, and disseminated mycosis in immunocompromised patients, oncology patients, transplant patients, patients with leukemia and lymphoma, and patients with the acquired immunodeficiency syndrome (AIDS)

Methodology Culture under aerobic conditions on several media

Additional Information Optimal isolation of fungi from fluid is accomplished by processing as much tissue as possible. **Swab specimens of body fluids should not be submitted for fungal culture.** Specimen selection tables are provided in the listings for Fungus Culture, Sputum and Fungus Culture, Skin. Depending upon the geographic area *Histoplasma capsulatum, Blastomyces dermatitidis,* and *Coccidioides immitis,* among the deep pathogenic fungi, are most frequently isolated, but from tissue more commonly than from fluid. Immunocompromised patients, transplant patients, and patients with acquired immunodeficiency syndrome (AIDS), are susceptible to opportunistic mycoses. The recovery of a recognized fungal pathogen from a fluid or draining sinus is significant. Isolates such as *Candida* sp and *Aspergillus* sp are often environmental in origin and must be interpreted in the clinical context.

Fungal peritonitis is clinically similar to bacterial peritonitis with pain, fever, and abdominal tenderness. Thirty-two fungal infections due to *Candida* sp (mostly *Candida albicans* and *Candida parapsilosis*), and rare single cases of *Aspergillus fumigatus* and the higher bacterium *Nocardia asteroides* have been reported in patients undergoing chronic dialysis. In a series of AIDS patients, bone marrow biopsy detected opportunistic fungal or mycobacterial infections in 20%. Eighty percent of the positive biopsies were associated with bone marrow granulomas. Fever, anemia, and neutropenia were often correlated with a positive biopsy. Neutrophil count <1000/mm^3 is associated with infection by *Candida, Aspergillus, Mucor, Rhizopus, Trichosporon,* and *Fusarium* sp. T-cell defects and/or impaired cell mediated immunity is associated with infection by *Candida, Cryptococcus neoformans, Histoplasma capsulatum, Coccidioides immitis,* and *Aspergillus* sp. Catheterization, arterial venous, or urinary and (Continued)

Fungus Culture, Body Fluid *(Continued)*

mechanical disruption of the skin is associated with *Candida* and *Rhodotorula* sp infections. Disruption of the natural barrier of the GI tract and respiratory tree by cytotoxic chemotherapy predispose to *Candida* sp infections.

Selected Readings

Gray LD and Roberts GD, "Laboratory Diagnosis of Systemic Fungal Diseases," *Infect Dis Clin North Am*, 1988, 2(4):779-803.

Lyons RW and Andriole VT, "Fungal Infections of the CNS," *Neurol Clin*, 1986, 4(1):159-70.

Musial CE, Cockerill FR 3d, and Roberts GD, "Fungal Infections of the Immunocompromised Host: Clinical and Laboratory Aspects," *Clin Microbiol Rev*, 1988, 1(4):349-64.

Fungus Culture, Bone Marrow see Fungus Culture, Body Fluid on previous page

Fungus Culture, Bronchial Aspirate

Synonyms Bronchial Aspirate Fungus Culture; Lower Respiratory Fungus Culture

Applies to Bronchoalveolar Lavage (BAL); Fungus Culture, Tracheal Aspirate; Fungus Culture, Transtracheal Aspirate; Percutaneous Transtracheal Fungus Culture; Tracheal Aspirate Fungus Culture; Transtracheal Aspirate Fungus Culture

Test Includes Culture, Gram's stain, KOH preparation

Special Instructions Requisition **must** state site of specimen

Specimen Bronchial aspirate, tracheal aspirate, transtracheal aspirate. These specimens are clinically equivalent to sputum (for microbiology purposes). **Do not submit specimen on a swab.**

Container Sterile tube, Lukens tube, or sputum container

Collection The specimen can be divided for fungus culture, mycobacteria culture and smear, and routine bacterial culture and Gram's stain only if the specimen is accompanied by properly completed requisitions for these procedures and if the specimen is of adequate volume for all tests requested. Specify fungal species suspected.

Storage Instructions Specimen must be delivered to the laboratory as soon as possible. Refrigerate specimen until delivery is possible.

Causes for Rejection Specimen on outside of container, insufficient numbers of completed requisitions for the procedures requested

Turnaround Time Physicians will be notified of all positive cultures. Negative cultures are reported after 4 weeks.

Reference Range No fungi grown

Use Isolate and identify fungi

Limitations A single negative culture does not rule out presence of fungal infection

Additional Information Saprophytic fungi (especially yeast) isolated from respiratory aspirates are not uncommon. If mycobacteria are isolated, the isolate will be identified and referred for susceptibility testing on request.

Fungus Culture, Bronchoscopy see Fungus Culture, Sputum on page 419

Fungus Culture, Cerebrospinal Fluid

Related Information

Cerebrospinal Fluid Analysis on page 354

Cryptococcal Antigen Serology, Serum or Cerebrospinal Fluid on page 379

India Ink Preparation on page 460

Viral Culture, Central Nervous System Symptoms on page 570

Synonyms Cerebrospinal Fluid Fungus Culture; CSF Fungus Culture; Fungus Culture, CSF; Fungus Culture, Spinal Fluid; Spinal Fluid Fungus Culture

Test Includes Culture for fungi, India ink, fungus smear, and cryptococcal antigen test if requested (and depending on laboratory protocol)

Patient Preparation Aseptic preparation of aspiration site

Special Instructions The laboratory should be informed of the specific source of specimen.

Specimen Cerebrospinal fluid

Container Sterile CSF tube

Collection Tubes should be numbered 1, 2, 3 with tube #1 representing the first portion of the sample collected. Contamination with normal flora from skin or other body surfaces must be avoided. The third tube collected during lumbar puncture is most suitable for culture because skin contaminants from the puncture usually are washed out with fluid collected in the first two tubes.

Storage Instructions The specimen should be transported immediately to the laboratory. If it cannot be processed immediately, it should be kept at room temperature or placed in an incubator. Do not refrigerate.

Turnaround Time Negative cultures are usually reported after 4 weeks

Reference Range No growth

Use Isolate and identify fungi, particularly *Cryptococcus neoformans*. Diagnosis is established by detection of cryptococcal antigen.

Limitations Recovery of fungi from cerebrospinal fluid is directly related to the volume of cerebrospinal fluid available. Recovery is <100% on one specimen. A minimum of 10 mL is recommended. *Cryptococcus* can be mistaken for small lymphocytes in the counting chamber.

Methodology Aerobic culture of centrifuged sediment on several fungal media

Additional Information India ink preparations are not very useful (sensitivity, <50%) in identifying the presence of *Cryptococcus neoformans*, the most common fungus isolated from cerebrospinal fluid. Cryptococcal antigen titers of serum and cerebrospinal fluid provide rapid diagnosis and have greater sensitivity than India ink preparation. The diagnosis of central nervous system fungal infections is frequently complicated by the overlapping array of signs and symptoms which may accompany other clinical entities such as tuberculous meningitis, pyogenic abscess, brain tumor, hypersensitivity or allergic reactions, collagen vascular disease, leptomeningeal malignancy, chemical meningitis, meningeal inflammation secondary to contiguous suppuration, Behçet's disease, Mollaret's meningitis, and the uveomeningitic syndromes.

Especially in immunocompromised hosts, aspergillosis, mucormycosis, and candidiasis are observed. Infections with species which cause phaeohyphomycosis are described. Nocardiosis can infect the meninges. *Cryptococcus neoformans* has been isolated from up to 10% of patients with acquired immunodeficiency syndrome (AIDS).

Selected Readings
Greenlee JE, "Approach to Diagnosis of Meningitis - Cerebrospinal Fluid Evaluation," *Infect Dis Clin North Am*, 1990, 4(4):583-98.

Tunkel AR, Wispelwey B, and Scheld WM, "Pathogenesis and Pathophysiology of Meningitis," *Infect Dis Clin North Am*, 1990, 4(4):555-81.

Fungus Culture, CSF *see* Fungus Culture, Cerebrospinal Fluid *on previous page*

Fungus Culture, Dermatophytes *see* Fungus Culture, Skin *on this page*

Fungus Culture, Gastric Aspirate *see* Fungus Culture, Sputum *on page 419*

Fungus Culture, Hair *see* Fungus Culture, Skin *on this page*

Fungus Culture, Nail *see* Fungus Culture, Skin *on this page*

Fungus Culture, Skin

Related Information
KOH Preparation *on page 467*
Methenamine Silver Stain *on page 487*
Periodic Acid-Schiff Stain *on page 518*
Skin Biopsy *on page 535*

Applies to Dermatophyte Fungus Culture; Fungus Culture, Dermatophytes; Fungus Culture, Hair; Fungus Culture, Nail; Hair Fungus Culture; Nail Fungus Culture

Patient Preparation Select fluorescent hairs or nonfluorescent hairs which are broken off and appear diseased and pluck them with sterile forceps. If diseased hair stubs are not apparent, scrape the edges of a skin lesion with a sterile scalpel. Cleanse skin lesions first with 70% alcohol to reduce bacteria and saprophytic fungi. Scrape from the outer edges of skin lesions. In infections of the nails, scrape out the friable material beneath the edge of the nails, or scrape or clip off portions of abnormal appearing nail and submit for examination and culture.

Special Instructions Careful choice of specimens for laboratory study is important. A Wood's lamp can occasionally be useful in the collection of specimens in tinea capitis infections because hairs infected by most members of the genus *Microsporum* frequently exhibit fluorescence under a Wood's lamp. However, in tinea capitis due to *Trichophyton* sp, infected hairs usually do not fluoresce. The laboratory should be informed of the specific site of the specimen. See table. (Continued)

Fungus Culture, Skin *(Continued)*

Selection of Specimens for the Diagnosis of Superficial Mycosis and Dermatomycosis

Diagnosis	Specimen of Choice
Superficial mycoses	
Piedra	Hair
Tinea nigra	Skin scraping
Tinea versicolor	Skin scraping
Dermatomycoses (cutaneous mycoses)	
Onychomycosis	Nail scraping
Tinea capitis	Hair (black dot)
Tinea corporis	Skin scraping
Tinea pedis	Skin scraping
Tinea cruris	Skin scraping
Candidiasis	
Thrush	Scraping of oral white patches
Diaper dermatitis	Scraping of pustules at margin
Paronychia	Scraping skin around nail
Cutaneous candidiasis	Scraping of pustules at margin
Erosio interdigitalis blastomycetia (coinfection with gram-negative rods)	Scrapings of interdigital space (routine culture also)
Congenital candidiasis	Scraping of scales, pustules and cutaneous debris, cultures of umbilical stump, mouth, urine and stool
Mucocutaneous candidiasis	Scraping of affected area

Specimen Skin scrapings, exudates, nail clippings, whole nail, debris under nail, hair

Container Petri dish, urine container, envelope

Collection Enclose hair specimens, skin scrapings, or nail clippings or scrapings in clean paper envelopes, urine container, or Petri dish. Label the specimen with the patient's name. Enclose these envelopes in larger heavy paper envelopes. Do not put specimens in cotton-plugged tubes, because the specimen may become trapped among the cotton fibers and lost. Do not put specimen into closed containers, such as rubber-stoppered tubes, because this keeps the specimen moist and allows overgrowth of bacteria and saprophytic fungi. The laboratory should be informed of the fungal species suspected.

Storage Instructions Keep specimen at room temperature until delivered to the laboratory

Turnaround Time Cultures positive for *Candida* sp are usually reported within 1 week. Cultures positive for dermatophytes are usually reported within 2-3 weeks. Negative cultures are usually reported after 1 month. Cultures in which suspicion of systemic fungal infection has been indicated are usually reported upon becoming positive, or negative after 4 weeks.

Reference Range No growth

Use Isolate and identify fungi

Limitations A single negative specimen does not rule out fungal infections. If infection with mycobacteria or aerobic organisms cannot be excluded clinically, a separate culture should be submitted as indicated.

Methodology Aerobic culture on selective media usually including nonselective Sabouraud's agar

Additional Information *Candida* sp may colonize skin. Clinical diagnosis of *Candida* infection involves consideration of predisposing factors such as occlusion, maceration altered cutaneous barrier function. Signs of *Candida* infection include bright erythema, fragile papulopustules, and satellite lesions.

Selected Readings

Cohn MS, "Superficial Fungal Infections. Topical and Oral Treatment of Common Types," *Postgrad Med*, 1992, 91(2):239-44, 249-52.

McKay M, "Cutaneous Manifestations of Candidiasis," *Am J Obstet Gynecol*, 1988, 158(4):991-3.

Meyer RD, "Cutaneous and Mucosal Manifestations of the Deep Mycotic Infections," *Acta Derm Venereol Suppl (Stockh)*, 1986, 121:57-72.

Stein DH, "Superficial Fungal Infections," *Pediatr Clin North Am*, 1983, 30(3):545-61.

Fungus Culture, Spinal Fluid *see* Fungus Culture, Cerebrospinal Fluid *on page 416*

Fungus Culture, Sputum

Related Information
Methenamine Silver Stain *on page 487*
Periodic Acid-Schiff Stain *on page 518*

Synonyms Sputum Fungus Culture

Applies to Bronchoscopy Fungus Culture; Fungus Culture, Bronchoscopy; Fungus Culture, Gastric Aspirate; Fungus Culture, Tracheal Aspirate; Fungus Culture, Transtracheal Aspirate; Gastric Aspirate Fungus Culture; Percutaneous Transtracheal Fungus Culture; Tracheal Aspirate Fungus Culture; Transtracheal Aspirate Fungus Culture

Patient Preparation The patient should be instructed to remove dentures, rinse mouth with water and cough deeply expectorating sputum into the sputum collection cup.

Special Instructions The laboratory should be informed of the specific source of specimen and the suspected clinical diagnosis should be stated.

Specimen First morning sputum. Microbiologically, this specimen is equivalent to the following: gastric aspirate, induced sputum, aspirated sputum, bronchial aspirate, tracheal aspirate, transtracheal aspirate. See table.

Selection of Specimens for the Diagnosis of Systemic and Subcutaneous Mycosis

Diagnosis	Specimen of Choice in Order of Usefulness	Diagnosis	Specimen of Choice in Order of Usefulness
Systemic Mycoses		**Systemic Mycoses (continued)**	
Aspergillosis	Sputum	Mycomycosis/	Sputum
	Bronchial aspirate	phycomycosis	Bronchial aspirate
	Biopsy (lung)		Biopsy (lung)
Blastomycosis	Skin scrapings	Paracoccidioidomycosis	Skin scrapings
	Abscess drainage (pus)	(South American	Mucosal scrapings
	Urine	blastomycosis)	Biopsy (lymph nodes)
	Sputum		Sputum
	Bronchial aspirate		Bronchial aspirate
Candidiasis	Sputum		
	Bronchial aspirate	**Subcutaneous Mycoses**	
	Blood		
	Cerebrospinal fluid	Chromoblastomycosis	Skin scrapings
	Urine		Biopsy (skin)
	Stool		Drainage (pus)
Coccidioidomycosis	Sputum	Maduromycosis	Drainage (pus)
	Bronchial aspirate	(mycetoma)	Abscess drainage
	Cerebrospinal fluid		Biopsy (lesion)
	Urine		
	Skin scrapings	Sporotrichosis	Drainage (pus)
	Abscess drainage (pus)		Abscess drainage
			Biopsy (skin, lymph node)
Cryptococcosis	Cerebrospinal fluid		
	Sputum		
	Abscess drainage (pus)		
	Skin scraping		
	Urine		

Container Sterile sputum cup, sputum trap, sterile tracheal aspirate tube or sterile bronchoscopy tube
(Continued)

Fungus Culture, Sputum *(Continued)*

Collection Every effort should be made to collect the specimen early in the day so that it may be processed by the laboratory for optimal recovery. A recommended screening procedure is three first morning specimens submitted on three successive days. The specimen can be divided for fungus culture, mycobacteria culture and smear, and routine bacterial culture and Gram's stain only if the specimen is of adequate volume for all tests requested.

Storage Instructions Refrigerate the specimen if storage is in excess of 1 hour

Causes for Rejection Specimens contaminated on the outside of the container pose excessive risk to laboratory personnel and may not be acceptable to the laboratory.

Turnaround Time Negative cultures are reported after 4 weeks

Reference Range No growth; yeast from the oropharynx may be present.

Use Establish the presence of potentially pathogenic fungi

Limitations The yield may be reduced by bacterial overgrowth during storage or on standing; therefore, fresh sputum is preferred. A single negative culture does not rule out the presence of fungal infection. If two specimens are received simultaneously, many laboratories will pool them and process them as one specimen unless specific instructions are provided.

Methodology Culture on selective and nonselective media

Additional Information Deeply coughed sputum, transtracheal aspirate, bronchial washing or brushing, or deep tracheal aspirate are preferred specimens. Oncology patients, transplant patients, and patients with the acquired immunodeficiency syndrome (AIDS) are particularly prone to infection with fungi.

Primary fungal pulmonary infections frequently result in granulomatous disease. Classically, *Histoplasma capsulatum*, *Coccidioides immitis*, *Cryptococcus neoformans*, and *Blastomyces dermatitidis* have been implicated. The incidence was largely related to geographic exposure and many cases occurred in seemingly normal hosts. Recently increasing numbers of reports of opportunistic fungal pulmonary infections due to a wide variety of etiologic agents which are ubiquitous in the environment, are being published. Definitive diagnosis depends upon the following: presence of clinical signs of pulmonary infection including rales, rhonchi and fever, and a chest x-ray picture revealing consolidation of granuloma; laboratory isolation of a potentially significant organism from a suitable specimen; histologic documentation of tissue invasion by the isolated organism. Many lists of documented etiologic agents of pulmonary fungal disease have been reported (see table).

Common Pulmonary Fungal Infections

Endemic Fungi	Opportunistic Fungi
Histoplasma capsulatum	Candida albicans
Blastomyces dermatitidis	Candida tropicalis
Coccidioides immitis	Aspergillus niger
Paracoccidioides brasiliensis	Aspergillus fumigatus
	Mucor
	Rhizopus
	Absidia
	Cryptococcus neoformans

From Haque AK, "Pathology of Common Pulmonary Fungal Infections," *J Thorac Imaging*, 1992, 7:1-11, with permission.

In practice a diagnosis sufficient for therapy can frequently be established by observation of hyphae, pseudohyphae or yeast cells in tissue sections; recovery of the organism from a normally sterile site; repeated isolation of the same suspect organism from the same or different sites; seroconversion (ie, the development of an immune response to the suspected organism). *Candida* and *Aspergillus* sp are the most frequently isolated usually pathogenic organisms. However, they are frequently present as the result of contamination from the patient's normal flora or airborne sources. Their presence may represent colonization rather than invasion. Recovery of *Candida* from blood (see Blood Culture, Fungus *on page 341*) is a major adjunct to definitive diagnosis. Even without invasion *Aspergillus* may cause IgE-mediated asthma, allergic alveolitis cell mediated hypersensitivity, mucoid impaction, and bronchocentric granulomatosis. Fungal tracheobronchitis has recently been recognized to present as a pseudomembranous form involving the circumference of the bronchial wall or as multiple or discrete plaques. The plaques or pseudomembranes are composed of necrotic tissue exudate and fungal hyphae.

Selected Readings
Rinaldi MG, "Invasive Aspergillosis," *Rev Infect Dis*, 1983, 5(6):1061-77.

Schuyler MR, "Allergic Bronchopulmonary Aspergillosis," *Clin Chest Med*, 1983, 4(1):15-22.

Stamm AM and Dismukes WE, "Current Therapy of Pulmonary and Disseminated Fungal Diseases," *Chest*, 1983, 83(6):911-7.

Zarabi MC and Salmassi S, "Antemortem Diagnosis of Systemic Aspergillosis: Ten Year Review and Report of a Case," *South Med J*, 1984, 77(5):584-8.

Fungus Culture, Surgical Specimen *see* Fungus Culture, Biopsy *on page 414*

Fungus Culture, Surgical Specimen *see* Fungus Culture, Body Fluid *on page 415*

Fungus Culture, Tissue *see* Fungus Culture, Biopsy *on page 414*

Fungus Culture, Tissue *see* Fungus Culture, Body Fluid *on page 415*

Fungus Culture, Tracheal Aspirate *see* Fungus Culture, Bronchial Aspirate *on page 416*

Fungus Culture, Tracheal Aspirate *see* Fungus Culture, Sputum *on page 419*

Fungus Culture, Transtracheal Aspirate *see* Fungus Culture, Bronchial Aspirate *on page 416*

Fungus Culture, Transtracheal Aspirate *see* Fungus Culture, Sputum *on page 419*

Fungus Culture, Urine

Related Information

Methenamine Silver Stain *on page 487*

Periodic Acid-Schiff Stain *on page 518*

Synonyms Urine Fungus Culture

Patient Preparation Usual preparation for clean catch midvoid urine specimen collection. See listing Urine Culture, Clean Catch *on page 565*.

Special Instructions The laboratory should be informed of the specific source of the specimen and the fungal species suspected.

Specimen Urine

Container Sterile plastic container or tube

Collection The specimen should be transported to laboratory within 2 hours of collection if not refrigerated. The patient must be instructed to thoroughly cleanse skin and collect midstream specimen.

Causes for Rejection Unrefrigerated specimen more than 2 hours old may be subject to overgrowth and may not yield valid results

Reference Range No growth

Use Isolate and identify fungi

Limitations A single negative culture does not rule out the presence of fungal infection.

Additional Information Patients with candiduria may or may not have candidemia; positive urine culture for fungi often may be followed by positive blood culture for fungi. Ascending infections occur in patients with diabetes, prolonged antimicrobial therapy, or following instrumentation. Urinary obstruction due to "fungus balls" may occur in diabetes and following renal transplantation. Candiduria associated with hematogenous infections is observed in patients with granulocytopenia, corticosteroid therapy, and with immunosuppression. The source is frequently the gastrointestinal tract or indwelling catheters particular with hyperalimentation. A blood fungus culture is useful in defining invasive disease. However, proof of invasive *Candida* infection requires direct cystoscopic or operative visualization of fungus balls, or pyelonephritis, or histological evidence of mucosa invasion. Urine is a useful specimen for culture in cryptococcosis, blastomycosis, and candidiasis. See table for fungus culture specimen selection in Fungus Culture, Sputum *on page 419*. The incidence of genitourinary fungal infections is increasing. They are usually associated with broad spectrum antibiotic therapy, corticosteroid therapy, underlying general debility, and AIDS. In addition to *Candida*, opportunistic pathogens in the genitourinary tract include *Aspergillus* and *Cryptococcus*. Endemic pathogens such as *Histoplasma*, *Blastomyces*, and *Coccidioides* are also encountered.

Selected Readings
Frangos DN and Nyberg LM Jr, "Genitourinary Fungal Infections," *South Med J*, 1986, 79(4):455-9.

(Continued)

Fungus Culture, Urine *(Continued)*

Roy JB, Geyer JR, and Mohr JA, "Urinary Tract Candidiasis: An Update," *Urology*, 1984, 23(6):533-7.

"Urinary Tract Candidosis," *Lancet*, 1988, 2(8618):1000-2.

Gallium Abscess Scan *see* Gallium Scan *on this page*

Gallium Scan

Applies to Gallium Abscess Scan; Gallium Tumor Scan; Soft Tissue Scan

Test Includes The patient receives an intravenous injection of gallium-67 citrate. Images are then acquired for some combination of 24, 48, and 72 hours after injection.

Patient Preparation Patient should have all RIA blood work performed, or at least drawn, prior to injection of any radioactive material. The patient does not need to be fasting or NPO for this procedure.

Special Instructions Requisition must state the current patient diagnosis in order to select the most appropriate radiopharmaceutical and/or imaging technique. Other Nuclear Medicine procedures (bone, liver, lung) should be completed prior to gallium injection. If abdominal abscess/infection is suspected, laxatives, and/or enemas may be ordered for the patient prior to delayed imaging at 48 or 72 hours. This will help clear normal intestinal gallium activity from the colon. **DURATION OF PROCEDURE:** 24-72 hours **RADIOPHARMACEUTICAL:** Gallium-67 citrate.

Technique The application of single-photon emission tomography (SPECT) techniques may contribute significantly to the diagnostic accuracy of this imaging study.

Turnaround Time A written report will be sent to the patient's chart and/or to the referring physician.

Normal Findings Gallium will localize to some degree in liver and spleen, bone, nasopharynx, lacrimal glands, and breast tissue. There is normally some secretion of gallium into the bowel. This may require laxatives and/or enemas for the patient to evacuate this normal activity before additional imaging of possible abdominal infection or abscess. Abnormal accumulation of gallium will usually be asymmetric, increase in later images, and remain in the same location (normal bowel luminal gallium activity will transit).

Use Gallium localizes at sites of active inflammation or infection as well as in some neoplasms. Gallium imaging is very sensitive in detection of abscesses, pneumonia, pyelonephritis, active sarcoidosis, and active tuberculosis. Even in immunocompromised patients (eg, those with AIDS), gallium imaging can detect early complications such as *Pneumocystis carinii* pneumonitis. The nonspecificity of gallium activity, however, requires that correlation with other radiographic studies and clinical findings be given close attention. Gallium imaging is very useful in the differential diagnosis and staging of some neoplasms, notably Hodgkin's disease, lymphoma, hepatocellular carcinoma, bronchogenic carcinoma, melanoma, and leukemia. Recent evidence has shown a correlation of gallium localization in the lungs with the activity of disease in pulmonary fibrosis and asbestosis. Gallium is also used in addition to bone scintigraphy for detecting osteomyelitis, especially in its chronic stages. A common indication for gallium imaging is as a screening procedure for infection in fever of unknown origin (FUO).

Limitations There is variable normal excretion of gallium via the intestinal tract. This contributes to the nonspecificity of gallium imaging in suspected abdominal or pelvic infections. Previous treatment with antibiotics or high doses of steroids may decrease the inflammatory response and result in false-negative gallium imaging.

Additional Information Other isotope studies may need to be postponed up to 7 days after a gallium scan has been done due to its slow elimination from soft tissue.

Selected Readings

Bisson G, Lamoureux G, and Bégin R, "Quantitative Gallium-67 Lung Scan to Assess the Inflammatory Activity in the Pneumoconioses," *Semin Nucl Med*, 1987, 17(1):72-80.

Israel O, Front D, Epelbaum R, et al, "Residual Mass and Negative Gallium Scintigraphy in Treated Lymphoma," *J Nucl Med*, 1990, 31(3):365-8.

Maderazo EG, Hickingbotham NB, Woronick CL, et al, "The Influence of Various Factors on the Accuracy of Gallium-67 Imaging for Occult Infection," *J Nucl Med*, 1988, 29(5):608-15.

Rossleigh MA, Murray IP, Mackey DW, et al, "Pediatric Solid Tumors: Evaluation by Gallium-67 SPECT Studies," *J Nucl Med*, 1990, 31(2):168-72.

Gallium Tumor Scan *see* Gallium Scan *on previous page*

Garamycin®, Blood *see* Gentamicin Level *on page 425*

Gastric Aspirate Fungus Culture *see* Fungus Culture, Sputum *on page 419*

Gastric Aspirate Mycobacteria Culture *see* Mycobacteria Culture, Sputum *on page 495*

Gastric Biopsy Culture for *Helicobacter pylori* *see* Helicobacter pylori Culture and Urease Test *on page 432*

Gastrointestinal Viruses by EM *see* Electron Microscopic (EM) Examination for Viruses, Stool *on page 403*

GC Culture *see* Neisseria gonorrhoeae Culture *on page 501*

GC Culture, Throat *see* Neisseria gonorrhoeae Culture *on page 501*

Genital Culture

Related Information

Abscess Aerobic and Anaerobic Culture *on page 304*
Chlamydia Culture *on page 359*
Genital Culture for *Ureaplasma urealyticum* *on next page*
Group B *Streptococcus* Antigen Test *on page 429*
Neisseria gonorrhoeae Culture *on page 501*
Trichomonas Preparation *on page 555*

Applies to Cervical Culture; Endocervical Culture; Prostatic Fluid Culture; Vaginal Culture

Test Includes Culture for aerobic organisms, *Candida* sp, and *Neisseria gonorrhoeae*. *Gardnerella* and *Mobiluncus*, Gram's stain, and fungal stain may require separate requests.

Special Instructions The laboratory should be informed of the specific source of specimen, age of patient, current antibiotic therapy, clinical diagnosis, and time of collection.

Specimen Swab of vagina, cervix, discharge, aspirated endocervical, endometrial, prostatic fluid, or urethral discharge. Specimens to be cultured for *N. gonorrhoeae* **must** be cultured at bedside (onto special medium at room temperature) and be in the laboratory within 30 minutes.

Container Sterile Culturette® or sterile tube

Collection The specimen should be transported to laboratory within 2 hours of collection. Refrigeration may reduce yield.

Turnaround Time Preliminary reports are usually available at 24 hours. Cultures with no growth are usually reported after 48 hours. Cultures from which pathogens are isolated usually require a minimum of 48 hours for completion.

Reference Range Normal flora; properly collected prostatic fluid and endocervical cultures are normally sterile.

Use Isolate and identify potentially pathogenic organisms. Infectious causes of abnormal vaginal discharge or vulvovaginitis include *Candida albicans*, *Trichomonas vaginalis*, *Gardnerella vaginalis*, *Mobiluncus* sp, *Chlamydia trachomatis*, herpes simplex virus, human papillomavirus, *Enterobius vermicularis* (pinworms), *Giardia lamblia* and other microorganisms. Normal vaginal secretions have a pH of 4.5 or less, characteristic appearance, and consist of clear mucus, epithelial cells, and have no unusual odor. Many bacterial organisms and perhaps *Candida albicans* are present in a stable symbiotic relationship. Culture may allow documentation of a change in balance of normal organism populations or detection of a specific pathogen. Also used to document presence of *Staphylococcus aureus* in cases of suspected toxic shock syndrome.

Limitations *Chlamydia* and *Ureaplasma urealyticum* are not recovered by this procedure.

Methodology Aerobic culture with selective (Thayer-Martin) and nonselective media incubated at 35°C to 37°C with CO_2

Additional Information Rapid growing aerobic organisms which predominate are usually identified. Susceptibility testing can be performed if indicated. Routine culture often includes culture for *N. gonorrhoeae*, *Candida albicans*, *Staphylococcus aureus*, group B streptococci, and *Gardnerella vaginalis*. Presence or absence of normal flora will usually be reported. Normal flora of the vagina is dependent upon age, glycogen content, pH, exogenous hormone therapy, etc. Normal vaginal flora includes anaerobes, corynebacteria, enteric gram-negative rods, enterococci, lactobacilli, *Moraxella* sp, staphylococci, streptococci (alpha and nonhemolytic), *Mycobacterium smegmatis*. The laboratory (Continued)

Genital Culture *(Continued)*

should be consulted to arrange for special toxin identification procedures if toxic shock syndrome is suspected and *Staphylococcus aureus* is recovered.

Vaginitis is one of the most commonly encountered complaints of female patients. The majority of cases (approximately 90%) are caused by *Candida*, *Gardnerella*, or *Trichomonas*. Diagnosis and effective treatment depend upon accurate identification of the etiologic agent, effective specific therapy, and restoration of the normal ecosystem of the vagina. Proper hygiene, dietary control, and management of stress also are important factors in control of recurrent vaginal infections.

Candida sp are frequently present as normal flora in vagina. A saline wet mount may demonstrate yeast cells or pseudohyphae and may provide rapid diagnostic information. The most common clinical presentation is a characteristic clumpy white cottage cheese appearance with vaginal or vulvar itching. Vaginitis frequently complicates pregnancy and diabetes, and is seen with broad spectrum antibiotic therapy as well as in conditions which lower host resistance.

Selected Readings

Faro S, "Bacterial Vaginitis," *Clin Obstet Gynecol*, 1991, 34(3):582-6.

Sobel JD, "Vaginal Infections in Adult Women," *Med Clin North Am*, 1990, 74(6):1573-602.

Spiegel CA, "Bacterial Vaginosis," *Clin Microbiol Rev*, 1991, 4(4):485-502.

Thomason JL, Gelbart SM, and Scaglione NJ, "Bacterial Vaginosis: Current Review With Indications for Asymptomatic Therapy," *Am J Obstet Gynecol*, 1991, 165(4 Pt 2):1210-7.

Zenilman JM, "Gonorrhea: Clinical and Public Health Issues," *Hosp Pract (Off Ed)*, 1993, 28(2A):29-35, 39-40, 43-50.

Genital Culture for *Mycoplasma* T-Strain *see* Genital Culture for *Ureaplasma urealyticum* on this page

Genital Culture for *Ureaplasma urealyticum*

Related Information

Genital Culture *on previous page*

Mycoplasma/Ureaplasma Culture *on page 499*

Neisseria gonorrhoeae Culture *on page 501*

Synonyms Genital Culture for *Mycoplasma* T-Strain; *Mycoplasma* T-Strain Culture, Genital; *Ureaplasma urealyticum* Culture, Genital

Applies to Cervical Culture for T-Strain *Mycoplasma*; Cervical Culture for *Ureaplasma urealyticum*; Urethral Culture for T-Strain *Mycoplasma*

Special Instructions *Ureaplasma* and *Mycoplasma* are sensitive to delays in processing and storage. Consult the laboratory prior to collecting the specimen for optimal handling instructions.

Specimen Culturette® swab of urethra or cervix

Container Culturette® swab

Storage Instructions Keep specimen refrigerated. **Organism is remarkably sensitive to drying**; swab must be placed promptly into Culturette® and hand delivered to the Microbiology Laboratory.

Turnaround Time 8 days if negative, up to 2 weeks if positive

Reference Range Frequently isolated from asymptomatic individuals

Use Establish the diagnosis of *Ureaplasma urealyticum* infection in suspected cases of nongonococcal urethritis and cervicitis

Limitations Culture may be negative in the presence of infection, and the presence of *Ureaplasma urealyticum* or *Mycoplasma hominis* does not always indicate infection, although there is a significant association with symptomatic disease.

Methodology Culture on selective media

Additional Information *Ureaplasma* and *Mycoplasma* can be isolated from urethral and genital swabs and from urine of sexually active individuals. Sixty percent or more of all women asymptomatically carry *U. urealyticum* in their genital tract. Usual prevalence of these organisms in patients with urethral symptoms also is high; thus, conclusions regarding the etiologic role of an isolate in a given patient are difficult to make. *U. urealyticum* is usually associated with cases of nongonococcal urethritis.

Selected Readings

Bell TA, "*Chlamydia trachomatis, Mycoplasma hominis,* and *Ureaplasma urealyticum* Infections of Infants," *Semin Perinatol*, 1985, 9(1):29-37.

Cassell GH, Waites KB, Watson HL, et al, "*Ureaplasma urealyticum* Intrauterine Infection: Role in Prematurity and Disease in Newborns," *Clin Microbiol Rev*, 1993, 6(1):69-87.

Taylor-Robinson D and McCormack WM, "The Genital *Mycoplasma*," *N Engl J Med*, 1980, 302(19):1003-67.

Genotyping, HCV *see* Hepatitis C Viral RNA Genotyping *on page 438*
Gen-Probe® for *Neisseria gonorrhoeae* *see* Neisseria gonorrhoeae by Nucleic Acid Probe *on page 500*

Gentamicin Level

Related Information
Antibiotic Level, Serum *on page 321*

Synonyms Garamycin®, Blood

Abstract Aminoglycoside antibiotics, including gentamicin, are used primarily to treat infections caused by aerobic gram-negative bacilli. Additionally, when used in combination with penicillins, they may have synergistic bactericidal activity against gram-positive cocci such as *Staphylococcus aureus* and *Enterococcus*. Gentamicin has a narrow therapeutic window, and its use in life-threatening infections makes it mandatory that effective levels be achieved without overdosage.

Specimen Serum, urine

Container Red top tube, plastic urine container

Sampling Time Peak: 30-60 minutes after end of 30 minute I.V. infusion or 60 minutes post I.M. dose; trough: immediately prior to next dose. Specimens should be drawn at steady-state, usually after fifth dose, if drug given every 8 hours, or after third dose, if drug given every 12 hours.

Storage Instructions Separate within 1 hour of collection and refrigerate or freeze until assayed. Must be frozen if a β-lactam antibiotic is also present because of potential inactivation of aminoglycosides.

Reference Range Therapeutic: peak: 4-10 µg/mL (SI: 8-21 µmol/L) (depends in part on the minimal inhibitory concentration of the drug against the organism being treated); trough: <2 µg/mL (SI: <4 µmol/L)

Possible Panic Range Toxic: peak: >12 µg/mL (SI: >25 µmol/L); trough: >2 µg/mL (SI: >4 µmol/L)

Use Peak levels are necessary to assure adequate therapeutic levels for organism being treated. Trough levels are necessary to reduce the likelihood of nephrotoxicity.

Limitations High peak levels may not have strong correlation with toxicity.

Methodology Enzyme immunoassay (EIA), fluorescence polarization immunoassay (FPIA), high performance liquid chromatography (HPLC)

Additional Information Gentamicin is cleared by the kidney and accumulates in renal tubular cells. Nephrotoxicity is most closely related to the length of time that trough levels exceed 2 µg/mL (SI: >4 µmol/L). Creatinine levels should be monitored every 2-3 days as an indicator of impending renal toxicity. The initial toxic result is nonoliguric renal failure that is usually reversible if the drug is discontinued. Continued administration of gentamicin may produce oliguric renal failure. Nephrotoxicity may occur in as many as 10% to 25% of patients receiving aminoglycosides; most of this toxicity can be avoided by monitoring levels and adjusting dosing schedules accordingly.

Aminoglycosides may also cause irreversible ototoxicity that manifests itself clinically as hearing loss. Aminoglycoside ototoxicity is relatively uncommon and clinical trials where levels were carefully monitored and dosing adjusted failed to show a correlation between auditory toxicity and plasma aminoglycoside levels. In situations where dosing is not monitored and adjusted, however, sustained high levels may be associated with ototoxicity. This association is far from clear cut, and new once-daily dosing regimens (and associated high peak serum concentrations) that fail to enhance toxicity further complicate this issue.

Selected Readings
Dipersio JR, "Gentamicin and Other Aminoglycosides," *Clinical Chemistry Theory, Analysis, and Correlation*, 2nd ed, Kaplan LA and Pesce AJ, eds, St Louis, MO: CV Mosby Co, 1989, 1102-8.
Edson RS and Terrell CL, "The Aminoglycosides," *Mayo Clin Proc*, 1991, 66(11):1158-64.
Pancoast SJ, "Aminoglycoside Antibiotics in Clinical Use," *Med Clin North Am*, 1987, 72(3):581-612.

German Measles Culture *see* Rubella Virus Culture *on page 532*
German Measles Serology *see* Rubella Serology *on page 531*
GFR *see* Creatinine Clearance *on page 378*
Giardia Antigen *see* Giardia Specific Antigen (GSA65) *on next page*
Giardia Immunoassay *see* Giardia Specific Antigen (GSA65) *on next page*

Giardia Screen *see Giardia Specific Antigen (GSA65) on this page*

Giardia Specific Antigen (GSA65)

Synonyms *Giardia* Antigen; *Giardia* Immunoassay; *Giardia* Screen

Test Includes A solid-phase immunoassay based on specific antibody to *Giardia* specific antigen (GSA65)

Specimen
- Fresh random stool, collected in a clean sealable plastic container - refrigerated or frozen until testing.
- Stool in 10% formalin - refrigerated or frozen.
- Stool in Cary-Blair medium - refrigerated or frozen.
- Rectal swabs, transported in Stewart's Culturette® or Ames Charcoal Culturette®. Swabs should not be allowed to dry out.
- Stool in PVA fixative **is not** acceptable.

Reference Range Negative

Use Diagnose giardiasis; monitor effectiveness of anti-*Giardia* therapy

Methodology Solid phase immunoassay

Additional Information A positive result indicates the presence of *Giardia* specific antigen (GGSA65). Secretion of GSA65 is present only when *Giardia* infection is present. GSA65 does not cross react with other enteric parasites, bacteria, or yeast. This test is more sensitive for the diagnosis of *Giardia* than the routine ova and parasite examination. It is not a substitute for the broad screen provided by the ova and parasite examination. An equivalent screening test (immunofluorescent antibody) is available in some laboratories.

Selected Readings

Maddison SE, "Serodiagnosis of Parasitic Diseases," *Clin Microbiol Rev*, 1991, 4(4):457-69.

Wolfe MS, "Giardiasis," *Clin Microbiol Rev*, 1992, 5(1):93-100.

Glomerular Filtration Rate *see Creatinine Clearance on page 378*

GMS Stain *see Methenamine Silver Stain on page 487*

Gomori-Methenamine Silver Stain *see Methenamine Silver Stain on page 487*

Gonorrhea Culture *see Neisseria gonorrhoeae Culture on page 501*

Gonorrhea Culture, Throat *see Neisseria gonorrhoeae Culture on page 501*

Gram's Stain

Related Information

Acid-Fast Stain, Modified, *Nocardia* Species *on page 307*
Actinomyces Culture, All Sites *on page 308*
Methenamine Silver Stain *on page 487*
Periodic Acid-Schiff Stain *on page 518*
Skin Biopsy *on page 535*

Synonyms Bacterial Smear; Smear, Gram's Stain

Patient Preparation Same as for routine culture of specific site

Special Instructions The laboratory should be informed of the specific site of specimen, age of patient, current antibiotic therapy, and clinical diagnosis.

Specimen Duplicate of specimen appropriate for routine culture of the specific site

Container Sterile specimen container, or sterile tube or appropriate tube for swab

Collection Collection procedure same as for routine culture of the specific site. Specimen must be collected to avoid contamination with skin, adjacent structures, and nonsterile surfaces.

Storage Instructions Same as for a culture of the specimen

Causes for Rejection Insufficient specimen volume

Turnaround Time Usually same day

Reference Range Depends on site of specimen

Use Determine the presence or absence of bacteria, yeast, neutrophils, and epithelial cells; establish the presence of potentially pathogenic organisms. The Gram's stain is essential in the evaluation of all suspected cases of bacterial meningitis.

Limitations Organism isolation and identification will usually be performed only if culture is requested. Request for Gram's stain will not lead to stain for mycobacteria (TB). For detection of tubercle bacilli, an acid-fast stain must also be requested. Certain organisms do not stain or do not stain well with Gram's stain, eg, *Legionella pneumophila* and *Campylobacter* sp. As many as 30% of cases of bacterial meningitis have a negative Gram's stain. Yield may be increased by use of the acridine orange stain (AO) particularly in cases of partially treated meningitis, but few laboratories elect to use this method. Gram's stain is **not** reliable for diagnosis of cervical, rectal, pharyngeal, or asymptomatic urethral gonococcal infection, except for gonococcal urethritis in males.

Methodology Gram's stain technique:

- Make a thin smear of the material for study and allow to air dry.
- Fix the material to the slide by passing the slide 3 or 4 times through the flame of a Bunsen burner so that the material does not wash off during the staining procedure. Some workers now recommend the use of alcohol for the fixation of material to be Gram's stained (flood the smear with methanol or ethanol for a few minutes or warm for 10 minutes at 60°C on a slide warmer).
- Place the smear on a staining rack and overlay the surface with crystal violet solution.
- After 1 minute (less time may be used with some solutions) of exposure to the crystal violet stain, wash thoroughly with distilled water or buffer.
- Overlay the smear with Gram's iodine solution for 1 minute. Wash again with water.
- Hold the smear between the thumb and forefinger and flood the surface with acetone-alcohol decolorizer until no violet color washes off. This usually takes 1-3 seconds.
- Wash with running water and again place the smear on the staining rack. Overlay the surface with safranin counterstain for 1 minute. Wash with running water.
- Use paper towels to blot the smear dry.
- Examine the stained smear under the 100x (oil) immersion objective of the microscope. Gram-positive bacteria stain dark blue; gram-negative bacteria appear pink-red.

Additional Information Gram's stains are usually scanned for the presence or absence of white blood cells (indicative of infection) and squamous epithelial cells (indicative of mucosal contamination). A sputum specimen showing more than 25 squamous epithelial cells per low powered field, regardless of the number of white blood cells, is indicative that the specimen is grossly contaminated with saliva and the culture results cannot be properly interpreted. Additional sputum specimens should be submitted to the laboratory if evidence of contamination by saliva is revealed.

The Gram's stain can be a reliable indicator to guide initial antibiotic therapy in community acquired pneumonia. It is imperative that a valid sputum specimen be obtained for Gram's stain. In a well designed trial, valid expectorated sputum was obtained in 41% (59 of 144 patients). The Gram's stain is reliable but not infallible.

Although mycobacteria have classically been considered to be gram-positive or faintly gram-positive, they are more correctly characterized as "gram-neutral" on routine stains. A careful search for mycobacteria should be undertaken when purulent sputum without stainable organisms is encountered.

Gram's stains revealing 1 bacterium per high powered (100x) field in an uncentrifuged urine specimen (or any fluid) suggest a colony count of 10^5 bacteria/mL. Bacteria in the majority of fields suggests 10^6 bacteria/mL, a level associated with significant bacteriuria.

Gram's stain is the most valuable immediately available diagnostic test in bacterial meningitis. Organisms are detectable in 60% to 80% of patients who have not been treated, and in 40% to 60% of those who have been given antibiotics. Its sensitivity relates to the number of organisms present. The sensitivity of the Gram's stain is greater in gram-positive infections, and is only positive in half of the instances of gram-negative meningitis. It is positive even less frequently with listeriosis meningitis or with anaerobic infections.

Culture and Gram's stain should always have priority over antigen detection methods.

Selected Readings

Gleckman R, DeVita J, Hibert D, et al, "Sputum Gram's Stain Assessment in Community-Acquired Bacteremic Pneumonia," *J Clin Microbiol*, 1988, 26(5):846-9.

Granoff DM, Murphy TV, Ingram DL, et al, "Use of Rapidly Generated Results in Patient Management," *Diagn Microbiol Infect Dis*, 1986, 4(3 Suppl):157S-66S.

Gray LD and Fedorko DP, "Laboratory Diagnosis of Bacterial Meningitis," *Clin Microbiol Rev*, 1992, 5(2):130-45.

(Continued)

Gram's Stain *(Continued)*

Provine H and Gardner P, "The Gram's Stained Smear and Its Interpretation," *Hosp Pract*, 1974, 9:85-91.

Riccardi NB and Felman YM, "Laboratory Diagnosis in the Problem of Suspected Gonococcal Infection," *JAMA*, 1979, 242(24):2703-5.

Smith AL, "Bacterial Meningitis," *Pediatr Rev*, 1993, 14:11-8.

Grocott's Modified Silver Stain *see* Methenamine Silver Stain *on page 487*

Gross and Microscopic Pathology *see* Histopathology *on page 448*

Group A Beta-Hemolytic *Streptococcus* Culture, Throat *see* Throat Culture for Group A Beta-Hemolytic *Streptococcus* *on page 550*

Group A *Streptococcus* Antigen Test

Related Information

Bacterial Antigens, Rapid Detection Methods *on page 335*

Throat Culture for Group A Beta-Hemolytic *Streptococcus* *on page 550*

Synonyms Coagglutination Test for Group A Streptococci; *Streptococcus* Group A Latex Screen; Throat Swab for Group A Streptococcal Antigen

Applies to Enzyme Immunoassay for Group A *Streptococcus* Antigen

Test Includes Latex agglutination test for group A *Streptococcus* (GAS) antigen

Special Instructions Some laboratories favor submission of dry swabs for antigen testing. Consult the laboratory for their specific recommendations.

Specimen Throat swab; many laboratories request two swabs, one for culture if the rapid screen is negative. Specimens negative by this test must be cultured to confirm the negative result.

Container Rayon or Dacron swabs rather than cotton swabs enhance the chance of detection.

Collection Rigorous swabbing of the tonsillar pilars and posterior throat increases the probability of detection of streptococcal antigen.

Use Detect the presence of group A streptococcal antigen in throat specimens

Limitations Many reviews have indicated a sensitivity of 75% to 80% and a specificity of 95% to 98% for the rapid methods. Sensitivity varies between manufacturers. Some kits are capable of detecting as few as 10 colony forming units (CFU) on culture while others require 100-1000 CFU on culture. Specimens which yield <10 colonies on culture usually are negative by rapid method. Adequate specimen collection on younger patients may be difficult, and thus, contribute to the false-negative rate. A positive result can be relied upon as a rational basis to begin therapy. **A negative result is only presumptive and a culture should be performed to reasonably exclude the diagnosis of group A streptococcal infection.** Careful attention to the details of the method and the use of appropriate controls are required to assume adequate performance. Group A streptococcal antigen disappears rapidly following antibiotic therapy. Thus a history of prior therapy should be sought when assessing pharyngitis.

Contraindications The test may become negative 4 hours after therapy has been started.

Methodology The streptococcal group carbohydrate antigen is extracted from the swab used for collection by use of acid or enzyme reagents. The extraction mixture is added to particles coated with antistreptococcal antibody. If the streptococcal antigen is present visible agglutination occurs due to antigen cross links with antibody coated latex within 10 minutes. Enzyme immunoassay methods (EIA) are also used.

Additional Information Rheumatic fever remains a concern in the United States and serious complications have been reported to be increasing in frequency; therefore, timely diagnosis and early institution of appropriate therapy remains important. Timely therapy may reduce the acute symptoms and overall duration of streptococcal pharyngitis. The sequelae of poststreptococcal glomerulonephritis and rheumatic fever are diminished by early therapy.

Selected Readings

Facklam RR, "Specificity Study of Kits for Detection of Group A Streptococci Directly From Throat Swabs," *J Clin Microbiol*, 1987, 25(3):504-8.

Kaplan EL, "The Rapid Identification of Group A Beta-Hemolytic Streptococci in the Upper Respiratory Tract - Current Status," *Pediatr Clin North Am*, 1988, 35(3):535-42, (review).

Nadler HL, "Group A Strep Detection," *Diagn Clin Test*, 1989, 27:3:35-41, (review of rapid methods).

"Rapid Diagnostic Tests for Group A Streptococcal Pharyngitis," *Med Lett Drugs Ther*, 1991, 33(843):40-1.

Group B *Streptococcus* Antigen Test

Related Information

Bacterial Antigens, Rapid Detection Methods *on page 335*

Genital Culture *on page 423*

Synonyms *Streptococcus agalactiae*, Latex Screen; *Streptococcus* Group B Latex Screen

Applies to CIE for Group B Streptococcal Antigen; Counterimmunoelectrophoresis for Group B Streptococcal Antigen; Group B *Streptococcus*, Counterimmunoelectrophoresis

Test Includes Latex screen for group B beta *Streptococcus* or counterimmunoelectrophoresis (CIE)

Special Instructions The specimen should be tested as soon as possible after collection.

Specimen Cerebrospinal fluid, serum, urine, endocervical, or amniotic fluid

Container Sterile container, red top tube

Storage Instructions If the specimen cannot be tested immediately it may be stored at 2°C to 8°C for 1 day or frozen at -20°C for longer storage.

Turnaround Time Routine: 24 hours; stat: 1 hour

Use Detect group B *Streptococcus* antigen in body fluids. Detection of group B *Streptococcus* antigen at the time of delivery is usually an indication for chemoprophylaxis.

Limitations Latex agglutination tests appear to have a slightly greater sensitivity than counterimmunoelectrophoresis (CIE) procedures. Sensitivity is relatively low, 15% to 21%, for rapid group B streptococcal antigen tests. False-positives are rare. Concentrated urine is a good specimen. Testing CSF and serum, as well as culture for the organism, should be considered to establish the definitive diagnosis.

Methodology Latex agglutination (LA), counterimmunoelectrophoresis (CIE). Polystyrene latex particles coated with antibodies specific for the group B *Streptococcus* antigen agglutinate in the presence of the homologous antigen. Controls for nonspecific agglutination of latex particles are generally used. The specimen is heat inactivated and cooled to room temperature before testing. Urine may be concentrated. The infection can be diagnosed by detection of the group B specific carbohydrate antigen of the organism's cell wall which may be present in body fluids, serum and cerebrospinal fluid and which is excreted in urine. Counterimmunoelectrophoresis is an alternate method for detection of the group B *Streptococcus* antigen but is rarely available.

Additional Information Group B *Streptococcus* is currently one of the most significant human pathogens in the neonatal period. The most common mode of acquisition by the neonate is exposure to the maternal genital flora *in utero* through ruptured membranes or by contamination during passage through the birth canal. Rapid identification of group B *Streptococcus* carriers is important in management of premature rupture of the membranes because the effectiveness of intrapartum prophylactic ampicillin may be compromised by awaiting the results of conventional cultures. Infection is manifested in two major forms, early onset septicemic infection manifest in the first few days of life and late onset meningitis which occurs during the first few months of life.

Isolates of group B *Streptococcus* resistant to erythromycin, intermediate to clindamycin, and resistant to cefoxitin, as well as strains with multiple antimicrobial resistance, have been reported. Susceptibility testing may be useful in selecting alternate antibiotic regimens.

Selected Readings

Brady K, Duff P, Schilhab JC, et al, "Reliability of a Rapid Latex Fixation Test for Detecting Group B Streptococci in the Genital Tract of Parturients at Term," *Obstet Gynecol*, 1989, 73(4):678-81.

Newton ER and Clark M, "Group B *Streptococcus* and Preterm Rupture of Membranes," *Obstet Gynecol*, 1988, 71(2):198-202.

Spence MR, "A Rapid Screening Test for the Diagnosis of Endocervical Group B Streptococci in Pregnancy: Microbiologic Results and Clinical Outcome," *Obstet Gynecol*, 1988, 71(2):284, (letter).

Stiller RJ, Blair E, Clark P, et al, "Rapid Detection of Vaginal Colonization With Group B Streptococci by Means of Latex Agglutination," *Am J Obstet Gynecol*, 1989, 160(3):566-8.

Group B *Streptococcus*, Counterimmunoelectrophoresis *see* Group B *Streptococcus* Antigen Test *on this page*

***Haemophilus influenzae* Susceptibility Testing** *see* Penicillinase Test *on page 517*

HAG *see Histoplasma capsulatum* Antigen Assay *on page 450*

Hair Fungus Culture *see* Fungus Culture, Skin *on page 417*

Hand, Left or Right, X-ray *see* Bone Films *on page 343*

Hands and Wrist Arthritis, X-ray *see* Bone Films *on page 343*

Hanging Drop Mount for *Trichomonas* *see Trichomonas* Preparation *on page 555*

Hank's Stain *see* Acid-Fast Stain, Modified, *Nocardia* Species *on page 307*

Hantavirus Pulmonary Syndrome *see* Hantavirus Serology *on this page*

Hantavirus Serology

Synonyms Muerto Canyon Strain Virus

Applies to Hantavirus Pulmonary Syndrome

Test Includes Detection of IgM and IgG antibody specific for the Muerto Canyon strain of hantavirus.

Abstract An outbreak of severe respiratory illness associated with respiratory failure, shock, and high mortality was recognized in May, 1993 in the southwestern part of the United States. The cause of the illness was identified as a unique hantavirus now known as the Muerto Canyon strain, and the disease is now called hantavirus pulmonary syndrome (HPS). Since the recognition of this disease, other cases have been recognized in 17 states, with most of the cases occurring west of the Mississippi. HPS begins with nonspecific symptoms such as fever and myalgia, which is followed in 3-6 days by progressive cough and shortness of breath. Common findings during this later stage include tachypnea, tachycardia, fever, and hypotension. Bilateral abnormalities on the chest radiograph are detected, and pleural effusions are common. Hemoconcentration, thrombocytopenia, prolonged activated partial thromboplastin time, an increased proportion of immature granulocytes on the peripheral blood smear, leukocytosis, and elevated levels of serum lactate dehydrogenase and aspartate aminotransferase are found. Serum antibodies are detectable at the time of clinical presentation.

Special Instructions Specimens should be sent to the CDC through state health departments.

Specimen Serum from acute phase of illness

Container Red top tube

Storage Instructions Serum can be stored at 4°C up to 1 week; serum should be stored at -70°C after 1 week and during shipping

Reference Range No detectable hantavirus IgM or less than a fourfold increase in IgG specific for the N and G1 proteins of the Muerto Canyon virus.

Use Confirm the diagnosis of hantavirus pulmonary syndrome

Limitations Assays for the detection of antibody to hantavirus are experimental and none have been approved by the Food and Drug Administration for use in the United States. All requests for testing must be sent to the CDC.

Methodology Western blot; enzyme-linked immunosorbent assay (ELISA)

Additional Information Hantaviruses are single-stranded RNA viruses of the family Bunyaviridae. The Muerto Canyon strain of hantavirus has been found in a proportion of the deer mouse (*Peromyscus maniculatus*) population which is prevalent in the western United States. Thus, this rodent species is thought to be the reservoir for the etiologic agent of HPS. Recommendations for prevention include avoidance of contact with the deer mouse and excreta from deer mice. Currently, no evidence exists for person-to-person transmission of HPS.

HPS can also be diagnosed by detection of hantavirus antigen in tissue by immunohistochemistry with a monoclonal antibody reactive with conserved hantaviral nucleoproteins. In addition, hantaviral nucleotide sequences can be detected in tissue using a reverse transcriptase polymerase chain reaction.

Selected Readings

Butler JC and Peters CJ, "Hantaviruses and Hantavirus Pulmonary Syndrome," *Clin Infect Dis*, 1994, 19(3):387-95.

Duchin JS, Koster FT, Peters CJ, et al, "Hantavirus Pulmonary Syndrome: A Clinical Description of 17 Patients With a Newly Recognized Disease. The Hantavirus Study Group," *N Engl J Med*, 1994, 330(14):949-55.

From the Centers for Disease Control and Prevention, "Progress in the Development of Hantavirus Diagnostic Assays - United States," *JAMA*, 1993, 270:1920-1.

Jenison S, Yamada T, Morris C, et al, "Characterization of Human Antibody Responses to Four Corners Hantavirus Infections Among Patients With Hantavirus Pulmonary Syndrome," *J Virol*, 1994, 68(5):3000-6.

HCV Branched DNA *see* Hepatitis C Viral RNA, Quantitative bDNA *on page 440*

HCV Genotyping *see* Hepatitis C Viral RNA Genotyping *on page 438*

HCV Monitor *see* Hepatitis C Viral RNA, Quantitative PCR *on page 441*

HCV PCR *see* Hepatitis C Viral RNA, Quantitative PCR *on page 441*

HCV RNA, bDNA *see* Hepatitis C Viral RNA, Quantitative bDNA *on page 440*

HCV Serology *see* Hepatitis C Serology *on page 437*

HCV Viral Load by bDNA *see* Hepatitis C Viral RNA, Quantitative bDNA *on page 440*

HCV Viral Load by PCR *see* Hepatitis C Viral RNA, Quantitative PCR *on page 441*

Head Lice Identification *see* Arthropod Identification *on page 334*

Head Studies, CT *see* Computed Transaxial Tomography, Head Studies *on page 374*

Helicobacter pylori Antigen, Direct

Related Information

Helicobacter pylori Culture and Urease Test *on next page*
Helicobacter pylori Culture, Gastric Biopsy *on page 433*
Helicobacter pylori Serology *on page 433*

Test Includes Extraction and direct assay for *Helicobacter pylori* antigen in stool

Specimen Fresh liquid, semiliquid, or formed stool; watery specimen is not appropriate for this test and should **not** be tested

Container Clean container, no preservative

Collection Do not place specimen in preservative, transport media, or collect on swab.

Storage Instructions Refrigerate specimen (up to 72 hours if necessary) at 4°C until testing. If testing will be delayed more than 72 hours, specimen should be frozen at -20°C or lower.

Reference Range Negative

Use Detect *Helicobacter pylori* antigens during active infection, monitor drug therapy

Limitations A positive result (antigen detected) is indicative of *H. pylori* presence (96% sensitivity); however some individuals may have *H. pylori* but no disease. A negative result (antigen not detected) indicates absence of *H. pylori* or an antigenic level below the assay limit of detection (184 ng *H. pylori* protein/mL of stool) (96% specificity). False-negative results may be obtained on specimens from patients who have ingested selected compounds (antimicrobial agents, proton pump inhibitors, and bismuth preparations) within 2 weeks prior to specimen collection. In such cases, another specimen should be collected more than 2 weeks after stopping the use of these agents. The test is not recommended for patients younger than 18 years of age.

Methodology Enzyme immunoassay (EIA) using a polyclonal antibody specific for *H. pylori* antigens

Additional Information *Helicobacter pylori* is associated with peptic ulcer disease (duodenal and gastric) and chronic active gastritis. *H. pylori* is also an independent risk factor for gastric cancer and primary malignant lymphoma of the stomach.

A positive result ≥7 days post therapy is indicative of treatment failure. A negative result ≥4 weeks post therapy indicates eradication of the infection. Repeat testing may be desirable to document sustained eradication beyond 4 weeks post therapy.

In patients highly suspected of having a *H. pylori* infection, this test could be an alternative to endoscopy, urea breath test, and serology.

Selected Readings

Dunn BE, Cohen H, and Blaser MJ, "*Helicobacter pylori*," *Clin Microbiol Rev*, 1997, 10(4):720-41.

Jolobe OM, "Treatment of *Helicobacter pylori* Infection," *Gut*, 1998, 43(1):148.

Makristhathis A, Pasching E, Schutze K, et al, "Detection of *Helicobacter pylori* in Stool Specimens by PCR and Antigen Enzyme Immunoassay, *J Clin Microbiol*, 1998, 36(9):2772-4.

Numans ME and Quartero AO, "*Helicobacter pylori* Infection," *Lancet*, 1997, 349(9055):879.

Trevisani L, Sartori S, Galvani F, et al, "Detection of *Helicobacter pylori* in Faeces With a New Enzyme Immunoassay Method: Preliminary Results," *Scand J Gastroenterol*, 1998, 33(8):893-4.

Versalovic J, "*Helicobacter pylori* Update," *Clin Microbiol Newslett*, 1998, 20(13):107-13.

Helicobacter pylori Culture and Urease Test

Related Information

Helicobacter pylori Antigen, Direct *on previous page*
Helicobacter pylori Culture, Gastric Biopsy *on next page*
Helicobacter pylori Serology *on next page*

Synonyms *Campylobacter pylori* Urease Test and Culture; CLO™ Test; Gastric Biopsy Culture for *Helicobacter pylori*; Urease Test and Culture, *Helicobacter pylori*

Test Includes Screening for the presence of urease activity indirectly indicating the presence of *Helicobacter pylori*, culture of the organism from gastric biopsy specimens

Specimen Gastric mucosal biopsy

Container Sterile container; **no fixative** for these microbiologic tests

Storage Instructions If specimen cannot be transported immediately to the laboratory, it should be placed in 0.5 mL transport medium (normal saline).

Turnaround Time 24 hours for urease final report; up to 7 days for culture

Reference Range Negative for urease activity, negative culture, biopsy negative for gastritis and negative for *H. pylori*

Use Establish the presence and possible etiologic role of *Helicobacter pylori* in cases of chronic gastric ulcer, chronic active gastritis, and a relationship with duodenal ulcers

Limitations Culture and urease testing alone, without biopsies, may allow occult neoplasms to go undetected.

Methodology Urease test: Gastric biopsies are incubated on slightly buffered medium. A change of phenol red to alkaline (pink color) persisting more than 5 minutes is considered positive and presumptively indicative of the presence of *Helicobacter pylori* even if the organism cannot be grown in culture. Specimens negative at 30 minutes should be re-examined periodically up to 24 hours. The sensitivity of urease testing leaves something to be desired and depends on the selected gold standard. It was only 62% at 24 hours in a 1991 report. This method is also is characterized by false-positive results.

Culture: Culture media may include enriched chocolate, Thayer-Martin with antibiotics, brain heart infusion (BHI) with 7% horse blood, and Mueller-Hinton with 5% sheep blood. The organism is microaerophilic and grows best in a reduced O_2 atmosphere or in a Campy-Pak™ system at 42°C. Cultures are usually observed for 7 days before being reported as negative.

Cytology: Touch cytology preparations (ie, imprints from biopsies) may provide a rapid diagnosis and preserve the biopsy specimen for histopathology or culture.

Smear: A direct smear can be Gram's stained.

Approximate sensitivities of methods for detection of *H. pylori*:

- 24-hour urease: 62%
- direct Gram's stain: 69%
- culture: 90%
- histology: 93%

Additional Information *Helicobacter pylori* is a major cause of chronic active gastritis. Its importance and etiologic relationship with duodenal ulcer requires further study. Seventy-eight percent to 100% of subjects who have duodenal ulcer have *H. pylori* infection, but 3% to 70% of patients without duodenal ulcer have *H. pylori* as well. The organism may be seen in biopsies stained with Gram's stain, hematoxylin-eosin (H & E), Giemsa or Warthin-Starry silver stain. It is most often recognized in biopsies of the antrum but may also be seen in the fundic mucosa, metaplastic gastric mucosa of esophagus (Barrett's esophagus), or duodenum. Biopsy may also establish the diagnosis of carcinoma or lymphoma. *H. pylori* was not found in the gastric mucosa of Meckel's diverticula. Gram's stains performed by a reuse imprint technique on biopsies from both the antrum and fundus yielded positives in 100% of 32 culture positive cases.

Most peptic ulcers related to *H. pylori* infection are reported as curable.

Breath isotope methods measuring bacterial urease by detection of labeled CO_2 and serologic tests for the detection of antibody are also useful but are rarely available. The breath test is preferred as a means of documenting presence of active infection and eradication of infection after therapy in the absence of endoscopy.

The serologic tests can be very helpful but are limited because they can remain positive for months following therapy. Use of specific IgA enhances the value of serology in monitoring therapy.

Past *H. pylori* infection increases risk of carcinoma of stomach. Chronic atrophic gastritis and intestinal metaplasia are related to *H. pylori* infection, which induces as well development of lymphoid tissue in the gastric mucosa. A possible role for *H. pylori* in the development of primary malignant lymphoma of stomach has been postulated.

Selected Readings

Blaser MJ, "*Helicobacter pylori*: Its Role in Disease," *Clin Infect Dis*, 1992, 15(3):386-91.

Cover TL and Blaser MJ, "*Helicobacter pylori* and Gastroduodenal Disease," *Annu Rev Med*, 1992, 43:135-45.

Debongnie JC, Delmee M, Mainguet P, et al, "Cytology: A Simple, Rapid, Sensitive Method in the Diagnosis of *Helicobacter pylori*," *Am J Gastroenterol*, 1992, 87(1):20-3.

Dooley CP and Cohen H, "The Clinical Significance of *Campylobacter pylori*," *Ann Intern Med*, 1988, 108(1):70-9.

Hoek FJ, Noach LA, Rauws EJ, et al, "Evaluation of the Performance of Commercial Test Kits for Detection of *Helicobacter pylori* Antibodies in Serum," *J Clin Microbiol*, 1992, 30(6):1525-8.

Murry DM, "Clinical Relevance of Infection by *Helicobacter pylori*," *Clin Microbiol Newslett*, 1993, 15(5):33-7.

Perez-Perez GI and Dunn BE, "Diagnosis of *C. pylori* Infection by Serologic Methods," *Campylobacter pylori in Gastritis and Peptic Ulcer Disease*, New York, NY: Igaku-Shoin, 1989, 163-74.

Peterson WL, "*Helicobacter pylori* and Peptic Ulcer Disease," *N Engl J Med*, 1991, 324(15):1043-8.

Helicobacter pylori Culture, Gastric Biopsy

Related Information

Helicobacter pylori Antigen, Direct *on page 431*

Helicobacter pylori Culture and Urease Test *on previous page*

Helicobacter pylori Serology *on this page*

Synonyms *Campylobacter pylori*, Gastric Biopsy Culture

Special Instructions Notify laboratory before biopsy to obtain additional instructions and transport media.

Specimen Gastric mucosal biopsy

Container Sterile container, no fixative

Collection Special instructions from laboratory

Storage Instructions Transport specimen to the laboratory immediately. If specimen cannot be transported immediately to the laboratory it should be placed in 0.5 mL transport medium (normal saline).

Causes for Rejection Excessive delay in transport.

Reference Range No *Helicobacter pylori* detected

Use Establish the presence and possible etiologic role of *Helicobacter pylori* in cases of chronic gastric ulcer, gastritis, duodenal ulcer, dyspepsia, etc

Limitations *C. pylori* infections can be very focal. A negative culture does not rule out *C. pylori* or disease that may have been caused by *C. pylori*.

Additional Information *Helicobacter pylori* has been implicated as a factor associated with chronic gastritis. The clinical significance of the organism in regard to gastric or duodenal ulcers, dyspepsia, and gastric carcinoma remains unclear. Other factors such as pepsin, nonsteroidal anti-inflammatory agents (NSAIDs), aspirin, ischemia, stress, alcohol, and bile salts as well as *H. pylori* all may have a role in altering the material mucosal barrier. The relative etiologic role of *H. pylori* remains a subject of speculation. Large numbers of small bacteria, *Helicobacter pylori*, can be cultured from, or seen microscopically (especially with Dieterle stain) in gastric biopsies from most patients with chronic gastritis and/or peptic ulcers. They can also be found in significant numbers of asymptomatic patients who have histologic gastritis, and from some individuals with no abnormality.

Helicobacter pylori Serology

Related Information

Helicobacter pylori Antigen, Direct *on page 431*

Helicobacter pylori Culture and Urease Test *on previous page*

Helicobacter pylori Culture, Gastric Biopsy *on this page*

Synonyms *Campylobacter pylori* Serology

Abstract Persons with peptic ulcer disease either are users of nonsteroidal anti-inflammatory agents or have infection with *H. pylori*. Patients with peptic ulcer (Continued)

Helicobacter pylori Serology *(Continued)*

disease associated with *H. pylori* have elevated levels of serum antibody against this bacterium. *H. pylori* is very strongly associated with duodenal and gastric ulcer and chronic active gastritis. It is an independent risk factor for gastric cancer. Antibodies persist as long as a year after treatment.

Specimen Serum or plasma

Container Red top tube; some laboratories use EDTA or heparin tubes

Collection Acute and convalescent samples may be helpful.

Reference Range Undetectable or lower than cutoff limits in commercial assays

Use Increased antibody levels are associated with *H. pylori* infection, chronic active gastritis, and peptic ulcer. Negative serological results provide evidence against these diagnoses.

Limitations Serologic findings provide evidence of past or present infection. A large number of people are infected with the organism but do not have apparent disease. Commercially available assays for diagnosis have sensitivities of 59% to 100% and specificities of 29% to 65%. (In contrast, the sensitivity and specificity of histopathologic examination of gastric mucosal biopsy are well above 90%.) If used to follow response to therapy, long-term follow-up is necessary.

Additional Information *Helicobacter pylori* causes chronic active gastritis. Strong evidence exists that it contributes to the pathogenesis of peptic ulcer diseases. It is linked to gastric carcinoma and lymphoma.

Large numbers of small, spiral-shaped bacteria, *H. pylori*, can be cultured from, or seen microscopically (especially with Dieterle or Giemsa stain) in gastric biopsies from most patients with chronic active gastritis and/or peptic ulcers. They can also be found in significant numbers of asymptomatic patients who have histologic gastritis, and from some individuals with no abnormality. Similarly, patients with chronic gastritis usually have elevated titers of IgG antibodies to *H. pylori*. The association of *H. pylori* infection in development of carcinoma and primary malignant lymphoma of stomach is recognized.

Strong correlation between carbon-13 labeled urea breath testing and serologic testing has been shown in symptom-free subjects.

Selected Readings

Blecker U, Lanciers S, Hauser B, et al, "Serology as a Valid Screening Test for *Helicobacter pylori* Infection in Asymptomatic Subjects," *Arch Pathol Lab Med*, 1995, 119(1):30-2.

Breslin NP and O'Morain CA, "Noninvasive Diagnosis of *Helicobacter pylori* Infection: A Review," *Helicobacter*, 1997, 2(3):111-7.

de Boer WA and van Zwet TA, "Diagnose and Treat *Helicobacter pylori* as Any Other Infectious Disease," *Am J Gastroenterol*, 1996, 91(10):2255-6.

Fennerty MB, "*Helicobacter pylori*," *Arch Intern Med*, 1994, 154(7):721-7.

Harris A, Danesh J, and Forman D, "*Helicobacter pylori* Infection," *Lancet*, 1997, 349(9055):879-80.

Mendall MA, "Serology for Diagnosis of *Helicobacter pylori* Infection," *Helicobacter*, 1997, 2(1):54-5.

Sung JJ, Chung SC, Ling TK, et al, "Antibacterial Treatment of Gastric Ulcers Associated With *Helicobacter pylori*," *N Engl J Med*, 1995, 332(3):139-42.

Helminths, Blood Preparation *see* Microfilariae, Peripheral Blood Preparation *on page 489*

Helper Cell/Suppressor Ratio *see* T4/T8 Ratio *on page 545*

Hemoflagellates *see* Microfilariae, Peripheral Blood Preparation *on page 489*

Hemogram *see* Complete Blood Count *on page 369*

Hemovac® Tip Culture *see* Intravenous Line Culture *on page 464*

Hepatitis A Profile

Test Includes Determination of IgG and IgM antibody to hepatitis A virus and confirmation of all new IgM positives by repeat testing

Specimen Serum

Container Red top tube or serum separator tube

Storage Instructions Transport specimen to the laboratory immediately. Separate serum and freeze.

Reference Range IgG: negative; IgM: negative

Use Determine recent or past infection with hepatitis A virus

Methodology Radioimmunoassay (RIA) or enzyme immunoassay (EIA)

Additional Information Hepatitis A is transmitted by the fecal-oral route, usually foodborne. Its incubation period is 2-7 weeks. Hepatitis A virus is a picornavirus, and antibody is made to capsid proteins. Fecal excretion of HAV peaks before symptoms develop. If hepatitis A antibody is IgM, the hepatitis A infection is probably acute. IgM antibody develops within a week of symptom onset, peaks in 3 months, and is usually gone after 6 months. Hepatitis A antibody of IgG type is indicative of old infection, is found in almost half of adults, and is not usually clinically relevant. Many cases of hepatitis A are subclinical, particularly in children. Presence of IgG antibody to HAV does not exclude acute hepatitis B or non-A, non-B hepatitis.

HEPATITIS A PROFILE

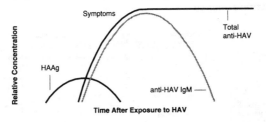

Selected Readings

Giacoia GP and Kasprisin DO, "Transfusion-Acquired Hepatitis A," *South Med J*, 1989, 82(11):1357-60.

Hollinger FB and Dreesman GR, "Hepatitis Viruses," *Manual of Clinical Laboratory Immunology*, 4th ed, Rose NR, de Macario EC, Fahey JL, et al, eds, Washington, DC: American Society for Microbiology, 1992, 634-50.

Lee HS and Vyas GN, "Diagnosis of Viral Hepatitis," *Clin Lab Med*, 1987, 7:741:57.

Mbithi JN, Springthorpe VS, Boulet JR, et al, "Survival of Hepatitis A Virus on Human Hands and Its Transfer on Contact With Animate and Inanimate Surfaces," *J Clin Microbiol*, 1992, 30(4):757-63.

Mishu B, Hadler SC, Boaz VA, et al, "Foodborne Hepatitis A: Evidence That Microwaving Reduces Risk?" *J Infect Dis*, 1990, 162(3):655-8.

Summers PL, DuBois DR, Houston Cohen WH, et al, "Solid-Phase Antibody Capture Hemadsorption Assay for Detection of Hepatitis A Virus Immunoglobulin M Antibodies," *J Clin Microbiol*, 1993, 31(5):1299-302.

Hepatitis B Profile

Related Information

Postexposure Prophylaxis for Hepatitis B *on page 1054*

Test Includes Detection of hepatitis B surface antigen (HB$_s$Ag), antibody to hepatitis B surface antigen (anti-HB$_s$), hepatitis B core antibody (anti-HB$_c$), and confirmation of all new positives by repeat testing

Specimen Serum

Container Red top tube or serum separator tube

Storage Instructions Transport specimen to the laboratory immediately. Do not store blood.

Causes for Rejection Recently administered radioisotopes if assay performed by RIA, excessive hemolysis

Reference Range Negative

Use Determine serological status to hepatitis B virus

Limitations Patients who are negative for HB$_s$Ag may still have acute type B viral hepatitis. There is sometimes a "window" stage when HB$_s$Ag has become negative and the patient has not yet developed the antibody (anti-HB$_s$Ag). On such occasions the anti-HB$_c$Ag (IgM) is usually positive, and the patient should be treated as potentially infectious until anti-HB$_s$Ag is detected, at which time immunity is probable. In cases with strong clinical suspicion of viral hepatitis, serologic testing should not be limited to detecting HB$_s$Ag but should include a battery of (Continued)

Hepatitis B Profile *(Continued)*

tests to evaluate different stages of acute and convalescent hepatitis. These should include a test for hepatitis A antibody (IgM), and HB_sAg, HB_sAb, HB_cAb (IgM), and hepatitis C virus (HCV).

Presence of HB_sAb is not an absolute indicator of resolved hepatitis infection, nor of protection from future infection. Since there are different serologic subtypes of hepatitis B virus, it is possible (and has been reported) for a patient to have antibody to one surface antigen type and to be acutely infected with virus of a different subtype. Thus, a patient may have coexisting HB_sAg and HB_sAb. Transfused individuals or hemophiliacs receiving plasma components may give false-positive tests for antibody to hepatitis B surface antigen. Individuals vaccinated with HBV vaccine will have antibodies to the surface protein.

HEPATITIS B PROFILE

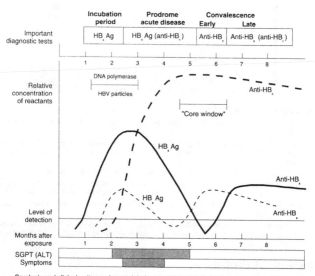

Serologic and clinical patterns observed during acute hepatitis B viral infection. From Hollinger FB and Dreesman GR, *Manual of Clinical Immunology*, 2nd ed, Rose NR and Friedman H, eds, Washington, DC: American Society for Microbiology, 1980, with permission.

Contraindications Patients on heparin therapy may demonstrate weak positive results.

Methodology Radioimmunoassay (RIA); enzyme immunoassay (EIA)

Additional Information Hepatitis B virus (HBV) is a DNA virus with a protein coat, surface antigen (HB_sAg), and a core consisting of nucleoprotein, (HB_cAg is the core antigen). There are eight different serotypes. Early in infection, HB_sAg, HBV DNA, and DNA polymerase can all be detected in serum.

Transmission is parenteral, sexual or perinatal. The incubation period of hepatitis B is 2-6 months. HB_sAg can be detected 1-7 weeks **before** liver enzyme elevation or the appearance of clinical symptoms. Three weeks after the onset of acute hepatitis about 50% of the patients will still be positive for HB_sAg, while at 17 weeks only 10% are positive. The best available markers for infectivity are HB_sAg and HB_eAg. The presence of HB_sAb and HB_eAb is associated with noninfectivity. The chronic carrier state is indicated by the persistence of HB_sAg and/or HB_eAg over long periods (6 months to years) without seroconversion to the corresponding antibodies. Such a condition has the potential to lead to serious liver damage but may be an isolated asymptomatic serologic phenomenon. Persistence of HB_sAg, without anti-HB_s, with combinations of positivity of anti-HB_{core}, HB_eAg, or anti-HB_e indicate infectivity and need for investigation for chronic persistent or chronic aggressive hepatitis. Chronic carrier states are found in up to 10% of cases. Some remain healthy, but evolution to chronic persistent hepatitis, chronic active hepatitis, cirrhosis, and hepatoma represent major problems of this disease.

Prevention of hepatitis B for those at risk is available via vaccination, as well as treatment for some chronic carriers. For prophylaxis information see appendix table Postexposure Prophylaxis for Hepatitis B *on page 1054.*

Selected Readings
Centers for Disease Control, "Screening Donors of Blood, Plasma, Organs, Tissues, and Semen for Evidence of Hepatitis B and Hepatitis C," *Lab Med,* 1991, 22(8):555-63.

Devine P, Taswell HF, Moore SB, et al, "Passively Acquired Antibody to Hepatitis B Surface Antigen. Pitfall in Evaluating Immunity to Hepatitis B Viral Infections," *Arch Pathol Lab Med,* 1989, 113(5):529-31.

Edwards MS, "Hepatitis B Serology - Help in Interpretation," *Pediatr Clin North Am,* 1988, 35(3):503-15.

Hollinger FB and Dreesman GR, "Hepatitis Viruses," *Manual of Clinical Laboratory Immunology,* 4th ed, Rose NR, de Macario EC, Fahey JL, et al, eds, Washington, DC: American Society for Microbiology, 1992, 634-50.

Lee HS and Vyas GN, "Diagnosis of Viral Hepatitis," *Clin Lab Med,* 1987, 7:741-57.

Hepatitis C Gene Product *see* Hepatitis C Serology *on this page*

Hepatitis C Serology

Related Information
Hepatitis C Viral RNA Genotyping *on next page*

Hepatitis C Viral RNA, Quantitative bDNA *on page 440*

Hepatitis C Viral RNA, Quantitative PCR *on page 441*

Synonyms HCV Serology

Applies to Anti-HCV (IgM); C 100-3; Hepatitis C Gene Product; Non-A, Non-B Hepatitis; Surrogate Tests for Non-A, Non-B Hepatitis

Test Includes Detection of antibody specific for hepatitis C in patient's serum

Abstract Most cases of post-transfusion non-A, non-B viral hepatitis are caused by HCV. Application of this test has caused a great decrease of post-transfusion hepatitis.

Patient Preparation Avoid recent administration of radioisotopes if assay is RIA

Specimen Serum

Container Red top tube

Causes for Rejection Recently administered radioisotopes if assay is RIA

Reference Range Negative

Use Differential diagnosis of acute hepatitis; screen blood units for transfusion safety

Limitations Since as many as 90% of commercial intravenous immunoglobulins test positive for hepatitis C antibody, a false-positive can result briefly after such transfusion.

Methodology Radioimmunoassay (RIA), enzyme-linked immunosorbent assay (ELISA)

Additional Information Before initiation of hepatitis B surface antigen testing in the 1970's, most significant post-transfusion hepatitis was due to hepatitis B. Following the development of sensitive and specific testing for hepatitis B, greater than 90% of post-transfusion hepatitis became so called "non-A, non-B." Hepatitis C virus is the most common cause of non-A, non-B hepatitis in the United States. Chiron Corporation has isolated a gene product (c100-3) of hepatitis C virus (HCV) and developed an assay for antibodies to it. The assay detects antibody to the flavivirus which is the etiologic agent of hepatitis C. Non-A, non-B, and non-C hepatitis can still occur, probably due to CMV, hepatitis E, and to other viruses that have not been identified.

For blood donors, hepatitis C serology correlates with surrogate tests for non-A, non-B hepatitis (ALT and anti-HB$_c$). Since hepatitis C serology identifies a broader group of infected individuals than surrogate testing, it reduces risk of HCV during transfusion. Studies in hemophiliacs indicate that antibody to HCV is a reliable marker of HCV. Recently, IgM anti-HCV core has been shown to be a useful acute marker for HCV infection. Transmission is by intravenous drug abuse, dialysis, and other needlesticks. Sexual transmission also occurs. Before screening for hepatitis C antibody was in place, non-A, non-B hepatitis was said to occur in as many as 10% of transfusions. With the introduction of first generation hepatitis C screening tests, the number has fallen to 1 in 3300 units. With the introduction of a more sensitive second generation hepatitis C test in 1992, safety has increased even more. Chronic carrier states develop in more than
(Continued)

Hepatitis C Serology *(Continued)*

half the patients, and chronic liver disease is a major problem. Substantial risk of chronic active hepatitis and cirrhosis exists in those who develop chronic non-A, non-B hepatitis, of whom, about 80% develop anti-HCV. A risk of hepatocellular carcinoma exists for these patients, as well as a risk of liver failure.

Selected Readings

Allain JP, Dailey SH, Laurian Y, et al, "Evidence for Persistent Hepatitis C Virus (HCV) Infection in Hemophiliacs," *J Clin Invest*, 1991, 88(5):1672-9.

Alter MJ, Hadler SC, Judson FN, et al, "Risk Factors for Acute Non-A, Non-B Hepatitis in the United States and Association With Hepatitis C Virus Infection," *JAMA*, 1990, 264(17):2231-5.

Alter MJ, Margolis HS, Krawczynski K, et al, "The Natural History of Community-Acquired Hepatitis C in the United States," *N Engl J Med*, 1992, 327(27):1899-905.

Centers for Disease Control, "Screening Donors of Blood, Plasma, Organs, Tissues, and Semen for Evidence of Hepatitis B and Hepatitis C," *Lab Med*, 1991, 22(8):555-63.

Clemens JM, Taskar S, Chau K, et al, "IgM Antibody Response in Acute Hepatitis C Viral Infection," *Blood*, 1992, 79(1):169-72.

Choo Q-L, Kuo G, Weiner AJ, et al, "Isolation of a cDNA Clone Derived From a Blood-Borne Non-A, Non-B Viral Hepatitis Genome," *Science*, 1989, 244(4902):359-62.

Cuthbert JA, "Hepatitis C: Progress and Problems," *Clin Microbiol Rev*, 1994, 7(4):505-32.

Dodd LG, McBride JH, Gitnick GL, et al, "Prevalence of Non-A, Non-B Hepatitis/Hepatitis C Virus Antibody in Human Immunoglobulins," *Am J Clin Pathol*, 1992, 97(1):108-13.

Dodd RY, "Hepatitis C Virus, Antibodies and Infectivity - Paradox, Pragmatism, and Policy," *Am J Clin Pathol*, 1992, 97(1):4-6, (editorial).

Gambino R, "NANB Hepatitis - A New Antibody Test for the Hepatitis C Virus," *Lab Report for Physicians*,™ 1988, 10:89-93.

Gretch DR, "Diagnostic Tests for Hepatitis C," *Hepatology*, 1997, 26(3 Suppl 1):43S-7S.

Hsieh TT, Yao DS, Sheen IS, et al, "Hepatitis C Virus in Peripheral Blood Mononuclear Cells," *Am J Clin Pathol*, 1992, 98(4):392-6.

Kuo G, Choo QL, Alter HJ, et al, "An Assay for Circulating Antibodies to a Major Etiologic Virus of Human Non-A, Non-B Hepatitis," *Science*, 1989, 244(4902):362-4.

Prince AM, Brotman B, Inchauspé G, et al, "Patterns and Prevalence of Hepatitis C Virus Infection in Post-Transfusion Non-A, Non-B Hepatitis," *J Infect Dis*, 1993, 167(6):1296-301.

Richards C, Holland P, Kuramoto K, et al, "Prevalence of Antibody to Hepatitis C Virus in a Blood Donor Population," *Transfusion*, 1991, 31(2):109-13.

Seeff LB, Buskell-Bales Z, Wright EC, et al, "Long-Term Mortality After Transfusion-Associated Non-A, Non-B Hepatitis," *N Engl J Med*, 1992, 327(27):1906-11.

Hepatitis C Viral RNA Genotyping

Related Information

Hepatitis C Serology *on previous page*
Hepatitis C Viral RNA, Quantitative bDNA *on page 440*
Hepatitis C Viral RNA, Quantitative PCR *on page 441*

Synonyms Genotyping, HCV; HCV Genotyping

Abstract Hepatitis C virus (HCV) is the primary cause of non-A, non-B hepatitis (NANBH) in the United States. Acute HCV infection is usually without symptoms; however, 85% of infected individuals develop chronic liver infection and frequently progress to cirrhosis and hepatocellular carcinoma. Alpha interferon therapy has been the treatment of choice, although only 20% of patients demonstrate a sustained response. Low pretreatment HCV RNA levels and the absence of cirrhosis prior to treatment are independent, favorable predictors of therapeutic response.

HCV genotype is also an independent predictor of therapeutic response. Subpopulations having genotype 1 respond less favorably than subpopulations having a genotype other than 1 (ie, genotypes 2-6). For example, in two recent studies demonstrating increased response following interferon and ribavirin combination therapy, the subpopulations having genotypes other than 1 had response rates more than twice that of subpopulations with genotype 1, 73% vs 30% (Davis GL, et al) and 66% vs 28% (McHutchison JG, et al). By combining genotype and HCV RNA levels, risk was further stratified. The subpopulation with both a genotype other than 1 and a low pretreatment HCV RNA level ($\leq 2 \times 10^6$ copies/mL) had a response rate of 100%. Thus, HCV genotype, alone or in combination with viral load, can stratify patients according to their likelihood of response to drug therapy.

Special Instructions Use of HCV genotyping should be limited to patients with detectable hepatitis C viral RNA

Specimen Serum

Container Red top tube; yellow top (ACD) tube and lavender top (EDTA) tube are also acceptable

Storage Instructions Separate serum (plasma) from cells within 1 hour of collection and freeze.

Use Predict the likelihood of therapeutic response in patients with hepatitis C infection

Methodology The method used by Quest Diagnostics Inc Nichols Institute includes reverse transcription-polymerase chain reaction (RT-PCR) and DNA sequencing of the NS5B region of the HCV genome (nucleotide positions 7975-8196) and detects HCV genotypes 1-6 and subtypes 1a, 1b, 1cE, 1cO, 2a, 2b, 2c, 3a, 3b, 3c, 3(10a), 4a, 4c, 4d, 4e, 4f, 4g, 4h, 5a, 6a, 6e, 6g, 6i, and 6l, as well as novel subtypes.

Additional Information A HCV genotype 1 indicates a poor potential for response to alpha interferon therapy when used alone or in combination with ribavirin. Conversely, genotypes other than 1 (2-6 and associated subtypes) indicate a significantly higher likelihood for sustained response. HCV genotype should be interpreted in conjunction with pretreatment HCV viral load, pretreatment cirrhosis status, and other clinical and laboratory findings. Any decision to withhold drug therapy must be made very carefully since individual patients may not respond as predicted.

Multiple HCV subtypes indicate multiple infections.

Distribution of HCV Genotypic Subtypes in the United States

HCV Subtype	Frequency
1a	58%
1b	21%
2b	13%
3a	5%
Other	3%

Worldwide HCV Genotypic Subtype Distribution

HCV Genotype	Predominant Geographic Location
1	North America, Europe, East Asia
2	North America, Europe, East Asia
3	North America, Europe, East Asia
4	Middle East, Central Africa
5	South Africa, Southeast Asia
6	South Africa, Southeast Asia

Selected Readings

Amoroso P, Rapicetta M, Tosti ME, et al, "Correlation Between Virus Genotype and Chronicity Rate in Acute Hepatitis C, *J Hepatol*, 1998, 28(6):939-44.

Bellobuono A, Mondazzi L, Tempini S, et al, "Prospective Comparison of Four Lymphoblastoid Interferon Alpha Schedules For Chronic Hepatitis C. A Multivariate Analysis of Factors Predictive of Sustained Response to Treatment," *Eur J Gastroenterol Hepatol*, 1997, 9(12):1169-77.

Brouwer JT, Nevens F, Kleter B, et al, "Efficacy of Interferon Dose and Prediction of Response in Chronic Hepatitis C: Benelux Study in 336 Patients," *J Hepatol*, 1998, 28(6):951-9.

Davis GL, Esteban-Mur R, Rustgi V, et al, "Interferon Alfa-2b Alone or in Combination With Ribavirin for the Treatment of Chronic Hepatitis C. International Hepatitis Interventional Therapy Group," *N Engl J Med*, 1998, 339(21):1493-9.

Gerken G, Knolle P, Jakobs S, et al, "Quantification and Genotyping of Serum HCV-RNA in Patients With Chronic Hepatitis C Undergoing Interferon Treatment," *Arch Virol*, 1997, 142(3):459-64.

Gross JB Jr, "Clinician's Guide to Hepatitis C," *Mayo Clin Proc*, 1998, 73(4):355-60.

Knolle PA, Kremp S, Hohler T, et al, "Viral and Host Factors in the Prediction of Response to Interferon-Alpha Therapy in Chronic Hepatitis C After Long-Term Follow-up," *J Viral Hepat*, 1998, 5(6):399-406.

Management of Hepatitis C," *NIH Consens Statement*, 1997, 15(3):1-41.

Martinot-Peignoux M, Boyer N, Pouteau M, et al, "Predictors of Sustained Response to Alpha Interferon Therapy in Chronic Hepatitis C," *J Hepatol*, 1998, 29(2):214-23.

McHutchison JG, Gordon SC, Schiff ER, et al, "Interferon Alfa-2b Alone or in Combination With Ribavirin as Initial Treatment for Chronic Hepatitis C. Hepatitis Interventional Therapy Group," *N Engl J Med*, 1998, 339(21):1485-92.

Poynard T, Marcellin P, Lee SS, et al, "Randomised Trial of Interferon Alpha2b Plus Ribavirin for 48 Weeks or for 24 Weeks Versus Interferon Alpha2b Plus Placebo for 48 weeks for Treatment of Chronic Infection With Hepatitis C Virus. International Hepatitis Interventional Therapy Group (IHIT)," *Lancet*, 1998, 352(9138):1426-32.

Simmonds P, Holmes EC, Cha TA, et al, "Classification of Hepatitis C Virus Into Six Major Genotypes and a Series of Subtypes by Phylogenetic Analysis of the NS-5 Region," *J Gen Virol*, 1993, 74(Pt 11):2391-9.

Hepatitis C Viral RNA, Quantitative bDNA

Related Information

Hepatitis C Serology *on page 437*

Hepatitis C Viral RNA Genotyping *on page 438*

Hepatitis C Viral RNA, Quantitative PCR *on next page*

Synonyms HCV Branched DNA; HCV RNA, bDNA; HCV Viral Load by bDNA

Abstract HCV RNA is a direct measurement of the level of hepatitis C virus. High levels of virus have been associated with lack of response to interferon treatment whereas low levels of virus have been associated with an increased rate of sustained response. Thus, quantitative HCV RNA testing can eliminate potentially ineffective and costly therapy by identifying nonresponders prior to initiation of therapy. Alanine aminotransferase (ALT), HCV RNA levels, or repeat liver biopsies can be used to assess response, or lack thereof, once therapy has been initiated. Patients who normalize ALT but do not have an appreciable change in HCV RNA within 3 months are less likely to benefit from further therapy. Quantitative HCV RNA levels need to be assessed in combination with all available clinical, biochemical, and liver biopsy information.

Specimen Serum

Container Red top tube

Storage Instructions Remove serum from clot within 1 hour of collection and freeze immediately.

Reference Range <0.2 million Eq/mL (lowest reportable value: 0.2 million Eq/mL); one equivalent (Eq) is approximately 1 copy of HCV RNA

Use Assess prognosis prior to initiation of antiviral therapy, predict response to alpha interferon therapy, monitor the effect of antiviral therapy, individualize antiviral therapy. HCV viral load is increased in active HCV infection, decreased likelihood of response to alpha interferon therapy (suggested by high initial viral load levels), insufficient therapeutic response (suggested by persistent elevation of viral load levels). HCV viral load is decreased in response to therapy and remission.

Limitations This test is for research use only. It is not to be used as a diagnostic procedure without confirmation of the diagnosis by another established product or procedure.

Methodology Branched DNA (bDNA) signal amplification in which viral RNA is captured on the surface of a microtiter well by synthetic oligonucleotides coating the well. The solid-phase bound viral RNA is hybridized to multiple-branched DNA molecules. Alkaline phosphatase-labeled probes are in turn hybridized to the branched DNA and reacted with a chemiluminescent substrate to produce a greatly amplified light signal. The amount of light emitted is directly proportional to the quantity of RNA in the specimen. This method demonstrates equal quantification of HCV genotypes 1-6.

Selected Readings

Alter HJ, "To C or Not to C: These Are the Questions," *Blood*, 1995, 85(7):1681-95.

Davis GL, Lau JY, Urdea MS, et al, "Quantitative Detection of Hepatitis C Virus RNA With a Solid-Phase Signal Amplification Method: Definition of Optimal Conditions for Specimen Collection and Clinical Application in Interferon-Treated Patients," *Hepatology*, 1994, 19(6):1337-41.

Detmer J, Lagier R, Flynn J, et al, "Accurate Quantitation of Hepatitis C Virus (HCV) RNA From All HCV Genotypes By Using Branched-DNA Technology," *J Clin Microbiol*, 1996, 34(4):901-7.

Fried MW and Hoofnagle JH, "Therapy of Hepatitis C," *Semin Liver Dis*, 1995, 15(1):82-91.

Gretch DR, dela Rosa C, Carithers RL Jr, et al, "Assessment of Hepatitis C Viremia Using Molecular Amplification Technologies: Correlations and Clinical Implications," *Ann Intern Med*, 1995, 123(5):321-9.

Lau JY, Davis GL, Kniffen J, et al, "Significance of Serum Hepatitis C Virus RNA Levels in Chronic Hepatitis C," *Lancet*, 1993, 341(8859):1501-4.

Lau JY, Mizokami M, Ohno T, et al, "Discrepancy Between Biochemical and Virological Responses to Interferon-Alpha in Chronic Hepatitis C," *Lancet*, 1993, 342(8881):1208-9.

Martinot-Peignoux M, Marcellin P, Ponteau M, et al, "Pretreatment Serum Hepatitis C Virus RNA Levels and Hepatitis C Virus Genotype are the Main and Independent Prognostic Factors of Sustained Response to Interferon Alfa Therapy in Chronic Hepatitis C, " *Hepatology*, 1995, 22(4 Pt 1):1050-6.

Nomura H, Kimura Y, Rikimaru N, et al, "Usefulness of HCV-RNA Assays in Efficacy Evaluation of Interferon Treatment for Chronic Hepatitis C: Amplicor HCV Assay and Branched DNA Probe Assay," *J Infect*, 1997, 34(3):249-55.

Shiratori Y, Kato N, Yokosuka O, et al, "Quantitative Assays for Hepatitis C Virus in Serum As Predictors of the Long-Term Response to Interferon," *J Hepatol*, 1997, 27(3):437-44.

Wada M, Kang KB, Nishigami T, et al, "Importance of Pretreatment Viral Load and Monitoring of Serum Hepatitis C Virus RNA in Predicting Response to Interferon-Alpha2a Treatment of Chronic Hepatitis C. Hanshin Chronic Hepatitis C Study Group," *J Interferon Cytokine Res*, 1997, 17(11):707-12.

Wilber JC and Polito A, "Serological and Virological Diagnostic Tests for Hepatitis C Virus Infection," *Semin Gastrointest Dis*, 1995, 6(1):13-9.

Hepatitis C Viral RNA, Quantitative PCR

Related Information
Hepatitis C Serology *on page 437*
Hepatitis C Viral RNA Genotyping *on page 438*
Hepatitis C Viral RNA, Quantitative bDNA *on previous page*
Polymerase Chain Reaction *on page 523*

Synonyms Amplicor™ HCV Monitor; HCV Monitor; HCV PCR; HCV Viral Load by PCR

Abstract HCV RNA is a direct measurement of the level of hepatitis C virus. High levels of virus have been associated with lack of response to interferon treatment whereas low levels of virus have been associated with an increased rate of sustained response. Thus, quantitative HCV RNA testing can eliminate potentially ineffective and costly therapy by identifying nonresponders prior to initiation of therapy. Alanine aminotransferase (ALT), HCV RNA levels, or repeat liver biopsies can be used to assess response, or lack thereof, once therapy has been initiated. Patients who normalize ALT but do not have an appreciable change in HCV RNA within 3 months are less likely to benefit from further therapy. Quantitative HCV RNA levels need to be assessed in combination with all available clinical, biochemical, and liver biopsy information.

Specimen Serum

Container Red top tube

Storage Instructions Remove serum from clot within 1 hour of collection and freeze. Do not thaw.

Reference Range Not detected (lowest reportable value: 500 copies/mL)

Use Indicate infectivity, confirm HCV antibody test results, assess prognosis prior to initiation of antiviral therapy, predict response to alpha interferon therapy, monitor the effect of antiviral therapy, individualize antiviral therapy. HCV viral load is increased in active HCV infection, decreased likelihood of response to alpha interferon therapy (suggested by high initial viral load levels), insufficient therapeutic response (suggested by persistent elevation of viral load levels). HCV viral load is decreased in response to therapy and remission.

Limitations This test is for research only. It is not to be used as a diagnostic procedure without confirmation of the diagnosis by another established product or procedure.

Methodology Reverse transcription-polymerase chain reaction (RT-PCR) in which viral RNA is extracted from serum. RNA is then reverse-transcribed into DNA and amplified with biotin-labeled HCV-specific primers by the polymerase chain reaction (PCR). An internal quantitation standard (IQS) is also amplified. The amplification products are hybridized to capture probes and detected with an avidin-HRP conjugate in a colorimetric assay. Viral copy numbers are quantified as the ratio of viral and IQS products.

This method is more sensitive than the branched DNA (bDNA) method.

Selected Readings
Alter HJ, "To C or Not to C: These Are the Questions," *Blood*, 1995, 85(7):1681-95.

Berger A, Braner J, Doerr HW, et al, "Quantification of Viral Load: Clinical Relevance for Human Immunodeficiency Virus, Hepatitis B Virus, and Hepatitis C Virus Infection," *Intervirology*, 1998, 41(1):24-34.

Fanning L, Kenny E, Sheehan M, et al, "Viral Load and Clinicopathological Features of Chronic Hepatitis C in a Homogeneous Patient Population," *Hepatology*, 1999, 29(3):904-7.

Fried MW and Hoofnagle JH, "Therapy of Hepatitis C," *Semin Liver Dis*, 1995, 15(1):82-91.

Gretch D, Corey L, Wilson J, et al, "Assessment of Hepatitis C RNA Levels by Quantitative Competitive RNA Polymerase Chain Reaction: High-Titer Viremia Correlates With Advanced Stage of Disease," *J Infect Dis*, 1994, 169(6):1219-25.

Gretch DR, dela Rosa C, Carithers RL Jr, et al, "Assessment of Hepatitis C Viremia Using Molecular Amplification Technologies: Correlations and Clinical Implications," *Ann Intern Med*, 1995, 123(5):321-9.

Lau JY, Davis GL, Kniffen J, et al, "Significance of Serum Hepatitis C Virus RNA Levels in Chronic Hepatitis C," *Lancet*, 1993, 341(8859):1501-4.

Martinot-Peignoux M, Marcellin P, Ponteau M, et al, "Pretreatment Serum Hepatitis C Virus RNA Levels and Hepatitis C Virus Genotype Are the Main and Independent Prognostic Factors of Sustained Response to Interferon Alfa Therapy in Chronic Hepatitis C," *Hepatology*, 1995, 22(4 Pt 1):1050-6.

Nomura H, Kimura Y, Rikimaru N, et al, "Usefulness of HCV-RNA Assays in Efficacy Evaluation of Interferon Treatment for Chronic Hepatitis C: Amplicor HCV Assay and Branched DNA Probe Assay," *J Infect*, 1997, 34(3):249-55.

(Continued)

Hepatitis C Viral RNA, Quantitative PCR

Shiratori Y, Kato N, Yokosuka O, et al, "Quantitative Assays for Hepatitis C Virus in Serum As Predictors of the Long-Term Response to Interferon," *J Hepatol*, 1997, 27(3):437-44.

Wada M, Kang KB, Nishigami T, et al, "Importance of Pretreatment Viral Load and Monitoring of Serum Hepatitis C Virus RNA in Predicting Response to Interferon-Alpha2a Treatment of Chronic Hepatitis C. Hanshin Chronic Hepatitis C Study Group," *J Interferon Cytokine Res*, 1997, 17(11):707-12.

Yun ZB, Reichard O, Chen M, et al, "Serum Hepatitis C Virus RNA Levels in Chronic Hepatitis C - Importance for Outcome of Interferon Alfa-2b Treatment," *Scand J Infect Dis*, 1994, 26(3):263-70.

Hepatitis D Serology

Synonyms Delta Agent Serology; Delta Hepatitis Serology

Abstract Hepatitis D virus (HDV) was first recognized in 1977 by Rizzetto and colleagues. HDV always occurs as a simultaneous coinfection with hepatitis B (HBV). Patients coinfected with HDV and HBV have fulminant hepatitis more often than patients infected with HBV alone. Testing for serological markers of HDV should be considered when a patient shows clinical signs of acute or fulminant hepatitis.

Patient Preparation Avoid recent administration of radioisotopes

Specimen Serum

Container Red top tube

Causes for Rejection Recently administered radioisotopes

Reference Range Negative

Use Differential diagnosis of chronic, recurrent, and acute viral hepatitis

Methodology Radioimmunoassay (RIA), enzyme-linked immunosorbent assay (ELISA)

Additional Information Hepatitis D virus ("delta" agent) is an incomplete RNA virus, or viroid, that can only infect livers already infected by hepatitis B virus. It may occur, therefore, as coinfection with acute HBV hepatitis or super imposed on chronic HBV infection. It cannot occur in an HB_sAg-negative individual. IgG and IgM antibodies to HDV develop 5-7 weeks after infection. IgM antibody is most useful in distinguishing those patients with active liver disease. HDAg can be detected in serum or liver biopsies but is technically demanding and offers little to diagnosis. False-positive EIA results have been reported in patients with lipemia or high titer rheumatoid factor. Studies of liver transplants in patients with end-stage liver disease due to hepatitis B/D have shown, through serial biopsies post-transplant, that HDV viral reinfection occurs within 1 week but without damage. Not until HBV proliferation occurs several weeks to months later does one find histologic and clinical changes.

Hepatitis D Superinfection

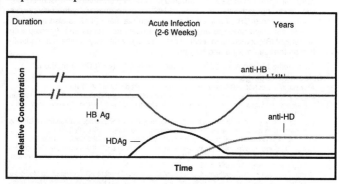

Reprinted from Abbott Diagnosis

Selected Readings
Craig JR, "Hepatitis Delta Virus - No Longer A Defective Virus," *Am J Clin Pathol*, 1992, 98(6):552-3, (editorial).

Davies SE, Lau JY, O'Grady JG, et al, "Evidence That Hepatitis D Virus Needs Hepatitis B Virus to Cause Hepatocellular Damage," *Am J Clin Pathol*, 1992, 98(6):554-8.

Govindarajan S, Valinluck B, Lake-Bakkar G, "Evaluation of a Commercial Anti-Delta EIA Test for Detection of Antibodies to Hepatitis Delta Virus," *Am J Clin Pathol*, 1991, 95(2):240-1.

Hepatitis D Coinfection

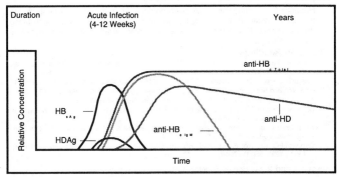

Reprinted from Abbott Diagnostics

Gupta S, Govindarajan S, Cassidy WM, et al, "Acute Delta Hepatitis: Serological Diagnosis With Particular Reference to Hepatitis Delta Virus RNA," *Am J Gastroenterol*, 1991, 86(9):1227-31.

Lee HS and Vyas GN, "Diagnosis of Viral Hepatitis," *Clin Lab Med*, 1987, 7(4):741-57.

Pohl C, Baroudy BM, Bergmann KF, et al, "A Human Monoclonal Antibody That Recognizes Viral Polypeptides and *In Vitro* Translation Products of the Genome of the Hepatitis D Virus," *J Infect Dis*, 1987, 156(4):622-9.

Polish LB, Gallagher M, Fields HA, et al, "Delta Hepatitis: Molecular Biology and Clinical and Epidemiological Features," *Clin Microbiol Rev*, 1993, 6(3):211-29.

Hepatitis E Antibody, IgG *see* Hepatitis E Serology *on page 443*

Hepatitis E Serology

Synonyms Anti-Hepatitis E Virus; Anti-HEV; Hepatitis E Antibody, IgG; HEV Antibody, IgG

Specimen Serum

Collection Samples from individuals with suspected HEV infection should be collected as early in the course of illness as possible.

Storage Instructions Refrigerate serum.

Reference Range Nonreactive

Use Diagnose acute hepatitis E viral (HEV) infection; differential diagnosis of enteric hepatitis. HEV IgG increased in HEV infection; HEV decreased in the absence of HEV infection, early in HEV infection (prior to seroconversion), and in past, resolved HEV infection

Limitations A nonreactive test result does not rule out acute HEV infection (prior to seroconversion) or past HEV infection

Methodology Enzyme immunoassay (EIA); anti-HEV antibodies in the patient serum bind to two recombinant HEV antigens coating the polystyrene well. Following a wash to remove unbound material, HRP-conjugated goat antihuman IgG is added to bind to the antigen-antibody complexes. After a second wash, *o*-phenylenediamine (OPD) substrate is added, resulting in production of a yellow-orange color. The amount of color produced is directly proportional to the amount of antibody present in the patient specimen. Results are reported as nonreactive or repeatedly reactive.

Additional Information This test is for research use only. It is not to be used as a diagnostic procedure without confirmation of the diagnosis by another established product or procedure.

Hepatitis E virus (HEV) is the major etiologic agent of enterically transmitted non-A, non-B hepatitis in developing countries. In the United States, it is usually diagnosed in recent travelers to endemic areas (India, Asia, Africa, and Central America). Like hepatitis A, HEV occurs in both sporadic and epidemic forms and causes an acute, moderately severe, but not chronic, hepatitis that is frequently cholestatic. Unlike hepatitis A virus, HEV progresses to fatal fulminant hepatitis in at least 10% to 20% of pregnant patients, especially in the third trimester. The infection may also manifest without jaundice or be present subclinically. (Continued)

Hepatitis E Serology (Continued)

Hepatitis E IgG antibodies have been detected in up to 93% of patients during the acute phase. In most patients, IgG antibodies are short lived, often being undetectable 6-12 months after onset; however, duration up to 4.5 years has been observed.

Selected Readings

Fields HA, Favorov MO, and Margolis II, "The Hepatitis E Virus: A Review," *J Clin Immunoassay*, 1993, 16:215-222.

"Hepatitis E Among U.S. Travelers, 1989-1992," *MMWR Morb Mortal Wkly Rep*, 1993, 42(1):1-4.

Purdy MA and Krawczynski K, "Hepatitis E," *Gastroenterol Clin North Am*, 1994, 23(3):537-46.

"Self-Learning Review, Hepatitis E," *Can Fam Physician*, 1998, 44:2648, 2652.

Ticchurst J, "Hepatitis E Virus," *Manual of Clinical Microbiology*, 6th ed, Murray PR, ed, Washington, DC: ASM Press, 1995, 1056-67.

Yang G and Vyas GN, "Immunodiagnosis of Viral Hepatitides A to E and Non-A to -E," *Clin Diagn Lab Immunol*, 1996, 3(3):247-56.

Yarbough PO, Tam AW, Fry KE, et al, "Hepatitis E Virus: Identification of Type-Common Epitopes," *J Virol*, 1991, 65(11):5790-7.

Herpes 1 and 2 *see* Herpes Simplex Antibody *on next page*

Herpes Culture *see* Herpes Simplex Virus Culture *on page 446*

Herpes Cytology

Related Information

Herpes Simplex Antibody *on next page*
Herpes Simplex Virus by Direct Immunofluorescence *on next page*
Herpes Simplex Virus Culture *on page 446*
Herpes Simplex Virus Isolation, Rapid *on page 447*
Skin Biopsy *on page 535*

Synonyms Herpetic Inclusion Bodies, Cytology; Inclusion Body Stain; Tzanck Smear; Viral Study, Herpes

Test Includes Preparation of cytological smears, staining of smears, and microscopic evaluation for viral inclusions

Special Instructions A stat Pap stain can be requested at the time of delivery if active herpes is suspected.

Specimen Direct scrape of lesion

Collection Firmly scrape lesion area with sterile tongue depressor, swab, scalpel, or Culturette®. Spread cellular material evenly on glass slides and fix immediately in 95% ethyl alcohol or inexpensive hairspray. Cells on a swab should be rolled onto a slide; scraped cells should be dabbed onto a slide. Cells should be obtained from a freshly unroofed lesion. Label frosted slide with patient's name. For lesions of skin or vulva, which are dry surfaces, it is helpful to moisten the lesion with saline before scraping it. **Do not air dry smears.**

Causes for Rejection Improper fixation, air drying artifact

Use To establish the presence of herpesvirus infection

Limitations Herpes inclusions may not be seen in 50% of active lesions. Viral cultures are the definitive method but may take 2 or more days.

Methodology Pap stained smear, immunoperoxidase stain for herpes viral antigen

Additional Information Diagnostic yield is increased by immunoperoxidase or immunofluorescent procedures, which become positive before characteristic viral cytopathic changes develop. Smears with a heavy inflammatory exudate may be difficult to interpret because of nonspecific staining. Smears must be done with and without the primary antibody and positive and negative controls must be run concurrently.

Selected Readings

Arvin AM and Prober CG, "Herpes Simplex Viruses," *Manual of Clinical Microbiology*, 5th ed, Balows A, Hausler WJ Jr, Herrmann KL, et al, eds, Washington, DC: American Society for Microbiology, 1991, 822-8.

Corey L and Holmes KK, "Genital Herpes Simplex Virus Infections: Current Concepts in Diagnosis, Therapy, and Prevention," *Ann Intern Med*, 1983, 98(6):973-83.

Corey L and Spear PG, "Infections With Herpes Simplex Viruses," *N Engl J Med*, 1986, 314(12):686-91 and 749-56.

Herpes Hominis 1 and 2 *see* Herpes Simplex Antibody *on next page*

Herpes Simplex 1 and 2 Culture *see* Herpes Simplex Virus Culture *on page 446*

Herpes Simplex Antibody

Related Information

Herpes Cytology *on previous page*
Herpes Simplex Virus by Direct Immunofluorescence *on this page*
Herpes Simplex Virus Culture *on next page*
Herpes Simplex Virus Isolation, Rapid *on page 447*

Synonyms Herpes 1 and 2; Herpes Hominis 1 and 2

Test Includes HSV 1 and 2

Specimen Serum

Container Red top tube or serum separator tube

Reference Range Interpretation depends on whether episode is initial or reinfection. IgG and IgM specific antibodies may give more useful information about an acute event.

Limitations Extensive background antibody in the population, and cross reaction of HSV 1 and HSV 2 responses make test useful only in epidemiology. The test is not generally useful except to determine rising titers.

Methodology Immunofluorescence, hemagglutination, complement fixation, enzyme immunoassay (EIA)

Additional Information A primary HSV 1 or HSV 2 infection will produce a classical rising antibody titer. However, because exposure to herpesvirus is almost universal (50% to 90% of adults have antibodies) the background of antibody makes the serologic response in any particular episode of recurrence difficult to interpret. This is made especially true by the fact the antibody to one virus type may be stimulated by infection with the heterologous virus type. Both false-positive and false-negatives are common with currently licensed enzyme immunoassays. Collecting the requisite paired sera to delineate which titers are rising or stable generally adds nothing to clinical management, and thus herpes serology cannot be recommended in routine clinical cases. However, in research settings or for epidemiologic studies serologic definition of the type of herpes infection have been worthwhile.

Herpes serology has not been proved clinically useful in determining whether caesarean delivery should be undertaken in pregnant patients with questionably active herpes. Pap smear or immunochemical demonstration of viral antigen is more useful for this. Nor is herpes serology usually helpful in the differential of a very sick infant with possible congenital herpes. Because of the fulminant course, even early IgM antibody may not be demonstrable in time to contribute to care.

Selected Readings

Ashley R, Cent A, Maggs V, et al, "Inability of Enzyme Immunoassays to Discriminate Between Infections With Herpes Simplex Virus Types 1 and 2," *Ann Intern Med*, 1991, 115(7):520-6.

Corey L, Adams HG, Brown ZA, et al, "Genital Herpes Simplex Virus Infections: Clinical Manifestations, Course, and Complications," *Ann Intern Med*, 1983, 98(6):958-72.

Corey L and Spear PG, "Infections With Herpes Simplex Viruses," *N Engl J Med*, 1986, 314(12):686-91 and 749-56.

Erlich KS, "Laboratory Diagnosis of Herpesvirus Infections," *Clin Lab Med*, 1987, 7(4):759-76.

Stewart JA, "Herpes Simples Virus," *Manual of Clinical Laboratory Immunology*, 4th ed, Rose NR, de Macario EC, Fahey JL, et al, eds, Washington, DC: American Society for Microbiology, 1992, 554-9.

Herpes Simplex Virus Antigen Detection *see* Herpes Simplex Virus by Direct Immunofluorescence *on this page*

Herpes Simplex Virus by Direct Immunofluorescence

Related Information

Herpes Cytology *on previous page*
Herpes Simplex Antibody *on this page*
Herpes Simplex Virus Culture *on next page*
Herpes Simplex Virus Isolation, Rapid *on page 447*
Skin Biopsy *on page 535*

Synonyms Herpes Simplex Virus Antigen Detection; HSV Antigen Detection, Direct

Test Includes Direct (nonculture) detection of HSV-infected cells

Special Instructions Make more than one slide preparation

Specimen Basal cells of a freshly unroofed lesion rolled onto a clean microscope slide

Sampling Time Preferably within 3 days of lesion eruption

(Continued)

Herpes Simplex Virus by Direct Immunofluorescence
(Continued)

Collection Make a preparation of cells taken from the suspected herpetic lesion onto a plain 1" x 3" glass slide. Cells from the bottom of an ulcer or vesicle should be scraped with a swab, scalpel or curette. Swabs should be **rolled (not smeared)** across a small area of the slide several times, and cells scraped with a scalpel should be gently dabbed onto the slide. The best specimen is a collection of the cells at the base of an intact vesicle. Cells from a diseased cornea can also be used. **The smear should be air dried at room temperature.**

Storage Instructions Do not store the specimen. Send it to the laboratory immediately.

Causes for Rejection Insufficient quantity of specimen on slide, poorly prepared or labeled slides

Turnaround Time Less than 1 day

Reference Range No herpes simplex virus-infected cells detected

Use Rapid detection of herpes simplex virus in oral or genital lesions

Limitations Some of the variables in this test include proper collection of specimens, stage and location of lesion, and community prevalence of the disease.

The efficiency of detection of HSV material depends in great part on the collection of a sufficiently large number of intact infected cells from the lesion. It is important to obtain cells from the base of an intact vesicle if at all possible. The presence of infected cells decreases as the lesion heals, and crusted lesions may have little or no herpes antigenic material remaining.

Methodology Immunoperoxidase or immunofluorescence staining of collected cells

Additional Information In certain situations, this direct antigen detection test can be more sensitive than cell culture; however, and in general, this test is only approximately 70% as sensitive as cell culture. In critical situations, clinicians should consider using both methods.

Air-dried preparations on slides can also be stained with Giemsa or Diff-Quik™ stains (Tzanck). Fixed preparations (usually 95% ethanol) can also be stained with the Papanicolaou or immunoperoxidase methods. Smears fixed with hairspray and subsequently stained with the Papanicolaou stain usually are excellent preparations.

Selected Readings

Arvin AM and Prober CG, "Herpes Simplex Viruses," *Manual of Clinical Microbiology*, 5th ed, Balows A, Hausler WJ Jr, Herrmann KL, et al, eds, Washington, DC: American Society for Microbiology, 1991, 822-8.

Drew WL, "Diagnostic Virology," *Clin Lab Med*, 1987, 7(4):721-40.

Smith TF, "Rapid Methods for the Diagnosis of Viral Infections," *Lab Med*, 1987, 18:16-20.

Herpes Simplex Virus Culture

Related Information

Herpes Cytology *on page 444*
Herpes Simplex Antibody *on previous page*
Herpes Simplex Virus by Direct Immunofluorescence *on previous page*
Herpes Simplex Virus Isolation, Rapid *on next page*

Synonyms Herpes Culture; Herpes Simplex 1 and 2 Culture; HSV 1 and 2 Culture; HSV Culture

Applies to Viral Culture, Eye; Viral Culture, Genital; Viral Culture, Skin

Test Includes Culture for HSV only; HSV also is usually detected in a routine/general virus culture

Special Instructions Special viral transport medium must be obtained from the laboratory prior to collection of specimen.

Specimen Specimen depends on type of infection:
- genital - vesicle fluid, lesion, endocervical
- conjunctivitis - conjunctival
- congenital - throat, vesicle, cerebrospinal fluid
- encephalitis - brain biopsy
- meningitis - cerebrospinal fluid
- respiratory/oral - throat, vesicle

Container Sterile container; cold viral transport medium for swabs

Collection All specimens should be kept cold and moist. As for most viral cultures, specimens should be collected in the acute stage of the disease, preferably within 3 days and no longer than 7 days after the onset of illness. Spinal fluid specimens should be submitted in the usual sterile tube; no special transport medium is necessary. All other specimens should be collected on a sterile swab as described and **the swab should be placed into cold viral transport medium immediately after collection.**

Endocervical: Swab cervix with enough force to obtain epithelial cells.

Vesicular lesion: Wash vesicles with sterile saline. Carefully open several vesicles and soak up vesicular fluid with swab. If vesicles are absent, vigorously swab base of lesion (specimen should be collected during first 3 days of eruption, because specimens collected later in the course of disease rarely yield virus).

Conjunctival: Using a moistened swab, firmly rub conjunctiva using sufficient force to obtain epithelial cells.

Throat, respiratory, oral: Rotate swab in both tonsillar crypts and against posterior oropharynx.

Storage Instructions Specimens should be delivered to the laboratory and handed to a technologist within 30 minutes of collection. Outpatient specimens: If transport is to be delayed more than 30 minutes after collection, specimen **must** be refrigerated (held at 4°C to 8°C) until it can be transported to the laboratory. Do not freeze specimen.

Causes for Rejection Dry specimen, specimen not refrigerated during transport, specimen fixed in formalin, unlabeled specimen

Turnaround Time Variable (1-14 days) and depends on culture method used and amount of virus in specimen

Reference Range No virus isolated

Use Aid in the diagnosis of HSV disease

Methodology Inoculation of specimen into cell cultures, incubation of cultures, observation of characteristic cytopathic effect, and identification by fluorescent monoclonal antibodies specific for type 1 or 2.

Additional Information HSV can only rarely be isolated from the CSF of patients with HSV 1 encephalitis. The virus is occasionally isolated from spinal fluid of patients with HSV 2 meningitis and of neonates with congenital herpes and from urine from patients with primary genital HSV infections concurrent with cystitis.

Serology for the detection of herpes simplex virus is available, but the results usually are of value only in the diagnosis of primary HSV infections. There is much cross-reaction between the antibodies to HSV 1 and HSV 2.

Selected Readings
Arvin AM and Prober CG, "Herpes Simplex Viruses," *Manual of Clinical Microbiology*, 5th ed, Balows A, Hausler WJ Jr, Herrmann KL, et al, eds, Washington, DC: American Society for Microbiology, 1991, 822-8.

Drew WL, "Diagnostic Virology," *Clin Lab Med*, 1987, 7(4):721-40.

Reichman RC, "Herpes Simplex Viruses," *Textbook of Human Virology*, Belshe RB, ed, Littleton, MA: PSG Publishing Co, 1984, 811-28.

Solomon AR, "New Diagnostic Tests for Herpes Simplex and Varicella Zoster Infections," *J Am Acad Dermatol*, 1988, 18(1 Pt 2):218-21.

Herpes Simplex Virus, Direct Detection see Virus Detection by DFA *on page 576*

Herpes Simplex Virus Isolation, Rapid

Related Information

Herpes Cytology *on page 444*
Herpes Simplex Antibody *on page 445*
Herpes Simplex Virus by Direct Immunofluorescence *on page 445*
Herpes Simplex Virus Culture *on previous page*

Synonyms HSV Shell Vial Method, Spin Amplification

Applies to Culture, HSV Only; HSV, Rapid Isolation; Skin Culture for HSV

Test Includes Inoculation of cell cultures in shell vials, 16-hour incubation, and immunofluorescence staining for HSV 1 and 2

Specimen Swab of genital, lip, or mucous membrane lesion; vesicular fluid; biopsy

Container Sterile container; cold viral transport medium for swabs

Collection All specimens should be kept cold and moist. As for most viral cultures, specimens should be collected in the acute stage of the disease, (Continued)

Herpes Simplex Virus Isolation, Rapid *(Continued)*

preferably within 3 days and no longer than 7 days after the onset of illness. Spinal fluid specimens should be submitted in the usual sterile tube; no special transport medium is necessary. All other specimens should be collected on a sterile swab as described and **the swab should be placed into cold viral transport medium immediately after collection**.

Endocervical: Swab cervix with enough force to obtain epithelial cells.

Vesicular lesion: Wash vesicles with sterile saline. Carefully open several vesicles and soak up vesicular fluid with swab. If vesicles are absent, vigorously swab base of lesion (specimen should be collected during first 3 days of eruption, because specimens collected later in the course of disease rarely yield virus).

Conjunctival: Using a moistened swab, firmly rub conjunctiva using sufficient force to obtain epithelial cells.

Throat, respiratory, oral: Rotate swab in both tonsillar crypts and against posterior oropharynx.

Turnaround Time Overnight to 2 days depending on method and capability of laboratory

Reference Range No HSV detected

Use Aid in the diagnosis of disease caused by HSV

Methodology Shell vial isolation technique with direct immunofluorescent staining for HSV 1 and HSV 2. Specimens are centrifuged onto cell cultures grown on coverslips in the bottoms of 1-dram shell vials. Centrifugation greatly accelerates virus attachment and penetration. After incubation, fluorescein-labeled monoclonal antibodies are applied to the infected cells to detect viral antigens that are expressed in the membranes of the cells. Characteristic fluorescent foci indicate the presence of virus.

Additional Information The rapid shell vial culture technique for the detection of HSV 1 and 2 has been reported to be as sensitive as conventional cell culture methods.

Selected Readings

Gleaves CA, Wilson DJ, Wold AD, et al, "Detection and Serotyping of Herpes Simplex Virus in MRC-5 Cells by Use of Centrifugation and Monoclonal Antibodies 16-Hr Postinoculation," *J Clin Microbiol*, 1985, 21(1):29-32.

Smith TF, "Rapid Methods for the Diagnosis of Viral Infections," *Lab Med*, 1987, 18:16-20.

Solomon AR, "New Diagnostic Tests for Herpes Simplex and Varicella Zoster Infections," *J Am Acad Dermatol*, 1988, 18(1 Pt 2):218-21.

Herpes Zoster Serology *see* Varicella-Zoster Virus Serology *on page 569*

Herpetic Inclusion Bodies, Cytology *see* Herpes Cytology *on page 444*

HEV Antibody, IgG *see* Hepatitis E Serology *on page 443*

HHV-6, IgM, IgG *see* Human Herpesvirus 6, IgG and IgM Antibodies, Quantitative *on page 458*

Hip Arthrogram *see* Arthrogram *on page 334*

Hip, Left or Right, and Pelvis, X-ray *see* Bone Films *on page 343*

Hip, Left or Right, X-ray *see* Bone Films *on page 343*

Hips Arthritis, X-ray *see* Bone Films *on page 343*

Histo Antigen *see* Histoplasma capsulatum Antigen Assay *on page 450*

Histopathology

Related Information

Aerobic Culture, Body Fluid *on page 310*
Biopsy Culture, Routine *on page 337*
Electron Microscopic (EM) Examination for Viruses, Stool *on page 403*
Fungus Culture, Biopsy *on page 414*
Fungus Culture, Body Fluid *on page 415*
Liver Biopsy *on page 474*
Lymph Node Biopsy *on page 482*
Methenamine Silver Stain *on page 487*
Muscle Biopsy *on page 491*
Mycobacteria Culture, Biopsy or Body Fluid *on page 493*
Periodic Acid-Schiff Stain *on page 518*
Skin Biopsy *on page 535*
Virus Detection by DFA *on page 576*

Synonyms Biopsy; Gross and Microscopic Pathology; Pathologic Examination; Surgical Pathology; Tissue Examination

Applies to Bronchial Biopsy; Endoscopic Biopsy; Lung Biopsy; Medical Legal Specimens

Test Includes Gross and microscopic examination and diagnosis. Imprints may be made if the tissue is fresh and unfixed and if indications for imprints exist.

Abstract Surgical pathology has been defined as the discipline which deals with the anatomic pathology of tissues removed from living patients. Smears, aspirates, special stains, immunocytochemistry, flow cytometry, and molecular pathology may be included.

Patient Preparation It is essential that each specimen be accompanied by an adequate description of what it is thought to represent, as well as an appropriate clinical history.

Special Instructions Consult the laboratory prior to beginning the procedure for specific instructions. Requisition should state operative diagnosis and source of specimen, as well as patient's name, age, sex, room or location, name of surgeon, and names of other physicians who will need a copy of the pathology report.

Specimen Fresh tissue, tissue fixed in phosphate-buffered formalin or other appropriate fixative. Each specimen container must be labeled to include source as well as patient's name. Each specimen from a different anatomic site must be placed in a separate, correctly labeled container, designated "left," "right," "proximal," "distal," "ventral," "dorsal," and so forth.

Container Jars of assorted sizes, containing formalin or another appropriate fixative; the neck of the container should not be smaller than its diameter. Fresh specimens should be submitted on a sterile gauze pad moistened with sterile saline and should not be left on countertops; they must be placed in the hands of a responsible person.

Collection Small biopsy specimens are to be placed immediately in fixative, unless special needs such as frozen section exist. Use approximately 5 to 20 times as much fixative solution as the bulk of the tissue. Small tissues such as those from bronchoscopic biopsy, bladder biopsy, and endometrium can be ruined in a very short time by drying out.

Storage Instructions Fixation in formalin solution or other appropriate fixative

Causes for Rejection Mislabeled specimen container, unlabeled specimen

Turnaround Time Biopsy reports commonly require a day or more. Delays are caused by need for clinical information, deeper sections, decalcification, or special stains.

Use Histopathologic diagnosis; evaluate extent of lesions and provision of classification and, when appropriate, grading in the case of tumors

Limitations Tissue fixed in formalin **cannot** be used for microbial culture, chemical estrogen or progesterone receptor assay, certain types of histochemistry, frozen sections, gene rearrangement, or optimal electron microscopy.

Additional Information A major advantage of conventional over frozen sections is that extensive sampling of the entire specimen can take place.

Cultures of tissue are best taken in the O.R., where a sterile field exists. A piece of tissue should be placed in an appropriate sterile container with requests for smear, culture, anaerobic culture, mycobacteria, and fungus culture if appropriate. It should be immediately taken to the Microbiology Laboratory. See test listings of suspected organism and specific site cultures.

Routine tissues are brought in fixative. Fixatives should be picked up prior to the biopsy. Commonly used fixatives include modified Zenker's fluid (for tiny specimens, eg, endometrial curettage, liver, and other needle biopsies, **not** skin), and formalin (for specimens thicker than 3 mm).

Bullets, shotgun pellets, and other metallic objects require special handling, but no fixative is needed. Of major importance in handling bullets and other specimens of possible forensic significance, including vaginal swabs obtained in rape cases, is the scrupulous maintenance of a chain-of-custody. Specimens must be accurately labeled, and transfer and receipt must be documented. Specimens must be kept under safeguards in the laboratory until turned over to law enforcement officials.

Bone biopsy for metabolic bone disease requires special handling. (Continued)

Histopathology *(Continued)*

Materials sometimes not sent for histopathologic examination, depending on the institution, include bullets, shotgun pellets, neonatal foreskins, grossly unremarkable placentas from uneventful deliveries, and orthopedic appliances. If a specimen is not sent to the Pathology Department, the surgeon should carefully describe the specimen in the operative report.

Histoplasma capsulatum **Antibody and Antigen** *see* Histoplasmosis Serology *on this page*

Histoplasma capsulatum Antigen Assay

Synonyms HAG; Histo Antigen; HPA

Test Includes Detection of *H. capsulatum* polysaccharide antigen

Special Instructions Specimens must be shipped to the *Histoplasma* Reference Laboratory, Room OPW 441, Wishard Memorial Hospital, 1001 W Tenth St, Indianapolis, IN 46202-2879. Information about testing, interpretation, and results can be obtained by calling 1-800-HISTO-DG.

Specimen Urine is the preferred specimen but can be done on blood, bronchoalveolar lavage, or other sterile body fluids

Container Sterile container for urine or body fluid, red top tube for blood

Storage Instructions Stable for 7 days at 4°C.

Reference Range Negative: <1.0 unit; indeterminate: 1.0-2.0 units; positive: >2.0 units

Use Assist in the diagnosis of disseminated histoplasmosis

Limitations Sensitivity of assay varies with the severity of infection: disseminated: 92%, acute pulmonary: 44%, chronic pulmonary: 21%, meningitis: 67%. Specificity of this assay is approximately 98%. False-positive results may occur with other systemic mycoses.

Methodology Enzyme immunoassay (EIA)

Additional Information The *Histoplasma* antigen is not only useful in the initial diagnosis but may be used to follow patients and for detection of relapse. Patients with suspected relapse experience a 2 unit rise in antigen, and patients with a definite relapse experience at least a 4 unit rise. Patients that are responding to therapy show a continual decline in antigen and approximately 70% of AIDS patients after 1 year of chronic suppressive therapy will have a urine HAG <4.0 units. Of note, there is significant run variability, and one should not compare previous reported results with the most recent result. The last specimen has been stored and is run concurrently with the newly obtained specimen. Results of the repeated last specimen and the new specimen are available with an interpretation of these results by the Histoplasmosis Reference Laboratory.

Selected Readings

Durkin MM, Connolly PA, and Wheat LJ, "Comparison of Radioimmunoassay and Enzyme-Linked Immunoassay Methods for Detection of *Histoplasma capsulatum* var *capsulatum* Antigen," *J Clin Microbiol*, 1997, 35(9):2252-5.

Lee BL, Tauber MG, and Aberg JA, "Histoplasmosis" *The AIDS Knowledge Base*, 3rd ed, Chapter 59, Philadelphia, PA: Lippincott, Williams & Wilkins, 1999.

Wheat J, Wheat H, Connolly P, et al, "Cross-Reactivity in *Histoplasma capsulatum* Variety *capsulatum* Antigen Assays of Urine Samples From Patients With Endemic Mycoses," *Clin Infect Dis*, 1997, 24(6):1169-71.

Histoplasmosis Immunodiffusion *see* Fungal Serology *on page 410*

Histoplasmosis Serology

Related Information

Periodic Acid-Schiff Stain *on page 518*

Applies to *Histoplasma capsulatum* Antibody and Antigen

Test Includes Reaction with yeast and mycelial antigens

Specimen Serum (antibody); urine (antigen)

Container Red top tube, plastic urine container

Collection Acute and convalescent sera are recommended, especially when acute titers are only presumptive

Reference Range Antibody: less than a fourfold change in titer between acute and convalescent samples; titers less than 1:4; negative CSF. Antigen: negative.

Use Diagnosis and prognosis of histoplasmosis

Limitations A negative result does not rule out histoplasmosis. Histoplasmin skin testing may interfere with results. Testing with both antigens must be performed.

There are cross reactions with other fungi. Anticomplementary sera cannot be tested for complement fixing antibodies. The latex agglutination test gives some false-positives, and must be confirmed with another procedure.

Contraindications Previous skin testing

Methodology Complement fixation (CF), immunodiffusion (ID), latex agglutination (LA), radioimmunoassay (RIA) (antigen), enzyme immunoassay (EIA)

Additional Information CF titers 1:8 or 1:16 are presumptive evidence of histoplasmosis. Titers ≥1:32 are highly suggestive of *H. capsulatum* infection but cannot be relied on as the sole means of diagnosis. Complement fixation and immunodiffusion each detect about 85% of disease. H and M bands on immunodiffusion indicate active disease. Complement fixation is less sensitive to disseminated or chronic disease. The latex agglutination test detects IgM antibodies and is positive early in disease, but not in late, chronic, or recurrent infection.

Tests for fungal antigen are now available and obviate some of the problems of ordinary serology - cross reactions, decreased immune response, need for paired specimens over time. The use of enzyme immunoassay and radioimmunoassay to detect *H. capsulatum* antigen has proven to be a useful approach in the diagnosis of histoplasmosis. Antigenuria or antigenemia is excellent evidence of disseminated disease.

In addition to histoplasmosis in immunologically intact individuals, this fungal infection is a serious opportunistic infection in patients with AIDS (occasionally as its first manifestation).

Selected Readings

Drutz DJ, "Antigen Detection in Fungal Infections," *N Engl J Med*, 1986, 314(2):115-7.

Kaufman L and Reiss E, "Serodiagnosis of Fungal Diseases," *Manual of Clinical Laboratory Immunology*, 4th ed, Rose NR, de Macario EC, Fahey JL, et al, eds, Washington, DC: American Society for Microbiology, 1992, 506-28.

Wheat LJ, Connolly-Stringfield PA, and Baker RL, "Disseminated Histoplasmosis in the Acquired Immune Deficiency Syndrome: Clinical Findings, Diagnosis and Treatment, and Review of the Literature," *Medicine (Baltimore)*, 1990, 69(6):361-74.

Wheat LJ, Kohler RB, and Tewari RP, "Diagnosis of Disseminated Histoplasmosis by Detection of *Histoplasma capsulatum* Antigen in Serum and Urine Specimens," *N Engl J Med*, 1986, 314(2):83-8.

HIV-1 Drug Resistance Testing *see* HIV Genotyping *on page 456*

HIV-1 Gene Sequencing *see* HIV Genotyping *on page 456*

HIV-1 Mutations Testing *see* HIV Genotyping *on page 456*

HIV-1 RNA, Expanded Range *see* HIV-1 RNA, Quantitative PCR, 2nd Generation *on next page*

HIV-1 RNA, Qualitative PCR *see* HIV-1 RNA, Quantitative PCR, 2nd Generation *on next page*

HIV-1 RNA, Quantitative bDNA, 3rd Generation

Related Information

HIV-1 RNA, Quantitative PCR, 2nd Generation *on next page*

HIV-1 Serology *on page 454*

HIV Genotyping *on page 456*

Synonyms bDNA Testing for HIV; HIV bDNA; HIV Branched DNA; HIV Viral Load

Special Instructions This test is intended for use only in individuals with known HIV-1 infection. Qualitative tests may be used for diagnosis.

Specimen Plasma

Container Lavender top (EDTA) tube

Storage Instructions Remove plasma from cells within 6 hours of collection and freeze.

Reference Range 50 copies/mL

Use Monitor progression of HIV infection, assess prognosis, monitor the effect of antiretroviral drug therapy HIV viral load is increased in acute HIV infection, increased risk of progression to AIDS, disease progression, clinical AIDS, and drug resistance. HIV viral load is decreased in response to therapy and remission.

Methodology Branched DNA (bDNA) signal amplification in which viral RNA is extracted, captured by solid-phase bound synthetic oligonucleotides and hybridized to target probes and multiple-branched DNA molecules. Alkaline phosphatase-labeled probes are in turn hybridized to the branched DNA and reacted with (Continued)

HIV-1 RNA, Quantitative bDNA, 3rd Generation
(Continued)

a chemiluminescent substrate to produce a greatly amplified light signal. The amount of light emitted is directly proportional to the quantity of RNA in the specimen.

Additional Information The measurement of HIV-1 RNA provides the most direct and accurate assessment of HIV viral load, or viremia, by quantifying the amount of HIV-1 RNA in plasma. Levels of HIV RNA are elevated during primary HIV-1 infection preceding seroconversion. During the years of clinical latency, patients maintain a relatively constant, individually variable level of RNA. As infection progresses and the immune system weakens, HIV-1 RNA levels increase. The plasma viral RNA level has been shown to be a better independent predictor of progression to AIDS and death than the number of CD4+ T-cells. Changes in RNA levels have been shown to be the most accurate indicator of the patient's response to therapy. Plasma HIV RNA levels must increase or decrease more than threefold (0.5 log) to be clinically significant in an individual patient.

Selected Readings

Cao Y, Ho DD, Todd J, et al, "Clinical Evaluation of Branched DNA Signal Amplification for Quantifying HIV Type 1 in Human Plasma," *AIDS Res Hum Retroviruses*, 1995, 11(3):353-61.

Carpenter CC, Fischl MA, Hammer SM, et al, "Antiretroviral Therapy for HIV Infection in 1998: Updated Recommendations of the International AIDS Society-USA Panel," *JAMA*, 1998, 280(1):78-86.

Dewar RL, Highbarger HC, Sarmiento MD, et al, "Aplication of Branched DNA Signal Amplification to Monitor Human Immunodeficiency Virus Type 1 Burden in Human Plasma," *J Infect Dis*, 1994, 170(5):1172-9.

Mellors JW, Kingsley LA, Rinaldo CR Jr, et al, "Quantitation of HIV-1 RNA in Plasma Predicts Outcome After Seroconversion," *Ann Intern Med*, 1995, 122(8):573-9.

Mellors JW, Rinaldo CR Jr, Gupta P, et al, "Prognosis in HIV-1 Infection Predicted by the Quantity of Virus in Plasma," *Science*, 1996, 272(5265):1167-70.

Pachl C, Todd JA, Kern DG, et al, "Rapid and Precise Quantification of HIV-1 RNA in Plasma Using a Branched DNA Signal Amplification Assay," *J Acquir Immune Defic Syndr Hum Retrovirol*, 1995, 8(5):446-54.

Perelson AS, Neumann AU, Markowitz M, et al, "HIV-1 Dynamics *in vivo*: Virion Clearance Rate, Infected Cell Life-Span, and Viral Generation Time," *Science*, 1996, 271(5255):1582-6.

Volberding PA, "HIV Quantification: Clinical Applications," *Lancet*, 1996, 347(8994):71-3.

HIV-1 RNA, Quantitative PCR, 1st Generation see HIV-1 RNA, Quantitative PCR, 2nd Generation *on this page*

HIV-1 RNA, Quantitative PCR, 2nd Generation

Related Information

HIV-1 RNA, Quantitative bDNA, 3rd Generation *on previous page*
HIV-1 Serology *on page 454*
HIV Genotyping *on page 456*
Human Immunodeficiency Virus Culture *on page 459*
p24 Antigen *on page 509*
Polymerase Chain Reaction *on page 523*

Synonyms HIV-1 RNA, Quantitative PCR, Ultrasensitive; HIV Polymerase Chain Reaction; HIV Viral Load; Human Immunodeficiency Virus 1 RNA, 2nd Generation

Applies to HIV-1 RNA, Expanded Range; HIV-1 RNA, Qualitative PCR; HIV-1 RNA, Quantitative PCR, 1st Generation

Abstract The measurement of HIV-1 RNA provides the most direct and accurate assessment of HIV viral load, or viremia, by quantifying the amount of HIV-1 RNA in plasma. Levels of HIV RNA are elevated during primary HIV-1 infection preceding seroconversion. During the years of clinical latency, patients maintain a lower, and relatively constant, level of RNA. As the infection progresses and the immune system weakens, HIV-1 RNA levels increase. The HIV RNA level and the number of CD4+ T-cells combined are a more accurate predictor of progression to AIDS and death than either marker alone. Change in the HIV RNA level is the most accurate individual marker of a patient's response to therapy. Levels must increase or decrease more than threefold (0.5 log) to be clinically significant in an individual patient.

Special Instructions This test is intended for use only in individuals with known HIV-1 infection. Qualitative tests may be used for diagnosis.

Specimen Plasma

Container Lavender top (EDTA) tube or yellow top (ACD) tube

Storage Instructions Remove plasma from cells within 6 hours of collection and freeze immediately.

Reference Range <40 copies/mL

Use Monitor the effect of antiretroviral drug therapy with maximum sensitivity, monitor progression of HIV infection, assess prognosis, individualize antiretroviral therapy

HIV viral load in increases in:
- acute HIV infection
- increased risk of progression to AIDS
- disease progression
- clinical AIDS
- drug resistance

HIV viral load is decreased in:
- response to therapy
- remission

Second generation assays can accurately quantify HIV RNA levels 10-fold lower than the first generation assay; thus, it is particularly useful for monitoring patients on combination antiretroviral therapy whom may routinely have HIV RNA levels <400 copies/mL. The first generation assay continues to be the method of choice for patients with viral loads >100,000 copies/mL. Qualitative HIV-1 RNA assays can detect as few as 10 copies/mL.

Limitations Results obtained from different anticoagulants (EDTA, ACD) are not interchangeable; therefore, use of only one anticoagulant is recommended for patient monitoring

Methodology Enhanced reverse transcription-polymerase chain reaction (RT-PCR); increased sensitivity as a result of sample pretreatment methods

Additional Information Second generation assays can accurately quantify HIV RNA levels 10-fold lower than the first generation assay; thus, it is particularly useful for monitoring patients on combination antiretroviral therapy whom may routinely have HIV RNA levels <400 copies/mL. The first generation assay continues to be the method of choice for patients with viral loads >100,000 copies/mL. Qualitative HIV-1 RNA assays can detect as few as 10 copies/mL.

HIV-1 Qualitative, Quantitative, and Genotyping Tests

Test Name	Sensitivity	Reference Range
HIV-1 DNA, Qualitative PCR	10 copies	Not detected
HIV-1 RNA, Qualitative PCR	10 copies	Not detected
HIV-1 RNA, Quantitative bDNA, 3rd Generation	50-500,000 copies/mL	<50 copies/mL; <1.60 log copies/mL
HIV-1 RNA, Quantitative PCR, 1st Generation	400-750,000 copies/mL	<400 copies/mL; <2.60 log copies/mL
HIV-1 RNA, Quantitative PCR, 2nd Generation	40-100,000 copies/mL	<40 copies/mL; <1.60 log copies/mL
HIV-1 RNA, Quantitative PCR, Expanded Range	40-7,500,000 copies/mL	<40 copies/mL; <1.60 log copies/mL
HIV-1 Genotyping for Drug Resistance to Protease Inhibitors (PrIs) and Reverse Transcriptase Inhibitors (RTs)	Do not genotype if viral load is <600 copies/mL; viral populations of >40% detected	No mutations detected None associated

Selected Readings

Carpenter CC, Fischl MA, Hammer SM, et al, "Antiretroviral Therapy for HIV Infection in 1998: Updated Recommendations of the International AIDS Society-U.S.A. Panel," *JAMA*, 1998, 280(1):78-86.

Detels R, Munoz A, McFarlane G, et al, "Effectiveness of Potent Antiretroviral Therapy on Time to AIDS and Death in Men With Known HIV Infection Duration. Multicenter AIDS Cohort Study Investigators," *JAMA*, 1998, 280(17):1497-503.

Ho DD, Neumann AU, Perelson AS, et al, "Rapid Turnover of Plasma Virions and CD4 Lymphocytes in HIV-1 Infection," *Nature*, 1995, 373(6510):123-6.

Holodniy M, Mole L, Winters M, et al, "Diurnal and Short-Term Stability of HIV Virus Load as Measured by Gene Amplification," *J Acquir Immune Defic Syndr*, 1994, 7(4):363-8.

Hughes MD, Johnson VA, Hirsch MS, et al, "Monitoring Plasma HIV-1 RNA Levels in Addition to CD4+ Lymphocyte Count Improves Assessment of Antiretroviral Therapeutic Response. ACTG 241 Protocol Virology Substudy Team," *Ann Intern Med*, 1997, 126(12):929-38.

(Continued)

HIV-1 RNA, Quantitative PCR, 2nd Generation
(Continued)

Mellors JW, Kingsley LA, Rinaldo CR Jr, et al, "Quantitation of HIV-1 RNA in Plasma Predicts Outcome After Seroconversion," *Ann Intern Med*, 1995, 122(8):573-9.

Mellors JW, Rinaldo CR Jr, Gupta P, et al, "Prognosis in HIV-1 Infection Predicted by the Quantity of Virus in Plasma," *Science*, 1996, 272(5265):1167-70.

O'Brien WA, Hartigan PM, Daar ES, et al, "Changes in Plasma HIV RNA Levels and CD4+ Lymphocyte Counts Predict Both Response to Antiretroviral Therapy and Therapeutic Failure. VA Cooperative Study Group on AIDS," *Ann Intern Med*, 1997, 126(12):939-45.

Paxton WB, Coombs RW, McElrath MJ, et al, "Longitudinal Analysis of Virologic Measures in Human Immunodeficiency Virus-Infected Subjects With ≥400 CD4 Lymphocytes: Implications for Applying Measurements to Individual Patients. National Institute of Allergy and Infectious Diseases AIDS Vaccine Evaluation Group," *J Infect Dis*, 1997, 175(2):247-54.

Saag MS, Holodniy M, Kuritzkes DR, et al, "HIV Viral Load Markers in Clinical Practice," *Nat Med*, 1996, 2(6):625-9.

Schockmel GA, Yerly S, and Perrin L, "Detection of·Low HIV-1 RNA Levels in Plasma," *J Acquir Immune Defic Syndr Hum Retrovirol*, 1997, 14(2):179-83.

Volberding PA, "HIV Quantification: Clinical Applications," *Lancet*, 1996, 347(8994):71-3.

HIV-1 RNA, Quantitative PCR, Ultrasensitive *see* HIV-1 RNA, Quantitative PCR, 2nd Generation *on page 452*

HIV-1 Serology

Related Information
HIV-1 RNA, Quantitative bDNA, 3rd Generation *on page 451*
HIV-1 RNA, Quantitative PCR, 2nd Generation *on page 452*
HIV Genotyping *on page 456*
Human Immunodeficiency Virus Culture *on page 459*
p24 Antigen *on page 509*

Synonyms Human Immunodeficiency Virus Serology

Test Includes Screening test with confirmation of repeated positives

Patient Preparation In some states test may not be done or results revealed without express written or informed consent of the patient.

Special Instructions Blood and body fluid precautions must be observed

Specimen Serum

Reference Range Negative

Use Diagnose AIDS, exposure to HIV-1; screen blood and blood products for transfusion

Methodology Enzyme-linked immunosorbent assay (ELISA), Western blot for confirmation

HIV-1 Infection Laboratory Tests

Test	Significance
HIV ELISA, EIA	Screening test for HIV infection. Sensitivity >99.9%. Reactive results must be confirmed by Western blot.
Western blot	Confirmatory test for HIV ELISA. Specificity when combined with ELISA >99.9%. Indeterminate results with early HIV infection, HIV-2 infection, autoimmune disease, pregnancy, and recent tetanus toxoid administration.
Absolute CD4 lymphocyte count	Most widely used predictor of HIV progression. Risk of progression is high with CD4 <200 cells/µL. Best short-term predictor for development of opportunistic infections.
CD4 lymphocyte percentage	Useful in conjunction with CD4 count. Risk of progression is high with percentage <20%.
β_2-Microglobulin	Cell surface protein indicative of macrophage-monocyte stimulation. Levels >3.5 mg/dL associated with rapid progression of disease. Limited usefulness.
p24 antigen	Indicates active HIV replication. Tends to be positive prior to seroconversion and with advanced disease. Relatively insensitive.
HIV DNA PCR	Most sensitive assay for diagnosing infection.
HIV RNA quantitative PCR or branched DNA	Most useful tests for determining prognosis and monitoring therapy.
HIV culture	Clinical research tool.

Chronology of Clinical and Laboratory Manifestations of HIV Infection

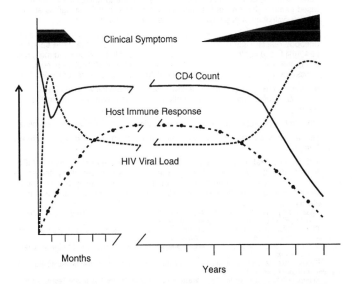

Primary infection may be asymptomatic or may be associated with transient flu-like symptoms which subside as the immune response develops. Rapid viral replication and high viral load levels are observed in the primary phase of infection. Prolonged "latent" period of dynamic host-virus quasi-equilibrium is associated with continuing viral replication and increased CD4 cell turnover. As the infection progresses, the host immune response wanes, viral replication increases, CD4 counts fall, and the clinical symptoms of AIDS manifest.

Limitations There is a 2- to 12-week or longer interval after infection before antibody becomes detectable. Positive screening tests must be confirmed by more specific follow-up procedures (usually Western blot). Antibody is not protective against disease. There are some cross reactions in some test systems due to histocompatibility antigen mismatches (in particular, antibodies to HLA-DR4). Cross-reactions have been observed to other viral antigens as well. A recent influenza vaccine resulted in reactivity against p24 antigen and give false-positive enzyme-linked immunosorbent assays.

Additional Information Human immunodeficiency virus (HIV, formerly HTLV-III), a lentivirus, is the etiologic agent of AIDS. Acute infection, spread by blood or sexual contact, is usually followed within days by a flu-like illness, or no symptoms. During this time, HIV antigen, usually p24 core protein, may be detectable in serum. This becomes negative in 2 weeks to a month. There then follows a period of weeks to months during which an individual is infected with HIV, which may or may not be replicating at a low rate, but screening tests for antibody to HIV are **negative**.

Present screening tests for HIV antibodies are ELISA or EIA procedures which use disrupted virus or recombinant antigen products. Different antibodies are detected. Sensitivity and specificity of these tests are both extremely high, but positive results on a screen should be repeated; if positive a second time they should be confirmed with a Western blot procedure. Because of the grave implications of a positive result, confirmation of positive results by testing a second sample may be indicated.

Some individuals may have reactive screening tests, restricted to one test system, and completely negative Western blots. This may be due to HLA antibodies reacting with residual human cell surface proteins incorporated in the test

HIV-1 Serology *(Continued)*

kit. False-positives have been reported in individuals who have received intravenous gamma globulin. Since these proteins are due to antibodies in the transfused gamma globulin, repeat analysis in 3 months (half-life for IgG is about 3 weeks), will show a negative or much weaker EIA result.

Western blot analysis can identify the exact viral products with which patient antibody reacts. Criteria for a positive blot include: two of the three bands for p24, gp41, and gp120/160 (Centers for Disease Control); or, one gag (p55, p24, p17), one pol (p64, p53, p31), and one env (gp41, gp120/160) (American Red Cross); or, p24, p31, and gp41 and/or gp120/160 (FDA license for Du Pont kit).

In donor screening programs, a low rate of false-positive (~0.0004%, 1 in 251,000) occurs. These cases usually lack Western blot reactivity to the p31 band.

HIV viral RNA testing is useful in the resolution of inconclusive Western blots.

HIV antibody can be detected in postmortem specimens of blood or vitreous humor.

Although **central nervous system involvement** is extremely common in AIDS, tests to detect HIV antigen or antibody in CSF lack both sensitivity and specificity. These tests do not help in differentiating neurologic symptoms secondary to HIV infection from those due to CNS neoplasm or opportunistic infection.

Selected Readings

Agbede OO, "HIV-1-Indeterminate Western Blot Results: Implications for Diagnosis and Subject Notification," *Clin Microbiol Newslett*, 1992, 14(16):121-5.

Brown AE, Jackson B, Fuller SA, et al, "Viral RNA in the Resolution of Human Immunodeficiency Virus Type 1 Diagnostic Serology," *Transfusion*, 1997, 37(9):926-9.

Burke DS, "Laboratory Diagnosis of Human Immunodeficiency Virus Infection," *Clin Lab Med*, 1989, 9(3):369-92.

Caliendo AM, "Methods, Interpretation, and Applications of HIV-1 Viral Load Measurements," *Clin Microbiol Newslett*, 1997, 19(1):1-7.

"Interpretive Criteria Used to Report Western Blot Results in HIV-1 Antibody Testing - United States," *MMWR Morb Mortal Wkly Rep*, 1991, 40(40):692-5.

Kleinman S, Busch MP, Hall L, et al, "False-Positive HIV-1 Test Results in a Low-Risk Screening Setting of Voluntary Blood Donation," *JAMA*, 1998, 280(12):1080-5.

Krieger JN, "Acquired Immunodeficiency Syndrome Antibody Testing and Precautions," *J Urol*, 1992, 147(3):713-6.

O'Gorman MR, Weber D, Landis SE, et al, "Interpretive Criteria of the Western Blot Assay for Serodiagnosis of Human Immunodeficiency Virus Type 1 Infection," *Arch Pathol Lab Med*, 1991, 115(1):26-30.

Sloand EM, Pitt E, Chiarello RJ, et al, "HIV Testing - State of the Art," *JAMA*, 1991, 266(20):2861-6.

Yen-Lieberman B, "Rapid and Alternative Specimen Source Testing for HIV Antibody," *Clin Microbiol Newslett*, 1998, 20(16):133-6.

HIV bDNA *see* HIV-1 RNA, Quantitative bDNA, 3rd Generation *on page 451*

HIV Branched DNA *see* HIV-1 RNA, Quantitative bDNA, 3rd Generation *on page 451*

HIV Core Antigen *see* p24 Antigen *on page 509*

HIV Culture *see* Human Immunodeficiency Virus Culture *on page 459*

HIV Genotyping

Related Information

HIV-1 RNA, Quantitative bDNA, 3rd Generation *on page 451*
HIV-1 RNA, Quantitative PCR, 2nd Generation *on page 452*
HIV-1 Serology *on page 454*
Human Immunodeficiency Virus Culture *on page 459*
p24 Antigen *on page 509*

Synonyms HIV-1 Drug Resistance Testing; HIV-1 Gene Sequencing; HIV-1 Mutations Testing

Special Instructions Testing for HIV-1 infected patients exhibiting resistance to antiretroviral therapy and having HIV-1 RNA levels >2000 copies/mL.

Specimen Plasma

Container Lavender top (EDTA) tube, yellow top (ACD) tube

Storage Instructions Remove plasma from cells within 6 hours of collection and freeze immediately.

Reference Range Reported mutations indicate resistance to the specified antiretroviral drug(s); however, multiple mutations may be required to confer resistance to a specific drug or drug combination. Conversely, the absence of mutations does not necessarily infer drug susceptibility. Mutations in minor viral populations (ie, those below a 40% prevalence threshold) may not be detected but may become predominant in the future. Therapeutic failure may also be due to patient noncompliance, suboptimal antiretroviral drug therapy, decreased drug bioavailability, or as yet uncharacterized mutations in the Pr and RT genes. Results should be interpreted in conjunction with the patient's past antiretroviral therapy and all other relevant clinical and laboratory findings.

Specimens with fewer than 2000 HIV-1 RNA copies/mL may fail to yield sufficient amounts of cDNA for sequence analysis. Viral genetic heterogeneity and endogenous inhibitors may also yield uninterpretable results.

Use Detect genotypic resistance to HIV antiretroviral therapy; determine cause of HIV antiretroviral drug failure; assist in drug selection prior to initial treatment or following therapeutic failure

Methodology
- Reverse transcription and PCR amplification of plasma HIV-1 RNA followed by automated DNA sequencing
- Amplification of the entire sequence of the Pr gene and the amino-terminal 240 amino acids of the RT gene
- Sequencing in three overlapping reactions with d-Rhodamine-labeled terminators using an Applied Biosystems Model 377 automated sequencer
- Interpretation aided by a computer software program that compares the patient's HIV-1 sequence to the consensus clade B HIV-1 sequence
- Report includes detected mutations and associated drug resistance
- Clinical sensitivity: Viral populations >40% of the individual's HIV-1 population

Additional Information In HIV-1 infected patients, a large number of mutated virions are produced daily due to the high replication rate of HIV and the absence of replication error control mechanisms. Certain mutations are associated with resistance to specific therapeutic agents, thus resulting in the presence of resistant viral strains. Selective pressure favors replication of these resistant strains. As sensitive strains are eradicated by antiretroviral therapy, a resistant strain may become the dominant population in an individual patient, resulting in drug resistance and subsequent therapeutic failure. Mutations may occur in both the reverse transcriptase gene and the protease gene.

HIV-1 genotyping identifies mutations in individual patient viral populations, some of which are associated with therapeutic resistance. In this test, mutations currently known to be associated with resistance are reported.

Selected Readings
Brown AJ and Richman DD, "HIV-1: Gambling on the Evolution of Drug Resistance?" *Nat Med*, 1997, 3(3):268-71.

Carpenter CC, Fischl MA, Hammer SM, et al, "Antiretroviral Therapy for HIV Infection in 1996. Recommendations of an International Panel. International AIDS Society-USA," *JAMA*, 1996, 276(2):146-54.

Cohen J, "The Daunting Challenge of Keeping HIV Suppressed," *Science*, 1997, 277(5322):32-3.

Deeks SG and Abrams DI, "Genotypic-Resistance Assays and Antiretroviral Therapy," *Lancet*, 1997, 349(9064):1489-90.

Deeks SG, Smith M, Holodniy M, et al, "HIV-1 Protease Inhibitors: A Review for Clinicians," *JAMA*, 1997, 277(2):145-53.

Havlir DV and Richman DD, "Viral Dynamics of HIV: Implications for Drug Development and Therapeutic Strategies," *Ann Intern Med*, 1996, 124(11):984-94.

Hirsch MS, Conway B, D'Aquila RT, et al, "Antiretroviral Drug Resistance Testing in Adults With HIV Infection: Implications for Clinical Management. International AIDS Society-USA Panel," *JAMA*, 1998, 279(24):1984-91.

Katzenstein D, "Combination Therapies for HIV Infection and Genomic Drug Resistance," *Lancet*, 1997, 350(9083):970-1.

Larder BA, Kohli A, Kellam P, et al, "Quantitative Detection of HIV-1 Drug Resistance Mutations by Automated DNA Sequencing," *Nature*, 1993, 365(6447):671-3.

Mayers DL, "Drug-Resistant HIV-1: The Virus Strikes Back," *JAMA*, 1998, 279(24):2000-2.

Molla A, Korneyeva M, Gao Q, et al, "Ordered Accumulation of Mutations in HIV Protease Confers Resistance to Ritonavir," *Nat Med*, 1996, 2(7):260-6.

Schinazi RF, Larder BA, and Mellors JW, "Mutations in Retroviral Genes Associated With Drug Resistance," *Intern Antiviral News*, 1996, 4:95-107.

Tack PC, Bremer JW, Harris AA, et al, "Genotypic Analysis of HIV-1 Isolates to Identify Antiretroviral Resistance Mutations From Source Patients Involved in Health Care Worker Occupational Exposures," *JAMA*, 1999, 281(12):1085-6.

Wainberg MA and Friedland G, "Public Health Implications of Antiretroviral Therapy and HIV Drug Resistance," *JAMA*, 1998, 279(24):1977-83.

HIV p24 Antigen *see* p24 Antigen *on page 509*

HIV Polymerase Chain Reaction *see* HIV-1 RNA, Quantitative PCR, 2nd Generation *on page 452*

HIV Viral Load *see* HIV-1 RNA, Quantitative bDNA, 3rd Generation *on page 451*

HIV Viral Load *see* HIV-1 RNA, Quantitative PCR, 2nd Generation *on page 452*

HPA *see Histoplasma capsulatum* Antigen Assay *on page 450*

HSV 1 and 2 Culture *see* Herpes Simplex Virus Culture *on page 446*

HSV Antigen Detection, Direct *see* Herpes Simplex Virus by Direct Immunofluorescence *on page 445*

HSV Culture *see* Herpes Simplex Virus Culture *on page 446*

HSV, Rapid Isolation *see* Herpes Simplex Virus Isolation, Rapid *on page 447*

HSV Shell Vial Method, Spin Amplification *see* Herpes Simplex Virus Isolation, Rapid *on page 447*

HTLV-I/II Antibody

Synonyms Human T-Cell Leukemia Virus Type I and Type II; Human T-Lymphotropic Virus Type I Antibody

Specimen Serum

Container Red top tube

Reference Range Negative

Use Screen blood and blood products for transfusion; differential diagnosis of spastic myelopathy and adult T-cell acute lymphoblastic leukemia (ALL). HTLV-II has been associated with chronic neuromuscular diseases.

Limitations The combined assay for Anti HTLV-I/II is used mainly to screen blood donors. The assay detects 80% of patients with antibody to HTLV-II. The 20% of blood donors who are not detected by the assay for HTLV-II are not at sufficiently high risk to transmit the disease to warrant a separate assay.

Methodology Screen: enzyme immunoassay (EIA); confirmation: Western blot (WB) or radioimmunoprecipitation (RIPA)

Additional Information Human T-lymphotropic virus type I (HTLV-I) is a pathogenic retrovirus which is irregularly distributed in the world. Infection is generally uncommon in the U.S. and Europe. The virus is most commonly found in Japan and the Carribean. The virus can be asymptomatic for prolonged periods (20 years) but is strongly associated with myelopathies and adult T-cell leukemia. Less than 5% of those with antibody to HTLV-I develop myelopathies or leukemias even after 20 years. Adult T-cell leukemia is an aggressive malignancy of T lymphocytes often associated with skin infiltrates and hypercalcemia. The virus is tropic for T4 lymphocytes and is passed by sexual contact, blood products, from mother to fetus, and by breast milk. Pretransfusion testing for antibody to HTLV-I is now mandated by blood banks, in order to avoid transfusion transmitted HTLV-I infection from asymptomatic infected donors. The clinical course of HTLV-I infection, and the meaning of a positive serology are not yet well understood. Indeed, a recent study of hemophiliacs who were transfused regularly with plasma or its derivatives found no evidence of HTLV-I/II antibody in 179 patients.

Selected Readings

Blattner WA, "Human T-Lymphotropic Viruses and Diseases of Long Latency," *Ann Intern Med*, 1989, 111(1):4-6.

CDCP and USPHS Working Group, "Guidelines for Counseling Persons Infected With Human T-Lymphotropic Virus Type I (HTLV-I) and Type II (HTLV-II)," *Ann Intern Med*, 1993, 118(6):448-54.

Sullivan MT, Williams AE, Fang CT, et al, "Transmission of Human T-Lymphotropic Virus Types I and II by Blood Transfusion," *Arch Intern Med*, 1991, 151(10):2043-8.

Zaaijer HL, Cuypers HT, Dudok de Wit C, et al, "Results of 1-Year Screening of Donors in the Netherlands for Human T-Lymphotropic Virus (HTLV) Type I: Significance of Western Blot Patterns for Confirmation of HTLV Infection," *Transfusion*, 1994, 34(10):877-80.

HTLV-III Culture *see* Human Immunodeficiency Virus Culture *on next page*

Human Herpesvirus 6, IgG and IgM Antibodies, Quantitative

Synonyms HHV-6, IgM, IgG

Specimen Serum

Container Red top tube or serum separator tube

Collection Specimens should be free from bacterial contamination and hemolysis

Storage Instructions Refrigerate serum

Causes for Rejection Gross lipemia

Use IgM HHV-6 may aid in the diagnosis of acute or recent infection with HHV-6. An increase in IgG HHV-6 (fourfold titer) between acute and convalescent samples is evidence for a recent HHV-6 infection.

Methodology Indirect fluorescent antibody (IFA)

Additional Information Human herpesvirus 6 (HHV-6) has recently been identified as the agent associated with both pediatric and adult infections. Most children have been infected by age 3 years. The acute infection in children is characterized clinically by an acute febrile illness, irritability, inflammation of tympanic membranes, and (uncommonly) a rash characteristic of roseola. When acute and convalescent (4-6 weeks later) serum samples are compared, a fourfold rise in HHV-6 IgG titer is typical. It has also been thought to be the etiological agent of exanthem subitum (roseola) in children.

In adults, HHV-6 has been associated with chronic fatigue and spontaneously resolving fever resembling a mononucleosis-like illness. During the acute episode an elevated IgM HHV-6 is useful. An increase in IgG HHV-6 between acute and convalescent serum sample is consistent with a recent HHV-6 infection. There is no antiviral agents directed toward this virus.

Selected Readings

Agbede O, "Human Herpesvirus 6: A Virus in Search of a Disease," *Clin Microbiol Newslett*, 1993, 15(4):25-7.

Irving WL and Cunningham AL, "Serological Diagnosis of Infection With Human Herpesvirus Type 6," *BMJ*, 1990, 300(6718):156-9.

Oren I and Sobel JD, "Human Herpesvirus Type 6: Review," *Clin Infect Dis*, 1992, 14(3):741-6.

Pruksananonda P, Hall CB, Insel RA, et al, "Primary Human Herpesvirus 6 Infection in Young Children," *N Engl J Med*, 1992, 326(22):1445-50.

Rathore MH, "Human Herpesvirus 6," *South Med J*, 1993, 86(11):1197-205.

Human Immunodeficiency Virus 1 RNA, 2nd Generation *see* HIV-1 RNA, Quantitative PCR, 2nd Generation *on page 452*

Human Immunodeficiency Virus Culture

Related Information

HIV-1 RNA, Quantitative PCR, 2nd Generation *on page 452*

HIV-1 Serology *on page 454*

HIV Genotyping *on page 456*

p24 Antigen *on page 509*

Synonyms AIDS Virus Culture; HIV Culture; HTLV-III Culture

Specimen Blood (20-40 mL), cerebrospinal fluid (10 mL), other body fluids, biopsies. All specimens **must** be labeled with the patient's name or code and **must** be transported to the laboratory in a **sealed** plastic bag with the request form attached. Some laboratories will not accept patient names associated with HIV specimens.

Container Green top (heparin) tube for blood, sterile container for CSF and other fluids

Collection Routine venipuncture. Invert the tubes several times after drawing the blood to be sure the blood is thoroughly mixed with the heparin.

Storage Instructions Do not store the specimen. Send it to the laboratory immediately. Some laboratories require specimen to be received into the laboratory the same day the specimen is received.

Causes for Rejection Dry specimen, specimen not refrigerated during transport, specimen fixed in formalin, unlabeled specimen

Turnaround Time Positive cultures are usually reported after 2 consecutive positive reverse transcriptase assays. Blood cultures are usually incubated 4 weeks and some laboratories incubate CSF cultures 8 weeks before termination as negative.

Reference Range No virus isolated

Use Aid in the diagnosis of disease caused by HIV, research studies, recover virus for phenotyping

Limitations A negative culture cannot be assumed to rule out the presence of the virus.

Methodology Growth of virus in lymphocyte culture and subsequent (indirect) testing for presence of virus in culture fluids by EIA reverse transcriptase assay

Selected Readings

Erice A, Sannerud KJ, Leske VL, et al, "Sensitive Microculture Method for Isolation of Human Immunodeficiency Virus Type 1 from Blood Leukocytes," *J Clin Microbiol*, 1992, 30(2):444-8.

Garcia Rodriguez MC, Bates I, de Jose I, et al, "Prognostic Value of Immunological Data, *in vitro* Antibody Production, and Virus Culture in Vertical Infection With HIV-1, *Arch Dis Child*, 1995, 72(6):498-501.

(Continued)

Human Immunodeficiency Virus Culture *(Continued)*

Jackson JB, "Human Immunodeficiency Virus Type 1 Antigen and Culture Assays," *Arch Pathol Lab Med*, 1990, 114(3):249-53.

Jackson JB and Balfour HH Jr, "Practical Diagnostic Testing for Human Immunodeficiency Virus," *Clin Microbiol Rev*, 1988, 1(1):124-38.

MacGregor RR, Dubin G, Frank I, et al, "Failure of Culture and Polymerase Chain Reaction to Detect Human Immunodeficiency Virus (HIV) in Seronegative Steady Sexual Partners of HIV-Infected Individuals," *Clin Infect Dis*, 1995, 21(1):122-7.

Markham PD and Salahuddin SZ, "*In Vitro* Cultivation of Human Leukocytes: Methods for the Expression and Isolation of Human Retroviruses," *BioTechniques*, 1987, 5:432-43.

Schleupner CJ, "Detection of HIV-1 Infection," *Principles and Practice of Infectious Diseases*, 4th ed, Mandell GL, Bennett JE, and Dolin R, eds, New York, NY: Churchill Livingstone, 1995, 1253-66.

Human Immunodeficiency Virus Serology *see* HIV-1 Serology *on page 454*

Human T-Cell Leukemia Virus Type I and Type II *see* HTLV-I/II Antibody *on page 458*

Human T-Lymphotropic Virus Type I Antibody *see* HTLV-I/II Antibody *on page 458*

Humerus, Left or Right, X-ray *see* Bone Films *on page 343*

Hyperalimentation Line Culture *see* Intravenous Line Culture *on page 464*

IgG Antibodies to Rubella *see* Rubella Serology *on page 531*

IgM Antibodies to Rubella *see* Rubella Serology *on page 531*

Iliac Arteries Ultrasound *see* Ultrasound, Peripheral Arteries and Veins *on page 561*

Immunofluorescent Studies, Biopsy

Related Information

Skin Biopsy *on page 535*

Synonyms Direct Immunofluorescent Studies, Biopsy

Test Includes Fluorescent stains for immunoglobulins, complement, fibrin, and routine histopathology

Special Instructions Consult the pathologist prior to biopsy procedure for specific instructions. Requisition **must** state operative diagnosis and source of specimen.

Specimen Biopsy of kidney, skin, muscle, and lung submitted fresh in saline-moistened gauze as soon as possible following removal

Container Jar with gauze pad moistened with sterile saline

Collection Container **must** be labeled with patient's full name, and date

Storage Instructions Transport specimen to the laboratory immediately.

Causes for Rejection Specimen allowed to dry

Reference Range Negative

Use Determine the presence of tissue deposits of IgG, IgM, IgA, C1q, C3, albumin, fibrinogen, and kappa and lambda light chains in immunological diseases of kidney (eg, immune complex glomerulonephritis and antiglomerular basement membrane glomerulonephritis), skin (pemphigus, bullous pemphigoid, dermatitis herpetiformis, lupus erythematosus), neoplasms (plasma cell myeloma, macroglobulinemia of Waldenström, malignant lymphoma), and lung (lupus erythematosus, Goodpasture's syndrome)

Additional Information Submit additional specimen in formalin for light microscopy. Electron microscopy is commonly needed in many of the same biopsies in which fluorescence is desired, but usually requires a different fixative than does light microscopy processing.

Inclusion Body Stain *see* Herpes Cytology *on page 444*

Inclusion Conjunctivitis *see* Ocular Cytology *on page 505*

India Ink Preparation

Related Information

Cryptococcal Antigen Serology, Serum or Cerebrospinal Fluid *on page 379*
Fungus Culture, Cerebrospinal Fluid *on page 416*
Methenamine Silver Stain *on page 487*
Periodic Acid-Schiff Stain *on page 518*

Synonyms Cerebrospinal Fluid India Ink Preparation; *Cryptococcus* Preparation; *Cryptococcus* Stain; Nigrosin Preparation

Patient Preparation Same as for culture of specific site

Specimen For all practical purposes, the only reasonably useful specimen is cerebrospinal fluid.

Container Sterile CSF tube

Collection The specimen may be divided for fungal culture, and mycobacteria culture and smear, and routine bacterial culture and Gram's stain only if the specimen is of adequate volume for all tests requested.

Storage Instructions Do not refrigerate.

Causes for Rejection Insufficient specimen volume

Turnaround Time Routine: 24 hours; stat: 2 hours

Reference Range No encapsulated yeast identified

Use Establish the presence of *Cryptococcus* sp or other fungi

Limitations This technique is only 30% to 50% sensitive in cases of cryptococcal meningitis. Cultures and rapid latex agglutination (LA) methods are more sensitive than direct preparations; therefore, the India ink preparation may be negative when the culture or LA test is positive. Immunologic tests for *Cryptococcus* antigen have a sensitivity of 90% to 100%. Many laboratories have abandoned the use of the India ink preparation in favor of LA.

Methodology Wet mount with India ink (nigrosin) for contrast. Centrifugation may concentrate organisms and improve sensitivity.

Additional Information *Cryptococcus neoformans* is the most common central nervous system fungus in both normal hosts and patients with the acquired immunodeficiency syndrome (AIDS). Pigeon droppings act as a year round reservoir for dispersion of encapsulated yeast cells.

Selected Readings

Berlin L and Pincus JH, "Cryptococcal Meningitis. False-Negative Antigen Test Results and Cultures in Nonimmunosuppressed Patients," *Arch Neurol*, 1989, 46(12):1312-6.

Ellis DH and Pfeiffer TJ, "Ecology, Life Cycle, and Infectious Propagule of *Cryptococcus neoformans*," *Lancet*, 1990, 336(8720):923-5.

McGinnis MR, "Detection of Fungi in Cerebrospinal Fluid," *Am J Med*, 1983, 75(1B):129-38.

Indium-111 Labeled Leukocyte Scan *see* Indium Leukocyte Scan *on this page*

Indium Leukocyte Scan

Synonyms Indium-111 Labeled Leukocyte Scan; Infection Scan; Infection Scintigraphy; Leukocyte Scintigraphy; WBC Scan; White Blood Cell Scan

Test Includes The patient receives an intravenous reinjection of radiolabeled leukocytes. The patient initially has a 60-80 mL sample of blood drawn for an *in vitro* process of labeling and separating the leukocyte component. Images are acquired at intervals between 2-24 hours after subsequent reinjection of radiolabeled cells.

Patient Preparation The patient does not need to be fasting or NPO for this procedure. Patient should have all RIA blood work performed, or at least drawn, prior to injection of any radioactive material.

Special Instructions Requisition must state the current patient diagnosis in order to select the most appropriate radiopharmaceutical and/or imaging technique. DURATION OF PROCEDURE: Two hours from blood draw to reinjection of labeled cells. 2-24 hours for imaging at intervals. RADIOPHARMACEUTICAL: Indium-111 labeled leukocytes

Causes for Rejection Other recent Nuclear Medicine procedure may interfere. If uncertain, call the Nuclear Medicine Department.

Turnaround Time A written report will be sent to the patient's chart and/or to the referring physician.

Normal Findings Radiolabeled leukocytes will localize to some degree in the liver, spleen, and bone marrow. Focal accumulations in soft tissue or asymmetric uptake in bone will be seen in infected or inflamed sites. For osteomyelitis, a bone scan is usually performed first for comparison with the radiolabeled leukocyte scan findings.

Use Radiolabeled leukocyte imaging is useful either in determining the site of an occult infection or in confirming the presence or absence of infection at a suspected site. This technique has largely replaced gallium-67 imaging for acute infections because of the better image resolution and greater specificity. Some chronic infections, eg, chronic osteomyelitis, may be better imaged with gallium-67. Radiolabeled leukocyte imaging is especially helpful in detecting postoperative infection sites and in documenting lack of residual infection after a course of therapy.

(Continued)

Indium Leukocyte Scan *(Continued)*

Limitations Leukocyte radiolabeling is a complex process and is usually performed on-site only where there are dedicated radiopharmacy laboratories. Most commercial radiopharmacies will also provide this service locally.

Additional Information An alternative method of leukocyte radiolabeling with technetium-99m (^{99m}Tc) HMPAO is now available. Early reports show possible advantages with earlier imaging times and better sensitivity for infections in extremities with utilization of higher doses of ^{99m}Tc versus indium-111.

Selected Readings

Abreu SH, "Skeletal Uptake of Indium-111 Labeled White Blood Cells," *Semin Nucl Med*, 1989, 19(2):152-5.

Datz FL and Thorne DA, "Effect of Antibiotic Therapy on the Sensitivity of Indium-111 Labeled Leukocyte Scans," *J Nucl Med*, 1986, 27(12):1849-53.

Froelich JW and Field SA, "The Role of Indium-111 White Blood Cells in Inflammatory Bowel Disease," *Semin Nucl Med*, 1988, 18(4):300-7.

Laitinen R, Tähtinen J, Lantto T, et al, "^{99m}Tc Labeled Leukocytes in Imaging of Patients With Suspected Acute Abdominal Inflammation," *Clin Nucl Med*, 1990, 15(9):597-602.

Roddie ME, Peters AM, Danpure HJ, et al, "Inflammation: Imaging With ^{99m}Tc HMPAO-Labeled Leukocytes," *Radiology*, 1988, 166(3):767-72.

Induced Sputum Technique for *Pneumocystis* *see* Pneumocystis carinii Test *on page 522*

Infant Botulism, Toxin Identification *see* Botulism, Diagnostic Procedure *on page 351*

Infection Scan *see* Indium Leukocyte Scan *on previous page*

Infection Scintigraphy *see* Indium Leukocyte Scan *on previous page*

Infectious Mononucleosis Serology

Related Information

Epstein-Barr Virus Serology *on page 406*

Synonyms Monospot™ Test; Monosticon® Dri-Dot® Test; Mono Test

Replaces Davidsohn Differential; Paul-Bunnell Test

Test Includes Screening for the presence of heterophil antibodies

Specimen Serum

Container Red top tube or serum separator tube

Reference Range Negative

Use Diagnosis of infectious mononucleosis

Limitations Correlation with clinical findings is imperative since false-positive and negative results have been reported. About 15% of the adult population with infectious mononucleosis will not develop heterophil antibodies. Failure to develop heterophil antibodies occurs even more frequently in children. In these instances, patients usually are tested for specific Epstein-Barr virus antibodies. Less than 2% false-positives have been reported with Hodgkin's disease, lymphoma, acute lymphocytic leukemia, infectious hepatitis, pancreatic carcinoma, cytomegalovirus, Burkitt's lymphoma, rheumatoid arthritis, malaria, and rubella.

Overall, the Monospot™ test has 99% specificity and 86% sensitivity.

Methodology Latex agglutination (LA) and enzyme immunoassay (EIA)

Additional Information The infectious mononucleosis heterophil antibody appears in the serum of patients by the sixth to tenth day of illness. Highest titers are usually found in the second to third week. Antibody levels may remain detectable for as little as 1 week or persist up to a year; usual persistence is 4-8 weeks. The level of antibody activity is not correlated with the severity of disease or the degree of lymphocytosis. A positive screening or differential test in the appropriate clinical and hematologic setting is sufficient to make the diagnosis of infectious mononucleosis.

If there is clinically a mononucleosis syndrome, but the screening test is negative, a differential absorption will add nothing. Instead, consider tests for EBV specific antibodies, CMV, and toxoplasmosis antibodies.

Selected Readings

Evans AS and Niederman JC, "EBV-IgA and New Heterophile Antibody Tests in Diagnosis of Infectious Mononucleosis," *Am J Clin Pathol*, 1982, 77(5):555-60.

Fleisher GR, Collins M, and Fager S, "Limitations of Available Tests for Diagnosis of Infectious Mononucleosis," *J Clin Microbiol*, 1983, 17(4):619-24.

Horwitz CA, Henle W, Henle G, et al, "Heterophil-Negative Infectious Mononucleosis and Mononucleosis-Like Illnesses," *Am J Med*, 1977, 63(6):947-57.

Sumaya CV and Jenson HB, "Epstein-Barr Virus," *Manual of Clinical Laboratory Immunology*, 4th ed, Rose NR, de Macario EC, Fahey JL, et al, eds, Washington, DC: American Society for Microbiology, 1992, 568-75.

Influenza A and B Serology

Related Information
Influenza Virus Culture *on this page*

Test Includes IgG and IgM antibody titers

Specimen Serum

Container Red top tube or serum separator tube

Collection Acute and convalescent sera drawn 10-14 days apart are required

Reference Range Less than a fourfold increase in titer in paired sera; IgG <1:10, IgM <1:10

Use Establish the diagnosis of influenza virus infection; epidemiologic surveillance and tracking; differentiate type A from B for treatment with amantadine

Methodology Complement fixation (CF), hemagglutination inhibition (HAI), single radial immunodiffusion (RID), enzyme immunoassay (EIA)

Additional Information Influenza virus is typed by specifying a neuraminidase and hemagglutinin. Although serologic diagnosis is seldom practical (or necessary) during an influenza epidemic, serologic typing is valuable for epidemiology, and for planning therapy. Since type A influenza can be treated with amantadine, but type B cannot, this distinction may need to be made. Presence of specific IgM antibody indicates acute infection.

Selected Readings
Bryan JA, "The Serologic Diagnosis of Viral Infections," *Arch Pathol Lab Med*, 1987, 111(11):1015-23.

Rota PA, Regnery HL, and Kendal AP, "Influenza Virus," *Manual of Clinical Laboratory Immunology*, 4th ed, Rose NR, de Macario EC, Fahey JL, et al, eds, Washington, DC: American Society for Microbiology, 1992, 576-81.

Shaw MW, Arden NH, and Maassab HF, "New Aspects of Influenza Viruses," *Clin Microbiol Rev*, 1992, 5(1):74-92.

Influenza Virus Culture

Related Information
Influenza A and B Serology *on this page*
Viral Culture, Throat *on page 574*

Test Includes Concurrent culture for other respiratory viruses (parainfluenza and respiratory syncytial virus)

Specimen Throat or nasopharyngeal swab, sputum, bronchial washings, bronchoalveolar lavage

Container Sterile container; cold virus transport medium for swabs

Sampling Time Specimens should be collected within 3 days of the onset of illness.

Storage Instructions Specimens should be placed into viral transport medium and kept cold at all times. Do not freeze specimens. Specimens should be delivered immediately to the laboratory.

Causes for Rejection Dry specimen, specimen not refrigerated during transport, specimen fixed in formalin, unlabeled specimen

Turnaround Time Variable (5-14 days) and depends on culture method used and the amount of virus in the specimen

Reference Range No virus isolated

Use Isolate and identify influenza virus as an etiologic agent in cases of influenza and viral pneumonia

Methodology Inoculation of specimens into cell cultures, incubation of cultures, observation of cultures for characteristic cytopathic effect, and identification/speciation by methods such as hemadsorption and fluorescent monoclonal antibodies specific for influenza virus A or B

Additional Information The shell vial technique to rapidly (within 24 hours) detect viruses has recently been adapted to detect influenza A and B viruses. Serology for the detection of influenza antibodies is available. A commercial and rapid (less than 15 minutes) enzyme immunoassay for the detection of influenza A virus in patient specimen is available.

Selected Readings
Guenthner SH and Linneman CC, "Indirect Immunofluorescence Assay for Rapid Diagnosis of Influenza Virus," *Lab Med*, 1988, 581-3.
(Continued)

Influenza Virus Culture *(Continued)*

Harmon MW and Kendal AP, "Influenza Viruses," *Manual of Clinical Microbiology*, 5th ed, Balows A, Hausler WJ Jr, Herrmann KL, et al, eds, Washington, DC: American Society for Microbiology, 1991, 868-77.

Shaw MW, Arden NH, and Maassab HF, "New Aspects of Influenza Viruses," *Clin Microbiol Rev*, 1992, 5(1):74-92.

Van Voris LP, Young JF, Bernstein JM, et al, "Influenza Viruses," *Textbook of Human Virology*, Belshe RB, ed, Littleton, MA: PSG Publishing Co, 1984, 267-97.

Waner JL, Todd SJ, Shalaby H, et al, "Comparison of Directigen FLU-A With Viral Isolation and Direct Immunofluorescence for the Rapid Detection and Identification of Influenza A Virus," *J Clin Microbiol*, 1991, 29(3):479-82.

Influenza Virus, Direct Detection *see* Virus Detection by DFA *on page 576*

Infusion Pyelogram *see* Urography *on page 567*

Insect Identification *see* Arthropod Identification *on page 334*

Intercellular Antibody Basement Membrane Antibody *see* Skin Biopsy, Immunofluorescence *on page 538*

Intrauterine Device Culture *see* Actinomyces Culture, All Sites *on page 308*

Intravenous Devices Culture *see* Intravenous Line Culture *on this page*

Intravenous Line Culture

Synonyms Arterial Line Culture; Catheter Culture, Intravenous; Catheter Tip Culture; Hemovac® Tip Culture; Hyperalimentation Line Culture; Intravenous Devices Culture; I.V. Catheter Culture; Shunt Culture; Swan-Ganz Tip Culture; Venous Catheter Culture

Test Includes Culture of foreign body organism identification, antibiotic susceptibilities of potential pathogens

Specimen Blood and distal 2" of I.V. catheter tip collected in a sterile manner (cut with sterile scissors and at a point just below the skin line)

Container Sterile container

Collection Aseptically prepare insertion site. Remove line without contact with adjacent skin and send only intra-arterial segment. Catheter tip aseptically removed and placed in sterile container. A procedure for quantitative comparative central and peripheral blood culture is as follows.

Separate blood samples (10 mL each) are obtained in a sterile manner from a peripheral blood vessel and from the central catheter. Aseptic technique at the catheter is as follows:

- The catheter is clamped and the needle adapter removed.
- The end of the catheter is swabbed once with 70% isopropyl alcohol and then with an iodine solution (allow to air dry).
- A sterile needle adapter is inserted into the end of the catheter.
- The clamp is removed and 2 mL of blood is drawn through a sterile syringe to clear the catheter.
- The blood for culture is then subsequently obtained in a separate sterile syringe.
- The catheter adapter is reattached to the intravenous tubing.

The paired blood specimens are placed in separate lysis centrifugation tubes after the stopper is swabbed three times with povidone-iodine. See also the listing Blood Culture, Aerobic and Anaerobic *on page 337*.

Storage Instructions Specimens should be transported to the laboratory within 1 hour of collection for optimal results. However, if specimens cannot be collected and delivered to the laboratory during regular hours specimen may be refrigerated overnight.

Reference Range No growth. For culture taken through a central catheter, a tenfold greater colony count than a simultaneous peripheral culture or >100 CFU/mL if only a central catheter culture is presumptive evidence of a colonized catheter. A culture of a catheter tip (rolled onto agar media) result ≥15 CFU also is presumptive evidence of a colonized catheter.

Use Identify a possible source of bacteremia or fungemia; particularly useful for the diagnosis of catheter-related sepsis (CRS) secondary to blood-borne seedling of catheters, and CRS associated with coagulase-negative staphylococci

Limitations Culture of blood obtained from intravenous lines is fraught with problems. Blood obtained from a line is easily contaminated and interpretation of results usually is difficult.

Methodology Quantitative or semiquantitative culture with or without lysis centrifugation. A very simple and equally effective semiquantitative technique is to roll the culture tip on a blood or chocolate agar plate. Greater than 15 CFU suggests infection; <15 CFU indicates a low probability of infection.

Additional Information Infections complicating therapy with indwelling central venous catheters pose a difficult problem. Catheter-related sepsis is defined when:

- Positive blood cultures collected through the central venous catheter can show a tenfold or greater colony count compared with peripheral quantitative blood culture or >100 CFU/mL if only central venous catheter blood culture is available
- A semiquantitative catheter tip culture result ≥15 CFU
- No obvious clinical or microbiologic source for the infection is apparent

Exit site infections are defined as purulent drainage or erythema at the catheter exit site. Tunnel infection is defined as spreading cellulitis with erythema, tenderness, and swelling of the skin surrounding the subcutaneous tunnel tract of the catheter. Successful therapy of catheter-related infection with antibiotics and local care has been reported. However, catheter removal almost always is required to achieve cure. *Staphylococcus aureus* and polymicrobial infections also are more difficult to eradicate. Intraluminal culture has been reported to correlate well with catheter tip cultures (87.5% identical) while skin puncture sites are usually less frequently identical (37.5%). See table.

Summary of Results of Prospective Studies Using Semiquantitative Techniques to Diagnose Vascular-Access Infections

Organism	No. With Same Organism in Semiquantitative Catheter Culture and Blood Culture
Coagulase-negative staphylococci	27
Staphylococcus aureus	26
Yeast	17
Enterobacter	7
Serratia	5
Enterococcus	5
Klebsiella	4
Streptococcus viridans group	3
Pseudomonas species	2
Proteus	2
Others: *Pseudomonas aeruginosa, Yersinia*	1 each

From Hampton A and Sheretz RJ, "Vascular-Access Infections in Hospitalized Patients," *Surg Clin North Am*, 1988, 68:57-72, with permission.

Selected Readings

Andremont A, Paulet R, Nitenberg G, et al, "Value of Semiquantitative Cultures of Blood Drawn Through Catheter Hubs for Estimating the Risk of Catheter Tip Colonization in Cancer Patients," *J Clin Microbiol*, 1988, 26(11):2297-9.

Fry DE, Fry RV, and Borzotta AP, "Nosocomial Blood-Borne Infection Secondary to Intravascular Devices," *Am J Surg*, 1994, 167(2):268-72.

Garrison RN and Wilson MA, "Intravenous and Central Catheter Infections," *Surg Clin North Am*, 1994, 74(3):557-70.

Henderson DK, "Bacteremia Due to Percutaneous Intravascular Devices," *Principles and Practice of Infectious Diseases*, 4th ed, Mandell GL, Bennett JE and, eds, New York, NY: Churchill Livingstone, 1995, 2587-99.

Maki DG, Weise CE, and Sarafin HW, "A Semiquantitative Culture Method for Identifying Intravenous-Catheter-Related Infection," *N Engl J Med*, 1977, 296(23):1305-9.

Reimer LG, "Catheter-Related Infections and Blood Cultures," *Clin Lab Med*, 1994, 14(1):51-8.

Widmer AF, Nettleman M, Flint K, et al, "The Clinical Impact of Culturing Central Venous Catheters. A Prospective Study," *Arch Intern Med*, 1992, 152(6):1299-302.

Intravenous Pyelogram *see* Urography *on page 567*

Iron Stain *see* Bone Marrow Aspiration and Biopsy *on page 343*

Itraconazole Level

Synonyms Sporanox® Level, Blood

Abstract Itraconazole is an orally administered antifungal agent with a broad spectrum of activity.

Specimen Serum

Container Red top tube

(Continued)

Itraconazole Level *(Continued)*

Sampling Time 4 hours after oral dose and approximately 1-2 weeks after therapy has begun so that a steady-state is achieved

Reference Range Therapeutic: varies with methodology; see Additional Information.

Use May be useful to ensure therapeutic levels if poor absorption is suspected, or in cases of therapeutic failure or relapse

Limitations *In vitro* susceptibility testing of fungi against itraconazole is method dependent and may not accurately predict clinical success. Consequently, monitoring levels and adjusting dosage to attain therapeutic concentrations as determined by minimum inhibitory concentrations may not be helpful. Assays for itraconazole are performed only in a few reference laboratories.

Methodology Bioassay, high performance liquid chromatography (HPLC)

Additional Information Serum levels as determined by bioassay are approximately 10 times the levels determined by HPLC, presumably because bioassay also detects an active metabolite. Consequently therapeutic levels vary with method. Concentrations >5 µg/mL (bioassay) were predictive of therapeutic success in invasive aspergillosis, whereas serum concentrations <1 µg/mL (bioassay) predicted therapeutic failure in cases of cryptococcal meningitis. Concentrations <0.25 µg/mL (HPLC) predicted failure to prevent aspergillosis in granulocytopenic patients. Absorption is often depressed in bone marrow transplant and in AIDS patients.

Selected Readings
Bodey GP, "Topical and Systemic Antifungal Agents," *Med Clin North Am*, 1988, 72(3):637-59.
British Society for Antimicrobial Chemotherapy Working Party, "Laboratory Monitoring of Antifungal Chemotherapy," *Lancet*, 1991, 337(8757):1577-80.
Terrell CL and Hughes CE, "Antifungal Agents Used for Deep-Seated Mycotic Infections," *Mayo Clin Proc*, 1992, 67(1):69-91.

IUD Culture *see* Actinomyces Culture, All Sites *on page 308*

I.V. Catheter Culture *see* Intravenous Line Culture *on page 464*

IVP *see* Urography *on page 567*

Ixodes dammini Identification *see* Arthropod Identification *on page 334*

Joint Fluid Culture *see* Aerobic Culture, Body Fluid *on page 310*

Joint Fluid Fungus Culture *see* Fungus Culture, Body Fluid *on page 415*

Joint Study *see* Arthrogram *on page 334*

Joint Tap *see* Arthrocentesis *on page 330*

Kahn Test *replaced by* RPR *on page 530*

Kanamycin (Kantrex®) Level *see* Amikacin Level *on page 315*

Ketoconazole Level

Synonyms Nizoral

Abstract Ketoconazole is an orally administered antifungal agent that is appropriately used for a variety of nonlife-threatening fungal infections. Determining serum levels rarely contributes significantly to patient care.

Specimen Serum

Container Red top tube

Sampling Time 2 hours after administration

Reference Range Therapeutic: 5-20 µg/mL, dependent on dose

Use Usually unnecessary. May be useful to ensure therapeutic levels if poor absorption is suspected, or in cases of therapeutic failure or relapse.

Limitations *In vitro* susceptibility testing of fungi against ketoconazole is method dependent and may not accurately predict clinical success. Consequently, monitoring levels and adjusting dosage to attain therapeutic concentrations as determined by minimum inhibitory concentrations may not be helpful. Assays for ketoconazole are performed only in a few reference laboratories.

Methodology Bioassay, high performance liquid chromatography (HPLC)

Additional Information Approximately 5% to 10% of patients receiving ketoconazole develop abnormally elevated serum transaminases, a transient and reversible state. Rarely, patients develop symptomatic hepatitis which is idiosyncratic and not dependent upon serum concentrations. Absorption is often depressed in bone marrow transplant and AIDS patients.

Selected Readings
Bodey GP, "Topical and Systemic Antifungal Agents," *Med Clin North Am*, 1988, 72(3):637-59.

British Society for Antimicrobial Chemotherapy Working Party, "Laboratory Monitoring of Antifungal Chemotherapy," *Lancet*, 1991, 337(8757):1577-80.

Terrell CL and Hughes CE, "Antifungal Agents Used for Deep-Seated Mycotic Infections," *Mayo Clin Proc*, 1992, 67(1):69-91.

Kidneys Ultrasound *see* Ultrasound, Kidneys *on page 561*

Kinyoun Stain *see* Acid-Fast Stain *on page 305*

Kirby-Bauer Susceptibility Test *see* Antimicrobial Susceptibility Testing, Aerobic and Facultatively Anaerobic Organisms *on page 323*

Kline Test *replaced by* RPR *on page 530*

Knee Arthrogram *see* Arthrogram *on page 334*

Knee, Left or Right, X-ray *see* Bone Films *on page 343*

Knees Arthritis, X-ray *see* Bone Films *on page 343*

KOH Preparation

Related Information

Fungus Culture, Skin *on page 417*
Methenamine Silver Stain *on page 487*
Periodic Acid-Schiff Stain *on page 518*
Skin Biopsy *on page 535*

Synonyms Potassium Hydroxide Preparation

Test Includes Potassium hydroxide, (KOH) hydrolysis of proteinaceous debris, cells, etc. Microscopic examination under 10x and 40x.

Patient Preparation Same as for culture of specific site

Special Instructions The laboratory should be informed of the specific source of the specimen and the clinical diagnosis.

Specimen Appropriate specimen for KOH preparation is a specimen composed mostly of keratin (hair, skin, nails).

Container Same as for culture of specific site

Collection The specimen may be divided for fungus culture and KOH preparation, mycobacteria culture and smear, and routine bacterial culture and Gram's stain only if the specimen is of adequate volume for all tests requested.

Causes for Rejection Insufficient specimen volume

Reference Range No fungus elements identified

Use Determine presence of fungi in skin, nails, or hair

Limitations Cultures are more sensitive than smears; therefore, the KOH preparation may be negative when culture is positive. The test may require overnight incubation for complete disintegration of hair, nail, or skin debris.

Methodology 10% KOH with gentle heat, alternately 20% KOH or 10% KOH and 40% dimethyl sulfoxide (DMSO)

Additional Information See the specimen selection tables provided in the listings, Fungus Culture, Skin *on page 417* and Fungus Culture, Sputum *on page 419*. For the diagnosis of keratomycosis direct examination may have a higher yield than culture because of the presence of dead organisms in the corneal tissue.

Recent reports have emphasized the changing pattern of tinea capitis, particularly the fact that infection due to *Trichophyton tonsurans* has become increasingly common. When present it causes a less discrete, more diffuse pattern of alopecia. It is negative by Wood's light examination. The "black dot," a remnant of a broken infected hair shaft, is a good source for diagnostic material which should be sought with a magnifying glass and collected with forceps. Scale and pulled hairs are also useful specimens. Diagnostic specimens should be collected before antifungal therapy is instituted. Topic steroids should not be prescribed until fungal infection is excluded.

Selected Readings

Cohn MS, "Superficial Fungal Infections. Topical and Oral Treatment of Common Types," *Postgrad Med*, 1992, 91(2):239-44, 249-52.

Gray LD and Roberts GD, "Laboratory Diagnosis of Systemic Fungal Diseases," *Infect Dis Clin North Am*, 1988, 2(4):779-803.

Hebert AA and Burton-Esterly N, "Bacterial and Candidal Cutaneous Infections in the Neonate," *Dermatol Clin*, 1986, 4(1):3-21.

Ishibashi Y, Hommura S, and Matsumoto Y, "Direct Examination vs Culture of Biopsy Specimens for the Diagnosis of Keratomycosis," *Am J Ophthalmol*, 1987, 103(5):636-40.

Stein DH, "Superficial Fungal Infections," *Pediatr Clin North Am*, 1983, 30(3):545-61.

Latex Agglutination, Bacterial Antigens, Cerebrospinal Fluid *see* Bacterial Antigens, Rapid Detection Methods *on page 335*

LE Antibodies *see* Skin Biopsy, Immunofluorescence *on page 538*

Legionella Antigen, Urine

Related Information

Legionella pneumophila Culture *on next page*

Synonyms Urine *Legionella* Antigen

Specimen Random urine

Container Sterile specimen container

Collection Early morning specimens yield highest bacterial counts from overnight incubation in the bladder, and are the best specimens. Colony count interpretation standards are based on controlled studies from first early morning collections. Forced fluids or random specimens dilute the urine and may cause reduced colony counts. Hair from perineum will contaminate the specimen. The stream from a male may be contaminated by bacteria from beneath the prepuce. Bacteria from vaginal secretions, vulva or distal urethra may contaminate. Organisms from hands or clothing might contaminate. Receptacle must be sterile.

Male: Wash your hands thoroughly with soap and water. Rinse them well and dry with a paper towel. Tear open the towelette packages so that the towels can be easily removed with one hand as they are needed. Open the urine container. Do not touch any of the inside surfaces of the container or the lid. Pull back the foreskin to completely expose the head of the penis. Wash the head of the penis thoroughly using first one towelette then the other. Discard the used towelettes into the toilet bowl. Pass a small amount of urine into the toilet bowl, then pass a sample into the container. Do not allow the container to touch the legs or the penis. Keep your fingers away from the rim and inner surface of the container. Fill the container half full. Replace the lid on the container. The urine specimen should be refrigerated within 10 minutes of collection or taken immediately to the laboratory.

Female: Wash your hands thoroughly with soap and water. Rinse them well and dry with a paper towel. Tear open the towelette packages so that the towels can be easily removed with one hand as they are needed. Open the urine container. Do not touch any of the inside surfaces of the container or the lid. Remove your undergarments and sit on the toilet seat with your legs spread widely apart. With one hand, spread your labia apart to expose the vulva. Keep this hand in place during the washing and urinating procedure. Use one towelette to wash the vulva well passing the towelette only from front to back, not back and forth. Repeat this procedure using the second towelette. Discard the used towelettes into the toilet bowl. Begin urinating into the toilet bowl then without stopping the stream, insert the container to collect the specimen. Do not allow the container to touch the legs, vulva, or clothing. Keep your fingers away from the rim and inner surface of the container. Fill the container approximately half full. Replace the lid on the container. The urine specimen should be refrigerated within 10 minutes of collection or taken immediately to the laboratory. Apply the completed patient label to the specimen cup. Most patients, with instruction, do better with privacy than an attendant can.

Catheterized specimen: Do not collect urine from the drainage bag when an indwelling catheter is in place because growth of bacteria can occur in the bag itself. Rather, clean catheter with an alcohol sponge, puncture with sterile needle, collect in sterile syringe. Catheter tips are contaminated by the urethra as they are withdrawn; do not culture them.

Storage Instructions Specimen may be refrigerated if unable to transport immediately.

Causes for Rejection Specimen received in inappropriate or unlabeled container, specimen not received on ice, contaminated specimen. If an unacceptable specimen is received, the nursing unit will be notified and another specimen requested before disposal of the original specimen.

Reference Range Negative

Use Determine the presence of *Legionella* antigen in urine

Methodology Radioimmunoassay (RIA)

Additional Information This test is sensitive and specific. However, this test should be confirmed by culture and serology for optimal chances of correct diagnosis.

Legionella **Assay** *see Legionella* DNA Probe *on next page*

Legionella DNA Probe

Synonyms DNA Probe for *Legionella*; *Legionella* Assay

Specimen Respiratory secretions, sputum, bronchial washing, pleural fluid, lung biopsy

Container Sterile container

Storage Instructions Specimen should be received in the laboratory as soon as possible.

Reference Range Negative for *Legionella*

Use Determine the presence of *Legionella* species

Limitations Inconclusive results can be obtained.

Methodology DNA probe

Additional Information Culture for *Legionella* is the confirmatory test and should be done on all specimens received for *Legionella* DNA probe assay. The sensitivity and specificity of the DNA probe test is 60% to 75% and 98%, respectively.

Legionella pneumophila **Antibodies** *see Legionella Serology on page 471*

Legionella pneumophila Culture

Related Information
Aerobic Culture, Sputum *on page 312*
Legionella Antigen, Urine *on previous page*
Legionella pneumophila Smear *on next page*

Synonyms Culture, *Legionella pneumophila*

Applies to Biopsy *Legionella* Culture; Bronchoscopic *Legionella* Culture; Pleural Fluid *Legionella* Culture; Transtracheal Aspiration *Legionella* Culture

Test Includes Culture and, frequently, direct fluorescent antibody (DFA) smear for *Legionella pneumophila*

Specimen Lung tissue, other body tissue, pleural fluid, other body fluid, transtracheal aspiration, bronchoalveolar lavage, and bronchial brushing

Container Sterile container

Collection Contamination with normal flora from skin or other body surfaces should be avoided.

Turnaround Time Reports on specimens from which *Legionella* has been isolated require approximately 2-5 days.

Reference Range No growth

Use Isolate and identify *Legionella pneumophila*

Limitations Sputum (expectorated), bronchial aspirates, and other specimens having normal flora are subject to bacterial overgrowth and are not as desirable as transtracheal aspirates, pleural fluid, and biopsy material for culture. Sensitivity of cultures is relatively low (50% to 80%); however specificity is 100%. A direct fluorescent antibody smear without culture can be performed, but DFA alone is not recommended. Cross reactions with *B. fragilis*, *Pseudomonas fluorescens*, and other species occur. Newer approaches utilizing monoclonal antibodies have enhanced the yield of fluorescent procedures.

Methodology Culture on selective and nonselective media (buffered charcoal yeast extract)

Additional Information Acute and convalescent sera for *Legionella* antibodies should also be considered to increase the chance of documenting the diagnosis. A fourfold rise to a titer of 1:128 is a diagnostic standard criterion. Seroconversion may be detected in many patients in the first weeks. Seroconversion 0-7 days after onset, 16%; 0-14 days, 52%; 0-21 days, 66%; 0-28 days, 71%. Twenty-five percent of patients may not have diagnostic titers. Methods to detect *Legionella* antigens in urine include radioimmunoassay, enzyme immunoassay, and latex agglutination. Sensitivity of these methods can be up to 80% under ideal conditions. Consult the laboratory regarding availability and selection of the most appropriate method. Nosocomial infections have been recognized with reservoirs, water distribution systems, cooling systems, and hot water systems of hospitals being reported. Twenty species in the Legionellaceae family of bacteria have been discovered since *Legionella pneumophila* was first recognized. Thirteen species have been implicated as causes of human pneumonia. See tables on next page.

(Continued)

Legionella pneumophila Culture *(Continued)*

Infections Caused by *Legionella*

Culture proven
Pneumonia
Empyema
Sinusitis
Prosthetic valve endocarditis
Wound infection
Associated with pneumonia
    Bowel abscesses
    Brain abscesses
    Empyema
    Lung abscesses
    Myocarditis
    Pericarditis
    Peritonitis
    Renal abscesses/pyelonephritis
    Vascular graft infections
Strong seroepidemiological evidence
Pontiac fever
Weak seroepidemiological evidence
Encephalopathy without pneumonia
Myocarditis without pneumonia
Pericarditis without pneumonia

From Edelstein PH, "Laboratory Diagnosis of Infections Caused by *Legionella*," *Eur J Clin Microbiol*, 1987, 6:4-10, with permission.

Clinical Clues to the Diagnosis of Legionnaires' Disease

- Gram's stain of respiratory secretions reveals numerous neutrophils, but few organisms
- Presence of hyponatremia (serum sodium ≤130 mmol/L)
- Failure to respond to β-lactam and aminoglycoside antibiotics
- Occurrence in hospital where potable water system is known to be contaminated with *Legionella*
- History of smoking and alcohol use
- Pleuritic chest pain
- Fever malaise, myalgia, headache

From Harrison TG and Taylor AG, "Timing of Seroconversion in Legionnaires' Disease," *Lancet*, Oct 1988, 795, with permission.

Selected Readings

Fang GD, Yu VL, and Vickers RM, "Disease Due to the Legionellaceae (Other Than *Legionella pneumophila*). Historical, Microbiological, Clinical, and Epidemiological Review," *Medicine (Baltimore)*, 1989, 68(Suppl 2):116-32.

Hart CA and Makin T, "*Legionella* in Hospitals: A Review," *J Hosp Infect*, 1991, 18(Suppl A):481-9.

Hoge CW and Brieman RF, "Advances in the Epidemiology and Control of *Legionella* Infections," *Epidemiol Rev*, 1991, 13:329-40.

Nguyen ML and Yu VL, "*Legionella* Infection," *Clin Chest Med*, 1991, 12(2):257-68.

Rodgers FG, "New Perspectives on *Legionella* Infections," *Infect Med*, 1994, 11(2):137, 141-7.

Legionella pneumophila Smear

Related Information

Legionella pneumophila Culture *on previous page*

Legionella Serology *on next page*

Synonyms Direct Fluorescent Antibody Smear for *Legionella pneumophila*; FA Smear for *Legionella pneumophila*

Test Includes Direct fluorescent antibody (DFA) microscopic examination of specimen smear

Specimen Lung tissue, other body tissue, pleural fluid, other body fluid, transtracheal aspirate, sputum, bronchial washing

Container Sterile container

Collection Contamination with normal flora from skin or other body surfaces should be avoided

Causes for Rejection Saliva sent rather than sputum specimen

Reference Range No *Legionella pneumophila* seen in direct FA microscopic examination

Use Determine the presence of *Legionella pneumophila* organisms in direct FA smear of specimen, providing rapid diagnosis

Limitations Staining for several serogroups may be necessary. Most methods include antibodies only to *L. pneumophilia* and not to other *Legionella* species.

Methodology Direct fluorescent antibody (DFA)

Additional Information Community acquired and nosocomial infections caused by multiple serogroups of *Legionella* are increasingly recognized. Although culture is now possible on buffered charcoal yeast extract agar, the demonstration of organisms in tissue or brushings is the fastest way to make the diagnosis. It also has the advantage of applicability to specimens contaminated with other bacteria. Development of monoclonal antibodies have increased sensitivity and specificity. False-positive reaction has been reported in a case of pleuropulmonary tularemia and in cases of *Campylobacter* infection. A combination of both culture and DFA is recommended.

Selected Readings

Andersen LP and Bangsborg J, "Crossreactions Between *Legionella* and *Campylobacter* Spp," *Lancet*, 1992, 340(8813):245.

Edelstein PH, Beer KB, Sturge JC, et al, "Clinical Utility of a Monoclonal Direct Fluorescent Reagent Specific for *Legionella pneumophila*: Comparative Study With Other Reagents," *J Clin Microbiol*, 1985, 22(3):419-21.

Friedman H, Wider R, and Klein T, "Immunodiagnostic Assays for Legionellosis," *Lab Management*, 1983, 21:19-23.

Hart CA and Makin T, "*Legionella* in Hospitals: A Review," *J Hosp Infect*, 1991, 18(Suppl A):481-9.

Hicklin MD, Thomason BM, Chandler FW, et al, "Pathogenesis of Acute Legionnaires' Disease Pneumonia." *Am J Clin Pathol*, 1980, 73(4):480-7.

Roy TM, Fleming D, and Anderson WH, "Tularemic Pneumonia Mimicking Legionnaires' Disease With False-Positive Direct Fluorescent Antibody Stains for *Legionella*," *South Med J*, 1989, 82(11):1429-31.

Legionella Serology

Related Information

Legionella pneumophila Smear *on previous page*

Synonyms *Legionella pneumophila* Antibodies; Legionnaires' Disease Antibodies

Specimen Serum

Container Red top tube

Collection A convalescent sample should be obtained 10-14 days after acute sample

Reference Range Negative. Less than a fourfold change in titer between acute and convalescent samples. Less than 1:256 in a single sample.

Use Detect antibody to *Legionella pneumophila*; support the clinical diagnosis of Legionnaires' disease

Limitations Testing for multiple serogroups may be necessary

Methodology Indirect fluorescent antibody assay using serogroup 1: Philadelphia, Knoxville, serogroup 2: Togus, serogroup 3: Los Angeles, serogroup 4: Bloomington. A polyvalent antigen which includes serogroup 1-6 may be utilized. IgG and IgM titers may be provided. Latex agglutination may be used in some laboratories.

Additional Information A fourfold rise in titer exceeding a titer of 1:128 from the acute to convalescent phase provides evidence of recent infection. A single titer ≥1:256 is evidence of infection at an undetermined time. However, due to the relatively high prevalence of antibodies to *Legionella pneumophila*, acute and convalescent titers are preferred to a single sample. Demonstration of a high titer in the proper clinical setting may allow timely institution of specific treatment, and may eliminate the need for an invasive procedure to obtain a specimen for culture or direct immunofluorescence. Demonstration of IgM antibody to serogroup I may allow rapid diagnosis. Recent availability of a latex agglutination test with 98.3% specificity and 97.6% sensitivity is well suited as a screening test. Serologic study is also valuable in evaluation of epidemic disease.

Selected Readings

Edelstein PH, "Detection of Antibodies to *Legionella*," *Manual of Clinical Laboratory Immunology*, 4th ed, Rose NR, de Macario EC, Fahey JL, et al, eds, Washington, DC: American Society for Microbiology, 1992, 459-66.

Holliday MG, "Use of Latex Agglutination Technique for Detecting *Legionella pneumophila* (Serogroup I) Antibodies," *J Clin Pathol*, 1990, 43(10):860-2.

(Continued)

Legionella Serology *(Continued)*

Rodgers FG, "New Perspectives on *Legionella* Infections," *Infect Med*, 1994, 11(2):137, 141-7.

Legionnaires' Disease Antibodies *see Legionella* Serology *on previous page*

Leptospira, Blood Culture *see Leptospira* Culture *on this page*

Leptospira Culture

Related Information

Darkfield Examination, Leptospirosis *on page 393*

Leptospira Serology *on this page*

Synonyms Culture for *Leptospira*

Applies to Blood Culture, *Leptospira*; *Leptospira*, Blood Culture

Patient Preparation Urine specimen: Thoroughly instruct patient in the proper collection technique for a midvoid urine specimen; avoid contamination with skin flora. See also Urine Culture, Clean Catch *on page 565* and Blood Culture, Aerobic and Anaerobic *on page 337* for detailed instructions.

Special Instructions The laboratory should be informed of the specific request for *Leptospira* culture, collection time, date, specific site of specimen, age of patient, current antibiotic therapy, date of onset of illness, and clinical diagnosis. Urine must be alkaline; *Leptospira* do not survive in acid urine. Repeated cultures may be required.

Specimen Urine, indicate midvoid, catheter or suprapubic puncture specimen; blood and cerebrospinal fluid may also be cultured

Container Sterile container or tube

Collection Specimen should be transported to laboratory within 1 hour of collection. For midvoid urine culture, patient should be instructed to clean skin thoroughly, do not collect first portion of stream, collect midportion of stream, and do not collect final portion of stream. Catheter or suprapubic puncture specimen may also be used.

Causes for Rejection Specimens delayed in transit to the laboratory have less than optimal yield.

Turnaround Time 4-8 weeks. Consult the laboratory prior to the collection of the specimen, so that appropriate processing of the specimen can be arranged.

Reference Range No *Leptospira* isolated

Use Confirm the clinical diagnosis of leptospirosis

Limitations Specimen will be cultured for *Leptospira*; other organisms may not be identified

Contraindications Leptospiremia occurs during the septicemic acute phase of infection. This phase last 4-7 days after which organisms are not recoverable from blood. Cultures of blood should **not** be ordered after the first week of illness.

Methodology Urine or blood is inoculated onto specially prepared media containing rabbit serum or albumin and fatty acids. Incubation is for 4-6 weeks in the dark at 28°C to 29°C. Cultures are examined with darkfield or phase microscopy at weekly intervals; growth occurs 1-3 cm below the surface.

Additional Information Leptospirosis in humans is usually associated with occupational exposure. Veterinarians, dairymen, swineherds, abattoir workers, miners, fish and poultry processors and those who work in a rat-infested environment are at increased risk. During the first week of disease, the most reliable means of detecting leptospires is by direct culturing of blood or spinal fluid on appropriate media. **Urine does not become positive for *Leptospira* until the second week of disease and then can remain positive for several months. Concentration of *Leptospira* in human urine is low and shedding may be intermittent. Therefore, repeated isolation attempts should be made. Serology (acute and early convalescent) is recommended. Darkfield examination yields many false-positives.**

Selected Readings

Sperber SJ and Schleupner CJ, "Leptospirosis: A Forgotten Cause of Aseptic Meningitis and Multisystem Febrile Illness," *South Med J*, 1989, 82(10):1285-8.

Leptospira Serology

Related Information

Darkfield Examination, Leptospirosis *on page 393*

Leptospira Culture *on this page*

Test Includes Testing of patient's serum for antibodies against *Leptospira biflexa* serovar *L. patoc*, and the following serovars of *Leptospira interrogans*: *L. copenhageni*, *L. canicola*, *L. pomona*, *L. autumnalis*, *L. grippotyphosa*, *L. wolffi*, and *L. djatzi*. Supplemental testing may be needed against serovars: *L. poi*, *L. castellonis*, *L. pyrogenes*, *L. borincana*, *L. szwajizak*, *L. bratislava*, *L. tarassovi*, *L. shermani*, *L. panama*, *L. celledoni*, *L. djasiman*, *L. cynopteri*, and *L. louisiana*.

Specimen Serum

Container Red top tube

Collection Acute and convalescent sera drawn 10-14 days apart are suggested

Causes for Rejection Inadequate labeling, excessive hemolysis, chylous serum or gross contamination of the specimen

Reference Range Negative. A fourfold increase in titer is diagnostic of infection.

Use Support the diagnosis of leptospirosis

Limitations The antigens used in the test are the ones most commonly causing disease, but there are many other serovars which might not be detected. To optimize yield, a battery of antigens are used.

Methodology Microscopic agglutination test, macroagglutination, complement fixation, hemagglutination, enzyme linked immunosorbent assay

Additional Information Leptospirosis is an acute febrile illness caused primarily by *Leptospira interrogans*, a large spirochete with over 180 serologic variants. Patients with extensive animal contact, either in the wild or with carcasses or excrement, are particularly at risk.

Although leptospires can be cultured from blood or urine during the first week of illness, this interval is often missed, and diagnosis must be based on the demonstration of rising antibody titers. Antibody appears at the end of the first week of illness and peaks at 3-4 weeks, after which it slowly disappears.

There has been an association between patients with leptospirosis and anticardiolipin antibodies which may induce vascular endothelial injury in severe cases.

Selected Readings
Ribeiro MA, Sakata EE, Silva MV, et al, "Antigens Involved in the Human Antibody Response to Natural Infections With *Leptospira interrogans serovar copenhageni*," *J Trop Med Hyg*, 1992, 95(4):239-45.

Rugman FP, Pinn G, Palmer MF, et al, "Anticardiolipin Antibodies in Leptospirosis," *J Clin Pathol*, 1991, 44(6):517-9.

Leptospirosis, Darkfield Examination see Darkfield Examination, Leptospirosis on page 393

Lesion Culture see Wound Culture on page 577

Leukocyte Esterase, Urine

Related Information
Nitrite, Urine on page 503

Synonyms Bacteria Screen, Urine; Esterase, Leukocyte, Urine

Test Includes Screening of urine for leukocyte esterase activity by dipstick; frequently a part of urinalysis

Abstract A rapid indirect test for detection of bacteriuria. It indicates presence of esterase from intact or lysed neutrophils.

Specimen Random clean catch urine; preferably midstream clean-catch collection

Container Plastic urine container

Storage Instructions If the specimen cannot be processed within 2 hours it should be refrigerated.

Causes for Rejection Improper labeling, specimen not refrigerated

Reference Range Negative

Use Detect leukocytes in urine. Leukocyte esterase indicates the presence of either intact or lysed white blood cells and therefore can be positive when WBCs are not found on microscopic examination. The lysis of leukocytes that occurs when urine is allowed to stand intensifies the color reaction from release of esterase.

Limitations Cephalexin; cephalothin; tetracycline; large amounts of oxalic acid (eg, iced tea drinkers); high glucose and high specific gravity may decrease or suppress positive results. Albumin and ascorbic acid inhibit the method. Tetracycline may cause decreased reactivity or false-negatives. Neutropenia can cause false-negative results.

(Continued)

Leukocyte Esterase, Urine (Continued)

Leukocyte esterase, even combined with nitrite, should not replace microscopy and culture in symptomatic patients. Urine culture is indicated for subjects with symptoms of urinary tract infection. False-positive results from trichomonads have been controversial; however, false-positives may occur in specimens contaminated with vaginal secretions. Leukocyte esterase is unacceptable as a screen unless combined at least with nitrite testing.

Methodology Indoxyl is released by leukocyte esterase if present in the urine specimen. The substrate on the strip is indoxyl carbonic acid ester. Indoxyl is oxidized by atmospheric oxygen to indigo blue. The reaction time is 1 minute, but high sensitivity requires interpretation 5 minutes after immersion in the sample.

Additional Information Some institutions now perform microscopic urinalysis only on specific request or on the observation of an abnormal macroscopic finding. The principal advantage of the method is the ability to identify the presence of leukocyte esterase in dilute urine specimens and in specimens which have been subject to standing with lysis of the white cells. When combined with the nitrite test it provides sensitivity for both tests of up to 92% and specificity of 95%, respectively, either test abnormal. When false-negatives occur they are usually due to gram-positive organism bacteriuria. Some laboratories have established a screening protocol in which culture is only performed if screening with leukocyte esterase or nitrate is positive. Dipstick screening has been compared to Gram's stains of unspun urine and to urine sediment microscopy and culture.

Leukocyte esterase has been used for detection of sexually transmitted disease particularly in males.

Selected Readings

High SR, Rowe JA, and Maksem JA, "Macroscopic Physiochemical Testing for Screening Urinalysis," *Lab Med*, 1988, 19:174-6.

Leukocyte Scintigraphy see Indium Leukocyte Scan on page 461

Lice Identification see Arthropod Identification on page 334

Liver Biopsy

Related Information

Histopathology on page 448

Synonyms Blind Liver Biopsy; Needle Biopsy of the Liver; Percutaneous Liver Biopsy

Applies to Percutaneous Needle Aspiration Biopsy Under Fluoroscopic, CT, or Ultrasound Guidance; Transjugular Needle Biopsy of the Liver

Test Includes Percutaneous biopsy of liver parenchyma in a "blind" fashion (ie, not under radiologic guidance). This is carried out at the bedside under local anesthesia. A specialized, thin-bore needle is advanced between the ribs overlying the region of hepatic dullness. Several 2 cm cores of deep liver tissue are excised. Fresh specimens may be sent for gross pathologic inspection, routine light microscopy, special stains for liver storage diseases, transmission and immune electron microscopy, immunohistochemistry (using monoclonal antibodies), DNA hybridization studies, and microbiologic culture. Liver biopsy is a valuable and time-honored means of diagnosing diffuse liver parenchymal disease as well as disseminated focal disease.

Patient Preparation Procedures and risks of the procedure are explained and consent is obtained. Formal consultation with gastroenterology staff is usually required. Procedure entails overnight hospitalization in most cases but some patients may be candidates for a "same day" outpatient biopsy. This latter group is in good general health, not jaundiced, and displays no signs of liver failure (ascites, encephalopathy). They need to stay within several minutes of the hospital for 1-2 days postbiopsy and must have supervision from family or friends. Scheduling arrangements for both in-hospital and outpatient liver biopsies are handled by gastroenterology team. All aspirin products and nonsteroidal agents must be discontinued at least 5 days beforehand. If taking oral anticoagulants (Coumadin®), hospitalization is required to convert to heparin therapy before biopsy. Patient is NPO after midnight the evening prior. Daily medications may be taken on the day of procedure pending physician approval. In some hospitals, patient drinks 1-2 glasses of milk in the early AM on procedure day to empty the gallbladder. Screening laboratory studies ordered 24-48 hours in advance commonly include CBC, PT/PTT, BUN, bleeding time, and type and crossmatch for possible transfusion. Electrolytes and liver function tests are optional. If pneumonia or pleural effusion suspected on examination, PA and lateral chest x-ray is obtained. Premedication with meperidine and/or diazepam may be administered at physician discretion. This is not routine in some centers due to possible toxicity.

Aftercare Protocols are individualized for each hospital. In general, patient is monitored in a recovery area with frequent vital signs postbiopsy. If no complications are apparent, patient is transferred back to hospital room by cart. Strict bedrest is enforced for 24 hours; for the first 2 hours patient is positioned on his right side. After 5 hours, patient may be allowed to sit up. Vitals (blood pressure, pulse) are checked every 15-30 minutes for 2 hours, every 30 minutes for the next 2 hours, and then every hour for 8 hours. Following this, vitals every 4 hours are permissible. Physician should be immediately notified if hypotension, tachycardia, fever, or uncontrolled pain occurs. Diet is restricted to clear liquids for several hours, then full liquids as tolerated. Acetaminophen is usually sufficient for pain control. Some physicians recheck hematocrit 24 hours after procedure before approving hospital discharge.

Special Instructions In the appropriate high-risk patient, antibiotic prophylaxis for infective endocarditis may be considered. Little data exists regarding the risk of bacteremia, however, much less endocarditis.

Complications Based on several large series, serious morbidity has been estimated at 0.1% to 0.2%. Fatality rates have ranged from 0% to 0.17%, both figures being derived from studies involving >20,000 biopsies each. The more commonly seen complications are:

- pain - the most common adverse event, noted in ≤50% of cases. Usually it is confined to the right shoulder, probably referred pain from diaphragmatic pleura. Analgesia is required in approximately 20% of patients with acetaminophen sufficient in most cases. Symptoms resolve in 1-2 days.
- hemorrhage - minor episodes are common. Self-limited oozing from the puncture site may persist for approximately 1 minute, but with loss of only 5-10 mL blood. Significant hemorrhage is less frequent but is the most common cause of death from liver biopsy. Several series have estimated an incidence of approximately 0.2%, but Sherlock (1984) reported 40 patients out of 6379 required transfusion for intraperitoneal bleeding. She felt these statistics may even underestimate the incidence since those with severe coagulopathies were excluded. Bleeding usually results from a tear of a distended portal or hepatic vein. Specific sites include the abdominal cavity (hemoperitoneum), liver capsule (capsular hematoma), liver parenchyma (intrahepatic hematoma), or biliary tree (hemobilia). Postulated risk factors are coagulopathy, amyloid liver, hepatocellular injury, hemangioma, and vascularized tumor. However, bleeding may be massive when no risk factors are present. Not all episodes require surgery. In a study 4 of 7532 patients needed surgical intervention while 12 others with severe hemorrhage were transfused and observed.
- bile leakage with peritonitis - associated with severe obstruction of the larger bile ducts. This is felt to result from laceration of a small, distended duct or from puncture of the gallbladder. With the widespread use of noninvasive imaging, the size of the bile ducts is known prebiopsy and the complication rate has declined.
- laceration of internal organs and viscera - right kidney, gallbladder, colon, pancreas, and others
- others: right-sided pneumothorax, arteriovenous fistula - 5.4% of all biopsies, drug toxicity

Equipment Several biopsy needles are available.

- Menghini needle - 1.9 mm diameter steel shaft with sharpened beveled tip and syringe; specimen is obtained using suction/aspiration into a 10 mL syringe. Requires only 1 second within the liver ("1-second technique") and patient need not hold his breath. Disadvantages are small samples and fragmentation of biopsy specimens.
- "Trucut" needle - disposable 2.05 mm diameter needle designed to cut out cores of tissue. Specimens are less fragmented, even in the cirrhotic liver, and thus a high success rate. However, dwell time in liver is longer (5-10 seconds), patient must cooperate more, and several steps are necessary.
- Vim-Silverman needle - sheath with inner cutting blade (similar to a "punch" biopsy). Trucut needle is a modernized Vim-Silverman.

(Continued)

Liver Biopsy *(Continued)*

Technique Patient lies supine in bed with right hand behind his head. Liver margins are estimated by percussion. Two approaches are popular, transthoracic (intercostal) or subcostal (anterior). With the former, biopsy site is identified along the midaxillary line in the center of hepatic dullness, usually the eighth or ninth intercostal space. This approach avoids other abdominal organs but always penetrates the pleura. With the subcostal approach, the biopsy site lies below the bottom rib anteriorly, and is used when a liver mass is easily palpable below the right costal margin. The risk of visceral laceration is higher and this approach is infrequently used; fine needle aspiration under CT guidance has become more popular. A wide area is prepped and draped in sterile fashion with operators in gowns, gloves, and masks. The skin is anesthetized with 1% lidocaine, then deeper structures are infiltrated - subcutaneous tissue, intercostal muscles, and diaphragm. Some operators make a small superficial incision with a No 11 blade at the needle entry site to facilitate needle insertion. Techniques differ with the type of biopsy needle selected. In general, the biopsy needle is advanced as far as the diaphragm (depth estimated by a finder needle). If a Menghini needle is used, suction is applied to the syringe, the needle is pushed rapidly through the pleura and into the liver parenchyma. A 2.5 cm core of liver is aspirated and needle withdrawn, all within 1 second. If other needles are used, patient may need to hold his breath at end expiration to decrease the risk of pneumothorax. Several passes of the biopsy needle are performed to minimize sampling bias.

Specimen At least 2-3 liver cores, each >2 cm in length. Initial specimen processing and transportation handled by gastroenterology team. A typical protocol would be as follows:

- tissue fixation - for light microscopy, specimen is routinely fixed in 10% buffered formalin within 1 minute. For transmission electron microscopy, 1 mm cubes of specimen are fixed immediately in glutaraldehyde with further processing in Pathology Laboratory.
- routine tissue stains including: H & E - general liver histology stain; reticulin stain - for connective tissue, especially cirrhosis, fibrosis, bridging necrosis; trichrome - fibrosis; iron stain - useful for hemosiderosis, hemochromatosis, bile pigments; diastase PAS stain - useful for alpha$_1$-antitrypsin globules, bile ducts, iron; orcein - for hepatitis B surface antigen (if present, fine granular brown material stains in hepatocytes). Also for copper-binding protein in Wilson's disease.
- cytologic preparation - fluid from aspirating syringe may be smeared on clean microscope slide, fixed, and sent to Cytology Laboratory
- microbiological culture - specimen sent without fixative in sterile container. Special stains (AFB, KOH, etc) and cultures (tuberculosis, viral, *Brucella*, parasites, fungi) as needed
- optional special stains, ie, congo red for amyloidosis, immunohistochemistry

Use Candidates for liver biopsy must be carefully selected. This procedure, by nature, is invasive and histologic findings may often be reported as "consistent with" a particular disease (without being pathognomonic) or simply "nondiagnostic". In most cases, noninvasive imaging studies such as CT scan or ultrasound are now obtained first. With these considerations in mind, indications for liver biopsy include:

- suspected cases of liver cirrhosis, in order to confirm the diagnosis pathologically; establish etiology if possible (alcohol, alpha$_1$-antitrypsin deficiency, primary biliary cirrhosis, Wilson's disease, hemochromatosis, etc); assess and stage level of activity; assess complications
- chronic hepatitis, with or without cirrhosis, to identify cases of chronic activity hepatitis (liver biopsy mandatory for diagnosis) and differentiate this entity from chronic persistent hepatitis and lobular hepatitis
- suspected liver disease in the known alcoholic patient, to confirm alcoholic liver disease, exclude alternative causes of liver disease (which may be present in ≤20% of cases), stage and assess disease activity
- diagnosis of hepatoma or metastatic neoplasms
- suspected multisystem disease with liver involvement, where traditional diagnostic techniques have not been fruitful (eg, sarcoidosis, amyloidosis, tuberculosis, glycogen storage disease)
- staging of lymphoma
- unexplained hepatomegaly

- cholestasis of unknown etiology, where prior studies for biliary obstruction are negative
- persistently elevated liver enzyme tests
- selected cases of fever of unknown origin
- selected cases of hepatitis of unknown etiology, in order to differentiate viral from drug-induced etiologies (not always possible) or to assess complications, such as cholestasis
- evaluation of response to treatment

Liver biopsy is less useful in:

- acute hepatitis A or B infection, unless the diagnosis is in question
- extrahepatic biliary obstruction, where percutaneous transhepatic cholangiography and ERCP are considered first-line procedures
- fluid-filled liver cysts detected on ultrasound or CT scan, probably more amenable to guided thin needle aspiration first

Contraindications Mahal et al (1979) noted that failure to heed accepted contraindications led directly to 22 bleeding episodes in 3800 percutaneous liver biopsies. Contraindications include:

- impaired hemostasis, accepted as prothrombin time more than 3 seconds over control, PTT more than 20 seconds over control, thrombocytopenia, and markedly prolonged bleeding time
- severe anemia (Hgb <9.5 g/dL)
- local infection near needle entry site, such as right sided pleural effusion or empyema, right lower lobe pneumonia, local cellulitis, infected ascites or peritonitis
- tense ascites (low yield technically, risk of leakage)
- high-grade extrahepatic biliary obstruction with jaundice (increased risk of bile peritonitis)
- septic cholangitis
- possible hemangioma
- possible echinococcal (hydatid) cyst
- lack of compatible blood for transfusion
- uncooperative patient

Selected Readings

Lefkowitch JH, "Pathologic Diagnosis of Liver Disease," *Hepatology: A Textbook of Liver Disease*, 2nd ed, Chapter 29, Zakim D and Boyer TD, eds, Philadelphia, PA: WB Saunders Co, 1990, 711-32.

Mahal AS, Knauer CM, and Gregory PB, "Bleeding After Liver Biopsy," *West J Med*, 1981, 134(1):11-4.

Perrault J, McGill DB, Ott BJ, et al, "Liver Biopsy: Complications in 1000 Inpatients and Outpatients," *Gastroenterology*, 1978, 78(1):103-6.

Schaffner F, "Needle Biopsy of the Liver," *Bockus Gastroenterology*, 4th ed, Chapter 49, Berk JE, ed, Philadelphia, PA: WB Saunders Co, 1985, 657-66.

Sherlock S, Dick R, and van Leeuwen DJ, "Liver Biopsy Today. The Royal Free Hospital Experience," *J Hepatol*, 1984, 1(1):75-85.

Sherlock S, "Needle Biopsy of the Liver," *Diseases of the Liver and Biliary System*, 7th ed, Chapter 3, Oxford, England: Blackwell Scientific Publications, 1985, 28-37.

Van Ness MM and Diehl AM, "Is Liver Biopsy Useful in the Evaluation of Patients With Chronically Elevated Liver Enzymes?" *Ann Intern Med*, 1989, 111(6):473-8.

Lower Respiratory Fungus Culture *see* Fungus Culture, Bronchial Aspirate *on page 416*

Lower Respiratory Mycobacteria Culture *see* Mycobacteria Culture, Sputum *on page 495*

LP *see* Lumbar Puncture *on this page*

Lumbar Puncture

Synonyms Cerebrospinal Fluid Tap; LP; Spinal Tap

Test Includes Collection of cerebrospinal fluid (CSF) for chemical, cellular, and microbiological analysis. Performed as a bedside procedure under local anesthesia, a needle is passed into the L4-L5 vertebral interspace and subarachnoid fluid is withdrawn.

Patient Preparation Procedure and risks are explained and consent is obtained. If patient is confused or obtunded, obtain consent from guardians. If a coagulopathy is suspected, obtain platelet count and prothrombin/partial thromboplastin time if time permits. No intravenous pain medications such as meperidine are required routinely. Likewise, sedatives or anxiolytics may serve to confuse later assessments of mental status.
(Continued)

Lumbar Puncture *(Continued)*

Aftercare Patient should be kept at strict bedrest for a minimum of 3 hours postprocedure to minimize post-LP headache. Regarding the optimal patient positioning, opinions vary. Some authors recommend the prone position post-LP based on a study involving >1000 subjects which demonstrated a 0.5% incidence of headache in patients kept prone versus 36.5% in the supine group. The frequency of obtaining vital signs and neurologic checks after the procedure should be based on the patient's overall status. Nursing staff should be familiar with potential LP complications, especially acute deteriorations in mental status (possible tonsillar herniation), sensory deficits, leg muscle weakness, and bladder and bowel incontinence (possible expanding spinal subdural hematoma). If no complications arise, activity may later be upgraded to *ad lib* as tolerated, with physician's approval.

Complications Although a wide range of complications has been reported, LP should generally be considered a safe procedure. The most common complication is "spinal headache" with an estimated incidence of 10% to 25%. This may be minimized by using a small gauge spinal needle and placing the patient in the prone position after the procedure. Another common complication is local bleeding, the "traumatic tap," which results from needle rupture of venous plexuses surrounding the spinal sack. Incidence may be as high as 20%. As long as no coagulation defect exists, the traumatic tap is clinically insignificant and rarely leads to spinal hematoma. Immediate painful paresthesias due to nerve root irritation is another common complication (≤13%), but usually resolves upon repositioning the spinal needle. Rare complications (<1%) include persistent pain or leg paresthesias; spinal epidural, subdural or subarachnoid hematomas; arachnoiditis from tracking in povidone-iodine on the needle; local infection (epidural or subdural empyema); transient cranial nerve palsies (especially CN VI when large volumes of CSF removed); rupture of nucleus pulposus; delayed formation of intraspinal epidermoid tumors (when stylet is not used); and vagal cardiac arrest. Note that the use of anticoagulants or presence of a coagulopathy significantly increases the risk of spinal hematoma formation (≤7%). Tonsillar herniation is an infrequent but potentially lethal complication of LP which occurs in patients with increased intracranial pressure. The exact incidence is not clear. In one series of patients with papilledema and increased intracranial pressure from a variety of causes, tonsillar herniation occurred after LP in <1.2% of cases. A particularly high risk group appears to be the patient with brain abscess or subdural empyema, with an estimated 10% to 20% incidence of LP-induced herniation and death. The herniation risk in patients with brain tumor is not known, although one study (which predated head CT scans) reported neurologic deterioration following LP in only 1 of 400 brain tumor cases. In general, due to incomplete data, a variety of clinical approaches have been adopted to avoid this fatal complication (see Additional Information).

Equipment Commercial LP trays are available. Common items include iodine, alcohol pads, sterile gloves and drapes, local anesthesia (usually 1% lidocaine) with appropriate needles and syringes, four sterile collecting tubes, 3-way stopcock with connecting tubing, manometer, and spinal needle with stylette. In general, a small bore spinal needle should be used, such as a 25-gauge, due to a lower incidence of spinal headache compared with a 20- or 22-gauge needle.

Technique In all cases, perform a careful fundoscopic and neurologic exam to rule out papilledema or a focal neurologic deficit. LP is then performed in one of two ways. In the standard method, patient is placed on a firm surface in the lateral recumbent position, curled with knees down in towards the chest and neck maximally flexed. The lumbar region should be close to the edge of the bed, with the plane of the back and shoulders as perpendicular to the bed as possible. Proper positioning is by far the most important step to ensure success and usually requires one or more assistants. The L4-L5 interspace is identified by drawing an imaginary line between the two posterior iliac crests. This area is cleaned, prepped, and draped. Skin and deeper subcutaneous tissues are infiltrated with lidocaine. The spinal needle with stylette is then passed into the L4-L5 interspace along the midline, bevel upwards. The needle is angled slightly cephalad along an imaginary line between the site of entry and the umbilicus. As the needle is advanced, the stylette should be frequently withdrawn and replaced every 1-2 mm in order to identify the first drop of CSF (and avoid overpenetration). Once CSF fluid is seen in the needle hub, the manometer is immediately attached to the needle via connecting tubing. Opening pressure should be measured promptly (do not wait more than 1 minute) with the patient's legs and hips extended. If the opening pressure is elevated (>180 mm CSF), try to eliminate factors that may cause false elevations. Instruct patient to straighten his legs, breathe evenly, avoid Valsalva maneuvers, and relax his abdominal muscles. If the opening pressure remains markedly elevated, close the 3-way stopcock, collect only the CSF already in the manometer, disconnect all the tubing, reinsert stylette, and consider neurosurgical consultation. If opening pressure is normal, CSF is then collected in tubes 1-4 in sequence. Manometer is reconnected afterwards and a closing pressure recorded. Stylette is replaced and both needle and stylette removed together. Pressure is held over the puncture site. An alternate approach may be needed in the patient whose vertebral landmarks are difficult to palpate. Initially, patient is placed in a seated position with neck and spine maximally flexed, arms resting on a bedside table. The L4-L5 interspace is identified as before and the remainder of the procedure is identical. This may be used with the obese patient or the patient with ankylosing spondylitis or severe scoliosis. Variations of this procedure have been described including: a lateral approach through the paravertebral muscles, the "hanging drop" technique used by anesthesiologists for identifying entry into the subdural space, and suboccipital puncture of the cisterna magna. These techniques are not necessary in the majority of cases.

Data Acquired Estimation of spinal fluid pressure as described. CSF fluid analytic tests are ordered based on clinical suspicion. Routine tests include cell count and CSF glucose level. Optional tests (not all samples): protein, VDRL, bacterial antigen detection battery, fungal antigens (such as *Cryptococcus*), culture (bacterial, fungal, viral, tuberculous), India ink preparation for *Cryptococcus*, infectious antibody titers, Gram's stain, acid-fast bacilli smear, and cytology. Specialized tests include oligoclonal bands and myelin basic protein (for multiple sclerosis). The interested reader should refer to the *Laboratory Test Handbook* for further details.

Specimen 10-12 mL maximum removed from the adult. Smaller volumes are sufficient for most routine tests (confirm with laboratory).

Container Sterile tubes, numbered 1 to 4

Collection Tube 1: CSF protein and glucose; tube 2: cell count and differential; tube 3: Gram's stain and cultures; tube 4: save for optional studies

Storage Instructions Specimen should be sent to laboratory immediately, preferably hand carried by physician.

Normal Findings (Adults) opening pressure: 80-180 mm of CSF in lateral recumbent position, somewhat higher in sitting position. Respiratory variation of 5-10 mm normal. Clarity: normally very clear. CSF glucose: 60% to 70% of blood glucose. This estimation does not hold for blood glucose levels >300 mg/dL where CSF glucose empirically fails to rise. CSF protein: 15-55 mg/dL. CSF cell count and differential: 0-5 mononuclear white blood cells/mm^3 (lymphocytes and monocytes). The presence of even 1 or 2 polymorphonuclear cells (PMNs) is abnormal. Red blood cells: 0. Gram's stain and culture: negative.

Critical Values Interpretation of CSF findings have been reviewed in detail elsewhere. As a rule, interpretation of abnormal CSF values must always be made in close conjunction with the individual patient's clinical presentation. Considerable overlap exists among the "classic" CSF patterns which are meant to characterize different disease entities. No constellation of CSF findings is entirely specific for a given disease. LP has its greatest value in the diagnosis of bacterial meningitis. A classic CSF "purulent profile" has been described for bacterial meningitis, characterized by elevated WBCs in CSF (often >500/mm^3), predominance of PMN cells on CSF differential (>5/mm^3, presumed high sensitivity, low specificity), depressed CSF glucose levels (<40 mg/dL, 58% sensitivity), low CSF glucose to blood glucose ratio (<0.3, sensitivity 70%). Gram's stain of CSF is positive in most cases (60% to 90%) as is the culture (80%). However, even acute bacterial meningitis may present in an atypical fashion, with predominant CSF lymphocytosis (10%), negative Gram's stain, or, rarely, normal CSF leukocyte counts. In addition, the "purulent profile" may also be seen in noninfectious conditions such as subarachnoid hemorrhage (≤20% of cases). In contrast, CSF findings in viral meningitis typically reveal <100 WBCs/mm^3, predominantly mononuclear cells on differential, normal glucose levels, normal or elevated protein levels, and negative Gram's stain. However, some overlap exists with the profile for bacterial meningitis and 10% of patients with viral meningitis may have mostly PMNs, especially early in the course. Viral cultures are positive in <50% of the cases at best and may be as low as 5% for (Continued)

Lumbar Puncture *(Continued)*

herpes simplex virus. Thus, viral cultures have a limited role and LP is most useful clinically in ruling out bacterial meningitis. Viral meningitis rarely presents with WBC counts in CSF >1000/mm^3, CSF protein levels >100 mg/dL, or glucose <40 mg/dL. Such patients should be treated as bacterial meningitis until proven otherwise. Fungal meningitis rarely presents a normal CSF picture but the abnormalities are very nonspecific (elevated protein, depressed glucose, and lymphocytic pleocytosis). For the diagnosis of cryptococcal meningitis, the cryptococcal antigen detection test is accurate very early on. Similar nonspecific CSF profiles are seen in tuberculous meningitis and sometimes may mimic bacterial meningitis. The acid-fast smear has notoriously low sensitivity (<25%) but acid-fast bacilli culture has a 90% sensitivity. Malignancy involving the meninges (primary or metastatic) often results in a CSF picture mimicking infectious meningitis. Typically, there is a CSF leukocytosis, elevated protein, and glucose may range from normal to markedly decreased. A completely normal CSF exam essentially rules out CNS malignancy. Sensitivity of CSF cytology varies considerably among studies and varies from 60% to 90%, independent of such factors as tumor type, metastases, or primary brain site. A significant 3% false-positive rate has been reported which has limited its role as a routine staging screen for patients with malignancy. LP may be useful in diagnosing selected cases of subarachnoid hemorrhage (SAH), especially those in which head CT scan is equivocal. Interpretation of LP results may be problematic since RBCs in CSF commonly arise from a traumatic tap. The presence of xanthochromia in CSF has traditionally been associated with SAH, but has also been found in nearly one-third of traumatic taps. Similarly, a decreased RBC count from tube 1-4 has usually meant a traumatic tap but studies have shown a specificity of only 56%. Because of these limitations and potential LP complications, head CT scan has supplanted LP as the major diagnostic test in cases of suspected SAH. The diagnosis of multiple sclerosis may be supported by special CSF studies including oligoclonal banding and myelin basic protein, but sensitivity and specificity are variable. Another demyelinating condition, Guillain-Barré syndrome, is characterized by an isolated CSF protein value >200 mg/dL, with the remainder of CSF parameters normal. The absence of an elevated protein level practically excludes Guillain-Barré. In general, LP is more useful in Guillain-Barré syndrome than multiple sclerosis.

Use Practitioners vary in their threshold for performing an LP. This procedure is clearly indicated in the following clinical settings:

- clinically suspected meningitis, either acute (where procedure is emergent), subacute, or chronic; also, suspected encephalitis or meningoencephalitis
- suspected central nervous system syphilis in clearly symptomatic patients (tertiary neurosyphilis)
- evaluation of potential CNS lymphoma, meningeal leukemia, and meningeal carcinomatosis
- staging of lymphoma, previously diagnosed from another site
- clinically suspected demyelinating disease such as multiple sclerosis or Guillain-Barré syndrome
- possible cases of subarachnoid hemorrhage

CSF findings in each of these indications is fairly distinctive and LP substantially aids in clinical diagnosis. In contrast, several diseases have abnormal, but nonspecific, CSF findings and LP has low sensitivity and specificity. These include brain abscess or subdural empyema, primary brain tumor, tumors metastatic to brain, subdural or epidural hematoma, connective tissue diseases with CNS involvement (such as CNS lupus or Sjögren's syndrome). Additional studies (such as head CT scan) are necessary to confirm each of these conditions. LP should usually be delayed in favor of other more accurate and less invasive tests. Controversial indications for LP include suspected spinal epidural abscess, evaluation of the acute stroke to identify those which are hemorrhagic, evaluation of dementia (arguably to exclude neurosyphilis or chronic meningitis), evaluation of the asymptomatic patient with a positive serologic test for syphilis (to exclude asymptomatic neurosyphilis).

Limitations When a "traumatic tap" occurs (iatrogenic trauma), white blood cells may be passively transferred to the CSF. In general, for every 700 RBCs found in the CSF, 1 WBC is also expected (applies to the traumatic tap **only**).

Contraindications Procedure is contraindicated if there is a local infection at the proposed site of needle entry due to the potential for infectious seeding of meninges (several literature case reports). The presence of a severe bleeding diathesis is a relative contraindication to LP and an increased risk of spinal subdural hematoma has been demonstrated. Elevated intracranial pressure is an absolute contraindication to LP because of the risk of uncal herniation (see Complications). The presence of septicemia is **not** considered a contraindication. Retrospective studies have failed to show an increased incidence of meningitis in septic patients undergoing LP compared with septic patients who do not undergo the procedure.

Additional Information Because of the risk of tonsillar herniation following LP, controversy exists concerning the routine use of head CT scan prior to LP. Data is incomplete and several clinical approaches are available. The conservative approach is to always perform a head CT prior to LP regardless of neurologic findings, so as never to overlook an intracranial mass lesion. Other clinicians follow a more flexible approach and argue that tonsillar herniation only occurs with demonstrable papilledema or focal neurologic deficits; thus, when both of these physical signs are absent LP may be safely performed without prior head CT. A middle ground approach has been advocated where head CT scan is performed prior to LP in the following situations: papilledema, focal neurologic deficits, recent history of sinusitis or otitis media, severe and progressive headache, and deterioration of mental status. In our institution, we generally adopt the conservative approach (acute meningitis is treated empirically prior to CT and LP).

Selected Readings

Brocker RJ, "Technique to Avoid Spinal Tap Headache," *JAMA*, 1958, 68:261-3.

Chun CH, Johnson JD, Hofstetter M, et al, "Brain Abscess: A Study of 45 Consecutive Cases," *Medicine (Baltimore)*, 1986, 65(6):415-31.

Dougherty JM and Roth RM, "Cerebral Spinal Fluid," *Emerg Med Clin North Am*, 1986, 4(2):281-97.

Eng RH and Seligman SJ, "Lumbar Puncture-Induced Meningitis," *JAMA*, 1981, 245(14):1456-9.

Fishman RA, *Cerebrospinal Fluid in Diseases of the Nervous System*, Philadelphia, PA: WB Saunders Co, 1980.

Keroack MA, "The Patient With Suspected Meningitis," *Emerg Med Clin North Am*, 1987, 5(4):807-26.

Korein J, Cravisto H, and Leicach M, "Re-evaluation of Lumbar Puncture: A Study of 129 Patients With Papilledema or Intracranial Hypertension," *Neurology*, 1959, 9:290-7.

Marton KI and Gean AD, "The Spinal Tap: A New Look at an Old Test," *Ann Intern Med*, 1986, 104(6):840-8.

Reik L, "Disorders That Mimic CNS Infections," *Neurol Clin*, 1986, 4(1):223-48.

Simon R and Brenner B, "Neurosurgical Procedures," *Emergency Medicine*, Chapter 149, Baltimore, MD: Williams & Wilkins, 1982, 156-67.

Lumbar Puncture Analysis *see* Cerebrospinal Fluid Analysis *on page 354*

Lung Biopsy *see* Histopathology *on page 448*

Lupus Band Test *see* Skin Biopsy, Immunofluorescence *on page 538*

Lyme Arthritis Serology *see* Lyme Disease Serology *on this page*

Lyme Borreliosis Antibody by Western Blot *see* Lyme Disease Serology by Western Blot *on next page*

Lyme Disease Immunoblot *see* Lyme Disease Serology by Western Blot *on next page*

Lyme Disease Serology

Related Information

Lyme Disease Serology by Western Blot *on next page*

Synonyms Borreliosis Serology; Lyme Arthritis Serology

Specimen Serum or cerebrospinal fluid

Container Red top tube

Reference Range Values vary among laboratories

Use Laboratory confirmation of Lyme disease

Limitations Some cases are seronegative; there are cross reactions including those with antibodies to EB virus, *Rickettsia*, and syphilis. There is significant inter- and intralaboratory variation in this assay which highlights limitations of currently available testing. Even the Western blot is not considered a definitive assay. Consequently serologic evidence should not be the sole criterion for a diagnosis of Lyme disease. Serology is a confirmation test and should only **confirm** a clinical diagnosis.

Methodology Enzyme immunoassay (EIA), enzyme-linked immunosorbent assay (ELISA), indirect immunofluorescent antibody (IFA), Western blot

Additional Information Lyme disease is a multisystem disorder. A characteristic rash and arthritis are the hallmark symptoms. It is widespread in the US and (Continued)

Lyme Disease Serology *(Continued)*

is caused by *Borrelia burgdorferi*, a spirochete transmitted by the bite of the tick *Ixodes dammini*. The disease has protean manifestations, can become chronic, and responds to antibiotics; prompt proper diagnosis is therefore important.

Assay is available for IgG and IgM antibody in both serum and CSF. In early disease a negative assay does not exclude the diagnosis because assay sensitivity is only 40% to 60%. Antibody response may be blunted by antibiotics. All patients with chronic disease will have positive assays.

Recent studies using recombinant outer surface protein A and B and flagellin hold out promise for better serologic testing in the near future.

Patients may harbor *B. burgdorferi* asymptomatically and have positive serology. Some individuals may have symptoms of other illnesses incorrectly attributed to Lyme disease and be given inappropriate and ineffective treatment.

Antibodies against Lyme disease antigens can interfere with the ANA test.

Selected Readings

Craven RB, Quan TJ, Bailey RE, et al, "Improved Serodiagnostic Testing for Lyme Disease: Results of a Multicenter Serologic Evaluation," *Emerg Infect Dis*, 1996, 2(2):136-40.

Duffey PS and Salugsugan J, "Serodiagnosis of Lyme Borreliosis," *Clin Microbiol Newslett*, 1993, 15(11):81-5.

Fikrig E, Huguenel ED, Berland R, et al, "Serological Diagnosis of Lyme Disease Using Recombinant Outer Surface Proteins A and B and Flagellin," *J Infect Dis*, 1992, 165(6):1127-32.

Gill JS and Johnson RC, "Immunologic Methods for the Diagnosis of Infections by *Borrelia burgdorferi* (Lyme Disease)," *Manual of Clinical Laboratory Immunology*, 4th ed, Rose NR, de Macario EC, Fahey JL, et al, eds, Washington, DC: American Society for Microbiology, 1992, 452-8.

Mitchell PD, "Lyme Borreliosis: A Persisting Diagnostic Dilemma," *Clin Microbiol Newslett*, 1993, 15(8):57-9.

Steere AC, "Lyme Disease," *N Engl J Med*, 1989, 321(9):586-96.

Lyme Disease Serology by Western Blot

Related Information

Lyme Disease Serology *on previous page*
Nitrite, Urine *on page 503*

Synonyms Borreliosis Serology; Lyme Disease Immunoblot

Applies to Lyme Borreliosis Antibody by Western Blot

Test Includes Confirmation Lyme disease antibody test

Specimen Serum

Container Red top tube

Storage Instructions Separate and freeze serum.

Causes for Rejection Inadequate labeling, excessive hemolysis, chylous serum

Reference Range Normal: number of bands is defined by individual laboratory

Use Confirm positive screening tests for Lyme disease

Limitations The Western blot assay is not sensitive for detecting early Lyme disease. Its utility is for confirming stage 2 and stage 3 Lyme disease and to identify false-positive results in patients suspected of late Lyme disease. This test is performed by reference laboratories. Each laboratory designates which bands are most significant. Significant interlaboratory variation exists.

Contraindications Negative screening test for Lyme disease

Methodology Western blot technique utilizing a mixture of proteins (antigens) that are extracted from *Borrelia burgdorferi* and separated by SDS-PAGE; subsequent reaction of serum with bands/proteins.

Selected Readings

Duffey PS and Salugsugan J, "Serodiagnosis of Lyme Borreliosis," *Clin Microbiol Newslett*, 1993, 15(11):81-5.

Gill JS and Johnson RC, "Immunologic Methods for the Diagnosis of Infections by *Borrelia burgdorferi* (Lyme Disease)," *Manual of Clinical Laboratory Immunology*, 4th ed, Rose NR, de Macario EC, Fahey JL, et al, eds, Washington, DC: American Society for Microbiology, 1992, 452-8.

Mitchell PD, "Lyme Borreliosis: A Persisting Diagnostic Dilemma," *Clin Microbiol Newslett*, 1993, 15(8):57-9.

Lymph Node Biopsy

Related Information

Histopathology *on page 448*
Skin Biopsy *on page 535*

Applies to Cell Sorting Fluorescence Activation

Test Includes Microscopic examination of frozen sections, paraffin and/or plastic sections, and often, touch preparations. Immunoperoxidase studies for immunoglobulin heavy and light chains are best done on snap frozen cryostat sections rather than paraffin sections.

Special Instructions The specimen should not be placed in fixative if it can be delivered immediately to the laboratory. Diagnostic difficulties in diseases of lymph nodes are compounded by poor fixation and improper handling. Lymph node biopsies should be immediately delivered to the Histology Laboratory uncut and in a small sterile jar or Petri dish. Requests for all examinations including Microbiology should accompany the specimen. All such specimens should be brought to the immediate attention of a pathologist. Bone marrow, blood studies, and other clinical information are commonly needed for appropriate work-up.

Specimen Lymph node or other tissues suspected of harboring lymphoma, ideally submitted fresh within minutes of the biopsy

Container Sterile saline moistened sponge or Petri dish

Collection Optimal selection of site of biopsy and the lymph nodes to be biopsied enhance ultimate correct diagnosis. Supraclavicular and cervical biopsies will most likely provide diagnostic specimens. The most accessible lymph nodes are not always the best choice. The whole, intact lymph node with its capsule, and adjacent fat or other tissue provides an optimal specimen.

The proper initial triage of the tissue is of utmost importance in establishing the correct diagnosis. Usually, sufficient tissue must be available for both permanent sections and for immunophenotypic analysis of frozen sections. Tissues allocated for immunotypic studies are also suitable for genotypic studies if necessary. Routine histopathologic study remains the gold standard in diagnostic hematopathology and optimal histology begins with proper fixation. Fine nuclear detail is best achieved using B5, zinc formalin, or a Zenker's-like fixative. These fixatives are also best for cell marker analysis in paraffin section. An ever expanding selection of antibodies is useful for establishing lineage of hematopoietic cells in paraffin section (see table). However, phenotypic indicators of clonal proliferation are most reliably established in frozen section. As morphologic detail in frozen sections is intrinsically limited, every precaution to minimize artifacts must be taken. Snap freezing small, thin slices of tissue using liquid nitrogen cooled isopentane yields tissues free of freezing artifacts. Special attention to fine details of cryostat sectioning is necessary to yield interpretable results. If a frozen section evaluation is necessary to initiate a "lymphoma protocol," the tissues used for this rapid diagnosis are often unsuitable for immunophenotypic analysis. If the size of biopsy is limiting, a routine frozen section evaluation should be discouraged as freezing distorts lymphoid tissue and may result in errors in final interpretation.

If tissues are to be sent to a reference laboratory for immunotyping, three basic options are available. First, the tissues may be snap frozen and stored at -70°C or colder until such time as immunotyping is considered necessary. If facilities for proper snap freezing and storage are not available, this option should be discouraged. Second, the tissues may be delivered in carrier media or saline soaked gauze immediately by courier to the reference laboratory, where experienced personnel will process the tissue. Third, tissues may be placed in a carrier media which may circumvent the need for immediate action for 24 hours without significantly compromising the immunologic studies.

Storage Instructions Snap frozen tissues should be maintained at -70°C or colder until immunophenotypic analysis can be performed. If the frozen tissues are to be transported to a reference laboratory, they should be shipped on dry ice, using an overnight courier if necessary. Tissues placed in carrier media should be maintained on wet ice or at room temperature and packaged in insulated containers to avoid large fluctuations in temperature during transit.

Causes for Rejection Desiccated specimen, formalin exposure, excessive freezing artifact

Use Diagnose various lymphadenopathies, including cat scratch disease, malignant lymphoma, and metastatic neoplasia

Limitations Formalin-fixed tissue cannot be used for culture or imprints and is suboptimal for electron microscopy.

Methodology Quality basic histology is of paramount importance in the evaluation of the lymph node biopsy. Interpretive errors are often due to deficient basic histology. Touch preparations should always be obtained and are often times (Continued)

Lymphocyte Markers Useful in Paraffin Section*

	LCA (CD45)	EMA	LN-2 (CD71w)	L26 (CD20)	UCHL-1 (CD45RO)	CD3	Leu-M1 (CD15)	Mono Ig's	Lysozyme	KP1 (CD68)	CAE
Non-Hodgkin's lymphoma											
B-cell lymphomas†	+	-	+	+	-	-	-	+	-	-	-
T-cell lymphomas§	+	-/+	-	-	+	+	-/+	-	-	-	-
Hodgkin's disease (NS, MC, LD)	-	-	+	-	-	-	+	-	-	-	-
Hodgkin's disease, LP	+	+/-	+	+	-	-	-	-	-	-	-
Myeloma/plasmacytoma	-/+	-/+	-	-	-	-	-	+	-	-	-
Granulocytic sarcoma#	+/-	-	-/+	-	-	-	+/-	-	+	+	+
True histiocytic lymphoma#	+/-	-/+	-/+	-	-	-	-	-	+	+	-

Abbreviations: LCA: leukocyte common antigen; EMA: epithelial membrane antigen; Mono Ig's: monoclonal immunoglobulins; CAE: chloroacetate esterase (an enzyme cytochemical stain rather than an immunostain); Hodgkin's disease (NS, MC, LD): nodular sclerosing, mixed cellularity, and lymphocyte depleted subtypes, respectively; LP: lymphocyte predominate subtype.
Designated reactions: +: characteristically positive; -: characteristically negative; +/-: characteristically positive but may be negative; -/+: characteristically negative but may be positive; -: characteristically negative.

Footnotes:

*Most lymphomas characteristically contain neoplastic and non-neoplastic lymphoid elements in variable proportions. Caution must be exercised in determining the phenotype of the neoplastic cells.

†Monoclonal immunoglobulins are best detected in frozen section. Large cell lymphomas and those with plasmacytic differentiation are more likely to display a convincing staining in paraffin section than other subtypes.

§T-cell clonal proliferation cannot be determined in paraffin section alone. The best phenotypic expression of clonal proliferation is aberrant expression of pan T-cell antigens which can be detected only by frozen section immunohistology, by flow cytometry using cell suspensions, or by gene rearrangement.

#Enzyme cytochemical profile using touch preparations is extremely useful in establishing these diagnoses.

invaluable for final diagnosis. Representative tissues should be allocated for immunotyping, taking the necessary precautions to minimize morphologic artifacts while maintaining maximal antigenicity. Immunoperoxidase stains on paraffin or frozen sections are accomplished according to the general procedures outlined in the test listing Immunoperoxidase Procedures. Immunologic markers on touch preparations and bone marrow smears are often best demonstrated by using an alkaline phosphatase enzyme detection system to minimize background staining. Cultures for infectious agents are sometimes indispensable.

Additional Information Correlation with peripheral blood, bone marrow, and other clinical laboratory studies is often desirable and sometimes mandatory. Flow cytometry on dissociated tissues or body fluids is often utilized instead of immunohistology for cell marker analysis. This methodology offers a more quantitative approach to cell markers but only at the critical expense of destroying the immunoarchitecture of tissues. In general, immunohistology provides the best approach for typing tissues while flow cytometry is best suited for blood, bone marrow, and other body fluids. Properly acquired and frozen tissue is suitable for gene probe analysis (gene rearrangement studies), which may be necessary to document B- or T-cell clonal proliferation in rare cases.

Selected Readings

Jaffe ES, "Surgical Pathology of the Lymph Nodes and Related Organs," *Major Problems in Pathology*, Vol 16, Philadelphia, PA: WB Saunders Co, 1985.

Knowles DM, *Neoplastic Hematopathology*, Baltimore, MD: Williams & Wilkins, 1992.

Wright DH and Isaacson PG, *Biopsy Pathology of the Lymphoreticular System*, Baltimore, MD: Williams & Wilkins, 1983.

Lymph Node Culture *see* Epstein-Barr Virus Culture *on page 406*

Lymphocyte Culture *see* Epstein-Barr Virus Culture *on page 406*

Lymphogranuloma Venereum Culture *see Chlamydia* Culture *on page 359*

Magnetic Resonance Scan, Brain

Applies to Magnetic Resonance Scan, Head

Patient Preparation Inpatient: Patient must be able to lie quietly while the scan is performed. The patient should be screened for metallic devices by nursing personnel. (See Contraindications.) This includes metal introduced into the patient either surgically or by trauma. All metallic objects must be removed from the patient including jewelry or any other metal objects which may be in the patient's bedding. Please remove dentures or other dental appliances. I.V.s which contain no metal are fine, but infusion pumps must be removed. Oxygen tanks and metallic backboards may come with the patient but will be removed prior to the patient entering the magnet room. Oxygen may be provided in the magnet room. Trauma, ICU, or CCU patients should be accompanied by a nurse. If the patient is restless, combative, or claustrophobic, proper sedation may be administered on the floor prior to the MRI, or at the MRI Center. Consult the MRI radiologists with questions on proper sedation. Outpatient: The patient should be screened for metallic devices. (See Contraindications.) If a question exists as to the patient's suitability for MRI, the MRI radiologist will assist you with your questions. If the patient is claustrophobic, oral or parenteral sedation may be necessary. If so, the patient should be accompanied by another adult to provide transportation home after the examination.

Aftercare If the patient received an MRI contrast agent (Magnevist®) and develops a delayed hypersensitivity reaction (ie, hives or shortness of breath), the referring physician or MRI radiologist should be contacted immediately.

Data Acquired Digital information with film reproduction

Use Diagnose intracranial abnormalities including tumors, ischemia, infection, multiple sclerosis or any abnormalities relating to the brain or calvarium. MRI is an excellent modality for assessment of congenital brain abnormalities or relating to the status of brain maturation in the pediatric population.

Limitations Generally, the greatest limitation of magnetic resonance imaging results from the patient's fear of the procedure. The patient must remain quiet and still for several scans, each lasting from several minutes to 10 minutes in length. Total examination time is usually 30-45 minutes and occasionally up to 1 hour. If the patient is restless during the examination, motion artifacts will be present on the images limiting their diagnostic value. If the patient is claustrophobic, mild oral sedation or occasionally parenteral sedation may be needed. Also the patient can be accompanied by a family member or friend during the examination which helps calm the patient's anxiety in many cases. Patients (Continued)

Magnetic Resonance Scan, Brain *(Continued)*

requiring life support equipment such as ventilators require special preparation. Please refer to Contraindications for further causes for rejection.

Contraindications Patients weighing more than 300 lb and patients unable to squeeze into the magnet cannot undergo MRI. An absolute contraindication for MRI is a cardiac pacemaker. Relative contraindications to magnetic resonance imaging include intracranial aneurysm clips, cochlear implants, insulin infusion and chemotherapy pumps, neurocutaneous stimulators and prosthetic heart valves, depending on date of manufacture and metallurgical composition. Please consult MRI physician if questions arise. Patients who have metallic foreign bodies within the eye or who have undergone recent surgery within the last 6 weeks requiring placement of a vascular surgical clip, should also not undergo MRI. The safety of MRI in pregnant patients has not been determined. In such cases, prior consultation with the MRI physician is required. Generally, patients who have undergone recent surgery not requiring vascular clips or who have had coronary artery bypass surgery in the past may undergo MRI. Patients who have shrapnel wounds or orthopedic prostheses can generally safely undergo MRI unless the metallic device is in the anatomic region to be scanned which results in degradation of the images. Patients with surgically implanted intravascular vena cava filters to prevent pulmonary embolism can usually be scanned if the device has been in place for at least 6 weeks. Patients requiring life support equipment including ventilators require special preparation. Please contact MRI physician ahead of time. Central venous lines, Swan-Ganz catheters, and nasogastric (NG) tubes usually present no problems. If the patient is positive when screened for metallic devices and you are uncertain of their significance, the MRI radiologist will provide additional information to assist you.

Methodology Unlike most conventional radiologic procedures, magnetic resonance imaging does not utilize ionizing radiation, but relies upon radio frequency or radio signals induced within the patient by the magnetic field to obtain images. There are no known biologic effects secondary to the magnetic fields currently used in clinical MRI. Prior to the scan, the patient will be asked to remove all metallic objects from their person, including loose change, hair pins, earrings, belts, etc. This is for safety reasons as the strong magnetic field could result in these and any other metal objects becoming projectiles resulting in injury to the patient or MRI personnel. Also the patient should not carry a purse or wallet into the magnetic room, as the magnetic field can permanently erase bank cards or credit cards. The magnet is open on both ends and music can be played for the patient if desired. Fresh air is constantly circulated through the magnet room and the patient is continually monitored by the MRI technologist. An intercom system is provided for communication between the patient and the technologist. For MRI of the brain, a special coil surrounds, but does not touch the patient's head. The patient will be asked to remain very still while scans are being obtained. In certain cases, an MRI contrast agent, Gadopentetate Dimeglumine (Magnevist®) may be necessary to increase the diagnostic accuracy of the MRI examination. This is administered intravenously, via an antecubital vein in a small volume (<20 mL). This contrast agent may be used in patients who are allergic to conventional iodinated contrast agents such as is used in IVPs or CT examination without difficulty. There are very few contraindications to its use. (See Contraindications.)

Additional Information In some cases, an MRI contrast agent (Magnevist®) may be needed to increase the diagnostic accuracy of the MRI. This contrast agent can be administered to patients with a previous history of allergies to conventional iodinated x-ray agents as it contains no iodine. Contraindications to its use include previous allergy to the contrast agent itself, renal failure, certain types of anemia, and Wilson's disease. The contrast agent is generally very safe and increases the diagnostic efficacy of the MRI.

Selected Readings

Topics in Magnetic Resonance Imaging, Rockville, MD: Aspen Publishers, Inc, 1989.

Magnetic Resonance Scan, Head *see* Magnetic Resonance Scan, Brain *on previous page*

Malarial Parasites *see* Peripheral Blood Smear, Thick and Thin *on page 519*

Malaria Smear *see* Peripheral Blood Smear, Thick and Thin *on page 519*

Mantoux Test *see* Tuberculin Skin Testing, Intracutaneous *on page 557*

Maximum Bactericidal Dilution *see* Serum Bactericidal Test *on page 533*

Mazzini *replaced by* RPR *on page 530*

MBD *see* Serum Bactericidal Test *on page 533*

Measles Antibody

Test Includes IgG and IgM levels

Specimen Serum or cerebrospinal fluid

Container Red top tube

Reference Range Less than fourfold rise in titer; absent or stable IgM titer; HI >1:10, NT >1:20 indicates immunity. Consult laboratory for more specific (custom) information.

Use Differential diagnosis of viral exanthemas, particularly in pregnant women; diagnosis of subacute sclerosing panencephalitis; document adequacy of measles immunization

Limitations Antibody sometimes present in multiple sclerosis

Methodology Hemagglutination inhibition, viral neutralization, enzyme-linked immunosorbent assay

Additional Information Measles (rubeola) is caused by a paramyxovirus. Despite vaccination programs, there have been several recent local epidemics. Revaccination appears to be of greater value at 11-12 years of age than at 4-6 years of age. Serologic study can be useful in establishing that an individual has effective immunity subsequent to vaccination. In many individuals **detectable** immunity does not persist.

In acute illness, hemagglutinating and neutralizing antibody peak two weeks after the rash appears. It is necessary to demonstrate rising titers over 2 weeks, or identify IgM antibody.

Very high serum titers in the absence of acute illness and/or high CSF titers are seen in subacute sclerosing panencephalitis.

Selected Readings

Markowitz LE, Albrecht P, Orenstein WA, et al, "Persistence of Measles Antibody After Revaccination," *J Infect Dis*, 1992, 166(1):205-8.

Wittler RR, Veit BC, McIntyre S, et al, "Measles Revaccination Response in a School-Age Population," *Pediatrics*, 1991, 88(5):1024-30.

Measles Culture, 3-Day *see* Rubella Virus Culture *on page 532*

Measles Virus, Direct Detection *see* Virus Detection by DFA *on page 576*

Medical Legal Specimens *see* Histopathology *on page 448*

Methenamine Silver Stain

Related Information

Acid-Fast Stain, Modified, *Nocardia* Species *on page 307*

Cryptococcal Antigen Serology, Serum or Cerebrospinal Fluid *on page 379*

Fungus Culture, Biopsy *on page 414*

Fungus Culture, Body Fluid *on page 415*

Fungus Culture, Skin *on page 417*

Fungus Culture, Sputum *on page 419*

Fungus Culture, Urine *on page 421*

Gram's Stain *on page 426*

Histopathology *on page 448*

India Ink Preparation *on page 460*

KOH Preparation *on page 467*

Periodic Acid-Schiff Stain *on page 518*

Pneumocystis carinii Test *on page 522*

Skin Biopsy *on page 535*

Synonyms GMS Stain; Gomori-Methenamine Silver Stain; Grocott's Modified Silver Stain; Silver Stain

Test Includes Staining of organisms in a smear or histologic section with silver precipitate.

Patient Preparation If aspirate or biopsy, aseptic preparation of site is needed.

Specimen Bronchoalveolar lavage (BAL), lung biopsy, aspirated specimen, histopathology specimen

Container Sterile suction trap, sterile container for culture, jar with formalin for histopathology, clean glass slides air-dried or fixed in 95% alcohol for smears

Collection Touch preparation smears may be prepared by touching 8-10 glass slides to the cut surface of the fresh lung tissue. The slides should be fixed (Continued)

Methenamine Silver Stain *(Continued)*

individually upon preparation in 95% alcohol. Each slide should be labeled with the patient's name on the frosted end.

Reference Range No organisms identified

Critical Values Fungi or *Pneumocystis carinii* detected

Use Rapid detection of *Pneumocystis* or fungi

Limitations Organisms may be present in low numbers making detection difficult. Cost and time may also be factors. The silver stain (GMS) requires approximately 1 hour, is technically demanding, and requires significant reagent preparation. Yeasts (*Candida* and *Histoplasma*) similar in size to *Pneumocystis carinii* may be confused with *Pneumocystis carinii* on silver-stained tissue sections. Culture for fungus is always recommended.

Methodology A black precipitate on the fungal or *Pneumocystis* cell walls is produced by the chromic acid oxidation of cell wall carbohydrate hydroxyl groups to aldehydes and the subsequent reaction of the aldehyde groups with the silver reagent. Fungi appear as yeast cells, pseudohyphae, or hyphae. *Pneumocystis* stains gray to black, has a characteristic cup shape appearance 5-8 μm in diameter, and may demonstrate intracystic bodies.

Additional Information Recent studies have suggested that a combination of Papanicolaou (PAP) stain and Diff-Quik stain (a modified Giemsa stain) may provide comparable results to the GMS stain more rapidly and at less cost. Neither method is as sensitive as immunofluorescence for the detection of *Pneumocystis*. Silver stains in conjunction with other stains and morphologic evaluation by a skilled observer can frequently speciate fungal organisms in tissue specimens.

Selected Readings

Delvenne P, Arrese JE, Thiry A, et al, "Detection of Cytomegalovirus, *Pneumocystis carinii*, and Aspergillus Species in Bronchoalveolar Lavage Fluid. A Comparison of Techniques," *Am J Clin Pathol*, 1993, 100(4):414-8.

Homer KS, Wiley EL, Smith AL, et al "Monoclonal Antibody to *Pneumocystis carinii*. Comparison With Silver Stain in Bronchial Lavage Specimens," *Am J Clin Pathol*, 1992, 97(5):619-24.

Naimey GL and Wuerker RB, "Comparison of Histologic Stains in the Diagnosis of *Pneumocystis carinii*," *Acta Cytol*, 1995, 39(6):1124-7.

Raab SS, Cheville JC, Bottles K, et al, "Utility of Gomori Methenamine Silver Stains in Bronchoalveolar Lavage Specimens," *Mod Pathol*, 1994, 7(5):599-604.

MHA-TP

Synonyms Microhemagglutination, *Treponema pallidum*; Serologic Test for Syphilis

Applies to Syphilis Serology

Patient Preparation Patient should be fasting, if possible.

Specimen Serum

Container Red top tube

Storage Instructions Refrigerate

Reference Range Less than 1:160

Use Confirmatory serologic test for syphilis

Limitations Moderate sensitivity in early (primary) stages of syphilis. False-positives may occur in systemic lupus, infectious mononucleosis, and lepromatous leprosy.

Methodology Hemagglutination

Additional Information This is a *Treponema*-specific test and should not be used as a screening test. It is as sensitive and specific as FTA-ABS in all stages of syphilis except primary, in which it is less sensitive (but more sensitive than the VDRL). It will be positive with treponemal infections other than syphilis (bejel, pinta, yaws). Like FTA-ABS, MHA-TP once positive remains so, and cannot be used to judge effect of treatment. The test is not applicable to CSF.

Selected Readings

Hart G, "Syphilis Tests in Diagnostic and Therapeutic Decision Making," *Ann Intern Med*, 1986, 104(3):368-76.

Romanowski B, Sutherland R, Fick GH, et al, "Serologic Response to Treatment of Infectious Syphilis," *Ann Intern Med*, 1991, 114(12):1005-9.

MIC *see* Antimicrobial Susceptibility Testing, Aerobic and Facultatively Anaerobic Organisms *on page 323*

MIC, Anaerobic Bacteria *see* Antimicrobial Susceptibility Testing, Anaerobic Bacteria *on page 327*

Microfilariae, Peripheral Blood Preparation

Related Information

Peripheral Blood Smear, Thick and Thin *on page 519*

Synonyms Blood Smear for Trypanosomal/Filarial Parasites; Filariasis Peripheral Blood Preparation; Helminths, Blood Preparation; Trypanosomiasis Peripheral Blood Preparation

Applies to Filarial Infestation; Hemoflagellates; Peripheral Blood Preparation

Test Includes Examination of both thick and thin smears, wet preparation

Special Instructions If patient has traveled to an endemic area, the date of travel, the area, and the parasite suspected should be specified.

Specimen Fresh blood fingerstick

Container Slides

Collection Recommended procedure is for specimen to be obtained as follows: *Loa loa*, 10 AM - 2 PM; *Mansonella* and *Onchocerca*, anytime; *Wuchereria* and *Brugia*, 10 PM - 4 AM

Causes for Rejection Specimen clotted

Reference Range No parasites identified

Use Diagnose trypanosomiasis or microfilariasis, or parasitic infestation of blood

Limitations One negative result does not rule out the possibility of parasitic infestation. Since some species of blood parasites can be found during the day and others are nocturnal, both day and night specimens enhance identification. Most filariae generate microfilariae which can be found in peripheral blood, but *Onchocerca volvulus* and *Dipetalonema streptocerca* give rise to microfilariae which do not circulate.

Methodology Fresh wet blood film, with a coverslip, in which motile microfilariae cause agitation of adjacent red cells. Stained smears are used as well.

Additional Information Biopsy of skin and subcutaneous mass is used in diagnosis of *D. streptocerca* and *O. volvulus*. Differential diagnosis of species of circulating microfilariae requires distinction between the presence or absence of a sheath, the pattern of nuclei in the tail and sometimes the history of geographic exposure and time of sampling.

Microhemagglutination, *Treponema pallidum* see MHA-TP *on previous page*

Microsporidia Diagnostic Procedures

Test Includes Examination of stool, fluid, wash, or biopsy for microsporidia (*Enterocytozoon, Encephalitozoon, Nosema, Septata, Pleistophora*, and others)

Special Instructions Even though the test is relatively simple to perform, very few laboratories offer this test at this time because demand for the test is relatively low. The laboratory must be notified that microsporidia are suspected. Consult laboratory before ordering test for advice on availability of test and instructions on specimen collection.

Specimen Many different types of specimens are appropriate. The specimen must be obtained from a mucosal surface or an epithelial-lined surface (the sites of microsporidia replication) that represents the probable site of infection. In general, there are two types of specimens: those for exfoliative cytology examination and those for histological examination. Both types of specimens often are very productive. The specimen that should be collected depends on the suspected type of infection.

- Intestinal infection: direct stool smear, biliary tract biopsy, small intestine wash, small intestine mucosal biopsy
- Ocular infection: corneal scraping or swab
- Respiratory infection: sputum, BAL, transbronchial biopsy, bronchial brushing, mucosal biopsy
- Sino-nasal infection: scraping, smear, mucosal biopsy
- Urinary tract infection: concentrated urine, mucosal biopsy

Container Clean, screw-cap container appropriate for the particular specimen

Collection Appropriate for the site. Transport specimen to the laboratory as soon as possible. Biopsies should be fixed in formalin as soon as possible.

Use A part of the differential diagnostic work-up of diarrhea and other microsporidia-associated diseases in immunocompromised patients, particularly AIDS patients ; establish the diagnosis of microsporidiosis. Microsporidia have been demonstrated in immunocompetent persons.

(Continued)

Microsporidia Diagnostic Procedures *(Continued)*

Limitations Detection of microsporidia is entirely dependent on the adequacy of the specimen, staining and preparation of the specimen, and experience of the person who examines the specimen.

Methodology Microsporidia do not stain well with either hematoxylin, eosin, or the Papanicolaou stains. There are several good stains for microsporidia; however, not all of these stains stain the five major species of microsporidia. Microsporidia in paraffin-embedded tissues stain well with a tissue Gram's stain (Brown and Hoop stain; Brown and Brenn stain). Microsporidia in plastic-embedded tissues stain well with toluidine blue and with methylene blue-azure II-basic fuchsin. Microsporidia in cytologic centrifugation, smears, and scrapings preparations usually stain well with Gram's stain for specimens with little or no bacterial contamination. In these preparations, most microsporidia and bacteria are dark purple; some microsporidia are gram-negative or gram-variable. Weber's modified trichrome (chromotroph-based) stain works well with specimens with bacterial contamination; microsporidia are magenta-pink and the background (including bacteria) is blue-green. Some laboratories use Giemsa stain to stain stool smears and body fluids. Most stains cause microsporidia to appear as extremely fat bacteria which have a uniform oval shape, do not show budding, contain polar densities, and have a central clear band or area. The identification of microsporidia to species is very important in the selection of treatment. Speciation is accomplished most commonly by electron microscopy and, where available, molecular biology techniques. Cross reactions between the antibodies to the different types of microsporidia prevent serology from being clinically useful. Immunofluorescence staining techniques which include labeled antibody to specific microsporidia appear to work well in detecting microsporidia in clinical specimens and to be able to differentiate infections due to certain microsporidia. Some microsporidia have been cultured *in vitro*, but routine culture for microsporidia is not yet practical.

Selected Readings

Garcia LS, Shimuzu RY, and Brucker DA, "Detection of Microsporidial Spores in Fecal Specimens From Patients Diagnosed With Cryptosporidiosis," *J Clin Microbiol*, 1994, 32:1739-41.

Shadduck JA and Greely E, "Microsporidia and Human Infections," *Clin Microbiol Rev*, 1989, 2:158-65.

Sun T, "Microsporidiosis in the Acquired Immunodeficiency Syndrome," *Infect Dis Newslett*, 1993, 12:20-2.

Weber R and Bryan RT, "Microsporidial Infections in Immunodeficient and Immunocompetent Patients," *Clin Infect Dis*, 1994, 19:517-21.

Weber R, Bryan RT, Owen RL, et al, "Improved Light-Microscopical Detection of Microsporidia Spores in Stool and Duodenal Aspirates. The Enteric Opportunistic Infections Working Group," *N Engl J Med*, 1992, 326(3):161-6.

MicroTrak® *see* Chlamydia trachomatis by DFA *on page 363*

Midstream Urine Culture *see* Urine Culture, Clean Catch *on page 565*

Minimum Inhibitory Concentration Susceptibility Test *see* Antimicrobial Susceptibility Testing, Aerobic and Facultatively Anaerobic Organisms *on page 323*

Mite Identification *see* Arthropod Identification *on page 334*

M-Mode Echo *see* Echocardiography, M-Mode *on page 395*

Monospot™ Test *see* Infectious Mononucleosis Serology *on page 462*

Monosticon® Dri-Dot® Test *see* Infectious Mononucleosis Serology *on page 462*

Mono Test *see* Infectious Mononucleosis Serology *on page 462*

M. pneumoniae Titer *see* Mycoplasma Serology *on page 499*

Mucicarmine Stain *see* Periodic Acid-Schiff Stain *on page 518*

Muerto Canyon Strain Virus *see* Hantavirus Serology *on page 430*

Mumps Serology

Related Information

Mumps Virus Culture *on next page*

Specimen Serum

Container Red top tube

Collection Acute and convalescent sera drawn 10-14 days apart are required.

Reference Range A fourfold or greater increase in titer is indicative of recent mumps infection in the complement fixation test; a positive IgM immunofluorescent test is indicative of infection; an increasing hemagglutination inhibition titer indicates mumps **or parainfluenza virus** infection; a positive neutralization test indicates **immunity** to mumps.

Use Support the diagnosis of mumps virus infection; document previous exposure to mumps virus; document immunity

Limitations Several test systems are not specific for mumps

Methodology Complement fixation (CF), enzyme-linked immunosorbent assay (ELISA), immunofluorescence, hemagglutination inhibition (HAI), hemolysis-in-gel, virus neutralization

Additional Information Mumps is caused by a paramyxovirus. Serologic study may be undertaken to confirm a diagnosis in acute disease or to demonstrate established immunity. For diagnosis in an acute illness measuring the ratio of IgG to IgM antibody is simplest and fastest. Immunity depends on neutralizing antibody, which must be demonstrated in cell culture.

Selected Readings
Drew WL, "Diagnostic Virology," *Clin Lab Med*, 1987, 7(4):721-40.
Ukkonen P, Väisänen O, and Penttinen K, "Enzyme-Linked Immunosorbent Assay for Mumps and Parainfluenza Type 1 Immunoglobulin G and Immunoglobulin M Antibodies," *J Clin Microbiol*, 1980, 11(4):319-23.

Mumps Virus Culture

Related Information
Mumps Serology *on previous page*

Test Includes Concurrent culture for other viruses

Specimen Saliva, urine, cerebrospinal fluid

Container Sterile container for urine and CSF; tube with cold viral transport medium for swabs

Sampling Time At or within 5 days of the onset of illness

Collection It is desirable to collect specimens as early in the disease as possible. Saliva within 2 days of onset; spinal fluid of patients with meningoencephalitis within 6 days after onset. Virus is also excreted in urine for as long as 14 days.

In young patients, saliva is collected by a suitable suction device or by swabbing, especially the area around the orifices of Stensen's duct. The swabs must immediately be placed into cold viral transport medium. Spinal fluid is obtained in the usual manner and put into a sterile tube. For urine specimens, preferably the first voided morning urine is collected in a sterile container. All specimens must immediately be placed on ice and sent to the laboratory.

Storage Instructions Specimens should be delivered immediately on ice to the laboratory.

Causes for Rejection Dry specimen, specimen not refrigerated during transport, specimen fixed in formalin, unlabeled specimen

Turnaround Time Variable (5-14 days) and depends on methods used and amount of virus in the specimen

Reference Range No virus isolated

Use Aid in the diagnosis of disease caused by mumps virus

Methodology Inoculation of specimen into cell cultures, incubation, observation of characteristic cytopathic effect, and identification by methods such as hemadsorption and fluorescent monoclonal antibodies

Additional Information Although virus isolation is the most certain means for establishing the laboratory diagnosis, serologic methods are also useful and technically easier. Demonstration of IgM antibodies in acute serum is diagnostic of primary infection.

Selected Readings
Swierkosz EM, "Mumps Virus," *Manual of Clinical Microbiology*, 5th ed, Balows A, Hausler WJ Jr, Herrmann KL, et al, eds, Washington, DC: American Society for Microbiology, 1991, 912-7.
Tolpin MD and Schauf V, "Mumps Virus," *Textbook of Human Virology*, Belshe RB, ed, Littleton, MA: PSG Publishing Co, 1984, 311-31.

Mumps Virus, Direct Detection *see* Virus Detection by DFA *on page 576*

Murex CMV DNA Hybrid Capture Assay *see* Cytomegalovirus DNA Hybrid Capture *on page 390*

Muscle Biopsy

Related Information
Histopathology *on page 448*

Synonyms Skeletal Muscle Biopsy

(Continued)

Muscle Biopsy (Continued)

Test Includes Examination of muscle biopsy by histopathology. The procedure frequently includes enzyme histochemistry and electron microscopy.

Abstract Diagnosis and classification of muscle disease.

Patient Preparation Clinical data is required and should include the patient's age and sex; the pattern, severity, and tempo of the muscle involvement; relevant laboratory results (ie, CPK, ESR); electromyographic (EMG) findings; and the presence of significant related conditions (ie, dermatitis, neoplasm, steroid/AZT therapy, AIDS).

Sampling Time The biopsy should be performed early in the day as the specimen will immediately require special handling and should arrive when histotechnical personnel are available. The requisition should state a brief clinical history, pertinent laboratory findings, the biopsy site, and the name of the referring physician.

Collection Selection of muscle biopsy site: The muscle biopsies should be one that is familiar to the pathologist (ie, quadriceps, deltoid, biceps, gastrocnemius), unusual muscle groups such as oculomotor or pharyngeal muscles should be avoided as they have several unique and potentially confusing features. The biopsy should be from a muscle that is involved by the disease but has not reached "end-stage" atrophy. Injection sites, sites used for EMG, and sites near the myotendinous junction should be avoided as these biopsies will commonly exhibit artifactual changes.

Surgical technique: Except for children or exceptional adult cases, the procedure is done with local anesthesia. Ideally, the biopsied muscle should not be allowed to contract because this creates severe microscopic artifacts. To achieve an isometric specimen, it is best to use a surgical muscle clamp that prevents contraction.

If no clamp is available, pinning the muscle specimen to a tongue blade to prevent contraction may be used instead. A portion of the muscle, in continuity with that held in the clamp, should extend from the clamp so it can be cut off for freezing and histochemistry. A small piece should be placed in 1% glutaraldehyde for epon-embedding for electron microscopy, if necessary. Deliver on a saline-moistened gauze pad immediately to the Pathology Department. The moistened gauze pad is used to prevent drying. The specimen must not become saturated as this will cause severe ice crystal artifact, when the biopsy is subsequently snap frozen. The tissue should **not** be placed in fixative or frozen. It should ideally reach the Pathology Laboratory within 30 minutes to maintain enzyme activity.

Storage Instructions A small portion of the fresh material is usually stored deep frozen for possible later use as tissue for biochemical assays (eg, quantitation of glycogen, enzymes, or dystrophin levels).

Use Detect/diagnose trichinosis infection; evaluate muscle disease in terms of neurogenic atrophy, muscular dystrophies, myositis (infectious and "idiopathic," or autoimmune), endocrine myopathies, congenital myopathies, and enzyme deficiencies. Sometimes even with no observable clinical muscle disease, a muscle biopsy may shed light on a systemic condition such as systemic vasculitis.

Methodology A portion of the clamped muscle is oriented, frozen in isopentane/liquid nitrogen, and transverse sections are obtained for H & E, trichrome, and various histochemical preparations, some of which are listed below:

- Adenosine triphosphate (ATPase): At differing pH's, used to differentiates type I, IIa, and IIb myofibers and reveals abnormal fiber type distributions and diseases that selectively involve certain myofiber types.
- Succinate dehydrogenase (SDH): Stains mitochondria and shows abnormal aggregates or loss. Nicotinamide adenine dinucleotide-tetrazolium reductase (NADH-TR) may be used for the same purpose but is less sensitive.
- Oil red O: Stains lipids to detect abnormal accumulations.
- Periodic acid-Schiff (PAS): Used to detected glycogen in glycogenoses (ie, McArdle's disease, Pompe's disease, etc).

Extra frozen sections should be obtained and held in case additional, more specific, enzyme preparations are needed (ie, cytochrome C oxidase, phosphofructokinase, phosphorylase).

The remaining muscle tissue is formalin-fixed, paraffin-embedded, and stained for H & E and trichrome. These preparations are used to detect small foci of myositis or vasculitis which may be missed on the cryostat-cut sections, which are, of necessity, much smaller.

Selected Readings

Brooke MH, "Disorders of Skeletal Muscle," *Neurology in Clinical Practice*, Bradley WG, Daroff RB, Fenichel GM, et al, eds, Boston, MA: Butterworth-Heinemann, 1991, 1843-86.

DeGirolami U, Smith TW, Chad D, et al, "Skeletal Muscle," *Principles and Practice of Surgical Pathology*, Silverberg SG, ed, New York, NY: Churchill Livingstone, 1990, 545-92.

Heffner RR Jr, "Muscle Biopsy in Neuromuscular Disorders," *Diagnostic Surgical Pathology*, Sternberg SS, ed, New York, NY: Raven Press, 1989, 119-39.

Heffner RR Jr, "Skeletal Muscle," *Histology for Pathologists*, Sternberg SS, ed, New York, NY: Raven Press, 1992, 81-108.

Plotz PH, "Not Myositis: A Series of Chance Encounters," *JAMA*, 1992, 268(15):2074-7.

Mychel-S® *see* Chloramphenicol Serum Level *on page 367*

Mycobacteria Culture, Biopsy *see* Mycobacteria Culture, Biopsy or Body Fluid *on this page*

Mycobacteria Culture, Biopsy or Body Fluid

Related Information

Antimycobacterial Susceptibility Testing *on page 329*
Histopathology *on page 448*
Mycobacteria Culture, Sputum *on page 495*

Synonyms AFB Culture, Biopsy; Mycobacteria Culture, Biopsy; TB Culture, Biopsy

Applies to Bone Marrow Mycobacteria Culture; Mycobacteria Culture, Bone Marrow; Mycobacteria Culture, Surgical Specimen; Mycobacteria Culture, Tissue; Surgical Specimen Mycobacteria Culture; Tissue Mycobacteria Culture; Wound Mycobacteria Culture

Patient Preparation Aseptic preparation of biopsy site

Special Instructions The laboratory should be informed of the specific source of specimen, age of patient, current antibiotic therapy, clinical diagnosis, and time of collection. Specimens may be divided for fungus culture and KOH preparation, mycobacteria culture and acid-fast smear, and routine bacterial culture and Gram's stain only if the specimen is of adequate volume for all tests requested.

Specimen Surgical tissue, bone marrow, biopsy material; **swab specimens are never adequate**

Container Sterile, screw cap container

Collection The portion of the surgical specimen submitted for culture should be separated from the portion submitted for histopathology by the surgeon or pathologist, utilizing sterile technique

Storage Instructions The specimen should be transported to laboratory as soon as possible after collection.

Causes for Rejection Specimen in fixative

Turnaround Time Negative cultures may be be reported after 8 weeks.

Reference Range No growth

Use Isolate and identify mycobacteria; establish the etiology of granulomatous disease, fever of unknown origin (FUO) particularly in immunocompromised patients and others with subtle defects of cellular immunity

Limitations Transbronchial biopsy cultures may be of assistance in documenting the diagnosis of tuberculosis in sputum smear negative cases; however, sputum culture and bronchial washing cultures have a higher percentage of positives.

If *Mycobacterium marinum* which may cause a localized cutaneous lesion that may be nodular, verrucous, ulcerative, or sporotrichoid and which may rarely involve deeper structure is suspected, the laboratory must be notified so that the culture may be incubated at an appropriate temperature (30°C). *Mycobacterium marinum* infection occurs in patients who have been exposed to the organism following an aquatic-related exposure involving a cutaneous abrasion or penetrating injury. Common histories include exposure while cleaning aquariums or clearing barnacles.

Methodology Culture on specialized selective media, usually including Löwenstein-Jensen (LJ) and frequently Middlebrook 7H11, incubated at 35°C with 5% to 10% CO_2 (30°C if *Mycobacterium marinum* is suspected). Mycobacteria isolated are usually definitively identified and may be tested for antimicrobial susceptibility).
(Continued)

Mycobacteria Culture, Biopsy or Body Fluid
(Continued)

Radiometric (Bactec®) and DNA probe methods are utilized by some laboratories to provide rapid detection and identification of mycobacteria.

Susceptibility testing may be required because of the often unpredictable susceptibilities of the atypical mycobacteria. Susceptibility testing of mycobacteria is frequently referred to specialized laboratories and may only be offered by specific request.

Additional Information Occult infections with **atypical** mycobacteria (not *M. tuberculosis*), particularly *Mycobacterium avium* and *Mycobacterium intracellulare*, occur in patients with acquired immune deficiency syndrome (AIDS). In some institutions, the incidence of isolation of non-*Mycobacterium tuberculosis* species, specifically *M. avium-intracellulare* (*M. avium* complex), may exceed the rate of isolation of *M. tuberculosis*. Mycobacteria have been recovered from culture of Kaposi's sarcomas and bone marrow specimens, in which the characteristic granulomatous reaction has been absent. Optimal isolation of mycobacteria from tissue is accomplished by processing as much tissue as possible for culture. Swabs should be submitted only when adequate tissue is not available. Tuberculous spondylitis represents 50% to 60% of all cases of skeletal tuberculosis. It is seen in children in developing countries and adults older than 50 years of age in the United States and Europe. Frequently several vertebrae are involved and adjacent psoas muscle abscesses or paravertebral abscesses are not uncommon. Colony counts obtained from bone biopsies are low; however, >90% are culture positive. The diagnosis of vertebral tuberculosis should be considered in all cases of unexplained spondylitis.

Cases of sternal wound infection and of early onset prosthetic valve endocarditis have been recognized. *M. fortuitum* is the most commonly implicated mycobacterial species in these infections. Local environmental strains rather than contaminated commercial surgical materials or devices are considered to be the source of the organisms.

Pleural effusions frequently yield positive cultures in cases of pulmonary tuberculosis. The diagnosis of peritoneal tuberculosis is difficult and is usually made at laparotomy or after a considerable delay. Tuberculosis should be considered in any patient with ascitic fluid and chronic abdominal pain.

Selected Readings
Brown JW 3d and Sanders CV, "*Mycobacterium marinum* Infections: A Problem of Recognition, Not Therapy?" Arch Intern Med, 1987, 147(5):817-8.
Woods GI and Washington JA, "Mycobacteria Other Than *Mycobacterium tuberculosis*: Review of Microbiologic and Clinical Aspects," Rev Infect Dis, 1987, 9(2):275-94.

Mycobacteria Culture, Bone Marrow *see* Mycobacteria Culture, Biopsy or Body Fluid *on previous page*

Mycobacteria Culture, Bronchial Aspirate *see* Mycobacteria Culture, Sputum *on next page*

Mycobacteria Culture, Cerebrospinal Fluid
Related Information
Acid-Fast Stain *on page 305*
Viral Culture, Central Nervous System Symptoms *on page 570*
Synonyms CSF Mycobacteria Culture; Mycobacteria Culture, CSF; Mycobacteria Culture, Spinal Fluid; Spinal Fluid Mycobacteria Culture
Test Includes Culture for mycobacteria and acid-fast stain if requested
Patient Preparation Usual sterile preparation
Specimen Cerebrospinal fluid
Container Sterile CSF tube
Collection The specimen may be divided for fungus culture and India ink preparation, cryptococcal antigen testing, fungus smear, mycobacteria culture and smear, and routine bacterial culture and Gram's stain if the specimen is of adequate volume for all tests requested. Transport specimen to the laboratory as soon as possible.
Storage Instructions Do not refrigerate.
Turnaround Time Negative cultures are often reported after 6-8 weeks.
Reference Range No growth
Use Isolate and identify mycobacteria

Limitations Culture of for *M. tuberculosis* is usually nonproductive even in cases of tuberculosis meningitis. Culture of CSF for *M. tuberculosis* should be ordered only if such is truly suspected. Recovery of mycobacteria is directly related to the volume of specimen available to the laboratory for culture. 5-10 mL is recommended for optimal yield. Recovery of organisms can require as much as 4-6 weeks.

Methodology Culture on selective media usually including Löwenstein-Jensen (LJ) and Middlebrook 7H11 broth media may also be used with or without radiometric methodology

Additional Information A culture for mycobacteria is indicated if patient is immunocompromised and the Gram's stain is negative and the white cell count is elevated. Tuberculous meningitis occurs in both children and adults. Early in the course neutrophils may predominate in the CSF. Lymphocytes, mononuclear cells, and granulocytes are found later. Rarely does the cell count exceed 1000 cells/mm^3. The CSF is clear and colorless early; later, a pellicle forms on standing. Low CSF glucose, <40 mg/dL, frequently is observed as is increased protein often >300 mg/dL. Other factors raising the index of suspicion include a positive tuberculin skin test (evidence of tuberculosis outside the CNS), previous active tuberculosis, significant recent exposure to tuberculosis, and suspicion of tuberculosis on imaging procedures. Acid-fast organisms can be identified on centrifuged sediments in 60% to 80% of cases.

Untreated tuberculous meningitis can be rapidly fatal. Blacks, Hispanics, and the elderly are most frequently affected. Alcohol abuse, drug abuse, steroid therapy, head trauma, pregnancy, and AIDS all may increase risk. Despite therapy, the mortality risk is high, approximately 30%. Evaluation of contacts is recommended.

Selected Readings
Ogawa SK, Smith MA, Brennessel DJ, et al, "Tuberculous Meningitis in an Urban Medical Center," *Medicine (Baltimore)*, 1987, 66(4):317-26.

Mycobacteria Culture, CSF *see* Mycobacteria Culture, Cerebrospinal Fluid *on previous page*

Mycobacteria Culture, Gastric Aspirate *see* Mycobacteria Culture, Sputum *on this page*

Mycobacteria Culture, Spinal Fluid *see* Mycobacteria Culture, Cerebrospinal Fluid *on previous page*

Mycobacteria Culture, Sputum

Related Information
Acid-Fast Stain *on page 305*
Mycobacteria Culture, Biopsy or Body Fluid *on page 493*

Synonyms AFB Culture, Sputum; TB Culture, Sputum

Applies to AFB Culture, Bronchial Aspirate; AFB Culture, Gastric Aspirate; Bronchoscopy Mycobacteria Culture; DNA Probe for Mycobacteria; Gastric Aspirate Mycobacteria Culture; Lower Respiratory Mycobacteria Culture; Mycobacteria Culture, Bronchial Aspirate; Mycobacteria Culture, Gastric Aspirate; Mycobacteria Culture, Tracheal Aspirate; Mycobacteria Culture, Transtracheal Aspirate; Mycobacteria, DNA Probe; Percutaneous Transtracheal Mycobacteria Culture; TB Culture, Bronchial Aspirate; TB Culture, Gastric Aspirate; Tracheal Aspirate Mycobacteria Culture; Transtracheal Aspirate Mycobacteria Culture

Test Includes Mycobacteria (AFB) culture and stain

Patient Preparation The patient should be instructed to remove dentures, rinse mouth with water, and then cough deeply expectorating sputum into the sputum collection cup.

Special Instructions Early morning specimen is preferred. Since at least 5 mL of sputum (**not saliva**) is required, the specimen may be collected over a 1- to 2-hour period in order to obtain sufficient quantity. However, 24-hour specimens are unacceptable because of bacterial overgrowth.

Specimen First morning sputum or induced sputum, fasting gastric aspirate, bronchial aspirate, tracheal aspirate, transtracheal aspirate, bronchial lavage

Container Sputum cup, sputum trap, sterile tracheal aspirate tube or sterile bronchoscopy tube

Sampling Time In children, the gastric aspirate should be done early in the morning as the child awakens before the stomach empties.

Collection A recommended screening procedure is three first morning specimens submitted on three successive days. The patient should be instructed to
(Continued)

Mycobacteria Culture, Sputum *(Continued)*

brush his/her teeth and/or rinse mouth well with water before attempting to collect the specimen to reduce the possibility of contaminating the specimen with food particles, oropharyngeal secretions, etc. After the specimen has been collected, the specimen should be examined to make sure it contains a sufficient quantity (at least 5 mL) of thick mucus (**not saliva**). If a two part collection system has been used, only the screw cap tube should be submitted to the laboratory. (The outer container is considered contaminated and its transport through the hospital constitutes a health hazard!) The specimen should be properly labeled and accompanied by a properly completed requisition. The specimen can be divided in the laboratory for fungal, mycobacterial, and routine cultures.

Storage Instructions The specimen should be refrigerated if it cannot be promptly processed. If a gastric aspirate cannot be processed immediately the pH should be neutralized for storage until it can be processed.

Causes for Rejection Specimens contaminated on the outside of the container pose excessive risk to laboratory personnel and may not be acceptable to the laboratory.

Turnaround Time Negative cultures are reported after 6-8 weeks.

Reference Range No growth

Use Isolate and identify mycobacteria

Limitations Bronchial washings are frequently diluted with topical anesthetics and irrigating fluids which may have an inhibitory effect on mycobacterial growth. Postbronchoscopy expectorated specimens may provide a better yield of organisms than those obtained during the procedure. Gastric aspirates yield organisms in <50% of cases of *M. tuberculosis* infection in children. Acid-fast stain of gastric aspirate has a sensitivity of 30%. Separate Cytology specimens must be submitted.

The relative yield of mycobacteria from clinical specimens is prebronchoscopy sputum > bronchial washings > postbronchoscopy sputum > bronchial biopsy.

Methodology Culture on selective media usually including Löwenstein-Jensen (LJ) and Middlebrook 7H11 with and without antibiotics. DNA probe technology using probes complementary to the ribosomal RNA of the *M. tuberculosis* complex (*M. tuberculosis, M. bovis*, BCG, *M. africanum*, and *M. microti*), as well as to *M. avium, M. intracellulare M. kansasii* and *M. gordonae* are available for culture confirmation. The probes can provide rapid confirmation of the species of mycobacteria isolated. Mycobacteria in clinical specimens can be detected by the radiometric Bactec® system which detects production of $^{14}CO_2$ from ^{14}C labeled palmitic acid supplemented Middlebrook 7H12 medium. Detection times are more rapid than with conventional culture methods. Gas-liquid chromatography can be used to rapidly speciate mycobacteria.

Additional Information Tuberculosis decreased in incidence in the United States in the 1970s and 1980s, however, high incidence populations exist in depressed inner city areas, some rural areas, amongst new immigrants, and in HIV-positive patients. The emergence of *M. tuberculosis* and *M. avium-intracellulare* infections complicating the acquired immunodeficiency syndrome has been striking. Primary pulmonary infections are common as case defining infections. Extrapulmonary mycobacterial infections are frequent in patients with an established diagnosis of AIDS.

See also listings Acid-Fast Stain *on page 305*, and Mycobacteria Culture, Biopsy or Body Fluid *on page 493* for additional discussion of mycobacterial disease in patients with the acquired immunodeficiency syndrome (AIDS).

Implication of *M. avium-intracellulare* as a pathogen usually requires at least one of the following criteria:

- Clinical evidence of a disease process that can be explained by atypical mycobacterial infection
- Repeated isolation of the same mycobacterial species from sputum over a period of weeks to months
- Exclusion of other possible etiologies
- Biopsy demonstrating acid-fast bacilli or diagnostic histopathologic changes

Endobronchial tuberculosis has been increasingly recognized because of its incidence in association with the acquired immunodeficiency syndrome and because it may mimic carcinoma.

Nosocomial transmission of multidrug-resistant *Mycobacterium tuberculosis* has been noted to occur from patient to patient and from patient to healthcare worker. Acid-fast bacilli isolation precautions and adherence to appropriate infection control procedures is recommended.

Selected Readings

Chaisson RE and Slutkin G, "Tuberculosis and Human Immunodeficiency Virus Infection," *J Infect Dis*, 1989, 159(1):96-100.

Inderlied CB, Kemper CA, and Bermudez LE, "The *Mycobacterium avium* Complex," *Clin Microbiol Rev*, 1993, 6(3):266-310.

Marmion BP, Williamson J, Worswick DA, et al, "Experience With Newer Techniques for the Laboratory Detection of *Mycoplasma pneumoniae* Infection: Adelaide, 1978-1992," *Clin Infect Dis*, 1993, 17(Suppl 1):S90-9.

Mehta JB and Morris F, "Impact of HIV Infection on Mycobacterial Disease," *Am Fam Physician*, 1992, 45(5):2203-11.

Pearson ML, Jereb JA, Frieden TR, et al, "Nosocomial Transmission of Multidrug-Resistant *Mycobacterium tuberculosis*. A Risk to Patients and Health Care Workers," *Ann Intern Med*, 1992, 117(3):191-6.

Stratton CW, "Mycobacterial Infections Other Than Tuberculosis in the AIDS Era," *Infect Dis Newslett*, 1992, 11(12):89-96.

Wellstood SA, "Diagnostic Mycobacteriology: Current Challenges and Technologies," *Lab Med*, 1993, 24(6):357-61.

Witebsky FG and Conville PS, "The Laboratory Diagnosis of Mycobacterial Diseases," *Infect Dis Clin North Am*, 1993, 7(2):359-76.

Mycobacteria Culture, Surgical Specimen *see* Mycobacteria Culture, Biopsy or Body Fluid *on page 493*

Mycobacteria Culture, Tissue *see* Mycobacteria Culture, Biopsy or Body Fluid *on page 493*

Mycobacteria Culture, Tracheal Aspirate *see* Mycobacteria Culture, Sputum *on page 495*

Mycobacteria Culture, Transtracheal Aspirate *see* Mycobacteria Culture, Sputum *on page 495*

Mycobacteria, DNA Probe *see* Mycobacteria Culture, Sputum *on page 495*

Mycobacteria, Susceptibility Testing *see* Antimycobacterial Susceptibility Testing *on page 329*

Mycobacterium **Smear** *see* Acid-Fast Stain *on page 305*

Mycoplasma genitalium **Culture** *see* Mycoplasma/Ureaplasma Culture *on page 499*

Mycoplasma hominis **Culture** *see* Mycoplasma/Ureaplasma Culture *on page 499*

Mycoplasma pneumoniae *see* Mycoplasma/Ureaplasma Culture *on page 499*

Mycoplasma pneumoniae **Culture** *see* Mycoplasma pneumoniae Diagnostic Procedures *on this page*

Mycoplasma pneumoniae Diagnostic Procedures

Related Information

Aerobic Culture, Sputum *on page 312*
Darkfield Examination, Leptospirosis *on page 393*
Mycoplasma Serology *on page 499*
Mycoplasma/Ureaplasma Culture *on page 499*

Synonyms *Mycoplasma pneumoniae* Culture

Test Includes Culture and identification of *Mycoplasma pneumoniae*

Abstract *Mycoplasma pneumoniae* commonly causes respiratory infections. Most involve the upper respiratory tract, but pneumonia and other manifestations can occur as well.

Specimen Throat or nasopharyngeal swabs

Collection Throat or nasopharyngeal swabs should be placed **immediately** in transport medium and sent immediately to the laboratory.

Turnaround Time 2-3 weeks

Reference Range No *Mycoplasma pneumoniae* identified

Use Aid in the diagnosis of pneumonia caused by *Mycoplasma pneumoniae*

Limitations The culture procedure is not often used because it is slow and insensitive; 2-3 weeks or more are often required for isolation and definitive identification of positive cultures.

Methodology Isolates are cultured in special broth and on special agar media and are identified by biochemical tests and ability to hemolyze erythrocytes. However, the most commonly used and currently recommended method of diagnosis is serology to measure acute and convalescent antibody levels to *M. pneumoniae*.

(Continued)

Mycoplasma pneumoniae Diagnostic Procedures
(Continued)

Additional Information *Mycoplasma pneumoniae* infection is acquired via the respiratory route from small-particle aerosols or large droplets of secretions. The organism can penetrate the mucociliary barrier of respiratory epithelium and produce cellular injury and ciliostasis which may account for the prolonged cough observed clinically. Most infections are observed in older children and young adults. Early infection in infancy or childhood may increase the severity of subsequent infections. Cold agglutinins and *Mycoplasma pneumoniae* complement fixation serology have been the mainstays of diagnosis because of the limitations and long turnaround time for cultures. However, immunofluorescence techniques and immunoassays to detect antibodies to *M. pneumoniae* are available and are the recommended diagnostic methods. DNA probes for *Mycoplasma* are not yet available for routine testing. Consult the laboratory for availability of specific tests and specific instructions for specimen collection. See table.

Mycoplasma pneumoniae Clinical Manifestations of Infection

Respiratory	Pneumonia
	Pharyngitis
	Otitis media
	Bullous myringitis
	Sinusitis
	Laryngotracheobronchitis
	Bronchiolitis
	Nonspecific upper respiratory symptoms
Neurologic	Meningoencephalitis
	Encephalitis
	Transverse myelitis
	Cranial neuropathy
	Poliomyelitis-like syndrome
	Psychosis
	Cerebral infarction
	Guillain-Barré syndrome
Cardiac	Pericarditis
	Myocarditis
	Complete heart block
	Congestive heart failure
	Myocardial infarction
Gastrointestinal	Pancreatitis
	Hepatic dysfunction
Hematologic	Autoimmune hemolytic anemia
	Bone marrow suppression
	Thrombocytopenia
	Disseminated intravascular coagulation
Musculoskeletal	Myalgias
	Arthralgias
	Arthritis
Genitourinary	Glomerulonephritis
	Tubulointerstitial nephritis
	Tubo-ovarian abscess
Immunologic	Depressed cellular immunity and neutrophil chemotaxis

From Broughton RA, "Infections Due to *Mycoplasma pneumoniae* in Childhood," *Pediatr Infect Dis J*, 1986, 71-85, with permission.

Selected Readings

Clyde WA Jr, "Clinical Overview of Typical *Mycoplasma pneumoniae* Infections," *Clin Infect Dis*, 1993, 17(Suppl 1)S32-6.

Mansel JK, Rosenow EC 3d, Smith TF, et al, "*Mycoplasma pneumoniae* Pneumonia," *Chest*, 1989, 95(3):639-46.

Martin RE and Bates JH, "Atypical Pneumonia," *Infect Dis Clin North Am*, 1991, 5(3):585-601.

"The Changing Role of Mycoplasmas in Respiratory Disease and AIDS," *Clin Infect Dis*, 1993, 17(Suppl 1):S1-315.

Wijnands GJ, "Diagnosis and Interventions in Lower Respiratory Tract Infections," *Am J Med*, 1992, 92(4SA):91S-7S.

Mycoplasma pneumoniae Titer *see Mycoplasma Serology on this page*

Mycoplasma Serology

Related Information

Mycoplasma pneumoniae Diagnostic Procedures *on page 497*

Synonyms Eaton Agent Titer; *M. pneumoniae* Titer; *Mycoplasma pneumoniae* Titer; PPLO Titer

Specimen Serum

Container Red top tube

Collection Acute and convalescent sera drawn 10-14 days apart are required

Reference Range Negative: IgG <1:10, IgM <1:10. A fourfold increase in titer in paired sera or a single complement fixation titer >1:256 suggests infection. Contact laboratory for specific cutoff values and significant titers.

Use Support the diagnosis of *Mycoplasma pneumoniae* infection

Limitations False-positives occur in pancreatitis.

Methodology Complement fixation, immunofluorescence, enzyme immunoassay

Additional Information *Mycoplasma pneumoniae* is the cause of the relatively common "primary atypical pneumonia." *Mycoplasma* is more difficult to culture than are bacteria; thus, serologic confirmation of the diagnosis is often desirable. The complement fixation test to detect antibody to a lipid antigen is more specific and more sensitive than is the cold agglutinin test. However, complement fixation requires paired sera, and is thus of limited clinical utility. Demonstration of specific IgG and IgM antibody by immunofluorescence is rapid, sensitive, and specific. IgM antibody indicates acute infection.

Selected Readings

Kenny GE, "Immunologic Methods for Mycoplasmas and Miscellaneous Bacteria," *Manual of Clinical Laboratory Immunology*, 4th ed, Rose NR, de Macario EC, Fahey JL, et al, eds, Washington, DC: American Society for Microbiology, 1992, 497-8.

Smith TF, "*Mycoplasma pneumoniae* Infections: Diagnosis Based on Immunofluorescence Titer of IgG and IgM Antibodies," *Mayo Clin Proc*, 1986, 61(10):830-1.

Waites KB, Bébéar C, Robertson JA, et al, "Laboratory Diagnosis of Mycoplasmal and Ureaplasmal Infections," *Clin Microbiol Newslet*, 1996, 18(14):105-11.

Mycoplasma T-Strain Culture, Genital *see Genital Culture for Ureaplasma urealyticum on page 424*

Mycoplasma/Ureaplasma Culture

Related Information

Genital Culture for *Ureaplasma urealyticum* on page 424

Mycoplasma pneumoniae Diagnostic Procedures *on page 497*

Synonyms PPLO Culture

Applies to Cervix, *Mycoplasma* Culture; *Mycoplasma genitalium* Culture; *Mycoplasma hominis* Culture; *Mycoplasma pneumoniae*; *Ureaplasma urealyticum* Culture; Urethra, *Mycoplasma* Culture; Urine, *Mycoplasma* Culture

Specimen The following specimens are appropriate: throat swabs (send two swabs), sputum, bronchial washings, tracheal aspiration, cerebrospinal fluid, heparinized blood, urethral swab, vaginal swab, cervical swab, placenta, and urine. Urine should **not** be clean catch midstream. Initial urine flow is best specimen.

Collection The laboratory **must** be contacted prior to collection for advice and for appropriate transport medium. Transport specimen to the laboratory within 1 hour. Do **not** use cotton swabs or swabs with wooden sticks.

Turnaround Time 1-6 weeks

Reference Range No *Mycoplasma* isolated

Use Isolate and identify *Mycoplasma*

Limitations Culture is frequently negative in presence of *Mycoplasma* infection.

Methodology Isolates are cultured in special broth and on special agar media and are identified by biochemical tests and ability to hemolyze erythrocytes. However, the most commonly used and currently recommended method of diagnosis is serology to measure acute and convalescent antibody levels to *M. pneumoniae*.

Additional Information *Mycoplasma pneumoniae* is the causative agent of mycoplasmal pneumonia or atypical pneumonia. This condition is generally mild, but may develop into severe illness. Other members of the *Mycoplasma* family are *M. hominis* and *Ureaplasma urealyticum*, which cause infection of the (Continued)

Mycoplasma/Ureaplasma Culture *(Continued)*

urogenital tract, namely pelvic inflammatory disease and 10% of the cases of nongonococcal urethritis. Both organisms can be isolated for identification and both respond to erythromycin and tetracycline.

Nail Fungus Culture *see Fungus Culture, Skin on page 417*

Nasopharyngeal Culture for *Bordetella pertussis* *see Bordetella pertussis Naso-pharyngeal Culture on page 349*

Nasopharyngeal Culture for *Corynebacterium diphtheriae* *see Throat Culture for Corynebacterium diphtheriae on page 549*

Nasopharyngeal Smear for *Bordetella pertussis* *see Bordetella pertussis Direct Fluorescent Antibody on page 349*

Nebcin®, Blood *see Tobramycin Level on page 551*

Needle Biopsy of the Liver *see Liver Biopsy on page 474*

Negri Bodies *see Rabies Detection on page 525*

Neisseria gonorrhoeae by Nucleic Acid Probe

Related Information

Neisseria gonorrhoeae Culture *on next page*

Synonyms DNA Hybridization Test for *Neisseria gonorrhoeae*; DNA Test for *Neisseria gonorrhoeae*; Gen-Probe® for *Neisseria gonorrhoeae*; *Neisseria gonorrhoeae* DNA Detection Test; PACE2®

Test Includes Direct detection of *Neisseria gonorrhoeae* nucleic acid in clinical specimens from the urogenital site. This test cannot be used in legal cases or child protection cases.

Patient Preparation When taking urethral specimens, the patient should not have urinated for 1 hour prior to collection.

Specimen Swab specimen collected from the genitourinary site of a male or female patient

Container Special transport medium is provided by the laboratory and should not be substituted. A kit containing a swab and special transport medium is made by Gen-Probe, Inc. and is recommended for this test.

Collection Currently the probe test for *Neisseria gonorrhoeae* is FDA approved only for genitourinary specimens. It has not yet been approved for testing of nongenital specimens (ie, ocular).

For a male, the urethra is swabbed by rotating the swab 2-3 cm into the urethra. This should provide enough specimen from the infected site to detect *N. gonorrhoeae* nucleic acid. The swab is then placed in the transport tube for shipment to the laboratory.

For females, the Gen-Probe® kit provides two swabs. The cervix or endocervix should be swabbed with one swab **first** to clean the area and then the **second** swab is used to collect the specimen. The swab is then put immediately into the transport tube and shipped to the laboratory. This is the same collection kit used for the *Chlamydia trachomatis* probe assay. A single swab specimen from each patient is sufficient to test for both *N. gonorrhoeae* and *C. trachomatis*.

Storage Instructions The specimens should be kept at room temperature or refrigerated. Do not freeze.

Causes for Rejection Contamination of specimen with urine

Turnaround Time Results are available within 24 hours of receipt of the specimen. However, most laboratories batch test every 2 or 3 days.

Reference Range Normal: Negative for *Neisseria gonorrhoeae* nucleic acid. A sexually active, asymptomatic female may harbor *N. gonorrhoeae* without overt clinical symptoms.

Use Rapid detection of *N. gonorrhoeae* in clinical urogenital specimens

Limitations Nucleic acid detection tests should not be done in child abuse cases. In these cases many laboratories perform more than one confirmatory test after culture of the isolate. The probe assay can be used to confirm the identification of organisms recovered by culture.

Methodology This test detects *N. gonorrhoeae* nucleic acid directly from swab specimens. This requires denaturation of the nucleic acid in the specimens by heating, hybridization with a specific nucleic acid probe, and detection of bound probe after several washing steps.

Additional Information Gonorrhea is a commonly reported sexually transmitted disease in the United States. The disease is manifest as acute urethritis in males and as cervicitis in females. *N. gonorrhoeae* can be isolated from asymptomatic females. Treatment of these individuals is critical because gonorrhea can result in more serious complications such as pelvic inflammatory disease, sterility, and ectopic pregnancy.

It is very important to control the spread of this disease between sexual partners, thus the use of a quick, reliable test system is essential. The DNA detection assay has a sensitivity and a specificity equal to traditional methods of organism isolation and identification. The current definitive method of detection for *N. gonorrhoeae* is the culture of the microorganism. However, this organism is fastidious and can be difficult to grow in culture when an established laboratory is not available. Loss of viability and overgrowth of contaminating microorganisms may limit recovery of *N. gonorrhoeae* by culture from clinical specimens that must be transported to a referral laboratory.

The major disadvantage of the probe method at the present time is that this test cannot be done in child abuse cases. These cases must be documented with the recovery of *N. gonorrhoeae* organism from the clinical specimen.

Selected Readings
Panke ES, Yang LI, Leist PA, et al, "Comparison of Gen-Probe DNA Probe Test and Culture for the Detection of *Neisseria gonorrhoeae* in Endocervical Specimens," *J Clin Microbiol*, 1991, 29(5):883-8.

Neisseria gonorrhoeae Culture

Related Information
Genital Culture *on page 423*
Genital Culture for *Ureaplasma urealyticum* *on page 424*
Neisseria gonorrhoeae by Nucleic Acid Probe *on previous page*
Penicillinase Test *on page 517*

Synonyms GC Culture; Gonorrhea Culture

Applies to Cervix Culture *Neisseria gonorrhoeae*; GC Culture, Throat; Gonorrhea Culture, Throat; Prostatic Fluid Culture *Neisseria gonorrhoeae*; Synovial Fluid Culture for *Neisseria gonorrhoeae*, Only; Throat Culture for *Neisseria gonorrhoeae*; Urethral Culture for *Neisseria gonorrhoeae*; Urine Culture, First Voided, for *Neisseria gonorrhoeae*; Vaginal Culture *Neisseria gonorrhoeae*

Selection of Culture Sites for the Isolation of *Neisseria gonorrhoeae*

Culture Site	Diagnostic Sensitivity (%)
Female (nonhysterectomized)	
Primary site	
Endocervical canal	86-96
Secondary sites	
Vagina	55-90
Urethra	60-86
Anal canal	70-85
Oropharynx	50-70
Female (hysterectomized)	
Primary site	
Urethra	88.9
Secondary sites	
Vagina	55.7
Anal canal	40.7
Male (heterosexuals)	
Primary site	
Urethra	94-98 (symptomatic)
	84 (asymptomatic)
Male (homosexuals)	
Primary sites	
Urethra	60-98
Anal canal	40-85
Oropharynx	50-70

From Ehret JM and Knapp JS, "Gonorrhea," *Clin Lab Med*, 1989, 9:445-80, with permission.

(Continued)

Neisseria gonorrhoeae Culture *(Continued)*

Patient Preparation Preparation same as for clean catch urine. See listing Urine Culture, Clean Catch *on page 565* for detailed information. *Neisseria gonorrhoeae* is very sensitive to lubricants and disinfectants. If possible avoid collecting urethral specimens until at least 1 hour after urinating.

Special Instructions The laboratory should be informed of the specific request for culture of *Neisseria gonorrhoeae* only, and the collection time, date, specific site of specimen, age of patient, current antibiotic therapy, and clinical diagnosis.

Specimen Body fluid, discharge, pus, swab of genital lesions, urethral discharge (best when available for men); endocervix (best when available for female); sediment of first 10 mL of centrifuged urine collected at least 2 hours after last micturition or first few drops of urine voided into a sterile cup for "first voided urine specimen" for asymptomatic males, or first void overnight urine, centrifuged. See table on previous page.

Container Swab with transport medium or sterile container if transported to laboratory within a few minutes; otherwise, direct planting on **room temperature** transgrow medium, Jembec™, NYC, or Thayer-Martin medium

Collection

Urethral discharge: Collect male urethral discharge by endourethral swab after stripping toward the orifice to express exudate.

Rectal swab: Collect anorectal specimens from the crypts just inside the anal ring. Direct visualization with anoscopy is useful. Insert the swab past the anal sphincter. Move the swab circumferentially around the anal crypts. Allow 15-30 seconds for organisms to adsorb onto the swab. Replace the swab and crush the media compartment. Prostatic fluid yields fewer positives than does culture of urethral discharge. Cultures from the urethra or vagina are indicated from females when endocervical culture is not possible.

Endocervical/cervical: Gently compress cervix between speculum blades to express any endocervical exudate. Swab in a circular pattern.

Bartholin gland: Express exudate from duct. Abscesses should be aspirated with needle and syringe.

Urethra in women: Massage the urethra against the pubic symphysis to express discharge or use endourethral swab.

Vagina: Obtain the specimen from the vaginal vault. Allow 15-30 seconds for organisms to adsorb onto the swab.

The specimen should be transported to laboratory within 1 hour of collection.

Storage Instructions Specimen **must not** be refrigerated or exposed to a cold environment. If the specimen is directly inoculated on Thayer-Martin medium it should be transported to the laboratory as soon as possible and placed directly in CO_2 incubator or candle jar.

Causes for Rejection Specimen not received in appropriate container, refrigerated specimens

Turnaround Time Preliminary reports are usually available at 24 hours. Cultures with no growth are commonly reported after 48 hours. Cultures from which *N. gonorrhoeae* is isolated require a minimum of 48 hours for completion.

Reference Range No *Neisseria gonorrhoeae* isolated

Use Isolate and identify *Neisseria gonorrhoeae*, establish the diagnosis of gonorrhea

Limitations See table on previous page. Cultures are usually screened only for *Neisseria gonorrhoeae*. No other organisms are usually identified. Overgrowth by *Proteus* and yeast may make it impossible to rule out presence of *N. gonorrhoeae*. The vancomycin in Thayer-Martin media may inhibit some stains of *N. gonorrhoeae*. Nongonococcal urethritis may be caused by *Ureaplasma urealyticum*, *Corynebacterium genitalium* type 1, *Trichomonas vaginalis*, *Chlamydia trachomatis*, herpes simplex virus, and rarely, *Candida albicans*.

Methodology Culture on selective medium, Thayer-Martin or NYC. Nucleic acid probes, monoclonal antibodies and enzyme-linked immunoassays are used as alternatives to culture in some laboratories. Advantages of the newer methods over traditional culture and smear techniques are not universally recognized.

Additional Information Thirty percent to 50% of patients infected with *N. gonorrhoeae* are also infected with *Chlamydia trachomatis*. In high prevalence populations, the recovery of *N. gonorrhoeae* is as follows: endocervix > urine sediment

> anal canal > pharynx. A serologic test for syphilis (VDRL, RPR, or ART), HIV, and cervical/vaginal cytology should be considered in patients suspected of having gonorrhea.

Selected Readings
Judson FN, "Gonorrhea," *Med Clin North Am*, 1990, 74(6):1353-66.

***Neisseria gonorrhoeae* DNA Detection Test** *see Neisseria gonorrhoeae by Nucleic Acid Probe on page 500*

***Neisseria gonorrhoeae* Susceptibility Testing** *see Penicillinase Test on page 517*

Nigrosin Preparation *see India Ink Preparation on page 460*

Nitrite, Urine

Related Information
Leukocyte Esterase, Urine *on page 473*
Lyme Disease Serology by Western Blot *on page 482*

Synonyms Bacteria Screen, Urine

Test Includes This test is usually part of a routine urinalysis

Abstract A rapid method for detection of bacteriuria. A positive test indicates the presence of bacteria which reduce urinary nitrate to nitrite.

Specimen Urine, first morning specimen is preferred; random urine is acceptable; preferably midstream, clean catch collection

Container Plastic urine container

Storage Instructions If the specimen cannot be processed within 2 hours it should be refrigerated.

Reference Range Negative

Use Detect the presence of potentially significant bacteriuria; aid to the diagnosis of cystitis, pyelonephritis, urinary tract infection

Limitations This test is not specific. The sensitivity of the nitrite test is decreased with high urine specific gravity and with high urine ascorbic acid content. False-negatives are relatively common and relate to varying retention times of urine in the bladder, varying urinary nitrate concentrations (diet dependent) and the presence and quantity of nitrate reducing organisms present. Storage of sample at room temperature for excessive periods (more than 2 hours) may lead to reduction of nitrite to nitrogen.

Some urinary tract infections are caused by organisms which do not contain reductase to convert nitrate to nitrite. These include infections caused by *Enterococcus faecalis* and other gram-positive cocci, *N. gonorrhoeae*, *M. tuberculosis*. Negative results are found when infecting organisms do not convert nitrate to nitrite. In addition, urine may not have been retained in the bladder for 4 hours or more to allow adequate reduction of nitrate to occur.

Methodology This reaction depends upon the conversion of nitrate to nitrite by the action of certain species of urinary bacteria. Nitrite from the urine reacts with p-arsanilic acid forming a diazonium compound. The diazonium compound couples with 1,2,3,4-tetrahydrobenzo(h)quinolin-3-ol.

Additional Information A positive nitrite test is strongly suggestive of urinary tract infection (ie, ≥10^5 organisms/mL). Therefore, when positive, a urine culture is recommended, but urine culture is indicated in any case if the patient is symptomatic. The use of nitrate and leukocyte esterase together is more extensively discussed in the listing Leukocyte Esterase, Urine *on page 473*.

Selected Readings
Damato JJ, Garis J, Hawley RJ, et al, "Comparative Leukocyte Esterase-Nitrite and BAC-T-SCREEN Studies Using Single and Multiple Urine Volumes," *Arch Pathol Lab Med*, 1988, 112(5):533-5.

Nits Identification *see Arthropod Identification on page 334*

Nizoral *see Ketoconazole Level on page 466*

Nocardia Culture, All Sites

Related Information
Acid-Fast Stain, Modified, *Nocardia* Species *on page 307*
Actinomyces Culture, All Sites *on page 308*

Test Includes Culture for *Nocardia* sp and direct microscopic examination of Gram's stain for branching gram-positive bacilli, modified acid-fast stain

Abstract *Nocardia asteroides*, *N. brasiliensis*, and *N. caviae* cause two disease entities, nocardiosis and mycetoma. The latter relates to trauma.
(Continued)

Nocardia Culture, All Sites *(Continued)*

Special Instructions Consultation with laboratory prior to collection of the specimen is recommended when nocardiosis is suspected clinically. Culture should be specifically ordered as Culture for *Nocardia*.

Specimen Pus, tissue, cerebrospinal fluid or other body fluid, aspirate, sputum. The usual portal of entry is the lung. Swabs are vastly inferior to aspirates and/or tissue specimens.

Collection Refer to listing for culture of specific site for complete collection and storage instructions (eg, Biopsy or Body Fluid Culture, Sputum Culture, or Wound Culture).

Turnaround Time Negative cultures are reported after 2-4 weeks.

Reference Range No *Nocardia* sp isolated

Critical Values *Nocardia* sp recovered from a central nervous system specimen

Use Establish the diagnosis of nocardiosis

Limitations *Nocardia* sp will not be recovered by routine culture techniques because of its relatively slow growth. Growth of *Nocardia* may be obscured by overgrowth of other organisms in mixed culture (ie, sputum). The diagnosis may not be made unless the laboratory is advised of the clinical suspicion of nocardiosis. *Nocardia* sp are not strongly gram-positive, but their branching pattern when visible is helpful. A modified acid-fast stain (see Acid-Fast Stain, Modified, *Nocardia* Species *on page 307*) is needed, since *Nocardia* are weakly acid-fast and may not be found with conventional acid-fast staining. Staining may be positive when cultures fail. Repeated sputum cultures may not yield a diagnosis of pulmonary nocardiosis. Bronchoscopic biopsy, transtracheal aspiration, or fine needle biopsy is often required.

Methodology Aerobic culture on blood agar and Löwenstein-Jensen (LJ) media with no antibiotics. Recent data supports the use of *Legionella* culture media (selective and nonselective buffered charcoal yeast agar) for recovery of *Nocardia*. *Nocardia* sp can also be cultured on noninhibitory fungal media. Cultures are usually held for 10-30 days. Cultures for *Nocardia* often need to be decontaminated similar to the decontamination process for *Mycobacterium*.

Additional Information *Nocardia* sp are aerobic, gram-positive bacteria which are filamentous, relatively slow growing, and variably acid fast. Human infection is seen most frequently in patients whose immune systems are suppressed by HIV infection, lymphoreticular malignancy, or chemotherapy. Nocardiosis frequently affects debilitated hosts and has been implicated in cases of infections in renal transplant patients, osteomyelitis, in patients on long-term steroid therapy and with peritonsillar abscess, and in cutaneous infections. The clinical picture may be similar to that observed with systemic mycobacterial or fungal infections. Infections may be acute, subacute, or chronic; and they may be disseminated or localized to cutaneous sites or the respiratory tract. Hematogenous dissemination occurs. Metastatic infection in brain, bone, skin, or subcutaneous infection in the presence of pulmonary involvement is suggestive of nocardiosis. *Nocardia asteroides* is the species most commonly recovered from clinical specimens and is usually associated with the respiratory tract; this species is phenotypically heterogeneous, and it has been proposed that the species be considered a complex which is subdivided. *Nocardia brasiliensis* and *Nocardia caviae* also produce human infections; of the two, *Nocardia brasiliensis* is far more common. The species found in mycetoma is usually *N. brasiliensis*.

Nocardia sp are variably acid-fast and may be frequently confused with *Actinomyces* sp or saprophytic fungi in Gram's stains of clinical specimens. Prognosis is dependent on early diagnosis, treatment with appropriate antimicrobials, and the course of the underlying disease. In management of high-risk patients, a strong index of suspicion for the diagnosis of nocardiosis must be maintained.

Selected Readings

Bennett JE, "Actinomycosis and Nocardiosis," *Harrison's Principles of Internal Medicine*, 12th ed, Chapter 152, Wilson JD, Braunwald E, Isselbacher KJ, et al, eds, New York, NY: McGraw-Hill Inc, 1991, 752-3.

Chazen G, "*Nocardia*," *Infect Control*, 1987, 8:260-3.

Hellyar AG, "Experience With *Nocardia asteroides* in Renal Transplant Recipients," *J Hosp Infect*, 1988, 12(1):13-8.

Javaly K, Horowitz HW, and Wormser GP, "Nocardiosis in Patients With Human Immunodeficiency Virus Infection. Report of 2 Cases and Review of the Literature," *Medicine (Baltimore)*, 1992, 71(3):128-38.

Kalb RE, Kaplan MH, and Grossman ME, "Cutaneous Nocardiosis. Case Reports and Review," *J Am Acad Dermatol*, 1985, 13:125-33.

Kerr E, Snell H, Black BL, et al, "Isolation of *Nocardia asteroides* From Respiratory Specimens by Using Selective Buffered Charcoal-Yeast Extract Agar," *J Clin Microbiol*, 1992, 30(5):1320-2.

McNeil MM and Brown JM, "The Medically Important Aerobic Actinomycetes: Epidemiology and Microbiology," *Clin Microbiol Rev*, 1994, 7(3):357-417.

McNeil MM, Brown JM, Jarvis WR, et al, "Comparison of Species Distribution and Antimicrobial Susceptibility of Aerobic Actinomycetes From Clinical Specimens," *Rev Infect Dis*, 1990, 12(5):778-83.

Schwartz JG and Tio FO, "Nocardial Osteomyelitis: A Case Report and Review of the Literature," *Diagn Microbiol Infect Dis*, 1987, 8:37-46, (review).

Vickers RM, Rihs JD, and Yu VL, "Clinical Demonstration of Isolation of *Nocardia asteroides* on Buffered Charcoal-Yeast Extract Media," *J Clin Microbiol*, 1992, 30(1):227-8.

Wallace RJ Jr, Brown BA, Tsukamura M, et al, "Clinical and Laboratory Features of *Nocardia nova*," *J Clin Microbiol*, 1991, 29(11):2407-11.

Wilson JP, Turner HR, Kirchner KA, et al, "Nocardial Infections in Renal Transplant Recipients," *Medicine (Baltimore)*, 1989, 68(1):38-57.

Nocardia Species Modified Acid-Fast Stain *see* Acid-Fast Stain, Modified, Nocardia Species *on page 307*

Non-A, Non-B Hepatitis *see* Hepatitis C Serology *on page 437*

Nucleic Acid Amplification *see* Polymerase Chain Reaction *on page 523*

Occult Blood, Semiquantitative, Urine *see* Urinalysis *on page 562*

Ocular Cytology

Synonyms *Chlamydia* Smear; Conjunctival Smear; Corneal Smear; Eye Smear for Cytology

Applies to Inclusion Conjunctivitis

Test Includes Papanicolaou stain and/or Giemsa stain

Specimen Direct smear of ocular lesion

Collection Swab lesion with cotton-tipped applicator or scrape with sterile ophthalmic spatula and smear on clean glass slides (2), **immediately** spray fix one slide, let other air dry. Label frosted end of slide with patient's name and date.

Causes for Rejection Inadequate fixation

Use Diagnose trachoma-inclusion conjunctivitis, adenovirus infection, vaccinia infection or herpetic conjunctivitis; evaluate possible dysplastic or malignant conjunctival lesions

Limitations The sensitivity of this test is very low. Positive results are only suggestive and should prompt subsequent culture.

Additional Information Diagnosis of viral and chlamydial infections is considerably improved by immunofluorescent and immunoperoxidase stains for organisms.

Selected Readings

Sanderson TL, Pustai W, Shelley L, et al, "Cytologic Evaluation of Ocular Lesions," *Acta Cytol*, 1980, 24(5):391-400.

Schumann GB, O'Dowd GJ, and Spinnler PA, "Eye Cytology," *Lab Med*, 1980, 11:533-40.

Ova and Parasite, Pinworm Preparation *see* Pinworm Preparation *on page 520*

Ova and Parasites, Stool

Related Information

Pinworm Preparation *on page 520*

Stool Culture *on page 540*

Synonyms Parasites, Stool; Parasitology Examination, Stool; Stool for Ova and Parasites

Test Includes Gross appearance, direct wet mounts, saline and iodine, concentration procedure, hematoxylin smear or trichrome smear

Patient Preparation Specimens obtained with a warm saline enema or Fleet® Phospho®-Soda are acceptable. Specimens obtained with mineral oil, bismuth, or magnesium compounds are unsatisfactory. Wait 1 week or more after barium procedures before collecting stools for examination.

Aftercare Warning: Any stool collected by or from the patient may harbor pathogens which are **immediately infective.**

Specimen Fresh or preserved random stool. If pinworm is suspected, a Scotch® Tape preparation should be submitted to the laboratory instead of stool. See also test listing Pinworm Preparation *on page 520.*

(Continued)

Ova and Parasites, Stool *(Continued)*

OVA AND PARASITES, AMEBAE

	AMEBAE						
	Entamoeba histolytica	Entamoeba hartmanni	Entamoeba coli	Entamoeba polecki[1]	Endolimax nana	Iodamoeba bütschlii	Dientamoeba fragilis[2]
Trophozoite							
Cyst							No cyst

[1] Rare, probably of animal origin
[2] Flagellate

Scale: 0   5   10μm

Amebae found in human stool specimens.

OVA AND PARASITES, COCCIDIA

CILIATE	COCCIDIA			BLASTOCYSTIS
Balantidium coli	Isospora belli	Sarocystis spp.	Cryptosporidium spp.	Blastocystis hominis
Trophozoite		immature oocyst	mature oocyst	mature oocyst	
Cyst		mature oocyst	single sporocyst		

0 20 40 μm   Scale: 0 10 20 30 μm   Scale: 0 10 20 μm

Ciliate, coccidia, and *B. hominis* found in human stool specimens.

OVA AND PARASITES, FLAGELLATES

	FLAGELLATES				
	Trichomonas hominis	Chilomastix mesnili	Giardia lamblia	Enteromonas hominis	Retortamonas intestinalis
Trophozoite					
Cyst	No cyst Scale: 0 5 10 μm				

Flagellates found in human stool specimens.

Container Plastic stool container. The collection procedure of choice is to provide patients with containers with polyvinyl alcohol (PVA) and formalin into which they can place stool. This procedure assures that the specimen will be well preserved. Degradation of parasites during transportation to the laboratory will be markedly reduced.

Collection The specimen should be delivered within 1 hour of collection to laboratory. Direct wet preparation exams for motile trophozoite observation can be performed on stools which arrive in the laboratory not longer than 1 hour after collection. The old recommended screening procedure is the automatic ordering of three random stool specimens; one collected every other day. The current, and much more clinically relevant, recommendation is a single specimen and obtaining its result; then the ordering of additional specimens if indicated. Specimens may be preserved in polyvinyl alcohol (PVA) fixative which is suitable for the preparation of permanent stains and formalin or merthiolate-iodine-formalin (MIF), which is suitable for concentration preparations and direct examination.

Storage Instructions Liquid specimens should be brought directly to laboratory. Wet mounts can be performed immediately and the specimen placed in PVA and/or MIF preservatives to maintain ova and trophozoite states when applicable.

Causes for Rejection Because of risk to laboratory personnel, specimens sent on diaper or tissue paper, specimen contaminating outside of transport container may not be acceptable to the laboratory. Specimen containing interfering substances, eg, castor oil, bismuth, Metamucil®, barium specimens delayed in transit and those contaminated with urine will not have optimal yield.

Turnaround Time Variable, depending on method

Reference Range No parasites seen

Use Establish the diagnosis of parasitic infestation

Limitations Note: One negative result does not rule out the possibility of parasitic infestation. Stool examination for *Giardia* may be negative in early stages of infection, in patients who shed organisms cyclically, and in chronic infections. The sensitivity of microscopic methods for the detection of *Giardia* vary. Tests for *Giardia* antigen and immunofluorescence tests have a higher yield.

Contraindications Administration of barium, bismuth, Metamucil®, castor oil, mineral oil, tetracycline therapy, administration of antiamebic drugs within 1 week prior to test. Purgation contraindicated for pregnancy, ulcerative colitis, cardiovascular disease, child younger than 5 years of age, appendicitis or possible appendicitis.

Methodology Wet mount and trichrome stain after concentration, immunofluorescence (IF), counterimmunoelectrophoresis (CIE), or enzyme-linked immunosorbent assay (ELISA) for the detection of *Giardia* antigens. The use of pooled preserved specimens to contain costs is acceptable.

Additional Information Parasite exams on stool from patients hospitalized ≥3 days are rarely, if ever, productive and should not be ordered unless special circumstances exist.

Amebas and certain other parasites cannot be seen in stools containing barium. Optimal diagnostic yield is obtained by the examination of fresh, warm stool by an experienced technologist, during usual laboratory hours. Amebic cysts, *Giardia* cysts, and helminth eggs are often recovered from formed stools. Mushy or liquid stools (either normally passed or obtained by purgation) often yield trophozoites. Purgation does not enhance the yield of *Giardia*. Stools which can be processed by the laboratory in less than 1 hour need not be preserved. Mushy, loose, or watery stools which cannot reach the laboratory within 1 hour should be preserved in formalin or merthiolate-iodine-formalin (MIF) and/or polyvinyl alcohol (PVA). Formalin will preserve protozoan cysts and larvae and the eggs of helminths. It is used for concentration procedures. PVA will preserve the trophozoite stage of protozoa. A trichrome stained smear may be prepared from PVA fixed material. PVA cannot be concentrated; therefore, they should always be accompanied by a portion of the specimen in formalin. Formed stools may be preserved in formalin, or refrigerated in a secure container until they can be transported to the laboratory. The collection/preservation kits will preserve protozoan cysts, helminth eggs and larvae. It is meant to be sent home with the patient and mailed back to the laboratory.

(Continued)

Ova and Parasites, Stool *(Continued)*

Parasites commonly identified in the stool of AIDS patients include *Cryptosporidium*, *Entamoeba histolytica*, *Giardia lamblia*, and Microsporidia.

Blastocystis hominis which is commonly observed in stool of healthy and symptomatic patients is not currently deemed to be pathogenic. The current consensus is that there is no convincing proof of a causal relationship between *B. hominis* and symptoms, that there is no correlation between resolution of symptoms with therapy or with the disappearance of the organism from stool, and that treatment directed at the indication of *B. hominis* is not indicated.

In a large children's hospital study of nosocomial diarrhea rotavirus, *C. difficile* and enteric adenovirus were recovered. Stool for ova and parasites and bacterial stool cultures yielded no pathogens.

Selected Readings

Brooke MM and Melvin DM, "Morphology of Diagnostic Stages of Intestinal Parasites of Humans," 2nd ed, *US Department of Health and Human Services*, Publication No (CDC) 84-8116, Atlanta, GA: Centers for Disease Control.

Miller RA and Minshew BH, "*Blastocystis hominis*: An Organism in Search of a Disease," *Rev Infect Dis*, 1988, 10(5):930-8.

Ova and Parasites, Urine or Aspirates

Synonyms Aspirates for Ova and Parasites; Parasites, Urine; Urine for Parasites; Urine for *Schistosoma haematobium*

Test Includes Wet preparation and concentration procedure

Special Instructions The laboratory should be informed of the parasite clinically suspected.

Specimen Freshly voided urine, sputum, aspirates, body fluid

Container Sterile urine container, sterile screw cap tube

Collection

Urine: The specimen should be less than 4 hours old and not refrigerated. The recommended screening procedure is to submit three first morning urines on successive days.

Sigmoidoscopic specimens: Mix material with 2-3 drops of PVA on a slide and allow to air dry. As an alternative, the material may be smeared on the slide and fixed immediately in Schaudinn's fixative. Please indicate on the requisition slip as sigmoidoscopic specimen and that the slide(s) has been fixed.

Material from suspected amebic abscess: Preserve in PVA fixative.

Sputum for ameba: Preserve in PVA fixative.

Sputum for nematode larvae or *Paragonimus* eggs: Preserve in formalin.

Duodenal aspirate: Centrifuge specimen if necessary (>0.5 mL) for 2 minutes at 1500 rpm. Examine sediment for motile organisms. Examination of motile organisms is best performed at the local facility. If specimen is to be sent to the laboratory, mix the sediment with 1-2 drops of PVA on a glass slide and allow to air dry. As an alternative, the material may be smeared on the slide and fixed immediately in Schaudinn's fixative.

Bone marrow aspirates: Submit alcohol fixed bone marrow films. Aspirates may also be submitted in EDTA tubes.

Storage Instructions Do **not** refrigerate. Transport to laboratory as soon as possible after collection.

Causes for Rejection Specimen more than 4 hours old, specimen sent on swab, specimen consisting entirely of saliva, specimen contaminated with urine and/or water, specimen containing interfering substances, eg, castor oil, bismuth, Metamucil®, barium (upper or lower GI); specimen refrigerated, specimen contaminated on outside of container, biopsy in formalin, specimen dried out

Turnaround Time Variable - depending upon procedure required

Reference Range No ova or parasites seen

Use Establish the diagnosis of parasitic infestation

Limitations The specimen will be examined for parasites only. One negative result does not rule out the possibility of parasitic infestation. Three specimens over 5- to 7-day period are desirable before a negative report is acceptable.

Methodology Saline preparation, iodine preparation, trichome stain

Additional Information Patient should have a geographic history consistent with schistosomiasis to warrant undertaking screening the urine.

Selected Readings

Tsang VC and Wilkins PP, "Immunodiagnosis of Schistosomiasis. Screen with FAST-ELISA and Confirm With Immunoblot," *Clin Lab Med*, 1991, 11(4):1029-39.

p24 Antigen

Related Information
HIV-1 RNA, Quantitative PCR, 2nd Generation *on page 452*
HIV-1 Serology *on page 454*
HIV Genotyping *on page 456*
Human Immunodeficiency Virus Culture *on page 459*

Synonyms HIV Core Antigen; HIV p24 Antigen

Applies to AIDS Antigen

Special Instructions Observe strict blood and body fluid precautions. In some states written or informed patient consent is a prerequisite for the test. Results may need to be kept confidential.

Specimen Serum or cerebrospinal fluid

Container Red top tube

Reference Range Negative

Use Diagnose recent acute infection with HIV; may also be of prognostic significance in AIDS, if antigen becomes positive during infection, after having been negative. (Can also be used to test viral culture supernatants.)

Limitations Test is not as sensitive as culture for detecting HIV infection.

Methodology Enzyme immunoassay (EIA)

Additional Information p24 antigen is a 24 kD protein product of the **gag** gene of HIV. As a viral, rather than host, product, it appears concomitant with initial infection, and then generally becomes undetectable during periods of viral latency. It reappears with renewed viral replication; the reappearance of p24 antigen in serum generally heralds progression of clinical disease in AIDS. Measuring antigen may also be useful in assessing therapy. It has not been recommended as a further screening test for blood products for transfusion. However, recent studies indicate that an acid dissociation procedure that disrupts the p24 antigen-antibody complexes can increase the sensitivity of the procedure up to fivefold. This may improve its diagnostic utility.

Selected Readings
Bollinger RC Jr, Kline RL, Francis HL, et al, "Acid Dissociation Increases the Sensitivity of p24 Antigen Detection for the Evaluation of Antiviral Therapy and Disease Progression in Asymptomatic HIV-Infected Persons," *J Infect Dis*, 1992, 165(5):913-6.

PA *see* Chest Films *on page 359*

PA and Lateral CXR *see* Chest Films *on page 359*

PACE2® *see Chlamydia trachomatis* by DNA Probe *on page 364*

PACE2® *see Neisseria gonorrhoeae* by Nucleic Acid Probe *on page 500*

Paracentesis

Synonyms Abdominal Paracentesis; Ascites Fluid Tap

Test Includes At the bedside, physician introduces a needle into the peritoneal space of a patient with free ascites, and samples the fluid for diagnostic and/or therapeutic purposes.

Patient Preparation Technique and risks of the procedure are explained. Premedications (eg, sedatives or narcotics) are not routinely required. Laboratory requisitions are completed in advance to avoid delay in fluid processing later. Prothrombin and partial thromboplastin times prior to paracentesis are ordered at physician discretion (some elect to transfuse fresh frozen plasma immediately prior to procedure if PT/PTT are prolonged).

Aftercare No special limitations exist for the patient postprocedure. If large amounts of ascites are removed (several liters), frequent blood pressure measurements are needed to monitor possible hypotension. Patients may ambulate postprocedure if vital signs remain stable. Occasionally, ascites fluid may leak persistently from the puncture site; in this instance, the patient should remain supine with the site angled directly upwards, until the leak stops spontaneously.

Special Instructions In clinical practice, paracentesis is at times performed on patients with significant hepatic encephalopathy. Additional personnel may be required for conferring with family members and for proper patient positioning during the procedure.

Complications The medical literature is divided on the incidence of complications from paracentesis. Earlier literature was more negative and tended to emphasize the possible complications, based on retrospective analysis. Some authors suggested that paracentesis itself was the cause of many cases of

(Continued)

Paracentesis *(Continued)*

ascites fluid infection. A recent prospective study concluded that paracentesis is a safe procedure, carrying <1% risk of major complications and <1% risk of minor complications. No deaths or bowel perforations were seen in 229 consecutive attempts. The most feared complication is needle perforation of an abdominal viscus or solid organ such as liver or spleen. Others include: intraperitoneal hemorrhage from laceration of an umbilical vein, scrotal or penile edema, abdominal wall hematoma, contamination of ascites by nonsterile technique. Hypotension can be seen when large amounts of ascites (>1500 mL) are removed rapidly.

Equipment Sterile gloves, drapes (optional), and adequate local anesthesia (26-gauge subcutaneous needle, 2% lidocaine). In clinical practice, various needles and angiocatheters are used. A 22-gauge, 1.5" metal needle with a plastic catheter is recommended. If a thick panniculus is encountered, a 3" to 5" 22-gauge needle may be substituted. Also required are a sterile 50 mL syringe and, if large volumes of ascites are to be removed, a sterile 1 L vacuum bottles with connecting tubing.

Technique Patient empties bladder prior to procedure. Physician confirms presence of ascites by physical examination with patient in a semirecumbent position. Preferred site of entry is in the midline, inferior to the umbilicus. If a midline scar is present from prior surgery or if percussion is not reliable, an area near the flank is selected. At times, physician may request patient to assume the hand-knees position if small amounts of ascites are present. The entry site is then caudad to the umbilicus. The site is prepped with iodine solution and skin and deeper tissues are infiltrated with lidocaine. The skin is retracted caudally and the 22-gauge needle (attached to syringe) is inserted into the anesthetized area and advanced while aspirating. When ascites fluid returns freely, the needle is held in position and not advanced further (avoiding bowel trauma). Multiple aliquots (50 mL) may be obtained in this manner. For larger volumes, the syringe is removed and connecting tubing is directly attached to the 22-gauge needle to allow drainage into vacuum bottles. Once the desired amount is collected, the needle is withdrawn quickly and the caudal skin retraction is released, allowing the skin to return to its normal position. This causes the entrance and exit needle sites to form a "Z-tract" which minimizes ascites leakage.

Data Acquired Ascites fluid is routinely analyzed for cell count and differential, chemistries including LD, albumin and protein, Gram's stain, bacterial culture, and cytology. Additional tests include special cultures for tuberculosis or fungi, ascites fluid pH, amylase, lipase, glucose, triglycerides, lactate, CEA, and hyaluronic acid.

Specimen When the procedure is performed therapeutically, the maximum volume of ascites that can be removed safely depends on the presence or absence of peripheral edema. It is recommended that in patients without edema, the upper limit should be 1500 mL. Patients with peripheral edema may tolerate larger volumes without hypotension (in one study, ≤5 L). When performed for diagnostic purposes, smaller volumes (50-100 mL) are adequate for routine studies. If malignancy or fastidious infection is suspected, larger volumes (>100 mL) will improve laboratory yield.

Container Lavender top tube for cell count; red top tube for routine chemistries; aerobic and anaerobic culture media bottles for bacteriology. For cytology, send sterile vacuum bottles with 5000 units of heparin added. If ascites fluid pH desired, send specimen to laboratory in an anaerobic syringe (gas bubbles removed) on ice.

Collection Some authorities recommend inoculating the bacterial culture media with ascites fluid immediately at bedside. The average concentration of bacteria in ascites fluid is very low in most cases of spontaneous peritonitis. In addition, a significant number of organisms may not survive in the time needed for specimen transport and plating in the Microbiology Laboratory. Bedside inoculation of appropriate media (standard blood culture bottles) may improve the chances of obtaining a positive bacterial culture several fold.

Normal Findings Ascites fluid is traditionally categorized as either "exudative" or "transudative" based on laboratory analysis. Transudative ascites is caused for the most part by cirrhosis physiology; that is, increased portal venous pressure or decreased portal venous colloid osmotic pressure. Examples of transudates include hepatic cirrhosis, congestive heart failure, constrictive pericarditis, Budd-

Chiari syndrome, inferior vena caval obstruction, and nephrotic syndrome. Exudative ascites is generally noncirrhotic in its pathophysiology and may be due to peritoneal membrane permeability defects. Examples of exudates include malignancy, spontaneous bacterial peritonitis (SBP), or other ascites infections (such as tuberculosis), vasculitis, pancreatitis, myxedema.

Critical Values Transudates are characteristically "low-protein" ascites and have been defined by ascites protein <3 g/dL; exudates >3 g/dL. Exceptions are common and other laboratory tests are often used in conjunction with the protein concentration. These include (for transudates): LD <200 units/L, protein ascites/serum ratio <0.5, LD ascites/serum ratio <0.6. Values outside these ranges support the diagnosis of an exudate. The "albumin gradient," defined as serum albumin minus ascites albumin, has recently been shown to accurately identify ascites caused by portal hypertension physiology (eg, cirrhosis). An albumin gradient >1.1 is considered transudative and is due to an oncotic (albumin) pressure gradient between the systemic arterial pressure and ascites fluid, as seen with elevated portal pressures. Exudates tend to have gradients <1.1. The early diagnosis of spontaneous bacterial peritonitis (SBP) prior to bacterial culture results can frequently be made on routine analysis of ascites fluid. Patients with SBP, or other ascites fluid infections, have ascites WBC count >500/mm^3 along with many polymorphonuclear (PMN) cells on the differential (>250/mm^3). In addition, two other laboratory indices suggestive of SBP are ascites pH <7.35 and ascites lactate <25 ng/dL. The clinical utility of these last two criteria has not been as well established as the standard PMN count. Many physicians will begin empiric antibiotics on the basis of PMN >250/mm^3 alone. Gram's stain of ascites fluid has low sensitivity for detecting SBP due to the low bacterial concentration, even on a centrifuged sample. Malignant ascites can be expected to have abnormal cytology in >50% of the cases. Indirect evidence of neoplasm include: grossly hemorrhagic fluid (may also be traumatic); ascites CEA >10 ng/mL with adenocarcinoma; ascites hyaluronic acid >0.25 mg/mL with mesothelioma; high ascites triglyceride levels with chronic chylous ascites (>80% of cases are lymphoma); ascites WBC count >500/mm^3 with peritoneal carcinomatosis (but PMN count low, <250/mm^3), pH <7.35, lactate <25 mg/dL. None of these values are considered diagnostic of malignancy and should be used only as supportive evidence.

Use Diagnostic indications include:

- patients with new onset of ascites
- ascites fluid of unknown etiology
- patients with clinically suspected ascites fluid infections (abdominal pain, unexplained fever, leukocytosis, declining mental status)

Therapeutic paracentesis is indicated when ascites fluid has accumulated enough to cause respiratory compromise, abdominal pain, or worsening of existing inguinal or umbilical hernias. Paracentesis should not be performed to diagnose the presence of ascites fluid. This should be known prior to the procedure (by physical examination or radiological imaging).

Limitations As described previously, the strict use of the ascites protein concentration alone in differentiating exudate from transudate has considerable potential for error. Multiple criteria should be considered, including the albumin gradient and relevant clinical findings.

Contraindications Severe coagulopathy not correctable by vitamin K, fresh frozen plasma, etc; inability of physician to demonstrate ascites fluid on physical examination; lack of patient cooperation. Recent literature suggests the following factors are **not** contraindications for paracentesis: morbid obesity, low grade coagulopathy, multiple abdominal surgical scars, and bacteremia.

Additional Information Paracentesis is a safe procedure when ascites is easily demonstrable on physical examination. When small amounts of ascites are present, a fluid wave may be difficult to demonstrate even when ≤1.5 L ascites are present. CT scan or abdominal ultrasound guided needle aspiration is particularly useful in these cases. Patients with ascites from cirrhosis may develop SBP and yet have minimal evidence of infection; some patients may be completely asymptomatic. A low threshold for performing paracentesis is recommended in this setting, despite the low-grade coagulopathy that frequently is seen.

Selected Readings

Bender MD and Ockner RK, "Ascites," *Gastrointestinal Disease*, 4th ed, Sleisenger MH and Fordtran JS, eds, Philadelphia, PA: WB Saunders Co, 1988.

(Continued)

Paracentesis *(Continued)*

Conn HO, "Bacterial Peritonitis: Spontaneous or Paracentric?" *Gastroenterology*, 1979, 77(5):1145-6.

Hoefs JC and Runyon BA, "Spontaneous Bacterial Peritonitis," *Dis Mon*, 1985, 31(9):1-48.

Kao HW, Rakov NE, Savage E, et al, "The Effect of Large Volume Paracentesis on Plasma Volume - A Cause of Hypovolemia?" *Hepatology*, 1985, 5(3):403-7.

Liebowitz HR, "Hazards of Abdominal Paracentesis in the Cirrhotic Patient," *N Y State J Med*, 1962, 62:1822-6, 1997-2004, 2223-9.

Mallory A and Schaefer JW, "Complications of Diagnostic Paracentesis in Patients With Liver Disease," *JAMA*, 1978, 239(7):628-30.

Pare P, Talbot J, and Hoefs JC, "Serum Ascites Albumin Concentration Gradient: A Physiologic Approach to the Differential Diagnosis of Ascites," *Gastroenterology*, 1983, 85(2):240-4.

Pinzello G, Simonetti RG, and Craxi A, "Spontaneous Bacterial Peritonitis: A Prospective Investigation in Predominantly Nonalcoholic Cirrhotic Patients," *Hepatology*, 1983, 3(4):545-9.

Rocco VK and Ware AJ, "Cirrhotic Ascites: Pathophysiology, Diagnosis, and Management," *Ann Intern Med*, 1986, 105(4):573-85.

Runyon BA, Umland ET, and Merlin T, "Inoculation of Blood Culture Bottles With Ascitic Fluid; Improved Detection of Spontaneous Bacterial Peritonitis," *Arch Intern Med*, 1987, 147(1):73-5.

Yang CY, Liaw YF, Chu CM, et al, "White Count, pH, and Lactate in the Diagnosis of Spontaneous Bacterial Peritonitis," *Hepatology*, 1985, 5(1):85-90.

Paracentesis Fluid Cytology *see* Cytology, Body Fluids *on page 386*

Parainfluenza 1, 2, and 3 Virus Culture *see* Parainfluenza Virus Culture *on this page*

Parainfluenza Virus Antigen by Direct Fluorescent Antibody

Related Information

Parainfluenza Virus Culture *on this page*

Parainfluenza Virus Serology *on next page*

Test Includes Testing of appropriate clinical materials for presence of parainfluenza virus antigen

Special Instructions Before ordering, contact laboratory to determine if this test is available. DFA test should be performed as soon as possible.

Specimen Appropriate specimens include nasopharyngeal wash (specimen of choice), respiratory secretions (next most useful), nasopharyngeal swabs (less useful), tracheal aspirates, sputum, appropriate autopsy and biopsy specimens

Collection Specimen should be received fresh, not in fixative

Reference Range Negative

Use Identify parainfluenza antigen in clinical specimens

Methodology Direct fluorescent antibody (DFA)

Additional Information This procedure does not depend on a changing antibody titer over time, and is diagnostic for the presence of virus (although the virus may not be the cause of the clinical illness in question). There is also a nonimmunologic cytologic change, ciliocytophthoria, which may be seen in sputum cytology and suggests parainfluenza infection.

Selected Readings

Waner JL, "Parainfluenza Viruses," *Manual of Clinical Microbiology*, 5th ed, Balows A, Hausler WJ Jr, Herrmann KL, et al, eds, Washington, DC: American Society for Microbiology, 1991, 878-82.

Parainfluenza Virus Culture

Related Information

Parainfluenza Virus Antigen by Direct Fluorescent Antibody *on this page*

Parainfluenza Virus Serology *on next page*

Viral Culture, Throat *on page 574*

Synonyms Parainfluenza 1, 2, and 3 Virus Culture

Test Includes Concurrent culture for other respiratory viruses (influenza, adenovirus, and respiratory syncytial viruses)

Specimen Throat or nasopharyngeal swab, nasopharyngeal washes and secretions

Container Sterile container; cold viral transport medium for swabs

Collection Place swabs into cold viral transport medium and keep cold. Infants and small children: soft catheters and suction devices (syringes and suction bulbs) can be used to collect nasal secretions (best specimens) as the catheter is withdrawn from far back in the nose. Another excellent method is to introduce 3-7 mL of sterile saline into the child's posterior nasal cavity and immediately aspirate the fluid.

Storage Instructions Keep specimens ice cold but **do not freeze specimens**.

Causes for Rejection Dry specimen, specimen not refrigerated during transport, specimen fixed in formalin, unlabeled specimen

Turnaround Time Variable (5-14 days) and depends on culture method and amount of virus in specimen

Reference Range No virus isolated

Use Aid in the diagnosis of disease caused by parainfluenza virus

Methodology Inoculation of specimens into cell cultures, incubation of cultures, observation of cultures for hemadsorption or characteristic cytopathic effect, and identification/speciation by fluorescent monoclonal antibodies specific for types 1, 2, or 3 or by virus neutralization

Additional Information Most virology laboratories hemadsorb all viral (especially respiratory) cultures at 14 days (prior to discarding the culture) to detect hemadsorbing viruses that have not produced cytopathic effect by that time. Positive hemadsorption tests are often reported preliminarily as "hemadsorbing virus present." This result suggests the presence of influenza, parainfluenza, measles, and/or mumps virus.

Serology for the detection of parainfluenza antibodies is available, but the results are often difficult to interpret.

Selected Readings
Waner JL, "Parainfluenza Viruses," *Manual of Clinical Microbiology*, 5th ed, Balows A, Hausler WJ Jr, Herrmann KL, et al, eds, Washington, DC: American Society for Microbiology, 1991, 878-82.

Wright PF, "Parainfluenza Viruses," *Textbook of Human Virology*, Belshe RB, ed, Littleton, MA: PSG Publishing Co, 1984, 299-309.

Parainfluenza Virus, Direct Detection *see* Virus Detection by DFA *on page 576*

Parainfluenza Virus Serology

Related Information
Parainfluenza Virus Antigen by Direct Fluorescent Antibody *on previous page*
Parainfluenza Virus Culture *on previous page*

Test Includes Antibody titers to parainfluenza virus types 1, 2, and 3

Specimen Serum

Container Red top tube or serum separator tube

Sampling Time Acute and convalescent sera drawn 10-14 days apart are recommended.

Causes for Rejection Inadequate labeling, gross contamination of specimen

Reference Range A single low titer or less than a fourfold change in titer in paired sera

Use Support the diagnosis of parainfluenza virus infection

Limitations Need for convalescent specimen delays diagnosis. Heterotypic rises in parainfluenza titers may occur in infections with other viruses. Infant antibody response may be undetectable.

Methodology Complement fixation (CF), hemagglutination inhibition (HAI), enzyme-linked immunosorbent assay (ELISA)

Additional Information Since the demonstration of a fourfold rise in antibody titer requires testing a convalescent specimen, serologic diagnosis is seldom useful in clinical management of an acute illness. This is especially so since the rise may occur even in an infection caused by some other virus. Serologic studies are of value in epidemiology. Rapid diagnosis during acute illness may be accomplished by demonstrating viral antigen in smears or tissue by immunofluorescence. Since parainfluenza virus may respond to ribavirin, prompt accurate diagnosis could become important, particularly in the immunocompromised host.

Selected Readings
Mufson MA and Belshe RB, "Respiratory Syncytial Virus and the Parainfluenza Viruses," *Manual of Clinical Laboratory Immunology*, 4th ed, Rose NR, de Macario EC, Fahey JL, et al, eds, Washington, DC: American Society for Microbiology, 1992.

Sperber SJ and Hayden FG, "Antiviral Chemotherapy and Prophylaxis of Viral Respiratory Disease," *Clin Lab Med*, 1987, 7(4):869-96.

Paranasal Sinuses, CT *see* Computed Transaxial Tomography, Paranasal Sinuses *on page 375*

Parasites, Stool *see* Ova and Parasites, Stool *on page 505*

Parasites, Urine *see* Ova and Parasites, Urine or Aspirates *on page 508*

Parasitology Examination, Stool *see* Ova and Parasites, Stool *on page 505*

Parvovirus B19 DNA, Qualitative PCR

Related Information

Parvovirus B19 Serology *on this page*
Polymerase Chain Reaction *on page 523*

Synonyms B19 DNA

Specimen Plasma, amniotic fluid, synovial fluid

Container Lavender top (EDTA) tube, yellow top (ACD) tube

Storage Instructions Separate plasma from cells and freeze.

Reference Range Not detected

Use Determine etiology of acute and chronic anemias, erythema infectiosum, and polyarthropathy; diagnose parvovirus infection as the causative agent for fetal hydrops; diagnose parvovirus infection in immunosuppressed individuals (HIV-infected individuals, transplant patients); diagnose parvovirus infection prior to seroconversion

Limitations Diagnosis of parvovirus infection should not rely solely on the result of a PCR test. A negative test result does not exclude the diagnosis of parvovirus infection. Sensitivity of test is 400 copies/mL.

Methodology Polymerase chain reaction (PCR) and enzyme immunoassay (EIA) in which DNA is extracted from the patient specimen and a viral DNA segment is then amplified by polymerase chain reaction (PCR). The amplified DNA is used as sample in an enzyme immunoassay utilizing a digoxigenin (DIG)-labeled probe specific for parvovirus B19. Results are reported as parvovirus B19 DNA detected, not detected, or indeterminate.

Additional Information Parvovirus B19 is an unenveloped single-stranded DNA virus which infects, replicates in and lyses red cell progenitors. Clinical symptoms of infection result from subsequent erythroid aplasia or from the host immune response. In children, the infection manifests as a nonspecific illness or with erythema infectiosum with a characteristic "slapped-cheek" malar rash. Parvovirus occasionally causes polyarthritis in adults and transient aplastic crisis may occur in patients with chronic hemolytic anemia (sickle cell, hereditary spherocytosis, beta thalassemia, etc). Although usually self-limiting, parvovirus infection may cause acute or chronic anemia in the immunocompromised host and is the leading cause of red cell aplasia in AIDS patients. In pregnant women, the infection may be transmitted to the fetus. Fetal anemia, hydrops fetalis, or fetal demise may occur in a small percentage of intrauterine infections.

In intense viremia develops 7-14 days after parvovirus infection. Clinical symptoms occur with the onset of specific IgM production, followed shortly by IgG production. Detection of parvovirus DNA is an earlier and more sensitive marker of viral infection than antiviral antibodies and should be used in conjunction with antiparvovirus IgM detection for optimal diagnostic sensitivity. Parvovirus DNA is especially useful for immunosuppressed patients in whom antibody levels may be undetectable.

Selected Readings

Alger LS, "Toxoplasmosis and Parvovirus B19," *Infect Dis Clin North Am*, 1997, 11(1):55-75.

Cassinotti P, Bas S, Siegl G, et al, "Association Between Human Parvovirus B19 Infection and Arthritis," *Ann Rheum Dis*, 1995, 54(6):498-500.

Clewley JP, "PCR Detection of Parvovirus B19," *Diagnostic Molecular Microbiology: Principles and Applications*, Persing DH, Smith TF, Tevover FC, et al, eds, Washington, DC: American Society for Microbiology, 1993, 367-73.

Clewley JP, "Polymerase Chain Reaction Assay of Parvovirus B19 DNA in Clinical Specimens," *J Clin Microbiol*, 1989, 27(12):2647-51.

Heegaard ED Myhre J, Hornsleth A, et al, "Parvovirus B19 Infections in Patients With Chronic Anemia," *Haematologica*, 1997, 82(4):402-5.

Jacobson SK, Daly JS, Thorne GM, et al, "Chronic Parvovirus B19 Infection Resulting in Chronic Fatigue Syndrome: Case History and Review," *Clin Infect Dis*, 1997, 24(6):1048-51.

Musiani M, Zerbini M, Gentilomi G, et al, "Parvovirus B19 Clearance From Peripheral Blood After Acute Infection," *J Infect Dis*, 1995, 172(5):1360-3.

Portmore AC, "Parvovirus (Erythema Infectiosum, Alplastic Crisis)," *Principles and Practice of Infectious Diseases*, 4th ed, Mandell GL, Bennett JE, and Dolan R, eds, New York, NY: Churchill Livingstone, 1995, 1439-46.

Torok TJ, Wang Q, Gray GW Jr, et al, "Prenatal Diagnosis of Intrauterine Infection With Parvovirus B19 by the Polymerase Chain Reaction Technique," *Clin Infect Dis*, 1992, 14(1):149-55.

Parvovirus B19 Serology

Related Information

Parvovirus B19 DNA, Qualitative PCR *on this page*

Synonyms Anti-B19 Parvovirus IgG Antibodies; Anti-B19 Parvovirus IgM Antibodies

Test Includes Assays for parvovirus B19 IgM and IgG antibodies

Specimen Blood

Container Red top tube

Storage Instructions Separate serum and freeze.

Use Diagnose parvovirus B19 infection

Methodology Radioimmunoassay (RIA) or immunoblot assay (Western blot) for the detection of IgM and IgG antibodies to parvovirus B19

Additional Information Parvovirus B19 is a DNA virus and can cause a wide spectrum of disease ranging from outbreaks of self-limiting erythema infectiosum (Fifth disease) to persistent bone marrow failure and fetal death. Intrauterine transfusion has been suggested when there is evidence of B19 parvovirus-associated hydrops and anemia. In most people the low-titer parvovirus B19 viremia, which begins approximately 1 week after exposure and lasts 7-10 days, is associated with mild symptoms and a subclinical red cell aplasia. Because the virus destroys erythroid precursor cells, which leads to a reduction in normal red blood cell production, infection with parvovirus B19 can cause a transient aplastic crisis in patients already at maximum red cell production and in those with increased red cell destruction (sickle cell disease, β-thalassemia, and spherocytosis). In immunocompromised patients, parvovirus B19 infection can cause life-threatening anemia. IgM antibodies are detectable 2 weeks after exposure. IgG antibody production usually occurs 18-24 days after exposure and is probably immune-complex mediated. The presence of IgM antibodies to parvovirus B19 provide definite evidence of recent infection.

Selected Readings

Cohen BJ, "Detection of Parvovirus B19-Specific IgM by Antibody Capture Radioimmunoassay," *J Virol Methods*, 1997, 66(1):1-4.

Gentilomi G, Musiani M, Zerbini M, et al, "Dot Immunoperoxidase Assay for Detection of Parvovirus B19 Antigens in Serum Samples," *J Clin Microbiol*, 1997, 35(6):1575-8.

Rodis JF, Quinn DL, Gary GW Jr, et al, "Management and Outcome of Pregnancies Complicated by Human B19 Parvovirus Infection: A Prospective Study," *Am J Obstet Gynecol*, 1991, 164(4 Pt 1):1363-4.

PAS Stain *see* Periodic Acid-Schiff Stain *on page 518*

Patella of Knee, Left or Right, X-ray *see* Bone Films *on page 343*

Pathologic Examination *see* Histopathology *on page 448*

Paul-Bunnell Test *replaced by* Infectious Mononucleosis Serology *on page 462*

PCR *see* Polymerase Chain Reaction *on page 523*

***Pediculus humanus* Identification** *see* Arthropod Identification *on page 334*

Pelvis AP, X-ray *see* Bone Films *on page 343*

Pelvis Stereo, X-ray *see* Bone Films *on page 343*

Pemphigus Antibodies *see* Skin Biopsy, Immunofluorescence *on page 538*

Penicillin Allergy Skin Testing

Synonyms Penicillin Skin Tests; Skin Tests for Penicillin Allergy

Test Includes Skin testing patients with suspected IgE-mediated penicillin allergy. The reagents used in this procedure are derivatives of the basic benzylpenicillin molecule. They are introduced into the epidermis by a skin prick or into the dermis by an intracutaneous (intradermal) injection. An immediate wheal-and-flare reaction confirms immediate hypersensitivity (Gell and Coombs' type I reaction). This is an important procedure in clinical practice and accurately identifies those individuals at high risk for a severe allergic reaction to penicillin.

Patient Preparation In some medical centers, penicillin skin testing is permitted only after formal consultation with the allergist performing the procedure. If the procedure appears necessary, the technique, risks, and benefits should be explained to the patient. As a preliminary screening measure, the physician should perform a brief dermatologic exam to ensure adequate areas of normal-appearing skin and to identify the rare patient with dermographism. Patient should be instructed to discontinue the following medications several days prior to testing: antihistamines, tricyclic antidepressants, hydroxyzine, phenothiazines. Newer antihistamines with extended half-lives may interfere with testing for over 1 week. All medication changes should be approved by the primary physician.

Aftercare If no complications have occurred, the patient may be discharged from the testing center following completion of the test. Skin sites should be kept clean but remain uncovered. Physician should be contacted immediately if (Continued)

Penicillin Allergy Skin Testing *(Continued)*

symptoms of wheezing, lightheadedness, or shortness of breath develop several hours later (the unusual case of the "late phase response").

Special Instructions If skin testing is performed by a nurse or physician-assistant, a physician should be immediately available for the rare case of anaphylactic shock. Emergency equipment must be in the testing area, including defibrillation equipment, intubation blades, lidocaine (and other cardiac medications), aqueous epinephrine for injection needles, syringes, and tourniquets.

Complications When properly performed, serious adverse reactions are unusual. The incidence of systemic reactions has been estimated at <1%, with the majority of these being mild or self-limited. Local complications are more common, but generally resolve within hours. These include subcutaneous hemorrhage, localized pruritus, and nonspecific irritant reactions. The risk of hepatitis B, local infection, or human immunodeficiency virus (HIV) transmission is diminishingly small since needles are not reused between patients. The "late response" is a rare but reported complication of allergy skin testing.

Equipment The reagents used for skin testing include:

- The "major determinant," a derivative of the benzylpenicillin molecule called benzylpenicillin-polylysine. It is standardized, commercially available, and routinely used.
- The "minor determinant mixture (MDM)," either benzylpenicillin itself or another derivative (such as penicilloate or penicilloyl-amine). The MDM has not yet been standardized and is not commercially available. Nonetheless, the MDM is widely employed by many allergists and is clinically relevant.

Both the major and minor determinants are administered in most cases. If the major determinant is used alone, 10% to 25% of allergic individuals could be missed. If the minor determinant is used alone, perhaps 5% to 10% of cases could remain undetected, including potential cases of anaphylaxis. In addition to these two reagents, positive (histamine) and negative (diluent) controls are often given. Standard tuberculin syringes, 27-gauge needles, and prick test equipment are also needed.

Technique Ideally, skin test reagents are applied first by the prick test, followed by an intradermal test if the prick test is negative. The prick test is carried out by placing a drop of the reagent in a predetermined location on the skin, usually the forearm. A small needle is passed through the drop and into the epidermis, then removed. For intracutaneous testing, each reagent is individually drawn up into a tuberculin syringe. Again, the volar aspect of the forearm is the preferred site for testing. The reagent (or control) is injected into the dermis, using a 27-gauge needle. A small bleb is raised, usually 0.01-0.02 mL.

Data Acquired Test sites are examined at 15-20 minutes for a local wheal-and-flare reaction. The largest diameter of the wheal and/or erythema is measured and recorded in millimeters.

Normal Findings No wheal or erythema after the major determinant, minor determinant, and diluent control. Administration of histamine control should result in a positive skin reaction, with induration >5 mm diameter.

Critical Values For both the prick test and the intracutaneous test, a wheal >5 mm in diameter (with erythema) is considered a positive test. For proper interpretation, the patient should be questioned regarding a history of penicillin allergy. If a reasonable history of penicillin allergy is obtained, a negative skin test essentially rules out a life-threatening allergic response to therapeutic doses of penicillin. No cases of anaphylaxis have been reported in patients who are skin test negative. However, ≤3% of patients who are skin test negative may develop minor reactions while on therapy, such as rash and pruritus. In the patient who has a positive skin test and a positive history of penicillin allergy, the odds of a serious allergic reaction to penicillin therapy are quite high, perhaps 50% to 70%. If skin tests are administered to patients who provide no history of penicillin allergy, the chances of a positive test are low (about 2%). Unfortunately, anaphylaxis during penicillin therapy has been reported in this patient population, although rare. Skin testing all patients prior to beta-lactam therapy, with or without a history of penicillin allergy, is not practical or cost-effective.

Use Theoretically, all patients about to receive a beta-lactam antibiotic should be skin tested. However, it has been demonstrated that such a comprehensive testing policy has a low yield and is not cost-effective. Most authorities recommend skin testing in the following situations:

- patients with a history of penicillin allergy who require penicillin as the drug of choice (eg, treatment of central nervous system syphilis)
- patients with a history of penicillin allergy who require a beta-lactam antibiotic (eg, semisynthetic penicillin, cephalosporin)
- patients with a history of multiple "antibiotic allergies;" skin testing can determine if a beta-lactam drug is a safe treatment option.

Limitations

- This procedure detects only IgE-mediated allergic reactions. Thus, a variety of adverse drug reactions may still occur in skin test negative patients, including serum sickness, drug fever, antibiotic associated colitis, interstitial nephritis, contact dermatitis, bone marrow suppression, and others.
- A number of factors can cause false-positive and false-negative results, as seen in other forms of skin testing.
- Test results apply to penicillin-type antibiotics (natural penicillins, semisynthetic penicillins), but not to cephalosporins, aztreonam, or imipenem.

Contraindications

- Documented history of penicillin-induced anaphylaxis, Stevens-Johnson syndrome, exfoliative dermatitis, or status asthmaticus. These conditions are life-threatening and contraindicate the use of penicillins in general; thus, there is little need to skin test.
- Recent use of medications known to inhibit the IgE-mediated skin response (wheal and flare); this includes antihistamines, hydroxyzine, tricyclic antidepressants, and phenothiazines

Selected Readings

Sarti W, "Routine Use of Skin Testing for Immediate Penicillin Allergy to 6764 Patients in an Outpatient Clinic," *Ann Allergy*, 1985, 55(2):157-61.

VanArsdel PP Jr, Martonick GJ, Johnson LE, et al, "The Value of Skin Testing for Penicillin Allergy Diagnosis," *West J Med*, 1986, 144(3):311-4.

Weiss ME and Adkinson NF Jr, "β-Lactam Allergy," *Principles and Practice of Infectious Diseases*, 4th ed, Mandell GL, Bennett JE, and Dolin R, eds, New York, NY: Churchill Livingstone, 1995, 272-8.

Weiss ME and Adkinson NF, "Immediate Hypersensitivity Reactions to Penicillin and Related Antibiotics," *Clin Allergy*, 1988, 18(6):515-40.

Penicillinase-Producing Organisms Susceptibility Testing *see* Penicillinase Test *on this page*

Penicillinase Test

Related Information

Antimicrobial Susceptibility Testing, Aerobic and Facultatively Anaerobic Organisms *on page 323*

Antimicrobial Susceptibility Testing, Anaerobic Bacteria *on page 327*

Neisseria gonorrhoeae Culture *on page 501*

Synonyms Beta-Lactamase Production Test; Cefinase (Nitrocefin) Testing; Cephalosporinase Production Testing; Penicillinase-Producing Organisms Susceptibility Testing

Applies to Beta-Lactam Ring; *Haemophilus influenzae* Susceptibility Testing; *Neisseria gonorrhoeae* Susceptibility Testing

Test Includes Rapid testing of isolated bacterial colonies for the production of beta-lactamase

Abstract Certain bacteria produce enzymes that inactivate beta-lactam antibiotics. Some enzymes can hydrolyze penicillin (penicillinases); others hydrolyze cephalosporins (cephalosporinases). In either case the detection of enzyme production by bacterial isolates is essential in determination of appropriate therapy.

Specimen *Haemophilus influenzae*, *Moraxella* (*Branhamella*) *catarrhalis*, *Neisseria gonorrhoeae*, enterococci, *Staphylococcus* species, or gram-negative anaerobic rods including *Bacteroides fragilis*

Use Rapid detection of beta-lactamase production from isolated colonies of *Haemophilus influenzae*, *Neisseria gonorrhoeae*, *Moraxella catarrhalis*, *S. aureus*, and enterococci sp. This test can be used to predict resistance to penicillins and some cephalosporins. Most isolates of *Staphylococcus aureus* produce beta-lactamases and thus, are often treated as beta-lactamase positive without testing for enzyme production.

Methodology The acidimetric method uses pH color indicators to detect increased acidity that results when the beta-lactam ring of penicillin is cleaved to yield a penicilloic acid. Penicilloic acid can also reduce iodine that can be detected as the decolorization of a starch-iodine mixture. This method is referred
(Continued)

Penicillinase Test *(Continued)*

to as the iodometric method. The most commonly used method is the use of a chromogenic cephalosporin reagent. The hydrolysis of the beta-lactam ring results in a color change that is quickly detected. The chromogenic assay can detect both penicillinases and cephalosporinases.

Additional Information The nitrocefin method is favored for anaerobes because it can detect both the cephalosporinases produced by *Bacteroides fragilis* and *Prevotella melaninogenica* (*Bacteroides melaninogenicus*), as well as, the penicillinases produced by other anaerobes. This is also the method recommended for testing *M. catarrhalis* and *S. aureus* isolates.

Plasmid-mediated production of beta-lactamase occurs in 5% to 15% of clinical isolates of *H. influenzae* type b. However, other mechanisms of resistance have also been reported. Routine testing of *H. influenzae* for beta-lactamase production is performed by most laboratories. Strains of *N. gonorrhoeae* producing beta-lactamase have been linked to contacts of patients acquiring the infection outside the United States and in prostitutes and sexual contacts of drug users. Incidence of penicillinase-producing *N. gonorrhoeae* has increased drastically in Florida, California, and New York. Routine testing of *N. gonorrhoeae* for beta-lactamase production is not routinely necessary in many parts of the United States, but should be considered in treatment failure cases and in areas in which resistance is endemic.

Selected Readings

Bell SM and Plowman D, "Mechanisms of Ampicillin Resistance in *Haemophilus influenzae* From Respiratory Tract," *Lancet*, 1980, 1(8163):279-80.

Handsfield HH, Rice RJ, Roberts MC, et al, "Localized Outbreak of Penicillinase-Producing *Neisseria gonorrhoeae* Paradigm for Introduction and Spread of Gonorrhea in a Community," *JAMA*, 1989, 261(16):2357-61.

Rosenblatt JE, "Susceptibility Testing of Anaerobic Bacteria," *Clin Lab Med*, 1989, 9(2):239-54, (review).

Stratton CW and Cooksey RC, "Susceptibility Tests: Special Tests," *Manual of Clinical Microbiology*, 5th ed, Balows A, Hausler WJ Jr, Herrmann KL, et al, eds, Washington, DC: American Society for Microbiology, 1991, 1153-65.

Penicillin Skin Tests *see* Penicillin Allergy Skin Testing *on page 515*

Percutaneous Biopsy of Musculoskeletal Lesions and Synovial Membranes *see* Bone Biopsy *on page 342*

Percutaneous Liver Biopsy *see* Liver Biopsy *on page 474*

Percutaneous Needle Aspiration Biopsy Under Fluoroscopic, CT, or Ultrasound Guidance *see* Liver Biopsy *on page 474*

Percutaneous Transtracheal Culture Routine *see* Aerobic Culture, Sputum *on page 312*

Percutaneous Transtracheal Fungus Culture *see* Fungus Culture, Bronchial Aspirate *on page 416*

Percutaneous Transtracheal Fungus Culture *see* Fungus Culture, Sputum *on page 419*

Percutaneous Transtracheal Mycobacteria Culture *see* Mycobacteria Culture, Sputum *on page 495*

Pericardial Fluid Culture *see* Aerobic Culture, Body Fluid *on page 310*

Pericardial Fluid Cytology *see* Cytology, Body Fluids *on page 386*

Pericardial Fluid Fungus Culture *see* Fungus Culture, Body Fluid *on page 415*

Periodic Acid-Schiff Stain

Related Information

Acid-Fast Stain, Modified, *Nocardia* Species *on page 307*
Antifungal Susceptibility Testing *on page 323*
Cryptococcal Antigen Serology, Serum or Cerebrospinal Fluid *on page 379*
Cryptococcus Serology *on page 380*
Cryptosporidium Diagnostic Procedures, Stool *on page 381*
Fungus Culture, Biopsy *on page 414*
Fungus Culture, Body Fluid *on page 415*
Fungus Culture, Skin *on page 417*
Fungus Culture, Sputum *on page 419*
Fungus Culture, Urine *on page 421*
Gram's Stain *on page 426*
Histopathology *on page 448*
Histoplasmosis Serology *on page 450*

India Ink Preparation *on page 460*
KOH Preparation *on page 467*
Methenamine Silver Stain *on page 487*
Skin Biopsy *on page 535*
Sporotrichosis Serology *on page 540*

Synonyms PAS Stain

Applies to Mucicarmine Stain

Test Includes Staining of organisms in smear or histologic section with periodic acid-Schiff stain (PAS)

Specimen Bronchoalveolar lavage (BAL), lung biopsy, aspirated specimen, histopathology specimen

Container Sterile suction trap, sterile container for culture, jar with formalin for histopathology, clean glass slides air-dried or fixed in 95% alcohol for smears

Collection Touch preparation smears may be prepared by touching 8-10 glass slides to the cut surface of the fresh lung tissue. The slides should be fixed individually upon preparation in 95% alcohol. Each slide should be labeled with the patient's name on the frosted end.

Reference Range No organisms identified

Critical Values Fungal elements identified

Use Detect fungal elements in clinical specimens, primarily tissue and sputum. Stains fungal elements well; hyphae and yeast can be distinguished relatively easily.

Limitations Takes 1 hour to prepare stain. *Nocardia* species do not stain reliably. *Blastomyces dermatitidis* may vary in appearance. Interpretation requires recognition of PAS-positive artifacts which may appear as yeast cells.

Methodology Periodic acid oxidation of the hydroxyl group in fungal cell wall carbohydrate and reaction with Schiff's reagent to stain the hyphae pink-red

Additional Information In addition to the PAS stain, the methenamine silver stain and the mucicarmine stain are useful for the identification of fungi in tissue. The mucicarmine stain stains the polysaccharide capsular material of *Cryptococcus neoformans* bright pink. See also the listings Skin Biopsy *on page 535* and Methenamine Silver Stain *on page 487*.

Peripheral Arteries and Veins Ultrasound *see* Ultrasound, Peripheral Arteries and Veins *on page 561*

Peripheral Blood Preparation *see* Microfilariae, Peripheral Blood Preparation *on page 489*

Peripheral Blood Smear, *Bartonella see* Peripheral Blood Smear, Thick and Thin *on this page*

Peripheral Blood Smear, Thick and Thin

Related Information

Microfilariae, Peripheral Blood Preparation *on page 489*

Synonyms Blood Smear for Malarial Parasites; Malarial Parasites; Malaria Smear; Thin and Thick Smears, Blood

Applies to Peripheral Blood Smear, *Bartonella*

Test Includes Examination of thick and thin smears

Abstract Malaria is still one of the most common infectious disease in the world. Its rapid diagnosis in the laboratory is extremely important. Although there are not many cases in the United States, with more world travel, it can be expected to increase.

Special Instructions If the patient has traveled to a malaria-endemic area the date and area traveled should be communicated to the laboratory. Most cases of malaria seen in the U.S. are found in foreign nationals traveling in the United States.

Specimen Fresh blood - fresh fingerstick smears (two or three of each thick and thin film type) made at bedside preferred, EDTA anticoagulated blood for saponin lysis. Contact laboratory for preparation of thick and thin smears.

Container Slides and lavender top (EDTA) tube

Collection Several samples should be taken during a 24-hour period until diagnosis is established or excluded.

Causes for Rejection Specimen clotted

Reference Range No organisms identified

Use Diagnose malaria, parasitic infestation of blood; evaluate febrile disease of unknown origin

(Continued)

Peripheral Blood Smear, Thick and Thin *(Continued)*

Limitations One negative result does not rule out the possibility of parasitic infestation. If protozoal, filarial, or trypanosomal infection is strongly suspected, test should be performed at least three times with samples obtained at different times in the fever cycle.

Malaria Species Infecting Human Red Cells

Plasmodium Species	Malaria	Length of Cycle (hours)
P. vivax	Tertian	45
P. falciparum	Malignant tertian	48
P. ovale	Ovale	48
P. malariae	Quartan	72

Methodology Microscopic examination of thick and thin Giemsa-stained smears. Thick films are more difficult to read and require considerable experience to interpret. Use of thick smears increases the number of cells examined in a given time period by a factor of about 12 because infected cells and organisms are concentrated. Screening by fluorescent microscopy using acridine orange and with gene probes have been described. Thin smears, although not as sensitive, are far superior for determining the species of *Plasmodium* on morphological grounds.

Additional Information Proper therapy depends upon identification of the specific variety of malaria parasite. Release of trophozoites and RBC debris results in a febrile response. Periodicity of fever correlates with type of malaria (see table). Organisms are most likely to be detected just before onset of fever which is predictable in many cases. Sampling immediately upon onset of fever is the most desirable time to obtain blood. Cases with a strong clinical history, which prove negative on initial laboratory screening, may require multiple sampling at different times in the fever cycle to document the diagnosis. Malarial parasites are destroyed in AS and SS patients. The cause of parasite death in AS cells is potassium loss, in SS cells Hb S aggregates destroy the parasites by physical penetration.

Changes in Infected RBCs Useful in Identification of Malaria Species

Plasmodium Species	Infected RBC Enlarged	Presence of Schüffner Dots	Presence of Maurer Dots	Multiple Parasites per RBC	Parasite With Double Chromatin Dots	Parasite With Sausage-Shaped Gametocytes
P. vivax	+	+	—	Rare	Rare	—
P. falciparum	—	—	+	+	+	+
P. ovale	±	+	—	—	—	—
P. malariae	—	—	+	—	—	—

Selected Readings

Krogstad DJ, Visvesvara GS, Walls KW, et al, "Blood and Tissue Protozoa," *Manual of Clinical Microbiology*, 5th ed, Balows A, Hausler WJ, Herrmann KL, et al, eds, Washington, DC: American Society for Microbiology, 1991, 727-50.

Pammenter MD, "Techniques for the Diagnosis of Malaria," *S Afr Med J*, 1988, 74(2):55-7.

Peritoneal Fluid Culture *see* Aerobic Culture, Body Fluid *on page 310*

Peritoneal Fluid Cytology *see* Cytology, Body Fluids *on page 386*

Peritoneal Fluid Fungus Culture *see* Fungus Culture, Body Fluid *on page 415*

Pertussis Culture *see* Bordetella pertussis Nasopharyngeal Culture *on page 349*

Pertussis Serology *see* Bordetella pertussis Serology *on page 351*

Phthirus pubis Identification *see* Arthropod Identification *on page 334*

Pinworm Preparation

Related Information

Ova and Parasites, Stool *on page 505*

Synonyms Enterobiasis Test; *Enterobius vermicularis* Preparation; Ova and Parasite, Pinworm Preparation; Scotch® Tape Test

Specimen Scotch® Tape slide preparation of perianal region

Container Scotch® Tape slide must be submitted in a covered container. Commercial kit products are also available for collection of pinworm specimens and are convenient, inexpensive, and highly recommended. **Caution**: Pinworm eggs are very infectious.

Collection The specimen is best obtained a few hours after the patient has retired (ie, 10 or 11 PM), or early in the morning before a bowel movement or bath. This collection procedure is essential if valid results are expected. Clear Scotch® Tape should be used. The nontransparent type is unsatisfactory. An 8 cm (3 in) piece of cellophane tape is placed over the end of a glass slide sticky side out. The anal folds are spread apart and the mucocutaneous junction is firmly pressed in all four quadrants. The tape is then pressed over the slide and the specimen is transported to the laboratory in a carefully sealed container. Refer to diagram.

PINWORM PREPARATION

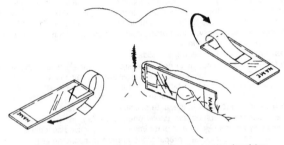

Cellophane tape slide preparation. Attach 3" piece of cellophane tape to undersurface of clear end of microscope slide, which has previously been identified (ground-glass end). Press sticky surface of tape against perianal skin. Then roll back tape onto slide, sticky surface down. Wash hands and nails well. From Bauer JD, *Clinical Laboratory Methods*, 9th ed, Mosby-Year Book Inc, St. Louis, MO: 1982, 989, with permission.

Causes for Rejection Use of nontransparent Scotch® Tape, Scotch® Tape on both sides of the slide, specimen which is not inside a covered container, use of frosted slide, tape sent sticky side up. Specimens which are not properly contained pose excessive risk to laboratory personnel and may not be acceptable to the laboratory.

Reference Range No pinworm eggs (*Enterobius vermicularis*) identified. Positives reported as few, moderate, or many eggs identified.

Use Detect cases of pinworm infestation (enterobiasis), *Enterobius vermicularis* parasitic infestation

Limitations Examination for pinworm only. One negative result does not rule out possibility of parasitic infestation. Stool specimens are not satisfactory for pinworm studies.

Contraindications Specimen collection at improper time

Additional Information The most satisfactory means of diagnosing pinworm infection is by the recovery of eggs or female worms from the perianal region. Only 5% to 10% of infected persons have demonstrable eggs in their stools. If feces is submitted for examination, only the surface should be sampled. Enterobiasis often is present in multiple family members. Therefore, it is recommended that all members of the family be tested. The responsible parent should be instructed how to collect samples using one kit per individual. Female worms or parts of them may be demonstrated on the tape by microscopic examination. Eggs, if present, may be immature, embryonated (with viable or dead larvae), or empty egg shells if the specimen is several days or more old. *Enterobius vermicularis* has been reported as a rare cause of appendicitis, salpingitis, epididymitis, and hepatic granuloma. Diagnosis at colonoscopy has also been reported.

Selected Readings
Bauer JD, "Parasitology," *Clinical Laboratory Methods*, 9th ed, St Louis, MO: CV Mosby Co, 1982, 987-9.

Pleural Fluid Culture *see* Aerobic Culture, Body Fluid *on page 310*
Pleural Fluid Cytology *see* Cytology, Body Fluids *on page 386*

Pleural Fluid Fungus Culture see Fungus Culture, Body Fluid on page 415

Pleural Fluid *Legionella* Culture see Legionella pneumophila Culture on page 469

Pleural Fluid "Tap" see Thoracentesis on page 546

Pneumocystis carinii Test

Related Information
Methenamine Silver Stain on page 487

Applies to Biopsy of Lung (Transbronchial) for *Pneumocystis*; Bronchial Aspiration for *Pneumocystis*; Bronchopulmonary Lavage for *Pneumocystis*; Induced Sputum Technique for *Pneumocystis*; Transthoracic Needle Aspiration for *Pneumocystis*

Test Includes Methenamine silver stain; toluidine blue stain and/or Giemsa and/or Wright's stain, or monoclonal antibodies to *Pneumocystis*

Abstract Diagnosis of *Pneumocystis* pneumonia in patients with or without AIDS.

Patient Preparation Induced sputum technique: Gargle with 30 mL 3% NaCl, then inhalation of 3% NaCl mist from an ultrasonic nebulizer for 5-15 minutes.

Specimen Lung biopsy, transthoracic needle aspirate, bronchopulmonary lavage or induced sputum technique

Container Sterile jar, clean glass slides

Collection When inoculating needle aspirate on slides, single drops should be applied. They may be alcohol-fixed or allowed to air dry without spreading. Biopsy specimens should be submitted in formalin. Jar must be labeled with patient's name, room number, date, and time. Slides must bear patient's name.

Causes for Rejection Inadequate specimen for diagnosis

Use Diagnose *Pneumocystis carinii* pneumonia (eg, in acquired immunodeficiency syndrome (AIDS) and other immunocompromised conditions)

Limitations *Pneumocystis* preparations applied to spontaneously expectorated sputum have an extremely low yield. However, in about 40% of individuals with AIDS and symptomatic pneumonia caused by other agents one may anticipate *P. carinii* in bronchoalveolar lavage fluid.

Methodology Methenamine silver stain (GMS), immunofluorescence, toluidine blue stain

Additional Information This organism is found in patients with clinical diffuse interstitial pneumonitis. Immunocompromised patients have a high incidence of *Pneumocystis carinii* infection (as high as 44% in some series). *Pneumocystis carinii* pneumonia may be, but is not always, rapidly progressive. It may be life-threatening, so that rapid diagnosis is important to allow prompt institution of therapy. *Pneumocystis carinii* is the most frequent cause of death in children with ALL in remission, such that some institutions routinely give prophylactic trimethoprim-sulfamethoxazole to their leukemic children undergoing antineoplastic therapy. It is also the most common infection and the most common cause of death in patients with AIDS.

Selected Readings
Cameron RB, Watts JC, and Kasten BL, "*Pneumocystis carinii* Pneumonia. An Approach to Rapid Laboratory Diagnosis," Am J Clin Pathol, 1979, 72(1):90-3.

Goodell B, Jacobs JB, Powell RD, et al, "*Pneumocystis carinii*: The Spectrum of Diffuse Interstitial Pneumonia in Patients With Neoplastic Diseases," Ann Intern Med, 1970, 72(3):337-40.

Kim HK and Hughes WT, "Comparison of Methods for Identification of *Pneumocystis carinii* in Pulmonary Aspirates," Am J Clin Pathol, 1973, 60(4):462-6.

Smith JW and Bartlett MS, "Diagnosis of *Pneumocystis* Pneumonia," Lab Med, 1979, 10:429.

Poliovirus Antibody see Poliovirus Serology on this page

Poliovirus Culture see Enterovirus Culture on page 405

Poliovirus Culture, Stool see Viral Culture, Stool on page 573

Poliovirus Serology

Synonyms Poliovirus Antibody

Specimen Serum

Container Red top tube

Collection Acute and convalescent sera drawn 10-14 days apart are required

Reference Range A fourfold increase in titer in paired sera is diagnostic; presence of neutralizing antibody indicates adequate immunization; normal <1:8

Use Support the diagnosis of poliovirus infection; document previous exposure to poliovirus (complement fixing antibodies); document immunization (neutralizing antibodies)

Methodology Viral neutralization, complement fixation (CF)

Additional Information Poliovirus may also be cultured, producing a characteristic cytopathic effect in cell culture. Culture is more suitable than serology for diagnosis of acute infection.

Selected Readings

Melnick JL, "Enteroviruses," *Manual of Clinical Laboratory Immunology*, 4th ed, Rose NR, de Macario EC, Fahey JL, et al, eds, Washington, DC: American Society for Microbiology, 1992, 631-3.

Polymerase Chain Reaction

Synonyms Nucleic Acid Amplification; PCR

Abstract The polymerase chain reaction is **not** a test; it is a method to amplify small quantities of the nucleic acid of a microorganism so the microorganism can be detected by other molecular biology means. The polymerase chain reaction is a molecular biology target amplification technique developed with much current and potential use in the medical laboratory. The technique was developed at the Cetus Corporation in Emeryville, California, and was first described for use in the prenatal diagnosis of sickle cell anemia. It may become as important as gene cloning itself. The PCR technique permits a numerous log-fold amplification of segments of DNA in several hours. The amplification is performed by multiple cycles of DNA polymerizing enzyme activity at the sites of known nucleotide sequences. (See figure on next page.) Thus, the nucleotide sequence of the gene to be amplified must be known so oligonucleotide primers flanking the region to be amplified can be synthesized. The method has continually expanding applications not only in prenatal diagnosis, but also for cancer and infectious disease detection and diagnosis.

Specimen The specimen for the PCR assay depends on the type of analysis. For example, prenatal diagnosis will require amniotic fluid or chorionic villus biopsy whole blood will be required for human immunodeficiency virus (HIV) detection, other specimens such as cerebrospinal fluid, sputum, serum, biopsies, or discharge from wounds for other infectious agents, or solid tissue by biopsy for cancer diagnosis.

Collection Varies with type of specimen. Methods of collecting, storing, and transporting vary greatly and depend on the microorganism sought and the laboratory performing the test. Consult the laboratory before ordering the test and collecting the specimen.

Use Uses in the laboratory include prenatal diagnosis of sickle cell anemia, hemophilia, cystic fibrosis, and muscular dystrophy, as well as oncogene activation in the case of lymphoma and chronic myelogenous leukemia. Numerous infectious agents such as *Mycobacterium* species, the agent of Lyme disease, and viruses, have been detected using this amplification technique.

Limitations The tests must be carefully monitored with appropriate controls (especially negative controls) due to the great sensitivity of the amplification technique which may lead to false-positive results.

Methodology The PCR technique requires knowledge of the base sequence of the target gene. From the sequence data, oligonucleotide primers, 25 nucleotides in length, can be constructed using oligonucleotide synthesizers. These primers flank a 100-2000 base sequence in the nucleic acid segment of interest. The primers are constructed so that the primers bind to opposite strands of the target double helix. A special thermostable DNA polymerase is used because it can withstand the many denaturing, reannealing, and polymerizing cycles without the need for replenishment. The reaction requires the target DNA, the primers, polymerase, and the four deoxynucleotide triphosphates. The mixture is heated several minutes to 95°C to separate the target DNA double strands. The primers are then allowed to bind to the target DNA at 50°C to 60°C and the polymerase reaction allowed to proceed for several minutes at 72°C. This cycle of denaturation, annealing, polymerization is repeated over and over as many as 25-35 times amplifying the sequence between the primers hundreds of thousands to millions of times (see figure on next page). The amplified DNA can then be detected by agarose electrophoresis followed by ethidium bromide staining. The amplified bands can be seen with a UV light and photographed for analysis.

DNA can be extracted from paraffin-embedded tissue for PCR analysis. Such tissue is best fixed in 10% formalin. Genotype can be ascertained by selective ultraviolet radiation fractionation.
(Continued)

Polymerase Chain Reaction (Continued)
Polymerase Chain Reaction Cycles

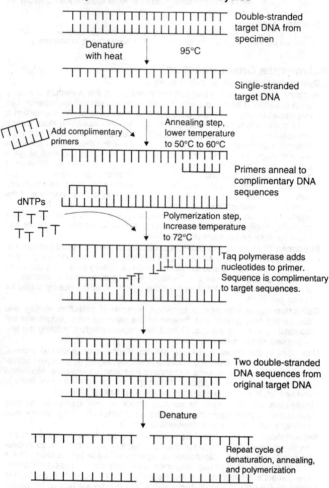

Double-stranded target DNA from specimen

Denature with heat — 95°C

Single-stranded target DNA

Add complimentary primers — Annealing step, lower temperature to 50°C to 60°C

Primers anneal to complimentary DNA sequences

dNTPs — Polymerization step, Increase temperature to 72°C

Taq polymerase adds nucleotides to primer. Sequence is complimentary to target sequences.

Two double-stranded DNA sequences from original target DNA

Denature

Repeat cycle of denaturation, annealing, and polymerization

Additional Information PCR is being expanded and refined. The procedure is automated with programmable heating blocks to cycle the reaction automatically. The technique has unprecedented amplification capability and is able to amplify nanogram quantities of target DNA and can, theoretically, be used to amplify the DNA from a single cell. Amplification reactions other than PCR are also being developed for use in the diagnostic laboratory.

Selected Readings

Crotty PL, Staggs RA, Porter PT, et al, "Quantitative Analysis in Molecular Diagnostics," *Hum Pathol*, 1994, 25(6):572-9.

Loda M, "Polymerase Chain Reaction-Based Methods for the Detection of Mutations in Oncogenes and Tumor Suppressor Genes," *Hum Pathol*, 1994, 25(6):564-71.

Mies C, "Molecular Biological Analysis of Paraffin-Embedded Tissues," *Hum Pathol*, 1994, 25(6):555-60.

Rogers BB, "Nucleic Acid Amplification and Infectious Disease," *Hum Pathol*, 1994, 25(6):590-3.

Shibata D, "Extraction of DNA From Paraffin-Embedded Tissue for Analysis by Polymerase Chain Reaction: New Tricks From an Old Friend," *Hum Pathol*, 1994, 25(6):561-3.

Popliteal Ultrasound *see* Ultrasound, Peripheral Arteries and Veins *on page 561*

Postexposure Prophylaxis for Hepatitis B *see page 1054*

Postreduction Films, X-ray *see* Bone Films *on page 343*

Potassium Hydroxide Preparation *see* KOH Preparation *on page 467*

pp65 Antigenemia *see* Cytomegalovirus Antigenemia *on page 386*

PPD Test *see* Tuberculin Skin Testing, Intracutaneous *on page 557*

PPLO Culture *see* Mycoplasma/Ureaplasma Culture *on page 499*

PPLO Titer *see* Mycoplasma Serology *on page 499*

Prostatic Fluid Culture *see* Genital Culture *on page 423*

Prostatic Fluid Culture *Neisseria gonorrhoeae* *see* Neisseria gonorrhoeae Culture *on page 501*

Proteus OX-19 *replaced by* Rocky Mountain Spotted Fever Serology *on page 529*

Pseudomembranous Colitis Toxin Assay *see* Clostridium difficile Toxin Assay *on page 367*

Pubic Lice Identification *see* Arthropod Identification *on page 334*

Purified Protein Derivative (PPD) Test *see* Tuberculin Skin Testing, Intracutaneous *on page 557*

Q Fever Serology

Synonyms *Coxiella burnetii* Titer

Special Instructions Acute and convalescent samples are recommended.

Specimen Serum

Container Red top tube

Reference Range Titer of less than 1:2; comparison of acute and convalescent titers is of greatest diagnostic value

Use Support the diagnosis of Q fever due to *Coxiella burnetii*

Limitations Reagents prepared from fresh isolates (phase I organisms) react differently from those from multiply-passaged organism (phase II)

Methodology Complement fixation (CF), indirect fluorescent antibody (IFA)

Additional Information Q fever shows no reaction in the Weil-Felix test with *Proteus* antigen, so serologic diagnosis must be based on specific rickettsial antigen. Convalescent sera react best with phase II organism (see above), but sera from chronic persistent infection react best with phase I organisms. Cross reactions with *Legionella* have been described.

Selected Readings
Eisemann CS and Osterman JV, "Rickettsia," Manual of Clinical Laboratory Immunology, 3rd ed, Rose NR, Friedman H, and Fahey JL, eds, Washington, DC: American Society for Microbiology, 1986, 847-58.
Hechemy KE, "The Immunoserology of Rickettsiae," Manual of Clinical Laboratory Immunology, 4th ed, Rose NR, de Macario EC, Fahey JL, et al, eds, Washington, DC: American Society for Microbiology, 1992, 667-75.
Reimer LG, "Q Fever," Clin Microbiol Rev, 1993, 6(3):193-8.

Rabbit Fever Antibodies *see* Tularemia Serology *on page 559*

Rabid Animals *see* Rabies Detection *on this page*

Rabies Detection

Related Information
Animal and Human Bites Guidelines *on page 1061*
Brain Biopsy *on page 352*

Synonyms Rabid Animals

Applies to Fluorescent Rabies Antibody Test; FRA Test; Negri Bodies

Test Includes Examination of animal brain for Negri bodies or inoculation of mice with suspension of brain tissue

Abstract Rabies has been a recognized disease in humans and animals for more than 25 centuries. Zinke is credited with first demonstrating the virus in 1804. Unlike many other viruses, the rabies virus is capable of infecting a number of different animal species, allowing it to propagate and survive in nature. Individuals with a high risk of contact with rabid animals (veterinarians, animal control officers, etc) should consider vaccination against rabies.

Specimen Head of large animal or entire small animal suspected of rabies. Use gloves and mask when handling an animal carcass suspected of rabies.

Container Sealed container

(Continued)

Rabies Detection *(Continued)*

Storage Instructions Ideally, animal brain should be examined in the fresh state. Transport using wet ice or place in absorbent material, then in two plastic bags, or, place half the brain in 50% glycerol, half in 10% formalin, depending on instructions from state laboratory. Local state laboratory must be consulted. Rabies virus may also be demonstrated by immunofluorescence in skin biopsies of patients suspected of having rabies (*vide infra*).

Causes for Rejection Unlabeled or improperly packaged specimen

Use Diagnose rabies; evaluate animal bites

Limitations Negri bodies are found in about 90% of rabid animals.

Contraindications Formalin fixation precludes fluorescent antibody application

Methodology Fluorescent antibody examination (but Negri bodies can be seen in H & E)

Additional Information Animals at risk for rabies include skunks, raccoons, dogs, cats, bats, cattle, foxes, and to a lesser extent, jackals, wolves, coyotes, mongooses, weasels, squirrels, and any escaped wild animal. Bites of rabbits, squirrels, hamsters, guinea pigs, gerbils, chipmunks, rats, mice, and other rodents have seldom if ever resulted in human rabies in the United States and are regarded as low risk. High risk species include bats, raccoons, skunks, and foxes among wild carnivorous animals.

Domestic animals should be kept alive if possible, to be quarantined. Animal bites, when unprovoked, are more likely to transmit rabies. Survival of animal for 10 days makes rabies unlikely. Signs of rabies among wild carnivorous animals cannot be reliably interpreted and any such animal that bites or scratches a person should be killed at once and the head submitted for rabies testing.

Rabies is a zoonosis caused by a neurotropic RNA virus which occurs in saliva, central nervous system, urine, and feces. Rabies virus produces Negri bodies (viral inclusions) in neurons.

The geographic area is important. Although a dog bite along the U.S.-Mexican border is considered a rabies exposure until proven otherwise, such bites in New York or Philadelphia are reported not to require prophylaxis. Most Americans dying of rabies were exposed in foreign countries. One patient, bitten by a rabid dog in Kenya, had even had pre-exposure prophylaxis with human diploid cell vaccine. This emphasizes the **necessity for postexposure therapy in appropriate cases.** Almost all rabies follows bite exposure. However, rabies virus can (rarely) enter through nonbite exposure, such as an open wound, or by inhalation of aerosolized bat urine (eg, cave explorers) or by corneal transplantation. The following table lists location of exposure to rabid canine bites and extent of exposure as it relates to mortality rates. The proportion of cases for which the source of exposure is not known has been increasing since 1960.

Representative Mortality Rates in Nonvaccinated Individuals Following Exposure to Rabid Canines

Location of Exposure	Extent of Exposure	Mortality (%)
Face	Bites (multiple and severe)	60
Other part of head	Bites (multiple and severe)	50
Face	Bite (single)	30
Fingers/hand	Bite (severe)	15
Face	Bites (multiple and superficial)	10
Hand	Bites (multiple and superficial)	5
Trunk/legs	Scratch	3
Hands/exposed skin	Bleeding and superficial wound	2
Skin covered by clothes	Superficial wound	0.5
Recent wound	Saliva	0.1
Wounds >24 h old	Saliva	0.0

From Whitley RJ and Middlebrooks M, "Rabies," *Infections of the Central Nervous System,* Chapter 7, Scheld WM, Whitley RJ, and Durack DT, eds, New York, NY: Raven Press, 1991, 134, with permission.

Antemortem rabies virus has been isolated from human saliva, brain tissues, CSF, urine sediment, and tracheal secretions. Rabies virus may also be demonstrated by immunofluorescent rabies antibody staining of skin biopsy tissue. The most reliable and reproducible of the immunofluorescent studies that can aid in patient diagnosis is biopsy of the neck skin. A 6-8 mm full thickness wedge or punch biopsy specimen from the neck containing as many hair follicles as possible should be sampled, snap frozen, and shipped frozen at -70°C to a reference laboratory. Consult with reference laboratory for shipping instructions. False-negative results do occur especially after the development of neutralizing antibodies.

Selected Readings

Bussereau F, Vincent J, Coudrier D, et al, "Monoclonal Antibodies to Mokola Virus for Identification of Rabies and Rabies-Related Viruses," *J Clin Microbiol*, 1988, 26(12):2489-94.

Center for Disease Control, "Compendium of Animal Rabies Control, 1990," *MMWR Morb Mortal Wkly Rep*, 1990, 39(RR-4):1-8.

Center for Disease Control, "Human Rabies - Oregon," *MMWR Morb Mortal Wkly Rep*, 1989, 38(19):335-7.

Center for Disease Control, "Rabies Prevention - United States, 1991 - Recommendations of the Immunization Practices Advisory Committee (ACIP)," *MMWR Morb Mortal Wkly Rep*, 1991, 40(RR-3):1-19.

Dietzschold B, Tollis M, Rupprecht CE, et al, "Antigenic Variation in Rabies and Rabies-Related Viruses: Cross-Protection Independent of Glycoprotein-Mediated Virus-Neutralizing Antibody," *J Infect Dis*, 1987, 156:815.

Fishbein DB and Baer GM, "Animal Rabies: Implications for Diagnosis and Human Treatment," *Ann Intern Med*, 1988, 109(12):935-7.

Fishbein DB and Bernard KW , "Rabies Virus," *Principles and Practice of Infectious Diseases*, Mandell GL, Bennett JE, and Dolin R, eds, New York, NY: Churchill Livingstone, 1995, 1527-43.

Mrak, RE and Young L, "Rabies Encephalitis in a Patient With No History of Exposure," *Hum Pathol*, 1992, 24(1):109-10.

Smith JS, Fishbein DB, Rupprecht CE, et al, "Unexplained Rabies in Three Immigrants in the United States. A Virologic Investigation," *N Engl J Med*, 1991, 324(4):205-11.

Whitley RJ and Middlebrooks M, "Rabies," *Infections of the Central Nervous System*, Scheld WM, Whitley RJ, and Durack DT, eds, New York, NY: Raven Press, 1991, 134.

Rabies Virus, Direct Detection see Virus Detection by DFA *on page 576*

Radionuclide Bone Scan see Bone Scan *on page 348*

Rapid Plasma Reagin Test see RPR *on page 530*

Rectal Swab Culture see Stool Culture *on page 540*

Rectal Swab Culture for Diarrheagenic, *E. coli* see Stool Culture, Diarrheagenic E. coli *on page 542*

Rectal Swab, Unusual Organism see Stool Culture, Uncommon Organisms *on page 543*

Renal Ultrasound see Ultrasound, Kidneys *on page 561*

Respiratory Syncytial Virus Antigen by EIA

Related Information

Respiratory Syncytial Virus Culture *on next page*
Respiratory Syncytial Virus Serology *on next page*

Synonyms RSV Testing

Test Includes Enzyme immunoassay for respiratory syncytial virus infection

Specimen Nasopharyngeal washes or aspirates, sputum, appropriate autopsy or biopsy specimens

Container Capped syringe

Collection Send specimen fresh, not in fixative. Tissues may be snap frozen.

Causes for Rejection Inadequate specimen

Reference Range No virus detected.

Use Identify respiratory syncytial virus, particularly in infants and young children

Limitations Inadequate specimen collection, improper sample handling/transport or low levels of virus shedding may yield false-negative result. Accordingly, a negative result does not totally eliminate the possibility of RSV infection.

Methodology Enzyme immunoassay (EIA)

Additional Information This test allows rapid diagnosis of the presence of respiratory syncytial virus. It avoids the necessity of obtaining acute and convalescent specimens over a 2-week period. It may be particularly useful in children younger than 6 months of age, whose antibody response to infection may not be diagnostic. However, it must be remembered that showing the virus is present is not equivalent to showing that it is causing a particular disease.

(Continued)

Respiratory Syncytial Virus Antigen by EIA *(Continued)*

Selected Readings

Hughes JH, Mann DR, and Hamparian VV, "Detection of Respiratory Syncytial Virus in Clinical Specimens by Viral Culture, Direct and Indirect Immunofluorescence, and Enzyme Immunoassay," *J Clin Microbiol*, 1988, 26(3):588-91.

Swenson PD and Kaplan MH, "Rapid Detection of Respiratory Syncytial Virus in Nasopharyngeal Aspirates by a Commercial Enzyme Immunoassay," *J Clin Microbiol*, 1986, 23(3):485-8.

Welliver RC, "Detection, Pathogenesis, and Therapy of Respiratory Syncytial Virus Infections," *Clin Microbiol Rev*, 1988, 1(1):27-39.

Respiratory Syncytial Virus Culture

Related Information

Respiratory Syncytial Virus Antigen by EIA *on previous page*
Respiratory Syncytial Virus Serology *on this page*
Viral Culture, Throat *on page 574*

Synonyms RSV Culture

Test Includes Concurrent culture for other respiratory viruses (influenza and parainfluenza viruses)

Specimen Throat or nasopharyngeal swab, nasopharyngeal washes and secretions

Container Sterile container; cold viral transport medium for swabs

Collection Place swabs into cold viral transport medium and keep cold. Infants and small children: soft catheters and suction devices (syringes and suction bulbs) can be used to collect nasal secretions (best specimens) as the catheter is withdrawn from far back in the nose. Another excellent method is to introduce 3-7 mL of sterile saline into the child's posterior nasal cavity and immediately aspirate the fluid.

Storage Instructions Respiratory syncytial virus is extremely labile. **Do not freeze** specimens and send specimens to the laboratory **as soon as possible.**

Causes for Rejection Dry specimen, specimen not refrigerated during transport, specimen fixed in formalin, unlabeled specimen

Turnaround Time Variable (1-14 days) depending on culture method and amount of virus in specimen

Reference Range No virus isolated

Use Aid in the diagnosis of respiratory disease caused by respiratory syncytial virus

Methodology Inoculation of specimen into cell cultures, incubation of cultures, observation of cultures for characteristic cytopathic effect in 2-7 days, and identification by fluorescent monoclonal antibodies specific for respiratory syncytial virus. The use of a rapid shell viral culture technique may yield positive culture results overnight.

Additional Information Serology is available to detect antibodies to respiratory syncytial virus. Many laboratories offer enzyme immunoassay (EIA) tests for the direct detection of RSV in patient specimens. In general, these tests are very rapid, sensitive, and specific.

Selected Readings

Hughes JH, Mann DR, and Hamparian VV, "Detection of Respiratory Syncytial Virus in Clinical Specimens by Viral Culture, Direct and Indirect Immunofluorescence, and Enzyme Immunoassay," *J Clin Microbiol*, 1988, 26(3):588-91.

Welliver RC, "Detection, Pathogenesis, and Therapy of Respiratory Syncytial Virus Infections," *Clin Microbiol Rev*, 1988, 1(1):27-39.

Respiratory Syncytial Virus, Direct Detection *see* Virus Detection by DFA *on page 576*

Respiratory Syncytial Virus Serology

Related Information

Respiratory Syncytial Virus Antigen by EIA *on previous page*
Respiratory Syncytial Virus Culture *on this page*

Synonyms RSV Titer

Specimen Serum

Container Red top tube

Reference Range IgG <1:5, IgM <1:5; less than fourfold rise in titer by CF

Use Establish the diagnosis of respiratory syncytial virus infection

Limitations Children younger than 6 months of age may not mount a diagnostic serologic response to infection

Methodology Complement fixation, enzyme linked immunosorbent assay

Additional Information Diagnosis by CF depends on demonstrating a rise in antibody titer over a 2- to 3-week period. As such, the test is seldom useful in planning clinical care in an acute illness. For rapid diagnosis the demonstration of viral antigen in nasopharyngeal washings or of IgM antibody is more useful.

Rhinovirus Culture *see* Viral Culture, Throat *on page 574*

***Rickettsia rickettsii* Serology** *see* Rocky Mountain Spotted Fever Serology *on this page*

Rocky Mountain Spotted Fever Serology

Related Information
Ehrlichia Serology *on page 397*

Synonyms *Rickettsia rickettsii* Serology

Replaces *Proteus* OX-19

Special Instructions Acute and convalescent specimens are recommended.

Specimen Serum

Container Red top tube

Reference Range Less than a fourfold increase in titer in paired sera; IgG <1:64, IgM <1:8

Use Establish the diagnosis of Rocky Mountain spotted fever

Limitations Cross reactions with other organism in the spotted fever group. False-positive reactions may occur during pregnancy, especially in the last two trimesters.

Methodology Complement fixation, immunofluorescence, hemagglutination, enzyme linked immunosorbent assay

Additional Information Rocky Mountain spotted fever occurs primarily in the southeastern and western United States from April through October, but is also endemic on Long Island. It is a disease of variable clinical manifestation (some cases present with few or no "spots"), and since there is good specific therapy, and serious outcome if untreated, all aids to diagnosis are important. Serologic diagnosis may be made promptly enough to direct therapy.

Hemagglutination and immunofluorescent tests are least subject to cross reactions with other *Rickettsia*. The complement fixation test can be used with different concentration of antigen to minimize cross reactions. Tests for IgM specific antibody are helpful in early disease, since they appear in 3-8 days. Patients treated with antibiotics early in illness may not develop serologic responses. A direct fluorescent test is also available to demonstrate the *Rickettsia* in tissue.

As many as 71% of patients with Rocky Mountain spotted fever also develop antibodies against cardiolipin and endothelial cells.

Selected Readings
Kaplowitz LG, Fischer JJ, and Sparling PF, "Rocky Mountain Spotted Fever: A Clinical Dilemma," *Current Clinical Topics in Infectious Disease - 2*, Remington JS and Swartz MN, eds, New York, NY: McGraw-Hill Book Co, 1981, 89-108.
Salgo MP, Telzak EE, Currie B, et al, "A Focus of Rocky Mountain Spotted Fever Within New York City," *N Engl J Med*, 1988, 318(21):1345-8.
Sexton DJ and Corey GR, "Rocky Mountain 'Spotless' and 'Almost Spotless' Fever: A Wolf in Sheep's Clothing," *Clin Infect Dis*, 1992, 15(3):439-48.

Rose Handlers Disease *see* Sporotrichosis Serology *on page 540*

Rotavirus Detection by EM *see* Electron Microscopic (EM) Examination for Viruses, Stool *on page 403*

Rotavirus, Direct Detection

Synonyms Rotavirus Rapid Detection

Applies to Viral Antigen Detection, Direct, Stool

Test Includes Direct (nonculture) detection of rotavirus in stool specimens

Specimen Stool from the acute, diarrheal phase of disease

Container Sterile container

Sampling Time As soon as possible after onset of disease, preferably 3 to 5 days after onset

Collection Several specimens during the course of illness should be submitted in an attempt to eliminate false-negative results.

Causes for Rejection Excessive transit time to laboratory, unlabeled specimen

Turnaround Time 1 day

Reference Range No virus detected

(Continued)

Rotavirus, Direct Detection *(Continued)*

Use Detect rotavirus in stools of patients suspected of having viral gastroenteritis

Limitations Quality of specimens cannot be evaluated, and specimens are collected randomly.

Methodology Commercially available (and often automated) enzyme immunoassays (EIA) are the preferred diagnostic methods. Commercial kits have not been standardized.

Additional Information Rotavirus is an extremely common cause of pediatric gastroenteritis. The illness is most common in winter, is highly contagious, involves 5-8 days of diarrhea, and is rarely fatal. Patients should also be evaluated for possible bacterial gastroenteritis.

Selected Readings

Christensen ML, "Human Viral Gastroenteritis," *Clin Microbiol Rev*, 1989, 2(1):51-89.

Gray LD, "Novel Viruses Associated With Gastroenteritis," *Clin Microbiol Newslett*, 1991, 13(18):137-44.

Yolken RH, "Enzyme Immunoassay for the Detection of Rotavirus Antigen and Antibody," *Manual of Clinical Laboratory Immunology*, 4th ed, Rose NR, de Macario EC, Fahey JL, et al, eds, Washington, DC: American Society for Microbiology, 1992, 651-60.

Rotavirus Rapid Detection *see Rotavirus, Direct Detection* on previous page

Routine Bone Marrow Culture *see Bone Marrow Culture, Routine* on page 347

Routine Culture, Rectal Swab *see Stool Culture* on page 540

RPR

Related Information

Darkfield Examination, Syphilis *on page 394*

FTA-ABS, Serum *on page 410*

VDRL, Cerebrospinal Fluid *on page 570*

Synonyms Rapid Plasma Reagin Test; Serologic Test for Syphilis; STS; Syphilis Screening Test

Applies to Syphilis Serology

Replaces Kahn Test; Kline Test; Mazzini; Wassermann

Test Includes Reactive specimens may be titered and/or an FTA-ABS test performed

Specimen Serum

Container Red top tube

Reference Range Negative

Use Screening test for syphilis

Limitations This is a nontreponemal test and is associated with false-positive reactions due to intercurrent infections, pregnancy, drug addiction, collagen-vascular diseases, and Gaucher's disease.

Methodology Cord agglutination test with reagin antibody

Additional Information This is a very sensitive (but nonspecific) screening test for syphilis and detects antibodies to reagin. These antibodies usually develop within 4-6 weeks of initial infection, peak during the secondary phase of disease, and then decrease. They also decrease with treatment. Greater than 90% of patients with primary syphilis will have positive tests. RPR titers are usually higher in HIV-infected patients than in those who do not have HIV infection.

Because of the many causes of false-positive tests any reactive serum should be tested by a treponemal-specific test (HAI or FTA-ABS). The RPR should not be done on cerebrospinal fluid.

False-negative tests may occur at birth in some infants with recently acquired congenital syphilis. Therefore, especially in areas where the disease is prevalent, a serologic test for syphilis should be included in evaluating febrile infants even if they had a negative screen at birth. False-negatives have also been due to the prozone effect. Therefore, pregnant women in areas with high syphilis prevalence should have dilution performed on negative screening tests.

Selected Readings

Dorfman DH and Glaser JH, "Congenital Syphilis Presenting in Infants After the Newborn Period," *N Engl J Med*, 1990, 323(19):1299-302.

Hart G, "Syphilis Tests in Diagnostic and Therapeutic Decision Making," *Ann Intern Med*, 1986, 104(3):368-76.

Huber TW, Storms S, Young P, et al, "Reactivity of Microhemagglutination, Fluorescent Treponemal Antibody Absorption, Venereal Disease Research Laboratory, and Rapid Plasma Reagin Tests in Primary Syphilis," *J Clin Microbiol*, 1983, 17(3):405-9.

van Voorst and Vader PC, "Syphilis Management and Treatment," *Dermatol Clin*, 1998, 16(4):699-711, xi.

Young H, "Syphilis. Serology," *Dermatol Clin*, 1998, 16(4):691-8.

RSV Culture *see* Respiratory Syncytial Virus Culture *on page 528*
RSV Testing *see* Respiratory Syncytial Virus Antigen by EIA *on page 527*
RSV Titer *see* Respiratory Syncytial Virus Serology *on page 528*
Rubella Antibodies *see* Rubella Serology *on this page*

Rubella Serology

Synonyms German Measles Serology; Rubella Antibodies
Applies to IgG Antibodies to Rubella; IgM Antibodies to Rubella
Test Includes Detection of serologic response to rubella infection or vaccination
Abstract German measles is a viral infection usually characterized by a macular exanthem, an incubation period of 14-21 days and lymphadenopathy, pharyngitis, and conjunctivitis. Severe transplacental infections occur in the first trimester.
Specimen Serum
Container Red top tube
Reference Range Absence of antibody indicates susceptibility to rubella. Presence of IgM antibody indicates acute infection or vaccination. Presence of IgG antibody requires interpretation.
Possible Panic Range Evidence of susceptibility in a pregnant woman recently exposed to rubella
Use Aid in diagnosis of congenital rubella infections; evaluate susceptibility to infections
Limitations Requires clinical correlation and judgment. Low levels of antibody are poorly detected by enzyme immunoassays.
Methodology Indirect fluorescent antibody (IFA), hemagglutination, enzyme-linked immunosorbent assay (ELISA), radioimmunoassay (RIA), complement fixation (CF), latex agglutination (LA), enzyme immunoassay (EIA)
Additional Information Rubella virus is the cause of German measles, usually a mild exanthem, often subclinical. However, when acquired *in utero*, rubella virus can cause the congenital rubella syndrome, and lead to fetal demise, cataracts, malformation, deafness, and mental retardation. For this reason the federal government and many states support programs to immunize women against rubella before they have children. There has been a resurgence of congenital rubella in the early 1990s and more widespread screening for rubella serology is recommended.

The role of serologic testing for antibodies to rubella is different in different clinical settings. The simplest and most straight forward application is in premarital assessment of immunity. If a woman has antibodies against rubella, even of low titer, demonstrated by any of multiple methods, she need not worry about infection during subsequent pregnancy. If she is not immune, and is not pregnant, she can receive rubella vaccine.

A second, more complex, role is in the management of a pregnant woman who has been exposed to rubella. Here the questions include susceptibility, present acute infection, and risk to the fetus. Several flowcharts are available to assess these possibilities, utilizing antibody titers, class of antibody, and changes in titer over time. Management of such a case requires individualized expert consultation. Of particular concern is that some enzyme-linked immunoassays are not as sensitive and specific as hemagglutination inhibition.

Still a third role is in the evaluation of an infant born with an illness which may be congenital rubella. Problems here include evaluating whether antibody is present, and whether it represents antibody passively acquired by transplacental passage or is indicative of true neonatal infection. In this setting determining the immunoglobulin class is particularly important; IgM antibody strongly supports congenital infection.

Selected Readings
Fayram SL, Akin S, Aarnaes SL, et al, "Determination of Immune Status in Patients With Low Antibody Titers for Rubella Virus," *J Clin Microbiol*, 1987, 25(1):178-80.

Lee SH, Ewert DF, Frederick PD, et al, "Resurgence of Congenital Rubella Syndrome in the 1990s. Report on Missed Opportunities and Failed Prevention Policies Among Women of Childbearing Age," *JAMA*, 1992, 267(19):2616-20.

Zhang T, Mauracher CA, Mitchell LA, et al, "Detection of Rubella Virus-Specific Immunoglobulin G (IgG), IgM, and IgA Antibodies by Immunoblot Assays," *J Clin Microbiol*, 1992, 30(4):824-30.

Rubella Virus Culture

Synonyms German Measles Culture; Measles Culture, 3-Day

Test Includes Isolation and identification of rubella virus in cell culture

Specimen Two throat swabs, 10 mL urine, cerebrospinal fluid, tissues, amniotic fluid

Container Sterile urine container

Sampling Time Virus is more likely to be isolated if specimen is collected within 5 days after onset of illness.

Storage Instructions Specimens should not be stored. Specimens should be delivered immediately to the laboratory. If unavoidable delays occur the specimen can be stored at 4°C for up to 3 days, but there is a loss of infectivity when culture is delayed.

Causes for Rejection Dry specimen, specimen not refrigerated during transport, specimen fixed in formalin, unlabeled specimen

Turnaround Time Positive cultures are detected in 3-7 days. Negative cultures are usually reported after 3 weeks.

Reference Range No virus isolated

Use Aid in the diagnosis of disease caused by rubella virus (eg, congenital viral infection)

Limitations Isolation of rubella virus is usually of little help in the diagnosis of rubella except in cases of severe rubella complications, epidemiological purposes, and fatality. Serological diagnosis is much more useful.

Methodology Cell culture, isolation, and confirmation/identification by antibody-specific neutralization

Additional Information The incidence of rubella has been reduced dramatically by the wide use of immunization in children. However, rubella can still occur in older people who were not vaccinated or people who have immigrated to the United States from countries where vaccination for rubella is not common. Pregnant women, who become infected with rubella, have a very high chance of the virus crossing the placenta and infecting the fetus. Congenital rubella infections have disastrous effects, causing fetal death, premature delivery, and severe congenital defects including deafness and congenital heart disease. Neonates with congenital rubella excrete rubella virus in nasopharyngeal secretions and urine for many months after birth. These children pose a risk to susceptible pregnant women. Serology is available for diagnostic purposes. Usually immune status can be determined by examining a single serum sample.

Selected Readings

Centers for Disease Control, "Increase in Rubella and Congenital Rubella Syndrome - United States, 1988-1990," *MMWR Morb Mortal Wkly Rep*, 1991, 40(6):93-9.

Chernesky MA and Mahony JB, "Rubella Virus," *Manual of Clinical Microbiology*, 5th ed, Balows A, Hausler WJ Jr, Herrmann KL, et al, eds, Washington, DC: American Society for Microbiology, 1991, 918-23.

Herrmann KL, "Rubella Virus," *Laboratory Diagnosis of Viral Infections*, Lennette EH, ed, New York, NY: Marcel Dekker Inc, 1992, 731-47.

Sabin-Feldman Dye Test *replaced by Toxoplasma Serology on page 552*

***Sarcoptes scabiei* Skin Scrapings Identification** *see Arthropod Identification on page 334*

Scanogram, X-ray *see Bone Films on page 343*

Scapula, Left or Right, X-ray *see Bone Films on page 343*

Schlichter Test *see Serum Bactericidal Test on next page*

Scotch® Tape Test *see Pinworm Preparation on page 520*

Screening Culture for Group A Beta-Hemolytic *Streptococcus* *see Throat Culture for Group A Beta-Hemolytic Streptococcus on page 550*

Sedimentation Rate *see Sedimentation Rate, Erythrocyte on this page*

Sedimentation Rate, Erythrocyte

Related Information

C-Reactive Protein *on page 378*

Synonyms Sedimentation Rate; Westergren Sedimentation Rate

Abstract This test is not a very specific in measuring inflammation and infection. It is used mainly to follow management of rheumatology patients.

Specimen Blood

Container Blue top (sodium citrate) tube or lavender top (EDTA) tube

Collection Specimen must be received within 4 hours of collection.

Causes for Rejection Insufficient blood, clotted, hemolyzed specimen

Reference Range Male: <50 years: 0-15 mm/hour, >50 years: 0-20 mm/hour; female: <50 years: 0-25 mm/hour, >50 years: 0-30 mm/hour by Westergren method

Use Evaluate the nonspecific activity of infections, inflammatory states, autoimmune disorders, and plasma cell dyscrasias

Limitations Anemia and paraproteinemia invalidate results; some procedural methods may be associated with hazardous exposure of medical technologists to fresh whole blood.

Methodology Red cell sedimentation rate expressed in mm/hour, utilizing Westergren type sedimentation tubes

Additional Information Elevations in fibrinogen, alpha- and beta-globulins (acute phase reactants), and immunoglobulins increase the sedimentation rate of red cells through plasma. The test is important in the diagnosis of temporal arteritis, as well as its management.

Selected Readings

Bottiger LE and Svedberg CA, "Normal Erythrocyte Sedimentation Rate and Age," *Br Med J*, 1967, 2(544):85-7.

Singer JI, Buchino JJ, and Chabali R, "Selected Laboratory in Pediatric Emergency Care," *Emerg Med Clin North Am*, 1986, 4(2):377-96.

Serologic Test for Syphilis *see* MHA-TP *on page 488*

Serologic Test for Syphilis *see* RPR *on page 530*

Serologic Test for Syphilis *see* FTA-ABS, Serum *on page 410*

Serologic Test for Syphilis, CSF *see* VDRL, Cerebrospinal Fluid *on page 570*

Serum Antibacterial Titer *see* Serum Bactericidal Test *on this page*

Serum Bactericidal Level *see* Serum Bactericidal Test *on this page*

Serum Bactericidal Test

Related Information

Antimicrobial Susceptibility Testing, Aerobic and Facultatively Anaerobic Organisms *on page 323*

C-Reactive Protein *on page 378*

Synonyms Antibacterial Activity, Serum; Bacterial Inhibitory Level, Serum; Maximum Bactericidal Dilution; MBD; Schlichter Test; Serum Antibacterial Titer; Serum Bactericidal Level; Serum Inhibitory Titer; Susceptibility Testing, Schlichter Test; Susceptibility Testing, Serum Bactericidal Dilution Method

Special Instructions If a serum bactericidal test is desired, the physician **must** request that the laboratory save the patient's isolate within 48 hours of submission of the specimen for initial culture. If the isolate has not been saved, the test cannot be performed. The laboratory **must** be informed of current antibiotic therapy including date and time of last dosage, route of administration on all antimicrobial agents patient is receiving and clinical diagnosis. Time of specimen collection should be indicated on requisition.

Specimen Serum or body fluid. Bacterial isolate causing infection prepared by laboratory.

Container Red top tube; sterile tube for body fluid

Sampling Time The peak level for intravenously (I.V.) administered drugs is obtained 30-60 minutes after the drug is absorbed and distributed. The trough level is obtained within 30 minutes or less of the next dose. For intramuscularly (I.M.) administered drugs and oral drugs, the peak should be drawn later at 2-4 hours. Vancomycin peak is drawn 2 hours post dose.

Collection Specimen should be transported to laboratory within 1 hour of collection.

Storage Instructions Separate serum using aseptic technique and freeze.

Causes for Rejection Isolate discarded before request for testing.

Turnaround Time 2-3 days

Reference Range Peak bactericidal activity should be observed at ≥1:8 dilution, trough at ≥1:2

Use Determine the maximum bactericidal dilution of the serum or body fluid, MBD, which is bactericidal for the patient's infecting organism; monitor total therapeutic effect. Frequently used to evaluate therapy in endocarditis, osteomyelitis, and suppurative arthritis. Serum bactericidal titers ≥1:8 are often recommended for the optimal treatment of infective endocarditis, osteomyelitis and suppurative arthritis.

(Continued)

Serum Bactericidal Test (Continued)

Limitations There is no universal agreement on the clinical utility and prognostic value of this test. The serum bactericidal assay has many ill-defined variables, ie, no widely accepted standard procedure, no consensus as to whether dilutions should be performed with serum or broth, the unknown inhibitory effect of serum if used as a diluent, etc. The use of pooled serum diluent may not accurately predict actual bactericidal titers in patients with abnormal protein binding.

Results will reflect the combined *in vitro* effect of all antimicrobial agents present in the patient's serum or body fluid on his/her infecting organism(s). Results are accurate to plus or minus 1 dilution, and are not necessarily equivalent to a serum assay. Maximum inhibitory concentration (MIC) may also be reported. An apparently adequate ratio may represent a highly susceptible organism responding to a relatively low blood level, or a moderately resistant organism responding to an unexpectedly high blood level. A serum inhibitory titer might suggest an adequate therapeutic level, but would give no clue to potential toxicity, when an extremely narrow margin exists between a therapeutically adequate dose and a possibly toxic one (eg, aminoglycosides).

Contraindications The bacterium isolated from patient is not available or fails to grow for the serum bactericidal test.

Methodology Serial dilution of patient's serum; each dilution is incubated with an inoculum of the patient's isolate. Subsequent steps are complicated and vary from laboratory to laboratory.

Additional Information It is preferable to perform this test with paired specimens, one obtained approximately 15 minutes before an antibiotic dose (predose trough), and one obtained 30-60 minutes after an antibiotic dose (postdose peak).

In patients with chronic osteomyelitis, the observation of peak levels <1:16 and trough levels <1:2 accurately predicted treatment failure. In acute osteomyelitis, peak levels >1:16 and trough levels >1:2 accurately predicted medical cure. The serum bactericidal test alone is not sufficient to predict outcome in endocarditis. The therapeutic outcome of endocarditis depends on many clinical factors including cardiac status, underlying medical disease, embolic complications, and clinical management of patient. In granulocytopenic patient, titers 1:8-1:16 or greater in patients on combination therapy was associated with a more favorable outcome.

The serum bactericidal test has been applied to detect antimicrobial activity in cerebrospinal fluid and joint fluid. It is also useful in determining whether serum antimicrobial activity remains adequate after a shift from parenteral to oral therapy.

Selected Readings
Jordan GW and Kawachi MM, "Analysis of Serum Bactericidal Activity in Endocarditis, Osteomyelitis, and Other Bacterial Infections," *Medicine (Baltimore)*, 1981, 60(1):49-61.

MacLowry JD, "Perspective: The Serum Dilution Test," *J Infect Dis*, 1989, 160(4):624-6.

Stratton CW, "Serum Bactericidal Test," *Clin Microbiol Rev*, 1988, 1(1):19-26.

Wolfson JS and Swartz MN, "Drug Therapy. Serum Bactericidal Activity as a Monitor of Antibiotic Therapy," *N Engl J Med*, 1985, 312(15):968-75.

Serum Inhibitory Titer *see* Serum Bactericidal Test *on previous page*

Shiga Toxin Test, Direct

Test Includes Direct assay for *E. coli* Shiga toxin in stool

Specimen Fresh stool

Container Clean container, no preservative

Storage Instructions Refrigerate specimen (up to 7 days if necessary) at 4°C until testing.

Reference Range Negative

Use Detect shiga-like cytotoxin in the stool of persons with diarrhea suspected of being caused by EHEC

Limitations The test detects Shiga toxin produced by *Shigella dysenteriae*; this Shiga toxin is almost identical to that produced by EHEC

Methodology Enzyme immunoassay (EIA) using a monoclonal antibody specific for the shiga-like toxin

Additional Information Most culture techniques for EHEC are able to detect only the O157:H7 serotype of *E. coli*, by far the most common serotype of

EHEC. However, many serotypes other than O157:H7 produce shiga-like toxin. Therefore, an obvious advantage of this enzyme immunoassay test over culture is the fact that this test can detect the presence of EHEC other than serotype O157:H7. The level of the detected toxin has not been shown to correlate with either the presence or the severity of EHEC-induced diarrhea. Therefore, the results of the test should be interpreted in relation to the clinical presentation and patient history. Consult the clinical microbiology laboratory to determine the availability of the test.

Skin Biopsy

Related Information

Applies to Skin Lesions

Abstract This section deals with sampling and procurement techniques and with a selected group of diagnostic skin problems.

Container 10% neutral formalin is satisfactory for submission of most specimens, but there are special requirements for culture, immunofluorescence, and electron microscopy.

Collection Techniques for procuring skin specimens:

Shave biopsy: A technique for obtaining superficial samples of predominantly epidermal or projecting lesions by cutting them flush with the adjacent skin as illustrated in Figure 1. This technique is usually used for nonmalignant lesions but may be useful for the patch phase of mycosis fungoides. **Since shave biopsy provides the most limited specimen, a serious potential for histopathologic misdiagnosis exists, especially in regard to melanocytic lesions.**

Punch biopsy: Very popular with dermatologists because it can be done easily, quickly, and repetitively at low cost in office practice. Biopsy punches, illustrated in Figure 2, range from 3-6 mm in size. The punch is pressed into the skin and rotated. It yields a plug or core of tissue which is cut from its base by scissors as the punch is withdrawn. It may be difficult to adequately sample subcutanea by punch. Punch biopsies may be submitted for culture. They may be particularly useful in the diagnosis of cutaneous myosis and mycobacterial disease. Pathologists prefer the largest possible sample.

Excisional biopsy: This usually implies total removal of a skin lesion, most commonly a tumor, with a scalpel as illustrated in Figure 3. It is a preferred technique for removal of pigmented lesions and tumors.
(Continued)

Skin Biopsy *(Continued)*

Figure 1. Shave Biopsy

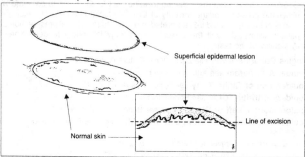

Superficial epidermal lesion

Line of excision

Normal skin

Figure 2. Punch Biopsy

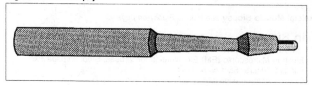

Figure 3. Excisional Biopsy by Scalpel

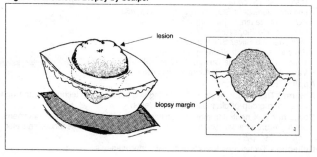

lesion

biopsy margin

Incisional biopsy: The removal of a portion of a lesion by scalpel as illustrated in Figure 4. It is performed when a non-neoplastic lesion (ie, necrobiosis lipoidica) is too large to be totally excised but definitive diagnosis mandates a large sample to evaluate overall architectural detail or, in the case of tumors, for which complete excision would require extensive surgery and/or would produce cosmetic deformity which would not be warranted until accurate histologic diagnosis is established.

Smears and/or aspirates: Stained with Wright or Giemsa type stains may suffice to demonstrate polys or eosinophils (as in toxic erythema or pustular melanosis of newborns). Gram's, acid-fast, PAS and GMS stains, and cultures are used to establish the presence of bacterial or fungal organisms. Finding multinucleated giant cells in smears in a proper clinical context suggests herpes or related viral infection. Aspirates may be adequate for cultures for bacteria, fungi, and viruses. Scrapings are often utilized in the diagnosis of dermatomycoses. Cytologic techniques (Tzanck smears) are rarely used in practice to evaluate acantholytic processes or tumors.

Figure 4. Incisional Biopsy by Scalpel

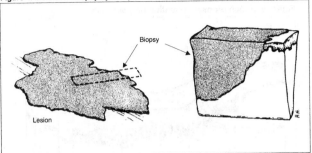

Curettings: Most frequently used when nodular basal cell carcinoma is suspected, and used as well for actinic and seborrheic keratoses. **Contraindicated for suspicious melanotic lesions.**

Storage Instructions Fixation in formalin solution or other appropriate fixative

Use Diagnosis of dermatologic disease including cutaneous manifestations of systemic or localized fungal, mycobacterial, or bacterial infections.

Additional Information Selected Problems in Dermatopathology:

A. Specimens of Pigmented Lesions and Tumors
1. In general, pigmented lesions and tumors should not be needled, aspirated, curetted, shaved or punched, but should be excised, *in toto*, whenever possible, to permit comprehensive evaluation and measurements appropriate for melanoma.

B. Specimens of Vesiculobullous Lesions
1. If the diagnostic impression is pemphigus or pemphigoid, fresh lesions are preferred. Figure 5 illustrates appropriate biopsy technique.

Figure 5. Punch Biopsy Pemphigus or Pemphigoid

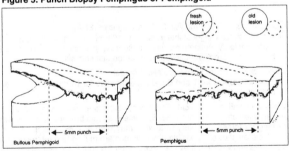

2. If the diagnostic impression is dermatitis herpetiformis, take the biopsy at the edge of the lesion (to study the change in the dermal papillae) as shown in Figure 6, rather than the lesion itself.
3. If the diagnostic impression is epidermolysis bullosa, the clinician should be aware of the availability of four special regional reference centers in the U.S. for special studies of mechanobullous lesion.
4. Immunofluorescent studies of vesiculobullous lesions: Vesiculobullous lesions which require biopsy should be considered for immunofluorescent studies (IF). In many laboratories, skin samples for immunofluorescent studies are separately submitted in vials of isopentane prior to snap freezing in liquid nitrogen by the laboratory. Some reference laboratories provide special solutions in which to store specimens for their analysis.

C. Specimens for Lupus Erythematosus (LE)
(Continued)

Skin Biopsy (Continued)

Figure 6. Punch Biopsy: Dermatitis Herpetiformis

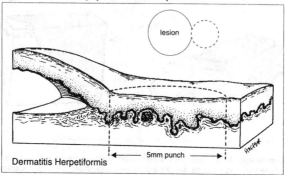

Dermatitis Herpetiformis — 5mm punch —

1. Direct immunofluorescence was first utilized on cutaneous biopsies in LE. The procedure (the lupus band test) was widely utilized to study SLE, DLE, and MCTD. Recent data suggests the band test is much less specific and sensitive than previously thought, that it is not clinically useful in discriminating SLE from other CT disorders or in predicting which patients with undifferentiated CT disease would develop SLE. Serologic evaluation is more sensitive, more efficient , and more cost effective in discriminating DLE and SLE.

Biopsy Site	SLE	DLE
Lesional Tissue	+	+
Uninvolved, Sun-exposed	+	-

D. Specimens of Epidermolysis Bullosa Acquisita (EBA)
   1. Recent studies suggest that from 5% to 10% of patients regarded as bullous pemphigoid by routine direct immunofluorescence can be shown to be EBA based on indirect immunofluorescence on salt-split skin.

E. Special Studies for Hematopoietic Disorders
   1. Special studies for T and B cells and markers for lymphocytes are considered elsewhere.

Pitfalls and artifacts to avoid: The biopsy technique should provide adequate and representative lesional tissue. Specimens should be handled gently without crushing by forceps. Cautery of lesions may burn or coagulate tissue making pathologic diagnosis impossible. If specimens are mailed to a reference laboratory in freezing weather, they may freeze after fixation. Formation of ice crystals may render interpretation hazardous if not impossible. Send in Lillie's "winter fixative" (acetic acid alcohol and formaldehyde).

Selected Readings
Dimino-Emme L and Gurevitch AW, "Cutaneous Manifestations of Disseminated Cryptococcosis," *J Am Acad Dermatol*, 1995, 32(5 Pt 2):844-50.

Skin Biopsy Antibodies see Skin Biopsy, Immunofluorescence on this page

Skin Biopsy For Bullous or Collagen Disease see Skin Biopsy, Immunofluorescence on this page

Skin Biopsy For Pemphigus see Skin Biopsy, Immunofluorescence on this page

Skin Biopsy, Immunofluorescence
Synonyms Basement Membrane Antibodies; Bullous Pemphigoid Antibodies; Dermatitis Herpetiformis Antibodies; Intercellular Antibody Basement Membrane

Antibody; LE Antibodies; Lupus Band Test; Pemphigus Antibodies; Skin Biopsy Antibodies; Skin Biopsy For Bullous or Collagen Disease; Skin Biopsy For Pemphigus

Test Includes Anti-IgG, anti-IgA, anti-IgM, anti-C3, anti-C1q, antialbumin, antifibrinogen, antikappa and lambda light chains immunofluorescence

Specimen 3 mm skin punch biopsy and serum

Container Covered Petri dish or screw cap glass vial, red top tube for blood

Collection Take biopsies from the following sites: If pemphigus or bullous pemphigoid is suspected and fresh lesions are present, take a 3 mm biopsy at the edge of the bulla. If only old lesions are available, take biopsy from adjacent area. If dermatitis herpetiformis is suspected or both bullous pemphigoid and dermatitis herpetiformis are suspected, take not only lesion biopsy, but also biopsy of uninvolved area around lesions. Repeated biopsies are sometimes necessary to confirm dermatitis herpetiformis. If systemic lupus erythematosus or discoid LE is suspected, take biopsy of sun-exposed normal skin, preferably of the wrist, for diagnosis of SLE. Biopsies from lesions may be positive in both SLE and discoid LE while normal appearing sun-exposed skin yields positive findings in SLE only. Lesions older than 6 weeks should be biopsied in SLE. In vasculitis lesions for biopsy should be less than 24 hours old. Biopsy must be kept moist on saline soaked gauze or filter paper. Deliver to the laboratory on wet ice immediately upon completion of biopsy.

Storage Instructions Do not put specimen in formalin, Zenker's solution, or other usual fixatives. Specimen may not be stored, it must be delivered (iced or on moist saline) immediately to the laboratory. Fixation in N-ethylmaleimide requires subsequent removal of fixative and frozen section. Consult the laboratory prior to obtaining specimen.

Causes for Rejection Specimen in formalin, drying out of specimen

Reference Range No deposition of immunoglobulins, complement, or fibrinogen

Use Detect immune complexes, complement, and immunoglobulin deposition in SLE, DLE, pemphigus, bullous pemphigoid, and dermatitis herpetiformis; differential diagnosis of bullous skin diseases

Limitations Many skin lesions which may clinically resemble SLE and DLE also have deposits of Ig at the basement membrane. These include psoriasis, polymorphous light eruption, and drug eruptions.

Contraindications Specimen should not be taken from heavily keratinized body areas if possible. Failure to demonstrate IgG in some biopsies may be due to a secondary change in the tissue due to infection and inflammatory reaction.

Methodology Direct fluorescent antibody (DFA), indirect fluorescent antibody (IFA)

Additional Information Distinctive patterns of IgG, IgA, IgM, and complement components in epidermis, basement membrane, and dermal vessels may contribute to the differential diagnosis of bullous skin diseases, and discoid and systemic lupus erythematosus.

- Pemphigus: Fixation of IgG or other immunoglobulin along intercellular bridges of squamous cells; C3 can be fixed.
- Bullous pemphigoid: Fixation of IgG and C3 along epidermal basement membrane.
- Dermatitis herpetiformis: Fixation of IgA immunoglobulin deposits near the epidermal-dermal junction of skin adjacent to bulla.
- Lupus erythematosus: Fixation of IgG or other immunoglobulin deposits and complement along the epidermal-dermal junction. IgG, IgM, and C3 are the most common.

Serum antibodies to the same skin components can also be demonstrated, using a tissue substrate (usually monkey or guinea pig esophagus), and these may correlate with disease activity. Steroid therapy can convert findings to negative in previously positive patients. In bullous disease antibody levels often reflect disease activity and rising titers may foretell clinical relapse.

Skin Culture for HSV *see* Herpes Simplex Virus Isolation, Rapid *on page 447*

Skin Lesions *see* Skin Biopsy *on page 535*

Skin Scrapings for *Sarcoptes scabiei* Identification *see* Arthropod Identification *on page 334*

Skin Test Battery *see* Anergy Skin Test Battery *on page 318*

Skin Tests for Histoplasmosis, Blastomycosis, Coccidioidomycosis *see* Fungal Skin Testing *on page 411*

Skin Tests for Penicillin Allergy see Penicillin Allergy Skin Testing on page 515

Smear, Gram's Stain see Gram's Stain on page 426

Soft Tissue Scan see Gallium Scan on page 422

Somatosensory Evoked Potentials see Electroencephalography on page 397

Spinal Fluid Analysis see Cerebrospinal Fluid Analysis on page 354

Spinal Fluid Cryptococcal Latex Agglutination see Cryptococcal Antigen Serology, Serum or Cerebrospinal Fluid on page 379

Spinal Fluid Fungus Culture see Fungus Culture, Cerebrospinal Fluid on page 416

Spinal Fluid Mycobacteria Culture see Mycobacteria Culture, Cerebrospinal Fluid on page 494

Spinal Fluid VDRL see VDRL, Cerebrospinal Fluid on page 570

Spinal Tap see Cerebrospinal Fluid Analysis on page 354

Spinal Tap see Lumbar Puncture on page 477

Spleen Cell Culture see Epstein-Barr Virus Culture on page 406

Sporanox® Level, Blood see Itraconazole Level on page 465

Sporothrix Antibodies see Sporotrichosis Serology on this page

Sporothrix schenckii see Sporotrichosis Serology on this page

Sporotrichosis Serology

Related Information

Fungus Culture, Biopsy on page 414
Fungus Culture, Body Fluid on page 415
Periodic Acid-Schiff Stain on page 518

Synonyms Sporothrix Antibodies

Applies to Rose Handlers Disease; Sporothrix schenckii

Test Includes Detection of serological response to Sporothrix schenckii

Abstract Sporotrichosis is a fungal disease classically beginning in a distal extremity, often at a site of inoculation, spreading proximally involving lymphatics. The organisms in tissue and in 37°C culture exist as yeast, which are often difficult or impossible to see in tissue sections. Extracutaneous disease includes monarticular arthritis. Pulmonary sporotrichosis is much less frequently found than osteoarticular infection.

Specimen Serum or cerebrospinal fluid

Container Red top tube; sterile CSF tube

Reference Range Latex agglutinating titer: <1:4; ELISA: <1:16 in serum, <1:8 in CSF

Use Diagnose sporotrichosis, especially extracutaneous disease

Limitations A negative test result does not rule out infection. Serial titers are not prognostically useful. There are occasional low titer false-positives from nonfungal disease. This test is not widely available.

Methodology Tube agglutination, latex agglutination (LA), enzyme-linked immunosorbent assay (ELISA)

Additional Information Titer ≥1:4 is presumptive evidence for sporotrichosis. Titers >1:128, rising titers, and persistent elevation are common with pulmonary or systemic disease. Positive reaction in CSF is diagnostic, and is particularly useful in chronic meningitis caused by this organism, which is difficult to culture.

Selected Readings

Bennett JE, "Sporothrix schenckii," Principles and Practice of Infectious Diseases, 3rd ed, Mandell GL, Douglas RG Jr, and Bennett JE, eds, New York, NY: Churchill Livingstone, 1990, 1972-5.
Scott EN, Kaufman L, Brown AC, et al, "Serologic Studies in the Diagnosis and Management of Meningitis Due to Sporothrix schenckii," N Engl J Med, 1987, 317:935-40.

Sputum Culture, Aerobic see Aerobic Culture, Sputum on page 312

Sputum Fungus Culture see Fungus Culture, Sputum on page 419

Sternoclavicular Joint, Left or Right, X-ray see Bone Films on page 343

Stool Culture

Related Information

Fecal Leukocyte Stain on page 408
Ova and Parasites, Stool on page 505

Synonyms Enteric Pathogens Culture, Routine; Stool for Culture

Applies to Rectal Swab Culture; Routine Culture, Rectal Swab

Test Includes Screening culture for *Salmonella*, *Shigella*, *Helicobacter*, and, if requested, *Staphylococcus*.

Special Instructions The laboratory should be informed of the specific pathogen suspected if not *Salmonella*, *Shigella*, or *Campylobacter*.

Specimen Fresh random stool, rectal swab

Container Plastic stool container, Culturette®

Collection If stool is collected in a clean bedpan, it must not be contaminated with urine, residual soap, or disinfectants. Swabs of lesions of the rectal wall during proctoscopy or sigmoidoscopy are preferred.

Rectal swab: Insert the swab past the anal sphincter, move the swab circumferentially around the rectum. Allow 15-30 seconds for organisms to adsorb onto the swab. Withdraw swab, place in Culturette® tube, and crush media compartment.

Storage Instructions Refrigerate if the specimen cannot be processed promptly.

Causes for Rejection Because of risk to laboratory personnel, specimens sent on diaper or tissue paper, specimen contaminating outside of transport container may not be acceptable to the laboratory. Specimen containing interfering substances (eg, castor oil, bismuth, Metamucil®, barium), specimens delayed in transit and those contaminated with urine may not have optimal yield.

Turnaround Time Minimum 48 hours if negative

Reference Range Negative for *Salmonella*, *Shigella*, and *Campylobacter*. In endemic areas the isolation of a pathogen may not indicate the cause or only cause of diarrhea.

Use Screen for common bacterial pathogenic organisms in the stool; diagnose typhoid fever, enteric fever, bacillary dysentery, *Salmonella* infection

Indications for stool culture include:
- Bloody diarrhea
- Fever
- Tenesmus
- Severe or persistent symptoms
- Recent travel to a third world country
- Known exposure to a bacterial agent
- Presence of fecal leukocytes

Limitations *Yersinia* species and *Vibrio* species may not be isolated unless specifically requested.

Contraindications A rectal swab culture is not as effective as a stool culture for detection of the carrier state.

Methodology Aerobic culture on selective media

Additional Information Stool cultures on patients hospitalized ≥3 days are not productive and should not be ordered unless special circumstances exist.

In enteric fever caused by *Salmonella typhi*, *S. choleraesuis*, or *S. enteritidis*, blood culture may be positive before stool cultures, and blood cultures are indicated early. Diarrhea is common in patients with the acquired immunodeficiency syndrome (AIDS). Diarrhea in AIDS is frequently caused by the classic bacterial pathogens; however, parasitic infestation is also common with *Giardia* and *Cryptosporidium*. Rectal swabs are useful for the diagnosis of *Neisseria gonorrhoeae* and *Chlamydia* infections.

In acute or subacute diarrhea, three common syndromes are recognized: gastroenteritis, enteritis, and colitis (dysenteric syndrome). With colitis, patients have fecal urgency and tenesmus. Stool are frequently small in volume and contain blood, mucus, and leukocytes. External hemorrhoids are common and painful. Diarrhea of small bowel origin is indicated by the passage of few large volume stools. This is due to accumulation of fluid in the large bowel before passage. Leukocytes indicate colonic inflammation rather than a specific pathogen. Bacterial diarrhea may be present in the absence of fecal leukocytes and fecal leukocytes may be present in the absence of bacterial or parasitic agents (ie, idiopathic inflammatory bowel disease). See table on next page. Although most bacterial diarrhea is transient (1-30 days) cases of persistent symptoms (10 months) have been reported. The etiologic agent in the reported case was *Shigella flexneri* diagnosed by culture of rectal swab. In infants younger than 1 year of age, a history of blood in the stool, more than 10 stools in 24 hours, and temperature >39°C have a high probability of having bacterial diarrhea.
(Continued)

Stool Culture *(Continued)*

Diarrhea Syndromes Classified by Predominant Features

Syndrome (anatomic site)	Features	Characteristic Etiologies
Gastroenteritis (stomach)	Vomiting	Rotavirus Norwalk virus Staphylococcal food poisoning *Bacillus cereus* food poisoning
Enteritis (small bowel)	Watery diarrhea Large-volume stools, few in number	Enterotoxigenic *Escherichia coli* *Vibrio cholerae* Any enteric microbe Inflammatory bowel disease
Dysentery, colitis (colon)	Small-volume stools containing blood and/or mucus and many leukocytes	*Shigella* *Campylobacter* *Salmonella* Invasive *E. coli* *Plesiomonas shigelloides* *Aeromonas hydrophila* *Vibrio parahaemolyticus* *Clostridium difficile* *Entamoeba histolytica* Inflammatory bowel disease

Selected Readings

Bishop WP and Ulshen MH, "Bacterial Gastroenteritis," *Pediatr Clin North Am*, 1988, 35(1):69-87.

Farmer RG, "Infectious Causes of Diarrhea in the Differential Diagnosis of Inflammatory Bowel Disease," *Med Clin North Am*, 1990, 74(1):29-38.

Gracey M, "Bacterial Diarrhea," *J Clin Gastroenterol*, 1986, 15(1):21-37.

Guerrant RL, Wanke CA, Barrett LJ, et al, "A Cost Effective and Effective Approach to the Diagnosis and Management of Acute Infectious Diarrhea," *Bull N Y Acad Med*, 1987, 63(6):484-99.

Pickering LK, "Therapy for Acute Infectious Diarrhea in Children," *J Pediatr*, 1991, 118(4 Pt 2):S118-28.

Radetsky M, "Laboratory Evaluation of Acute Diarrhea," *Pediatr Infect Dis*, 1986, 5(2):230-8.

Stool Culture, Diarrheagenic *E. coli*

Related Information

Fecal Leukocyte Stain *on page 408*

Applies to Enterohemorrhagic *E. coli*, Stool Culture; Enteroinvasive *E. coli*, Stool Culture; Enteropathogenic *E. coli*, Stool Culture; Enterotoxigenic *E. coli*, Stool Culture; EPEC, Stool Culture; Rectal Swab Culture for Diarrheagenic, *E. coli*; Stool Culture, EPEC; Verocytotoxin Producing *E. coli*, Stool Culture

Special Instructions Routine stool culture is usually performed on all requests for enteropathogenic *E. coli*

Specimen Rectal swab, fresh stool

Container Plastic stool container, Culturette®

Collection If stool is collected in sterile bedpan, must not be contaminated with urine or residual soap or disinfectants. Swabs of lesions of the rectal wall during proctoscopy or sigmoidoscopy preferred.

Rectal swab: Insert the swab past the anal sphincter, move the swab circumferentially around the anus. Allow 15-30 seconds for organisms to adsorb onto the swab. Withdraw swab, place in Culturette® tube, and crush media compartment.

Storage Instructions Do not refrigerate

Causes for Rejection Because of risk to laboratory personnel, specimen sent on diaper or tissue paper, specimen contaminating outside of transport container may not be acceptable to the laboratory. Specimen containing interfering substances (eg, castor oil, bismuth, Metamucil®, barium), specimens delayed in transit, and those contaminated with urine may not have optimal yield.

Turnaround Time Preliminary report available at 24 hours; minimum 72 hours for final reports

Reference Range Normal colonic flora

Use Establish diarrheagenic *E. coli* as the cause of clinical illness

Limitations Many laboratories are not equipped to perform elaborate diagnostic procedures needed to definitively characterize diarrheagenic *E. coli*. Clinical diagnosis and exclusion of other more readily characterized pathogens form the practical basis of presumptive diagnosis of diarrheagenic E. coli illness.

Methodology Cultures may be screened for sorbitol-negative (colorless) colonies on sorbitol-MacConkey agar; EHEC is confirmed by serotyping. Culture filtrate can be incubated with Vero cells. Changes observed in the presence of toxin include rounding up at 36 hours and destruction of the monolayer with detachment at 72 hours. Shiga-like toxin is most frequently associated with the O157:H7 serotype.

Additional Information Factors common to diarrheagenic E. coli include the presence of critical virulence factors encoded in plasmids, characteristic interaction with intestinal mucosa, production of enterotoxin or cytotoxin, and the observation that within each category the strains fall into certain O:H serotypes. See table.

Four Major Categories of Diarrheagenic E. coli

Category	Abbreviation	Clinical Manifestation
Enterotoxigenic	ETEC	Travelers diarrhea and infant diarrhea in less developed countries
Enteropathogenic	EPEC	Infant diarrhea
Enterohemorrhagic	EHEC	Hemorrhagic colitis Hemolytic uremic syndrome Thrombotic thrombocytopenia purpura
Enteroinvasive	EIEC	Dysentery

Hemorrhagic colitis can be differentiated from other causes of diarrhea by its progression from watery to bloody diarrhea over a few days time. The fecal leukocytes are markedly increased. Fever is usually absent. The disease is mediated by the production of a Shiga-like toxin which interferes with colonic brush border cells, protein synthesis, and ultimately causes cell death. Enterohemorrhagic E. coli (EHEC), differ from other strains of bacteria in the large amount of toxin they produce. Virtually all O157:H7 organisms produce this toxin.

Enterotoxigenic E. coli (ETEC) infection is acquired by ingesting contaminated food or water. The organisms colonize the proximal small intestine and there they elaborate enterotoxins. Clinical features of ETEC infection include watery diarrhea, nausea, abdominal cramps, and low grade fever. Enterotoxigenic E. coli is the most common agent of travelers diarrhea. Symptoms start early in the visit, typically on day 3. The illness may typically last 3-4 days.

Enteropathogenic E. coli (EPEC) produce a cytotoxin similar or identical to that produced by Shigella dysenteriae type 1. The clinical symptoms of EPEC infection include fever, malaise, vomiting, and diarrhea with large amounts of mucus but not grossly bloody. EPEC diarrhea in infants may persist for longer than 14 days and is frequently severe.

Enteroinvasive E. coli (EIEC) invade and proliferate within epithelial cells and cause eventual cell death, like Shigella. Clinical illness is characterized by fever, severe abdominal cramps, malaise, toxemia, and watery diarrhea. The illness progresses to gross dysentery with scant stools consisting of blood and mucus. The methylene blue stain of stool reveals sheets of leukocytes.

Selected Readings
Bishop WP and Ulshen MH, "Bacterial Gastroenteritis," Pediatr Clin North Am, 1988, 35(1):69-87.

Doyle MP, "Pathogenic Escherichia coli, Yersinia enterocolitica, and Vibrio parahaemolyticus," Lancet, 1990, 336(8723):1111-5.

Griffin PM, Ostroff SM, and Tauxe RV, "Illness Associated With Escherichia coli O157:H7 Infections - A Broad Clinical Spectrum," Ann Intern Med, 1988, 109(9):705-12.

Levine MM, "Escherichia coli That Cause Diarrhea: Enterotoxigenic, Enteropathogenic, Enteroinvasive, Enterohemorrhagic, and Enteroadherent," J Infect Dis, 1987, 155(3):377-89.

Sack RB, "Enterohemorrhagic Escherichia coli," N Engl J Med, 1987, 317(24):1535-7, (editorial).

Stool Culture, EPEC see Stool Culture, Diarrheagenic E. coli on previous page

Stool Culture, Uncommon Organisms

Applies to Rectal Swab, Unusual Organism; Vibrio cholerae, Stool Culture; Vibrio parahaemolyticus, Stool Culture; Yersinia enterocolitica, Stool Culture

Special Instructions Laboratory must be contacted prior to collecting specimen

Specimen Rectal swab or fresh stool

Container Culturette® or plastic stool container

(Continued)

Stool Culture, Uncommon Organisms *(Continued)*

Collection If collected in sterile bedpan, must not be contaminated with urine or residual soap or disinfectants. Specimen must be less than 3 hours old.

Storage Instructions Do not refrigerate.

Causes for Rejection Specimen more than 3 hours old, rectal swabs in which the medium compartment is not broken, insufficient specimen volume, specimen contaminated with urine and/or water, specimen containing interfering substances (eg, castor oil, bismuth, Metamucil®, barium); specimen refrigerated; more than two specimens submitted to the laboratory per day; specimen not submitted as sealed swab or in a sealed plastic stool container. **Diapers are not acceptable.**

Reference Range No organisms detected.

Use Identify an etiologic agent in cases of diarrhea

Limitations Special media necessary for the isolation of these specific pathogens may have to be prepared **prior** to collection of specimen.

Stool for Culture *see Stool Culture on page 540*

Stool for Ova and Parasites *see Ova and Parasites, Stool on page 505*

Stool Viral Culture *see Viral Culture, Stool on page 573*

Strep Throat Screening Culture *see Throat Culture for Group A Beta-Hemolytic Streptococcus on page 550*

Streptococcus agalactiae, Latex Screen *see Group B Streptococcus Antigen Test on page 429*

Streptococcus Group A Latex Screen *see Group A Streptococcus Antigen Test on page 428*

Streptococcus Group B Latex Screen *see Group B Streptococcus Antigen Test on page 429*

Streptodornase *see Antideoxyribonuclease-B Titer, Serum on page 322*

Streptozyme

Related Information

Antideoxyribonuclease-B Titer, Serum *on page 322*
Antistreptolysin O Titer, Serum *on page 330*

Test Includes Screening for anti-NADase, anti-DNase B, antistreptokinase, antistreptolysin O (ASO), antihyaluronidase. Sheep red blood cells are sensitized with these the five streptococcal exoenzymes.

Specimen Serum

Container Red top tube

Reference Range <100 streptozyme units

Use Screen for antibodies to streptococcal antigens: NADase, DNase B, streptokinase, streptolysin O, and hyaluronidase

Limitations A single determination is less useful than a series. May not be as sensitive in children as in adults.

Methodology Hemagglutination

Additional Information Streptozyme is a screening test for antibodies to several streptococcal antigens. It has the advantages of detecting several antibodies in a single assay (although which one has been detected cannot be ascertained), of being technically quick and easy, and of being unaffected by several factors producing false-positives in the ASO test. A serially rising titer is more significant than a single determination.

A disadvantage of the test is that borderline antibody elevations, which could be clinically significant particularly in children, may not be detected.

Selected Readings

Ayoub EM and Harden E, "Immune Response to Streptococcal Antigens: Diagnostic Methods," *Manual of Clinical Laboratory Immunology*, 4th ed, Rose NR, de Macario EC, Fahey JL, et al, eds, Washington, DC: American Society for Microbiology, 1992, 427-34.

el-Kholy A, Hafez K, and Krause RM, "Specificity and Sensitivity of the Streptozyme Test for the Detection of Streptococcal Antibodies," *Appl Microbiol*, 1974, 27(4):748-52.

Klein GC and Jones WL, "Comparison of the Streptozyme Test With the Antistreptolysin O, Antideoxyribonuclease B, and Antihyaluronidase Tests," *Appl Microbiol*, 1971, 21(2):257-9.

STS *see RPR on page 530*

Sudden Death Syndrome *see Botulism, Diagnostic Procedure on page 351*

Sulfur Granule, Culture *see Actinomyces Culture, All Sites on page 308*

Surgical Pathology *see Histopathology on page 448*

T4/T8 Ratio

Synonyms Helper Cell/Suppressor Ratio

Test Includes Quantitation of T4 and T8 cells

Specimen Blood

Container Yellow top (ACD) tube or green top (heparin) tube

Collection Routine venipuncture

Storage Instructions Maintain specimen at room temperature.

Causes for Rejection Excessive hemolysis, lipemia

Use Evaluate patients with suspected AIDS

Limitations Not diagnostic for AIDS

Methodology Flow cytometry

Additional Information Normal immunity requires a balance between thymus-derived helper cells (T4) and suppressor cells (T8). The quantitation of the T4 (helper) and T8 (suppressor) is helpful in the evaluation of a patient with suspected AIDS. In AIDS, the T4 cells are severely reduced, and the T4/T8 ratio is <1.

Teichoic Acid Antibody

Specimen Serum

Container Red top tube

Reference Range Titer ≤1:2. Less than a fourfold rise between acute and convalescent serum. (Reference ranges vary among laboratories.)

(Continued)

Teichoic Acid Antibody *(Continued)*

Use Assess therapy in chronic infections caused by *Staphylococcus aureus*

Limitations Clinical utility is not well established and is equivocal. Technical variability.

Methodology Gel diffusion assay, enzyme linked immunosorbent assay

Additional Information Teichoic acid is a component of the cell wall of gram-positive bacteria. Antibodies to teichoic acid can be demonstrated in some patients with infections due to such organisms, particularly staphylococcal endocarditis and osteomyelitis. Serial determinations of teichoic acid antibodies have been used by some to assess the adequacy of therapy for these conditions, but this or other clinical applications are not yet established.

Selected Readings
Herzog C, Wood HC, Noel I, et al, "Comparison of a New Enzyme-Linked Immunosorbent Assay Method With Counterimmunoelectrophoresis for Detection of Teichoic Acid Antibodies in Sera From Patients With *Staphylococcus aureus* Infections," *J Clin Microbiol*, 1984, 19(4):511-15.

Jacob E, Durham LC, Falk MC, et al, "Antibody Response to Teichoic Acid and Peptidoglycan in *Staphylococcus aureus* Osteomyelitis," *J Clin Microbiol*, 1987, 25(1):122-7.

Temporomandibular Joint Arthrogram *see* Arthrogram *on page 334*

Thin and Thick Smears, Blood *see* Peripheral Blood Smear, Thick and Thin *on page 519*

Thoracentesis

Synonyms Pleural Fluid "Tap"

Test Includes At the bedside, a physician utilizes a needle and catheter system to withdraw fluid from a patient with radiographically demonstrable pleural effusion for diagnostic or therapeutic purposes.

Patient Preparation Technique and risks of procedure are explained and consent is obtained. Chest x-ray is routinely performed prior to procedure, including a PA, lateral, and lateral decubitus view, and should be available for physician review. Recent prothrombin, partial thromboplastin time, and platelet count on the chart. Laboratory requisitions completed in advance. Premedication for pain (such as parenteral meperidine) is rarely required and local anesthesia during the procedure is usually sufficient.

Aftercare Immediately postprocedure, a "stat" chest x-ray is performed, usually at end-expiration. Vital signs must be monitored closely, especially if >1 L fluid is removed. Hypoxemia is a known complication of thoracentesis and some patients may require temporary supplemented oxygen. If dyspnea or hypotension develops, physician must be contacted promptly. Otherwise, if vital signs and postprocedure chest x-ray are satisfactory, patient activity may be ad lib.

Complications Although numerous complications have been reported, diagnostic thoracentesis is generally at low risk. Complications may be classified as traumatic or nontraumatic. Nontraumatic complications are related to predictable physiologic responses and include:
- syncope
- cough
- hypotension, either immediate (vasovagal reaction) or delayed (fluid shifts)
- noncardiogenic pulmonary edema (following rapid expansion of a collapsed lung, especially on removal of large volumes of a chronic effusion)
- hypoxemia; PaO_2 may drop by 10 mm Hg within minutes and not return to baseline until the following day. Some authorities recommend supplemental oxygen routinely.

Traumatic complications are iatrogenic and include:
- pneumothorax, simple or tension (requiring chest tube); lateral decubitus radiograph demonstrating a pleural effusion <10 mm thick substantially increases the risk of pneumothorax
- hemothorax
- laceration of intercostal artery, potentially lethal
- puncture of liver or spleen
- miscellaneous, subcutaneous emphysema, air embolism, infection

Of note, the recovery of a grossly bloody pleural effusion (RBC >100,000/mm³) does not automatically imply needle trauma since blood may be seen in several pleural diseases as well. To differentiate this, traumatic effusions tend to clot rapidly and become more clear as serial samples are withdrawn; bloody effusions from pleural disease generally are slow to clot due to defibrination over time. In doubtful cases, a hematocrit should be obtained on the bloody effusion and compared with plasma hematocrit.

Equipment Several complete thoracentesis kits are available commercially. Alternatively, individual components commonly found in most clinics and hospitals may be assembled separately. Common items include sterile drapes, iodine, alcohol pads, gauze, local anesthesia (1% lidocaine), at least four sterile tubes, syringes, and anaerobic culture media. Two red top tubes and two lavender top (EDTA containing) tubes may be used in place of the four sterile tubes. If cytologic studies are planned, heparin (1:1000) is needed as an additive. If pleural fluid pH is planned, a heparinized syringe and ice bag are needed. Several needle and catheter assemblies are available. For diagnostic thoracentesis (only 50-100 mL fluid removed), a 2" angiocatheter is convenient (18- or 20-gauge needle within catheter). For therapeutic thoracentesis with >1 L removed, a catheter within needle arrangement is effective. A 12" long plastic catheter (16-gauge) within a 14-gauge needle allows more complete pleural space drainage. Also required are liter-sized vacuum bottles and connecting tubing for collection of large volumes of fluid. Commercial thoracentesis kits represent variations of the above and are most useful when >1 L fluid is to be removed.

Technique Ideally, patient is positioned so that he is seated and leaning forward slightly, arms crossed in front and resting comfortably on a bedside table. The highest level of pleural effusion is determined by physical examination and a mark is placed one intercostal space below. The area is prepped and draped, and the skin and subcutaneous tissues are infiltrated with local anesthetic. Generally, the site is located 5-10 cm lateral to the spine, near the posterior axillary line. At this point technique varies with equipment used. If a catheter within needle is used, the needle (14-gauge) is passed bevel down over the superior aspect of the rib in the anesthetized intercostal space (avoiding the neurovascular bundle). Once the needle has penetrated the parietal pleura and fluid easily aspirated, the smaller plastic catheter (16-gauge) can be advanced its entire length into the pleural space. The needle is then completely withdrawn through the skin. Pleural fluid can be aspirated through the plastic catheter into a 50 mL syringe. Multiple samples of 50 mL may be obtained in this fashion. Alternatively, the catheter may be attached to sterile connecting tubing and fluid collected with liter-sized vacuum bottles. Once the desired amount is obtained, the catheter is pulled out completely and pressure held over the puncture site. If an angiocatheter is used (needle within catheter), the technique is similar. Immediately after collection, serum is drawn for LDH, protein, and further additional studies depending on the clinical situation (see Additional Information).

Specimen For diagnostic thoracentesis, 50-100 mL is adequate for routine studies. If cytology desired, larger volumes have been recommended (100-250 mL), although occasionally as little as 5 mL have been sufficient. For therapeutic thoracentesis, removal of 1000-1500 mL is generally well tolerated.

Container Lavender top tube for cell count, red top tube for chemistries, sterile syringe adequate for transport to Microbiology Laboratory. For cytology samples add 5000-10,000 units of heparin to syringe or vacuum bottle and label. For pleural fluid pH send specimen in anaerobic syringe (air bubbles removed) on ice immediately to acute care (blood gas) laboratory.

Collection Samples should be hand carried to respective laboratories immediately.

Causes for Rejection Lack of heparin additive to cytology (or cell count, if plain glass tube used in place of lavender top tube), improper collection technique for pH (not on ice)

Normal Findings Pleural effusions are traditionally classified as either "transudates" or "exudates" based on the underlying mechanism of pleural fluid formation. This is the first and most crucial step in pleural fluid analysis. Transudates are ultrafiltrates of plasma which result from alterations in the osmotic or hydrostatic focus across pleural membranes. The pleural surface itself is usually disease-free. Examples include congestive heart failure (elevated hydrostatic pressure), nephrotic syndrome, and other hypoproteinemic states (decreased oncotic pressure), cirrhosis, myxedema, sarcoidosis, and Meig's syndrome. Exudates occur when the pleural membrane is involved in a disease process which increases pleural capillary permeability or obstructs lymphatics. Causes of exudates include pulmonary infections (pneumonia, empyema, abscess), malignancy (mesothelioma or metastases), collagen vascular diseases, pulmonary (Continued)

Thoracentesis *(Continued)*

embolism, gastrointestinal diseases (pancreatitis, esophageal rupture), hemothorax, chylothorax, and miscellaneous causes such as postmyocardial infarction syndrome, uremia, and postradiation. In general, discovering a transudate allows therapy to be focused on the underlying systemic disease causing the effusion (eg, cirrhosis). Further studies of the pleural space are not necessary. Discovering an exudate, however, is more ominous and mandates additional, thorough diagnostic testing to rule out entities such as occult malignancy and pleural space infection.

Critical Values The following biochemical criteria were found by Light to accurately predict an exudate:

- pleural fluid protein to serum protein ratio >0.5
- pleural fluid LDH to serum LDH ratio >0.6
- pleural fluid LDH >200 units/L (or >two-thirds the upper limit of normal serum LDH)

Exudates satisfy one or more of these three criteria. Effusions are classified as transudates only if none of the these criteria are met. Misclassification rate is <1%, based on several prospective studies. In the past, specific gravity (SG) was used as the sole criteria for separating transudates (SG <1.016) from exudates (SG >1.016). Despite its appeal as a simple and inexpensive test, it is no longer recommended due to its high misclassification rate (≤30%). Similarly, older criteria using pleural fluid protein alone to differentiate transudates (protein <3.0 mg/dL) from exudates (>3 mg/dL) carries a misclassification rate near 15% and should no longer be used.

Use The major diagnostic indication is the presence of pleural fluid of unclear etiology. In those instances where the etiology of a pleural effusion is clinically apparent, thoracentesis may be deferred at physician's discretion. For example, the patient with recurrent congestive heart failure who presents with typical left ventricular failure and pleural effusion may appropriately undergo a trial of diuresis prior to thoracentesis. The major therapeutic indication for thoracentesis is respiratory compromise secondary to a large pleural effusion. Less commonly, the procedure may be used to evacuate trapped air in the pleural space (rather than fluid) as with a tension pneumothorax.

Contraindications Platelet count <50,000/mm³; severe, uncorrectable coagulopathy; effusions <10 mm thick on decubitus radiograph (or effusions not freely movable on decubitus radiograph); inability to define rib landmarks (necessary for proper needle placement); an uncooperative patient, unable to sit immobile. Other high-risk situations, not necessarily representing contraindications, include: mechanical ventilation with positive end expiratory pressure (PEEP); severe emphysema with blebs; patients who have undergone pneumonectomy with pleural effusion located on the side of the remaining lung. In these instances, ultrasound or CT guided aspiration of pleural fluid may be more prudent; a common complication such as pneumothorax could have profound consequences.

Additional Information Supplemental tests are available for more specific evaluation of the exudate. To minimize expense, test selection should be based on the differential diagnosis of an individual case. Malignant effusions are often grossly bloody with RBCs from 5000-100,000/mm³. Cytologic exam is initially positive for malignancy in approximately 60% of cases of later documented pleural malignancy; if three separate samples are sent, yield improves to 90%. Pleural fluid pH is often <7.3 and glucose is low (<60 mg/dL) in 15% of cases. In patients with empyema, enormous numbers of polymorphonuclear cells are present in pleural fluid. Parapneumonic effusions are sterile effusions secondary to pneumonia and require pleural pH measurement for optimal management. A pH <7.2, in the absence of systemic acidosis, indicates that the effusion will behave clinically like an empyema and will require chest tube drainage for resolution. Note that pleural fluid pH <7.2 may occur in other conditions (malignancy, TB, rheumatoid arthritis) which do not necessarily require tube thoracotomy. Tuberculosis effusions are characterized by WBC count >10,000/mm³ with >50% small lymphocytes. This latter finding is highly suggestive of either TB or malignancy and may warrant pleural biopsy. Mesothelial cells are absent in tuberculous effusions; some authors feel that the presence >1% mesothelial cells effectively rules out TB. AFB stains alone are initially positive in only 25% of proven cases. Rheumatoid effusions characteristically have low glucose levels and a value >30 mg/dL makes the diagnosis doubtful. Pleural pH levels are quite low (often <7). Rheumatoid factor testing on pleural fluid is nonspecific and not clinically useful. In suspected lupus effusions, the finding of lupus erythematosus (LE) cells in pleural fluid is pathognomonic for systemic lupus erythematosus. Effusions associated with both pancreatitis and esophageal rupture have similar laboratory profiles. Amylase levels are elevated >160 units/L with both esophageal rupture (salivary amylase) and pancreatitis (pancreatic amylase). Pleural fluid pH is low in both cases, and may be <7 with esophageal rupture.

Selected Readings

Brandstetter RD and Cohen RP, "Hypoxemia After Thoracentesis: A Predictable and Treatable Condition," 1979, 242(10):1060-1.

Corwin RW and Irwin RS, "Thoracentesis," *Intensive Care Med*, 3rd ed, Rippe JM, Irwin RS, Alpert JS, et al, eds, Boston, MA: Little, Brown and Co, 1985, 121-7.

Hausheer FH and Yarbro JW, "Diagnosis and Treatment of Malignant Pleural Effusion," *Semin Oncol*, 1985, 12(1):54-75.

Health and Public Policy Committee, American College of Physicians, "Diagnostic Thoracentesis and Pleural Biopsy in Pleural Effusions," *Ann Intern Med*, 1985, 103(5):799-802.

Grogan DR, Irwin RS, Channick R, et al, "Complications Associated With Thoracentesis. A Prospective, Randomized Study Comparing Three Different Methods," *Arch Intern Med*, 1990, 150(4):873-7.

Jay SJ, "Pleural Effusions: Preliminary Evaluation - Recognition of the Transudate," *Postgrad Med*, 1986, 80(5):164-7, 170-7.

Light RW, "Management of Parapneumonic Effusions," *Arch Intern Med*, 1981, 141(10):1339-41.

Light RW, Girard WM, Jenkinson SG, et al, "Parapneumonic Effusions," *Am J Med*, 1980, 69(4):507-12.

Light RW, Macgregor MI, and Luchsinger PC, "Pleural Effusions: The Diagnostic Separation of Transudates and Exudates," *Ann Intern Med*, 1972, 77(4):507-13.

McVay PA and Toy PT, "Lack of Increased Bleeding After Paracentesis and Thoracentesis in Patients With Mild Coagulation Abnormalities," *Transfusion*, 1991, 31(2):164-71.

Paradis IL and Caldwell EJ, "Diagnostic Approach to Pleural Effusion," *J Maine Med Assoc*, 1977, 68(10):378-82.

Prakash UB, "Malignant Pleural Effusions," *Postgrad Med*, 1986, 80(5):201-9.

Sahn SA, "The Differential Diagnosis of Pleural Effusions," *West J Med*, 1982, 137(2):99-108.

Thoracentesis Fluid Cytology *see* Cytology, Body Fluids *on page 386*

Thoracentesis Fluid Fungus Culture Bone Marrow Fungus Culture *see* Fungus Culture, Body Fluid *on page 415*

Three-Phase Bone Scan *see* Bone Scan *on page 348*

Throat Culture for *Bordetella pertussis* *replaced by* Bordetella pertussis Nasopharyngeal Culture *on page 349*

Throat Culture for *Corynebacterium diphtheriae*

Synonyms *Corynebacterium diphtheriae* Culture, Throat; Diphtheria Culture

Applies to Nasopharyngeal Culture for *Corynebacterium diphtheriae*

Abstract Diphtheria causes pseudomembranes. It may be found in the anterior nasal mucosa, but classically it is a disease of the oropharynx. It may spread to or begin in the larynx and can involve the tracheobronchial tree. The major effects of the exotoxin are on the heart and nervous system.

Aftercare Observe for laryngospasm following collection of specimen.

Special Instructions The laboratory should be notified before collection of specimens so that special isolation media can be made available. The laboratory should be informed of the specific site of specimen, age of patient, current antibiotic therapy, and clinical diagnosis.

Specimen Throat swab, nasopharyngeal swab

Container Sterile Mini-Tip Culturette® or flexible calcium alginate swab, Calgiswab®, is recommended for obtaining nasopharyngeal culture.

Collection The tongue should be depressed while both the tonsillar crypts and nasopharynx and throat lesions are swabbed. If a pseudomembrane is present, the swab should be taken from the membrane and beneath its edge if possible. Separate swabs for throat and nasopharynx are desirable. Avoid swabbing the tongue and uvula. Specimen must be transported to the laboratory immediately following collection.

Storage Instructions Refrigerate the specimen if it cannot be promptly processed.

Turnaround Time Preliminary reports are usually available at 24 hours. Cultures with no growth are usually reported after 72 hours. Final reports on specimens from which *C. diphtheriae* has been isolated usually take at least 4 days.

Reference Range No *C. diphtheriae* isolated

Use Isolate *C. diphtheriae* from patients suspected of having diphtheria. The organisms remain superficial in the respiratory tract and skin, but the potent exotoxin is responsible for the virulence of the disease.

(Continued)

Throat Culture for *Corynebacterium diphtheriae* (Continued)

Limitations Cultures should be taken from nasopharynx, as well as, the throat; culture of both sites increases the chance of recovery of the organism. Stain results are presumptive and are commonly reported out as "gram-positive pleomorphic bacilli suggestive of *C. diphtheriae*". Definitive diagnosis depends on isolation of the organism because of the similar appearance of other organisms commonly found in the oropharynx.

Contraindications Lack of clinical symptoms or signs of diphtheria, valid history of immunization

Methodology Culture on selective medium (Löeffler's), cystine tellurite agar, and blood agar smear stained with Löeffler's methylene blue stain and/or Gram's stain. *C. diphtheriae* may appear as V, Y, or L figures. Metachromatic granules which stain deep blue may also be seen.

Additional Information Routine throat culture should be ordered in addition. *C. diphtheriae* may occasionally cause skin infections, wound infections, pulmonary infections, and endocarditis and may be recovered from the oropharynx of healthy carriers. *C. diphtheriae* is spread through respiratory secretions by convalescent and healthy carriers. The clinical presentation includes a grayish pseudomembrane, overlying superficial ulcers in the oropharynx. The organism is noninvasive, however, the exotoxin elaborated in the throat affects primarily the heart and nervous system. Mortality is 10% to 30%. Only strains of *C. diphtheriae* infected by B-phage are capable of producing toxin. Nontoxigenic strains are commonly recovered and are capable of producing pharyngitis. Confirmation of exotoxin production requires animal testing and is rarely done for clinical testing. *C. ulcerans* may also produce a diphtheria-like disease.

Selected Readings

Farizo KM, Strebel PM, Chen RT, et al, "Fatal Respiratory Disease Due to *Corynebacterium diphtheriae*: Case Report and Review of Guidelines for Management, Investigation, and Control," *Clin Infect Dis*, 1993, 16(1):59-68.

Larsson P, Brinkhoff B, and Larsson L, "*Corynebacterium diphtheriae* in the Environment of Carriers and Patients," *J Hosp Infect*, 1987, 10:282-6.

MacGregor RR, "*Corynebacterium diphtheriae*," *Principles and Practice of Infectious Diseases*, 3rd ed, Mandell GL, Douglas RG Jr, and Bennett JE, eds, New York, NY: Churchill Livingstone, 1990, 1574-81.

Rappuoli R, Perugini M, and Falsen E, "Molecular Epidemiology of the 1984-1986 Outbreak of Diphtheria in Sweden," *N Engl J Med*, 1988, 318:12-4.

Walters RF, "Diphtheria Presenting in the Accident and Emergency Department," *Arch Emerg Med*, 1987, 4:47-51.

Throat Culture for Group A Beta-Hemolytic *Streptococcus*

Related Information

Group A *Streptococcus* Antigen Test *on page 428*

Synonyms Beta-Hemolytic Strep Culture, Throat; Group A Beta-Hemolytic *Streptococcus* Culture, Throat; Screening Culture for Group A Beta-Hemolytic *Streptococcus*; Strep Throat Screening Culture

Patient Preparation Do not swab throat in cases of acute epiglottitis unless provisions to establish an alternate airway are readily available.

Special Instructions The laboratory should be informed of the specific site of specimen, age of patient, current antibiotic therapy, and clinical diagnosis.

Specimen Throat swab

Container Sterile Culturette®; Dacron or rayon swabs are acceptable.

Collection The tongue should be depressed while both tonsillar pillars and the oropharynx are swabbed. Exudates should be swabbed and the tongue and uvula should be avoided.

Turnaround Time Reports are usually available within 24 hours. Cultures with no beta-hemolytic streptococci are usually reported after 24 or 48 hours. Reports on specimens from which beta-hemolytic streptococci group A have been isolated require a minimum of 24-48 hours for completion.

Reference Range No beta-hemolytic *Streptococcus pyogenes* isolated

Use Isolate and identify group A beta-hemolytic streptococci; establish the diagnosis of strep throat

Limitations Cultures are usually screened for beta-hemolytic strep group A only. The group A designation in most laboratories is presumptive and is based on rapid commercially available tests. No other organisms are usually reported.

Interpretation of throat cultures requires a significant level of experience and technical proficiency in order to avoid false-positives and false-negatives.

Methodology Culture on blood agar plate, latex agglutination screen

Additional Information *Streptococcus pyogenes* (group A beta-hemolytic strep) is generally susceptible to penicillin and its derivatives; therefore, susceptibility need not be routinely determined. The principal reason for considering an alternative drug for individual patients is allergy to penicillin. Erythromycin or a cephalosporin might be substituted in these cases. Patients allergic to penicillins may also be allergic to cephalosporins.

Use of rapid tests providing confirmation of the presence of group A streptococci is common. The sensitivity of the rapid methods is 80% to 95% in overt clinical pharyngitis. The screening method is far less sensitive in cases where concomitant cultures yield <10 colonies.

In the late 1980s, a resurgence of serious *Streptococcus pyogenes* infection was observed. Complications including rheumatic fever, sepsis, severe soft tissue invasion, and toxic shock-like syndrome (TSLS) are reported to be most common with the M1 serotype and that a unique invasive clone has become the predominant cause of severe streptococcal infections.

Selected Readings

Cleary PP, Kaplan EL, Handley JP, et al, "Clonal Basis for Resurgence of Serious *Streptococcus pyogenes* Disease in the 1980s," *Lancet*, 1992, 339(8792):518-21.

Kaplan EL, "The Rapid Identification of Group A Beta-Hemolytic Streptococci in the Upper Respiratory Tract," *Pediatr Clin North Am*, 1988, 35(3):535-42.

Lieu TA, Fleisher GR, and Schwartz JS, "Cost-Effectiveness of Rapid Latex Agglutination Testing and Throat Culture for Streptococcal Pharyngitis," *Pediatrics*, 1990, 85(3):246-56.

Throat Culture for *Neisseria gonorrhoeae* see Neisseria gonorrhoeae Culture on page 501

Throat Swab for Group A Streptococcal Antigen see Group A *Streptococcus* Antigen Test on page 428

Throat Viral Culture see Viral Culture, Throat on page 574

Thumb, Left or Right, X-ray see Bone Films on page 343

Tibia and Fibula, Left or Right, X-ray see Bone Films on page 343

Tick Identification see Arthropod Identification on page 334

Tissue Anaerobic Culture see Anaerobic Culture on page 316

Tissue Culture, *Brucella* see Biopsy Culture, Routine on page 337

Tissue Culture, Routine see Biopsy Culture, Routine on page 337

Tissue Examination see Histopathology on page 448

Tissue Fungus Culture see Fungus Culture, Body Fluid on page 415

Tissue Mycobacteria Culture see Mycobacteria Culture, Biopsy or Body Fluid on page 493

Tobramycin Level

Related Information

Antibiotic Level, Serum on page 321

Synonyms Nebcin®, Blood

Abstract Aminoglycoside antibiotics, including tobramycin, are used primarily to treat infections caused by aerobic gram-negative bacilli. Tobramycin has a narrow therapeutic window, and its use in life-threatening infections makes it mandatory that effective levels be achieved without overdosing.

Specimen Serum

Container Red top tube

Sampling Time Peak: 30 minutes after I.V. infusion; trough: immediately before next dose. Levels should be drawn at steady-state, usually 24-36 hours after starting treatment, depending on dosing schedule.

Storage Instructions Separate serum and refrigerate; must be frozen if a β-lactam is also present

Reference Range Therapeutic: peak: 4-10 µg/mL (SI: 8-21 µmol/L) (depends in part on the minimal inhibitory concentration of the drug against the organism being treated); trough: <2 µg/mL (SI: <4 µmol/L)

Possible Panic Range Toxic: peak: >12 µg/mL (SI: >25 µmol/L); trough: >2 µg/mL (SI: >4 µmol/L)

Use Peak levels are necessary to assure adequate therapeutic levels for organism being treated. Trough levels are necessary to reduce the likelihood of nephrotoxicity.

(Continued)

Tobramycin Level *(Continued)*

Limitations High peak levels may not have strong correlation with toxicity.

Methodology Immunoassay, fluorescence polarization immunoassay (FPIA)

Additional Information Tobramycin is cleared by the kidney, and accumulates in renal tubular cells. Nephrotoxicity is most closely related to the length of time that trough levels exceed 2 µg/mL (SI: >4 µmol/L). Creatinine levels should be monitored every 2-3 days as this serves as a useful indicator of impending renal toxicity. The initial toxic result is nonoliguric renal failure that is usually reversible if the drug is discontinued. Continued administration of tobramycin may produce oliguric renal failure. Nephrotoxicity may occur in as many as 10% to 25% of patients receiving aminoglycosides; most of this toxicity can be eliminated by monitoring levels and adjusting dosing schedules accordingly.

Aminoglycosides may also cause irreversible ototoxicity that manifests itself clinically as hearing loss. Aminoglycoside ototoxicity is relatively uncommon and clinical trials where levels were carefully monitored and dosing adjusted failed to show a correlation between auditory toxicity and plasma aminoglycoside levels. In situations where dosing is not adjusted, however, sustained high levels may be associated with ototoxicity. This association is far from clear cut, and new once-daily dosing regimens (and associated high peak serum concentrations) that fail to enhance toxicity further complicates the understanding of this issue.

Selected Readings

Edson RS and Terrell CL, "The Aminoglycosides," *Mayo Clin Proc*, 1991, 66(11):1158-64.

Gilbert DN, "Once-Daily Aminoglycoside Therapy," *Antimicrob Agents Chemother*, 1991, 35(3):399-405.

Pancoast SJ, "Aminoglycoside Antibiotics in Clinical Use," *Med Clin North Am*, 1987, 72(3):581-612.

Townsend PL, Fink MP, Stein KL, et al, "Aminoglycoside Pharmacokinetics: Dosage Requirements and Nephrotoxicity in Trauma Patients," *Crit Care Med*, 1989, 17(2):154-7.

Toes of Foot, Left or Right, X-ray *see* Bone Films *on page 343*

Toxin Assay, *Clostridium difficile* *see Clostridium difficile* Toxin Assay *on page 367*

Toxoplasma Antigen by ELISA

Related Information

Toxoplasma Serology *on this page*

Synonyms Toxoplasmosis Antibodies; Toxoplasmosis Titer

Test Includes Detection of *Toxoplasma* antigen by ELISA. IgG and IgM antibodies to *Toxoplasma gondii* may also be included. This test may also be available as a component of the TORCH serology battery.

Special Instructions Collection of convalescent specimen 10-14 days after acute specimen is collected facilitates interpretation of the results.

Specimen Serum

Container Red top tube

Storage Instructions Separate serum and refrigerate if the specimen cannot be delivered to the laboratory within 2 hours of collection.

Causes for Rejection Excessive hemolysis, chylous serum, gross contamination of the specimen.

Reference Range IgG: negative: ≤0.79; equivocal: 0.80-0.99; low positive: 1.00-2.49; midpositive: 2.50-4.59; high positive: ≥4.60. IgM: negative: ≤0.24; equivocal: 0.25-0.35; positive: ≥0.36.

Use Support the diagnosis of toxoplasmosis; document past exposure

Limitations Very limited availability

Methodology Enzyme-linked immunosorbent assay (ELISA)

Additional Information Toxoplasmosis infection in an immunocompromised patient is serious and can produce fatal cerebritis or disseminated illness. The majority of exposed individuals who are immunocompetent develop antibody without clinical disease.

Toxoplasma Serology

Related Information

Toxoplasma Antigen by ELISA *on this page*

Synonyms Toxoplasmosis Titer

Replaces Sabin-Feldman Dye Test

Test Includes IgG and IgM antibodies to *Toxoplasma*. IgA anti-*Toxoplasma* may also be available.

Special Instructions Acute and convalescent specimens are recommended.

Specimen Serum

Container Red top tube

Reference Range Titer: <1:64 by immunofluorescence; <1:256 by indirect hemagglutination; significance of titers varies by laboratory and methodology.

Use Support the diagnosis of toxoplasmosis; document past exposure and/or immunity to *Toxoplasma gondii*

Limitations Diagnosis of neonatal infection may be difficult because the clinical course of infection outstrips demonstrable antibody response

Methodology Indirect fluorescent antibody (IFA), indirect hemagglutination (IHA), enzyme-linked immunosorbent assay (ELISA)

Additional Information *Toxoplasma gondii* is endemic in cats and is excreted by them. Humans are easily exposed to cyst forms, either in caring for pets or in casual environmental contact. The majority of individuals develop antibody without any clinical disease. A self-limited lymphadenitis is the most common clinical presentation in symptomatic infection.

Congenital toxoplasmosis and infection in an immunocompromised host (AIDS) are more serious, and can produce a fatal cerebritis or disseminated illness. Congenital toxoplasmosis can now be diagnosed *in utero* by detection of IgM antibody in fetal blood.

The diagnosis of toxoplasmosis is supported by high or rising IgG antibody titer, or the demonstration of IgM antibody. The recent availability of IgA anti-*Toxoplasma* may be useful in detection of congenital toxoplasmosis. However, IgM is still the established technique.

Selected Readings

Bessieres MH, Roques C, Berrebi A, et al, "IgA Antibody Response During Acquired and Congenital Toxoplasmosis," *J Clin Pathol*, 1992, 45(7):605-8.

Daffos F, Forestier F, Capella-Pavlovsky M, et al, "Prenatal Management of 746 Pregnancies at Risk for Congenital Toxoplasmosis," *N Engl J Med*, 1988, 318(5):271-5.

Wilson M and McAuley JB, "Laboratory Diagnosis of Toxoplasmosis," *Clin Lab Med*, 1991, 11(4):923-39.

Toxoplasmosis Antibodies see Toxoplasma Antigen by ELISA on previous page

Toxoplasmosis Titer see Toxoplasma Antigen by ELISA on previous page

Toxoplasmosis Titer see Toxoplasma Serology on previous page

Tracheal Aspirate Culture see Aerobic Culture, Sputum on page 312

Tracheal Aspirate Fungus Culture see Fungus Culture, Bronchial Aspirate on page 416

Tracheal Aspirate Fungus Culture see Fungus Culture, Sputum on page 419

Tracheal Aspirate Mycobacteria Culture see Mycobacteria Culture, Sputum on page 495

Transesophageal Echocardiography

Synonyms Esophageal Echo; TEE

Test Includes Transesophageal echocardiography (TEE) has been developed to solve one of the limitations of echocardiography, that is, the poor imaging quality seen in some patients in whom the bony structures as well as increased lung interface degrade the quality of the images obtained with conventional echocardiography. By placing an echo transducer at the tip of a gastroscope and advancing it into the esophagus, the heart can be imaged from behind without any lung or chest cage interference. Additionally, the closer proximity to the heart allows for utilization of higher frequency transducers which provide higher resolution images. Transesophageal echocardiography has provided a new window through which the heart can be examined with far greater detail than was once thought possible. The mild inconvenience of having to pass a transesophageal probe has been by far outweighed by the enhanced images obtained with it. Presently, transesophageal echocardiography includes 2-D echocardiography, pulsed Doppler, and color flow imagings. Continuous wave Doppler should be incorporated in the near future.

Special Instructions To minimize the risk of aspiration, a period of 6-8 hours fasting is recommended. An intravenous line to keep a vein open for administration of I.V. antibiotics is needed, and sedation as required is advised. Patients with prosthetic valves, native valve stenosis or insufficiency, and congenital heart disease should receive I.V. antibiotic prophylaxis as recommended by the American Heart Association. After the antibiotics have been given the patient should be expected to be in the laboratory for approximately 1 hour to allow for (Continued)

Transesophageal Echocardiography *(Continued)*

the performance of the procedure and recovery from sedation and analgesic when used. There is no need for repeated antibiotic prophylaxis after initial dose is completed. Most patients will be able to resume full activity after the procedure, but outpatients are advised to have a companion drive them back home to minimize risks from sedation and analgesics when used.

Technique A patient arriving at the Echo Laboratory is greeted by the laboratory personnel, a fasting period of 6-8 hours is confirmed, the reasons indicated for the test are reviewed, vital signs are obtained, symptomatic status is determined, history of allergies is determined, and a detailed explanation of the procedure is made. SBE antibiotic prophylaxis is completed as recommended by the AHA. The patient is asked to undress from the waist up and is gowned with the opening in the front. Electrocardiographic and blood pressure monitorization will be made throughout the procedure. The laboratory should be prepared for cardiopulmonary resuscitation. A local anesthetic is given to the back of the throat through a spray, and a fast-acting hypnotic and analgesic is given I.V. (currently we use Versed® 0.5-2 mg I.V. and Demend® 25-100 mg I.V.). The patient is then placed on left lateral decubitus and the esophageal probe is passed. A dental suction set minimizes flow of saliva out of the mouth. Patient stays awake and comfortable throughout the procedure in most cases. A systematic and complete study should be performed on each patient. Additionally, the area of specific concern should be evaluated with further detail. A complete study will include 2-D imaging and color flow Doppler study of all cardiac chambers, valves, and great vessels. The study is initiated with the probe placed most distally, which provides a short axis view of the left ventricle as the probe is removed a view equivalent to an apical 4-chamber is obtained. This allows for the best view of the mitral and tricuspid valves. Further removal of the probe allows for visualization of the outflow tract of the left ventricle and aortic valve, after this the left atrium atrial appendage, interatrial septum, and pulmonary veins can be studied. Finally, with further removal of the probe, the aortic arch is visualized. The color Doppler is turned on during the study to evaluate normal and abnormal flow patterns. A continuous video recording is obtained throughout the study for later study and analysis. After completion of the study, the transesophageal probe is removed and the patient is kept under observation until regaining a prestudy status.

Normal Findings Transesophageal echocardiography has provided a new window to the heart, but the operator must recognize and become familiar with the different orientation of the cardiac structures and tomographic planes as seen from a different perspective. Also, there is a limitation in the number of tomographic planes than can be obtained through TEE since the motion of the probe is somewhat limited in the esophagus. With these limitations in mind, the interpretation of images through TEE is similar to that described in the section of color Doppler echocardiography.

Use Transesophageal echocardiography currently is being used intraoperatively to follow cardiac function during cardiac and noncardiac surgery, in the intensive care units to follow and evaluate critically ill patients, and in the study of ambulatory patients to better evaluate a variety of cardiovascular disorders. Transesophageal echocardiography has been found most useful in the evaluation of prosthetic valve dysfunction, particularly mitral valve prosthesis, in the quantitation and diagnostic characterization of native mitral valve insufficiency, in the evaluation of left atrial thrombosis and masses, in the evaluation of bacterial endocarditis and its complications, and in the evaluation of intracardiac shunts.

Contraindications TEE is contraindicated in patients with esophageal obstructions or with respiratory failure if not intubated.

Selected Readings

Seward JB, Khandheria BK, Oh JK, et al, "Transesophageal Echocardiography: Technique, Anatomic Correlations, Implementation, and Clinical Applications," *Mayo Clin Proc*, 1988, 63(7):649-80.

Transjugular Needle Biopsy of the Liver *see* Liver Biopsy *on page 474*

Transthoracic Needle Aspiration for *Pneumocystis* *see* Pneumocystis carinii Test *on page 522*

Transtracheal Aspirate Anaerobic Culture *see* Anaerobic Culture *on page 316*

Transtracheal Aspirate Culture *see* Aerobic Culture, Sputum *on page 312*

Transtracheal Aspirate Fungus Culture *see* Fungus Culture, Bronchial Aspirate *on page 416*

Transtracheal Aspirate Fungus Culture *see* Fungus Culture, Sputum *on page 419*

Transtracheal Aspirate Mycobacteria Culture *see* Mycobacteria Culture, Sputum *on page 495*

Transtracheal Aspiration *Legionella* Culture *see Legionella pneumophila* Culture *on page 469*

***Treponema pallidum* Antibodies, CSF** *see* FTA-ABS, Cerebrospinal Fluid *on page 409*

***Treponema pallidum* Darkfield Examination** *see* Darkfield Examination, Syphilis *on page 394*

TRIC Agent Culture *see Chlamydia* Culture *on page 359*

***Trichinella* Antibody** *see Trichinella* Serology *on this page*

Trichinella Serology

Synonyms *Trichinella* Antibody; Trichinosis Serology

Applies to *Trichinella spiralis*

Specimen Serum

Container Red top tube

Reference Range Negative; Interpretation of positive results vary by method and by laboratory. Consult laboratory for specific interpretations.

Use Screen for antibodies to *Trichinella spiralis* to establish the diagnosis of trichinosis

Limitations Low titers may represent antibody from previous rather than current infection. The bentonite flocculation test cannot be used for testing lightly infected pigs. The test may have a high false-negative rate of 15% to 22% during the first period of the infection.

Methodology Bentonite flocculation test (BFT), indirect fluorescent antibody (IFA), complement fixation (CF), latex agglutination (LA), enzyme-linked immunosorbent assay (ELISA)

Additional Information The bentonite flocculation test is sensitive and specific. Antibody becomes detectable 3 weeks after infection, rises for several weeks, and then declines slowly so that most individuals will test negative in 2-3 years. Immunofluorescence is more sensitive for light infection in pigs. In humans, diagnosis can also be made by finding cysts in a muscle biopsy.

Selected Readings

Bruschi F, Tassi C, and Pozio E, "Parasite-Specific Antibody Response in *Trichinella* sp. 3 Human Infection: A One Year Follow-up," *Am J Trop Med Hyg*, 1990, 43(2):186-93.

Kagan IG, "Serodiagnosis of Parasitic Diseases," *Manual of Clinical Laboratory Immunology*, 3rd ed, Rose NR, Friedman H, and Fahey JL, eds, Washington, DC: American Society for Microbiology, 1986, 474-5.

Trichinella spiralis *see Trichinella* Serology *on this page*

Trichinosis Serology *see Trichinella* Serology *on this page*

***Trichomonas* Culture** *see Trichomonas* Preparation *on this page*

***Trichomonas* Pap Smear** *see Trichomonas* Preparation *on this page*

Trichomonas Preparation

Related Information

Genital Culture *on page 423*

Synonyms Hanging Drop Mount for *Trichomonas*; *Trichomonas vaginalis* Wet Preparation; Trich Prep; Wet Preparation for *Trichomonas vaginalis*

Applies to Cervical *Trichomonas* Smear; *Trichomonas* Culture; *Trichomonas* Pap Smear; *Trichomonas* Wet Preparation, Urine; Urethral *Trichomonas* Smear; Urine *Trichomonas* Wet Mount; Vaginal *Trichomonas* Smear

Test Includes Wet mount and microscopic examination. Pap smear and/or culture may also be performed.

Special Instructions The laboratory should be informed of the specific source of the specimen.

Specimen Vaginal, cervical, or urethral swabs, prostatic fluid, urine sediment

Container Sterile tube containing 1 mL of sterile nonbacteriostatic saline

Collection The specimen should be collected using a speculum without lubricant. The mucosa of the posterior vagina may be swabbed or the secretions may be collected with a pipette. The swab should be expressed into the saline for

(Continued)

Trichomonas Preparation *(Continued)*

transport to the laboratory. The specimen should be examined as soon as possible.

Storage Instructions Transport the specimen to the laboratory as soon as possible after collection. Do not refrigerate.

Causes for Rejection Specimen dried out

Turnaround Time Same day; culture in Kupferberg's medium is examined for 5 days

Reference Range Negative: no trichomonads identified; positive: demonstration of actively motile flagellates or positive culture

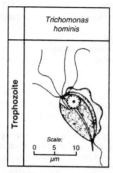

From Brooks MM and Melvin DM, *Morphology of Diagnostic Stages of Intestinal Parasites of Humans,* 2nd ed, Atlanta, GA: U.S. Department of Health and Human Services, Publication No. 84-8116, Centers for Disease Control, 1984, with permission.

Use Establish the presence of *Trichomonas vaginalis*

Limitations The specimen will be examined for *Trichomonas vaginalis* only. A separate swab (Culturette®) must be collected for culture of bacteria or fungus cultures, if required. One negative result does not rule out the possibility of *Trichomonas vaginalis* infection. The sensitivity of the wet mount procedure is low (50% to 70%); therefore, the wet mount is negative in 30% to 50% of women with trichomoniasis.

Contraindications Douching within 3 days prior to specimen collection

Methodology Wet mount microscopic examination, Pap smear, direct immunofluorescent technique with monoclonal antibody. Culture may be performed using Kupferberg's liquid medium or Hirsch charcoal agar.

Additional Information The absence of the classical yellow, frothy discharge does not exclude trichomoniasis. Culture usually yield positive results when wet preparations are negative. Cultures are the gold standard and are sensitive; however, they are expensive and have limited availability. The high rate of false-negatives, 48.4%, and false-positives observed with stained preparations (Pap smears) requires that confirmation by wet mount or culture be considered when the reported results are inconsistent with the clinical findings. Immunofluorescence tests are being adopted which have increased sensitivity. The false-positives observed when immunofluorescent methods are compared to culture may represent failure of culture in patients with few organisms. Culture is not available in many laboratories.

In a series of 600 "high risk" women, 88 *Trichomonas* infected patients were observed. Co-infection was noted as follows: *Ureaplasma urealyticum* 96%, *Gardnerella vaginalis* 91%, *Mycoplasma hominis* 89%, bacterial vaginosis 57%, *Neisseria gonorrhoeae* 29%, and *Chlamydia trachomatis* 15%. *Candida albicans* and other *Candida* sp are frequently implicated in vulvovaginitis. A vaginal pH above 5 is suggestive of *Trichomonas*.

In males a milky white fluid discharge and urethral irritation present for more than 4 weeks is frequently associated with urethritis caused by *T. vaginalis*.

Selected Readings

Bennett JR, "The Emergency Department Diagnosis of *Trichomonas vaginalis*," *Ann Emerg Med*, 1989, 18(5):564-6.

Clay JC, Veeravahu M, and Smyth RW, "Practical Problems of Diagnosing Trichomoniasis in Women," *Genitourin Med*, 1988, 64(2):115-7.

Krieger JN, Tam MR, Stevens CE, et al, "Diagnosis of Trichomoniasis, Comparison of Conventional Wet-Mount Examination With Cytologic Studies, Cultures, and Monoclonal Antibody Staining of Direct Specimens," *JAMA*, 1988, 259(8):1223-7.

Pastorek JG 2d, "Common Types of Vaginitis," *Hosp Med*, 1992, 73-88.

Sobel JD, "Vaginal Infections in Adult Women," *Med Clin North Am*, 1990, 74(6):1573-602.

***Trichomonas vaginalis* Wet Preparation** see *Trichomonas* Preparation on page 555

***Trichomonas* Wet Preparation, Urine** see *Trichomonas* Preparation on page 555

Trich Prep see *Trichomonas* Preparation on page 555

Trypanosomiasis Peripheral Blood Preparation see Microfilariae, Peripheral Blood Preparation on page 489

Tuberculin Skin Testing see Tuberculin Skin Testing, Intracutaneous on this page

Tuberculin Skin Testing, Intracutaneous

Related Information

Anergy Skin Test Battery on page 318
Fungal Skin Testing on page 411

Synonyms Mantoux Test; PPD Test; Purified Protein Derivative (PPD) Test; Tuberculin Skin Testing

Test Includes Intradermal injection of culture extracts of *Mycobacterium tuberculosis* (MTB). This is an *in vivo* means of evaluating delayed hypersensitivity to MTB. Skin test sites are examined at 24, 48, and 72 hours for signs of induration and erythema. A positive skin test indicates prior exposure to MTB (either recent or remote), with an adequate cell-mediated immune response.

Patient Preparation The procedure is explained to the patient. Inquiries should be made regarding past PPD reactions. No specific skin preparation is necessary; however, patients with severe skin disease, such as psoriasis, should be examined beforehand to ensure that there are suitable areas of normal appearing skin. Although testing need not be performed by a physician, one should be immediately available for systemic reactions.

Aftercare If no adverse reaction has occurred within several minutes, the patient may be discharged from the testing center. In some centers, patients are given written instructions on measurement and recording of a positive skin reaction at home. Other centers prefer patients to return to the test center at 48 and 72 hours for formal skin test reading by a nurse or physician. Test sites should be kept clean for 72 hours. No bathing restrictions are necessary. Patient should contact physician if a severe local reaction develops or if fever and dyspnea occurs.

Special Instructions If skin testing is performed in a separate department, requisition should state:
- the strength of tuberculin test (1 TU, 5 TU, 250 TU)
- whether an anergy skin battery is also desired (see Anergy Skin Test Battery on page 318)

Complications In general, adverse reactions are uncommon. Rare complications include fever, lymphangitis, adenopathy, and local ulcers or vesicles. If local lesions develop, these should be treated with dry sterile dressings. The use of topical ointments is optional.

Equipment Culture extracts of MTB (tuberculins) are available for injection in preparations termed "purified protein derivatives" or PPD. Commercial preparations of PPD are available in different doses, standard test dose being 5 tuberculin unit dose (5 TU). Also required are a disposable glass or plastic tuberculin syringe, a short 1/4" to 1/2" 26- or 27-gauge needle.

Technique The standard 5 TU tuberculin test is performed as follows. A skin site on the volar surface of the forearm is cleaned. 0.1 mL 5 TU PPD is drawn up into a tuberculin syringe and the needle is inserted bevel upwards intradermally and a discrete wheel (5-10 mL) is produced. If the test is improperly performed, a second dose can be given at an alternate location. Test sites are examined at
(Continued)

Tuberculin Skin Testing, Intracutaneous *(Continued)*

24, 48, and 72 hours for the presence of induration, by palpation and inspection. The largest transverse diameter of induration is measured along the long axis of the forearm. Areas of erythema are disregarded. The following should be **carefully** recorded in the chart: Strength of PPD used, date of testing, date of reading, and size of induration. The applied method described also applies to testing with nonstandard tuberculin doses (1 TU or 250 TU).

Normal Findings No reaction to the 5 TU PPD test, but a normal skin reaction to anergy skin testing.

Critical Values Interpretation of the tuberculin skin test is highly dependent on the background diseases of the person being tested. There is no single cutoff point for interpreting a positive or negative test. In 1990, the Centers for Disease Control recommended the following scheme for interpreting results of the 5 TU PPD test.

1. A skin reaction ≥5 mm is positive in those persons with:
   - HIV infection
   - chest x-ray with fibrotic lesions likely to be old healed TB
   - recent close contact with a patient with known infectious TB
2. A skin reaction of ≥10 mm is positive in the following groups.
   - Persons with medical risk factors known to increase the risk of active TB once infection has occurred (silicosis, diabetes mellitus, corticosteroids and other immunosuppressive therapies, hematologic disease, lymphoproliferate diseases, end-stage renal disease, intestinal bypass, postgastrectomy, carcinomas of head and neck, being 10% below ideal body weight)
   - Foreign born from areas (such as Asia, Africa, Latin America) where the prevalence of TB is high
   - Low income, high-risk minorities (African-American, Hispanics, American Indians)
   - I.V. drug users
   - Residents of long-term care facilities (jails, nursing homes)
3. A skin reaction ≥15 mm is positive in all other persons, including otherwise healthy persons.

Use In general, the tuberculin skin test is used to evaluate individuals with suspected MTB infection. Testing is routinely indicated in the following situations:
- patient with clinical signs and symptoms of active tuberculosis, either pulmonary or extrapulmonary
- patient with a chest radiograph compatible with past tuberculosis
- individuals who have been recently exposed to a proven (index) case of active tuberculosis; this includes close household contacts and healthcare workers with significant exposure
- individuals who have a history of tuberculosis in the remote past, never treated
- selected patients who are to start a prolonged course of steroids (or other immunosuppressives), particularly if there has been past exposure to MTB; this includes most solid organ transplantation candidates
- patients at increased risk for developing tuberculosis on the basis of their underlying disease (eg, silicosis, gastrectomy)
- routine surveillance of persons with ongoing exposure to MTB, such as nursing personnel, respiratory therapists, etc
- immigrants from areas where MTB is endemic
- epidemiologic and public health surveys (eg, nursing homes, innercity residents, etc)

Some clinicians will skin test any patient with a serious underlying illness, such as hepatitis, cirrhosis, AIDS, peptic ulcer disease, cardiomyopathy, severe pulmonary disease, end-stage renal failure, carcinoma, leukemia, and others. A positive tuberculin skin test in patients with these conditions is usually an indication for prolonged isoniazid prophylaxis.

Limitations For best results, trained personnel are necessary for administering and reading the test.

Contraindications Testing is contraindicated in the rare patient with known sensitivity to tuberculin. This includes severe local reactions (extensive erythema, vesiculations, ulcers) and anaphylaxis. Note that the development of local skin erythema (only) on a prior tuberculin skin test does not usually constitute a true hypersensitivity reaction. Some clinicians feel that the Mantoux test is contraindicated in the patient who has had a clearly documented positive PPD test in the past. The incidence and significance of this complication has not been studied formally; some physicians fear a hyperimmune local response when the patient is rechallenged with tuberculin.

Additional Information The tuberculin test is a measure of delayed (cellular) immunity to MTB. As such, a positive test indicates only exposure to MTB and does not distinguish current from past infections. False-positive tests may be seen with exposure to nontuberculous (atypical) *Mycobacterium* or previous inoculation with BCG vaccine. False-negative tests are common and can be difficult to interrupt. Causes for false-negative tests relate not only to the technique of administration, but also the age and immune status of the person being tested. Insignificant reactions are commonly seen secondary to anergy from immunosuppressive therapy, neoplastic disease, various bacterial or viral infections, and vaccinations. Thus, the tuberculin test is often performed along with skin tests for common antigens, such as *Candida* and mumps, to assess possible anergic states. In addition, hypersensitivity to tuberculin may diminish gradually with age. A "booster phenomenon" has been described in the elderly whereby waning tuberculin sensitivity is augmented by repeating 5 TU skin testing at 1 week intervals. Although controversy exists concerning the interpretation of both the booster phenomenon and of the standard tuberculin test itself, this test remains an invaluable aid in diagnosing tuberculous infection.

Selected Readings

Huebner RE, Schein MF, and Bass JB Jr, "The Tuberculin Skin Test," *Clin Infect Dis*, 1993, 17(6):968-75.

Reichman LB, "Tuberculin Skin Testing, The State of the Art," *Chest*, 1979, 76(6 Suppl):764-70.

Snider DE Jr, "Bacille Calmette-Guérin Vaccinations and Tuberculin Skin Tests," *JAMA*, 1985, 253(23):3438-9.

Stead WW and To T, "The Significance of the Tuberculin Skin Test in Elderly Persons," *Ann Intern Med*, 1987, 107(6):837-42.

The American Thoracic Society, "The Tuberculin Skin Test," *Am Rev Respir Dis*, 1981, 124:356-63.

Thompson NJ, Glassroth JL, Snider DE Jr, "The Booster Phenomenon in Serial Tuberculin Testing," *Am Rev Respir Dis*, 1979, 119(4):587-97.

Tularemia Serology

Synonyms *Francisella tularensis* Antibodies; Rabbit Fever Antibodies

Abstract *Francisella tularensis*, found in wild rabbits and in a number of other animals, may be transmitted to man by direct contact and by ticks and deer flies.

Specimen Serum

Container Red top tube

Collection Paired sera collected 2-3 weeks apart is recommended.

Reference Range Less than a fourfold increase in titer or single agglutination titer ≤1:40.

Critical Values Presumptive evidence for tularemia is provided by a single agglutination titer ≥1:160; a fourfold increase in titer is more convincing.

Use Investigation of illness characterized by an ulcerative lesion at a site of inoculation, with regional lymphadenopathy, fever, and pneumonia. Liver and spleen are affected. Conjunctivitis may occur. **Agglutinins represent the key laboratory evaluation in many cases.**

Limitations There is serologic cross reactivity with *Brucella* sp, *Proteus* OX-19, and *Yersinia* sp. IgM and IgG titers may remain elevated for over a decade after infection, limiting the value of unpaired specimens.

Methodology Agglutination, hemagglutination, enzyme-linked immunosorbent assay (ELISA)

Additional Information Although laboratory diagnosis of tularemia is often established by serologic methods, *F. tularensis* may be recovered in culture from a variety of clinical specimens. Blood cultures are often negative. *F. tularensis* is an extremely hazardous infectious agent responsible for several laboratory acquired infections. **If tularemia is clinically suspected, contact the laboratory so that appropriate precautions can be taken.**

Antibodies to *F. tularensis* develop 2-3 weeks after infection and peak at 4-5 weeks. Although *F. tularensis* antibodies may develop as a result of infection with cross-reacting organisms, titers are usually highest to the homologous agent.

(Continued)

Tularemia Serology *(Continued)*

Selected Readings

Fortier AH, Green SJ, Polsinelli T, et al, "Life and Death of an Intracellular Pathogen: *Francisella tularensis* and the Macrophage," *Immunol Ser*, 1994, 60:349-61.

Stewart SJ, "*Francisella*," *Manual of Clinical Microbiology*, 6th ed, Chapter 43, Murray PR, Baron EJ, Pfaller MA, et al, eds, Washington, DC: American Society for Microbiology, 1995, 545-55.

TWAR Strain *Chlamydia* *see Chlamydia pneumoniae Serology on page 361*

Tzanck Smear *see Herpes Cytology on page 444*

UA *see Urinalysis on page 562*

Ultrasound, Abdomen

Synonyms Abdomen Ultrasound

Applies to Follow-up Ultrasound Abdomen; Follow-up Ultrasound Retroperitoneal; Ultrasound Retroperitoneal

Test Includes Liver, spleen, gallbladder, pancreas, and biliary tree

Patient Preparation The patient should not have had a barium study within the 3 days prior to study. The examinations may be up to 1 hour each. An emergency exam or an unpredictably long preceding exam may result in additional delay. **Note**: Ultrasound exam is to be scheduled before endoscopy, endoscopic retrograde cholangiopancreatography, colonoscopy, or a barium study. If barium study was done, bowel preparation is needed before doing ultrasound examination. **No** barium studies should have been done for **at least** 2 days preceding exam. NPO after midnight before day of examination.

Special Instructions All outpatient examinations are by appointment only. All inpatients are placed on the daily schedule as time permits and are performed as scheduled. Nonemergent examinations are given secondary priority and therefore may not be able to be performed the same day scheduled. Patients will generally be asked to stay after the examination until films are reviewed by the radiologist. Instruct the patient that ultrasound uses sound waves to image the different organs. There is **no** radiation involved, therefore, it is not harmful to the patient.

Equipment Standard B-mode real time ultrasonic imager with 2-5 MHz transducer

Technique A gel is applied to the skin and a handheld transducer is swept across the abdomen to image the appropriate organs. Sound waves are used for the imaging and no radiation exposure is present. Images are recorded on x-ray film.

Data Acquired Transverse, sagittal, and oblique images of upper abdominal organs

Causes for Rejection Bowel gas, barium, eating or drinking, unresponsive or poorly responsive patient, open wound(s) overlying area of study

Turnaround Time A typed report will generally be issued within 36 hours. A preliminary verbal report generally can be given to the referring physician on request.

Normal Findings Absence of abnormal masses, fluid collections, enlarged structures, or calcifications

Use Determine the presence of neoplasms, cystic lesions, enlarged lymph nodes, bile ducts, abdominal abscesses, pancreatic mass or pseudocysts, gallbladder calculi, or any malignancies

Contraindications Open wound or incision overlying examination area, recent barium study

Additional Information Request for this study will result in imaging of liver, gallbladder, pancreas, and spleen. Individual study of any of these organs can be ordered as a specific examination (eg, gallbladder, ultrasound). Solid and cystic abnormalities of each of these organs may be detected as well as adenopathy or retroperitoneal masses. It is not uncommon to be unable to visualize the pancreas and/or retroperitoneum in its entirety due to overlying bowel gas. Common abnormalities detected by this modality include cholelithiasis, biliary tree dilatation, primary carcinomas of liver, gallbladder, and pancreas as well as metastatic disease to any organ studied. Ascites is also readily detected as well as inflammatory masses or collections.

Selected Readings

Bernardino ME, "The Liver: Anatomy and Examination Techniques," *Radiology*, Taveras JT and Ferrucci JT, eds, Philadelphia, PA: JB Lippincott, 1988.

Cooperberg PL and Rowley VA, "Abdominal Sonographic Examination Technique," *Radiology*, Taveras JT and Ferrucci JT, eds, Philadelphia, PA: JB Lippincott, 1988.

Goldberg BB, *Abdominal Ultrasonography*, New York, NY: John Wiley and Sons Inc, 1984.

Ultrasound, Kidneys

Synonyms Kidneys Ultrasound; Renal Ultrasound

Test Includes Kidneys

Patient Preparation The examination may be long, up to 1 hour including waiting time. An emergency examination or an unpredictably long preceding examination may result in additional delay. **Note**: Ultrasound exam to be scheduled before a barium study. If barium study was done, bowel preparation is needed before doing ultrasound examination.

Special Instructions All outpatient examinations are by appointment only. All inpatients are placed on the daily schedule as time permits and are performed as scheduled. Nonemergent examinations are given secondary priority and therefore may not be able to be performed the same day scheduled. Patients will generally be asked to stay after the examination until films are reviewed by the radiologist.

Equipment Standard B-mode real time ultrasonic imager with 2-5 MHz transducer.

Technique A gel is applied to the skin and a handheld transducer is swept across the area of interest to image the appropriate organs. Sound waves are used for the imaging and no radiation exposure is present. Images are recorded on x-ray film.

Data Acquired Longitudinal and transverse images of each kidney

Causes for Rejection Patient unable to cooperate with positioning and respiratory maneuvers; bowel gas, barium, obesity

Turnaround Time A typed report will generally be issued within 36 hours. A preliminary verbal report generally can be given to the referring physician on request.

Use Evaluate cysts and neoplasms, calcifications, abscess, and hydronephrosis and hydroureter

Additional Information Rapid, sensitive evaluation for the presence of hydronephrosis. Useful in confirming the cystic nature of lesions. Detection of hydroureter is often problematic.

Selected Readings

Goldberg BB, *Abdominal Ultrasonography*, New York, NY: John Wiley and Sons Inc, 1984.

Grant DC, "Ultrasound of the Genitourinary Tract," *Radiology*, Taveras JT and Ferrucci JT, eds, Philadelphia, PA: JB Lippincott, 1988.

Ultrasound, Peripheral Arteries and Veins

Synonyms Iliac Arteries Ultrasound; Peripheral Arteries and Veins Ultrasound; Popliteal Ultrasound

Test Includes Peripheral arteries and/or veins

Patient Preparation The examination may be long, up to 1 hour including waiting time. An emergency examination or an unpredictably long preceding examination may result in additional delay.

Special Instructions Specific vessels of interest to be studied as well as location must be specified. All outpatient examinations are by appointment only. All inpatients are placed on the daily schedule as time permits and are performed as scheduled. Nonemergent examinations are given secondary priority and therefore may not be able to be performed the same day scheduled. Patients will generally be asked to stay after the examination until films are reviewed by the radiologist.

Equipment Standard B-mode real time ultrasonic imager with Doppler capability with 5-10 MHz transducer.

Technique A gel is applied to the skin and a handheld transducer is swept across the area of interest to image the appropriate organs. Sound waves are used for the imaging and no radiation exposure is present. Images are recorded on x-ray film.

Turnaround Time A typed report will generally be issued within 36 hours. A preliminary verbal report generally can be given to the referring physician on request.

Normal Findings Presence of appropriate flow, compressibility of venous structures

(Continued)

Ultrasound, Peripheral Arteries and Veins *(Continued)*

Use Determine aneurysm, cysts, pseudoaneurysm, deep vein thrombosis (DVT), arterial insufficiency

Additional Information Examination is valuable in the detection of pseudoaneurysms, aneurysms, arterial insufficiency, and deep venous thrombosis (DVT)

Ultrasound Retroperitoneal *see* Ultrasound, Abdomen *on page 560*

Undulant Fever, Culture *see* Blood Culture, *Brucella on page 340*

Unidimensional Echo *see* Echocardiography, M-Mode *on page 395*

Urea Clearance *replaced by* Creatinine Clearance *on page 378*

Urea Nitrogen Clearance *replaced by* Creatinine Clearance *on page 378*

***Ureaplasma urealyticum* Culture** *see* Mycoplasma/Ureaplasma Culture *on page 499*

***Ureaplasma urealyticum* Culture, Genital** *see* Genital Culture for *Ureaplasma urealyticum on page 424*

Urease Test and Culture, *Helicobacter pylori* *see* Helicobacter pylori Culture and Urease Test *on page 432*

Urethral *Chlamydia* Culture *see* Chlamydia Culture *on page 359*

Urethral Culture for *Neisseria gonorrhoeae* *see* Neisseria gonorrhoeae Culture *on page 501*

Urethral Culture for T-Strain *Mycoplasma* *see* Genital Culture for *Ureaplasma urealyticum on page 424*

Urethral *Trichomonas* Smear *see* Trichomonas Preparation *on page 555*

Urethra, *Mycoplasma* Culture *see* Mycoplasma/Ureaplasma Culture *on page 499*

Urinalysis

Synonyms UA

Applies to Casts, Urine; Crystals, Urine; Occult Blood, Semiquantitative, Urine; Urine Crystals

Test Includes Opacity, color, appearance, specific gravity, pH, protein, glucose, occult blood, ketones, bilirubin, and in some laboratories, urobilinogen and microscopic examination of urine sediment. Some laboratories include screening for leukocyte esterase and nitrite and do not perform a microscopic examination unless one of the chemical screening (macroscopic) tests is abnormal or unless a specific request for microscopic examination is made.

Abstract The examination of urine is one of the oldest practices in medicine. A carefully performed urinalysis still provides a wealth of information about the patient, both in terms of differential diagnosis, and by exclusion of many conditions when the urinalysis is "normal."

Patient Preparation Instructions should be given in method of collection. Both males and females need instruction in cleansing the urethral meatus. "Midstream collections" are performed by initiating urination into the toilet, then bringing the collection device into the urine stream to catch the midportion of the void.

Specimen Urine

Container Plastic urine container

Collection A voided specimen is usually suitable. If the specimen is likely to be contaminated by vaginal discharge or hemorrhage, a clean catch specimen is desirable. If the specimen is collected by catheter, it should be so labeled. The timing of urine collection will vary with the purpose of the test. To check for casts or renal concentration ability, a first voided morning specimen may be preferred. For screening purposes, this is also the best time, as a later and more dilute specimen may make small increases in protein, RBC, or WBC excretion harder to detect. The upright position increases protein excretion by hemodynamic factors. Midmorning urine is likely to give the highest albumin excretion, but early morning urine is best when attempting to detect Bence Jones protein.

Storage Instructions Transport specimen to the laboratory as soon as possible after collection. If the specimen cannot be processed immediately by the laboratory it should be refrigerated. Refrigeration preserves formed elements in the urine, but may precipitate crystals not originally present.

Causes for Rejection Specimen delayed in transport, fecal contamination, decomposition, or bacterial overgrowth

Reference Range See table. **Crystals** are interpreted by the physician. Warm, freshly voided urine sediment from normal subjects almost never contains crystals, despite maximal concentration. Xanthine, cystine, and uric acid crystal (and stone) formation is favored by a consistently acid urine (pH <5.5-6). Calcium oxalate and apatite stones are associated with no particular disturbance of urine pH. Calcium carbonate, calcium phosphate, and especially magnesium ammonium phosphate stones are associated with pH >7. Urine pH >7.5 may briefly follow meals (alkaline tide) but more commonly indicate systemic alkali intake (NaHCO$_3$, etc) or urine infected by bacteria which split urea to ammonia.

Urinalysis

Test	Reference Range
Specific gravity	1.003-1.029
pH	4.5-7.8
Protein	Negative
Glucose	Negative
Ketones	Negative
Bilirubin	Negative
Occult blood	Negative
Leukocyte esterase	Negative
Nitrite	Negative
Urobilinogen	0.1-1.0 EU/dL
WBCs	0-4/hpf
RBCs	male: 0-3/hpf female: 0-5/hpf
Casts	0-4/lpf hyaline
Bacteria	Negative

hpf = high power field

lpf = low power field

EU = Ehrlich units

Possible Panic Range The presence of massive amounts of oxalate crystals in fresh urine should be reported promptly to the physician, as this finding may represent ethylene glycol intoxication.

Use Screen for abnormalities of urine; diagnose and manage renal diseases, urinary tract infection, urinary tract neoplasms, systemic diseases, and inflammatory or neoplastic diseases adjacent to the urinary tract

Limitations Insufficient volume, less than 2 mL, may limit the extent of procedures performed. Metabolites of Pyridium® may interfere with the dipstick reactions by producing color interference. High vitamin C intake may cause an underestimate of glucosuria, or a false-negative nitrate test. Survival of WBCs is decreased by low osmolality, alkalinity, and lack of refrigeration. Formed elements in the urine including casts disintegrate rapidly, therefore the specimen should be analyzed as soon as possible after collection. Specific gravity is affected by glucosuria, mannitol infusion, or prior administration of iodinated contrast material for radiologic studies (IVP dye). Some brands of test strips give a "trace positive" protein indication if not stored in dry atmosphere (cap of test strip bottle not on tight). Ambient humidity exposure of the test strips over time also causes some reduction of sensitivity for occult blood and nitrate and increased sensitivity for glucose (false-positive). This can be detected by using tap water as a negative control. False-positive tests for protein can also be due to contamination of the urine by an ammonium-containing cleansing solution. Problems relevant to the sensitivity of protein detection have led to development of methods described in the listing Microalbuminuria.

Methodology The chemical portion of the urinalysis is done by test strip, with confirming chemical method for protein (sulfosalicylic acid precipitation).

Additional Information

MICROSCOPY:

Crystalluria is frequently observed in urine specimens stored at room temperature or refrigerated. Such crystals are diagnostically useful when observed in
(Continued)

Urinalysis (Continued)

warm, fresh urine by a physician evaluating microhematuria, nephrolithiasis, or toxin ingestion.

In abundance, **calcium oxalate** and/or **hippurate crystals** may suggest ethylene glycol ingestion (especially if known to be accompanied by neurological abnormalities, appearance of drunkenness, hypertension, and a high anion gap acidosis.) Urine is usually supersaturated in calcium oxalate, often in calcium phosphate, and acid urine is often saturated in uric acid. Yet crystalluria is uncommon (in warm, fresh urine) because of the normal presence of crystal inhibitors, the lack of available nidus, and the time factor. When properly observed in fresh urine, crystals may provide a clue to the composition of renal stones even not yet passed, the nidus for such stones, or, as such, have been associated with microhematuria.

Uric acid crystals are reddish brown, rectangular, rhomboidal, or flower-like structures of narrow rectangular petals. **Ammonium urates**, in alkaline urine, are irregular blobs and crescents, sometimes resembling fragmented red cell shapes.

Calcium oxalate crystals are fairly uniform small double pyramids, base to base, which under the microscope look like little crosses on a square.

Calcium phosphate crystallizes in urine as flowers of narrow rectangular needles.

Cystine crystals, uniquely in urine, form large irregular hexagonal plates, which may dissolve if alkalinized. They occur only in the urine of subjects with cystinuria.

Calcium magnesium ammonium phosphate, or "triple phosphate," forms unique "coffin lid" angularly domed rectangles which may be present in massive quantities in alkaline urine. They usually are associated with urine infected by urea splitting bacteria which cause "infection," or "triple phosphate" stones.

Leukocyturia may indicate inflammatory disease in the genitourinary tract, including bacterial infection, glomerulonephritis, chemical injury, autoimmune diseases, or inflammatory disease adjacent to the urinary tract such as appendicitis or diverticulitis.

White cell casts indicate the renal origin of leukocytes, and are most frequently found in acute pyelonephritis. White cell casts are also found in glomerulonephritis such as lupus nephritis, and in acute and chronic interstitial nephritis. When nuclei degenerate, such leukocyte casts resemble renal tubular casts.

Red cell casts indicate renal origin of hematuria and suggest glomerulonephritis, including lupus nephritis. Red cell casts may also be found in subacute bacterial endocarditis, renal infarct, vasculitis, Goodpasture's syndrome, sickle cell disease, and in malignant hypertension. Degenerated red cell casts may be called **"hemoglobin casts"**. Orange to red casts may be found with myoglobinuria as well.

Dysmorphic red cells are observed in glomerulonephritis. "Dysmorphic" red cells refer to heterogeneous sizes, hypochromia, distorted irregular outlines and frequently small blobs extruding from the cell membrane. Phase contrast microscopy best demonstrates RBC and WBC morphology. Nonglomerular urinary red blood cells resemble peripheral circulating red blood cells. Schramek et al have used the presence or absence of dysmorphic red cells to direct the degree of work-up for hematuria and for follow-up.

Crenated RBCs provide no implication regarding RBC source.

Dark brown or smoky urine suggests a renal source of hematuria.

A **pink or red urine** suggests an extrarenal source.

Hyaline casts occur in physiologic states (eg, after exercise) and many types of renal diseases. They are best seen in phase contrast microscopy or with reduced illumination.

Renal tubular (epithelial) casts are most suggestive of tubular injury, as in acute tubular necrosis. They are also found in other disorders, including eclampsia, heavy metal poisoning, ethylene glycol intoxication, and acute allograft rejection.

Granular casts: Very finely granulated casts may be found after exercise and in a variety of glomerular and tubulointerstitial diseases.; coarse granular casts are abnormal and are present in a wide variety of renal diseases.

"Dirty brown" granular casts are typical of acute tubular necrosis.

Waxy casts are found especially in chronic renal diseases, and are associated with chronic renal failure; they occur in diabetic nephropathy, malignant hypertension, and glomerulonephritis, among other conditions. They are named for their waxy or glossy appearance. They often appear brittle and cracked.

Fatty casts are generally found in the nephrotic syndromes, diabetic nephropathy, other forms of chronic renal diseases, and glomerulonephritis. The fat droplets originate in renal tubular cells when they exceed their capacity to reabsorb protein of glomerular origin. Their inclusions have the features and significance of oval fat bodies.

Broad casts originate from dilated, chronically damaged tubules or the collecting ducts. They can be granular or waxy. **Broad waxy casts** are called "renal failure casts."

Spermatozoa may be seen in male urine related to recent or retrograde ejaculation. In female urine, the presence of spermatozoa may provide evidence of vaginal contamination following recent intercourse.

Automation of the urinalysis is routine in many laboratories. Some authors wish to abandon microscopic evaluation of the urine, which is not easily automated, on urine samples testing "normal" by dipstick screening. A urine sample that is normal to inspection and dipstick will be normal to microscopic exam 95% of the time.

One instrument for automating the entire urinalysis, the Yellow IRIS®, includes a module that automates the microscopic sediment exam. This has been found to be more consistent than the manual method for routine urinalysis and has increased the number of abnormal urines detected.

Selected Readings

Carlson D and Statland BE, "Automated Urinalysis," *Clin Lab Med*, 1988, 8(3):449-61.

Cohen HT and Spiegel DM, "Air-Exposed Urine Dipsticks Give False-Positive Results for Glucose and False-Negative Results for Blood," *Am J Clin Pathol*, 1991, 96(3):398-400.

Freeman JA and Beeler MF, *Laboratory Medicine/Urinalysis and Medical Microscopy*, 2nd ed, Philadelphia, PA: Lea & Febiger, 1983.

Haber MH, "Quality Assurance in Urinalysis," *Clin Lab Med*, 1988, 8(3):431-47.

Haber MH, *Urinary Sediment: A Textbook Atlas*, American Society of Clinical Pathologists, 1981.

Kiel DP and Moskowitz MA, "The Urinalysis: A Critical Appraisal," *Med Clin North Am*, 1987, 71(4):607-24.

Mariani AJ, Luangphinith S, Loo S, et al, "Dipstick Chemical Urinalysis: An Accurate Cost-Effective Screening Test," *J Urol*, 1984, 132(1):64-6.

Rizzoni G, Braggion F, and Zacchello G, "Evaluation of Glomerular and Nonglomerular Hematuria by Phase Contrast Microscopy," *J Pediatr*, 1983, 103:370-4.

Roe CE, Carlson DA, Daigneault RW, et al, "Evaluation of the Yellow IRIS®. An Automated Method for Urinalysis," *Am J Clin Pathol*, 1986, 86(5):661-5.

Schramek P, Schuster FX, Georgopoulos M, et al, "Value of Urinary Erythrocyte Morphology in Assessment of Symptomless Microhaematuria," *Lancet*, 1989, 2(8675):1316-9.

Schumann GB, "Cytodiagnostic Urinalysis for the Nephrology Practice," *Semin Nephrol*, 1986, 6(4):308-45.

Schumann GB, *Urine Sediment Examination*, Baltimore, MD: Williams and Wilkins, 1980.

Scott JH, "Abnormal Urinalysis in Appendicitis," *J Urol*, 1983, 129:1015.

Segasothy M, Lau TM, Birch DF, et al, "Immunocytologic Dissection of the Urine Sediment Using Monoclonal Antibodies," *Am J Clin Pathol*, 1988, 90(6):691-6.

Sheets C and Lyman JL, "Urinalysis," *Emerg Med Clin North Am*, 1986, 4(2):263-80.

Shenoy UA, "Current Assessment of Microhematuria and Leukocyturia," *Clin Lab Med*, 1985, 5:317-29, (review).

Wargotz ES, Hyde JE, Karcher DS, et al, "Urine Sediment Analysis by the Yellow IRIS® Automated Urinalysis Workstation," *Am J Clin Pathol*, 1987, 88(6):746-8.

Wenz B and Lampasso JA, "Eliminating Unnecessary Urine Microscopy - Results and Performance Characteristics of an Algorithm Based on Chemical Reagent Strip Testing," *Am J Clin Pathol*, 1989, 92(1):78-81.

Yager HM and Harrington JT, "Urinalysis and Urinary Electrolytes," *The Principles and Practice of Nephrology*, Chapter 28, Jacobson HR, Striker GE, and Klahr S, eds, Philadelphia, PA: BC Decker Inc, 1991, 167-77.

Urine Crystals *see* Urinalysis *on page 562*

Urine Culture *see* Urine Culture, Clean Catch *on this page*

Urine Culture, Clean Catch

Synonyms CMVS, Culture; Midstream Urine Culture; Urine Culture; Urine Culture, Midvoid Specimen

(Continued)

Urine Culture, Clean Catch *(Continued)*

Applies to Urine Culture, Foley Catheter

Patient Preparation Thoroughly instruct patient for proper collection of "clean catch" specimen. Wash hands thoroughly. Wash penis or vulva using downward strokes four times with four soapy sponges, then once with sponge wet with warm water. Urethral meatus and perineum must be washed. Each sponge must be discarded after one use. Urinate about 30 mL (1 ounce) of urine directly into toilet or bedpan and take middle portion of urine sample. Screw cap securely on container without touching the inside rim. Apply the completed patient label to the specimen cup. Most patients, with instruction, do better with privacy than with an attendant.

Specimen Random urine

Container Plastic urine container or sterile tube

Collection Early morning specimens yield highest bacterial counts from overnight incubation in the bladder. Forced fluids dilute the urine and may cause reduced colony counts. Hair from perineum will contaminate the specimen. The stream from a male may be contaminated by bacteria from beneath the prepuce. Bacteria from vaginal secretions, vulva or distal urethra may also contaminate the specimen as may organisms from hands or clothing. Receptacle must be sterile.

Storage Instructions The specimen should be refrigerated if it cannot be promptly transported to the laboratory. A transport stabilizer may be used to preserve the specimen if refrigeration is not available.

Causes for Rejection Unrefrigerated specimen more than 2 hours old may be subject to overgrowth, may not yield valid results, and will be rejected.

Turnaround Time Preliminary reports are usually available at 24 hours. Cultures with no growth are usually reported after 24 hours. Reports on specimens from which an organism or organisms have been isolated require a minimum of 48 hours for completion.

Reference Range No growth. Significant bacteriuria is usually considered to be 10^4 CFU/mL (colony forming units). A break point of 10^2 maximizes diagnostic sensitivity. Urethral contamination particularly in women may cause colony counts of 10^3 or 10^4; thus, a breakpoint of 10^2 CFU/mL causes inclusion of a large number of normal women without significant bacteriuria.

Use Isolate and identify potentially pathogenic organisms causing urinary tract infection

Limitations Bacteria present in numbers <1000 organisms/mL may not be detected by routine methods.

Methodology Quantitative aerobic culture

Additional Information A single culture is about 80% accurate in the female; two containing the same organism with count of 10^5 or more represents 95% chance of true bacteriuria; three such specimens mean virtual certainty of true bacteriuria. Urinary tract infection is significantly higher in women who use diaphragm-spermicide contraception, perhaps secondary to increased vaginal pH and a higher frequency of vaginal colonization with *E. coli*. A single clean voided specimen from an adult male may be considered diagnostic with proper preparation and care in specimen collection. If the patient is receiving antimicrobial therapy at the time the specimen is collected, any level of bacteriuria may be significant. When more than two organisms are recovered, the likelihood of contamination is high; thus, the significance of definitive identification of the organisms and susceptibility testing in this situation is severely limited. A repeat culture with proper specimen collection patient preparation is often indicated. Periodic screening of diabetics and pregnant women for asymptomatic bacteriuria has been recommended. Cultures of specimens from Foley catheters yielding multiple organisms with high colony counts may represent colonization of the catheter and not true significant bacteriuria. Most laboratories limit the number of organisms which will be identified when recovered from urine to two and similarly do not routinely perform susceptibility tests on isolates from presumably contaminated specimens.

Failure to recover aerobic organisms from patients with pyuria or positive Gram's stains of urinary sediment may indicate the presence of mycobacteria or anaerobes.

Selected Readings
Stamm WE, Counts GW, Running KR, et al, "Diagnosis of Coliform Infection in Acutely Dysuric Women," *N Engl J Med*, 1982, 307(8):462-8.
Stamm WE, Hooton TM, Johnson JR, et al, "Urinary Tract Infections: From Pathogenesis to Treatment," *J Infect Dis*, 1989, 159(3):400-6.

Urine Culture, First Voided, for *Neisseria gonorrhoeae* *see* Neisseria gonorrhoeae Culture *on page 501*

Urine Culture, Foley Catheter *see* Urine Culture, Clean Catch *on page 565*

Urine Culture, Midvoid Specimen *see* Urine Culture, Clean Catch *on page 565*

Urine for Parasites *see* Ova and Parasites, Urine or Aspirates *on page 508*

Urine for *Schistosoma haematobium* *see* Ova and Parasites, Urine or Aspirates *on page 508*

Urine Fungus Culture *see* Fungus Culture, Urine *on page 421*

Urine *Legionella* Antigen *see* Legionella Antigen, Urine *on page 468*

Urine, *Mycoplasma* Culture *see* Mycoplasma/Ureaplasma Culture *on page 499*

Urine *Trichomonas* Wet Mount *see* Trichomonas Preparation *on page 555*

Urodynamic Testing of Bladder Function *see* Cystometrogram, Simple *on page 382*

Urography

Synonyms Infusion Pyelogram; Intravenous Pyelogram; IVP

Test Includes Intravenous administration of a contrast material. The contrast material is concentrated and excreted by the kidneys. Appropriate radiographs are exposed during the concentration and excretion of the contrast material for evaluation of the morphology and function of the urinary tract.

Patient Preparation Patients are encouraged to take nothing by mouth after midnight the night before the examination. This degree of fluid restriction will not produce significant dehydration but will improve the overall quality of the examination. If the urography examination is to be performed in the afternoon, a light liquid breakfast may be consumed. Views on the necessity and the usefulness of cathartics in the preparation of patients for urography vary. Some physicians advocate the routine use of 10 oz of magnesium citrate the evening before the examination. Alternatives would include a mild laxative such as 1¼ oz of a standard extract of senna fruit the evening before the examination.

Aftercare Encourage hydration by fluid ingestion.

Special Instructions All patients undergoing this examination should be questioned specifically with regard to drug allergies, particularly iodine. A recent serum creatinine is requested on patients 60 years of age or older, those with significant atherosclerotic disease, those with a known diagnosis of diabetes mellitus or with known pre-existing renal disease.

Complications Reactions to contrast material and specific treatment for such reactions are beyond the scope of this handbook. An appropriately equipped emergency cart should be immediately available should resuscitation be necessary.

Equipment Overhead radiography tube with float top table. Tomographic capabilities are desirable.

Use This examination accurately demonstrates normal anatomy and a wide range of abnormalities involving the urinary tract.

Limitations Urography should be performed prior to barium studies of the gastrointestinal tract. The presence of barium within the abdomen will compromise the urographic examination.

Contraindications Allergy to iodine or a previous serious adverse reaction, advanced renal failure. A known diagnosis of multiple myeloma constitutes a relative contraindication. Every attempt should be made to hydrate patients with this diagnosis or with the diagnosis of diabetes mellitus prior to performance of a urogram as these patients run an increased risk of acute renal failure.

Selected Readings
Hattery RR, Williamson B Jr, Hartman GW, et al, "Intravenous Urographic Technique," *Radiology*, 1988, 167(3):593-9.
Miller DL, Chang R, Wells WT, et al, "Intravascular Contrast Media: Effect of Dose on Renal Function," *Radiology*, 1988, 167(3):607-11.

Vaginal Culture *see* Genital Culture *on page 423*

Vaginal Culture *Neisseria gonorrhoeae* *see* Neisseria gonorrhoeae Culture *on page 501*

Vaginal *Trichomonas* Smear *see* Trichomonas Preparation *on page 555*

Vancocin®, Blood see Vancomycin Level *on this page*

Vancoled®, Blood see Vancomycin Level *on this page*

Vancomycin Level

Related Information

Antibiotic Level, Serum *on page 321*

Synonyms Vancocin®, Blood; Vancoled®, Blood

Abstract Vancomycin is an antimicrobial agent with potent activity against most gram-positive bacteria. Its use has occasionally been associated with nephrotoxicity and/or ototoxicity, though the frequency of these toxicities has decreased as vancomycin preparations have become more purified.

Specimen Serum, body fluid

Container Red top tube, sterile fluid container

Sampling Time Peak: 30 minutes following dose; trough: immediately prior to next dose

Storage Instructions Separate serum using aseptic technique and place in freezer

Causes for Rejection Specimen more than 4 hours old

Reference Range Therapeutic concentration: peak: 20-40 µg/mL (SI: 14-27 µmol/L) (depends in part on minimum inhibitory concentration of organism being treated); trough: 5-10 µg/mL (SI: 3.4-6.8 µmol/L)

Possible Panic Range Toxic: >80 µg/mL (>54 µmol/L)

Use Monitor therapeutic levels and potential toxicities, particularly in patients with impaired renal function and in patients also being treated with aminoglycoside antibiotics

Methodology High performance liquid chromatography (HPLC), gas-liquid chromatography (GLC), immunoassay

Additional Information Vancomycin is currently being used in its intravenous form to treat a variety of gram-positive bacterial infections, particularly those due to methicillin-resistant staphylococci. Additionally, vancomycin is often used in its oral form to treat pseudomembranous colitis due to *Clostridium difficile*. When administered orally, serum vancomycin levels are undetectable due to poor absorption from the gastrointestinal tract. When administered intravenously, vancomycin may be ototoxic and nephrotoxic, though nephrotoxicity is rare with newer preparations. Ototoxicity is seen primarily in patients with extremely high serum concentrations (80-100 µg/mL; SI: 54-68 µmol/L) and rarely occurs when serum concentrations are maintained at ≤30 µg/mL (SI: 20 µmol/L). Both oto- and nephrotoxicity are enhanced by concurrent administration of aminoglycosides.

Selected Readings

Fogarty KA and McClain WJ, "Vancomycin: Current Perspectives and Guidelines for Use in the NICU," *Neonatal Netw*, 1989, 7(5):31-5.

Ingerman MJ and Santoro J, "Vancomycin. A New Old Agent," *Infect Dis Clin North Am*, 1989, 3(3):641-51.

Levine JF, "Vancomycin: A Review," *Med Clin North Am*, 1987, 71(6):1135-45.

Wilhelm MP, "Vancomycin," *Mayo Clin Proc*, 1991, 66(11):1165-70.

Varicella-Zoster Serology see Varicella-Zoster Virus Serology *on next page*

Varicella-Zoster Virus Culture

Related Information

Skin Biopsy *on page 535*

Varicella-Zoster Virus Serology *on next page*

Synonyms Chickenpox Culture; Shingles Culture

Applies to Viral Culture, Rash; Viral Culture, Skin

Test Includes Culture for VZV only; VZV also is usually detected in a routine/general virus culture

Specimen Swab specimens of the base of fresh, unroofed lesions, vesicle fluid, vesicle scrapings. In addition, acute and convalescent sera should be collected at appropriate times to document a clinically significant rise in antibody titer.

Container Cold viral transport medium

Sampling Time Specimens should be collected during the acute phase of the disease (within 3 days of lesion eruption).

Collection Unroofed lesions should be cleaned before specimens are taken. Vesicle fluid from several vesicles can be pooled and added to viral transport medium. Alternatively, the bases of several freshly unroofed lesions can be vigorously sampled with a sterile swab which subsequently should be placed into cold viral transport medium and sent to the laboratory as soon as possible.

Storage Instructions Keep specimens cold and moist. **Do not freeze specimens.**

Causes for Rejection Dry specimen, specimen not refrigerated during transport, specimen fixed in formalin, unlabeled specimen

Turnaround Time Variable (1-14 days) and depends on cell culture method used and amount of virus in the specimen

Reference Range No virus isolated

Use Aid in the diagnosis of disease caused by varicella-zoster virus (ie, chickenpox and shingles)

Methodology Inoculation of specimens into cell cultures, incubation of cultures, observation of characteristic cytopathic effect, and identification by fluorescent monoclonal antibody

Additional Information Varicella-zoster virus is a single virus which causes two diseases: **chickenpox** (varicella) in children and, after reactivation from latency, **shingles** (zoster) in adults.

Disease caused by VZV is usually self-limited. However, the disease can be life-threatening in pregnant persons, immunocompromised persons, and children who receive cancer therapy. In addition, congenital chickenpox can result in neonatal systemic disease and/or congenital malformations.

Serology for the detection of VZV antibodies is available. Rapid turnaround time of serological tests can be especially important in detecting the presence of antibody (prior exposure) in pregnant persons who have been exposed to persons with chickenpox because VZIG (varicella immune globulin) should be given within 3 days (maximum) of exposure.

Cell culture of VZV is considered less sensitive than direct antigen detection of VZV by immunofluorescence.

Selected Readings

Drew WL, "Diagnostic Virology," *Clin Lab Med*, 1987, 7(4):721-40.

Solomon AR, "New Diagnostic Tests for Herpes Simplex and Varicella-Zoster Infections," *J Am Acad Dermatol*, 1988, 18(1 Pt 2):218-21.

Strommen GL, Pucino F, Tight RR, et al, "Human Infection With Herpes Zoster: Etiology, Pathophysiology, Diagnosis, Clinical Course, and Treatment," *Pharmacotherapy*, 1988, 8(1):52-68.

Varicella-Zoster Virus, Direct Detection see Virus Detection by DFA on page 576

Varicella-Zoster Virus Serology

Related Information

Skin Biopsy on page 535
Varicella-Zoster Virus Culture on previous page

Synonyms Chickenpox Titer; Zoster Titer

Applies to Herpes Zoster Serology; Varicella-Zoster Serology

Special Instructions Acute and convalescent sera drawn 10-14 days apart are recommended.

Specimen Serum

Container Red top tube

Reference Range A single low titer or less than a fourfold increase in titer in paired sera by complement fixation; undetectable antibody by FAMA test

Use Establish the diagnosis of varicella-zoster infection; determine adult susceptibility to infection

Limitations Complement fixation test is insensitive and has heterologous reactions with herpesvirus

Methodology Fluorescent antibody to membrane antigen (FAMA), hemagglutination (HA), complement fixation (CF), enzyme-linked immunosorbent assay (ELISA)

Additional Information Although most cases of varicella or zoster are clinically unambiguous, serology may be occasionally useful in the differential diagnosis of other blistering illnesses or when infection shows an unusual complication, such as hepatitis. It may also be important to establish whether an individual is susceptible when clinical history is unclear, or when VZIG (varicella immune globulin) may be needed, as in the immunocompromised host or cancer patient on toxic chemotherapy.

(Continued)

Varicella-Zoster Virus Serology *(Continued)*

Zoster is more common with aging and may occur in the face of significant antibody titers, demonstrating that cell-mediated immunity is also significant.

Selected Readings

Landry ML, Cohen SD, Mayo DR, et al, "Comparison of Fluorescent Antibody to Membrane Antigen Test, Indirect Immunofluorescence Assay, and a Commercial Enzyme-Linked Immunosorbent Assay for Determination of Antibody to Varicella-Zoster Virus," *J Clin Microbiol*, 1987, 25(5):832-5.

Straus SE, Ostrove JM, Inchauspe G, et al, "Varicella-Zoster Virus Infections: Biology, Natural History, Treatment, and Prevention," *Ann Intern Med*, 1988, 108(2):221-36.

Weller TH, "Varicella and Herpes Zoster: Changing Concepts of the Natural History, Control, and Importance of a Not-So-Benign Virus," *N Engl J Med*, 1983, 309(22):1362-8.

VCA Titer *see* Epstein-Barr Virus Serology *on page 406*

VDRL, Cerebrospinal Fluid

Related Information

Cerebrospinal Fluid Analysis *on page 354*
Darkfield Examination, Syphilis *on page 394*
FTA-ABS, Cerebrospinal Fluid *on page 409*
FTA-ABS, Serum *on page 410*
RPR *on page 530*

Synonyms Cerebrospinal Fluid VDRL; CSF VDRL; Serologic Test for Syphilis, CSF; Spinal Fluid VDRL; VDRL, CSF

Test Includes Titer of reactive specimens

Specimen Cerebrospinal fluid

Container Clean, sterile container or glass tube

Reference Range Nonreactive

Use Test for syphilis, neurosyphilis

Limitations VDRL, CSF is the only laboratory test for neurosyphilis approved by the Center for Disease Control. It is quite specific and has acceptable sensitivity.

Methodology Flocculation test detects reagin, antibody to nontreponemal antigen

Additional Information A positive VDRL in a spinal fluid uncontaminated by serum is essentially diagnostic of neurosyphilis. However, a negative test may occur in 30% of patients with tabes dorsalis. The CSF VDRL may take years to become nonreactive after adequate therapy. In AIDS patients, serial CSF VDRL determinations may be needed when neurosyphilis is suspected. By requiring either a positive serum RPR or FTA-ABS, seropositivity of CSF VDRL could increase to 90%.

Selected Readings

Albright RE Jr, Christenson RH, Emlet JL, et al, "Issues in Cerebrospinal Fluid Management. CSF Venereal Disease Research Laboratory Testing," *Am J Clin Pathol*, 1991, 95(3):397-401.

Davis LE and Schmitt JW, "Clinical Significance of Cerebrospinal Fluid Tests for Neurosyphilis," *Ann Neurol*, 1989, 25(1):50-5.

Hart G, "Syphilis Tests in Diagnostic and Therapeutic Decision Making," *Ann Intern Med*, 1986, 104(3):368-76.

VDRL, CSF *see* VDRL, Cerebrospinal Fluid *on this page*

Venous Catheter Culture *see* Intravenous Line Culture *on page 464*

Ventricular Fluid Culture *see* Aerobic Culture, Cerebrospinal Fluid *on page 311*

Verocytotoxin Producing *E. coli*, Stool Culture *see* Stool Culture, Diarrheagenic *E. coli* on page 542

***Vibrio cholerae*, Stool Culture** *see* Stool Culture, Uncommon Organisms *on page 543*

***Vibrio parahaemolyticus*, Stool Culture** *see* Stool Culture, Uncommon Organisms *on page 543*

Viral Antigen Detection, Direct, Stool *see* Rotavirus, Direct Detection *on page 529*

Viral Culture, Brain *see* Viral Culture, Central Nervous System Symptoms *on this page*

Viral Culture, Bronchial Wash *see* Viral Culture, Throat *on page 574*

Viral Culture, Central Nervous System Symptoms

Related Information

Cerebrospinal Fluid Analysis *on page 354*
Fungus Culture, Cerebrospinal Fluid *on page 416*
Mycobacteria Culture, Cerebrospinal Fluid *on page 494*

Applies to Viral Culture, Brain; Viral Culture, CSF

Test Includes Isolation and identification of virus

Abstract Viral meningitis is by far the most important cause of aseptic meningitis. The latter includes multiple entities, both infectious and noninfectious. Most instances of aseptic meningitis are caused by viruses, especially enteroviruses, most often in the late summer. Subjects are usually children and young adults. Enteroviruses include polioviruses, Coxsackie viruses, and echoviruses. Aseptic meningitis syndrome is characterized by an acute disease with signs and symptoms of meningeal inflammation associated with pleocytosis (usually mononuclear), variable increase in protein content, normal glucose level, and no demonstrable organism by smear and routine culture of the cerebrospinal fluid (CSF).

By definition, the cerebrospinal fluid in aseptic meningitis will show a pleocytosis of white blood cells but no growth on bacterial culture.

Specimen Cerebrospinal fluid (do not put into virus transport medium), brain biopsy, lesions, throat or throat washings, stool, urine

Container Sterile tube for CSF; sterile screw cap container for biopsy, tissue, urine, or throat washing; sterile viral transport medium for swab specimens

Sampling Time As soon as possible after the onset of illness

Collection Always consult the laboratory for specific details prior to collecting specimen. Specimen should be collected during the acute phase of the disease, as follows:

Cerebrospinal fluid: Collect 1 mL CSF aseptically in a sterile dry screw cap vial. **Keep cold and bring to laboratory immediately.**

The following may be relevant to CNS viral infection: Specimens useful for diagnosis of CNS viral infections:

Eye swab or scraping: Use a Virocult® or Culturette® swab to collect conjunctival material or take conjunctival scrapings with a fine sterile spatula and transfer the scraping to a viral transport medium. **Keep cold and bring to laboratory immediately.**

Skin lesions: Open the vesicle and absorb exudate into a dry swab, and/or vigorously scrape base of freshly exposed lesion with a swab to obtain cells which contain viruses. If enough vesicle fluid is available, aspirate the fluid with a fine gauge needle and tuberculin syringe, and place the fluid into cold viral transport medium. Use Virocult® or Culturette® swabs for specimen collection. **Keep cold and bring to laboratory immediately.** The clinical appearance of herpes zoster or the vesicles of herpes simplex may suggest the diagnosis.

Throat swab: Carefully rub the posterior wall of the nasopharynx with a dry, sterile swab. Avoid touching the tongue or buccal mucosa. Use Virocult® or Culturette® swabs for specimen collection. **Keep cold and bring to laboratory immediately.** Coxsackie, mumps, adenovirus, herpes type 1, Epstein-Barr virus may be recovered from throat washings.

Feces: Collect 4-8 g of feces (about the size of a thumbnail), and place in a clean, leakproof container. Do **not** dilute the specimen (into virus transport medium) or use preservatives. **Keep cold and bring to laboratory immediately.** Enteroviruses, adenovirus.

Urine: Collect clean-catch, midstream urine in a leakproof, sterile, plastic container. **Keep cold and bring to laboratory immediately.** Mumps virus, cytomegalovirus.

Genital swab: See skin. **Keep cold and bring to laboratory immediately.**

Storage Instructions Keep all specimens cold and moist. Transport to laboratory immediately. Enteroviruses are relatively stable from -70°C to 4°C but are labile if allowed to dry or to be at room temperature for several hours.

Causes for Rejection Dry specimen, specimen not refrigerated during transport, specimen fixed in formalin, unlabeled specimen

Turnaround Time Variable (1-14 days) and depends on culture method used and amount of virus in specimen

Reference Range No virus isolated

Use Determine etiological agent of viral CNS diseases (eg, meningitis (aseptic), meningoencephalitis, polio, and encephalitis)

Limitations The CSF findings in tuberculous meningitis may simulate those of viral meningitis, especially herpes simplex and mumps.

(Continued)

Viral Culture, Central Nervous System Symptoms
(Continued)

Methodology Inoculation of specimen into cell cultures, incubation of cultures, observation of characteristic cytopathic effect, and identification/speciation by methods such as hemadsorption and fluorescent monoclonal antibodies. If specific viruses such as HSV, CMV, VZV, or adenovirus are suspected, the laboratory might be able to use rapid (1-2 days) culture (shell vial) methods to detect these viruses. Suckling mice are usually inoculated with the specimen if group A Coxsackie virus is suspected. The mice are observed for the development of flaccid paralysis. Bacterial culture, Gram's stain, cell count, glucose, and protein are needed to rule out bacterial meningitis, with antigen agglutination when indicated.

Additional Information Arthropod-borne (arbo) viruses and reoviruses are not considered culturable and may be detected indirectly by viral serology.

The seasonal peak of viral meningitis in late summer is widely recognized and clinically significant in differential diagnosis. Meningitis caused by HIV, Epstein-Barr virus, CMV, or herpes simplex lacks seasonal variation. The significance of seasonal curves for viral meningitis (more frequent in summer) versus bacterial meningitis is greater than most physicians recognize.

Mumps meningitis is usually self limited and benign. As with lymphocytic choriomeningitis and herpes simplex meningoencephalitis, hypoglycorrhachia may be found.

In the differential diagnosis between viral and bacterial meningitis, much higher WBC count ($>1180 \times 10^6$/L) and protein (>220 mg/dL) may be found in many cases of bacterial meningitis. In Spanos' series, no patient with acute viral meningitis had glucose <30.6 mg/dL but 43% with acute bacterial meningitis did. Although aseptic meningitis is usually characterized by mononuclear cells, PMNs may predominate early.

Five patients with mixed viral-bacterial meningitis among 276 patients with viral and/or bacterial culture proven meningitis are described.

A high frequency of negative lumbar punctures in babies presenting with fever but without other specific findings is recognized. In a series of children with high fever, 57% of patients with bacterial meningitis and 37% of those with aseptic meningitis had vomiting. In a study of 171 children with febrile convulsions, only one had bacterial meningitis and four had aseptic meningitis.

Complications of lumbar puncture (LP) are between 0.19% and 0.43%, reaching up to 35.5% when minor complications are included. Instances of meningitis and local infection are described following LP in subjects with bacteremia, who may be at risk for meningeal seeding during the puncture.

Nonviral aseptic causes of aseptic meningitis include meningeal carcinomatosis, collagen diseases, sarcoidosis, drugs including antineoplastic agents, immunosuppressants, materials used in radiology units, Mollaret's meningitis, and many other entities.

Selected Readings

Chonmaitree T, Baldwin CD, and Lucia HL, "Role of the Virology Laboratory in Diagnosis and Management of Patients With Central Nervous System Disease," *Clin Microbiol Rev*, 1989, 2(1):1-14.

Connolly KJ and Hammer SM, "The Acute Aseptic Meningitis Syndrome," *Infect Dis Clin North Am*, 1990, 4(4):599-622.

Greenlee JE, "Approach to Diagnosis of Meningitis - Cerebrospinal Fluid Evaluation," *Infect Dis Clin North Am*, 1990, 4(4):583-98.

Hammer SM and Connolly KJ, "Viral Aseptic Meningitis in the United States: Clinical Features, Viral Etiologies, and Differential Diagnosis," *Curr Clin Top Infect Dis*, 1992, 12:1-25.

Mishu B, "A Rabies Primer for Clinicians," *Infect Dis Newslett*, 1993, 12(1):1-4.

Viral Culture, CSF *see* Viral Culture, Central Nervous System Symptoms *on page 570*

Viral Culture, Cytomegalovirus *see* Cytomegalovirus Culture *on page 388*

Viral Culture, Eye *see* Herpes Simplex Virus Culture *on page 446*

Viral Culture, Genital *see* Herpes Simplex Virus Culture *on page 446*

Viral Culture, Nasopharyngeal *see* Viral Culture, Throat *on page 574*

Viral Culture, Pulmonary Biopsy *see* Viral Culture, Throat *on page 574*

Viral Culture, Rash *see* Varicella-Zoster Virus Culture *on page 568*

Viral Culture, Skin *see* Herpes Simplex Virus Culture *on page 446*

Viral Culture, Skin see Varicella-Zoster Virus Culture on page 568

Viral Culture, Stool

Synonyms Stool Viral Culture

Applies to Adenovirus Culture, Stool; Coxsackie Virus Culture, Stool; Echovirus Culture, Stool; Enterovirus Culture, Stool; Poliovirus Culture, Stool

Test Includes Isolation and identification of viruses

Specimen Stool or rectal swab. Freshly passed stool is much more preferable than a rectal swab.

Container Stool: screw cap container. Do not use cardboard or waxed containers. Swab: cold viral transport medium

Collection Collect stools into a clean and dry container. Insert swab gently into rectum and hold there for 10-15 seconds, moisten with contents of Culturette® bulb, and send to laboratory.

Storage Instructions Keep specimens cold

Causes for Rejection Dry specimen, specimen not refrigerated during transport, specimen fixed in formalin, unlabeled specimen

Turnaround Time Variable (usually 1-14 days) and depends on cell culture methods and amount of virus in the specimen

Reference Range No virus isolated

Use Identify carriage or excretion of a virus in stool; isolate and identify an enterovirus which could be the cause of meningitis

Limitations Children convalescing from upper respiratory illness or aseptic meningitis can shed virus in the stool for weeks; children recently vaccinated against polio can shed poliovirus in the stool for months after vaccination; sampling errors; presence of nonculturable, disease-causing virus (eg, encephalitis, hepatitis, and gastroenteritis viruses)

Methodology Inoculation of specimen into cell cultures, incubation of cultures, observation of characteristic cytopathic effect, and identification/speciation by methods such as hemadsorption and fluorescent monoclonal antibodies. If specific viruses such as HSV, CMV, VZV, or adenovirus are suspected, the laboratory might be able to use rapid (1-2 days) culture (shell vial) methods to detect these viruses.

Additional Information See table for viruses most likely to be isolated from stool specimens. The viruses most likely to be isolated from stool specimen are

Viruses Typically Isolated From Clinical Specimens

Specimen	Virus*
Blood	CMV, enteroviruses†,#, HSV#, VZV#
CSF and CNS tissues	Enteroviruses, mumps virus, HSV, CMV
Dermal lesions	HSV, VZV, adenovirus, enteroviruses
Eye	HSV, VZV, adenovirus, enteroviruses, CMV, Chlamydia
Genital	HSV, CMV, Chlamydia
Mucosal	HSV, VZV
Oral	HSV, VZV
Rectal	HSV, VZV, enterovirus
Respiratory tract	
upper	Adenovirus, rhinovirus, influenza, parainfluenza, enteroviruses, RSV, reovirus, HSV
lower	Adenovirus, influenza, parainfluenza, RSV, CMV•
Stool	Enteroviruses, adenoviruses
Tissues	CMV, HSV, enteroviruses
Urine	CMV, adenovirus, enteroviruses, mumps

*Abbreviations:

  HSV — herpes simplex virus

  CMV — cytomegalovirus

  VZV — varicella-zoster virus

  RSV — respiratory syncytial virus

†Enteroviruses: coxsackie virus, poliovirus, echovirus, and enterovirus.

#Rarely isolated.

•Usually in immunocompromised hosts.

(Continued)

Viral Culture, Stool *(Continued)*

those which are extremely hardy and which do not have a lipid membrane envelope (ie, adenovirus and enterovirus (polio, Coxsackie, and echoviruses)).

Selected Readings

Lennette DA, "Preparation of Specimens for Virological Examination," *Manual of Clinical Microbiology*, 5th ed, Balows A, Hausler WJ Jr, Herrmann KL, et al, eds, Washington, DC: American Society for Microbiology, 1991, 818-21.

Viral Culture, Throat

Related Information

Adenovirus Culture *on page 309*
Influenza Virus Culture *on page 463*
Parainfluenza Virus Culture *on page 512*
Respiratory Syncytial Virus Culture *on page 528*

Synonyms Throat Viral Culture; Viral Culture, Bronchial Wash; Viral Culture, Nasopharyngeal; Viral Culture, Pulmonary Biopsy; Viral Culture, Throat Swab

Applies to Rhinovirus Culture

Test Includes Isolation and identification of virus most likely to cause respiratory disease

Patient Preparation Local anesthesia might be necessary

Specimen Throat swab; throat washing; nasopharyngeal washing, aspirates, or secretions; sputum; bronchial washings or lavage; lung biopsy

Container Cold and sterile viral transport medium for swabs; sterile cup for feces, washings, aspirates, and sputum

Sampling Time As soon as possible after onset of illness

Collection Methods are the same as those used for collecting most respiratory specimens (see Specimen). If respiratory syncytial virus or parainfluenza virus is suspected, see collection techniques in Parainfluenza Virus Culture *on page 512.*

Storage Instructions Keep specimen cold and moist. Transport to laboratory immediately.

Causes for Rejection Dry specimen, specimen not refrigerated during transport, specimen fixed in formalin, unlabeled specimen

Turnaround Time Variable (1-14 days) and depends on culture method and amount of virus in specimen

Reference Range No virus isolated

Use Determine etiological agent of viral respiratory infections (eg, pneumonia, pneumonitis, croup, and influenza)

Limitations Sampling errors; presence of nonculturable, disease-causing virus (eg, encephalitis, hepatitis, and gastroenteritis viruses); invasive procedures. Many persons carry and shed viruses which might not be related to the patient's illness.

Methodology Inoculation of specimen into cell cultures, incubation of cultures, observation of characteristic cytopathic effect, and identification/speciation by methods such as hemadsorption and the use of fluorescent monoclonal antibodies. If specific viruses such as HSV, CMV, VZV, or adenovirus are suspected, the laboratory might be able to use rapid (1-2 days) culture (shell vial) methods to detect these viruses. Most laboratories use hemadsorption to help determine the presence of a respiratory virus in cell culture and usually will report "hemadsorbing virus present." Some laboratories are capable of using specific virus-neutralizing antibodies to determine the particular type of virus which caused the observed hemadsorption. This final identification can require as many as several days and often is done only by reference laboratories.

Additional Information Viruses to be considered as causes of viral respiratory illness include the following: influenza virus, parainfluenza virus, rhinovirus, RSV, adenovirus, CMV, and reovirus. See table in the listing Viral Culture, Stool *on page 573*. Contact the Virology Laboratory and inform the staff if influenza or parainfluenza is suspected.

Selected Readings

Lennette DA, "Preparation of Specimens for Virological Examination," *Manual of Clinical Microbiology*, 5th ed, Balows A, Hausler WJ Jr, Herrmann KL, et al, eds, Washington, DC: American Society for Microbiology, 1991, 818-21.

Ruben FL and Cate TR, "Influenza Pneumonia," *Semin Respir Infect*, 1987, 2(2):122-9.

Welliver RC, "Detection, Pathogenesis, and Therapy of Respiratory Syncytial Virus Infections," *Clin Microbiol Rev*, 1988, 1(1):27-39.

Viral Culture, Throat Swab *see* Viral Culture, Throat *on previous page*

Viral Direct Detection by Fluorescent Antibody *see* Virus Detection by DFA *on next page*

Viral Serology

Test Includes Detection of IgG and/or IgM formed in response to infection by a specific virus

Special Instructions For the determination of immune status, a single specimen is sufficient. For the determination of acute disease, both acute and convalescent specimens must be tested.

Specimen Serum

Container Red top tube

Collection Two specimens should be collected, an acute specimen obtained as soon as possible after the onset of symptoms and a convalescent specimen obtained 10-14 days later. Both specimens should be tested when the convalescent specimen is obtained.

Reference Range Varies greatly and depends on the antibody being tested

Use Determine the immune status of a patient; help in the diagnosis of a viral infection when culture for the virus or methods for the detection of viral antigen(s) are not available or do not exist

Limitations Serological tests for antibodies to viruses can provide valuable diagnostic information. The detection of virus-specific IgM or more than a fourfold rise (from acute disease to convalescence) in virus-specific IgG titer can confirm acute infection, and viral serology is the only laboratory method for the laboratory diagnosis of many viral diseases. On the other hand, such tests can be fraught with many problems: The results obtained by testing a single specimen are rarely (only if the titer is obviously and extremely high), if ever, useful; for the results of viral serological test to be clinically relevant, both acute and convalescent serum must be tested at the same time; and false-positive results can result if interfering rheumatoid factor is in the specimen or when virus-specific antibody is attracted to Fc receptors in cell substrates used in viral serology assays.

Methodology Several methods are used to detect and semiquantitate antibodies to viruses: indirect fluorescent antibody (IFA), enzyme immunoassay (EIA), complement fixation (CF), and Western blot (WB)

Additional Information For viral serology studies to be effective, specific serological tests for specific viruses must be ordered. Orders for "TORCH titers", "TORCH serology", "viral studies", "virus serology", "encephalitis titers", etc are useless, confusing, and wasteful orders which usually lead to results of equally useless value. Laboratories usually issue reports of antibody levels in terms of titers (usually determined by dilution and immunofluorescence) or index values (usually determined by enzyme immunoassay), each of which when interpreted alone usually is not of much clinical value. A fourfold rise in titer or an appropriately higher index value after testing of acute and convalescent specimens is considered clinically relevant and significant. IgM antibody levels are not always observed/detected immediately following a primary viral infection. With the

Viral Serology Tests Available

Infectious Disease or Medical Condition	Viruses and/or Serology Panels to Be Considered
AIDS	Human immunodeficiency virus
CNS infections	Western, eastern, California, St Louis equine encephalitis, lymphocytic choriomeningitis, measles, mumps, Epstein-Barr, rabies
Exanthems	Measles, rubella, parvovirus
Vesicles	Herpes simplex, varicella-zoster
Hepatitis A/B/C/E	Hepatitis A/B/C/E
Heterophil-negative syndrome	Cytomegalovirus, Epstein-Barr
Myocarditis-pericarditis	Coxsackie, influenza, cytomegalovirus
Respiratory	Influenza, parainfluenza, respiratory syncytial virus, adenovirus
Determination of immune status (single specimen)	Measles, mumps, rubella, varicella-zoster, cytomegalovirus, hepatitis B

(Continued)

Viral Serology *(Continued)*

herpes viruses (HSV, CMV, VZV, and EBV), IgM can appear more than once and suggest a reinfection or reactivation. Complement fixation tests detect both IgG and IgM at the same time, but the test is not able to differentiate between the two classes of antibodies.

See table on previous page for a list of viruses for which serological testing methods exist. The table also shows infectious diseases and medical conditions in which testing for specific antibodies to multiple viruses (panels/batteries) might be indicated. Some laboratories offer these or similar serology panels.

Selected Readings
Thompson RB, "Laboratory Methods in Basic Virology," *Bailey and Scott's Diagnostic Microbiology,* 9th ed, Baron EJ, Peterson LP, and Finegold SM, eds, St Louis, MO: Mosby-Year Book Inc, 1994, 634-88.

Viral Study, Herpes *see* Herpes Cytology *on page 444*

Virus Detection by DFA

Related Information
Histopathology *on page 448*

Synonyms Direct Detection of Virus; Direct Fluorescent Antibody Test for Virus; Viral Direct Detection by Fluorescent Antibody; Virus Fluorescent Antibody Test

Applies to Herpes Simplex Virus, Direct Detection; Influenza Virus, Direct Detection; Measles Virus, Direct Detection; Mumps Virus, Direct Detection; Parainfluenza Virus, Direct Detection; Rabies Virus, Direct Detection; Respiratory Syncytial Virus, Direct Detection; Varicella-Zoster Virus, Direct Detection

Test Includes Direct (nonculture) detection of virus-infected cells

Special Instructions Make at least four impression smears or place four frozen sections on four separate slides. Cell suspensions should be centrifuged, resuspended to slight turbidity, and applied to prewelled slides.

Specimen Impression smears of tissues, lesion scrapings and swabs, frozen sections, cell suspensions, upper respiratory tract swabs

Causes for Rejection Insufficient material, slides broken or badly scratched, fixative used on slide preparation (generally, the laboratory is responsible for fixing specimens)

Turnaround Time Less than 1 day

Reference Range No virus detected

Use Rapid diagnosis of HSV, VZV, RSV, parainfluenza, influenza, and rabies infections

Limitations Only a few viruses (HSV, VZV, RSV, influenza, parainfluenza, measles, mumps, and rabies virus) can be detected in this manner. It is possible for the test to be negative in the presence of viral infection. Expertly trained and experienced personnel, excellent quality reagents and adequate numbers of cells are required. **Contact laboratory prior to requesting test to determine if laboratory offers this/these tests.**

Methodology Monoclonal antibody reagents and immunofluorescence microscopy are used to detect viruses/viral antigens in specimen cells.

Additional Information Generally, this test is not as sensitive as cell culture.

Selected Readings
Drew WL, "Controversies in Viral Diagnosis," *Rev Infect Dis,* 1986, 8(5):814-24.
Drew WL, "Diagnostic Virology," *Clin Lab Med,* 1987, 7(4):721-40.
Smith TF, "Rapid Methods for the Diagnosis of Viral Infections," *Lab Med,* 1987, 18:16-20.

Virus Fluorescent Antibody Test *see* Virus Detection by DFA *on page 576*

Wassermann *replaced by* RPR *on page 530*

WBC Scan *see* Indium Leukocyte Scan *on page 461*

Westergren Sedimentation Rate *see* Sedimentation Rate, Erythrocyte *on page 532*

Wet Preparation for *Trichomonas vaginalis* *see* Trichomonas Preparation *on page 555*

White Blood Cell Scan *see* Indium Leukocyte Scan *on page 461*

Whole Body Bone Scan *see* Bone Scan *on page 348*

Whooping Cough Culture *see* Bordetella pertussis Nasopharyngeal Culture *on page 349*

Wound Culture

Related Information

Abscess Aerobic and Anaerobic Culture *on page 304*

Synonyms Lesion Culture

Test Includes Culture for aerobic organisms and usually Gram's stain

Patient Preparation Sterile preparation of the aspiration site

Special Instructions The laboratory should be informed of the specific site of specimen, the age of patient, current antibiotic therapy, clinical diagnosis, and time of collection. The submission of biopsy specimens or specimens from normally sterile sites should be clearly indicated to the laboratory. Procedures for laboratory work-up of wound cultures which may contain contamination from the skin surface are different than those from sites which are expected to be sterile. Drainage cultured by aspiration away from a sinus tract may provide more useful information.

Specimen Tissue or aspirated pus/fluid properly obtained from a wound site or abscess

Container Sterile tube or screw-cap container. **Swab specimens are extremely inadequate for almost all specimens except for throat, cervix, and other small openings.**

Collection The specimen should be transported to laboratory as soon as possible after collection. Contamination with normal flora from skin, rectum, vaginal tract, or other body surfaces must be avoided.

Storage Instructions Refrigerate the specimen if it cannot be promptly processed.

Causes for Rejection Specimens delayed in transit to the laboratory may have less than optimal yields.

Turnaround Time Preliminary reports are usually available at 24 hours. Cultures with no growth are usually reported after 72 hours. Reports on specimens from which pathogens are isolated require a minimum of 48 hours for completion.

Reference Range No growth. A simultaneous Gram's stain should always be performed to facilitate interpretation. Gram-negative organisms, frequently colonize wounds and mixed culture results are common.

Use Isolate and identify potentially pathogenic organisms

Limitations Only rapid-growing, nonfastidious aerobic organisms will be screened for and identified by routine methods. Often only organisms which predominate will be completely identified. Unless specifically requested by the physician or mandated by the specimen source (ie, genital specimen) fastidious organisms such as *N. gonorrhoeae* may not be isolated. Fungal and mycobacterial pathogens should be considered and appropriate cultures requested if indicated.

Contraindications Culture of contaminated open wounds which have not been cleansed or debrided

Additional Information Susceptibility testing is performed if laboratory personnel determine such is appropriate; such testing is not always performed

Classification of Soft-Tissue Infections

Tissue Level	Common Surgical Pathogens				
	S. pyogenes	*S. aureus*	*C. perfringens*	Mixed Bacteria	
				Staph & Strep	Enteric
Epidermis	Ecthyma contagiosum	Scalded-skin syndrome		Possibly impetigo	
Dermis and subdermis	Erysipelas/cellulitis	Folliculitis/abscess	Abscess/cellulitis	Meleny's ulcer (synergistic gangrene)	Tropical ulcer
Fascial planes	Strep gangrene	Carbuncle	Fasciitis	Necrotizing fasciitis	
Muscle tissue	Strep myositis	Muscular abscess/ pyomyositis	Myonecrosis	Nonclostridial myonecrosis	

From Ahrenholz DH, "Necrotizing Soft Tissue Infections," *Surg Clin North Am*, 1988, 68:198-214, with permission.

(Continued)

Wound Culture *(Continued)*

automatically when "culture and sensitivity" is ordered by a physician. If anaerobes are suspected a properly collected specimen for anaerobic culture should also be submitted. See table on previous page.

Effective treatment of wound infection usually includes drainage, removal of foreign bodies, infected prosthetic devices, and retained foreign objects such as suture material. Suction irrigation may be helpful in resolving wound infections. Species commonly recovered from wounds include *Escherichia coli*, *Proteus* sp, *Klebsiella* sp, *Pseudomonas* sp, *Enterobacter* sp, enterococci, streptococci, staphylococci, *Bacteroides* sp, and *Clostridium* sp.

Selected Readings

Erlich KS and Rumack JS, "Evaluation and Management of Nonhealing Infected Wounds in Diabetics," *Infect Med*, 1993, 10(8):21-7.

Gerding DN, Piziak VK, and Rowbotham JL, "Saving the Diabetic Foot," *Patient Care*, 1991.

Goldstein EJ, "Management of Human and Animal Bite Wounds," *J Am Acad Dermatol*, 1989, 21(6):1275-9.

Pollock AV and Evans M, "Microbiologic Prediction of Abdominal Surgical Wound Infection," *Arch Surg*, 1987, 122(1):33-7.

Wound Fungus Culture *see* Fungus Culture, Body Fluid *on page 415*

Wound Mycobacteria Culture *see* Mycobacteria Culture, Biopsy or Body Fluid *on page 493*

Wrist Arthrogram *see* Arthrogram *on page 334*

Wrist, Left or Right, X-ray *see* Bone Films *on page 343*

Yersinia enterocolitica, Stool Culture *see* Stool Culture, Uncommon Organisms *on page 543*

Ziehl-Neelsen Stain *see* Acid-Fast Stain *on page 305*

Zoster Titer *see* Varicella-Zoster Virus Serology *on page 569*

ANTIMICROBIAL THERAPY

A-200™ Shampoo [OTC] *see* Pyrethrins *on page 885*

Abacavir (a BAK a veer)

Related Information
HIV Therapeutic Information *on page 1008*

U.S. Brand Names Ziagen®

Use Treatment of HIV infections in combination with other antiretroviral agents

Pregnancy Risk Factor C

Pregnancy/Breast-Feeding Implications
Clinical effects on the fetus: Administer during pregnancy only if benefits to mother outweigh risks to the fetus

Breast-feeding/lactation: HIV-infected mothers are discouraged from breast-feeding to decrease potential transmission of HIV

Health professional are encouraged to contact the antiretroviral pregnancy registry to monitor outcomes of pregnant women exposed to abacavir (1-800-258-4263)

Contraindications Prior hypersensitivity to abacavir (or carbovir) or any component; do not rechallenge patients who have experienced hypersensitivity to abacavir

Warnings/Precautions Should always be used as a component of a multidrug regimen. Fatal hypersensitivity reactions have occurred. **Patients exhibiting symptoms of fever, skin rash, fatigue, and GI symptoms (eg, abdominal pain, nausea, vomiting) should discontinue therapy immediately and call for medical attention.** Ziagen® **should not** be restarted because more severe symptoms may occur within hours, including **life-threatening hypotension and death**. To report these events on abacavir hypersensitivity, a registry has been established (1-800-270-0425). Use with caution in patients with hepatic dysfunction; prior liver disease, prolonged use, and obesity may be risk factors for development of lactic acidosis and severe hepatomegaly with steatosis.

Adverse Reactions Note: Hypersensitivity reactions, which may be fatal, occur in ~5% of patients (see Warnings/Precautions). Symptoms may include anaphylaxis, fever, rash, fatigue, diarrhea, abdominal pain, nausea and vomiting. Less common symptoms may include edema, lethargy, malaise, myalgia, shortness of breath, mouth ulcerations, conjunctivitis, lymphadenopathy, hepatic failure and renal failure.

Rates of adverse reactions were defined during combination therapy with lamivudine. Adverse reaction rates attributable to abacavir alone are not available.

Adults:
  Central nervous system: Insomnia (7%)
  Endocrine & metabolic: Hyperglycemia, hypertriglyceridemia (25%)
  Gastrointestinal: Nausea (47%), vomiting (16%), diarrhea (12%), anorexia (11%), pancreatitis
  Hepatic: Elevated transaminases
  Neuromuscular & skeletal: Weakness
Children:
  Central nervous system: Fever (19%), headache (16%)
  Dermatologic: Rash (11%)
  Gastrointestinal: Nausea (38%), vomiting (38%), diarrhea (16%), anorexia (9%)

Stability Store at room temperature; do not freeze oral solution. Oral solution may be refrigerated.

Mechanism of Action Nucleoside reverse transcriptase inhibitor. Abacavir is a guanosine analogue which is phosphorylated to carbovir triphosphate which interferes with HIV viral RNA dependent DNA polymerase resulting in inhibition of viral replication.

Pharmacodynamics/Kinetics
Distribution: V_d: 0.86 L/kg
Protein binding: 27% to 33%
Metabolism: Hepatic, via alcohol dehydrogenase and glucuronyl transferase to inactive carboxylate and glucuronide metabolites
Bioavailability: 83%
Half-life: 1.5 hours
Time to maximum peak: 0.7-1.7 hours

Elimination: Primarily in urine, as metabolites, (1.2% unchanged); fecal elimination accounted for only 16% of the total dose

Usual Dosage Oral:

Children: 3 months to 16 years: 8 mg/kg twice daily (maximum 300 mg twice daily) in combination with other antiretroviral agents

Adults: 300 mg twice daily in combination with other antiretroviral agents

Administration May be taken with or without food.

Patient Information If you have experienced any of the following: fever, skin rash, fatigue, nausea, vomiting, diarrhea, or abdominal pain, contact your physician **immediately**. If you are instructed to stop the medication, **do not take this medication in the future.**

Additional Information A medication guide is available and should be dispensed with each prescription or refill for abacavir. A warning card is also available and patients should be instructed to carry this card with them.

Dosage Forms

Solution, oral (strawberry-banana flavored): 20 mg/mL (240 mL)

Tablet: 300 mg

Selected Readings

Havlir DV and Lange JM, "New Antiretrovirals and New Combinations," *AIDS*, 1998, 12(Suppl A):S165-74.

Schmit JC and Weber B, "Recent Advances in Antiretroviral Therapy and HIV Infection Monitoring," *Intervirology*, 1997, 40(5-6)304-21.

"Three New Drugs for HIV Infection," *Med Lett Drugs Ther*, 1998, 40(1041):114-6.

Weverling GJ, Lange JM, Jurriaans S, et al, "Alternative Multidrug Regimen Provides Improved Suppression of HIV-1 Replication Over Triple Therapy," *AIDS*, 1998, 12(11):F117-22.

ABCD *see* Amphotericin B Cholesteryl Sulfate Complex *on page 596*

Abelcet™ *see* Amphotericin B, Lipid Complex *on page 600*

ABLC *see* Amphotericin B, Lipid Complex *on page 600*

Absorbine® Antifungal [OTC] *see* Tolnaftate *on page 956*

Absorbine® Antifungal Foot Powder [OTC] *see* Miconazole *on page 822*

Absorbine® Jock Itch [OTC] *see* Tolnaftate *on page 956*

Absorbine Jr.® Antifungal [OTC] *see* Tolnaftate *on page 956*

Acel-Imune® *see* Diphtheria, Tetanus Toxoids, and Acellular Pertussis Vaccine *on page 708*

Acetasol® HC Otic *see* Acetic Acid, Propylene Glycol Diacetate, and Hydrocortisone *on this page*

Acetic Acid, Propylene Glycol Diacetate, and Hydrocortisone

(a SEE tik AS id, PRO pa leen GLY kole dye AS e tate, & hye droe KOR ti sone)

U.S. Brand Names Acetasol® HC Otic; VōSol® HC Otic

Generic Available Yes

Use Treatment of superficial infections of the external auditory canal caused by organisms susceptible to the action of the antimicrobial, complicated by inflammation

Adverse Reactions Transient burning or stinging may be noticed occasionally when the solution is first instilled into the acutely inflamed ear

Usual Dosage Adults: Instill 4 drops in ear(s) 3-4 times/day

Dosage Forms Solution, otic: Acetic acid 2%, propylene glycol diacetate 3%, and hydrocortisone 1% (10 mL)

Achromycin® Ophthalmic *see* Tetracycline *on page 944*

Achromycin® Topical *see* Tetracycline *on page 944*

Aciclovir *see* Acyclovir *on this page*

ActHIB® *see* Haemophilus b Conjugate Vaccine *on page 756*

ACV *see* Acyclovir *on this page*

Acycloguanosine *see* Acyclovir *on this page*

Acyclovir (ay SYE kloe veer)

U.S. Brand Names Zovirax®

Canadian Brand Names Avirax™

Synonyms Aciclovir; ACV; Acycloguanosine

Generic Available Yes

(Continued)

Acyclovir (Continued)

Use Treatment of initial and prophylaxis of recurrent mucosal and cutaneous herpes simplex (HSV-1 and HSV-2) infections; herpes simplex encephalitis; herpes zoster; genital herpes infection; varicella-zoster infections in healthy, nonpregnant persons >13 years of age, children >12 months of age who have a chronic skin or lung disorder or are receiving long-term aspirin therapy, and immunocompromised patients; for herpes zoster, acyclovir should be started within 72 hours of the appearance of the rash to be effective; acyclovir will not prevent postherpetic neuralgias

Drug of Choice or Alternative for

Organism(s)

Herpes Simplex Virus *on page 170*

Varicella-Zoster Virus *on page 294*

Pregnancy Risk Factor C

Contraindications Hypersensitivity to acyclovir

Warnings/Precautions Use with caution in patients with pre-existing renal disease or in those receiving other nephrotoxic drugs concurrently; maintain adequate urine output during the first 2 hours after I.V. infusion; use with caution in patients with underlying neurologic abnormalities, serious hepatic or electrolyte abnormalities, or substantial hypoxia

Adverse Reactions

>10%:

Local: Inflammation at injection site

1% to 10%:

Central nervous system: Headache, lethargy, dizziness, seizures, confusion, agitation, coma

Dermatologic: Rash

Gastrointestinal: Nausea, vomiting

Neuromuscular & skeletal: Tremor

Renal: Impaired renal function

<1%: Mental depression, insomnia, anorexia, LFT elevation, sore throat, hallucinations, leukopenia, thrombocytopenia, anemia

Overdosage/Toxicology

Symptoms of overdose include seizures, somnolence, confusion, elevated serum creatinine, and renal failure

In the event of an overdose, sufficient urine flow must be maintained to avoid drug precipitation within the renal tubules. Hemodialysis has resulted in up to 60% reductions in serum acyclovir levels.

Drug Interactions Increased CNS side effects with zidovudine and probenecid

Stability Incompatible with blood products and protein-containing solutions; reconstituted solutions remain stable for 24 hours at room temperature; do not refrigerate reconstituted solutions as they may precipitate; in patients who require fluid restriction, a concentration of up to 10 mg/mL has been infused, however, concentrations >10 mg/mL (usual recommended concentration: <7 mg/mL in D_5W) increase the risk of phlebitis

Mechanism of Action Acyclovir is converted to acyclovir monophosphate by virus-specific thymidine kinase then further converted to acyclovir triphosphate by other cellular enzymes. Acyclovir triphosphate inhibits DNA synthesis and viral replication by competing with deoxyguanosine triphosphate for viral DNA polymerase and being incorporated into viral DNA.

Pharmacodynamics/Kinetics

Absorption: Oral: 15% to 30%; food does not appear to affect absorption

Distribution: Widely distributed throughout the body including brain, kidney, lungs, liver, spleen, muscle, uterus, vagina, and CSF

Protein binding: <30%

Metabolism: Small amount of hepatic metabolism

Half-life, terminal phase:

Neonates: 4 hours

Children 1-12 years: 2-3 hours

Adults: 3 hours

Time to peak serum concentration:

Oral: Within 1.5-2 hours

I.V.: Within 1 hour

Elimination: Primary route is the kidney (30% to 90% of a dose excreted unchanged); hemodialysis removes ~60% of the dose while removal by peritoneal dialysis is to a much lesser extent (supplemental dose recommended)

Usual Dosage

Dosing weight should be based on the smaller of lean body weight or total body weight

Treatment of herpes simplex virus infections: Children >12 years and Adults: I.V.:

Mucocutaneous HSV or severe initial herpes genitalis infection: 750 mg/m^2/day divided every 8 hours or 5 mg/kg/dose every 8 hours for 5-10 days

HSV encephalitis: 1500 mg/m^2/day divided every 8 hours or 10 mg/kg/dose for 10 days

Treatment of genital herpes simplex virus infections: Adults:

Oral: 200 mg every 4 hours while awake (5 times/day) for 10 days if initial episode; for 5 days if recurrence (begin at earliest signs of disease)

Topical: $1/2$" ribbon of ointment for a 4" square surface area every 3 hours (6 times/day)

Treatment of varicella-zoster virus (chickenpox) infections:

Oral:

Children: 10-20 mg/kg/dose (up to 800 mg) 4 times/day for 5 days; begin treatment within the first 24 hours of rash onset

Adults: 600-800 mg/dose every 4 hours while awake (5 times/day) for 7-10 days or 1000 mg every 6 hours for 5 days

I.V.: Children and Adults: 1500 mg/m^2/day divided every 8 hours or 10 mg/kg/dose every 8 hours for 7 days

Treatment of herpes zoster (shingles) infections:

Oral:

Children (immunocompromised): 250-600 mg/m^2/dose 4-5 times/day for 7-10 days

Adults (immunocompromised): 800 mg every 4 hours (5 times/day) for 7-10 days

I.V.:

Children and Adults (immunocompromised): 10 mg/kg/dose or 500 mg/m^2/dose every 8 hours

Older Adults (immunocompromised): 7.5 mg/kg/dose every 8 hours

If nephrotoxicity occurs: 5 mg/kg/dose every 8 hours

Prophylaxis in immunocompromised patients:

Varicella zoster or herpes zoster in HIV-positive patients: Adults: Oral: 400 mg every 4 hours (5 times/day) for 7-10 days

Bone marrow transplant recipients: Children and Adults: I.V.:

Allogeneic patients who are HSV seropositive: 150 mg/m^2/dose (5 mg/kg) every 12 hours; with clinical symptoms of herpes simplex: 150 mg/m^2/dose every 8 hours

Allogeneic patients who are CMV seropositive: 500 mg/m^2/dose (10 mg/kg) every 8 hours; for clinically symptomatic CMV infection, consider replacing acyclovir with ganciclovir

Chronic suppressive therapy for recurrent genital herpes simplex virus infections: Adults: 200 mg 3-4 times/day or 400 mg twice daily for up to 12 months, followed by re-evaluation

Dosing adjustment in renal impairment:

Oral: HSV/varicella-zoster:

Cl_{cr} 10-25 mL/minute: Administer dose every 8 hours

Cl_{cr} <10 mL/minute: Administer dose every 12 hours

I.V.:

Cl_{cr} 25-50 mL/minute: 5-10 mg/kg/dose: Administer every 12 hours

Cl_{cr} 10-25 mL/minute: 5-10 mg/kg/dose: Administer every 24 hours

Cl_{cr} <10 mL/minute: 2.5-5 mg/kg/dose: Administer every 24 hours

Hemodialysis: Dialyzable (50% to 100%); administer dose postdialysis

Peritoneal dialysis: Dose as for Cl_{cr} <10 mL/minute

Continuous arteriovenous or venovenous hemofiltration (CAVH/CAVHD) effects: Dose as for Cl_{cr} <10 mL/minute

Administration Infuse over 1 hour; maintain adequate hydration of patient; check and rotate infusion sites for phlebitis

Monitoring Parameters Urinalysis, BUN, serum creatinine, liver enzymes, CBC

(Continued)

Acyclovir (Continued)

Patient Information Patients are contagious only when viral shedding is occurring; recurrences tend to appear within 3 months of original infection; acyclovir is **not** a cure; avoid sexual intercourse when lesions are present; may take with food

Nursing Implications Wear gloves when applying ointment for self-protection

Additional Information Sodium content of 1 g: 96.6 mg (4.2 mEq)

Dosage Forms
Capsule: 200 mg
Powder for Injection: 500 mg (10 mL); 1000 mg (20 mL)
Ointment, topical: 5% [50 mg/g] (3 g, 15 g)
Suspension, oral (banana flavor): 200 mg/5 mL
Tablet: 400 mg, 800 mg

Selected Readings
"Drugs for Non-HIV Viral Infections," *Med Lett Drugs Ther*, 1994, 36(919):27.
Dunkle LM, Arvin AM, Whitley RJ, et al, "A Controlled Trial of Acyclovir for Chickenpox in Normal Children," *N Engl J Med*, 1991, 325(22):1539-44.
Keating MR, "Antiviral Agents," *Mayo Clin Proc*, 1992, 67(2):160-78.
Wallace MR, Bowler WA, Murray NB, et al, "Treatment of Adult Varicella With Oral Acyclovir," *Ann Intern Med*, 1992, 117(5):358-63.
Whitley RJ and Gnann JW Jr, "Acyclovir: A Decade Later," *N Engl J Med*, 1992, 327(11):782-3.

Adamantanamine Hydrochloride see Amantadine on page 586

Adefovir (a DEF o veer)

U.S. Brand Names Preveon®

Use Investigational as of 8/1/98; treatment of HIV infections in combination with at least two other antiretroviral agents; also has some activity against hepatitis B virus and herpes viruses

Pregnancy Risk Factor Not available

Contraindications Hypersensitivity to adefovir, pregnancy

Warnings/Precautions Use with caution in patients with renal insufficiency

Adverse Reactions Percentage unknown: Rise in hemoglobin, GI symptoms, urethritis, transaminase elevations, hot flashes

Mechanism of Action Acyclic nucleotide reverse transcriptase inhibitor which interferes with HIV viral RNA dependent DNA polymerase resulting in inhibition of viral replication

Pharmacodynamics/Kinetics
Distribution: V_d: 0.4 L/kg
Metabolism: Oral adefovir dipivoxil is converted to adefovir in intestine
Protein binding: <3%
Bioavailability: <12%
Half-life: 1.6 hours; 16-18 hours intracellularly
Elimination: As adefovir, unchanged in urine

Usual Dosage Oral:
HIV: 30-120 mg once daily
Hepatitis B: 125 mg once daily

Additional Information Product information was not available at the time of this writing; Preveon® expanded access program: 1-800-GILEAD-5

Selected Readings
Schmit JC and Weber B, "Recent Advances in Antiretroviral Therapy and HIV Infection Monitoring," *Intervirology*, 1997, 40(5-6)304-21.
"Three New Drugs for HIV Infection," *Med Lett Drugs Ther*, 1998, 40(1041):114-6.

Adenine Arabinoside see Vidarabine on page 973

Aftate® for Athlete's Foot [OTC] see Tolnaftate on page 956

Aftate® for Jock Itch [OTC] see Tolnaftate on page 956

Agenerase® see Amprenavir on page 609

AgNO₃ see Silver Nitrate on page 918

AK-Chlor® Ophthalmic see Chloramphenicol on page 667

AK-Cide® Ophthalmic see Sulfacetamide Sodium and Prednisolone on page 928

AK-Neo-Dex® Ophthalmic see Neomycin and Dexamethasone on page 835

AK-Poly-Bac® Ophthalmic see Bacitracin and Polymyxin B on page 619

AK-Spore® H.C. Ophthalmic Ointment see Bacitracin, Neomycin, Polymyxin B, and Hydrocortisone on page 620

AK-Spore® H.C. Ophthalmic Suspension *see* Neomycin, Polymyxin B, and Hydrocortisone *on page 836*

AK-Spore® H.C. Otic *see* Neomycin, Polymyxin B, and Hydrocortisone *on page 836*

AK-Spore® Ophthalmic Ointment *see* Bacitracin, Neomycin, and Polymyxin B *on page 619*

AK-Spore® Ophthalmic Solution *see* Neomycin, Polymyxin B, and Gramicidin *on page 836*

AK-Sulf® Ophthalmic *see* Sulfacetamide Sodium *on page 927*

AKTob® Ophthalmic *see* Tobramycin *on page 953*

AK-Tracin® Ophthalmic *see* Bacitracin *on page 618*

AK-Trol® *see* Neomycin, Polymyxin B, and Dexamethasone *on page 836*

Alatrovafloxacin Mesylate *see* Trovafloxacin *on page 960*

Albendazole (al BEN da zole)

U.S. Brand Names Albenza®

Generic Available No

Use Treatment of parenchymal neurocysticercosis and cystic hydatid disease of the liver, lung, and peritoneum; albendazole has activity against *Ascaris lumbricoides* (roundworm), *Ancylostoma duodenale* and *Necator americanus* (hookworms), *Enterobius vermicularis* (pinworm), *Hymenolepis nana* and *Taenia* sp (tapeworms), *Opisthorchis sinensis* and *Opisthorchis viverrini* (liver flukes), *Strongyloides stercoralis* and *Trichuris trichiura* (whipworm); activity has also been shown against the liver fluke *Clonorchis sinensis*, *Giardia lamblia*, *Cysticercus cellulosae*, *Echinococcus granulosus*, *Echinococcus multilocularis*, and *Toxocara* sp.

Drug of Choice or Alternative for
Organism(s)
Microsporidia *on page 195*

Pregnancy Risk Factor C

Pregnancy/Breast-Feeding Implications Albendazole has been shown to be teratogenic in laboratory animals and should not be used during pregnancy, if at all possible

Contraindications Patients with hypersensitivity to albendazole or its components; pregnant women, if possible

Warnings/Precautions Discontinue therapy if LFT elevations are significant; may restart treatment when decreased to pretreatment values. Becoming pregnant within 1 month following therapy is not advised. Corticosteroids should be administered 1-2 days before albendazole therapy in patients with neurocysticercosis to minimize inflammatory reactions and steroid and anticonvulsant therapy should be used concurrently during the first week of therapy for neurocysticercosis to prevent cerebral hypertension. If retinal lesions exist in patients with neurocysticercosis, weigh risk of further retinal damage due to albendazole-induced changes to the retinal lesion vs benefit of disease treatment.

Adverse Reactions N = neurocysticercosis; H = hydatid disease
Central nervous system: Dizziness, vertigo, fever (≤1%); headache (11% - N; 1% - H); increased intracranial pressure
Dermatologic: Alopecia/rash/urticaria (<1%)
Gastrointestinal: Abdominal pain (6% - H, 0% - N); nausea/vomiting (3% to 6%)
Hematologic: Leukopenia (reversible) (<1%); granulocytopenia/agranulocytopenia/pancytopenia (rare)
Hepatic: Increased LFTs (~15% - H, <1% - N)
Miscellaneous: Allergic reactions (<1%)

Drug Interactions
Decreased effect: Carbamazepine may accelerate albendazole metabolism
Increased effect: Dexamethasone increases plasma levels of albendazole metabolites; praziquantel may increase plasma concentrations of albendazole by 50%; albendazole inhibits hepatic cytochrome P-450 1A and may consequently interact by increasing the concentrations of many drugs which are metabolized by this route; food (especially fatty meals) increases the oral bioavailability by 4-5 times

Mechanism of Action Active metabolite, albendazole, causes selective degeneration of cytoplasmic microtubules in intestinal and tegmental cells of intestinal helminths and larvae; glycogen is depleted, glucose uptake and cholinesterase secretion are impaired, and desecratory substances accumulate intracellulary.

(Continued)

Albendazole *(Continued)*

ATP production decreases causing energy depletion, immobilization, and worm death.

Pharmacodynamics/Kinetics

Absorption: Oral absorption is poor (<5%); may increase up to 4-5 times when administered with a fatty meal

Distribution: Well distributed inside hydatid cysts; excellent CSF concentrations

Protein binding: 70%

Metabolism: Extensive first-pass metabolism; metabolic pathways include rapid sulfoxidation (major), hydrolysis, and oxidation

Half-life: 8-12 hours

Time to peak serum concentration: 2-2.4 hours

Elimination: Active and inactive metabolites excreted in urine

Usual Dosage Oral:

Neurocysticercosis:

<60 kg: 15 mg/kg/day in 2 divided doses (maximum: 800 mg/day) with meals for 8-30 days

≥60 kg: 400 mg twice daily for 8-30 days

Note: Give concurrent anticonvulsant and steroid therapy during first week

Hydatid:

<60 kg: 15 mg/kg/day in 2 divided doses with meals (maximum: 800 mg/day) for three 28-day cycles with 14-day drug-free interval in-between

≥60 kg: 400 mg twice daily for 3 cycles as above

Strongyloidiasis/tapeworm:

≤2 years: 200 mg/day for 3 days; may repeat in 3 weeks

>2 years and Adults: 400 mg/day for 3 days; may repeat in 3 weeks

Giardiasis: Adults: 400 mg/day for 3 days

Hookworm, pinworm, roundworm:

≤2 years: 200 mg as a single dose; may repeat in 3 weeks

>2 years and Adults: 400 mg as a single dose; may repeat in 3 weeks

Administration Give with meals; administer anticonvulsant and steroid therapy during first week of neurocysticercosis therapy

Monitoring Parameters Monitor fecal specimens for ova and parasites for 3 weeks after treatment; if positive, retreat; monitor LFTs, and clinical signs of hepatotoxicity; CBC at start of each 28-day cycle and every 2 weeks during therapy

Patient Information Take with a high fat diet

Dosage Forms Tablet: 200 mg

Selected Readings

de Silva N, Guyatt H, and Bundy D, "Anthelmintics. A Comparative Review of Their Clinical Pharmacology," *Drugs*, 1997, 53(5):769-88.

Liu LX and Weller PF, "Antiparasitic Drugs," *N Engl J Med*, 1996, 334(18):1178-84.

Albenza® *see* Albendazole *on previous page*

Aldara™ *see* Imiquimod *on page 769*

Amantadine (a MAN ta deen)

U.S. Brand Names Symadine®; Symmetrel®

Canadian Brand Names Endantadine®; PMS-Amantadine

Synonyms Adamantanamine Hydrochloride; Amantadine Hydrochloride

Generic Available Yes

Use Symptomatic and adjunct treatment of parkinsonism; prophylaxis and treatment of influenza A viral infection; treatment of drug-induced extrapyramidal symptoms

Drug of Choice or Alternative for

Organism(s)

Influenza Virus *on page 181*

Pregnancy Risk Factor C

Contraindications Hypersensitivity to amantadine hydrochloride or any component

Warnings/Precautions Use with caution in patients with liver disease, a history of recurrent and eczematoid dermatitis, uncontrolled psychosis or severe psychoneurosis, seizures and in those receiving CNS stimulant drugs; reduce dose in renal disease; when treating Parkinson's disease, do not discontinue abruptly. In many patients, the therapeutic benefits of amantadine are limited to a few months. Elderly patients may be more susceptible to the CNS effects (using 2 divided daily doses may minimize this effect).

Adverse Reactions

1% to 10%:

Cardiovascular: Orthostatic hypotension, peripheral edema

Central nervous system: Insomnia, depression, anxiety, irritability, dizziness, hallucinations, headache

Dermatologic: Livedo reticularis

Gastrointestinal: Nausea, anorexia, constipation, xerostomia

<1%: Congestive heart failure, slurred speech, confusion, fatigue, rash, decreased libido, urinary retention, vomiting, weakness, visual disturbances, dyspnea

Overdosage/Toxicology

Symptoms of overdose include nausea, vomiting, slurred speech, blurred vision, lethargy, hallucinations, seizures, myoclonic jerking

Following GI decontamination, treatment should be directed at reducing the CNS stimulation and at maintaining cardiovascular function. Seizures can be treated with diazepam while a lidocaine infusion may be required for the cardiac dysrhythmias.

Drug Interactions

Increased effect: Drugs with anticholinergic or CNS stimulant activity

Increased toxicity/levels: Hydrochlorothiazide plus triamterene, amiloride

Stability Protect from freezing

Mechanism of Action As an antiviral, blocks the uncoating of influenza A virus preventing penetration of virus into host; antiparkinsonian activity may be due to its blocking the reuptake of dopamine into presynaptic neurons and causing direct stimulation of postsynaptic receptors

Pharmacodynamics/Kinetics

Onset of antidyskinetic action: Within 48 hours

Absorption: Well absorbed from GI tract

Distribution: To saliva, tear film, and nasal secretions; in animals, tissue (especially lung) concentrations higher than serum concentrations, crosses blood-brain barrier

V_d:

Normal: 4.4 ± 0.2 L/kg

Renal failure: 5.1 ± 0.2 L/kg

Protein binding:

Normal renal function: ~67%

Hemodialysis patients: ~59%

Metabolism: Not appreciable, small amounts of an acetyl metabolite identified

Half-life: 10-28 hours

Impaired renal function: 7-10 days

Time to peak: 1-4 hours

Elimination: 80% to 90% excreted unchanged in urine by glomerular filtration and tubular secretion

Usual Dosage

Children:

1-9 years: (<45 kg): 5-9 mg/kg/day in 1-2 divided doses to a maximum of 150 mg/day

10-12 years: 100-200 mg/day in 1-2 divided doses

Prophylaxis: Administer for 10-21 days following exposure if the vaccine is concurrently given or for 90 days following exposure if the vaccine is unavailable or contraindicated and re-exposure is possible

Adults:

Drug-induced extrapyramidal reactions: 100 mg twice daily; may increase to 300 mg/day, if needed

Parkinson's disease: 100 mg twice daily as sole therapy; may increase to 400 mg/day if needed with close monitoring; initial dose: 100 mg/day if with other serious illness or with high doses of other anti-Parkinson drugs

Influenza A viral infection: 200 mg/day in 1-2 divided doses

Prophylaxis: Minimum 10-day course of therapy following exposure if the vaccine is concurrently given or for 90 days following exposure if the vaccine is unavailable or contraindicated and re-exposure is possible

Elderly patients should take the drug in 2 daily doses rather than a single dose to avoid adverse neurologic reactions; see Warnings/Precautions

(Continued)

Amantadine *(Continued)*

Dosing interval in renal impairment:
Cl_{cr} 50-60 mL/minute: Administer 200 mg alternating with 100 mg/day
Cl_{cr} 30-50 mL/minute: Administer 100 mg/day
Cl_{cr} 20-30 mL/minute: Administer 200 mg twice weekly
Cl_{cr} 10-20 mL/minute: Administer 100 mg 3 times/week
Cl_{cr} <10 mL/minute: Administer 200 mg alternating with 100 mg every 7 days
Hemodialysis: Slightly hemodialyzable (5% to 20%); no supplemental dose is needed
Peritoneal dialysis: No supplemental dose is needed
Continuous arteriovenous or venovenous hemofiltration (CAVH/CAVHD): No supplemental dose is needed

Monitoring Parameters Renal function, mental status, blood pressure

Patient Information Do not abruptly discontinue therapy, it may precipitate a parkinsonian crisis; may impair ability to perform activities requiring mental alertness or coordination; must take throughout flu season or for at least 10 days following vaccination for effective prophylaxis; take second dose of the day in early afternoon to decrease incidence of insomnia

Nursing Implications If insomnia occurs, the last daily dose should be given several hours before retiring; assess parkinsonian symptoms prior to and throughout course of therapy

Dosage Forms
Capsule, as hydrochloride: 100 mg
Syrup, as hydrochloride: 50 mg/5 mL (480 mL)

Selected Readings
Arden NH, Patriarca PA, Fasano MB, et al, "The Roles of Vaccination and Amantadine Prophylaxis in Controlling an Outbreak of Influenza A (H3N2) in a Nursing Home," *Arch Intern Med*, 1988, 148(4):865-8.
Douglas RG Jr, "Prophylaxis and Treatment of Influenza," *N Engl J Med*, 1990, 322(7):443-50.
"Drugs for Non-HIV Viral Infections," *Med Lett Drugs Ther*, 1994, 36(919):27.
Keating MR, "Antiviral Agents," *Mayo Clin Proc*, 1992, 67(2):160-78.
Somani SK, Degelau J, Cooper SL, et al, "Comparison of Pharmacokinetic and Safety Profiles of Amantadine 50- and 100-mg Daily Doses in Elderly Nursing Home Residents," *Pharmacotherapy*, 1991, 11(6):460-6.

Amantadine Hydrochloride *see* Amantadine *on page 586*
AmBisome® *see* Amphotericin B, Liposomal *on page 602*

Amikacin *(am i KAY sin)*

Related Information
Aminoglycoside Dosing and Monitoring *on page 1058*
Antimicrobial Activity Against Selected Organisms *on page 983*
Tuberculosis Guidelines *on page 1114*

U.S. Brand Names Amikin® Injection
Canadian Brand Names Amikin®
Synonyms Amikacin Sulfate
Generic Available No

Use Treatment of serious infections due to organisms resistant to gentamicin and tobramycin including *Pseudomonas, Proteus, Serratia,* and other gram-positive bacilli (bone infections, respiratory tract infections, endocarditis, and septicemia); documented infection of mycobacterial organisms susceptible to amikacin.

Drug of Choice or Alternative for
Organism(s)
Mycobacterium avium-intracellulare on page 201

Pregnancy Risk Factor C

Contraindications Hypersensitivity to amikacin sulfate or any component; cross-sensitivity may exist with other aminoglycosides

Warnings/Precautions Dose and/or frequency of administration must be monitored and modified in patients with renal impairment; drug should be discontinued if signs of ototoxicity, nephrotoxicity, or hypersensitivity occur; ototoxicity is proportional to the amount of drug given and the duration of treatment; tinnitus or vertigo may be indications of vestibular injury and impending bilateral irreversible damage; renal damage is usually reversible

Adverse Reactions

1% to 10%:
 Central nervous system: Neurotoxicity
 Otic: Ototoxicity (auditory), ototoxicity (vestibular)
 Renal: Nephrotoxicity
<1%: Hypotension, headache, drowsiness, drug fever, rash, nausea, vomiting, eosinophilia, paresthesia, tremor, arthralgia, weakness, dyspnea

Overdosage/Toxicology

Symptoms of overdose include ototoxicity, nephrotoxicity, and neuromuscular toxicity

Treatment of choice following a single acute overdose appears to be the maintenance of good urine output of at least 3 mL/kg/hour. Dialysis is of questionable value in the enhancement of aminoglycoside elimination. If required, hemodialysis is preferred over peritoneal dialysis in patients with normal renal function.

Drug Interactions

Decreased effect of aminoglycoside: High concentrations of penicillins and/or cephalosporins (in vitro data)

Increased toxicity of aminoglycoside: Indomethacin I.V., amphotericin, loop diuretics, vancomycin, enflurane, methoxyflurane; increased toxicity of depolarizing and nondepolarizing neuromuscular blocking agents and polypeptide antibiotics with administration of aminoglycosides

Stability Stable for 24 hours at room temperature and 2 days at refrigeration when mixed in D_5W, $D_5^1/_4NS$, $D_5^1/_2NS$, NS, LR

Mechanism of Action Inhibits protein synthesis in susceptible bacteria by binding to 30S ribosomal subunits

Pharmacodynamics/Kinetics

Absorption: I.M.: May be delayed in the bedridden patient

Distribution: Crosses the placenta; primarily distributes into extracellular fluid (highly hydrophilic); penetrates the blood-brain barrier when meninges are inflamed

 Relative diffusion of antimicrobial agents from blood into cerebrospinal fluid (CSF): Good only with inflammation (exceeds usual MICs); ratio of CSF to blood level (%):
  Normal meninges: 10-20
  Inflamed meninges: 15-24

Half-life (dependent on renal function):
 Infants:
  Low birthweight (1-3 days): 7-9 hours
  Full term >7 days: 4-5 hours
 Children: 1.6-2.5 hours
 Adults:
  Normal renal function: 1.4-2.3 hours
  Anuria: End stage renal disease: 28-86 hours

Time to peak serum concentration: I.M.: Within 45-120 minutes

Elimination: 94% to 98% excreted unchanged in urine via glomerular filtration within 24 hours; clearance dependent on renal function and patient age

Usual Dosage Individualization is critical because of the low therapeutic index

Use of ideal body weight (IBW) for determining the mg/kg/dose appears to be more accurate than dosing on the basis of total body weight (TBW)
 In morbid obesity, dosage requirement may best be estimated using a dosing weight of IBW + 0.4 (TBW - IBW)

Initial and periodic peak and trough plasma drug levels should be determined, particularly in critically ill patients with serious infections or in disease states known to significantly alter aminoglycoside pharmacokinetics (eg, cystic fibrosis, burns, or major surgery)

Infants, Children, and Adults: I.M., I.V.: 5-7.5 mg/kg/dose every 8 hours

Some clinicians suggest a daily dose of 15-20 mg/kg for all patients with normal renal function. This dose is at least as efficacious with similar, if not less, toxicity than conventional dosing. (See also Aminoglycoside Dosing and Monitoring on page 1058.)

Dosing interval in renal impairment: Some patients may require larger or more frequent doses if serum levels document the need (ie, cystic fibrosis or febrile granulocytopenic patients)

(Continued)

Amikacin *(Continued)*

Cl$_{cr}$ ≥60 mL/minute: Administer every 8 hours
Cl$_{cr}$ 40-60 mL/minute: Administer every 12 hours
Cl$_{cr}$ 20-40 mL/minute: Administer every 24 hours
Cl$_{cr}$ <20 mL/minute: Loading dose, then monitor levels

Hemodialysis: Dialyzable (50% to 100%); administer dose postdialysis or administer $^2/_3$ normal dose as a supplemental dose postdialysis and follow levels

Peritoneal dialysis: Dose as Cl$_{cr}$ <10 mL/minute: Follow levels

Continuous arteriovenous or venovenous hemodiafiltration (CAVH/CAVHD) effects: Dose as for Cl$_{cr}$ 10-40 mL/minute and follow levels

Administration Administer I.M. injection in large muscle mass

Monitoring Parameters Urinalysis, BUN, serum creatinine, appropriately timed peak and trough concentrations, vital signs, temperature, weight, I & O, hearing parameters

Reference Range

Sample size: 0.5-2 mL blood (red top tube) or 0.1-1 mL serum (separated)

Therapeutic levels:

Peak:
Life-threatening infections: 25-30 µg/mL
Serious infections: 20-25 µg/mL
Urinary tract infections: 15-20 µg/mL

Trough:
Serious infections: 1-4 µg/mL
Life-threatening infections: 4-8 µg/mL

Toxic concentration: Peak: >35 µg/mL; Trough: >10 µg/mL

Timing of serum samples: Draw peak 30 minutes after completion of 30-minute infusion or at 1 hour following initiation of infusion or I.M. injection; draw trough within 30 minutes prior to next dose

Test Interactions Penicillin may decrease aminoglycoside serum concentrations *in vitro*

Patient Information Report loss of hearing, ringing or roaring in the ears, or feeling of fullness in head

Nursing Implications Aminoglycoside levels measured from blood taken from silastic central catheters can sometimes give falsely high readings (draw levels from alternate lumen or peripheral stick, if possible)

Additional Information Sodium content of 1 g: 29.9 mg (1.3 mEq)

Dosage Forms Injection, as sulfate: 50 mg/mL (2 mL, 4 mL); 250 mg/mL (2 mL, 4 mL)

Selected Readings

Begg EJ and Barclay ML, "Aminoglycosides - 50 Years On," *Br J Clin Pharmacol*, 1995, 39(6):597-603.

Cunha BA, "Aminoglycosides: Current Role in Antimicrobial Therapy," *Pharmacotherapy*, 1988, 8(6):334-50.

Edson RS and Terrell CL, "The Aminoglycosides," *Mayo Clin Proc*, 1999, 74(5):519-28.

Gilbert DN, "Once-Daily Aminoglycoside Therapy," *Antimicrob Agents Chemother*, 1991, 35(3):399-405.

Iseman MD, "Treatment of Multidrug-Resistant Tuberculosis," *N Engl J Med*, 1993, 329(11):784-91.

Lortholary O, Tod M, Cohen Y, et al, "Aminoglycosides," *Med Clin North Am*, 1995, 79(4):761-87.

McCormack JP and Jewesson PJ, "A Critical Reevaluation of the "Therapeutic Range" of Aminoglycosides," *Clin Infect Dis*, 1992, 14(1):320-39

Van der Auwera P, "Pharmacokinetic Evaluation of Single Daily Dose Amikacin," *J Antimicrob Chemother*, 1991, 27(Suppl C):63-71.

Amikacin Sulfate *see Amikacin on page 588*

Amikin® *see Amikacin on page 588*

Amikin® Injection *see Amikacin on page 588*

Aminobenzylpenicillin *see Ampicillin on page 604*

Aminoglycoside Dosing and Monitoring *see page 1058*

Aminoglycosides

Related Information

Antimicrobial Activity Against Selected Organisms *on page 983*

Refer to

Amikacin *on page 588*
Gentamicin *on page 747*
Kanamycin *on page 790*
Neomycin *on page 833*

Netilmicin *on page 837*
Streptomycin *on page 924*
Tobramycin *on page 953*

Drug of Choice or Alternative for

Disease/Syndrome(s)

Cholangitis, Acute *on page 21*
Fever, Neutropenic *on page 30*
Pneumonia, Hospital-Acquired *on page 46*
Sepsis *on page 48*
Urinary Tract Infection, Catheter-Associated *on page 52*

Organism(s)

Alcaligenes Species *on page 65*
Bordetella bronchiseptica *on page 80*
Pseudomonas aeruginosa *on page 235*
Yersinia enterocolitica *on page 299*

Aminosalicylate Sodium (a MEE noe sa LIS i late SOW dee um)

U.S. Brand Names Sodium P.A.S.
Canadian Brand Names Tubasal®
Synonyms PAS
Generic Available Yes
Use Adjunctive treatment of tuberculosis used in combination with other anti-tubercular agents; has also been used in Crohn's disease
Pregnancy Risk Factor C
Contraindications Hypersensitivity to aminosalicylate sodium
Warnings/Precautions Use with caution in patients with hepatic or renal dysfunction, patients with gastric ulcer, patients with CHF, and patients who are sodium restricted

Adverse Reactions
1% to 10%: Gastrointestinal: Nausea, vomiting, diarrhea, abdominal pain
<1%: Vasculitis, fever, skin eruptions, goiter with or without myxedema, leukopenia, agranulocytosis, thrombocytopenia, hemolytic anemia, jaundice, hepatitis

Overdosage/Toxicology
Acute overdose results in crystalluria and renal failure, nausea, and vomiting
Alkalinization of the urine with sodium bicarbonate and forced diuresis can prevent crystalluria and nephrotoxicity

Drug Interactions Decreased digoxin absorption; may increase anticoagulant effects of warfarin; diphenhydramine may decrease aminosalicylate absorption.
Mechanism of Action Aminosalicylic acid is a highly specific bacteriostatic agent active against *M. tuberculosis*. Structurally related to para-aminobenzoic acid (PABA) and its mechanism of action is thought to be similar to the sulfonamides, a competitive antagonism with PABA; disrupts plate biosynthesis in sensitive organisms

Pharmacodynamics/Kinetics
Absorption: Readily absorbed >90%
Metabolism: >50% acetylated in liver
Elimination: >80% excreted through kidneys as parent drug and metabolites; elimination is reduced with renal dysfunction

Usual Dosage Oral:
Children: 150 mg/kg/day in 3-4 equally divided doses
Adults: 150 mg/kg/day in 2-3 equally divided doses (usually 12-14 g/day)
Dosing adjustment in renal impairment:
Cl_{cr} 10-50 mL/minute: Administer 50% to 75% of dose
Cl_{cr} <10 mL/minute: Administer 50% of dose
Administer after hemodialysis

Administration Administer with food or meals
Patient Information Notify physician if persistent sore throat, fever, unusual bleeding or bruising, persistent nausea, vomiting, or abdominal pain occurs; do not stop taking before consulting your physician; take with food or meals; do not use products that are brown or purple; store in a cool, dry place away from sunlight. Take with food.
Nursing Implications Do not give if discolored
Additional Information Sodium content of 1 g: 108.1 mg (4.7 mEq)
Dosage Forms Tablet: 500 mg
(Continued)

Aminosalicylate Sodium *(Continued)*

Selected Readings

Davidson PT and Le HQ, "Drug Treatment of Tuberculosis - 1992," *Drugs*, 1992, 43(5):651-73.

"Drugs for Tuberculosis," *Med Lett Drugs Ther*, 1993, 35(908):99-101.

Iseman MD, "Treatment of Multidrug-Resistant Tuberculosis," *N Engl J Med*, 1993, 329(11):784-91.

Amoxicillin *(a moks i SIL in)*

Related Information

Antimicrobial Activity Against Selected Organisms *on page 983*

U.S. Brand Names Amoxil®; Biomox®; Polymox®; Trimox®; Wymox®

Canadian Brand Names Apo®-Amoxi; Novamoxin®; Nu-Amoxi; Pro-Amox®

Synonyms Amoxicillin Trihydrate; Amoxycillin; *p*-Hydroxyampicillin

Generic Available Yes

Use Treatment of otitis media, sinusitis, and infections caused by susceptible organisms involving the respiratory tract, skin, and urinary tract; prophylaxis of bacterial endocarditis in patients undergoing surgical or dental procedures; approved in combination for eradication of *H. pylori*

Drug of Choice or Alternative for

Disease/Syndrome(s)

Bronchitis *on page 20*

Otitis Media, Acute *on page 41*

Pharyngitis *on page 43*

Sinusitis, Community-Acquired, Acute *on page 48*

Urinary Tract Infection, Uncomplicated *on page 53*

Organism(s)

Haemophilus influenzae on page 157

Helicobacter pylori on page 160

Streptococcus agalactiae on page 266

Pregnancy Risk Factor B

Contraindications Hypersensitivity to amoxicillin, penicillin, or any component

Warnings/Precautions In patients with renal impairment, doses and/or frequency of administration should be modified in response to the degree of renal impairment; a high percentage of patients with infectious mononucleosis have developed rash during therapy with amoxicillin; a low incidence of cross-allergy with other beta-lactams and cephalosporins exists

Adverse Reactions

1% to 10%:

Central nervous system: Fever

Dermatologic: Urticaria, rash

Miscellaneous: Allergic reactions (includes serum sickness, rash, angioedema, bronchospasm, hypotension, etc)

<1%: Seizures, anxiety, confusion, hallucinations, depression (with large doses or patients with renal dysfunction), nausea, vomiting, leukopenia, neutropenia, thrombocytopenia, jaundice, interstitial nephritis

Overdosage/Toxicology

Symptoms of penicillin overdose include neuromuscular hypersensitivity (agitation, hallucinations, asterixis, encephalopathy, confusion, and seizures) and electrolyte imbalance with potassium or sodium salts, especially in renal failure

Hemodialysis may be helpful to aid in the removal of the drug from the blood, otherwise most treatment is supportive or symptom directed

Drug Interactions

Decreased effect: Efficacy of oral contraceptives may be reduced

Increased effect: Disulfiram, probenecid may increase amoxicillin levels

Increased toxicity: Allopurinol theoretically has an additive potential for amoxicillin rash

Stability Oral suspension remains stable for 7 days at room temperature or 14 days if refrigerated; unit dose antibiotic oral syringes are stable for 48 hours

Mechanism of Action Inhibits bacterial cell wall synthesis by binding to one or more of the penicillin binding proteins (PBPs); which in turn inhibits the final transpeptidation step of peptidoglycan synthesis in bacterial cell walls, thus inhibiting cell wall biosynthesis. Bacteria eventually lyse due to ongoing activity of cell wall autolytic enzymes (autolysins and murein hydrolases) while cell wall assembly is arrested.

Pharmacodynamics/Kinetics

Absorption: Oral: Rapid and nearly complete; food does not interfere

Distribution: Widely distributed to most body fluids and bone; penetration into cells, eyes, and across normal meninges is poor

Protein binding: 17% to 20%

Ratio of CSF to blood:
    Normal meninges: <1%
    Inflamed meninges: 8% to 90%

Metabolism: Partial

Half-life:
    Neonates, full-term: 3.7 hours
    Infants and Children: 1-2 hours
    Adults with normal renal function: 0.7-1.4 hours
    Patients with Cl_{cr} <10 mL/minute: 7-21 hours

Time to peak: 2 hours (capsule) and 1 hour (suspension)

Elimination: Renal excretion (80% as unchanged drug); lower in neonates

Usual Dosage Oral:

Children: 20-50 mg/kg/day in divided doses every 8 hours
    Subacute bacterial endocarditis prophylaxis: 50 mg/kg 1 hour before procedure

Adults: 250-500 mg every 8 hours or 500-875 mg twice daily; maximum dose: 2-3 g/day

Endocarditis prophylaxis: 2 g 1 hour before procedure

Helicobacter pylori: 250-500 mg 3 times/day or 500-875 mg twice daily; clinically effective treatment regimens include triple therapy with amoxicillin or tetracycline, metronidazole, and bismuth subsalicylate; amoxicillin, metronidazole, and an H_2-receptor antagonist; amoxicillin, lansoprazole, and clarithromycin.

Dosing interval in renal impairment:

Cl_{cr} 10-50 mL/minute: Administer every 12 hours

Cl_{cr} <10 mL/minute: Administer every 24 hours

Dialysis: Moderately dialyzable (20% to 50%) by hemo- or peritoneal dialysis

Continuous arteriovenous or venovenous hemofiltration (CAVH): Dose as per Cl_{cr} <10 mL/minute; ~50 mg of amoxicillin per liter of filtrate removed

Dietary Considerations Food: May be taken with food

Monitoring Parameters With prolonged therapy, monitor renal, hepatic, and hematologic function periodically; assess patient at beginning and throughout therapy for infection; monitor for signs of anaphylaxis during first dose

Test Interactions May interfere with urinary glucose tests using cupric sulfate (Benedict's solution, Clinitest®); may inactivate aminoglycosides *in vitro*

Patient Information Report diarrhea promptly; entire course of medication (10-14 days) should be taken to ensure eradication of organism; may interfere with oral contraceptives; females should report symptoms of vaginitis; pediatric drops may be placed on child's tongue or added to formula, milk, etc

Additional Information There is an increasing incidence of amoxicillin-resistant *H. influenzae* and *E. coli*; this should be taken into consideration when choosing treatment regimens

Dosage Forms

Capsule, as trihydrate: 250 mg, 500 mg

Powder for oral suspension, as trihydrate: 125 mg/5 mL (5 mL, 80 mL, 100 mL, 150 mL, 200 mL); 250 mg/5 mL (5 mL, 80 mL, 100 mL, 150 mL, 200 mL)

Powder for oral suspension, drops, as trihydrate: 50 mg/mL (15 mL, 30 mL)

Tablet, chewable, as trihydrate: 125 mg, 250 mg

Tablet, film coated: 500 mg, 875 mg

Selected Readings

Donowitz GR and Mandell GL, "Beta-Lactam Antibiotics," *N Engl J Med*, 1988, 318(7):419-26 and 318(8):490-500.

Wright AJ, "The Penicillins," *Mayo Clin Proc*, 1999, 74(3):290-307.

Amoxicillin and Clavulanate Potassium

(a moks i SIL in & klav yoo LAN ate poe TASS ee um)

Related Information

Antimicrobial Activity Against Selected Organisms *on page 983*

U.S. Brand Names Augmentin®

Canadian Brand Names Clavulin®

(Continued)

Amoxicillin and Clavulanate Potassium *(Continued)*

Synonyms Amoxicillin and Clavulanic Acid

Generic Available No

Use Treatment of otitis media, sinusitis, and infections caused by susceptible organisms involving the lower respiratory tract, skin and skin structure, and urinary tract; spectrum same as amoxicillin with additional coverage of beta-lactamase producing *B. catarrhalis*, *H. influenzae*, *N. gonorrhoeae*, and *S. aureus* (not MRSA).

Drug of Choice or Alternative for

Disease/Syndrome(s)

Bronchitis *on page 20*

Sinusitis, Community-Acquired, Acute *on page 48*

Organism(s)

Capnocytophaga Species *on page 93*

Haemophilus ducreyi on page 156

Haemophilus influenzae on page 157

Moraxella catarrhalis on page 196

Pasteurella multocida on page 224

Pregnancy Risk Factor B

Contraindications Known hypersensitivity to amoxicillin, clavulanic acid, or penicillin; concomitant use of disulfiram

Warnings/Precautions In patients with renal impairment, doses and/or frequency of administration should be modified in response to the degree of renal impairment; high percentage of patients with infectious mononucleosis have developed rash during therapy; a low incidence of cross-allergy with cephalosporins exists; incidence of diarrhea is higher than with amoxicillin alone Hepatic dysfunction, although rare, is more common in elderly and/or males and occurs more frequently with prolonged treatment.

Adverse Reactions

1% to 10%:

Dermatologic: Rash, urticaria

Gastrointestinal: Nausea, vomiting, diarrhea

Genitourinary: Vaginitis

<1%: Headache, abdominal discomfort, flatulence

Overdosage/Toxicology

Symptoms of penicillin overdose include neuromuscular hypersensitivity (agitation, hallucinations, asterixis, encephalopathy, confusion, and seizures) and electrolyte imbalance with potassium or sodium salts, especially in renal failure

Hemodialysis may be helpful to aid in the removal of the drug from the blood, otherwise most treatment is supportive or symptom directed

Drug Interactions

Decreased effect: Efficacy of oral contraceptives may be reduced

Increased effect: Disulfiram, probenecid may increase amoxicillin levels, increased effect of anticoagulants

Increased toxicity: Allopurinol theoretically has an additive potential for amoxicillin rash

Stability Discard unused suspension after 10 days; reconstituted oral suspension should be kept in refrigerator; unit dose antibiotic oral syringes are stable for 48 hours

Mechanism of Action Clavulanic acid binds and inhibits beta-lactamases that inactivate amoxicillin resulting in amoxicillin having an expanded spectrum of activity. Amoxicillin inhibits bacterial cell wall synthesis by binding to one or more of the penicillin binding proteins (PBPs); which in turn inhibits the final transpeptidation step of peptidoglycan synthesis in bacterial cell walls, thus inhibiting cell wall biosynthesis. Bacteria eventually lyse due to ongoing activity of cell wall autolytic enzymes (autolysins and murein hydrolases) while cell wall assembly is arrested.

Pharmacodynamics/Kinetics Amoxicillin pharmacokinetics are not affected by clavulanic acid

Absorption: Oral: Rapid and nearly complete; food does not interfere

Distribution: Both distribute into pleural fluids, lungs, and peritoneal fluid; high urine concentrations are attained; also into synovial fluid, liver, prostate, muscle, and gallbladder; penetrates into middle ear effusions, maxillary sinus secretions, tonsils, sputum, and bronchial secretions; crosses the placenta; low concentrations occur in breast milk

Protein binding: 17% to 20%

Metabolism: Partial (Clavulanic acid is hepatically metabolized)

Half-life:

Neonates, full-term: 3.7 hours

Infants and Children: 1-2 hours

Adults with normal renal function: ~1 hour for both agents

Patients with Cl_{cr} <10 mL/minute: 7-21 hours

Time to peak: 2 hours (capsule) and 1 hour (suspension)

Elimination: Amoxicillin excreted primarily (80%) unchanged and clavulanic acid is excreted 30% to 40% unchanged in the urine (lower in neonates)

Usual Dosage Oral:

Children ≤40 kg: 20-40 mg (amoxicillin)/kg/day in divided doses every 8 hours or 45 mg/kg in divided doses every 12 hours

Children >40 kg and Adults: 250-500 mg every 8 hours or 875 mg every 12 hours

Note: Augmentin® 200 suspension or chewable tablets 200 mg dosed every 12 hours is considered equivalent to Augmentin® "125" dosed every 8 hours; Augmentin® 400 suspension and chewable tablets may be similarly dosed every 12 hours and are equivalent to Augmentin® "250" every 8 hours

Dosing interval in renal impairment:

Cl_{cr} 10-30 mL/minute: Administer every 12 hours

Cl_{cr} <10 mL/minute: Administer every 24 hours

Hemodialysis: Moderately dialyzable (20% to 50%)

Amoxicillin/clavulanic acid: Administer dose after dialysis

Peritoneal dialysis: Moderately dialyzable (20% to 50%)

Amoxicillin: Administer 250 mg every 12 hours

Clavulanic acid: Dose for Cl_{cr} <10 mL/minute

Continuous arteriovenous or venovenous hemofiltration (CAVH) effects:

Amoxicillin: ~50 mg of amoxicillin/L of filtrate is removed

Clavulanic acid: Dose for Cl_{cr} <10 mL/minute

Monitoring Parameters Assess patient at beginning and throughout therapy for infection; with prolonged therapy, monitor renal, hepatic, and hematologic function periodically; monitor for signs of anaphylaxis during first dose

Test Interactions May interfere with urinary glucose tests using cupric sulfate (Benedict's solution, Clinitest®); may inactivate aminoglycosides *in vitro*

Patient Information Report diarrhea promptly; entire course of medication (10-14 days) should be taken to ensure eradication of organism; females should report onset of symptoms of candidal vaginitis; may interfere with the effects of oral contraceptives

Nursing Implications Two 250 mg tablets are not equivalent to a 500 mg tablet (both tablet sizes contain equivalent clavulanate); potassium content: 0.16 mEq of potassium per 31.25 mg of clavulanic acid

Dosage Forms

Suspension, oral:

125 (banana flavor): Amoxicillin trihydrate 125 mg and clavulanate potassium 31.25 mg per 5 mL (75 mL, 150 mL)

200: Amoxicillin 200 mg and clavulanate potassium 28.5 mg per 5 mL (50 mL, 75 mL, 100 mL)

250 (orange flavor): Amoxicillin trihydrate 250 mg and clavulanate potassium 62.5 mg per 5 mL (75 mL, 150 mL)

400: Amoxicillin 400 mg and clavulanate potassium 57 mg per 5 mL (50 mL, 75 mL, 100 mL)

Tablet:

250: Amoxicillin trihydrate 250 mg and clavulanate potassium 125 mg

500: Amoxicillin trihydrate 500 mg and clavulanate potassium 125 mg

875: Amoxicillin trihydrate 875 mg and clavulanate potassium 125 mg

Tablet, chewable:

125: Amoxicillin trihydrate 125 mg and clavulanate potassium 31.25 mg

200: Amoxicillin trihydrate 200 mg and clavulanate potassium 28.5 mg

250: Amoxicillin trihydrate 250 mg and clavulanate potassium 62.5 mg

400: Amoxicillin trihydrate 400 mg and clavulanate potassium 57 mg

Selected Readings

Donowitz GR and Mandell GL, "Beta-Lactam Antibiotics," *N Engl J Med*, 1988, 318(7):419-26 and 318(8):490-500.

(Continued)

Amoxicillin and Clavulanate Potassium *(Continued)*

Todd PA and Benfield P, "Amoxicillin/Clavulanic Acid. An Update of Its Antibacterial Activity, Pharmacokinetic Properties and Therapeutic Use," *Drugs*, 1990, 39(2):264-307.
Wright AJ, "The Penicillins," *Mayo Clin Proc*, 1999, 74(3):290-307.

Amoxicillin and Clavulanic Acid *see* Amoxicillin and Clavulanate Potassium *on page 593*

Amoxicillin Trihydrate *see* Amoxicillin *on page 592*

Amoxil® *see* Amoxicillin *on page 592*

Amoxycillin *see* Amoxicillin *on page 592*

Amphocin® *see* Amphotericin B (Conventional) *on next page*

Amphotec® *see* Amphotericin B Cholesteryl Sulfate Complex *on this page*

Amphotericin B Cholesteryl Sulfate Complex

(am foe TER i sin bee kole LES te ril SUL fate KOM plecks)

U.S. Brand Names Amphotec®

Synonyms ABCD; Amphotericin B Colloidal Dispersion

Use Treatment of invasive aspergillosis in patients who have failed amphotericin B deoxycholate treatment, or who have renal impairment or experience unacceptable toxicity which precludes treatment with amphotericin B deoxycholate in effective doses.

Drug of Choice or Alternative for

Organism(s)

Aspergillus Species *on page 70*

Pregnancy Risk Factor B

Pregnancy/Breast-Feeding Implications Breast-feeding/lactation: Due to limited data, consider discontinuing nursing during therapy

Contraindications Hypersensitivity to amphotericin B or its components

Warnings/Precautions Anaphylaxis has been reported; facilities for cardiopulmonary resuscitation should be available; infusion reactions, sometimes, severe, usually subside with continued therapy; in addition, amphotericin B colloidal dispersion may cause fever, chills, hypotension, nausea, or tachypnea, usually beginning 1 to 3 hours after infusion

Adverse Reactions

>10%

Central nervous system: Chills, fever

Renal: Increased serum creatinine

1% to 10%:

Cardiovascular: Hypotension, tachycardia

Central nervous system: Headache

Dermatologic: Rash

Endocrine & metabolic: Hypokalemia, hypomagnesemia

Gastrointestinal: Nausea, diarrhea, abdominal pain

Hematologic: Thrombocytopenia

Hepatic: LFT change

Neuromuscular & skeletal: Rigors

Respiratory: Dyspnea

Overdosage/Toxicology

Symptoms of overdosage include renal dysfunction, anemia, thrombocytopenia, granulocytopenia, fever, nausea, vomiting

Treatment is supportive

Drug Interactions

Increased nephrotoxicity: Aminoglycosides, cyclosporine, other nephrotoxic drugs

Potentiation of hypokalemia: Corticosteroids, corticotropin

Increased digitalis and neuromuscular blocking agent toxicity due to hypokalemia

Decreased effect: Pharmacologic antagonism may occur with azole antifungal agents (eg, miconazole, ketoconazole)

Pulmonary toxicity has occurred with concomitant administration of amphotericin B and leukocyte transfusions

Stability Amphotec® must be reconstituted with sterile water for injection. Do not reconstitute lyophilized powder with saline, dextrose, or bacteriostatic water. Do not admix the reconstituted liquid with saline, electrolytes, or other medications. After reconstitution, the drug should be refrigerated at 2°C to 8°C (36°F to 48°F) and used within 24 hours. Do not freeze. After further dilution with 5% Dextrose for Injection, the infusion should be stored in a refrigerator (2°C to 8°C) and used within 24 hours.

Mechanism of Action Binds to ergosterol altering cell membrane permeability in susceptible fungi and causing leakage of cell components with subsequent cell death

Pharmacodynamics/Kinetics

Distribution: V_d: Total amphotericin B increases with increasing doses of total amphotericin B (with 4 mg/kg/day = 4 L/kg); predominantly distributed in the liver; concentrations in kidneys and other tissues are lower than observed with conventional amphotericin B

Half-life: 28-29 hours

Plasma concentration: Total amphotericin B remains between 1-3 mcg/mL

Elimination: Clearance: 0.1 L/hour/kg (with 4 mg/kg/day)

Usual Dosage Children and Adults: I.V.:

Premedication: For patients who experience chills, fever, hypotension, nausea, or other nonanaphylactic infusion-related immediate reactions, premedicate with the following drugs, 30-60 minutes prior to drug administration: a nonsteroidal (eg, ibuprofen, choline magnesium trisalicylate, etc) with or without diphenhydramine; or acetaminophen with diphenhydramine; or hydrocortisone 50-100 mg. If the patient experiences rigors during the infusion, meperidine may be administered.

Range: 3-4 mg/kg/day (infusion of 1 mg/kg/hour); maximum: 7.5 mg/kg/day

Monitoring Parameters Liver function tests, electrolytes, BUN, Cr, temperature, CBC, I/O, signs of hypokalemia (muscle weakness, cramping, drowsiness, EKG changes)

Additional Information Controlled trials which compare the original formulation of amphotericin B to the newer liposomal formulations are lacking. Thus, comparative data discussing differences among the formulations should be interpreted cautiously.

Dosage Forms Suspension for injection: 5 mg/mL (20 mL)

Selected Readings

Hiemenz JW and Walsh TJ, "Lipid Formulations of Amphotericin B: Recent Progress and Future Directions," *Clin Infect Dis*, 1996, 22 Suppl 2:S133-44.

Patel R, "Antifungal Agents. Part I. Amphotericin B Preparations and Flucytosine," *Mayo Clin Proc*, 1998, 73(12):1205-25.

Slain D, "Lipid-Based Amphotericin B for the Treatment of Fungal Infections," *Pharmacotherapy*, 1999, 19(3):306-23.

Amphotericin B Colloidal Dispersion *see* Amphotericin B Cholesteryl Sulfate Complex *on page 596*

Amphotericin B (Conventional)

(am foe TER i sin bee kon VEN shun al)

U.S. Brand Names Amphocin®; Fungizone®

Synonyms Amphotericin B Desoxycholate

Generic Available Yes

Use Treatment of severe systemic and central nervous system infections caused by susceptible fungi such as *Candida* species, *Histoplasma capsulatum*, *Cryptococcus neoformans*, *Aspergillus* species, *Blastomyces dermatitidis*, *Torulopsis glabrata*, and *Coccidioides immitis*; fungal peritonitis; irrigant for bladder fungal infections; and topically for cutaneous and mucocutaneous candidal infections.

Also used in fungal infection in patients with bone marrow transplantation, amebic meningoencephalitis, ocular aspergillosis (intraocular injection), candidal cystitis (bladder irrigation), chemoprophylaxis (low-dose I.V.), immunocompromised patients at risk of aspergillosis (intranasal/nebulized), refractory meningitis (intrathecal), coccidioidal arthritis (intra-articular/I.M.). Low-dose amphotericin B 0.1-0.25 mg/kg/day has been administered after bone marrow transplantation to reduce the risk of invasive fungal disease. Alternative routes of administration and extemporaneous preparations have been used when standard antifungal therapy is not available. Examples include inhalation, intraocular injection, subconjunctival application, intracavitary administration into various joints and the pleural space.

Drug of Choice or Alternative for

Disease/Syndrome(s)

Meningitis, Postsurgical *on page 36*

(Continued)

Amphotericin B (Conventional) *(Continued)*

Organism(s)

Aspergillus Species *on page 70*
Blastomyces dermatitidis on page 78
Candida Species *on page 91*
Coccidioides immitis on page 109
Cryptococcus neoformans on page 117
Dematiaceous Fungi *on page 125*
Dermatophytes *on page 127*
Fusarium Species *on page 150*
Histoplasma capsulatum on page 173
Malassezia furfur on page 192
Mucor Species *on page 198*
Penicillium marneffei on page 226
Prototheca Species *on page 233*
Sporothrix schenckii on page 253

Pregnancy Risk Factor B

Contraindications Hypersensitivity to amphotericin or any component

Warnings/Precautions Anaphylaxis has been reported with other amphotericin B-containing drugs. During the initial dosing, the drug should be administered under close clinical observation. Avoid additive toxicity with other nephrotoxic drugs; drug-induced renal toxicity usually improves with interrupting therapy, decreasing dosage, or increasing dosing interval. I.V. amphotericin is used primarily for the treatment of patients with progressive and potentially fatal fungal infections; topical preparations may stain clothing. Infusion reactions are most common 1-3 hours after starting the infusion and diminish with continued therapy. Use amphotericin B with caution in patients with decreased renal function. Pulmonary reactions may occur in neutropenic patients receiving leukocyte transfusions; separation of the infusions as much as possible is advised.

Adverse Reactions

>10%:

Central nervous system: Chills, headache, malaise, generalized pain, rigors, hyperpyrexia

Endocrine & metabolic: Hypokalemia, hypomagnesemia

Gastrointestinal: Anorexia

Hematologic: Anemia

Renal: Nephrotoxicity

1% to 10%:

Cardiovascular: Hypotension, hypertension, flushing

Central nervous system: Delirium, arachnoiditis, pain along lumbar nerves

Gastrointestinal: Nausea, vomiting

Genitourinary: Urinary retention

Hematologic: Leukocytosis

Local: Thrombophlebitis

Neuromuscular & skeletal: Paresthesia (especially with I.T. therapy)

Renal: Renal tubular acidosis, renal failure

<1%: Cardiac arrest, convulsions, maculopapular rash, coagulation defects, thrombocytopenia, agranulocytosis, leukopenia, acute liver failure, vision changes, hearing loss, anuria, dyspnea, bone marrow suppression

Overdosage/Toxicology

Symptoms of overdose include renal dysfunction, anemia, thrombocytopenia, granulocytopenia, cardiac arrest, fever, nausea, and vomiting

Treatment is supportive

Drug Interactions

Increased nephrotoxicity: Aminoglycosides, cyclosporine, other nephrotoxic drugs

Potentiation of hypokalemia: Corticosteroids, corticotropin

Increased digitalis and neuromuscular blocking agent toxicity due to hypokalemia

Decreased effect: Pharmacologic antagonism may occur with azole antifungal agents (eg, miconazole, ketoconazole)

Pulmonary toxicity has occurred with concomitant administration of amphotericin B and leukocyte transfusions

Stability

Reconstitute only with sterile water without preservatives, not bacteriostatic water. **Benzyl alcohol, sodium chloride, or other electrolyte solutions may cause precipitation.**

For I.V. infusion, an in-line filter (>1 micron mean pore diameter) may be used

Short-term exposure (<24 hours) to light during I.V. infusion does **not** appreciably affect potency

Reconstituted solutions with sterile water for injection and kept in the dark remain stable for 24 hours at room temperature and 1 week when refrigerated

Stability of parenteral admixture at room temperature (25°C): 24 hours; at refrigeration (4°C): 2 days

Standard diluent: Dose/250-500 mL D_5W

Mechanism of Action Binds to ergosterol altering cell membrane permeability in susceptible fungi and causing leakage of cell components with subsequent cell death

Pharmacodynamics/Kinetics

Distribution: Minimal amounts enter the aqueous humor, bile, CSF (inflamed or noninflamed meninges), amniotic fluid, pericardial fluid, pleural fluid, and synovial fluid

Protein binding, plasma: 90% infusion

Half-life, biphasic:

Initial: 15-48 hours

Terminal: 15 days

Time to peak: Within 1 hour following a 4- to 6-hour dose

Elimination: 2% to 5% of dose eliminated in biologically active form in urine; approximately 40% eliminated over 7-day period and may be detected in urine for at least 7 weeks after discontinued use

Usual Dosage

I.V.:

Premedication: For patients who experience chills, fever, hypotension, nausea, or other nonanaphylactic infusion-related immediate reactions, premedicate with the following drugs, 30-60 minutes prior to drug administration: a nonsteroidal (eg, ibuprofen, choline magnesium trisalicylate, etc) with or without diphenhydramine; or acetaminophen with diphenhydramine; or hydrocortisone 50-100 mg. If the patient experiences rigors during the infusion, meperidine may be administered.

Infants and Children:

Test dose (not required): I.V.: 0.1 mg/kg/dose to a maximum of 1 mg; infuse over 30-60 minutes. Many clinicians believe a test dose is unnecessary.

Maintenance dose: 0.25-1 mg/kg/day given once daily; infuse over 2-6 hours. Once therapy has been established, amphotericin B can be administered on an every-other-day basis at 1-1.5 mg/kg/dose; cumulative dose: 1.5-2 g over 6-10 week

Adults:

Test dose (not required): 1 mg infused over 20-30 minutes. Many clinicians believe a test dose is unnecessary.

Maintenance dose: Usual: 0.25-1.5 mg/kg/day; 1-1.5 mg/kg over 4-6 hours every other day may be given once therapy is established; aspergillosis, mucormycosis, rhinocerebral phycomycosis often require 1-1.5 mg/kg/day; do not exceed 1.5 mg/kg/day

Duration of therapy varies with nature of infection: Usual duration is 4-12 weeks or cumulative dose of 1-4 g

I.T.: Meningitis, coccidioidal or cryptococcal:

Children: 25-100 mcg every 48-72 hours; increase to 500 mcg as tolerated

Adults: Initial: 25-300 mcg every 48-72 hours; increase to 500 mcg to 1 mg as tolerated; maximum total dose: 15 mg has been suggested

Oral: 1 mL (100 mg) 4 times/day

Topical: Apply to affected areas 2-4 times/day for 1-4 weeks of therapy depending on nature and severity of infection

Bladder irrigation: Candidal cystitis: Irrigate with 50 mcg/mL solution instilled periodically or continuously for 5-10 days or until cultures are clear

Dosing adjustment in renal impairment: If renal dysfunction is due to the drug, the daily total can be decreased by 50% or the dose can be given every other day; I.V. therapy may take several months

(Continued)

Amphotericin B (Conventional) *(Continued)*

Dialysis: Poorly dialyzed; no supplemental dosage necessary when using hemo- or peritoneal dialysis or CAVH/CAVHD

Administration in dialysate: Children and Adults: 1-2 mg/L of peritoneal dialysis fluid either with or without low-dose I.V. amphotericin B (a total dose of 2-10 mg/kg given over 7-14 days); precipitate may form in ionic dialysate solutions

Monitoring Parameters Renal function (monitor BUN and creatinine frequently during therapy), electrolytes (especially potassium and magnesium), liver function tests, temperature, PT/PTT, CBC; monitor input and output; monitor for signs of hypokalemia (muscle weakness, cramping, drowsiness, EKG changes, etc)

Reference Range Therapeutic: 1-2 µg/mL (SI: 1-2.2 µmol/L)

Patient Information Amphotericin cream may slightly discolor skin and stain clothing; good personal hygiene may reduce the spread and recurrence of lesions; avoid covering topical applications with occlusive bandages; most skin lesions require 1-3 weeks of therapy; report any cramping, muscle weakness, or pain at or near injection site

Nursing Implications May be infused over 2-6 hours

Additional Information Renal toxicity may be minimized by sodium loading (500 mL NS with each dose), or pentoxifylline

Dosage Forms

Cream: 3% (20 g)

Lotion: 3% (30 mL)

Ointment, topical: 3% (20 g)

Powder for injection, lyophilized, as desoxycholate: 50 mg

Suspension, oral: 100 mg/mL (24 mL with dropper)

Selected Readings

Bianco JA, Almgren J, Kern DL, et al, "Evidence That Oral Pentoxifylline Reverses Acute Renal Dysfunction in Bone Marrow Transplant Recipients Receiving Amphotericin B and Cyclosporine," *Transplantation*, 1991, 51(4):925-7.

Branch RA, "Prevention of Amphotericin B-Induced Renal Impairment. A Review on the Use of Sodium Supplementation," *Arch Intern Med*, 1988, 148(11):2389-94.

Cruz JM, Peacock JE Jr, Loomer L, et al, "Rapid Intravenous Infusion of Amphotericin B: A Pilot Study," *Am J Med*, 1992, 93:123-30.

Gallis HA, Drew RH, and Pickard WW, "Amphotericin B: 30 Years of Clinical Experience," *Rev Infect Dis*, 1990, 12(2):308-29.

Kauffman CA and Carver PL, "Antifungal Agents in the 1990s. Current Status and Future Developments," *Drugs*, 1997, 53(4):539-49.

Lyman CA and Walsh TJ, "Systemically Administered Antifungal Agents. A Review of Their Clinical Pharmacology and Therapeutic Applications," *Drugs*, 1992, 44(1):9-35.

Patel R, "Antifungal Agents. Part I. Amphotericin B Preparations and Flucytosine," *Mayo Clin Proc*, 1998, 73(12):1205-25.

Slain D, "Lipid-Based Amphotericin B for the Treatment of Fungal Infections," *Pharmacotherapy*, 1999, 19(3):306-23.

Amphotericin B Desoxycholate *see* Amphotericin B (Conventional) *on page 597*

Amphotericin B, Lipid Complex

(am foe TER i sin bee LIP id KOM plex)

U.S. Brand Names Abelcet™

Synonyms ABLC

Generic Available No

Use Treatment of aspergillosis or any type of progressive fungal infection in patients who are refractory to or intolerant of conventional amphotericin B therapy

Orphan drug: Cryptococcal meningitis

Drug of Choice or Alternative for

Organism(s)

Aspergillus Species *on page 70*

Candida Species *on page 91*

Pregnancy Risk Factor B

Pregnancy/Breast-Feeding Implications Breast-feeding/lactation: Due to limited data, consider discontinuing nursing during therapy

Contraindications Hypersensitivity to amphotericin or any component in the formulation

Warnings/Precautions Anaphylaxis has been reported with other amphotericin B-containing drugs. Facilities for cardiopulmonary resuscitation should be available during administration due to the possibility of anaphylactic reaction. If severe respiratory distress occurs, the infusion should be immediately discontinued. During the initial dosing, the drug should be administered under close clinical observation. Acute reactions (including fever and chills) may occur 1-2 hours after starting an intravenous infusion. These reactions are usually more common with the first few doses and generally diminish with subsequent doses. Pulmonary reactions may occur in neutropenic patients receiving leukocyte transfusions; separation of the infusions as much as possible is advised.

Adverse Reactions

>10%:
Central nervous system: Chills, fever
Renal: Increased serum creatinine

1% to 10%:
Cardiovascular: Hypotension, cardiac arrest
Central nervous system: Headache, pain
Dermatologic: Rash
Endocrine & metabolic: Bilirubinemia, hypokalemia, acidosis
Gastrointestinal: Nausea, vomiting, diarrhea, gastrointestinal hemorrhage, abdominal pain
Renal: Renal failure
Respiratory: Respiratory failure, dyspnea, pneumonia

Drug Interactions

Increased nephrotoxicity: Aminoglycosides, cyclosporine, other nephrotoxic drugs
Potentiation of hypokalemia: Corticosteroids, corticotropin
Increased digitalis and neuromuscular blocking agent toxicity due to hypokalemia
Decreased effect: Pharmacologic antagonism may occur with azole antifungal agents (eg, miconazole, ketoconazole)
Pulmonary toxicity has occurred with concomitant administration of amphotericin B and leukocyte transfusions

Stability 100 mg vials in 20 mL of suspension in single-use vials (no preservative is present). Intact vials should be stored at 2°C to 8°C (35°F to 46°F) and protected from exposure to light; do not freeze intact vials. Shake the vial gently until there is no evidence of any yellow sediment at the bottom. Withdraw the appropriate dose and filter the contents (5 micron filter) prior to dilution. Dilute into D_5W to a final concentration of 1 mg/mL. For pediatric patients and patients with cardiovascular disease, the drug may be diluted with D_5W to a final concentration of 2 mg/mL.

Do not dilute with saline solutions or mix with other drugs or electrolytes - compatibility has not been established

Do not use an in-line filter <5 microns

Diluted solution is stable for up to 15 hours at 2°C to 8°C (38°F to 46°F) and an additional 6 hours at room temperature

Mechanism of Action Binds to ergosterol altering cell membrane permeability in susceptible fungi and causing leakage of cell components with subsequent cell death

Pharmacodynamics/Kinetics

Distribution: V_d: Increases with increasing doses; reflects increased uptake by tissues (131 L/kg with 5 mg/kg/day)
Half-life: ~24 hours
Clearance: Increases with increasing doses [400 mL/hour/kg (with 5 mg/kg/day)]

Usual Dosage Children and Adults: I.V.:

Premedication: For patients who experience chills, fever, hypotension, nausea, or other nonanaphylactic infusion-related immediate reactions, premedicate with the following drugs, 30-60 minutes prior to drug administration: a nonsteroidal (eg, ibuprofen, choline magnesium trisalicylate, etc) with or without diphenhydramine; or acetaminophen with diphenhydramine; or hydrocortisone 50-100 mg. If the patient experiences rigors during the infusion, meperidine may be administered.

Range: 2.5-5 mg/kg/day as a single infusion

Dosing adjustment in renal impairment: None necessary; effects of renal impairment are not currently known

(Continued)

Amphotericin B, Lipid Complex *(Continued)*

Hemodialysis: No supplemental dosage necessary

Peritoneal dialysis: No supplemental dosage necessary

Continuous arteriovenous or venovenous hemofiltration (CAVH/CAVHD): No supplemental dosage necessary

Monitoring Parameters Renal function (monitor frequently during therapy), electrolytes (especially potassium and magnesium), liver function tests, PT/PTT, CBC, temperature; monitor input and output; monitor for signs of hypokalemia (muscle weakness, cramping, drowsiness, EKG changes, etc)

Additional Information As a modification of dimyristoyl phosphatidylcholine:dimyristoyl phosphatidylglycerol 7:3 (DMPC:DMPG) liposome, amphotericin B lipid complex has a higher drug to lipid ratio and the concentration of amphotericin B is 33 M; ABLC is a ribbon-like structure, not a liposome

Dosage Forms Injection: 5 mg/mL (20 mL)

Selected Readings

De Marie S, "Clinical Use of Liposomal and Lipid-Complexed Amphotericin B," *J Antimicrob Chemother*, 1994, 33(5):907-16.

Hiemenz JW and Walsh TJ, "Lipid Formulations of Amphotericin B: Recent Progress and Future Directions," *Clin Infect Dis*, 1996, 22 Suppl 2:S133-44.

Kline S, Larsen TA, Fieber L, et al, "Limited Toxicity of Prolonged Therapy With High Doses of Amphotericin B Lipid Complex," *Clin Infect Dis*, 1995, 21(5):1154-8.

Patel R, "Antifungal Agents. Part I. Amphotericin B Preparations and Flucytosine," *Mayo Clin Proc*, 1998, 73(12):1205-25.

Rapp RP, Gubbins PO, and Evans ME, "Amphotericin B Lipid Complex," *Ann Pharmacother*, 1997, 31(10):1174-86.

Slain D, "Lipid-Based Amphotericin B for the Treatment of Fungal Infections," *Pharmacotherapy*, 1999, 19(3):306-23.

Amphotericin B, Liposomal *(am foe TER i sin bee lye po SO mal)*

U.S. Brand Names AmBisome®

Synonyms L-AmB

Generic Available No

Use Empirical therapy for presumed fungal infection in febrile, neutropenic patients. Treatment of patients with *Aspergillus* species, *Candida* species and/or *Cryptococcus* species infections refractory to amphotericin B desoxycholate, or in patients where renal impairment or unacceptable toxicity precludes the use of amphotericin B desoxycholate. Treatment of visceral leishmaniasis. In immunocompromised patients with visceral leishmaniasis treated with amphotericin B, liposomal, relapse rates were high following initial clearance of parasites.

Pregnancy Risk Factor B

Contraindications In those patients who have demonstrated or have known hypersensitivity to amphotericin B or any other constituents of the product unless, in the opinion of the treating physician, the benefit of therapy outweighs the risk

Warnings/Precautions Anaphylaxis has been reported with amphotericin B desoxycholate and other amphotericin B-containing drugs. Facilities for cardiopulmonary resuscitation should be available during administration due to the possibility of anaphylactic reaction. As with any amphotericin B-containing product the drug should be administered by medically trained personnel. During the initial dosing period, patients should be under close clinical observation. Amphotericin B, liposomal has been shown to be significantly less toxic than amphotericin B desoxycholate; however, adverse events may still occur. If severe respiratory distress occurs, the infusion should be immediately discontinued and the patient should not receive further infusions. Acute reactions (including fever and chills) may occur 1-2 hours after starting an intravenous infusion. These reactions are usually more common with the first few doses and generally diminish with subsequent doses.

Adverse Reactions

>10%:

Central nervous system: Chills, fever

Renal: Increased serum creatinine

Miscellaneous: Multiple organ failure

1% to 10%:

Cardiovascular: Hypotension, cardiac arrest

Central nervous system: Headache, pain

Dermatologic: Rash

Endocrine & metabolic: Bilirubinemia, hypokalemia, acidosis

Gastrointestinal: Nausea, vomiting, diarrhea, gastrointestinal hemorrhage, abdominal pain

Renal: Renal failure

Respiratory: Respiratory failure, dyspnea, pneumonia

Overdosage/Toxicology

The toxicity due to overdose has not been defined. Repeated daily doses up to 7.5 mg/kg have been administered in clinical trials with no reported dose-related toxicity.

If overdosage should occur, cease administration immediately. Symptomatic supportive measures should be instituted. Particular attention should be given to monitoring renal function.

Drug Interactions

Increased nephrotoxicity: Aminoglycosides, cyclosporine, other nephrotoxic drugs

Potentiation of hypokalemia: Corticosteroids, corticotropin

Increased digitalis and neuromuscular blocking agent toxicity due to hypokalemia

Decreased effect: Pharmacologic antagonism may occur with azole antifungal agents (eg, miconazole, ketoconazole)

Pulmonary toxicity has occurred with concomitant administration of amphotericin B and leukocyte transfusions

Stability Follow package insert instructions carefully for preparation. Must be reconstituted using sterile water for injection, USP (without a bacteriostatic agent). Do not reconstitute with saline or add saline to the reconstituted concentration, or mix with other drugs. The use of any solution other than those recommended, or the presence of a bacteriostatic agent in the solution, may cause precipitation.

Must be diluted with 5% dextrose injection to a final concentration of 1-2 mg/mL prior to administration. Lower concentrations (0.2-0.5 mg/mL) may be appropriate for infants and small children to provide sufficient volume for infusion.

Injection should commence within 6 hours of dilution with 5% dextrose injection.

An in-line membrane filter may be used for the intravenous infusion; provided, THE MEAN PORE DIAMETER OF THE FILTER SHOULD NOT BE LESS THAN 1 MICRON.

Mechanism of Action Binds to ergosterol altering cell membrane permeability in susceptible fungi and causing leakage of cell components with subsequent cell death

Pharmacodynamics/Kinetics

Distribution: V_d: 131 L/kg

Half-life, terminal elimination: 174 hours

Poorly dialyzed

Usual Dosage Children and Adults: I.V.:

Premedication: For patients who experience chills, fever, hypotension, nausea, or other nonanaphylactic infusion-related immediate reactions, premedicate with the following drugs, 30-60 minutes prior to drug administration: a nonsteroidal (eg, ibuprofen, choline magnesium trisalicylate, etc) with or without diphenhydramine; or acetaminophen with diphenhydramine; or hydrocortisone 50-100 mg. If the patient experiences rigors during the infusion, meperidine may be administered.

Empirical therapy: Recommended initial dose of 3 mg/kg/day

Systemic fungal infections (*Aspergillus*, *Candida*, *Cryptococcus*): Recommended initial dose of 3-5 mg/kg/day

Treatment of visceral leishmaniasis: Amphotericin B, liposomal achieved high rates of acute parasite clearance in immunocompetent patients when total doses of 12-30 mg/kg were administered. Most of these immunocompetent patients remained relapse-free during follow-up periods of 6 months or longer. While acute parasite clearance was achieved in most of the immunocompromised patients who received total doses of 30-40 mg/kg, the majority of these patients were observed to relapse in the 6 months following the completion of therapy.

Dosing adjustment in renal impairment: None necessary; effects of renal impairment are not currently known

Hemodialysis: No supplemental dosage necessary

Peritoneal dialysis effects: No supplemental dosage necessary

(Continued)

Amphotericin B, Liposomal *(Continued)*

Continuous arteriovenous or venovenous hemofiltration (CAVH/CAVHD): No supplemental dosage necessary

Administration Should be administered by intravenous infusion, using a controlled infusion device, over a period of approximately 2 hours. Infusion time may be reduced to approximately 1 hour in patients in whom the treatment is well-tolerated. If the patient experiences discomfort during infusion, the duration of infusion may be increased. Administer at a rate of 2.5 mg/kg/hour; infusion bag or syringe should be shaken before start of infusion. If infusion time exceeds 2 hours, the contents of the infusion bag should be mixed every 2 hours by shaking.

Monitoring Parameters Renal function (monitor frequently during therapy), electrolytes (especially potassium and magnesium), liver function tests, PT/PTT, CBC, temperature; monitor input and output; monitor for signs of hypokalemia (muscle weakness, cramping, drowsiness, EKG changes, etc)

Additional Information Amphotericin B, liposomal is a true single bilayer liposomal drug delivery system. Liposomes are closed, spherical vesicles created by mixing specific proportions of amphophilic substances such as phospholipids and cholesterol so that they arrange themselves into multiple concentric bilayer membranes when hydrated in aqueous solutions. Single bilayer liposomes are then formed by microemulsification of multilamellar vesicles using a homogenizer. Amphotericin B, liposomal consists of these unilamellar bilayer liposomes with amphotericin B intercalated within the membrane. Due to the nature and quantity of amphophilic substances used, and the lipophilic moiety in the amphotericin B molecule, the drug is an integral part of the overall structure of the amphotericin B liposomal liposomes. Amphotericin B, liposomal contains true liposomes that are less than 100 nm in diameter.

Dosage Forms Injection: 50 mg

Selected Readings

Hiemenz JW and Walsh TJ, "Lipid Formulations of Amphotericin B: Recent Progress and Future Directions," *Clin Infect Dis*, 1996, 22 Suppl 2:S133-44.

Patel R, "Antifungal Agents. Part I. Amphotericin B Preparations and Flucytosine," *Mayo Clin Proc*, 1998, 73(12):1205-25.

Slain D, "Lipid-Based Amphotericin B for the Treatment of Fungal Infections," *Pharmacotherapy*, 1999, 19(3):306-23.

Ampicillin *(am pi SIL in)*

Related Information

Antimicrobial Activity Against Selected Organisms *on page 983*

U.S. Brand Names Marcillin®; Omnipen®; Omnipen®-N; Polycillin®; Polycillin-N®; Principen®; Totacillin®; Totacillin®-N

Canadian Brand Names Ampicin® Sodium; Apo®-Ampi Trihydrate; Jaa Amp® Trihydrate; Nu-Ampi Trihydrate; Pro-Ampi® Trihydrate; Taro-Ampicillin® Trihydrate

Synonyms Aminobenzylpenicillin; Ampicillin Sodium; Ampicillin Trihydrate

Generic Available Yes

Use Treatment of susceptible bacterial infections (nonbeta-lactamase-producing organisms); susceptible bacterial infections caused by streptococci, pneumococci, nonpenicillinase-producing staphylococci, *Listeria*, meningococci; some strains of *H. influenzae*, *Salmonella*, *Shigella*, *E. coli*, *Enterobacter*, and *Klebsiella*

Drug of Choice or Alternative for

Disease/Syndrome(s)

Endocarditis, Subacute Native Valve *on page 28*

Meningitis, Community-Acquired, Adult *on page 34*

Meningitis, Neonatal (<2 months of age) *on page 35*

Urinary Tract Infection, Catheter-Associated *on page 52*

Urinary Tract Infection, Pyelonephritis *on page 53*

Organism(s)

Actinomyces Species *on page 61*

Borrelia burgdorferi on page 84

Calymmatobacterium granulomatis on page 89

Enterococcus Species *on page 137*

Escherichia coli, Nonenterohemorrhagic *on page 147*

Gardnerella vaginalis on page 151

HACEK Group *on page 155*

Pregnancy Risk Factor B

Contraindications Known hypersensitivity to ampicillin or other penicillins

Warnings/Precautions Dosage adjustment may be necessary in patients with renal impairment; a low incidence of cross-allergy with other beta-lactams exists; high percentage of patients with infectious mononucleosis have developed rash during therapy with ampicillin. Appearance of a rash should be carefully evaluated to differentiate a nonallergic ampicillin rash from a hypersensitivity reaction. Ampicillin rash occurs in 5% to 10% of children receiving ampicillin and is a generalized dull red, maculopapular rash, generally appearing 3-14 days after the start of therapy. It normally begins on the trunk and spreads over most of the body. It may be most intense at pressure areas, elbows, and knees.

Adverse Reactions

>10%: Local: Pain at injection site

1% to 10%:

Dermatologic: Rash (appearance of a rash should be carefully evaluated to differentiate, if possible; nonallergic ampicillin rash from hypersensitivity reaction; incidence is higher in patients with viral infections, *Salmonella* infections, lymphocytic leukemia, or patients that have hyperuricemia)

Gastrointestinal: Diarrhea, vomiting, oral candidiasis, abdominal cramps

Miscellaneous: Allergic reaction (includes serum sickness, urticaria, angioedema, bronchospasm, hypotension, etc)

<1%: Penicillin encephalopathy, seizures (with large I.V. doses or patients with renal dysfunction), anemia, hemolytic anemia, thrombocytopenia, thrombocytopenic purpura, eosinophilia, leukopenia, granulocytopenia, decreased lymphocytes, interstitial nephritis (rare)

Overdosage/Toxicology

Symptoms of penicillin overdose include neuromuscular hypersensitivity (agitation, hallucinations, asterixis, encephalopathy, confusion, and seizures) and electrolyte imbalance with potassium or sodium salts, especially in renal failure

Hemodialysis may be helpful to aid in the removal of the drug from the blood, otherwise most treatment is supportive or symptom directed

Drug Interactions

Decreased effect: Efficacy of oral contraceptives may be reduced

Increased effect: Disulfiram, probenecid may increase penicillin levels, increased effect of anticoagulants

Increased toxicity: Allopurinol theoretically has an additive potential for amoxicillin (ampicillin) rash

Stability Oral suspension is stable for 7 days at room temperature or for 14 days under refrigeration; solutions for I.M. or direct I.V. should be used within 1 hour; solutions for I.V. infusion will be inactivated by dextrose at room temperature; if dextrose-containing solutions are to be used, the resultant solution will only be stable for 2 hours versus 8 hours in the 0.9% sodium chloride injection. D_5W has limited stability.

Minimum volume: Concentration should not exceed 30 mg/mL due to concentration-dependent stability restrictions. Manufacturer may supply as either the anhydrous or the trihydrate form.

Stability of parenteral admixture in NS at room temperature (25°C): 8 hours

Stability of parenteral admixture in NS at refrigeration temperature (4°C): 2 days

Standard diluent: 500 mg/50 mL NS; 1 g/50 mL NS; 2 g/100 mL NS

Mechanism of Action Inhibits bacterial cell wall synthesis by binding to one or more of the penicillin binding proteins (PBPs); which in turn inhibits the final transpeptidation step of peptidoglycan synthesis in bacterial cell walls, thus inhibiting cell wall biosynthesis. Bacteria eventually lyse due to ongoing activity of cell wall autolytic enzymes (autolysins and murein hydrolases) while cell wall assembly is arrested.

Pharmacodynamics/Kinetics

Absorption: Oral: 50%

(Continued)

Ampicillin *(Continued)*

Distribution: Distributes into bile; penetration into CSF occurs with inflamed meninges only, good only with inflammation (exceeds usual MICs)

Normal meninges: Nil

Inflamed meninges: 5-10

Protein binding: 15% to 25%

Half-life:

Neonates:

2-7 days: 4 hours

8-14 days: 2.8 hours

15-30 days: 1.7 hours

Children and Adults: 1-1.8 hours

Anuria/end stage renal disease: 7-20 hours

Time to peak: Oral: Within 1-2 hours

Elimination: ~90% of the drug excreted unchanged in the urine within 24 hours

Usual Dosage

Neonates: I.M., I.V.:

Postnatal age ≤7 days:

≤2000 g: Meningitis: 50 mg/kg/dose every 12 hours; other infections: 25 mg/kg/dose every 12 hours

>2000 g: Meningitis: 50 mg/kg/dose every 8 hours; other infections: 25 mg/kg/dose every 8 hours

Postnatal age >7 days:

<1200 g: Meningitis: 50 mg/kg/dose every 12 hours; other infections: 25 mg/kg/dose every 12 hours

1200-2000 g: Meningitis: 50 mg/kg/dose every 8 hours; other infections: 25 mg/kg/dose every 8 hours

>2000 g: Meningitis: 50 mg/kg/dose every 6 hours; other infections: 25 mg/kg/dose every 6 hours

Infants and Children: I.M., I.V.: 100-400 mg/kg/day in doses divided every 4-6 hours

Meningitis: 200 mg/kg/day in doses divided every 4-6 hours; maximum dose: 12 g/day

Children: Oral: 50-100 mg/kg/day in doses divided every 6 hours; maximum dose: 2-3 g/day

Adults:

Oral: 250-500 mg every 6 hours

I.M.: 500 mg to 1.5 g every 4-6 hours

I.V.: 500 mg to 3 g every 4-6 hours; maximum dose: 12 g/day

Sepsis/meningitis: 150-250 mg/kg/24 hours divided every 3-4 hours

Dosing interval in renal impairment:

Cl_{cr} 30-50 mL/minute: Administer every 6-8 hours

Cl_{cr} 10-30 mL/minute: Administer every 8-12 hours

Cl_{cr} <10 mL/minute: Administer every 12 hours

Hemodialysis: Moderately dialyzable (20% to 50%); administer dose after dialysis

Peritoneal dialysis: Moderately dialyzable (20% to 50%)

Administer 250 mg every 12 hours

Continuous arteriovenous or venovenous hemofiltration (CAVH) effects: Dose as for Cl_{cr} 10-50 mL/minute; ~50 mg of ampicillin per liter of filtrate is removed

Dietary Considerations Food: Decreases drug absorption rate; decreases drug serum concentration. Take on an empty stomach 1 hour before or 2 hours after meals.

Administration Administer orally on an empty stomach (ie, 1 hour prior to, or 2 hours after meals) to increase total absorption

Monitoring Parameters With prolonged therapy monitor renal, hepatic, and hematologic function periodically; observe signs and symptoms of anaphylaxis during first dose

Test Interactions May interfere with urinary glucose tests using cupric sulfate (Benedict's solution, Clinitest®); may inactivate aminoglycosides *in vitro*

Patient Information Food decreases rate and extent of absorption; take oral on an empty stomach, if possible (ie, 1 hour prior to, or 2 hours after meals); report diarrhea promptly; entire course of medication should be taken to ensure eradication of organism; females should report onset of symptoms of candidal vaginitis; may interfere with the effects of oral contraceptives

Nursing Implications Ampicillin and gentamicin should not be mixed in the same I.V. tubing or administered concurrently

Additional Information
Sodium content of 5 mL suspension (250 mg/5 mL): 10 mg (0.4 mEq)
Sodium content of 1 g: 66.7 mg (3 mEq)

Dosage Forms
Capsule, as anhydrous: 250 mg, 500 mg
Capsule, as trihydrate: 250 mg, 500 mg
Powder for injection, as sodium: 125 mg, 250 mg, 500 mg, 1 g, 2 g, 10 g
Powder for oral suspension, as trihydrate: 125 mg/5 mL (5 mL unit dose, 80 mL, 100 mL, 150 mL, 200 mL); 250 mg/5 mL (5 mL unit dose, 80 mL, 100 mL, 150 mL, 200 mL); 500 mg/5 mL (5 mL unit dose, 100 mL)
Powder for oral suspension, drops, as trihydrate: 100 mg/mL (20 mL)

Selected Readings
Donowitz GR and Mandell GL, "Beta-Lactam Antibiotics," *N Engl J Med*, 1988, 318(7):419-26 and 318(8):490-500.
Wright AJ, "The Penicillins," *Mayo Clin Proc*, 1999, 74(3):290-307.

Ampicillin and Sulbactam (am pi SIL in & SUL bak tam)

Related Information
Antimicrobial Activity Against Selected Organisms *on page 983*

U.S. Brand Names Unasyn®

Synonyms Sulbactam and Ampicillin

Generic Available No

Use Treatment of susceptible bacterial infections involved with skin and skin structure, intra-abdominal infections, gynecological infections; spectrum is that of ampicillin plus organisms producing beta-lactamases such as *S. aureus, H. influenzae, E. coli,* and anaerobes

Drug of Choice or Alternative for
Disease/Syndrome(s)
Cholangitis, Acute *on page 21*
Osteomyelitis, Diabetic Foot *on page 38*
Pelvic Inflammatory Disease *on page 41*
Peritonitis, Spontaneous Bacterial *on page 43*
Pneumonia, Aspiration, Community-Acquired *on page 44*
Pneumonia, Community-Acquired *on page 45*

Organism(s)
Acinetobacter Species *on page 58*
Bacteroides Species *on page 75*
Pasteurella multocida on page 224

Pregnancy Risk Factor B

Contraindications Hypersensitivity to ampicillin, sulbactam or any component, or penicillins

Warnings/Precautions Dosage adjustment may be necessary in patients with renal impairment; a low incidence of cross-allergy with other beta-lactams exists; high percentage of patients with infectious mononucleosis have developed rash during therapy with ampicillin. Appearance of a rash should be carefully evaluated to differentiate a nonallergic ampicillin rash from a hypersensitivity reaction. Ampicillin rash occurs in 5% to 10% of children receiving ampicillin and is a generalized dull red, maculopapular rash, generally appearing 3-14 days after the start of therapy. It normally begins on the trunk and spreads over most of the body. It may be most intense at pressure areas, elbows, and knees.

Adverse Reactions
>10%: Local: Pain at injection site (I.M.)
1% to 10%:
Dermatologic: Rash
Gastrointestinal: Diarrhea
Local: Pain at injection site (I.V.)
Miscellaneous: Allergic reaction (may include serum sickness, urticaria, bronchospasm, hypotension, etc)
<1%: Chest pain, fatigue, malaise, headache, chills, penicillin encephalopathy, seizures (with large I.V. doses or patients with renal dysfunction), itching, nausea, vomiting, enterocolitis, pseudomembranous colitis, hairy tongue, dysuria, vaginitis, leukopenia, neutropenia, thrombocytopenia, decreased hemoglobin and hematocrit, increased liver enzymes, thrombophlebitis, increased BUN/creatinine, interstitial nephritis (rare)

(Continued)

Ampicillin and Sulbactam *(Continued)*

Overdosage/Toxicology
Symptoms of penicillin overdose include neuromuscular hypersensitivity (agitation, hallucinations, asterixis, encephalopathy, confusion, and seizures) and electrolyte imbalance with potassium or sodium salts, especially in renal failure

Hemodialysis may be helpful to aid in the removal of the drug from the blood, otherwise most treatment is supportive or symptom directed

Drug Interactions
Decreased effect: Efficacy of oral contraceptives may be reduced

Increased effect: Disulfiram, probenecid results in increased ampicillin levels

Increased toxicity: Allopurinol theoretically has an additive potential for ampicillin rash

Stability I.M. and direct I.V. administration: Use within 1 hour after preparation; reconstitute with sterile water for injection or 0.5% or 2% lidocaine hydrochloride injection (I.M.); sodium chloride 0.9% (NS) is the diluent of choice for I.V. piggyback use, solutions made in NS are stable up to 72 hours when refrigerated whereas dextrose solutions (same concentration) are stable for only 4 hours

Mechanism of Action The addition of sulbactam, a beta-lactamase inhibitor, to ampicillin extends the spectrum of ampicillin to include some beta-lactamase producing organisms; inhibits bacterial cell wall synthesis by binding to one or more of the penicillin binding proteins (PBPs); which in turn inhibits the final transpeptidation step of peptidoglycan synthesis in bacterial cell walls, thus inhibiting cell wall biosynthesis. Bacteria eventually lyse due to ongoing activity of cell wall autolytic enzymes (autolysins and murein hydrolases) while cell wall assembly is arrested.

Pharmacodynamics/Kinetics
Distribution: Into bile, blister and tissue fluids; poor penetration into CSF with uninflamed meninges; higher concentrations attained with inflamed meninges

Protein binding:
Ampicillin: 28%
Sulbactam: 38%

Half-life: Ampicillin and sulbactam are similar: 1-1.8 hours and 1-1.3 hours, respectively in patients with normal renal function

Elimination: ~75% to 85% of both drugs are excreted unchanged in the urine within 8 hours following administration

Usual Dosage Unasyn® (ampicillin/sulbactam) is a combination product. Each 3 g vial contains 2 g of ampicillin and 1 g of sulbactam. Sulbactam has very little antibacterial activity by itself, but effectively extends the spectrum of ampicillin to include beta-lactamase producing strains that are resistant to ampicillin alone. Therefore, dosage recommendations for Unasyn® are based on the ampicillin component.

I.M., I.V.:
Children (3 months to 12 years): 100-200 mg ampicillin/kg/day (150-300 mg Unasyn®) divided every 6 hours; maximum dose: 8 g ampicillin/day (12 g Unasyn®)

Adults: 1-2 g ampicillin (1.5-3 g Unasyn®) every 6-8 hours; maximum dose: 8 g ampicillin/day (12 g Unasyn®)

Dosing interval in renal impairment:
Cl_{cr} 15-29 mL/minute: Administer every 12 hours
Cl_{cr} 5-14 mL/minute: Administer every 24 hours

Monitoring Parameters With prolonged therapy, monitor hematologic, renal, and hepatic function; monitor for signs of anaphylaxis during first dose

Test Interactions May interfere with urinary glucose tests using cupric sulfate (Benedict's solution, Clinitest®); may inactivate aminoglycosides *in vitro*

Nursing Implications Ampicillin and gentamicin should not be mixed in the same I.V. tubing or administered concurrently

Additional Information Sodium content of 1.5 g injection: 115 mg (5 mEq)

Dosage Forms Powder for injection: 1.5 g [ampicillin sodium 1 g and sulbactam sodium 0.5 g]; 3 g [ampicillin sodium 2 g and sulbactam sodium 1 g]

Selected Readings
Donowitz GR and Mandell GL, "Beta-Lactam Antibiotics," *N Engl J Med*, 1988, 318(7):419-26 and 318(8):490-500.

Itokazu GS and Danziger LH, "Ampicillin-Sulbactam and Ticarcillin-Clavulanic Acid: A Comparison of Their *In Vitro* Activity and Review of Their Clinical Efficacy," *Pharmacotherapy*, 1991, 11(5):382-414.

Wright AJ, "The Penicillins," *Mayo Clin Proc*, 1999, 74(3):290-307.

Ampicillin Sodium *see* Ampicillin *on page 604*

Ampicillin Trihydrate *see* Ampicillin *on page 604*

Ampicin® Sodium *see* Ampicillin *on page 604*

Amprenavir (am PRE na veer)

Related Information

HIV Therapeutic Information *on page 1008*

U.S. Brand Names Agenerase®

Use Treatment of HIV infections in combination with at least two other antiretroviral agents

Pregnancy Risk Factor Unknown

Contraindications Hypersensitivity to amprenavir or any component; concurrent therapy with rifampin, astemizole, bepridil, cisapride, dihydroergotamine, ergotamine, midazolam, and triazolam; severe previous allergic reaction to sulfonamides

Warnings/Precautions Because of hepatic metabolism and effect on cytochrome P-450 enzymes, amprenavir should be used with caution in combination with other agents metabolized by this system (see Contraindications and Drug Interactions). Use with caution in patients with diabetes mellitus, sulfonamide allergy, hepatic impairment, or hemophilia. Redistribution of fat may occur (eg, buffalo hump, peripheral wasting, cushingoid appearance). Additional vitamin E supplements should be avoided. Concurrent use of sildenafil should be avoided.

Adverse Reactions Protease inhibitors cause dyslipidemia which includes elevated cholesterol and triglycerides and a redistribution of body fat centrally to cause "protease paunch", buffalo hump, facial atrophy, and breast enlargement. These agents also cause hyperglycemia.

>10%:

Gastrointestinal: Nausea (38% to 73%), vomiting (20% to 29%), diarrhea (33% to 56%)

Dermatologic: Rash (28%)

Endocrine & metabolic: Hyperglycemia (37% to 41%), hypertriglyceridemia (38% to 27%)

Miscellaneous: Perioral tingling/numbness

1% to 10%:

Central nervous system: Depression (4% to 15%), headache, paresthesia, fatigue

Gastrointestinal: Taste disorders (1% to 10%)

Dermatologic: Stevens-Johnson syndrome (1% of total, 4% of patients who develop a rash)

Drug Interactions CYP3A4 inhibitor and substrate

Increased effect/toxicity: Abacavir, clarithromycin, indinavir, ketoconazole, and zidovudine increase the AUC of amprenavir. Nelfinavir had no effect on AUC, but increased the C_{min} of amprenavir. Amprenavir increased the AUC of ketoconazole, rifabutin, and zidovudine during concurrent therapy. Amprenavir may enhance the toxicity of astemizole, bepridil, cisapride, dihydroergotamine, ergotamine, midazolam, and triazolam - concurrent therapy with these drugs and amprenavir is contraindicated. May increase serum concentration of HMG-CoA reductase inhibitors, diltiazem, nicardipine, nifedipine, nimodipine, alprazolam, clorazepate, diazepam, flurazepam, itraconazole, dapsone, erythromycin, loratadine, sildenafil, carbamazepine, and pimizide. May also increase the toxic effect of amiodarone, lidocaine, quinidine, warfarin, and tricyclic antidepressants. Serum concentration monitoring of these drugs is necessary.

Mechanism of Action Binds to the protease activity site and inhibits the activity of the enzyme. HIV protease is required for the cleavage of viral polyprotein precursors into individual functional proteins found in infectious HIV. Inhibition prevents cleavage of these polyproteins, resulting in the formation of immature, noninfectious viral particles

Pharmacodynamics/Kinetics

Absorption: 1-2 hours

Distribution: 430 L

(Continued)

Amprenavir *(Continued)*

Protein binding: 90%
Metabolism: Hepatic, via cytochrome P-450 isoenzymes (primarily CYP3A4)
Elimination: Biliary (75%) and urine (14%) as metabolites

Usual Dosage Oral:

Capsules:

Children 4-12 years and older (<50 kg): 20 mg/kg twice daily or 15 mg/kg 3 times daily; maximum: 2400 mg/day

Children >13 years (>50 kg) and Adults: 1200 mg twice daily

Solution: Children 4-12 years or older (up to 18 years weighing <50 kg): 22 mg/kg twice daily or 17 mg/kg 3 times daily; maximum: 2400/day

Dosage adjustment in hepatic impairment:

Child-Pugh score between 5-8: 450 mg twice daily

Child-Pugh score between 9-12: 300 mg twice daily

Patient Information Advise prescriber of any previous reactions to sulfonamides. Do not take this medication with antacids or high-fat meals. Do not take additional vitamin E supplements. Consult pharmacist or physician prior to taking any other medications due to the potential for drug interactions. For women using oral contraceptives, an alternative method of contraception should be used.

Additional Information Capsules contain 109 Int. units of vitamin E per capsule; oral solution contains 46 Int. units of vitamin E per mL

Dosage Forms

Capsules: 50 mg, 150 mg

Solution: 15 mg/mL

Selected Readings

Kaul DR, Cinti SK, Carver PL, et al, "HIV Protease Inhibitors: Advances in Therapy and Adverse Reactions, Including Metabolic Complications," *Pharmacotherapy*, 1999, 19(3):281-98.

Anadrol® *see* Oxymetholone *on page 853*

Anapolon® *see* Oxymetholone *on page 853*

Ancef® *see* Cefazolin *on page 632*

Ancobon® *see* Flucytosine *on page 734*

Ancotil® *see* Flucytosine *on page 734*

Androderm® Transdermal System *see* Testosterone *on page 939*

Andro-L.A.® Injection *see* Testosterone *on page 939*

Androlone® *see* Nandrolone *on page 829*

Androlone®-D *see* Nandrolone *on page 829*

Andropository® Injection *see* Testosterone *on page 939*

Ansamycin *see* Rifabutin *on page 900*

Antibiotic® Otic *see* Neomycin, Polymyxin B, and Hydrocortisone *on page 836*

Antifungal, Topical

Refer to

Amphotericin B (Conventional) *on page 597*

Butenafine *on page 624*

Ciclopirox *on page 675*

Clotrimazole *on page 688*

Econazole *on page 717*

Ketoconazole *on page 791*

Naftifine *on page 828*

Nystatin *on page 845*

Nystatin and Triamcinolone *on page 846*

Oxiconazole *on page 852*

Sulconazole *on page 926*

Tolnaftate *on page 956*

Drug of Choice or Alternative for Organism(s)

Candida Species *on page 91*

Dermatophytes *on page 127*

Antimicrobial Activity Against Selected Organisms *see page 983*

Antiminth® [OTC] *see* Pyrantel Pamoate *on page 883*

Antirabies Serum (Equine) (an tee RAY beez SEER um EE kwine)

Synonyms ARS
Generic Available No
Use Rabies prophylaxis
Pregnancy Risk Factor C
Adverse Reactions 1% to 10%:
  Central nervous system: Pain (local)
  Dermatologic: Urticaria
  Miscellaneous: Serum sickness
Mechanism of Action Affords passive immunity against rabies
Usual Dosage 1000 units/55 lb in a single dose, infiltrate up to 50% of dose around the wound
Nursing Implications Take careful history of asthma, angioneurotic edema, or other allergies
Additional Information Because of a significantly lower incidence of adverse reactions, Rabies Immune Globulin, Human is preferred over Antirabies Serum Equine
Dosage Forms Injection: 125 units/mL (8 mL)

Antituberculars

Refer to
  Capreomycin on page 625
  Cycloserine on page 696
  Ethambutol on page 727
  Ethionamide on page 728
  Isoniazid on page 782
  Pyrazinamide on page 884
  Rifampin on page 902
  Rifampin and Isoniazid on page 905
  Rifampin, Isoniazid, and Pyrazinamide on page 905
  Streptomycin on page 924

Drug of Choice or Alternative for Organism(s)
  Mycobacterium bovis on page 203
  Mycobacterium tuberculosis on page 207

Aplisol® see Tuberculin Tests on page 962
Aplitest® see Tuberculin Tests on page 962
Apo®-Amoxi see Amoxicillin on page 592
Apo®-Ampi Trihydrate see Ampicillin on page 604
Apo®-Cefaclor see Cefaclor on page 627
Apo®-Cephalex see Cephalexin on page 660
Apo®-Cloxi see Cloxacillin on page 689
Apo®-Doxy see Doxycycline on page 713
Apo®-Doxy Tabs see Doxycycline on page 713
Apo®-Erythro E-C see Erythromycin on page 722
Apo®-Metronidazole see Metronidazole on page 817
Apo®-Minocycline see Minocycline on page 823
Apo®-Nitrofurantoin see Nitrofurantoin on page 842
Apo®-Pen VK see Penicillin V Potassium on page 865
Apo®-Sulfamethoxazole see Sulfamethoxazole on page 932
Apo®-Sulfatrim see Co-Trimoxazole on page 692
Apo®-Tetra see Tetracycline on page 944
Apo®-Zidovudine see Zidovudine on page 977
APPG see Penicillin G Procaine on page 862
Aqueous Procaine Penicillin G see Penicillin G Procaine on page 862
Aqueous Testosterone see Testosterone on page 939
Ara-A see Vidarabine on page 973
Arabinofuranosyladenine see Vidarabine on page 973
Aralen® Phosphate see Chloroquine Phosphate on page 672
Aralen® Phosphate With Primaquine Phosphate see Chloroquine and Primaquine on page 671

ARS *see* Antirabies Serum (Equine) *on previous page*

Atovaquone (a TOE va kwone)

U.S. Brand Names Mepron™

Use Acute oral treatment of mild to moderate *Pneumocystis carinii* pneumonia (PCP) in patients who are intolerant to co-trimoxazole; prophylaxis of PCP in patients intolerant to co-trimoxazole; treatment/suppression of *Toxoplasma gondii* encephalitis, primary prophylaxis of HIV-infected persons at high risk for developing *Toxoplasma gondii* encephalitis

Drug of Choice or Alternative for

Organism(s)

Pneumocystis carinii on page 228

Pregnancy Risk Factor C

Contraindications Life-threatening allergic reaction to the drug or formulation

Warnings/Precautions Has only been indicated in mild to moderate PCP; use with caution in elderly patients due to potentially impaired renal, hepatic, and cardiac function

Adverse Reactions Note: Adverse reaction statistics have been compiled from studies including patients with advanced HIV disease; consequently, it is difficult to distinguish reactions attributed to atovaquone from those caused by the underlying disease or a combination, thereof.

>10%:
Central nervous system: Headache, fever, insomnia, anxiety
Dermatologic: Rash
Gastrointestinal: Nausea, diarrhea, vomiting
Respiratory: Cough
1% to 10%:
Central nervous system: Dizziness
Dermatologic: Pruritus
Endocrine & metabolic: Hypoglycemia, hyponatremia
Gastrointestinal: Abdominal pain, constipation, anorexia, dyspepsia, elevated amylase
Hematologic: Anemia, neutropenia, leukopenia
Hepatic: Elevated liver enzymes
Neuromuscular & skeletal: Weakness
Renal: Increased BUN/creatinine
Miscellaneous: Oral moniliasis

Drug Interactions

Decreased effect: Rifamycins used concurrently decrease the steady-state plasma concentrations of atovaquone
Note: Possible increased toxicity with other highly protein bound drugs

Stability Do not freeze

Mechanism of Action Has not been fully elucidated; may inhibit electron transport in mitochondria inhibiting metabolic enzymes

Pharmacodynamics/Kinetics

Absorption: Decreased significantly in single doses >750 mg; increased three-fold when administered with a high-fat meal
Distribution: Enterohepatically recirculated
Protein binding: >99.9%
Bioavailability: ~30%
Half-life: 2.9 days
Elimination: In feces

Usual Dosage Adults: Oral: 750 mg twice daily with food for 21 days

Patient Information Take only prescribed dose; take each dose with a meal, preferably one with high fat content

Dosage Forms

Sachet: 750 mg/5 mL (42 sachets/box)
Suspension, oral (citrus flavor): 750 mg/5 mL (210 mL)

Selected Readings

Artymowicz RJ and James VE, "Atovaquone: A New Antipneumocystis Agent," *Clin Pharm*, 1993, 12(8):563-70.
El-Sadr WM, Murphy RL, Yurik TM, et al, "Atovaquone Compared With Dapsone for the Prevention of *Pneumocystic carinii* in Patients With HIV Infection Who Cannot Tolerate Trimethoprim, Sulfonamides, or Both," *N Engl J Med*, 1998, 339(26):1889-95.
Haile LG and Flaherty JF, "Atovaquone: A Review," *Ann Pharmacother*, 1993, 27(12):1488-94.

Hughes W, Leoung G, Kramer F, et al, "Comparison of Atovaquone (566C80) With Trimethoprim-Sulfamethoxazole to Treat *Pneumocystis carinii* Pneumonia in Patients With AIDS," *N Engl J Med*, 1993, 328(21):1521-7.

Spencer CM and Goa KL, "Atovaquone. A Review of Its Pharmacological Properties and Therapeutic Efficacy in Opportunistic Infections," *Drugs*, 1995, 50(1):176-96.

Atridox™ *see* Doxycycline *on page 713*

Attenuvax® *see* Measles Virus Vaccine, Live, Attenuated *on page 807*

Augmentin® *see* Amoxicillin and Clavulanate Potassium *on page 593*

Aureomycin® *see* Chlortetracycline *on page 674*

AVC™ **Cream** *see* Sulfanilamide *on page 933*

AVC™ **Suppository** *see* Sulfanilamide *on page 933*

Avirax™ *see* Acyclovir *on page 581*

Avlosulfon® *see* Dapsone *on page 698*

Ayercillin® *see* Penicillin G Procaine *on page 862*

Azactam® *see* Aztreonam *on page 615*

Azidothymidine *see* Zidovudine *on page 977*

Azithromycin (az ith roe MYE sin)

Related Information
Antimicrobial Activity Against Selected Organisms *on page 983*

U.S. Brand Names Zithromax™

Synonyms Azithromycin Dihydrate

Generic Available No

Use
Children: Treatment of acute otitis media due to *H. influenzae*, *M. catarrhalis*, or *S. pneumoniae*; pharyngitis/tonsillitis due to *S. pyogenes*

Adults:

Treatment of mild to moderate upper and lower respiratory tract infections, infections of the skin and skin structure, and sexually transmitted diseases due to susceptible strains of *C. trachomatis*, *M. catarrhalis*, *H. influenzae*, *S. aureus*, *S. pneumoniae*, *Mycoplasma pneumoniae*, and *C. psittaci*; community-acquired pneumonia, pelvic inflammatory disease (PID)

For preventing or delaying the onset of infection with *Mycobacterium avium* complex (MAC)

Prophylaxis of bacterial endocarditis in patients who are allergic to penicillin and undergoing surgical or dental procedures

Drug of Choice or Alternative for

Disease/Syndrome(s)
Pneumonia, Community-Acquired *on page 45*
Sinusitis, Community-Acquired, Acute *on page 48*
Urethritis, Nongonococcal *on page 51*

Organism(s)
Legionella pneumophila *on page 185*
Moraxella catarrhalis *on page 196*
Mycobacterium avium-intracellulare *on page 201*
Mycoplasma pneumoniae *on page 211*
Ureaplasma urealyticum *on page 292*

Pregnancy Risk Factor B

Contraindications Hepatic impairment, known hypersensitivity to azithromycin, other macrolide antibiotics, or any azithromycin components; use with pimozide

Warnings/Precautions Use with caution in patients with hepatic dysfunction; hepatic impairment with or without jaundice has occurred chiefly in older children and adults; it may be accompanied by malaise, nausea, vomiting, abdominal colic, and fever; discontinue use if these occur; may mask or delay symptoms of incubating gonorrhea or syphilis, so appropriate culture and susceptibility tests should be performed prior to initiating azithromycin; pseudomembranous colitis has been reported with use of macrolide antibiotics; safety and efficacy have not been established in children <6 months of age with acute otitis media and in children <2 years of age with pharyngitis/tonsillitis

Adverse Reactions
1% to 10%: Gastrointestinal: Diarrhea, nausea, abdominal pain, cramping, vomiting (especially with high single-dose regimens)

<1%: Ventricular arrhythmias, fever, headache, dizziness, rash, angioedema, hypertrophic pyloric stenosis, vaginitis, eosinophilia, elevated LFTs, cholestatic jaundice, thrombophlebitis, ototoxicity, nephritis, allergic reactions

(Continued)

Azithromycin *(Continued)*

Overdosage/Toxicology
Symptoms of overdose include nausea, vomiting, diarrhea, prostration
Treatment is supportive and symptomatic

Drug Interactions CYP3A3/4 enzyme inhibitor
Decreased peak serum levels: Aluminum- and magnesium-containing antacids by 24% but not total absorption

Increased effect/toxicity: Azithromycin may increase levels of tacrolimus, phenytoin, ergot alkaloids, alfentanil, astemizole, terfenadine, bromocriptine, carbamazepine, cyclosporine, digoxin, disopyramide, and triazolam; azithromycin did not affect the response to warfarin or theophylline although caution is advised when administered together

Avoid use with pimozide due to significant risk of cardiotoxicity

Mechanism of Action Inhibits RNA-dependent protein synthesis at the chain elongation step; binds to the 50S ribosomal subunit resulting in blockage of transpeptidation

Pharmacodynamics/Kinetics
Absorption: Rapid from the GI tract

Distribution: Extensive tissue distribution; distributes well into skin, lungs, sputum, tonsils, and cervix; penetration into the CSF is poor

Protein binding: 7% to 50% (concentration-dependent)

Metabolism: In the liver

Bioavailability: 37%, decreased by food

Half-life, terminal: 68 hours

Peak serum concentration: 2.3-4 hours

Elimination: 4.5% to 12% of dose is excreted in urine; 50% of dose is excreted unchanged in bile

Usual Dosage
Oral:

Children ≥6 months: Otitis media and community-acquired pneumonia: 10 mg/kg on day 1 (maximum: 500 mg/day) followed by 5 mg/kg/day once daily on days 2-5 (maximum: 250 mg/day)

Children ≥2 years: Pharyngitis, tonsillitis: 12 mg/kg/day once daily for 5 days (maximum: 500 mg/day)

Children: *M. avium*-infected patients with acquired immunodeficiency syndrome: Not currently FDA approved for use; 10-20 mg/kg/day once daily (maximum: 40 mg/kg/day) has been used in clinical trials; prophylaxis for first episode of MAC: 5-12 mg/kg/day once daily (maximum: 500 mg/day)

Adolescents ≥16 years and Adults:

Respiratory tract, skin and soft tissue infections: 500 mg on day 1 followed by 250 mg/day on days 2-5 (maximum: 500 mg/day)

Uncomplicated chlamydial urethritis/cervicitis or chancroid: Single 1 g dose

Gonococcal urethritis/cervicitis: Single 2 g dose

Prophylaxis of disseminated *M. avium* complex disease in patient with advanced HIV infection: 1200 mg once weekly (may be combined with rifabutin)

Prophylaxis for bacterial endocarditis: 500 mg 1 hour prior to the procedure

I.V.: Adults:

Community-acquired pneumonia: 500 mg as a single dose for at least 2 days, follow I.V. therapy by the oral route with a single daily dose of 500 mg to complete a 7-10 day course of therapy

Pelvic inflammatory disease (PID): 500 mg as a single dose for 1-2 days, follow I.V. therapy by the oral route with a single daily dose of 250 mg to complete a 7 day course of therapy

Dietary Considerations Food: Rate and extent of GI absorption decreased; take on an empty stomach
Azithromycin suspension, not tablet form, has significantly increased absorption (46%) with food

Administration Do not administer the suspension with food; tablet may be taken without regard to food

Monitoring Parameters Liver function tests, CBC with differential

Patient Information Take suspension 1 hour prior to a meal or 2 hours after; do not take with aluminum- or magnesium-containing antacids; tablet form may be taken with food to decrease GI effects

Additional Information Capsules are no longer being produced in the United States

Dosage Forms

Powder for injection: 500 mg

Powder for oral suspension, as dihydrate: 100 mg/5 mL (15 mL); 200 mg/5 mL (15 mL, 22.5 mL); 1 g (single-dose packet)

Tablet, as dihydrate: 250 mg, 600 mg

Selected Readings

Amsden GW, "Erythromycin, Clarithromycin, and Azithromycin: Are the Differences Real?" *Clin Ther*, 1996, 18(1):56-72.

Drew RH and Gallis HA, "Azithromycin-Spectrum of Activity, Pharmacokinetics, and Clinical Applications," *Pharmacotherapy*, 1992, 12(3):161-73.

Goldman MP and Longworth DL, "The Role of Azithromycin and Clarithromycin in Clinical Practice," *Cleve Clin J Med*, 1993, 60(5):359-64.

Tartaglione TA, "Therapeutic Options for the Management and Prevention of *Mycobacterium avium* Complex Infection in Patients With the Acquired Immunodeficiency Syndrome," *Pharmacotherapy*, 1996, 16(2):171-82.

Zuckerman JM and Kaye KM, "The Newer Macrolides. Azithromycin and Clarithromycin," *Infect Dis Clin North Am*, 1995, 9(3):731-45.

Azithromycin Dihydrate *see* Azithromycin *on page 613*

Azo-Sulfisoxazole *see* Sulfisoxazole and Phenazopyridine *on page 936*

AZT *see* Zidovudine *on page 977*

AZT + 3TC *see* Zidovudine and Lamivudine *on page 979*

Azthreonam *see* Aztreonam *on this page*

Aztreonam (AZ tree oh nam)

Related Information

Antimicrobial Activity Against Selected Organisms *on page 983*

U.S. Brand Names Azactam®

Synonyms Azthreonam

Generic Available No

Use Treatment of patients with urinary tract infections, lower respiratory tract infections, septicemia, skin/skin structure infections, intra-abdominal infections, and gynecological infections caused by susceptible gram-negative bacilli; often useful in patients with allergies to penicillins or cephalosporins

Drug of Choice or Alternative for Organism(s)

Acinetobacter Species *on page 58*

Alcaligenes Species *on page 65*

Klebsiella Species *on page 183*

Serratia Species *on page 250*

Pregnancy Risk Factor B

Contraindications Hypersensitivity to aztreonam or any component

Warnings/Precautions Rare cross-allergenicity to penicillins and cephalosporins; requires dosing adjustment in renal impairment

Adverse Reactions

1% to 10%:

Dermatologic: Rash

Gastrointestinal: Diarrhea, nausea, vomiting

Local: Thrombophlebitis, pain at injection site

<1%: Hypotension, seizures, confusion, headache, vertigo, insomnia, dizziness, fever, breast tenderness, pseudomembranous colitis, aphthous ulcer, abnormal taste, halitosis, numb tongue, vaginitis, hepatitis, jaundice, elevated liver enzymes, thrombocytopenia, eosinophilia, leukopenia, neutropenia, myalgia, weakness, diplopia, tinnitus, sneezing, anaphylaxis

Overdosage/Toxicology

Symptoms of overdose include seizures

If necessary, dialysis can reduce the drug concentration in the blood

Stability Reconstituted solutions are colorless to light yellow straw and may turn pink upon standing without affecting potency; use reconstituted solutions and I.V. solutions (in NS and D_5W) within 48 hours if kept at room temperature or 7 days if kept in refrigerator

Stability of I.V. infusion solution: 48 hours at room temperature (25°C) and 7 days at refrigeration (4°C)

Mechanism of Action Inhibits bacterial cell wall synthesis by binding to one or more of the penicillin binding proteins (PBPs); which in turn inhibits the final (Continued)

Aztreonam *(Continued)*

transpeptidation step of peptidoglycan synthesis in bacterial cell walls, thus inhibiting cell wall biosynthesis. Bacteria eventually lyse due to ongoing activity of cell wall autolytic enzymes (autolysins and murein hydrolases) while cell wall assembly is arrested. Monobactam structure makes cross-allergenicity with beta-lactams unlikely.

Pharmacodynamics/Kinetics

Absorption: I.M.: Well absorbed; I.M. and I.V. doses produce comparable serum concentrations

Distribution: Relative diffusion of antimicrobial agents from blood into cerebrospinal fluid (CSF): Good only with inflammation (exceeds usual MICs); widely distributed to most body fluids and tissues including breast milk; crosses placenta

V_d:
Neonates: 0.26-0.36 L/kg
Children: 0.2-0.29 L/kg
Adults: 0.2 L/kg

Ratio of CSF to blood level (%):
Inflamed meninges: 8-40
Normal meninges: ~1

Protein binding: 56%

Metabolism: Partial

Half-life:
Neonates:
<7 days, ≤2.5 kg: 5.5-9.9 hours
<7 days, >2.5 kg: 2.6 hours
1 week to 1 month: 2.4 hours
Children 2 months to 12 years: 1.7 hours
Adults: Normal renal function: 1.7-2.9 hours
End stage renal disease: 6-8 hours

Time to peak: Within 60 minutes (I.M., I.V. push) and 90 minutes (I.V. infusion)

Elimination: 60% to 70% excreted unchanged in urine and partially in feces

Usual Dosage

Neonates: I.M., I.V.:
Postnatal age ≤7 days:
<2000 g: 30 mg/kg/dose every 12 hours
>2000 g: 30 mg/kg/dose every 8 hours
Postnatal age >7 days:
<1200 g: 30 mg/kg/dose every 12 hours
1200-2000 g: 30 mg/kg/dose every 8 hours
>2000 g: 30 mg/kg/dose every 6 hours

Children >1 month: I.M., I.V.: 90-120 mg/kg/day divided every 6-8 hours
Cystic fibrosis: 50 mg/kg/dose every 6-8 hours (ie, up to 200 mg/kg/day); maximum: 6-8 g/day

Adults:
Urinary tract infection: I.M., I.V.: 500 mg to 1 g every 8-12 hours
Moderately severe systemic infections: 1 g I.V. or I.M. or 2 g I.V. every 8-12 hours
Severe systemic or life-threatening infections (especially caused by *Pseudomonas aeruginosa*): I.V.: 2 g every 6-8 hours; maximum: 8 g/day

Dosing adjustment in renal impairment: Adults:
Cl_{cr} >50 mL/minute: 500 mg to 1 g every 6-8 hours
Cl_{cr} 10-50 mL/minute: 50% to 75% of usual dose given at the usual interval
Cl_{cr} <10 mL/minute: 25% of usual dosage given at the usual interval

Hemodialysis: Moderately dialyzable (20% to 50%); administer dose postdialysis or supplemental dose of 500 mg after dialysis

Peritoneal dialysis: Administer as for Cl_{cr} <10 mL/minute

Continuous arteriovenous or venovenous hemofiltration (CAVH/CAVHD): Dose as for Cl_{cr} 10-50 mL/minute

Administration
Administer by IVP over 3-5 minutes or by intermittent infusion over 20-60 minutes at a final concentration not to exceed 20 mg/mL

Monitoring Parameters
Periodic liver function tests; monitor for signs of anaphylaxis during first dose

Test Interactions
May interfere with urine glucose tests containing cupric sulfate (Benedict's solution, Clinitest®)

Additional Information Although marketed as an agent similar to aminoglycosides, aztreonam is a monobactam antimicrobial with almost pure gram-negative aerobic activity; it cannot be used for gram-positive infections; aminoglycosides are often used for synergy in gram-positive infections

Dosage Forms Powder for injection: 500 mg (15 mL, 100 mL); 1 g (15 mL, 100 mL); 2 g (15 mL, 100 mL)

Selected Readings

Brogden RN and Heel RC, "Aztreonam. A Review of Its Antibacterial Activity, Pharmacokinetic Properties and Therapeutic Use," *Drugs*, 1986, 31(2):96-130.

Donowitz GR and Mandell GL, "Beta-Lactam Antibiotics," *N Engl J Med*, 1988, 318(7):419-26 and 318(8):490-500.

Hellinger WC and Brewer NS, "Carbapenems and Monobactams: Imipenem, Meropenem, and Aztreonam," *Mayo Clin Proc*, 1999, 74(4):420-34.

Johnson DH and Cunha BA, "Aztreonam," *Med Clin North Am*, 1995, 79(4):733-43.

Bacampicillin (ba kam pi SIL in)

U.S. Brand Names Spectrobid®

Canadian Brand Names Penglobe®

Synonyms Bacampicillin Hydrochloride; Carampicillin Hydrochloride

Generic Available No

Use Treatment of susceptible bacterial infections involving the urinary tract, skin structure, upper and lower respiratory tract; activity is identical to that of ampicillin

Pregnancy Risk Factor B

Contraindications Hypersensitivity to bacampicillin or any component or penicillins

Warnings/Precautions Use with caution in patients allergic to cephalosporins; modify dosage in patients with renal impairment; high percentage of patients with infectious mononucleosis develop a rash during amoxicillin therapy

Adverse Reactions

1% to 10%: Gastrointestinal: Gastric upset, diarrhea, nausea

<1%: Rash, pseudomembranous colitis, agranulocytosis, mild increase in AST, hypersensitivity reactions

Overdosage/Toxicology

Signs and symptoms: Neuromuscular sensitivity, many beta-lactam containing antibiotics have the potential to cause neuromuscular hyperirritability or convulsive seizures

Treatment: Hemodialysis may be helpful to aid in the removal of the drug from the blood, otherwise most treatment is supportive or symptom directed

Drug Interactions

Decreased effect of oral contraceptives

Increased levels with probenecid; allopurinol theoretically has has an additive potential for amoxicillin/ampicillin rash

Stability Reconstituted suspension is stable for 10 days when stored in the refrigerator

Mechanism of Action Interferes with bacterial cell wall synthesis during active multiplication causing cell wall death and resultant bactericidal activity against susceptible bacteria

Pharmacodynamics/Kinetics

Protein binding: 15% to 25%

Metabolism: Hydrolyzed to ampicillin

Bioavailability: 80% to 98%

Half-life: 65 minutes, prolonged in patients with impaired renal function

Time to peak serum concentration: Area under the serum concentration time curve is 40% higher for bacampicillin than after equivalent ampicillin doses

Usual Dosage Oral:

Children <25 kg: 25-50 mg/kg/day in divided doses every 12 hours

Children >25 kg and Adults: 400-800 mg every 12 hours

Dosing interval in renal impairment:

Cl_{cr} 10-30 mL/minute: Administer every 24 hours

Cl_{cr} <10 mL/minute: Administer every 36 hours

Monitoring Parameters Renal, hepatic, and hematologic function tests

Test Interactions False-positive urine glucose with Clinitest®

Patient Information Take oral suspension 1 hour before or 2 hours after a meal; report diarrhea promptly; entire course of medication (10-14 days) should be taken to ensure eradication of organism; should be taken in equal intervals

(Continued)

Bacampicillin *(Continued)*

around-the-clock to maintain adequate blood levels; may interfere with oral contraceptives, females should report symptoms of vaginitis

Nursing Implications Assess patient at beginning and throughout therapy for infection; observe for signs and symptoms of anaphylaxis

Additional Information Each mg of bacampicillin is equivalent to ampicillin 700 mcg

Dosage Forms

Powder for oral suspension, as hydrochloride: 125 mg/5 mL [chemically equivalent to ampicillin 87.5 mg per 5 mL] (70 mL)

Tablet, as hydrochloride: 400 mg [chemically equivalent to ampicillin 280 mg]

Bacampicillin Hydrochloride *see* Bacampicillin *on previous page*

Baciguent® Topical [OTC] *see* Bacitracin *on this page*

Bacigvent *see* Bacitracin *on this page*

Baci-IM® Injection *see* Bacitracin *on this page*

Bacillus Calmette-Guérin (BCG) Live *see* BCG Vaccine *on page 620*

Bacitin *see* Bacitracin *on this page*

Bacitracin *(bas i TRAY sin)*

U.S. Brand Names AK-Tracin® Ophthalmic; Baciguent® Topical [OTC]; Baci-IM® Injection

Canadian Brand Names Bacigvent; Bacitin

Generic Available Yes

Use Treatment of susceptible bacterial infections mainly has activity against gram-positive bacilli; due to toxicity risks, systemic and irrigant uses of bacitracin should be limited to situations where less toxic alternatives would not be effective; oral administration has been successful in antibiotic-associated colitis and has been used for enteric eradication of vancomycin-resistant enterococci (VRE)

Pregnancy Risk Factor C

Contraindications Hypersensitivity to bacitracin or any component; I.M. use is contraindicated in patients with renal impairment

Warnings/Precautions Prolonged use may result in overgrowth of nonsusceptible organisms; I.M. use may cause renal failure due to tubular and glomerular necrosis; **do not administer intravenously** because severe thrombophlebitis occurs

Adverse Reactions 1% to 10%:

Cardiovascular: Hypotension, edema of the face/lips, tightness of chest

Central nervous system: Pain

Dermatologic: Rash, itching

Gastrointestinal: Anorexia, nausea, vomiting, diarrhea, rectal itching

Hematologic: Blood dyscrasias

Miscellaneous: Diaphoresis

Overdosage/Toxicology Symptoms of overdose include nephrotoxicity (parenteral), nausea, vomiting (oral)

Drug Interactions Increased toxicity: Nephrotoxic drugs, neuromuscular blocking agents, and anesthetics (increases neuromuscular blockade)

Stability For I.M. use; bacitracin sterile powder should be dissolved in 0.9% sodium chloride injection containing 2% procaine hydrochloride; once reconstituted, bacitracin is stable for 1 week under refrigeration (2°C to 8°C); sterile powder should be stored in the refrigerator; do not use diluents containing parabens

Mechanism of Action Inhibits bacterial cell wall synthesis by preventing transfer of mucopeptides into the growing cell wall

Pharmacodynamics/Kinetics

Duration of action: 6-8 hours

Absorption: Poor from mucous membranes and intact or denuded skin; rapidly absorbed following I.M. administration; not absorbed by bladder irrigation, but absorption can occur from peritoneal or mediastinal lavage

Distribution: Relative diffusion of antimicrobial agents from blood into cerebrospinal fluid (CSF): Nil even with inflammation

Protein binding: Minimally bound to plasma proteins

Time to peak serum concentration: I.M.: Within 1-2 hours

Elimination: Slow elimination into urine with 10% to 40% of dose excreted within 24 hours

Usual Dosage Children and Adults (**do not administer I.V.**):

Infants: I.M.:
≤2.5 kg: 900 units/kg/day in 2-3 divided doses
>2.5 kg: 1000 units/kg/day in 2-3 divided doses

Children: I.M.: 800-1200 units/kg/day divided every 8 hours

Adults: Antibiotic-associated colitis: Oral: 25,000 units 4 times/day for 7-10 days

Topical: Apply 1-5 times/day

Ophthalmic, ointment: Instill 1/4" to 1/2" ribbon every 3-4 hours into conjunctival sac for acute infections, or 2-3 times/day for mild to moderate infections for 7-10 days

Irrigation, solution: 50-100 units/mL in normal saline, lactated Ringer's, or sterile water for irrigation; soak sponges in solution for topical compresses 1-5 times/day or as needed during surgical procedures

Administration For I.M. administration, confirm any orders for parenteral use; pH of urine should be kept >6 by using sodium bicarbonate; bacitracin sterile powder should be dissolved in 0.9% sodium chloride injection containing 2% procaine hydrochloride; do not use diluents containing parabens

Monitoring Parameters I.M.: Urinalysis, renal function tests

Patient Information Ophthalmic ointment may cause blurred vision; do not share eye medications with others

Ophthalmic administration: Tilt head back, place medication in conjunctival sac and close eyes; apply light finger pressure on lacrimal sac for 1 minute following instillation

Topical bacitracin should not be used for longer than 1 week unless directed by a physician

Additional Information 1 unit is equivalent to 0.026 mg

Dosage Forms
Injection: 50,000 units
Ointment:
Ophthalmic: 500 units/g (1 g, 3.5 g, 3.75 g)
Topical: 500 units/g (0.94 g, 15 g, 30 g, 454 g)

Selected Readings
Kelly CP, Pothoulakis C, and LaMont JT, "*Clostridium difficile* colitis," *N Engl J Med*, 1994, 330(4):257-62.

Bacitracin and Polymyxin B (bas i TRAY sin & pol i MIKS in bee)

Related Information
Bacitracin *on previous page*
Polymyxin B *on page 877*

U.S. Brand Names AK-Poly-Bac® Ophthalmic; Betadine® First Aid Antibiotics + Moisturizer [OTC]; Polysporin® Ophthalmic; Polysporin® Topical

Canadian Brand Names Bioderm®; Polytopic

Use Treatment of superficial infections caused by susceptible organisms

Usual Dosage Children and Adults:
Ophthalmic ointment: Instill 1/2" ribbon in the affected eye(s) every 3-4 hours for acute infections or 2-3 times/day for mild to moderate infections for 7-10 days
Topical ointment/powder: Apply to affected area 1-4 times/day; may cover with sterile bandage if needed

Dosage Forms
Ointment:
Ophthalmic: Bacitracin 500 units and polymyxin B sulfate 10,000 units per g (3.5 g)
Topical: Bacitracin 500 units and polymyxin B sulfate 10,000 units per g in white petrolatum (15 g, 30 g)
Powder: Bacitracin 500 units and polymyxin B sulfate 10,000 units per g (10 g)

Bacitracin, Neomycin, and Polymyxin B
(bas i TRAY sin, nee oh MYE sin, & pol i MIKS in bee)

Related Information
Bacitracin *on previous page*
Neomycin *on page 833*
Polymyxin B *on page 877*
(Continued)

Bacitracin, Neomycin, and Polymyxin B *(Continued)*

U.S. Brand Names AK-Spore® Ophthalmic Ointment; Medi-Quick® Topical Ointment [OTC]; Mycitracin® Topical [OTC]; Neomixin® Topical [OTC]; Neosporin® Ophthalmic Ointment; Neosporin® Topical Ointment [OTC]; Ocutricin® Topical Ointment; Septa® Topical Ointment [OTC]; Triple Antibiotic® Topical

Canadian Brand Names Neotopic

Use Helps prevent infection in minor cuts, scrapes and burns; short-term treatment of superficial external ocular infections caused by susceptible organisms

Usual Dosage Children and Adults:

Ophthalmic ointment: Instill ½" ribbon into the conjunctival sac every 3-4 hours for acute infections or 2-3 times/day for mild to moderate infections for 7-10 days

Topical: Apply 1-4 times/day to affected areas and cover with sterile bandage if necessary

Dosage Forms Ointment:

Ophthalmic: Bacitracin 400 units, neomycin sulfate 3.5 mg, and polymyxin B sulfate 10,000 units and per g

Topical: Bacitracin 400 units, neomycin sulfate 3.5 mg, and polymyxin B sulfate 5000 units per g

Bacitracin, Neomycin, Polymyxin B, and Hydrocortisone

(bas i TRAY sin, nee oh MYE sin, pol i MIKS in bee, & hye droe KOR ti sone)

Related Information

Bacitracin *on page 618*
Neomycin *on page 833*
Neomycin, Polymyxin B, and Hydrocortisone *on page 836*
Polymyxin B *on page 877*

U.S. Brand Names AK-Spore® H.C. Ophthalmic Ointment; Cortisporin® Ophthalmic Ointment; Cortisporin® Topical Ointment; Neotricin HC® Ophthalmic Ointment

Use Prevention and treatment of susceptible superficial topical infections

Usual Dosage Children and Adults:

Ophthalmic:

Ointment: Instill ½" ribbon to inside of lower lid every 3-4 hours until improvement occurs

Topical: Apply sparingly 2-4 times/day

Dosage Forms Ointment:

Ophthalmic: Bacitracin 400 units, neomycin sulfate 3.5 mg, polymyxin B sulfate 10,000 units, and hydrocortisone 10 mg per g (3.5 g)

Topical: Bacitracin 400 units, neomycin sulfate 3.5 mg, polymyxin B sulfate 10,000 units, and hydrocortisone 10 mg per g (15 g)

Bacticort® Otic *see* Neomycin, Polymyxin B, and Hydrocortisone *on page 836*

Bactocill® *see* Oxacillin *on page 849*

BactoShield® Topical [OTC] *see* Chlorhexidine Gluconate *on page 670*

Bactrim™ *see* Co-Trimoxazole *on page 692*

Bactrim™ DS *see* Co-Trimoxazole *on page 692*

Bactroban® *see* Mupirocin *on page 825*

Bactroban® Nasal *see* Mupirocin *on page 825*

Barc® Liquid [OTC] *see* Pyrethrins *on page 885*

BCG Vaccine (bee see jee vak SEEN)

U.S. Brand Names TheraCys®; TICE® BCG

Synonyms Bacillus Calmette-Guérin (BCG) Live

Generic Available No

Use In the United States, tuberculosis control efforts are directed toward early identification, treatment of cases, and preventive therapy with isoniazid. BCG vaccine is not recommended for adults at high risk for tuberculosis in the United States. BCG vaccination may be considered for infants and children who are skin test-negative to 5 tuberculin units and who cannot be given isoniazid preventive therapy but have close contact with untreated or ineffectively treated active tuberculosis patients or who belong to groups in which other control measures have not been successful; not for administration in patients with HIV or other more severely immunocompromised patients; immunotherapy for bladder cancer

Pregnancy Risk Factor C

Contraindications Tuberculin-positive individual, hypersensitivity to BCG vaccine or any component, immunocompromized and burn patients; pregnancy, unless there is unavoidable exposure to infectious tuberculosis

Warnings/Precautions Protection against tuberculosis is only relative, not permanent, nor entirely predictable; for live bacteria vaccine, proper aseptic technique and disposal of all equipment in contact with BCG vaccine as a biohazardous material is recommended

Adverse Reactions

1% to 10%: Genitourinary: Bladder infection, prostatitis, dysuria, urinary frequency

Miscellaneous: Flu-like syndrome

<1%: Skin ulceration, abscesses, hematuria, anaphylactic shock in infants, lymphadenitis, disseminated BCG

Drug Interactions Decreased effect: Antimicrobial or immunosuppressive drugs may impair response to BCG or increase risk of infection; antituberculosis drugs

Stability Refrigerate, protect from light, use within 2 (TICE® BCG) hours of mixing

Mechanism of Action Live culture preparation of Bacillus Calmette-Guérin (BCG) strain of *Mycobacterium bovis* is a substrain of Pasteur Institute strain; *M. bovis* is immunologically similar to *M. tuberculosis*, and therefore, simulates natural infection with *M. tuberculosis*, promoting cell-mediated immunity against tuberculosis. BCG live, when used intravesically for treatment of bladder carcinoma *in situ*, is thought to cause a local, chronic inflammatory response involving macrophage and leukocyte infiltration of the bladder which leads to destruction of superficial tumor cells of the urothelium.

Usual Dosage Children >1 month and Adults:

Immunization against tuberculosis (TICE® BCG): 0.2-0.3 mL percutaneous; initial lesion usually appears after 10-14 days consisting of small red papule at injection site and reaches maximum diameter of 3 mm in 4-6 weeks; conduct postvaccinal tuberculin test (ie, 5 TU of PPD) in 2-3 months; if test is negative, repeat vaccination

Immunotherapy for bladder cancer:

Intravesical treatment: Instill into bladder for 2 hours

TheraCys®: One dose diluted in 50 mL NS (preservative free) instilled into bladder once weekly for 6 weeks followed by one treatment at 3, 6, 12, 18, and 24 months after initial treatment

TICE® BCG: One dose diluted in 50 mL NS (preservative free) instilled into the bladder once weekly for 6 weeks followed by once monthly for 6-12 months

Administration Should only be given intravesicularly or percutaneously; **do not administer I.V., S.C., or intradermally;** can be used for bladder irrigation

Test Interactions PPD intradermal test

Patient Information Notify physician of persistent pain on urination or blood in urine

Nursing Implications Should only be given intravesicularly or percutaneously; do not give I.V., S.C., or intradermally; can be used for bladder irrigation

Dosage Forms Powder for injection, lyophilized:

Connaught Strain (TheraCys®): 3.4 ±3 x 10^8 CFU equivalent to approximately 27 mg

Tice Strain (TICE® BCG): 1-8 x 10^8 CFU equivalent to approximately 50 mg (2 mL)

Beepen-VK® *see* Penicillin V Potassium *on page 865*

Benzamycin® *see* Erythromycin and Benzoyl Peroxide *on page 725*

Benzathine Benzylpenicillin *see* Penicillin G Benzathine, Parenteral *on page 859*

Benzathine Penicillin G *see* Penicillin G Benzathine, Parenteral *on page 859*

Benzene Hexachloride *see* Lindane *on page 797*

Benzylpenicillin Benzathine *see* Penicillin G Benzathine, Parenteral *on page 859*

Benzylpenicillin Potassium *see* Penicillin G, Parenteral, Aqueous *on page 860*

Benzylpenicillin Sodium *see* Penicillin G, Parenteral, Aqueous *on page 860*

Betadine® First Aid Antibiotics + Moisturizer [OTC] *see* Bacitracin and Polymyxin B *on page 619*

Betapen®-VK *see* Penicillin V Potassium *on page 865*

Betasept® [OTC] *see* Chlorhexidine Gluconate *on page 670*

Biavax®ₙ *see* Rubella and Mumps Vaccines, Combined *on page 913*

Biaxin™ *see* Clarithromycin *on page 681*

Bicillin® C-R *see* Penicillin G Benzathine and Procaine Combined *on page 858*

Bicillin® C-R 900/300 *see* Penicillin G Benzathine and Procaine Combined *on page 858*

Bicillin® L-A *see* Penicillin G Benzathine, Parenteral *on page 859*

Biltricide® *see* Praziquantel *on page 880*

Biocef *see* Cephalexin *on page 660*

Bioderm® *see* Bacitracin and Polymyxin B *on page 619*

Biomox® *see* Amoxicillin *on page 592*

Bio-Tab® Oral *see* Doxycycline *on page 713*

Bismuth Subsalicylate (BIZ muth sub sa LIS i late)

U.S. Brand Names Devrom® [OTC]; Pepto-Bismol® [OTC]

Synonyms BSS

Generic Available Yes

Use Symptomatic treatment of mild, nonspecific diarrhea; indigestion, nausea, control of traveler's diarrhea; as an adjunct in the treatment of *Helicobacter pylori*-associated peptic ulcer disease

Drug of Choice or Alternative for Organism(s)

 Helicobacter pylori on page 160

Pregnancy Risk Factor C (D in 3rd trimester)

Contraindications Do not use subsalicylate in patients with influenza or chickenpox because of risk of Reye's syndrome; do not use in patients with known hypersensitivity to salicylates; history of severe GI bleeding; history of coagulopathy

Warnings/Precautions Subsalicylate should be used with caution if patient is taking aspirin; use with caution in children, especially those <3 years of age and those with viral illness; may be neurotoxic with very large doses

Adverse Reactions

 >10%: Gastrointestinal: Discoloration of the tongue (darkening), grayish black stools

 <1%: Impaction may occur in infants and debilitated patients, anxiety, confusion, slurred speech, headache, mental depression, muscle spasms, weakness, loss of hearing, confusion, buzzing in ears

Overdosage/Toxicology

 Symptoms of overdose include tinnitus (subsalicylate), fever; most toxic symptoms occur following subacute or chronic intoxications.

 Chelation with dimercaprol in doses of 3 mg/kg or penicillamine 100 mg/kg/day for 5 days can hasten recovery from bismuth-induced encephalopathy. When associated with methemoglobinemia, bismuth intoxications should be treated with methylene blue 1-2 mg/kg in a 1% sterile aqueous solution I.V. push over 4-6 minutes. This may be repeated within 60 minutes if necessary, up to a total dose of 7 mg/kg. Seizures usually respond to I.V. diazepam.

Drug Interactions

 Decreased effect of tetracyclines

 Increased toxicity of aspirin, warfarin, hypoglycemics

Mechanism of Action Bismuth subsalicylate exhibits both antisecretory and antimicrobial action. This agent may provide some anti-inflammatory action as well. The salicylate moiety provides antisecretory effect and the bismuth exhibits antimicrobial directly against bacterial and viral gastrointestinal pathogens. Bismuth has some antacid properties.

Pharmacodynamics/Kinetics

 Absorption: Bismuth is minimally absorbed across the GI tract while the salt (eg, salicylate) may be readily absorbed

 Distribution: Locally in the gut

 Protein binding: Subsalicylate: High (to albumin)

 Metabolism: Following oral administration, undergoes chemical dissociation to various bismuth salts

 Elimination: Fecal

Usual Dosage Oral:
Subsalicylate:
Nonspecific diarrhea:
Children: Up to 8 doses/24 hours:
3-6 years: 1/3 tablet or 5 mL every 30 minutes to 1 hour as needed
6-9 years: 2/3 tablet or 10 mL every 30 minutes to 1 hour as needed
9-12 years: 1 tablet or 15 mL every 30 minutes to 1 hour as needed
Adults: 2 tablets or 30 mL every 30 minutes to 1 hour as needed up to 8 doses/24 hours
Prevention of traveler's diarrhea: 2.1 g/day or 2 tablets 4 times/day before meals and at bedtime
Helicobacter (*Campylobacter*) *pylori*: Chew 2 tablets 4 times/day with meals and at bedtime with other agents in selected regimen (eg, an H_2 antagonist, tetracycline and metronidazole) for 14 days

Subgallate: 1-2 tablets 3 times/day with meals

Dosing comments in renal impairment: Should possibly be avoided with renal failure
Patient Information Chew tablet well or shake suspension well before using; may darken stools; if diarrhea persists for more than 2 days, consult a physician
Dosage Forms
Liquid, as subsalicylate (Pepto-Bismol®, Bismatrol®): 262 mg/15 mL (120 mL, 240 mL, 360 mL, 480 mL); 524 mg/15 mL (120 mL, 240 mL, 360 mL)
Tablet:
Chewable, as subsalicylate (Pepto-Bismol®, Bismatrol®): 262 mg
Chewable, as subgallate (Devrom®): 200 mg
Selected Readings
Graham DY, Lew GM, Evans DG, et al, "Effect of Triple Therapy (Antibiotics Plus Bismuth) on Duodenal Ulcer Healing," *Ann Intern Med*, 1991, 115(4):266-9.
Graham DY, Lew GM, Klein PD, et al, "Effect of Treatment of *Helicobacter pylori* Infection on the Long-Term Recurrence of Gastric or Duodenal Ulcer," *Ann Intern Med*, 1992, 116(9):705-8.
Ormand JE and Talley NJ, "*Helicobacter pylori*: Controversies and an Approach to Management," *Mayo Clin Proc*, 1990, 65(3):414-26.

Bismuth Subsalicylate, Metronidazole, and Tetracycline

(BIZ muth sub sa LIS i late, me troe NI da zole, & tet ra SYE kleen)
Related Information
Bismuth Subsalicylate *on page 622*
Metronidazole *on page 817*
Tetracycline *on page 944*
U.S. Brand Names Helidac™
Use In combination with an H_2 antagonist, used to treat and decrease rate of recurrence of active duodenal ulcer associated with *H. pylori* infection
Usual Dosage Adults: Chew 2 bismuth subsalicylate 262.4 mg tablets, swallow 1 metronidazole 250 mg tablet, and swallow 1 tetracycline 500 mg capsule plus an H_2 antagonist 4 times/day at meals and bedtime for 14 days; follow with 8 oz of water
Dosage Forms
Tablet:
Bismuth subsalicylate: Chewable: 262.4 mg
Metronidazole: 250 mg
Capsule: Tetracycline: 500 mg

Bleph®-10 Ophthalmic *see* Sulfacetamide Sodium *on page 927*

Blephamide® Ophthalmic *see* Sulfacetamide Sodium and Prednisolone *on page 928*

Blis-To-Sol® [OTC] *see* Tolnaftate *on page 956*

Botulinum Toxoid, Pentavalent Vaccine (Against Types A, B, C, D, and E Strains of *C. botulinum*)

(BOT yoo lin num TOKS oyd pen ta VAY lent vak SEEN)
Drug of Choice or Alternative for
Organism(s)
Clostridium botulinum on page 103
(Continued)

Botulinum Toxoid, Pentavalent Vaccine (Against Types A, B, C, D, and E Strains of *C. botulinum*) *(Continued)*

Additional Information For advice on vaccine administration and contraindications, contact the Division of Immunization, CDC, Atlanta, GA 30333 (404-639-3356).

Breezee® Mist Antifungal [OTC] *see* Miconazole *on page 822*
Breezee® Mist Antifungal [OTC] *see* Tolnaftate *on page 956*
BSS *see* Bismuth Subsalicylate *on page 622*

Butenafine (byoo TEN a fine)
U.S. Brand Names Mentax®
Synonyms Butenafine Hydrochloride
Use Topical treatment of tinea pedis (athlete's foot) and tinea cruris (jock itch)
Pregnancy Risk Factor B
Contraindications Hypersensitivity to butenafine or components
Warnings/Precautions Only for topical use (not ophthalmic, vaginal, or internal routes); patients sensitive to other allylamine antifungals may cross-react with butenafine
Adverse Reactions
>1%: Dermatologic: Burning, stinging, irritation, erythema, pruritus (2%)
<1%: Contact dermatitis
Mechanism of Action Butenafine exerts antifungal activity by blocking squalene epoxidation, resulting in inhibition of ergosterol synthesis (antidermatophyte and *Sporothrix schenckii* activity). In higher concentrations, the drug disrupts fungal cell membranes (anticandidal activity).
Pharmacodynamics/Kinetics
Absorption: Minimal systemic absorption when topically applied
Metabolism: Hepatic; principle metabolite via hydroxylation
Half-life: 35 hours
Time to peak serum concentration: 6 hours (10 ng/mL)
Usual Dosage Children >12 years and Adults: Topical: Apply once daily for 4 weeks to the affected area and surrounding skin
Monitoring Parameters Culture and KOH exam, clinical signs of tinea pedis
Patient Information Report any signs of rash or allergy to your physician immediately; do not apply other topical medications on the same area as butenafine unless directed by your physician
Dosage Forms Cream, as hydrochloride: 1% (2 g, 15 g, 30 g)
Selected Readings
McNeely W and Spencer CM, "Butenafine," *Drugs*, 1998, 55(3):405-12.
"Topical Butenafine for Tinea Pedis," *Med Lett Drugs Ther*, 1997, 39(1004):63-4.

Butenafine Hydrochloride *see* Butenafine *on page 624*

Butoconazole (byoo toe KOE na zole)
Synonyms Butoconazole Nitrate
Generic Available No
Use Local treatment of vulvovaginal candidiasis
Pregnancy Risk Factor C (For use only in 2nd or 3rd trimester)
Contraindications Known hypersensitivity to butoconazole
Warnings/Precautions In pregnancy, use only during second or third trimesters; if irritation or sensitization occurs, discontinue use
Adverse Reactions
1% to 10%: Genitourinary: Vulvar/vaginal burning
<1%: Genitourinary: Vulvar itching, soreness, edema, or discharge; urinary frequency
Stability Do not store at temperatures >40°C/104°F; avoid freezing
Mechanism of Action Increases cell membrane permeability in susceptible fungi (*Candida*)
Pharmacodynamics/Kinetics
Absorption: Following intravaginal application small amounts of drug are absorbed systemically (25%) within 2-8 hours

Half-life: 21-24 hours
Elimination: Into urine and feces in approximate equal amounts

Usual Dosage Adults:
Nonpregnant: Insert 1 applicatorful (~5 g) intravaginally at bedtime for 3 days, may extend for up to 6 days if necessary
Pregnant: **Use only during second or third trimesters**

Patient Information May cause burning or stinging on application; if symptoms of vaginitis persist, contact physician

Dosage Forms Cream, vaginal, as nitrate: 2% with applicator (28 g)

Butoconazole Nitrate see Butoconazole on previous page

Capastat® Sulfate see Capreomycin on this page

Capreomycin (kap ree oh MYE sin)

Related Information
Tuberculosis Guidelines on page 1114

U.S. Brand Names Capastat® Sulfate

Synonyms Capreomycin Sulfate

Generic Available No

Use Treatment of tuberculosis in conjunction with at least one other anti-tuberculosis agent

Pregnancy Risk Factor C

Contraindications Known hypersensitivity to capreomycin sulfate

Warnings/Precautions Use in patients with renal insufficiency or pre-existing auditory impairment must be undertaken with great caution, and the risk of additional eighth nerve impairment or renal injury should be weighed against the benefits to be derived from therapy. Since other parenteral antituberculous agents (eg, streptomycin) also have similar and sometimes irreversible toxic effects, particularly on eighth cranial nerve and renal function, simultaneous administration of these agents with capreomycin is not recommended. Use with nonantituberculous drugs (ie, aminoglycoside antibiotics) having ototoxic or nephrotoxic potential should be undertaken only with great caution.

Adverse Reactions
>10%:
Otic: Ototoxicity [subclinical hearing loss (11%), clinical loss (3%)], tinnitus
Renal: Nephrotoxicity (36%), increased BUN
1% to 10%: Hematologic: Eosinophilia (dose-related, mild)
<1%: Vertigo, hypokalemia, leukocytosis, thrombocytopenia (rare); pain, induration, and bleeding at injection site; hypersensitivity (urticaria, rash, fever)

Overdosage/Toxicology
Symptoms of overdose include renal failure, ototoxicity, thrombocytopenia
Treatment is supportive

Drug Interactions
Increased effect/duration of nondepolarizing neuromuscular blocking agents
Additive toxicity (nephro- and ototoxicity, respiratory paralysis): Aminoglycosides (eg, streptomycin)

Mechanism of Action Capreomycin is a cyclic polypeptide antimicrobial. It is administered as a mixture of capreomycin IA and capreomycin IB. The mechanism of action of capreomycin is not well understood. Mycobacterial species that have become resistant to other agents are usually still sensitive to the action of capreomycin. However, significant cross-resistance with viomycin, kanamycin, and neomycin occurs.

Pharmacodynamics/Kinetics
Absorption: Oral: Poor absorption necessitates parenteral administration
Half-life: Dependent upon renal function and varies with creatinine clearance; 4-6 hours
Time to peak serum concentration: I.M.: Within 1 hour
Elimination: Essentially excreted unchanged in the urine; no significant accumulation after ≥30 day of 1 g/day dosing in patients with normal renal function

Usual Dosage I.M.:
Infants and Children: 15 mg/kg/day, up to 1 g/day maximum
Adults: 15-20 mg/kg/day up to 1 g/day for 60-120 days, followed by 1 g 2-3 times/week

Dosing interval in renal impairment: Adults:
Cl_{cr} >100 mL/minute: Administer 13-15 mg/kg every 24 hours
(Continued)

Capreomycin *(Continued)*

Cl$_{cr}$ 80-100 mL/minute: Administer 10-13 mg/kg every 24 hours
Cl$_{cr}$ 60-80 mL/minute: Administer 7-10 mg/kg every 24 hours
Cl$_{cr}$ 40-60 mL/minute: Administer 11-14 mg/kg every 48 hours
Cl$_{cr}$ 20-40 mL/minute: Administer 10-14 mg/kg every 72 hours
Cl$_{cr}$ <20 mL/minute: Administer 4-7 mg/kg every 72 hours

Reference Range 10 µg/mL

Patient Information Report any hearing loss to physician immediately; do not discontinue without notifying physician

Nursing Implications The solution for injection may acquire a pale straw color and darken with time; this is not associated with a loss of potency or development of toxicity

Dosage Forms Injection, as sulfate: 100 mg/mL (10 mL)

Selected Readings

Davidson PT and Le HQ, "Drug Treatment of Tuberculosis - 1992," *Drugs*, 1992, 43(5):651-73.
"Drugs for Tuberculosis," *Med Lett Drugs Ther*, 1993, 35(908):99-101.
Iseman MD, "Treatment of Multidrug-Resistant Tuberculosis," *N Engl J Med*, 1993, 329(11):784-91.

Capreomycin Sulfate *see* Capreomycin *on previous page*

Carampicillin Hydrochloride *see* Bacampicillin *on page 617*

Carbenicillin *(kar ben i SIL in)*

Related Information

Antimicrobial Activity Against Selected Organisms *on page 983*

U.S. Brand Names Geocillin®

Canadian Brand Names Geopen®

Synonyms Carindacillin; Indanyl Sodium

Generic Available No

Use Treatment of serious urinary tract infections and prostatitis caused by susceptible gram-negative aerobic bacilli

Pregnancy Risk Factor B

Contraindications Hypersensitivity to carbenicillin or any component or penicillins

Warnings/Precautions Do not use in patients with severe renal impairment (Cl$_{cr}$ <10 mL/minute); dosage modification required in patients with impaired renal and/or hepatic function; oral carbenicillin should be limited to treatment of urinary tract infections. Use with caution in patients with history of hypersensitivity to cephalosporins.

Adverse Reactions

>10%: Gastrointestinal: Diarrhea

1% to 10%: Gastrointestinal: Nausea, bad taste, vomiting, flatulence, glossitis

<1%: Headache, skin rash, urticaria, anemia, thrombocytopenia, leukopenia, neutropenia, eosinophilia, hyperthermia, itchy eyes, vaginitis, hypokalemia, hematuria, thrombophlebitis

Overdosage/Toxicology

Symptoms of overdose include neuromuscular hypersensitivity, convulsions; many beta-lactam containing antibiotics have the potential to cause neuromuscular hyperirritability or convulsive seizures

Hemodialysis may be helpful to aid in the removal of the drug from the blood, otherwise most treatment is supportive or symptom directed

Drug Interactions

Decreased effect with administration of aminoglycosides within 1 hour; may inactivate both drugs

Increased duration of half-life with probenecid

Mechanism of Action Inhibits bacterial cell wall synthesis by binding to one or more of the penicillin binding proteins (PBPs); which in turn inhibits the final transpeptidation step of peptidoglycan synthesis in bacterial cell walls, thus inhibiting cell wall biosynthesis. Bacteria eventually lyse due to ongoing activity of cell wall autolytic enzymes (autolysins and murein hydrolases) while cell wall assembly is arrested.

Pharmacodynamics/Kinetics

Absorption: Oral: 30% to 40%

Distribution: Crosses the placenta; small amounts appear in breast milk; distributes into bile, low concentrations attained in CSF

Half-life:
Children: 0.8-1.8 hours
Adults: 1-1.5 hours, prolonged to 10-20 hours with renal insufficiency
Time to peak serum concentration: Within 0.5-2 hours in patients with normal renal function; serum concentrations following oral absorption are inadequate for treatment of systemic infections
Elimination: ~80% to 99% excreted unchanged in urine

Usual Dosage Oral:
Children: 30-50 mg/kg/day divided every 6 hours; maximum dose: 2-3 g/day

Adults: 1-2 tablets every 6 hours for urinary tract infections or 2 tablets every 6 hours for prostatitis

Dosing interval in renal impairment: Adults:
Cl_{cr} 10-50 mL/minute: Administer 382-764 mg every 12-24 hours
Cl_{cr} <10 mL/minute: Administer 382-764 mg every 24-48 hours
Moderately dialyzable (20% to 50%)

Monitoring Parameters Renal, hepatic, and hematologic function tests

Reference Range Therapeutic: Not established; Toxic: >250 µg/mL (SI: >660 µmol/L)

Test Interactions May interfere with urinary glucose tests using cupric sulfate (Benedict's solution, Clinitest®); may inactivate aminoglycosides *in vitro*; false-positive urine or serum proteins

Patient Information Tablets have a bitter taste; take with a full glass of water; take all medication for 7-14 days, do not skip doses; may interfere with oral contraceptives

Additional Information Sodium content of 382 mg tablet: 23 mg (1 mEq)

Dosage Forms Tablet, film coated: 382 mg

Selected Readings
Donowitz GR and Mandell GL, "Beta-Lactam Antibiotics," *N Engl J Med*, 1988, 318(7):419-26 and 318(8):490-500.
Wright AJ, "The Penicillins," *Mayo Clin Proc*, 1999, 74(3):290-307.

Cardioquin® *see* Quinidine *on page 888*

Carindacillin *see* Carbenicillin *on previous page*

Ceclor® *see* Cefaclor *on this page*

Ceclor® CD *see* Cefaclor *on this page*

Cedax® *see* Ceftibuten *on page 652*

Cefaclor (SEF a klor)

Related Information
Antimicrobial Activity Against Selected Organisms *on page 983*

U.S. Brand Names Ceclor®; Ceclor® CD

Canadian Brand Names Apo®-Cefaclor

Generic Available No

Use Infections caused by susceptible organisms including *Staphylococcus aureus* and *H. influenzae*; treatment of otitis media, sinusitis, and infections involving the respiratory tract, skin and skin structure, bone and joint, and urinary tract

Drug of Choice or Alternative for
Organism(s)
Haemophilus influenzae on page 157

Pregnancy Risk Factor B

Contraindications Hypersensitivity to cefaclor, any component, or cephalosporins

Warnings/Precautions Modify dosage in patients with severe renal impairment; prolonged use may result in superinfection; a low incidence of cross-hypersensitivity to penicillins exists

Adverse Reactions
1% to 10%:
Gastrointestinal: Diarrhea (1.5%)
Hematologic: Eosinophilia (2%)
Hepatic: Elevated transaminases (2.5%)
Dermatologic: Rash (maculopapular, erythematous, or morbilliform) (1% to 1.5%)
<1%: Anaphylaxis, urticaria, pruritus, angioedema, serum-sickness, arthralgia, hepatitis, cholestatic jaundice, Stevens-Johnson syndrome, nausea, vomiting, (Continued)

Cefaclor *(Continued)*

pseudomembranous colitis, vaginitis, hemolytic anemia, neutropenia, interstitial nephritis, CNS irritability, hyperactivity, agitation, nervousness, insomnia, confusion, dizziness, hallucinations, somnolence, seizures, prolonged PT

Reactions reported with other cephalosporins include fever, abdominal pain, superinfection, renal dysfunction, toxic nephropathy, hemorrhage, cholestasis

Overdosage/Toxicology

After acute overdose, most agents cause only nausea, vomiting, and diarrhea, although neuromuscular hypersensitivity and seizures are possible, especially in patients with renal insufficiency; many beta-lactam antibiotics have the potential to cause neuromuscular hyperirritability or seizures

Hemodialysis may be helpful to aid in the removal of the drug from the blood but not usually indicated, otherwise most treatment is supportive or symptom directed following GI decontamination

Drug Interactions

Increased effect: Probenecid may decrease cephalosporin elimination

Increased toxicity: Furosemide, aminoglycosides may be a possible additive to nephrotoxicity

Stability Refrigerate suspension after reconstitution; discard after 14 days; do not freeze

Mechanism of Action Inhibits bacterial cell wall synthesis by binding to one or more of the penicillin-binding proteins (PBPs) which in turn inhibits the final transpeptidation step of peptidoglycan synthesis in bacterial cell walls, thus inhibiting cell wall biosynthesis. Bacteria eventually lyse due to ongoing activity of cell wall autolytic enzymes (autolysins and murein hydrolases) while cell wall assembly is arrested.

Pharmacodynamics/Kinetics

Absorption: Oral: Well absorbed, acid stable

Distribution: Widely distributed throughout the body and reaches therapeutic concentration in most tissues and body fluids, including synovial, pericardial, pleural, and peritoneal fluids; also bile, sputum, and urine; also bone, myocardium, gallbladder, skin and soft tissue; crosses the placenta and appears in breast milk

Protein binding: 25%

Metabolism: Partially

Half-life: 0.5-1 hour, prolonged with renal impairment

Time to peak:

Capsule: 60 minutes

Suspension: 45 minutes

Elimination: 80% excreted unchanged in urine

Usual Dosage Oral:

Children >1 month: 20-40 mg/kg/day divided every 8-12 hours; maximum dose: 2 g/day (total daily dose may be divided into two doses for treatment of otitis media or pharyngitis)

Adults: 250-500 mg every 8 hours

Extended release tablets: 500 mg every 12 hours for 7 days for acute bacterial exacerbations of or secondary infections with chronic bronchitis or 375 mg every 12 hour for 10 days for pharyngitis or tonsillitis or for uncomplicated skin and skin structure infections

Dosing adjustment in renal impairment: Cl_{cr} <50 mL/minute: Administer 50% of dose

Hemodialysis: Moderately dialyzable (20% to 50%)

Monitoring Parameters Assess patient at beginning and throughout therapy for infection; monitor for signs of anaphylaxis during first dose

Test Interactions Positive direct Coombs', false-positive urinary glucose test using cupric sulfate (Benedict's solution, Clinitest®, Fehling's solution), false-positive serum or urine creatinine with Jaffé reaction

Patient Information Chilling of the oral suspension improves flavor (do not freeze); report persistent diarrhea; entire course of medication (10-14 days) should be taken to ensure eradication of organism; may interfere with oral contraceptives; females should report symptoms of vaginitis

Dosage Forms

Capsule: 250 mg, 500 mg

Powder for oral suspension (strawberry flavor): 125 mg/5 mL (75 mL, 150 mL); 187 mg/5 mL (50 mL, 100 mL); 250 mg/5 mL (75 mL, 150 mL); 375 mg/5 mL (50 mL, 100 mL)

Tablet, extended release: 375 mg, 500 mg

Selected Readings

Donowitz GR and Mandell GL, "Beta-Lactam Antibiotics," *N Engl J Med*, 1988, 318(7):419-26 and 318(8):490-500.
Marshall WF and Blair JE, "The Cephalosporins," *Mayo Clin Proc*, 1999, 74(2):187-95.
Smith GH, "Oral Cephalosporins in Perspective," *DICP*, 1990, 24(1):45-51.

Cefadroxil (sef a DROKS il)

Related Information
Antimicrobial Activity Against Selected Organisms *on page 983*

U.S. Brand Names Duricef®; Ultracef®

Synonyms Cefadroxil Monohydrate

Generic Available No

Use Treatment of susceptible gram-positive bacilli and cocci (not enterococcus); some gram-negative bacilli including *E. coli*, *Proteus*, and *Klebsiella* may be susceptible

Pregnancy Risk Factor B

Contraindications Hypersensitivity to cefadroxil or other cephalosporins

Warnings/Precautions Modify dosage in patients with severe renal impairment; prolonged use may result in superinfection; use with caution in patients with a history of penicillin allergy especially IgE-mediated reactions (eg, anaphylaxis, urticaria); may cause antibiotic-associated colitis or colitis secondary to *C. difficile*

Adverse Reactions
1% to 10%: Gastrointestinal: Diarrhea

<1%: Anaphylaxis, rash (maculopapular and erythematous), erythema multiforme, Stevens-Johnson syndrome, serum sickness, arthralgia, urticaria, pruritus, angioedema, pseudomembranous colitis, abdominal pain, dyspepsia, nausea, vomiting, elevated transaminases, cholestasis, vaginitis, neutropenia, agranulocytosis, thrombocytopenia, fever

Reactions reported with other cephalosporins include toxic epidermal necrolysis, abdominal pain, superinfection. renal dysfunction, toxic nephropathy, aplastic anemia, hemolytic anemia, hemorrhage, prolonged prothrombin time, increased BUN, increased creatinine, eosinophilia, pancytopenia, seizures

Overdosage/Toxicology
After acute overdose, most agents cause only nausea, vomiting, and diarrhea, although neuromuscular hypersensitivity and seizures are possible, especially in patients with renal insufficiency; many beta-lactam antibiotics have the potential to cause neuromuscular hyperirritability or seizures

Hemodialysis may be helpful to aid in the removal of the drug from the blood but not usually indicated, otherwise most treatment is supportive or symptom directed following GI decontamination

Drug Interactions
Increased effect: Probenecid may decrease cephalosporin elimination

Increased toxicity: Furosemide, aminoglycosides may be a possible additive to nephrotoxicity

Stability Refrigerate suspension after reconstitution; discard after 14 days

Mechanism of Action Inhibits bacterial cell wall synthesis by binding to one or more of the penicillin-binding proteins (PBPs) which in turn inhibits the final transpeptidation step of peptidoglycan synthesis in bacterial cell walls, thus inhibiting cell wall biosynthesis. Bacteria eventually lyse due to ongoing activity of cell wall autolytic enzymes (autolysins and murein hydrolases) while cell wall assembly is arrested.

Pharmacodynamics/Kinetics
Absorption: Oral: Rapid and well absorbed from GI tract

Distribution: Widely distributed throughout the body and reaches therapeutic concentrations in most tissues and body fluids, including synovial, pericardial, pleural, and peritoneal fluids; also bile, sputum, and urine; also bone, the myocardium, gallbladder, skin and soft tissue; crosses the placenta and appears in breast milk

Protein binding: 20%

Half-life: 1-2 hours; 20-24 hours in renal failure

(Continued)

Cefadroxil *(Continued)*

Time to peak serum concentration: Within 70-90 minutes
Elimination: >90% of dose excreted unchanged in urine within 8 hours

Usual Dosage Oral:
Children: 30 mg/kg/day divided twice daily up to a maximum of 2 g/day
Adults: 1-2 g/day in 2 divided doses

Prophylaxis against bacterial endocarditis: 2 g 1 hour prior to the procedure

Dosing interval in renal impairment:
Cl_{cr} 10-25 mL/minute: Administer every 24 hours
Cl_{cr} <10 mL/minute: Administer every 36 hours

Monitoring Parameters Observe for signs and symptoms of anaphylaxis during first dose

Test Interactions Positive direct Coombs', false-positive urinary glucose test using cupric sulfate (Benedict's solution, Clinitest®, Fehling's solution), false-positive creatinine with Jaffé reaction

Patient Information Report persistent diarrhea; entire course of medication (10-14 days) should be taken to ensure eradication of organism; may interfere with oral contraceptives; females should report symptoms of vaginitis

Dosage Forms
Capsule, as monohydrate: 500 mg
Suspension, oral, as monohydrate: 125 mg/5 mL, 250 mg/5 mL, 500 mg/5 mL (50 mL, 100 mL)
Tablet, as monohydrate: 1 g

Selected Readings
Donowitz GR and Mandell GL, "Beta-Lactam Antibiotics," *N Engl J Med*, 1988, 318(7):419-26 and 318(8):490-500.
Marshall WF and Blair JE, "The Cephalosporins," *Mayo Clin Proc*, 1999, 74(2):187-95.
Smith GH, "Oral Cephalosporins in Perspective," *DICP*, 1990, 24(1):45-51.

Cefadroxil Monohydrate *see* Cefadroxil *on previous page*

Cefadyl® *see* Cephapirin *on page 664*

Cefamandole (sef a MAN dole)

Related Information
Antimicrobial Activity Against Selected Organisms *on page 983*

U.S. Brand Names Mandol®

Synonyms Cefamandole Nafate

Generic Available No

Use Treatment of susceptible bacterial infection; mainly respiratory tract, skin and skin structure, bone and joint, urinary tract and gynecologic, septicemia; surgical prophylaxis. Active against methicillin-sensitive staphylococci, many streptococci, and various gram-negative bacilli including *E. coli*, some *Klebsiella*, *P. mirabilis*, *H. influenzae*, and *Moraxella*.

Pregnancy Risk Factor B

Contraindications Hypersensitivity to cefamandole nafate, any component, or cephalosporins

Warnings/Precautions Modify dosage in patients with severe renal impairment; prolonged use may result in superinfection; although rare, cefamandole may interfere with hemostasis via destruction of vitamin K producing intestinal bacteria, prevention of activation of prothrombin by the attachment of a methyltetrazolethiol side chain, and by an immune-mediated thrombocytopenia. Use with caution in patients with a history of penicillin allergy especially IgE-mediated reactions (eg, anaphylaxis, urticaria); may cause antibiotic-associated colitis or colitis secondary to *C. difficile*.

Adverse Reactions
Contains MTT side chain which may lead to increased risk of hypoprothrombinemia and bleeding

1% to 10%:
Gastrointestinal: Diarrhea
Local: Thrombophlebitis

<1%: Anaphylaxis, rash (maculopapular and erythematous), urticaria, pseudomembranous colitis, nausea, vomiting, elevated transaminases, cholestasis, eosinophilia, neutropenia, thrombocytopenia, increased BUN, increased creatinine, fever, prolonged PT

Reactions reported with other cephalosporins include toxic epidermal necrolysis, Stevens-Johnson syndrome, abdominal pain, superinfection, renal dysfunction, toxic nephropathy, aplastic anemia, hemolytic anemia, hemorrhage, pancytopenia, vaginitis, seizures

Overdosage/Toxicology

Symptoms of overdose include neuromuscular hypersensitivity and convulsions, especially in patients with renal insufficiency; many beta-lactam antibiotics have the potential to cause neuromuscular hyperirritability or seizures

Hemodialysis may be helpful to aid in the removal of the drug from the blood, otherwise most treatment is supportive or symptom directed

Drug Interactions

Disulfiram-like reaction has been reported when taken within 72 hours of alcohol consumption

Increased cefamandole plasma levels: Probenecid

Increased nephrotoxicity: Aminoglycosides, furosemide

Hypoprothrombinemic effect increased: Warfarin and heparin

Stability After reconstitution, CO_2 gas is liberated which allows solution to be withdrawn without injecting air; solution is stable for 24 hours at room temperature and 96 hours when refrigerated; for I.V., infusion in NS and D_5W is stable for 24 hours at room temperature, 1 week when refrigerated, or 26 weeks when frozen

Mechanism of Action Inhibits bacterial cell wall synthesis by binding to one or more of the penicillin-binding proteins (PBPs) which in turn inhibits the final transpeptidation step of peptidoglycan synthesis in bacterial cell walls, thus inhibiting cell wall biosynthesis. Bacteria eventually lyse due to ongoing activity of cell wall autolytic enzymes (autolysins and murein hydrolases) while cell wall assembly is arrested.

Pharmacodynamics/Kinetics

Distribution: Well throughout the body, except CSF; poor penetration even with inflamed meninges

Protein binding: 56% to 78%

Half-life: 30-60 minutes

Time to peak serum concentration: I.M.: Within 1-2 hours

Elimination: Extensive enterohepatic circulation; high concentrations in bile; majority of drug excreted unchanged in urine

Usual Dosage I.M., I.V.:

Children: 50-150 mg/kg/day in divided doses every 4-8 hours

Adults: Usual dose: 500-1000 mg every 4-8 hours; in life-threatening infections: 2 g every 4 hours may be needed

Dosing interval in renal impairment:

Cl_{cr} 25-50 mL/minute: 1-2 g every 8 hours

Cl_{cr} 10-25 mL/minute: 1 g every 8 hours

Cl_{cr} <10 mL/minute: 1 g every 12 hours

Hemodialysis: Moderately dialyzable (20% to 50%)

Monitoring Parameters Monitor for signs of bruising or bleeding; observe for signs and symptoms of anaphylaxis during first dose

Test Interactions Positive Coombs' test, false-positive urinary glucose test using cupric sulfate (Benedict's solution, Clinitest®, Fehling's solution), false-positive creatinine with Jaffé reaction

Nursing Implications Do not admix with aminoglycosides in same bottle/bag; observe for signs and symptoms of anaphylaxis during first dose

Additional Information Sodium content of 1 g: 76 mg (3.3 mEq); contains the n-methylthiotetrazole side chain

Dosage Forms Powder for injection, as nafate: 500 mg (10 mL); 1 g (10 mL, 100 mL); 2 g (20 mL, 100 mL); 10 g (100 mL)

Selected Readings

Donowitz GR and Mandell GL, "Beta-Lactam Antibiotics," *N Engl J Med*, 1988, 318(7):419-26 and 318(8):490-500.

Gentry LO, Zeluff BJ, and Cooley DA, "Antibiotic Prophylaxis in Open-Heart Surgery: A Comparison of Cefamandole, Cefuroxime, and Cefazolin," *Ann Thorac Surg*, 1988, 46(2):167-71.

Marshall WF and Blair JE, "The Cephalosporins," *Mayo Clin Proc*, 1999, 74(2):187-95.

Cefamandole Nafate *see* Cefamandole *on previous page*

Cefazolin (sef A zoe lin)

Related Information
Antimicrobial Activity Against Selected Organisms *on page 983*

U.S. Brand Names Ancef®; Kefzol®; Zolicef®

Synonyms Cefazolin Sodium

Generic Available Yes

Use Treatment of gram-positive bacilli and cocci (except enterococcus); some gram-negative bacilli including *E. coli*, *Proteus*, and *Klebsiella* may be susceptible

Drug of Choice or Alternative for
Disease/Syndrome(s)
Catheter Infection, Intravascular *on page 21*
Urinary Tract Infection, Perinephric Abscess *on page 52*

Pregnancy Risk Factor B

Contraindications Hypersensitivity to cefazolin sodium, any component, or cephalosporins

Warnings/Precautions Modify dosage in patients with severe renal impairment; prolonged use may result in superinfection; use with caution in patients with a history of penicillin allergy especially IgE-mediated reactions (eg, anaphylaxis, urticaria); may cause antibiotic-associated colitis or colitis secondary to *C. difficile*

Adverse Reactions
1% to 10%:
Gastrointestinal: Diarrhea
Local: Pain at injection site
<1%: Anaphylaxis, rash, pruritus, Stevens-Johnson syndrome, oral candidiasis, nausea, vomiting, abdominal cramps, anorexia, pseudomembranous colitis, eosinophilia, neutropenia, leukopenia, thrombocytopenia, thrombocytosis, elevated transaminases, phlebitis, vaginitis, fever, seizures

Other reactions with cephalosporins include toxic epidermal necrolysis, abdominal pain, cholestasis, superinfection, renal dysfunction, toxic nephropathy, aplastic anemia, hemolytic anemia, hemorrhage, prolonged prothrombin time, pancytopenia

Overdosage/Toxicology
Symptoms of overdose include neuromuscular hypersensitivity, convulsions especially with renal insufficiency; many beta-lactam antibiotics have the potential to cause neuromuscular hyperirritability or seizures
Hemodialysis may be helpful to aid in the removal of the drug from the blood, otherwise most treatment is supportive or symptom directed

Drug Interactions
Increased effect: High-dose probenecid decreases clearance
Increased toxicity: Aminoglycosides increase nephrotoxic potential

Stability
Store intact vials at room temperature and protect from temperatures exceeding 40°C
Reconstituted solutions of cefazolin are light yellow to yellow
Protection from light is recommended for the powder and for the reconstituted solutions
Reconstituted solutions are stable for 24 hours at room temperature and 10 days under refrigeration
Stability of parenteral admixture at room temperature (25°C): 48 hours
Stability of parenteral admixture at refrigeration temperature (4°C): 14 days
Standard diluent: 1 g/50 mL D_5W; 2 g/50 mL D_5W

Mechanism of Action Inhibits bacterial cell wall synthesis by binding to one or more of the penicillin-binding proteins (PBPs) which in turn inhibits the final transpeptidation step of peptidoglycan synthesis in bacterial cell walls, thus inhibiting cell wall biosynthesis. Bacteria eventually lyse due to ongoing activity of cell wall autolytic enzymes (autolysins and murein hydrolases) while cell wall assembly is arrested.

Pharmacodynamics/Kinetics
Distribution: Widely distributed into most body tissues and fluids including gallbladder, liver, kidneys, bone, sputum, bile, pleural and synovial fluids; CSF penetration is poor; crosses the placenta and small amounts appear in breast milk

Protein binding: 74% to 86%

Metabolism: Hepatic is minimal

Half-life: 90-150 minutes (prolonged with renal impairment)

Time to peak serum concentration: I.M.: Within 0.5-2 hours

Elimination: 80% to 100% is excreted unchanged in urine

Usual Dosage I.M., I.V.:

Children >1 month: 25-100 mg/kg/day divided every 6-8 hours; maximum: 6 g/day

Adults: 250 mg to 2 g every 6-12 (usually 8) hours, depending on severity of infection; maximum dose: 12 g/day

Dosing adjustment in renal impairment:

Cl_{cr} 10-30 mL/minute: Administer every 12 hours

Cl_{cr} <10 mL/minute: Administer every 24 hours

Hemodialysis: Moderately dialyzable (20% to 50%); administer dose postdialysis or administer supplemental dose of 0.5-1 g after dialysis

Peritoneal dialysis: Administer 0.5 g every 12 hours

Continuous arteriovenous or venovenous hemofiltration (CAVH/CAVHD): Dose as for Cl_{cr} 10-30 mL/minute; removes 30 mg of cefazolin per liter of filtrate per day

Monitoring Parameters Renal function periodically when used in combination with other nephrotoxic drugs, hepatic function tests, CBC; monitor for signs of anaphylaxis during first dose

Test Interactions Positive direct Coombs', false-positive urinary glucose test using cupric sulfate (Benedict's solution, Clinitest®, Fehling's solution), false-positive serum or urine creatinine with Jaffé reaction

Nursing Implications Do not admix with aminoglycosides in same bottle/bag; observe for signs and symptoms of anaphylaxis during first dose

Additional Information Sodium content of 1 g: 47 mg (2 mEq)

Dosage Forms

Infusion, premixed, as sodium, in D_5W (frozen) (Ancef®): 500 mg (50 mL); 1 g (50 mL)

Injection, as sodium (Kefzol®): 500 mg, 1 g

Powder for injection, as sodium (Ancef®, Zolicef®): 250 mg, 500 mg, 1 g, 5 g, 10 g, 20 g

Selected Readings

Donowitz GR and Mandell GL, "Beta-Lactam Antibiotics," *N Engl J Med*, 1988, 318(7):419-26 and 318(8):490-500.

Gentry LO, Zeluff BJ, and Cooley DA, "Antibiotic Prophylaxis in Open-Heart Surgery: A Comparison of Cefamandole, Cefuroxime, and Cefazolin," *Ann Thorac Surg*, 1988, 46(2):167-71.

Marshall WF and Blair JE, "The Cephalosporins," *Mayo Clin Proc*, 1999, 74(2):187-95.

Peterson CD, Lake KD, Arom KV, et al, "Antibiotic Prophylaxis in Open-Heart Surgery Patients: Comparison of Cefamandole and Cefuroxime," *Drug Intell Clin Pharm*, 1987, 21(9):728-32.

Cefazolin Sodium *see Cefazolin on previous page*

Cefdinir (SEF di ner)

U.S. Brand Names Omnicef®

Synonyms CFDN

Use Treatment of community-acquired pneumonia, acute exacerbations of chronic bronchitis, acute bacterial otitis media, acute maxillary sinusitis, pharyngitis/tonsillitis, and uncomplicated skin and skin structure infections.

Pregnancy Risk Factor B

Contraindications Hypersensitivity to cephalosporins or related antibiotics

Warnings/Precautions Administer cautiously to penicillin-sensitive patients. There is evidence of partial cross-allerginicity and cephalosporins cannot be assumed to be an absolutely safe alternative to penicillin in the penicillin-allergic patient. Serum sickness-like reactions have been reported. Signs and symptoms occur after a few days of therapy and resolve a few days after drug discontinuation with no serious sequelae. Pseudomembranous colitis occurs; consider its diagnosis in patients who develop diarrhea with antibiotic use.

Adverse Reactions

1% to 10%

Dermatologic: Cutaneous moniliasis (1%)

Gastrointestinal: Diarrhea (8%), rash (3%), vomiting (1%), increased GGT (1%)

<1%: Abdominal pain, leukopenia, nausea, vaginal moniliasis, vaginitis, dyspepsia, maculopapular rash, increased AST, Stevens-Johnson syndrome, (Continued)

Cefdinir (Continued)

exfoliative dermatitis, erythema multiforme, toxic epidermal necrolysis, erythema nodosum, conjunctivitis, stomatitis, hepatitis, cholestasis, hepatic failure, jaundice, increased amylase, anaphylaxis, shock, edema, laryngeal edema, hemorrhagic colitis, enterocolitis, pseudomembranous colitis, pancytopenia, granulocytopenia, leukopenia, thrombocytopenia, ITP, hemolytic anemia, respiratory failure, asthma exacerbation, eosinophilic pneumonia, idiopathic interstitial pneumonia, fever, acute renal failure, nephropathy, coagulopathy, DIC, upper gastrointestinal bleeding. Peptic ulcer, ileus, loss of consciousness, vasculitis, cardiac failure, chest pain, myocardial infarction, hypertension, involuntary movements, rhabdomyolysis

Other reactions with cephalosporins include dizziness, fever, headache, encephalopathy, asterixis, neuromuscular excitability, seizures, aplastic anemia, interstitial nephritis, toxic nephropathy, angioedema, hemorrhage, prolonged PT, serum-sickness reactions, and superinfection

Overdosage/Toxicology

After acute overdose, most agents cause only nausea, vomiting, and diarrhea, although neuromuscular hypersensitivity and seizures are possible, especially in patients with renal insufficiency

Hemodialysis may be helpful to aid in the removal of the drug from the blood but not usually indicated, otherwise most treatment is supportive or symptom directed following GI decontamination

Drug Interactions

Increased effect: Probenecid increases the effects of cephalosporins by decreasing the renal elimination in those which are secreted by tubular secretion

Increased toxicity: Anticoagulant effects may be increased when administered with cephalosporins

Stability Oral suspension should be mixed with 39 mL water for the 60 mL bottle and 65 mL of water for the 120 mL bottle. After mixing, the suspension can be stored at room temperature (25°C/77°F). The suspension may be used for 10 days. The suspension should be shaken well before each administration.

Mechanism of Action Inhibits bacterial cell wall synthesis by binding to one or more of the penicillin-binding proteins (PBPs) which in turn inhibits the final transpeptidation step of peptidoglycan synthesis in bacterial cell walls, thus inhibiting cell wall biosynthesis. Bacteria eventually lyse due to ongoing activity of cell wall autolytic enzymes (autolysins and murein hydrolases) while cell wall assembly is arrested.

Usual Dosage Oral:

Children: 7 mg/kg/dose twice daily or 14 mg/kg/dose once daily for 10 days (maximum: 600 mg/day)

Adolescents and Adults: 300 mg twice daily or 600 mg once daily for 10 days

Dosing adjustment in renal impairment: Cl_{cr} <30 mL/minute: 300 mg once daily

Hemodialysis removes cefdinir; recommended initial dose: 300 mg (or 7 mg/kg/dose) every other day. At the conclusion of each hemodialysis session, 300 mg (or 7 mg/kg/dose) should be given. Subsequent doses (300 mg or 7 mg/kg/dose) should be administered every other day.

Dosage Forms

Capsule: 300 mg

Suspension, oral: 125 mg/5 mL (60 mL, 100 mL)

Selected Readings

Marshall WF and Blair JE, "The Cephalosporins," *Mayo Clin Proc*, 1999, 74(2):187-95.

Cefepime (SEF e pim)

U.S. Brand Names Maxipime®

Synonyms Cefepime Hydrochloride

Use Treatment of uncomplicated and complicated urinary tract infections including pyelonephritis caused by typical urinary tract pathogens, uncomplicated skin and skin structure infections caused by *Streptococcus pyogenes*, moderate to severe pneumonia caused by pneumococcus, *Pseudomonas aeruginosa*, and other gram-negative organisms, and complicated intra-abdominal infections (in combination with metronidazole). Also active against methicillin-susceptible staphylococci, *Enterobacter* sp, and many other gram-negative bacilli. Use in pediatrics (2 months to 16 years): empiric therapy for febrile neutropenic patients, uncomplicated skin/soft tissue infections, pneumonia, and complicated/ uncomplicated urinary tract infections.

Drug of Choice or Alternative for
Disease/Syndrome(s)
Fever, Neutropenic on page 30

Pregnancy Risk Factor B

Contraindications Hypersensitivity to cefepime or its components, or other cephalosporins

Warnings/Precautions Modify dosage in patients with severe renal impairment; prolonged use may result in superinfection; use with caution in patients with a history of penicillin or cephalosporin allergy, especially IgE-mediated reactions (eg, anaphylaxis, urticaria); may cause antibiotic-associated colitis or colitis secondary to C. difficile

Adverse Reactions
>10%: Hematologic: Positive Coombs' test without hemolysis
1% to 10%:
Dermatologic: Rash, pruritus
Gastrointestinal: : Diarrhea, nausea, vomiting
Central nervous system: Fever (1%), headache (1%)
Local: Pain, erythema at injection site
<1%: Leukopenia, neutropenia, agranulocytosis, thrombocytopenia, myoclonus, seizures, encephalopathy, neuromuscular excitability

Other reactions with cephalosporins include toxic epidermal necrolysis, Stevens-Johnson syndrome, erythema multiforme, renal dysfunction, toxic nephropathy, aplastic anemia, hemolytic anemia, hemorrhage, prolonged PT, pancytopenia, vaginitis, superinfection

Overdosage/Toxicology
Symptoms of overdose include neuromuscular hypersensitivity, convulsions; many beta-lactam antibiotics have the potential to cause neuromuscular hyperirritability or seizures
Hemodialysis may be helpful to aid in the removal of the drug from the blood; however, most often treatment is supportive and symptom directed

Drug Interactions
Increased effect: High-dose probenecid decreases clearance
Increased toxicity: Aminoglycosides increase nephrotoxic potential

Stability Cefepime is compatible and stable with normal saline, D_5W, and a variety of other solutions for 24 hours at room temperature and 7 days refrigerated

Mechanism of Action Inhibits bacterial cell wall synthesis by binding to one or more of the penicillin-binding proteins (PBPs) which in turn inhibits the final transpeptidation step of peptidoglycan synthesis in bacterial cell walls, thus inhibiting cell wall biosynthesis. Bacterial eventually lyse due to ongoing activity of cell wall autolytic enzymes (autolysis and murein hydrolases) while cell wall assembly is arrested.

Pharmacodynamics/Kinetics
Absorption: I.M.: Rapid and complete; T_{max}: 0.5-1.5 hours
Distribution: V_d: Adults: 14-20 L; penetrates into inflammatory fluid at concentrations ~80% of serum levels and into bronchial mucosa at levels ~60% of those reached in the plasma, crosses blood-brain barrier
Protein binding, plasma: 16% to 19%
Metabolism: Very little
Half-life: 2 hours
Elimination: 85% eliminated as unchanged drug in urine

Usual Dosage I.V.:
Children:
Febrile neutropenia: 50 mg/kg every 8 hours for 7-10 days
Uncomplicated skin/soft tissue infections, pneumonia, and complicated/ uncomplicated UTI: 50 mg/kg twice daily
Adults:
Most infections: 1-2 g every 12 hours for 5-10 days; higher doses or more frequent administration may be required in pseudomonal infections
Urinary tract infections, uncomplicated: 500 mg every 12 hours
Monotherapy for febrile neutropenic patients: 2 g every 8 hours for 7 days or until the neutropenia resolves
(Continued)

Cefepime *(Continued)*

Dosing adjustment in renal impairment:

Cefepime

Creatinine Clearance (mL/minute)	Recommended Maintenance Schedule		
>60 Normal recommended dosing schedule	500 mg every 12 hours	1 g every 12 hours	2 g every 12 hours
30-60	500 mg every 24 hours	1 g every 24 hours	1 g every 24 hours
11-29	500 mg every 24 hours	500 mg every 24 hours	1 g every 24 hours
<10	250 mg every 24 hours	250 mg every 24 hours	500 mg every 24 hours

Hemodialysis: Removed by dialysis; administer supplemental dose of 250 mg after each dialysis session

Peritoneal dialysis: Removed to a lesser extent than hemodialysis; administer 250 mg every 48 hours

Continuous arteriovenous or venovenous hemofiltration (CAVH/CAVHD): Dose as normal Cl_{cr} (eg, >30 mL/minute)

Administration May be administered either I.M. or I.V.

Monitoring Parameters Obtain specimen for culture and sensitivity prior to the first dose; monitor for signs of anaphylaxis during first dose

Test Interactions Positive direct Coombs', false-positive urinary glucose test using cupric sulfate (Benedict's solution, Clinitest®, Fehling's solution), false-positive serum or urine creatinine with Jaffé reaction, false-positive urinary proteins and steroids

Patient Information Report side effects such as diarrhea, dyspepsia, headache, blurred vision, and lightheadedness to your physician

Nursing Implications Do not admix with aminoglycosides in the same bottle/bag; observe for signs and symptoms of bacterial infection, including defervescence; observe for anaphylaxis during first dose

Dosage Forms

Infusion, piggy-back: 1 g (100 mL); 2 g (100 mL)
Infusion (ADD-vantage®): 1 g
Injection: 500 mg, 1 g, 2 g

Selected Readings

Barradell LB and Bryson HM, "Cefepime. A Review of Its Antibacterial Activity, Pharmacokinetic Properties, and Therapeutic Use," *Drugs*, 1994, 47(3):471-505.

Cunha BA and Gill MV, "Cefepime," *Med Clin North Am*, 1995, 79(4):721-32.

Marshall WF and Blair JE, "The Cephalosporins," *Mayo Clin Proc*, 1999, 74(2):187-95.

Okamoto MP, Nakahiro RK, Chin A, et al, "Cefepime: A New Fourth-Generation Cephalosporin," *Am J Hosp Pharm*, 1994, 51(4):463-77.

Sanders CC, "Cefepime: The Next Generation?" *Clin Infect Dis*, 1993, 17(3):369-79.

Wynd MA and Paladino JA, "Cefepime: A Fourth-Generation Parenteral Cephalosporin," *Ann Pharmacother*, 1996, 30(12):1414-24.

Cefepime Hydrochloride *see Cefepime on page 634*

Cefixime *(sef IKS eem)*

Related Information

Antimicrobial Activity Against Selected Organisms *on page 983*

U.S. Brand Names Suprax®

Generic Available No

Use Treatment of urinary tract infections, otitis media, respiratory infections due to susceptible organisms including *S. pneumoniae* and *S. pyogenes*, *H. influenzae* and many Enterobacteriaceae; documented poor compliance with other oral antimicrobials; outpatient therapy of serious soft tissue or skeletal infections due to susceptible organisms; single-dose oral treatment of uncomplicated cervical/urethral gonorrhea due to *N. gonorrhoeae*

Drug of Choice or Alternative for

Organism(s)

Neisseria gonorrhoeae on page 215

Pregnancy Risk Factor B

Contraindications Hypersensitivity to cefixime or cephalosporins

Warnings/Precautions Prolonged use may result in superinfection; modify dosage in patients with renal impairment; use with caution in patients with a history of penicillin allergy especially IgE-mediated reactions (eg, anaphylaxis, urticaria); may cause antibiotic-associated colitis or colitis secondary to *C. difficile*

Adverse Reactions

>10%: Gastrointestinal: Diarrhea (16%)

1% to 10%: Gastrointestinal: Abdominal pain, nausea, dyspepsia, flatulence

<1%: Rash, urticaria, pruritus, erythema multiforme, Stevens-Johnson syndrome, serum sickness -like reaction, fever, vomiting, pseudomembranous colitis, transaminase elevations, increased BUN, increased creatinine, headache, dizziness, thrombocytopenia, leukopenia, eosinophilia, prolonged PT, vaginitis, candidiasis

Other reactions with cephalosporins include anaphylaxis, seizures, toxic epidermal necrolysis, renal dysfunction, toxic nephropathy, interstitial nephritis, cholestasis, aplastic anemia, hemolytic anemia, hemorrhage, pancytopenia, neutropenia, agranulocytosis, colitis, superinfection

Overdosage/Toxicology

After acute overdose, most agents cause only nausea, vomiting, and diarrhea, although neuromuscular hypersensitivity and seizures are possible, especially in patients with renal insufficiency; many beta-lactam antibiotics have the potential to cause neuromuscular hyperirritability or seizures

Hemodialysis may be helpful to aid in the removal of the drug from the blood but not usually indicated, otherwise most treatment is supportive or symptom directed following GI decontamination

Drug Interactions

Increased effect: Probenecid may decrease cephalosporin elimination

Increased toxicity: Furosemide, aminoglycosides may be a possible additive to nephrotoxicity

Stability After reconstitution, suspension may be stored for 14 days at room temperature

Mechanism of Action Inhibits bacterial cell wall synthesis by binding to one or more of the penicillin binding proteins (PBPs); which in turn inhibits the final transpeptidation step of peptidoglycan synthesis in bacterial cell walls, thus inhibiting cell wall biosynthesis. Bacteria eventually lyse due to ongoing activity of cell wall autolytic enzymes (autolysins and murein hydrolases) while cell wall assembly is arrested.

Pharmacodynamics/Kinetics

Absorption: Oral: 40% to 50%

Distribution: Widely distributed throughout the body and reaches therapeutic concentration in most tissues and body fluids, including synovial, pericardial, pleural, and peritoneal fluids; also bile, sputum, and urine; also bone, myocardium, gallbladder, and skin and soft tissue

Protein binding: 65%

Half-life:

Normal renal function: 3-4 hours

Renal failure: Up to 11.5 hours

Time to peak serum concentrations: Within 2-6 hours; peak serum concentrations are 15% to 50% higher for the oral suspension versus tablets; presence of food delays the time to reach peak concentrations

Elimination: 50% of absorbed dose excreted as active drug in urine and 10% in bile

Usual Dosage Oral:

Children: 8 mg/kg/day divided every 12-24 hours

Adolescents and Adults: 400 mg/day divided every 12-24 hours

Uncomplicated cervical/urethral gonorrhea due to *N. gonorrhoeae*: 400 mg as a single dose

For *S. pyogenes* infections, treat for 10 days; use suspension for otitis media due to increased peak serum levels as compared to tablet form

Dosing adjustment in renal impairment:

Cl_{cr} 21-60 mL/minute or with renal hemodialysis: Administer 75% of the standard dose

(Continued)

Cefixime *(Continued)*

Cl$_{cr}$ <20 mL/minute or with CAPD: Administer 50% of the standard dose
Moderately dialyzable (10%)

Administration Oral: May be administered with or without food; administer with food to decrease GI distress

Monitoring Parameters With prolonged therapy, monitor renal and hepatic function periodically; observe for signs and symptoms of anaphylaxis during first dose

Test Interactions Positive direct Coombs', false-positive urinary glucose test using cupric sulfate (Benedict's solution, Clinitest®, Fehling's solution), false-positive serum or urine creatinine with Jaffé reaction, false-positive urine ketones

Patient Information Report diarrhea promptly; entire course of medication (10-14 days) should be taken to ensure eradication of organism; may interfere with oral contraceptives, females should report symptoms of vaginitis

Additional Information Otitis media should be treated with the suspension since it results in higher peak blood levels than the tablet

Dosage Forms

Powder for oral suspension (strawberry flavor): 100 mg/5 mL (50 mL, 100 mL)
Tablet, film coated: 200 mg, 400 mg

Selected Readings

Donowitz GR and Mandell GL, "Beta-Lactam Antibiotics," *N Engl J Med*, 1988, 318(7):419-26 and 318(8):490-500.

Markham A and Brogden RN, "Cefixime. A Review of Its Therapeutic Efficacy in Lower Respiratory Tract Infections," *Drugs*, 1995, 49(6):1007-22.

Marshall WF and Blair JE, "The Cephalosporins," *Mayo Clin Proc*, 1999, 74(2):187-95.

Schatz BS, Karavokiros KT, Taeubel MA, et al, "Comparison of Cefprozil, Cefpodoxime Proxetil, Loracarbef, Cefixime, and Ceftibuten," *Ann Pharmacother*, 1996, 30(3):258-68.

Smith GH, "Oral Cephalosporins in Perspective," *DICP*, 1990, 24(1):45-51.

Cefizox® *see* Ceftizoxime *on page 654*

Cefmetazole *(sef MET a zole)*

Related Information

Antimicrobial Activity Against Selected Organisms *on page 983*

U.S. Brand Names Zefazone®

Synonyms Cefmetazole Sodium

Generic Available No

Use Second generation cephalosporin, useful for susceptible aerobic and anaerobic gram-positive and gram-negative bacteria; surgical prophylaxis, specifically colorectal and OB-GYN

Pregnancy Risk Factor B

Contraindications Hypersensitivity to cefmetazole or any component or cephalosporins

Warnings/Precautions Modify dosage in patients with severe renal impairment; prolonged use may result in superinfection; use with caution in patients with a history of penicillin allergy especially IgE-mediated reactions (eg, anaphylaxis, urticaria); may cause antibiotic-associated colitis or colitis secondary to *C. difficile*

Adverse Reactions

Contains MTT side chain which may lead to increased risk of hypoprothrombinemia and bleeding

1% to 10%:
Gastrointestinal: Diarrhea, nausea
Dermatologic: Rash

<1%: Pain at injection site, phlebitis, pseudomembranous colitis, epigastric pain, candidiasis, bleeding, shock, hypotension, headache, hot flashes, dyspnea, epistaxis, respiratory distress, fever, vaginitis

Other reactions with cephalosporins include anaphylaxis, seizures, toxic epidermal necrolysis, erythema multiforme, Stevens-Johnson syndrome, renal dysfunction, interstitial nephritis, toxic nephropathy, cholestasis, aplastic anemia, hemolytic anemia, hemorrhage, pancytopenia, neutropenia, agranulocytosis, colitis, superinfection

Overdosage/Toxicology

Symptoms of overdose include neuromuscular hypersensitivity, convulsions especially with renal insufficiency; many beta-lactam antibiotics have the potential to cause neuromuscular hyperirritability or seizures

Hemodialysis may be helpful to aid in the removal of the drug from the blood, otherwise most treatment is supportive or symptom directed

Drug Interactions

Increased effect: Probenecid may decrease cephalosporin elimination

Increased toxicity: Furosemide, aminoglycosides may be a possible additive to nephrotoxicity

Stability Reconstituted solution and I.V. infusion in NS or D_5W solution are stable for 24 hours at room temperature, 7 days when refrigerated, or 6 weeks when frozen; after freezing, thawed solution is stable for 24 hours at room temperature or 7 days when refrigerated

Mechanism of Action Inhibits bacterial cell wall synthesis by binding to one or more of the penicillin-binding proteins (PBPs) which in turn inhibits the final transpeptidation step of peptidoglycan synthesis in bacterial cell walls, thus inhibiting cell wall biosynthesis. Bacteria eventually lyse due to ongoing activity of cell wall autolytic enzymes (autolysins and murein hydrolases) while cell wall assembly is arrested.

Pharmacodynamics/Kinetics

Absorption: I.M.: Well absorbed

Distribution: Widely distributed

Protein binding: 65%

Metabolism: <15%

Half-life: 72 minutes

Elimination: Renal

Usual Dosage Adults: I.V.:

Infections: 2 g every 6-12 hours for 5-14 days

Prophylaxis: 2 g 30-90 minutes before surgery **or** 1 g 30-90 minutes before surgery; repeat 8 and 16 hours later

Dosing interval in renal impairment:

Cl_{cr} 50-90 mL/minute: Administer every 12 hours

Cl_{cr} 10-50 mL/minute: Administer every 16-24 hours

Cl_{cr} <10 mL/minute: Administer every 48 hours

Monitoring Parameters Monitor prothrombin times; observe for signs and symptoms of anaphylaxis during first dose

Test Interactions Positive direct Coombs', false-positive urinary glucose test using cupric sulfate (Benedict's solution, Clinitest®, Fehling's solution), false-positive serum or urine creatinine with Jaffé reaction

Patient Information Do not drink alcohol for at least 24 hours after receiving dose; report persistent diarrhea; may interfere with oral contraceptives, females should report symptoms of vaginitis

Nursing Implications Do not admix with aminoglycosides in same bottle/bag

Additional Information Sodium content of 1 g: 47 mg (2 mEq)

Dosage Forms Powder for injection, as sodium: 1 g, 2 g

Selected Readings

Donowitz GR and Mandell GL, "Beta-Lactam Antibiotics," *N Engl J Med*, 1988, 318(7):419-26 and 318(8):490-500.

Jones RN, "Review of the *In vitro* Spectrum and Characteristics of Cefmetazole (CS-1170)," *J Antimicrob Chemother*, 1989, 23(Suppl D):1-12.

Marshall WF and Blair JE, "The Cephalosporins," *Mayo Clin Proc*, 1999, 74(2):187-95.

Plouffe JF, "Cefmetazole Versus Cefoxitin in Prevention of Infections After Abdominal Surgery," *J Antimicrob Chemother*, 1989, 23(Suppl D):85-8.

Cefmetazole Sodium *see Cefmetazole on previous page*

Cefobid® *see Cefoperazone on page 641*

Cefonicid (se FON i sid)

Related Information

Antimicrobial Activity Against Selected Organisms *on page 983*

U.S. Brand Names Monocid®

Synonyms Cefonicid Sodium

Generic Available No

Use Treatment of susceptible bacterial infection; mainly respiratory tract, skin and skin structure, bone and joint, urinary tract and gynecologic, septicemia; active

(Continued)

Cefonicid *(Continued)*

against methicillin-sensitive staphylococci, many streptococci, and various gram-negative bacilli including *E. coli*, some *Klebsiella*, *P. mirabilis*, *H. influenzae*, and *Moraxella*.

Pregnancy Risk Factor B

Contraindications Hypersensitivity to cefonicid sodium, any component, or cephalosporins

Warnings/Precautions Modify dosage in patients with severe renal impairment; prolonged use may result in superinfection; use with caution in patients with a history of penicillin allergy especially IgE-mediated reactions (eg, anaphylaxis, urticaria); may cause antibiotic-associated colitis or colitis secondary to *C. difficile*

Adverse Reactions

1% to 10%:

Hematologic: Increased eosinophils (2.9%), increased platelets (1.7%)

Hepatic: Altered liver function tests (increased transaminases, LDH, alkaline phosphatase) (1.6%)

Local: Pain, burning at injection site (5.7%)

<1%: Fever, rash, pruritus, erythema, anaphylactoid reactions, diarrhea, pseudomembranous colitis, abdominal pain, increased transaminases, increased BUN, increased creatinine, interstitial nephritis, neutropenia, decreased WBC, thrombocytopenia

Other reactions with cephalosporins include anaphylaxis, seizures, Stevens-Johnson syndrome, toxic epidermal necrolysis, renal dysfunction, toxic nephropathy, cholestasis, aplastic anemia, hemolytic anemia, hemorrhage, pancytopenia, agranulocytosis, colitis, superinfection

Overdosage/Toxicology

Symptoms of overdose include neuromuscular hypersensitivity, convulsions especially with renal insufficiency; many beta-lactam antibiotics have the potential to cause neuromuscular hyperirritability or seizures

Hemodialysis may be helpful to aid in the removal of the drug from the blood, otherwise most treatment is supportive or symptom directed

Drug Interactions

Increased effect: Probenecid may decrease cephalosporin elimination

Increased toxicity: Furosemide, aminoglycosides may be a possible additive to nephrotoxicity

Stability Reconstituted solution and I.V. infusion in NS or D_5W solution are stable for 24 hours at room temperature or 72 hours if refrigerated

Mechanism of Action Inhibits bacterial cell wall synthesis by binding to one or more of the penicillin-binding proteins (PBPs) which in turn inhibits the final transpeptidation step of peptidoglycan synthesis in bacterial cell walls, thus inhibiting cell wall biosynthesis. Bacteria eventually lyse due to ongoing activity of cell wall autolytic enzymes (autolysins and murein hydrolases) while cell wall assembly is arrested.

Pharmacodynamics/Kinetics

Absorption: I.M.: Well absorbed

Distribution: Widely distributed into most body tissues with low concentrations in CSF and eye

Protein binding: 98%

Metabolism: None

Half-life: 3.5-5.8 hours

Elimination: Unchanged in urine

Cefonicid

Cl_{cr} (mL/min/1.73 m^2)	Dose (mg/kg) for Each Dosing Interval
60-79	10-24 q24h
40-59	8-20 q24h
20-39	4-15 q24h
10-19	4-15 q48h
5-9	4-15 q3-5d
<5	3-4 q3-5d

Usual Dosage Adults: I.M., I.V.: 0.5-2 g every 24 hours
Prophylaxis: Preop: 1 g/hour

Dosing interval in renal impairment: See table on previous page.

Monitoring Parameters Observe for signs and symptoms of anaphylaxis during first dose

Test Interactions Positive direct Coombs', false-positive urinary glucose test using cupric sulfate (Benedict's solution, Clinitest®, Fehling's solution), false-positive serum or urine creatinine with Jaffé reaction

Additional Information Sodium content of 1 g: 85.1 mg (3.7 mEq)

Dosage Forms Powder for injection, as sodium: 500 mg, 1 g, 10 g

Selected Readings
Donowitz GR and Mandell GL, "Beta-Lactam Antibiotics," *N Engl J Med*, 1988, 318(7):419-26 and 318(8):490-500.
Gustaferro CA and Steckelberg JM, "Cephalosporin Antimicrobial Agents and Related Compounds," *Mayo Clin Proc*, 1991, 66(10):1064-73.
Marshall WF and Blair JE, "The Cephalosporins," *Mayo Clin Proc*, 1999, 74(2):187-95.

Cefonicid Sodium *see* Cefonicid *on page 639*

Cefoperazone (sef oh PER a zone)

Related Information
Antimicrobial Activity Against Selected Organisms *on page 983*

U.S. Brand Names Cefobid®

Synonyms Cefoperazone Sodium

Generic Available No

Use Treatment of susceptible bacterial infection; mainly respiratory tract, skin and skin structure, bone and joint, urinary tract and gynecologic as well as septicemia. Active against a variety of gram-negative bacilli, some gram-positive cocci, and has some activity against *Pseudomonas aeruginosa*.

Pregnancy Risk Factor B

Contraindications Hypersensitivity to cefoperazone or any component or cephalosporins

Warnings/Precautions Modify dosage in patients with severe renal or hepatic impairment; prolonged use may result in superinfection; although rare, cefoperazone may interfere with hemostasis via destruction of vitamin K-producing intestinal bacteria, prevention of activation of prothrombin by the attachment of a methyltetrazolethiol side chain, and by an immune-mediated thrombocytopenia; use with caution in patients with a history of penicillin allergy especially IgE-mediated reactions (eg, anaphylaxis, urticaria); may cause antibiotic-associated colitis or colitis secondary to *C. difficile*

Adverse Reactions
Contains MTT side chain which may lead to increased risk of hypoprothrombinemia and bleeding

1% to 10%:
Dermatologic: Rash (maculopapular or erythematous) (2%)
Gastrointestinal: Diarrhea (3%)
Hematologic: Decreased neutrophils (2%), decreased hemoglobin or hematocrit (5%), eosinophilia (10%)
Hepatic: Increased transaminases (5% to 10%)
<1%: Hypoprothrombinemia, bleeding, pseudomembranous colitis, nausea, vomiting, elevated BUN, elevated creatinine, pain at injection site, induration at injection site, phlebitis, drug fever

Other reactions with cephalosporins include anaphylaxis, seizures, Stevens-Johnson syndrome, toxic epidermal necrolysis, renal dysfunction, toxic nephropathy, cholestasis, aplastic anemia, hemolytic anemia, pancytopenia, agranulocytosis, colitis, superinfection

Overdosage/Toxicology
Symptoms of overdose include neuromuscular hypersensitivity, convulsions especially with renal insufficiency; many beta-lactam antibiotics have the potential to cause neuromuscular hyperirritability or seizures
Hemodialysis may be helpful to aid in the removal of the drug from the blood, otherwise most treatment is supportive or symptom directed

Drug Interactions
Disulfiram-like reaction has been reported when taken within 72 hours of alcohol consumption
(Continued)

Cefoperazone *(Continued)*

Increased nephrotoxicity: Aminoglycosides, furosemide

Stability Reconstituted solution and I.V. infusion in NS or D$_5$W solution are stable for 24 hours at room temperature, 5 days when refrigerated or 3 weeks, when frozen; after freezing, thawed solution is stable for 48 hours at room temperature or 10 days when refrigerated

Mechanism of Action Inhibits bacterial cell wall synthesis by binding to one or more of the penicillin-binding proteins (PBPs) which in turn inhibits the final transpeptidation step of peptidoglycan synthesis in bacterial cell walls, thus inhibiting cell wall biosynthesis. Bacteria eventually lyse due to ongoing activity of cell wall autolytic enzymes (autolysins and murein hydrolases) while cell wall assembly is arrested.

Pharmacodynamics/Kinetics

Distribution: Widely distributed in most body tissues and fluids; highest concentrations in bile; low penetration in CSF; variable when meninges are inflamed; crosses placenta; small amounts into breast milk

Half-life: 2 hours, higher with hepatic disease or biliary obstruction

Time to peak serum concentration: I.M.: Within 1-2 hours

Elimination: Principally in bile (70% to 75%); 20% to 30% recovered unchanged in urine within 6-12 hours

Usual Dosage I.M., I.V.:

Children (not approved): 100-150 mg/kg/day divided every 8-12 hours; up to 12 g/day

Adults: 2-4 g/day in divided doses every 12 hours; up to 12 g/day

Dosing adjustment in hepatic impairment: Reduce dose 50% in patients with advanced liver cirrhosis; maximum daily dose: 4 g

Monitoring Parameters Monitor for coagulation abnormalities and diarrhea; observe for signs and symptoms of anaphylaxis during first dose

Test Interactions Positive direct Coombs', false-positive urinary glucose test using cupric sulfate (Benedict's solution, Clinitest®, Fehling's solution), false-positive serum or urine creatinine with Jaffé reaction

Nursing Implications Do not admix with aminoglycosides in same bottle/bag

Additional Information Sodium content of 1 g: 34.5 mg (1.5 mEq); contains the n-methylthiotetrazole side chain

Dosage Forms

Injection, as sodium, premixed (frozen): 1 g (50 mL); 2 g (50 mL)

Powder for injection, as sodium: 1 g, 2 g

Selected Readings

Donowitz GR and Mandell GL, "Beta-Lactam Antibiotics," *N Engl J Med*, 1988, 318(7):419-26 and 318(8):490-500.

Klein NC and Cunha BA, "Third-Generation Cephalosporins," *Med Clin North Am*, 1995, 79(4):705-19.

Marshall WF and Blair JE, "The Cephalosporins," *Mayo Clin Proc*, 1999, 74(2):187-95.

Cefoperazone Sodium *see* Cefoperazone *on previous page*

Cefotan® *see* Cefotetan *on page 644*

Cefotaxime *(sef oh TAKS eem)*

Related Information

Antimicrobial Activity Against Selected Organisms *on page 983*

U.S. Brand Names Claforan®

Synonyms Cefotaxime Sodium

Generic Available No

Use Treatment of susceptible infection in respiratory tract, skin and skin structure, bone and joint, urinary tract, gynecologic as well as septicemia, and documented or suspected meningitis. Active against most gram-negative bacilli (not *Pseudomonas*) and gram-positive cocci (not enterococcus). Active against many penicillin-resistant pneumococci.

Drug of Choice or Alternative for

Disease/Syndrome(s)

Brain Abscess *on page 19*

Peritonitis, Spontaneous Bacterial *on page 43*

Pneumonia, Community-Acquired *on page 45*

Organism(s)

Neisseria gonorrhoeae on page 215

Pregnancy Risk Factor B

Contraindications Hypersensitivity to cefotaxime, any component, or cephalosporins

Warnings/Precautions Modify dosage in patients with severe renal impairment; prolonged use may result in superinfection; a potentially life-threatening arrhythmia has been reported in patients who received a rapid bolus injection via central line. Use caution in patients with colitis; minimize tissue inflammation by changing infusion sites when needed. Use with caution in patients with a history of penicillin allergy especially IgE-mediated reactions (eg, anaphylaxis, urticaria); may cause antibiotic-associated colitis or colitis secondary to *C. difficile*.

Adverse Reactions

1% to 10%:
Dermatologic: Rash, pruritus
Gastrointestinal: Diarrhea, nausea, vomiting, colitis
Local: Pain at injection site

<1%: Anaphylaxis, urticaria, arrhythmias (after rapid IV injection via central catheter), pseudomembranous colitis, neutropenia, thrombocytopenia, eosinophilia, headache, fever, transaminase elevations, interstitial nephritis, increased BUN, increased creatinine, increased transaminases, phlebitis, candidiasis, vaginitis,

Other reactions with cephalosporins include seizures, Stevens-Johnson syndrome, toxic epidermal necrolysis, renal dysfunction, toxic nephropathy, cholestasis, aplastic anemia, hemolytic anemia, hemorrhage, pancytopenia, agranulocytosis, colitis, superinfection

Overdosage/Toxicology

Usually well tolerated even in overdose, convulsions possible many beta-lactam antibiotics have the potential to cause neuromuscular hyperirritability or seizures

Hemodialysis may be helpful to aid in the removal of the drug from the blood, otherwise most treatment is supportive or symptom directed

Drug Interactions

Increased effect: Probenecid may decrease cephalosporin elimination

Increased toxicity: Furosemide, aminoglycosides may be a possible additive to nephrotoxicity

Stability Reconstituted solution is stable for 12-24 hours at room temperature and 7-10 days when refrigerate and for 13 weeks when frozen; for I.V. infusion in NS or D$_5$W, solution is stable for 24 hours at room temperature, 5 days when refrigerated, or 13 weeks when frozen in Viaflex® plastic containers; thawed solutions previously of frozen premixed bags are stable for 24 hours at room temperature or 10 days when refrigerated

Mechanism of Action Inhibits bacterial cell wall synthesis by binding to one or more of the penicillin-binding proteins (PBPs) which in turn inhibits the final transpeptidation step of peptidoglycan synthesis in bacterial cell walls, thus inhibiting cell wall biosynthesis. Bacteria eventually lyse due to ongoing activity of cell wall autolytic enzymes (autolysins and murein hydrolases) while cell wall assembly is arrested.

Pharmacodynamics/Kinetics

Distribution: Widely distributed to body tissues and fluids including aqueous humor, ascitic and prostatic fluids, and bone; penetrates CSF best when meninges are inflamed; crosses the placenta and appears in breast milk

Metabolism: Partially in the liver to active metabolite, desacetylcefotaxime

Half-life:
Cefotaxime:
Premature neonates <1 week: 5-6 hours
Full-term neonates <1 week: 2-3.4 hours
Adults: 1-1.5 hours (prolonged with renal and/or hepatic impairment)
Desacetylcefotaxime: 1.5-1.9 hours (prolonged with renal impairment)

Time to peak serum concentration: I.M.: Within 30 minutes

Elimination: Renal excretion of parent drug and metabolites

Usual Dosage

Neonates: I.V.:
0-1 week: 50 mg/kg every 12 hours
1-4 weeks: 50 mg/kg every 8 hours

Infants and Children 1 month to 12 years: I.M., I.V.: <50 kg: 50-180 mg/kg/day in divided doses every 4-6 hours

(Continued)

Cefotaxime *(Continued)*

Meningitis: 200 mg/kg/day in divided doses every 6 hours
Children >12 years and Adults:
  Gonorrhea: I.M.: 1 g as a single dose
  Uncomplicated infections: I.M., I.V.: 1 g every 12 hours
  Moderate/severe infections: I.M., I.V.: 1-2 g every 8 hours
  Infections commonly needing higher doses (eg, septicemia): I.V.: 2 g every 6-8 hours
  Life-threatening infections: I.V.: 2 g every 4 hours
  Preop: I.M., I.V.: 1 g 30-90 minutes before surgery
  C-section: 1 g as soon as the umbilical cord is clamped, then 1 g I.M., I.V. at 6- and 12-hours intervals

Dosing interval in renal impairment:
  Cl_{cr} 10-50 mL/minute: Administer every 8-12 hours
  Cl_{cr} <10 mL/minute: Administer every 24 hours
Hemodialysis: Moderately dialyzable

Dosing adjustment in hepatic impairment: Moderate dosage reduction is recommended in severe liver disease

Continuous arteriovenous or venovenous hemodiafiltration (CAVH) effects: Administer 1 g every 12 hour

Administration Can be administered IVP over 3-5 minutes or I.V. retrograde or I.V. intermittent infusion over 15-30 minutes

Monitoring Parameters Observe for signs and symptoms of anaphylaxis during first dose; CBC with differential (especially with long courses)

Test Interactions Positive direct Coombs', false-positive urinary glucose test using cupric sulfate (Benedict's solution, Clinitest®, Fehling's solution), false-positive serum or urine creatinine with Jaffé reaction

Nursing Implications Do not admix with aminoglycosides in same bottle/bag

Additional Information Sodium content of 1 g: 50.6 mg (2.2 mEq)

Dosage Forms
  Infusion, as sodium, premixed, in D_5W (frozen): 1 g (50 mL); 2 g (50 mL)
  Powder for injection, as sodium: 500 mg, 1 g, 2 g, 10 g

Selected Readings
Brogden RN and Spencer CM, "Cefotaxime. A Reappraisal of Its Antibacterial Activity and Pharmacokinetic Properties, and a Review of Its Therapeutic Efficacy When Administered Twice Daily for the Treatment of Mild to Moderate Infections," *Drugs*, 1997, 53(3):483-510.
Donowitz GR and Mandell GL, "Beta-Lactam Antibiotics," *N Engl J Med*, 1988, 318(7):419-26 and 318(8):490-500.
Klein NC and Cunha BA, "Third-Generation Cephalosporins," *Med Clin North Am*, 1995, 79(4):705-19.
Marshall WF and Blair JE, "The Cephalosporins," *Mayo Clin Proc*, 1999, 74(2):187-95.

Cefotaxime Sodium *see Cefotaxime on page 642*

Cefotetan *(SEF oh tee tan)*

Related Information
  Antimicrobial Activity Against Selected Organisms *on page 983*

U.S. Brand Names Cefotan®

Synonyms Cefotetan Disodium

Generic Available No

Use Less active against staphylococci and streptococci than first generation cephalosporins, but active against anaerobes including *Bacteroides fragilis*; active against gram-negative enteric bacilli including *E. coli*, *Klebsiella*, and *Proteus*; used predominantly for respiratory tract, skin and skin structure, bone and joint, urinary tract and gynecologic as well as septicemia; surgical prophylaxis; intra-abdominal infections and other mixed infections

Drug of Choice or Alternative for
  Disease/Syndrome(s)
    Osteomyelitis, Diabetic Foot *on page 38*
    Pelvic Inflammatory Disease *on page 41*
    Peritonitis, Spontaneous Bacterial *on page 43*
  Organism(s)
    Bacteroides Species *on page 75*

Pregnancy Risk Factor B

Contraindications Hypersensitivity to cefotetan, any component, or cephalosporins

Warnings/Precautions Modify dosage in patients with severe renal impairment; prolonged use may result in superinfection; although cefotetan contains the methyltetrazolethiol side chain, bleeding has not been a significant problem; use with caution in patients with a history of penicillin allergy especially IgE-mediated reactions (eg, anaphylaxis, urticaria); may cause antibiotic-associated colitis or colitis secondary to *C. difficile*

Adverse Reactions

Contains MTT side chain which may lead to increased risk of hypoprothrombinemia and bleeding

1% to 10%:

Gastrointestinal: Diarrhea (1.3%)

Hepatic: Increased transaminases (1.2%)

Miscellaneous: Hypersensitivity reactions (1.2%)

<1%: Anaphylaxis, urticaria, rash, pruritus, pseudomembranous colitis, nausea, vomiting, eosinophilia, thrombocytosis, agranulocytosis, hemolytic anemia, leukopenia, thrombocytopenia, prolonged PT, bleeding, elevated BUN, elevated creatinine, nephrotoxicity, phlebitis, fever

Other reactions with cephalosporins include: Seizures, Stevens-Johnson syndrome, toxic epidermal necrolysis, renal dysfunction, toxic nephropathy, cholestasis, aplastic anemia, hemolytic anemia, hemorrhage, pancytopenia, agranulocytosis, colitis and superinfection

Overdosage/Toxicology

Symptoms of overdose include neuromuscular hypersensitivity, convulsions especially with renal insufficiency; many beta-lactam antibiotics have the potential to cause neuromuscular hyperirritability or seizures

Hemodialysis may be helpful to aid in the removal of the drug from the blood, otherwise most treatment is supportive or symptom directed

Drug Interactions

Disulfiram-like reaction has been reported when taken within 72 hours of alcohol consumption

Increased cefamandole plasma levels: Probenecid

Increased nephrotoxicity: Aminoglycosides, furosemide

Stability Reconstituted solution is stable for 24 hours at room temperature and 96 hours when refrigerated; for I.V. infusion in NS or D_5W solution and after freezing, thawed solution is stable for 24 hours at room temperature or 96 hours when refrigerated; frozen solution is stable for 12 weeks

Mechanism of Action Inhibits bacterial cell wall synthesis by binding to one or more of the penicillin-binding proteins (PBPs) which in turn inhibits the final transpeptidation step of peptidoglycan synthesis in bacterial cell walls, thus inhibiting cell wall biosynthesis. Bacteria eventually lyse due to ongoing activity of cell wall autolytic enzymes (autolysins and murein hydrolases) while cell wall assembly is arrested.

Pharmacodynamics/Kinetics

Distribution: Widely distributed to body tissues and fluids including bile, sputum, prostatic and peritoneal fluids; low concentrations enter CSF; crosses the placenta and appears in breast milk

Protein binding: 76% to 90%

Half-life: 3-5 hours

Time to peak serum concentration: I.M.: Within 1.5-3 hours

Elimination: Primarily excreted unchanged in urine with 20% excreted in bile

Usual Dosage I.M., I.V.:

Children: 20-40 mg/kg/dose every 12 hours

Adults: 1-6 g/day in divided doses every 12 hours; usual dose: 1-2 g every 12 hours for 5-10 days; 1-2 g may be given every 24 hours for urinary tract infection

Dosing interval in renal impairment:

Cl_{cr} 10-30 mL/minute: Administer every 24 hours

Cl_{cr} <10 mL/minute: Administer every 48 hours

Hemodialysis: Slightly dialyzable (5% to 20%)

Continuous arteriovenous or venovenous hemodiafiltration (CAVH) effects: Administer 750 mg every 12 hours

Monitoring Parameters Observe for signs and symptoms of anaphylaxis during first dose

(Continued)

Cefotetan *(Continued)*

Test Interactions Positive direct Coombs', false-positive urinary glucose test using cupric sulfate (Benedict's solution, Clinitest®, Fehling's solution), false-positive serum or urine creatinine with Jaffé reaction

Nursing Implications Do not admix with aminoglycosides in same bottle/bag

Additional Information Sodium content of 1 g: 34.5 mg (1.5 mEq); contains the n-methylthiotetrazole side chain

Dosage Forms Powder for injection, as disodium: 1 g (10 mL, 100 mL); 2 g (20 mL, 100 mL); 10 g (100 mL)

Selected Readings

"Antimicrobial Prophylaxis in Surgery," *Med Lett Drugs Ther,* 1993, 35(906):91-4.

Donowitz GR and Mandell GL, "Beta-Lactam Antibiotics," *N Engl J Med,* 1988, 318(7):419-26 and 318(8):490-500.

Marshall WF and Blair JE, "The Cephalosporins," *Mayo Clin Proc,* 1999, 74(2):187-95.

Cefotetan Disodium *see* Cefotetan *on page 644*

Cefoxitin *(se FOKS i tin)*

Related Information

Antimicrobial Activity Against Selected Organisms *on page 983*

U.S. Brand Names Mefoxin®

Synonyms Cefoxitin Sodium

Generic Available No

Use Less active against staphylococci and streptococci than first generation cephalosporins, but active against anaerobes including *Bacteroides fragilis*; active against gram-negative enteric bacilli including *E. coli, Klebsiella,* and *Proteus*; used predominantly for respiratory tract, skin and skin structure, bone and joint, urinary tract and gynecologic as well as septicemia; surgical prophylaxis; intra-abdominal infections and other mixed infections

Drug of Choice or Alternative for

Disease/Syndrome(s)

Osteomyelitis, Diabetic Foot *on page 38*

Pelvic Inflammatory Disease *on page 41*

Peritonitis, Spontaneous Bacterial *on page 43*

Organism(s)

Bacteroides Species *on page 75*

Pregnancy Risk Factor B

Contraindications Hypersensitivity to cefoxitin, any component, or cephalosporins

Warnings/Precautions Use with caution in patients with history of colitis; cefoxitin may increase resistance of organisms by inducing beta-lactamase; modify dosage in patients with severe renal impairment; prolonged use may result in superinfection; use with caution in patients with a history of penicillin allergy especially IgE-mediated reactions (eg, anaphylaxis, urticaria); may cause antibiotic-associated colitis or colitis secondary to *C. difficile*

Adverse Reactions

1% to 10%: Gastrointestinal: Diarrhea

<1%: Anaphylaxis, dyspnea, fever, rash, exfoliative dermatitis, toxic epidermal necrolysis, pruritus, angioedema, nausea, hypotension, vomiting, dyspnea, pseudomembranous colitis, phlebitis, interstitial nephritis, increased BUN, increased creatinine, leukopenia, thrombocytopenia, hemolytic anemia, bone marrow suppression, eosinophilia, increased transaminases, jaundice, thrombophlebitis, increased nephrotoxicity (with aminoglycosides), exacerbation of myasthenia gravis, prolonged PT

Other reactions with cephalosporins include: Seizures, Stevens-Johnson syndrome, toxic epidermal necrolysis, erythema multiforme, urticaria, serum-sickness reactions, renal dysfunction, toxic nephropathy, cholestasis, aplastic anemia, hemolytic anemia, hemorrhage, pancytopenia, agranulocytosis, colitis, vaginitis, superinfection

Overdosage/Toxicology

Symptoms of overdose include neuromuscular hypersensitivity, convulsions especially with renal insufficiency; many beta-lactam antibiotics have the potential to cause neuromuscular hyperirritability or seizures

Hemodialysis may be helpful to aid in the removal of the drug from the blood, otherwise most treatment is supportive or symptom directed

Drug Interactions

Increased effect: Probenecid may decrease cephalosporin elimination

Increased toxicity: Furosemide, aminoglycosides may be a possible additive to nephrotoxicity

Stability Reconstituted solution is stable for 24 hours at room temperature and 48 hours when refrigerated; I.V. infusion in NS or D_5W solution is stable for 24 hours at room temperature, 1 week when refrigerated, or 26 weeks when frozen; after freezing, thawed solution is stable for 24 hours at room temperature or 5 days when refrigerated

Mechanism of Action Inhibits bacterial cell wall synthesis by binding to one or more of the penicillin-binding proteins (PBPs) which in turn inhibits the final transpeptidation step of peptidoglycan synthesis in bacterial cell walls, thus inhibiting cell wall biosynthesis. Bacteria eventually lyse due to ongoing activity of cell wall autolytic enzymes (autolysins and murein hydrolases) while cell wall assembly is arrested.

Pharmacodynamics/Kinetics

Distribution: Widely distributed to body tissues and fluids including pleural, synovial, ascitic fluid, and bile; poorly penetrates into CSF even with inflammation of the meninges; crosses the placenta and small amounts appear in breast milk

Protein binding: 65% to 79%

Half-life: 45-60 minutes, increases significantly with renal insufficiency

Time to peak serum concentration: I.M.: Within 20-30 minutes

Elimination: Rapidly excreted as unchanged drug (85%) in urine

Usual Dosage I.M., I.V.:

Infants >3 months and Children:

Mild to moderate infection: 80-100 mg/kg/day in divided doses every 4-6 hours

Severe infection: 100-160 mg/kg/day in divided doses every 4-6 hours

Maximum dose: 12 g/day

Adults: 1-2 g every 6-8 hours (I.M. injection is painful); up to 12 g/day

Dosing interval in renal impairment:

Cl_{cr} 30-50 mL/minute: Administer every 8-12 hours

Cl_{cr} 10-30 mL/minute: Administer every 12-24 hours

Cl_{cr} <10 mL/minute: Administer every 24-48 hours

Hemodialysis: Moderately dialyzable (20% to 50%)

Continuous arteriovenous or venovenous hemodiafiltration (CAVH) effects: Dose as for Cl_{cr} 10-50 mL/minute

Monitoring Parameters Monitor renal function periodically when used in combination with other nephrotoxic drugs; observe for signs and symptoms of anaphylaxis during first dose

Test Interactions Positive direct Coombs', false-positive urinary glucose test using cupric sulfate (Benedict's solution, Clinitest®, Fehling's solution), false-positive serum or urine creatinine with Jaffé reaction

Additional Information Sodium content of 1 g: 53 mg (2.3 mEq)

Dosage Forms

Infusion, as sodium, premixed, in D_5W (frozen): 1 g (50 mL); 2 g (50 mL)

Powder for injection, as sodium: 1 g, 2 g, 10 g

Selected Readings

"Antimicrobial Prophylaxis in Surgery," *Med Lett Drugs Ther*, 1993, 35(906):91-4.

Donowitz GR and Mandell GL, "Beta-Lactam Antibiotics," *N Engl J Med*, 1988, 318(7):419-26 and 318(8):490-500.

Marshall WF and Blair JE, "The Cephalosporins," *Mayo Clin Proc*, 1999, 74(2):187-95.

Cefoxitin Sodium *see Cefoxitin on previous page*

Cefpodoxime (sef pode OKS eem)

Related Information

Antimicrobial Activity Against Selected Organisms *on page 983*

U.S. Brand Names Vantin®

Synonyms Cefpodoxime Proxetil

Generic Available No

Use Treatment of susceptible acute, community-acquired pneumonia caused by *S. pneumoniae* or nonbeta-lactamase producing *H. influenzae*; acute uncomplicated gonorrhea caused by *N. gonorrhoeae*; uncomplicated skin and skin structure infections caused by *S. aureus* or *S. pyogenes*; acute otitis media caused (Continued)

Cefpodoxime *(Continued)*

by *S. pneumoniae*, *H. influenzae*, or *M. catarrhalis*; pharyngitis or tonsillitis; and uncomplicated urinary tract infections caused by *E. coli*, *Klebsiella*, and *Proteus*

Pregnancy Risk Factor B

Contraindications Hypersensitivity to cefpodoxime or cephalosporins

Warnings/Precautions Modify dosage in patients with severe renal impairment; prolonged use may result in superinfection; a low incidence of cross-hypersensitivity to penicillins exists

Adverse Reactions

>10%:

Dermatologic: Diaper rash (12.1%)

Gastrointestinal: Diarrhea in infants and toddlers (15.4%)

1% to 10%:

Central nervous system: Headache (1.1%)

Dermatologic: Rash (1.4%)

Gastrointestinal: Diarrhea (7.2%), nausea (3.8%), abdominal pain (1.6%), vomiting (1.1% to 2.1%)

Genitourinary: Vaginal infections (3.1%)

<1%: Anaphylaxis, chest pain, hypotension, fungal skin infection, pseudomembranous colitis, vaginal candidiasis, pruritus, flatulence, decreased salivation, malaise, fever, decreased appetite, cough, epistaxis, dizziness, fatigue, anxiety, insomnia, flushing, weakness, nightmares, taste alteration, eye itching, tinnitus, purpuric nephritis

Other reactions with cephalosporins include seizures, Stevens-Johnson syndrome, toxic epidermal necrolysis, erythema multiforme, urticaria, serum-sickness reactions, renal dysfunction, interstitial nephritis toxic nephropathy, cholestasis, aplastic anemia, hemolytic anemia, hemorrhage, pancytopenia, agranulocytosis, colitis, vaginitis, superinfection

Overdosage/Toxicology

After acute overdose, most agents cause only nausea, vomiting, and diarrhea, although neuromuscular hypersensitivity and seizures are possible, especially in patients with renal insufficiency; many beta-lactam antibiotics have the potential to cause neuromuscular hyperirritability or seizures

Hemodialysis may be helpful to aid in the removal of the drug from the blood but not usually indicated, otherwise most treatment is supportive or symptom directed following GI decontamination

Drug Interactions

Decreased effect: Antacids and H_2-receptor antagonists (reduce absorption and serum concentration of cefpodoxime)

Increased effect: Probenecid may decrease cephalosporin elimination

Increased toxicity: Furosemide, aminoglycosides may be a possible additive to nephrotoxicity

Stability After mixing, keep suspension in refrigerator, shake well before using; discard unused portion after 14 days

Mechanism of Action Inhibits bacterial cell wall synthesis by binding to one or more of the penicillin-binding proteins (PBPs) which in turn inhibits the final transpeptidation step of peptidoglycan synthesis in bacterial cell walls, thus inhibiting cell wall biosynthesis. Bacteria eventually lyse due to ongoing activity of cell wall autolytic enzymes (autolysins and murein hydrolases) while cell wall assembly is arrested.

Pharmacodynamics/Kinetics

Absorption: Oral: Rapidly and well absorbed (50%), acid stable; enhanced in the presence of food or low gastric pH

Distribution: Good tissue penetration, including lung and tonsils; penetrates into pleural fluid

Protein binding: 18% to 23%

Metabolism: Oral: De-esterified in the GI tract to the active metabolite, cefpodoxime

Half-life: 2.2 hours (prolonged with renal impairment)

Time to peak: Within 1 hour (oral)

Elimination: Primarily eliminated by the kidney with 80% of dose excreted unchanged in urine in 24 hours

Usual Dosage Oral:

Children >5 months to 12 years:

Acute otitis media: 10 mg/kg/day as a single dose or divided every 12 hours (400 mg/day)

Pharyngitis/tonsillitis: 10 mg/kg/day in 2 divided doses (maximum: 200 mg/day)

Children ≥13 years and Adults:

Acute community-acquired pneumonia and bacterial exacerbations of chronic bronchitis: 200 mg every 12 hours for 14 days and 10 days, respectively

Skin and skin structure: 400 mg every 12 hours for 7-14 days

Uncomplicated gonorrhea (male and female) and rectal gonococcal infections (female): 200 mg as a single dose

Pharyngitis/tonsillitis: 100 mg every 12 hours for 10 days

Uncomplicated urinary tract infection: 100 mg every 12 hours for 7 days

Dosing adjustment in renal impairment: Cl_{cr} <30 mL/minute: Administer every 24 hours

Monitoring Parameters Observe for signs and symptoms of anaphylaxis during first dose

Test Interactions Positive direct Coombs', false-positive urinary glucose test using cupric sulfate (Benedict's solution, Clinitest®, Fehling's solution), false-positive serum or urine creatinine with Jaffé reaction

Patient Information Take with food; chilling improves flavor (do not freeze); report persistent diarrhea; entire course of medication (10-14 days) should be taken to ensure eradication of organism; may interfere with oral contraceptives; females should report symptoms of vaginitis

Dosage Forms

Granules for oral suspension, as proxetil (lemon creme flavor): 50 mg/5 mL (100 mL); 100 mg/5 mL (100 mL)

Tablet, film coated, as proxetil: 100 mg, 200 mg

Selected Readings

Adam D, Bergogne-Berezin E, and Jones RN, "Symposium on Cefpodoxime Proxetil: A New Third Generation Oral Cephalosporin," *Drugs*, 1991, 42(Suppl 3):1-66.

Cohen R, "Clinical Experience With Cefpodoxime Proxetil in Acute Otitis Media," *Pediatr Infect Dis J*, 1995, 14(Suppl 4):S12-8.

Marshall WF and Blair JE, "The Cephalosporins," *Mayo Clin Proc*, 1999, 74(2):187-95.

Schatz BS, Karavokiros KT, Taeubel MA, et al, "Comparison of Cefprozil, Cefpodoxime Proxetil, Loracarbef, Cefixime, and Ceftibuten," *Ann Pharmacother*, 1996, 30(3):258-68.

Cefpodoxime Proxetil *see* Cefpodoxime *on page 647*

Cefprozil (sef PROE zil)

U.S. Brand Names Cefzil®

Generic Available No

Use Treatment of otitis media and infections involving the respiratory tract and skin and skin structure; active against methicillin-sensitive staphylococci, many streptococci, and various gram-negative bacilli including *E. coli*, some *Klebsiella*, *P. mirabilis*, *H. influenzae*, and *Moraxella*

Pregnancy Risk Factor B

Contraindications Hypersensitivity to cefprozil or any component or cephalosporins

Warnings/Precautions Modify dosage in patients with severe renal impairment; prolonged use may result in superinfection; use with caution in patients with a history of penicillin allergy especially IgE-mediated reactions (eg, anaphylaxis, urticaria); may cause antibiotic-associated colitis or colitis secondary to *C. difficile*

Adverse Reactions

1% to 10%:

Central nervous system: Dizziness (1%)

Dermatologic: Diaper rash (1.5%)

Gastrointestinal: Diarrhea (2.9%), nausea (3.5%), vomiting (1%), abdominal pain (1%)

Genitourinary: Vaginitis, genital pruritus (1.6%)

Hepatic: Increased transaminases (2%)

Miscellaneous: Superinfection

<1%: Anaphylaxis, angioedema, pseudomembranous colitis, rash, urticaria, erythema multiforme, serum sickness, Stevens-Johnson syndrome, hyperactivity, headache, insomnia, confusion, somnolence, leukopenia, eosinophilia, (Continued)

Cefprozil *(Continued)*

thrombocytopenia, elevated BUN, elevated creatinine, arthralgia, cholestatic jaundice, fever

Other reactions with cephalosporins include: Seizures, toxic epidermal necrolysis, renal dysfunction, interstitial nephritis, toxic nephropathy, aplastic anemia, hemolytic anemia, hemorrhage, pancytopenia, agranulocytosis, colitis, vaginitis, superinfection

Overdosage/Toxicology

After acute overdose, most agents cause only nausea, vomiting, and diarrhea, although neuromuscular hypersensitivity and seizures are possible, especially in patients with renal insufficiency; many beta-lactam antibiotics have the potential to cause neuromuscular hyperirritability or seizures

Hemodialysis may be helpful to aid in the removal of the drug from the blood but not usually indicated, otherwise most treatment is supportive or symptom directed following GI decontamination

Drug Interactions

Increased effect: Probenecid may decrease cephalosporin elimination

Increased toxicity: Furosemide, aminoglycosides may be a possible additive to nephrotoxicity

Mechanism of Action Inhibits bacterial cell wall synthesis by binding to one or more of the penicillin-binding proteins (PBPs) which in turn inhibits the final transpeptidation step of peptidoglycan synthesis in bacterial cell walls, thus inhibiting cell wall biosynthesis. Bacteria eventually lyse due to ongoing activity of cell wall autolytic enzymes (autolysins and murein hydrolases) while cell wall assembly is arrested.

Pharmacodynamics/Kinetics

Absorption: Oral: Well absorbed (94%)

Distribution: Low distribution into breast milk

Protein binding: 35% to 45%

Half-life, elimination: 1.3 hours (normal renal function)

Peak serum levels: 1.5 hours (fasting state)

Elimination: 61% excreted unchanged in urine

Usual Dosage Oral:

Infants and Children >6 months to 12 years: Otitis media: 15 mg/kg every 12 hours for 10 days

Pharyngitis/tonsillitis:

Children 2-12 years: 7.5 -15 mg/kg/day divided every 12 hours for 10 days (administer for >10 days if due to *S. pyogenes*); maximum: 1 g/day

Children >13 years and Adults: 500 mg every 24 hours for 10 days

Uncomplicated skin and skin structure infections:

Children 2-12 years: 20 mg/kg every 24 hours for 10 days; maximum: 1 g/day

Children >13 years and Adults: 250 mg every 12 hours, or 500 mg every 12-24 hours for 10 days

Secondary bacterial infection of acute bronchitis or acute bacterial exacerbation of chronic bronchitis: 500 mg every 12 hours for 10 days

Dosing adjustment in renal impairment: Cl_{cr} <30 mL/minute: Reduce dose by 50%

Hemodialysis: Reduced by hemodialysis; administer dose after the completion of hemodialysis

Monitoring Parameters Assess patient at beginning and throughout therapy for infection; monitor for signs of anaphylaxis during first dose

Test Interactions Positive direct Coombs', false-positive urinary glucose test using cupric sulfate (Benedict's solution, Clinitest®, Fehling's solution), false-positive serum or urine creatinine with Jaffé reaction

Patient Information Chilling improves flavor (do not freeze); report persistent diarrhea; entire course of medication (10-14 days) should be taken to ensure eradication of organism; may interfere with oral contraceptives; females should report symptoms of vaginitis

Dosage Forms

Powder for oral suspension, as anhydrous: 125 mg/5 mL (50 mL, 75 mL, 100 mL); 250 mg/5 mL (50 mL, 75 mL, 100 mL)

Tablet, as anhydrous: 250 mg, 500 mg

Selected Readings

Gainer RB 2nd, "Cefprozil: A New Cephalosporin; Its Use in Various Clinical Trials," *South Med J*, 1995, 88(3):338-46.

Marshall WF and Blair JE, "The Cephalosporins," *Mayo Clin Proc*, 1999, 74(2):187-95.

Schatz BS, Karavokiros KT, Taeubel MA, et al, "Comparison of Cefprozil, Cefpodoxime Proxetil, Loracarbef, Cefixime, and Ceftibuten," *Ann Pharmacother*, 1996, 30(3):258-68.

Ceftazidime (SEF tay zi deem)

Related Information
Antimicrobial Activity Against Selected Organisms *on page 983*

U.S. Brand Names Ceptaz™; Fortaz®; Tazicef®; Tazidime®

Canadian Brand Names Ceptaz™

Generic Available No

Use Treatment of documented susceptible *Pseudomonas aeruginosa* infection and infections due to other susceptible aerobic gram-negative organisms; empiric therapy of a febrile, granulocytopenic patient

Drug of Choice or Alternative for
Disease/Syndrome(s)
Fever, Neutropenic *on page 30*
Meningitis, Postsurgical *on page 36*
Otitis Externa, Severe (Malignant) *on page 40*
Pneumonia, Hospital-Acquired *on page 46*
Sepsis *on page 48*
Sinusitis, Hospital-Acquired *on page 49*
Organism(s)
Burkholderia cepacia on page 87
Pseudomonas aeruginosa on page 235
Stenotrophomonas maltophilia on page 265

Pregnancy Risk Factor B

Contraindications Hypersensitivity to ceftazidime, any component, or cephalosporins

Warnings/Precautions Modify dosage in patients with severe renal impairment; prolonged use may result in superinfection; use with caution in patients with a history of penicillin allergy especially IgE-mediated reactions (eg, anaphylaxis, urticaria); may cause antibiotic-associated colitis or colitis secondary to *C. difficile*

Adverse Reactions
1% to 10%:
Gastrointestinal: Diarrhea (1.3%)
Local: Pain at injection site (1.4%)
Miscellaneous: Hypersensitivity reactions (2%)
<1%: Anaphylaxis, fever, headache, dizziness, paresthesia, pruritus, rash, Stevens-Johnson syndrome, toxic epidermal necrolysis, erythema multiforme, angioedema, nausea, vomiting, pseudomembranous colitis, eosinophilia, thrombocytosis, leukopenia, hemolytic anemia, elevated transaminases, increased BUN, increased creatinine, phlebitis, candidiasis, vaginitis, encephalopathy, asterixis, neuromuscular excitability

Other reactions with cephalosporins include seizures, urticaria, serum-sickness reactions, renal dysfunction, interstitial nephritis, toxic nephropathy, elevated BUN, elevated creatinine, cholestasis, aplastic anemia, hemolytic anemia, pancytopenia, agranulocytosis, colitis, prolonged PT, hemorrhage, superinfection

Overdosage/Toxicology
Symptoms of overdose include neuromuscular hypersensitivity, convulsions especially with renal insufficiency; many beta-lactam antibiotics have the potential to cause neuromuscular hyperirritability or seizures
Hemodialysis may be helpful to aid in the removal of the drug from the blood, otherwise most treatment is supportive or symptom directed

Drug Interactions
Increased effect: Probenecid may decrease cephalosporin elimination; aminoglycosides: *in vitro* studies indicate additive or synergistic effect against some strains of Enterobacteriaceae and *Pseudomonas aeruginosa*
Increased toxicity: Furosemide, aminoglycosides may be a possible additive to nephrotoxicity

Stability Reconstituted solution and I.V. infusion in NS or D_5W solution are stable for 24 hours at room temperature, 10 days when refrigerated, or 12 weeks when
(Continued)

Ceftazidime *(Continued)*

frozen; after freezing, thawed solution is stable for 24 hours at room temperature or 4 days when refrigerated; 96 hours under refrigeration, after mixing

Mechanism of Action Inhibits bacterial cell wall synthesis by binding to one or more of the penicillin-binding proteins (PBPs) which in turn inhibits the final transpeptidation step of peptidoglycan synthesis in bacterial cell walls, thus inhibiting cell wall biosynthesis. Bacteria eventually lyse due to ongoing activity of cell wall autolytic enzymes (autolysins and murein hydrolases) while cell wall assembly is arrested.

Pharmacodynamics/Kinetics

Distribution: Widely distributes throughout the body including bone, bile, skin, CSF (diffuses into CSF with higher concentrations when the meninges are inflamed), endometrium, heart, pleural and lymphatic fluids

Protein binding: 17%

Half-life: 1-2 hours (prolonged with renal impairment)

Neonates <23 days: 2.2-4.7 hours

Time to peak serum concentration: I.M.: Within 1 hour

Elimination: By glomerular filtration with 80% to 90% of the dose excreted as unchanged drug within 24 hours

Usual Dosage

Neonates 0-4 weeks: I.V.: 30 mg/kg every 12 hours

Infants and Children 1 month to 12 years: I.V.: 30-50 mg/kg/dose every 8 hours; maximum dose: 6 g/day

Adults: I.M., I.V.: 500 mg to 2 g every 8-12 hours

Urinary tract infections: 250-500 mg every 12 hours

Dosing interval in renal impairment:

Cl_{cr} 30-50 mL/minute: Administer every 12 hours

Cl_{cr} 10-30 mL/minute: Administer every 24 hours

Cl_{cr} <10 mL/minute: Administer every 48-72 hours

Hemodialysis: Dialyzable (50% to 100%)

Continuous arteriovenous or venovenous hemodiafiltration (CAVH) effects: Dose as for Cl_{cr} 30-50 mL/minute

Administration Any carbon dioxide bubbles that may be present in the withdrawn solution should be expelled prior to injection; administer around-the-clock to promote less variation in peak and trough serum levels; ceftazidime can be administered IVP over 3-5 minutes, or I.V. retrograde or I.V. intermittent infusion over 15-30 minutes; do not admix with aminoglycosides in same bottle/bag; final concentration for I.V. administration should not exceed 100 mg/mL

Monitoring Parameters Observe for signs and symptoms of anaphylaxis during first dose

Test Interactions Positive direct Coombs', false-positive urinary glucose test using cupric sulfate (Benedict's solution, Clinitest®, Fehling's solution), false-positive serum or urine creatinine with Jaffé reaction

Additional Information Sodium content of 1 g: 54 mg (2.3 mEq)

Dosage Forms

Infusion, premixed (frozen) (Fortaz®): 1 g (50 mL); 2 g (50 mL)

Powder for injection: 500 mg, 1 g, 2 g, 6 g

Selected Readings

Donowitz GR and Mandell GL, "Beta-Lactam Antibiotics," *N Engl J Med*, 1988, 318(7):419-26 and 318(8):490-500.

Klein NC and Cunha BA, "Third-Generation Cephalosporins," *Med Clin North Am*, 1995, 79(4):705-19.

Marshall WF and Blair JE, "The Cephalosporins," *Mayo Clin Proc*, 1999, 74(2):187-95.

Rains CP, Bryson HM, and Peters DH, "Ceftazidime. An Update of Its Antibacterial Activity, Pharmacokinetic Properties and Therapeutic Efficacy," *Drugs*, 1995, 49(4):577-617.

Vlasses PH, Bastion WA, Behal R, et al, "Ceftazidime Dosing in the Elderly: Economic Implications," *Ann Pharmacother*, 1993, 27(7-8):967-71.

Ceftibuten *(sef TYE byoo ten)*

U.S. Brand Names Cedax®

Use Oral cephalosporin for bronchitis, otitis media, and pharyngitis/tonsillitis due to *H. influenzae* and *M. catarrhalis*, both beta-lactamase-producing and -nonproducing strains, as well as *S. pneumoniae* (weak) and *S. pyogenes*.

Pregnancy Risk Factor B

Contraindications In patients with known allergy to the cephalosporin group of antibiotics

Warnings/Precautions Modify dosage in patients with severe renal impairment, prolonged use may result in superinfection; use with caution in patients with a history of penicillin allergy, especially IgE-mediated reactions (eg, anaphylaxis, urticaria); may cause antibiotic-associated colitis or colitis secondary to *C. difficile*

Adverse Reactions

1% to 10%:

Central nervous system: Headache (3%), dizziness (1%)

Gastrointestinal: Nausea (4%), diarrhea (3%), dyspepsia (2%), vomiting (1%), abdominal pain (1%)

Hematologic: Increased eosinophils (3%), decreased hemoglobin (2%), thrombocytosis

Hepatic: Increased ALT (1%), increased bilirubin (1%)

Renal: Increased BUN (4%)

<1%: Anorexia, agitation, constipation, diaper rash, dry mouth, dyspnea, dysuria, fatigue, candidiasis, rash, urticaria, irritability, paresthesia, nasal congestion, insomnia, rigors, increased transaminases, increased creatinine, leukopenia

Other reactions with cephalosporins include anaphylaxis, fever, paresthesia, pruritus, Stevens-Johnson syndrome, toxic epidermal necrolysis, erythema multiforme, angioedema, pseudomembranous colitis, hemolytic anemia, candidiasis, vaginitis, encephalopathy, asterixis, neuromuscular excitability, seizures, serum-sickness reactions, renal dysfunction, interstitial nephritis, toxic nephropathy, cholestasis, aplastic anemia, hemolytic anemia, pancytopenia, agranulocytosis, colitis, prolonged PT, hemorrhage, superinfection

Overdosage/Toxicology

After acute overdose, most agents cause only nausea, vomiting, and diarrhea, although neuromuscular hypersensitivity and seizures are possible, especially in patients with renal insufficiency; many beta-lactam antibiotics have the potential to cause neuromuscular hyperirritability or seizures

Hemodialysis may be helpful to aid in the removal of the drug from the blood but not usually indicated, otherwise most treatment is supportive or symptom directed following GI decontamination

Drug Interactions

Increased effect: High-dose probenecid decreases clearance

Increased toxicity: Aminoglycosides increase nephrotoxic potential

Stability Reconstituted suspension is stable for 14 days in the refrigerator

Mechanism of Action Inhibits bacterial cell wall synthesis by binding to one or more of the penicillin-binding proteins (PBPs) which in turn inhibits the final transpeptidation step of peptidoglycan synthesis in bacterial cell walls, thus inhibiting cell wall biosynthesis. Bacteria eventually lyse due to ongoing activity of cell wall autolytic enzymes (autolysins and murein hydrolases) while cell wall assembly is arrested.

Pharmacodynamics/Kinetics

Absorption: Rapid (T_{max}: 2-3 hours); food decreases peak concentrations, delays T_{max} and lowers the AUC (total amount of drug absorbed)

Distribution: V_d:

Children: 0.5 L/kg

Adults: 0.21 L/kg

Half-life: 2 hours

Elimination: In urine

Usual Dosage Oral:

Children <12 years: 9 mg/kg/day for 10 days; maximum daily dose: 400 mg

Children ≥12 years and Adults: 400 mg once daily for 10 days; maximum: 400 mg

Dosage adjustment in renal impairment:

Cl_{cr} 30-49 mL//minute: Administer 4.5 mg/kg or 200 mg every 24 hours

Cl_{cr} <29 mL/minute: Administer 2.25 mg/kg or 100 mg every 24 hours

Monitoring Parameters Observe for signs and symptoms of anaphylaxis during first dose; with prolonged therapy, monitor renal, hepatic, and hematologic function periodically

Test Interactions Positive direct Coombs', false-positive urinary glucose test using cupric sulfate (Benedict's solution, Clinitest®, Fehling's solution), false-positive serum or urine creatinine with Jaffé reaction

(Continued)

Ceftibuten (Continued)

Patient Information Must be administered at least 2 hours before meals or 1 hour after a meal; shake suspension well before use; suspension may be kept for 14 days if stored in refrigerator; discard any unused portion after 14 days; report prolonged diarrhea; entire course of medication should be taken to ensure eradication of organism; take at the same time each day to maintain adequate blood levels; may interfere with oral contraceptive; females should report symptoms of vaginitis

Additional Information Oral suspension contains 1 g of sucrose per 5 mL

Dosage Forms

Capsule: 400 mg

Powder for oral suspension (cherry flavor): 90 mg/5 mL (30 mL, 60 mL, 120 mL); 180 mg/5 mL (30 mL, 60 mL, 120 mL)

Selected Readings

Guay DR, "Ceftibuten: A New Expanded-Spectrum Oral Cephalosporin," *Ann Pharmacother*, 1997, 31(9):1022-33.

Owens RC Jr, Nightingale CH, and Nicolau DP, "Ceftibuten: An Overview," *Pharmacotherapy*, 1997, 17(4):707-20.

Schatz BS, Karavokiros KT, Taeubel MA, et al, "Comparison of Cefprozil, Cefpodoxime Proxetil, Loracarbef, Cefixime, and Ceftibuten," *Ann Pharmacotherapy*, 1996, 30(3):258-68.

Wiseman LR and Balfour JA, "Ceftibuten: A Review of Its Antibacterial Activity Pharmacokinetic Properties and Clinical Efficacy," *Drugs*, 1994, 47(5):784-808.

Ceftin® Oral *see* Cefuroxime *on page 658*

Ceftizoxime (sef ti ZOKS eem)

Related Information

Antimicrobial Activity Against Selected Organisms *on page 983*

U.S. Brand Names Cefizox®

Synonyms Ceftizoxime Sodium

Generic Available No

Use Treatment of susceptible bacterial infection; mainly respiratory tract, skin and skin structure, bone and joint, urinary tract and gynecologic, as well as septicemia. Active against many gram-negative bacilli (not *Pseudomonas*), some gram-positive cocci (not *Enterococcus*), and some anaerobes

Drug of Choice or Alternative for

Organism(s)

Neisseria gonorrhoeae on page 215

Pregnancy Risk Factor B

Contraindications Hypersensitivity to ceftizoxime, any component, or cephalosporins

Warnings/Precautions Modify dosage in patients with severe renal impairment, prolonged use may result in superinfection; use with caution in patients with a history of penicillin allergy, especially IgE-mediated reactions (eg, anaphylaxis, urticaria); may cause antibiotic-associated colitis or colitis secondary to *C. difficile*

Adverse Reactions

1% to 10%:

Central nervous system: Fever

Dermatologic: Rash, pruritus

Hematologic: Eosinophilia, thrombocytosis

Hepatic: Elevated transaminases, alkaline phosphatase

Local: Pain, burning at injection site

<1%: Anaphylaxis, diarrhea, nausea, vomiting, injection site reactions, phlebitis, paresthesia, numbness, increased bilirubin, increased BUN, increased creatinine, anemia, leukopenia, neutropenia, thrombocytopenia, vaginitis

Other reactions reported with cephalosporins include Stevens-Johnson syndrome, toxic epidermal necrolysis, erythema multiforme, pseudomembranous colitis, angioedema, hemolytic anemia, candidiasis, encephalopathy, asterixis, neuromuscular excitability, seizures, serum-sickness reactions, renal dysfunction, interstitial nephritis, toxic nephropathy, cholestasis, aplastic anemia, hemolytic anemia, pancytopenia, agranulocytosis, colitis, prolonged PT, hemorrhage, superinfection

Overdosage/Toxicology
Symptoms of overdose include neuromuscular hypersensitivity, convulsions especially with renal insufficiency; many beta-lactam antibiotics have the potential to cause neuromuscular hyperirritability or seizures

Hemodialysis may be helpful to aid in the removal of the drug from the blood, otherwise most treatment is supportive or symptom directed

Drug Interactions
Increased effect: Probenecid may decrease cephalosporin elimination

Increased toxicity: Furosemide, aminoglycosides may be a possible additive to nephrotoxicity

Stability Reconstituted solution is stable for 24 hours at room temperature and 96 hours when refrigerated; for I.V. infusion in NS or D_5W solution is stable for 24 hours at room temperature, 96 hours when refrigerated or 12 weeks when frozen; after freezing, thawed solution is stable for 24 hours at room temperature or 10 days when refrigerated

Mechanism of Action Inhibits bacterial cell wall synthesis by binding to one or more of the penicillin-binding proteins (PBPs) which in turn inhibits the final transpeptidation step of peptidoglycan synthesis in bacterial cell walls, thus inhibiting cell wall biosynthesis. Bacteria eventually lyse due to ongoing activity of cell wall autolytic enzymes (autolysins and murein hydrolases) while cell wall assembly is arrested.

Pharmacodynamics/Kinetics
Distribution: V_d: 0.35-0.5 L/kg; widely distributed into most body tissues and fluids including gallbladder, liver, kidneys, bone, sputum, bile, and pleural and synovial fluids; has good CSF penetration; crosses placenta; small amounts excreted in breast milk

Protein binding: 30%

Half-life: 1.6 hours, increases to 25 hours when Cl_{cr} falls to <10 mL/minute

Time to peak serum concentration: I.M.: Within 0.5-1 hour

Elimination: Excreted unchanged in urine

Usual Dosage I.M., I.V.:
Children ≥6 months: 150-200 mg/kg/day divided every 6-8 hours (maximum of 12 g/24 hours)

Adults: 1-2 g every 8-12 hours, up to 2 g every 4 hours or 4 g every 8 hours for life-threatening infections

Dosing adjustment in renal impairment: Adults:
Cl_{cr} 10-30 mL/minute: Administer 1 g every 12 hours
Cl_{cr} <10 mL/minute: Administer 1 g every 24 hours
Moderately dialyzable (20% to 50%)
Continuous arteriovenous or venovenous hemodiafiltration (CAVH) effects: Dose as for Cl_{cr} 10-50 mL/minute

Monitoring Parameters Observe for signs and symptoms of anaphylaxis during first dose

Test Interactions Positive direct Coombs', false-positive urinary glucose test using cupric sulfate (Benedict's solution, Clinitest®, Fehling's solution), false-positive serum or urine creatinine with Jaffé reaction

Nursing Implications Do not admix with aminoglycosides in same bottle/bag

Additional Information Sodium content of 1 g: 60 mg (2.6 mEq)

Dosage Forms
Injection, as sodium, in D_5W (frozen): 1 g (50 mL); 2 g (50 mL)
Powder for injection, as sodium: 500 mg, 1 g, 2 g, 10 g

Selected Readings
Donowitz GR and Mandell GL, "Beta-Lactam Antibiotics," *N Engl J Med*, 1988, 318(7):419-26 and 318(8):490-500.
Klein NC and Cunha BA, "Third-Generation Cephalosporins," *Med Clin North Am*, 1995, 79(4):705-19.
Marshall WF and Blair JE, "The Cephalosporins," *Mayo Clin Proc*, 1999, 74(2):187-95.

Ceftizoxime Sodium *see Ceftizoxime on previous page*

Ceftriaxone (sef trye AKS one)
Related Information
Antimicrobial Activity Against Selected Organisms *on page 983*
U.S. Brand Names Rocephin®
Synonyms Ceftriaxone Sodium
Generic Available No
(Continued)

Ceftriaxone *(Continued)*

Use Treatment of lower respiratory tract infections, skin and skin structure infections, bone and joint infections, intra-abdominal and urinary tract infections, sepsis and meningitis due to susceptible organisms; documented or suspected infection due to susceptible organisms in home care patients and patients without I.V. line access; treatment of documented or suspected gonococcal infection or chancroid; emergency room management of patients at high risk for bacteremia, periorbital or buccal cellulitis, salmonellosis or shigellosis, and pneumonia of unestablished etiology (<5 years of age); treatment of Lyme disease, depends on the stage of the disease (used in Stage II and Stage III, but not stage I; doxycycline is the drug of choice for Stage I)

Drug of Choice or Alternative for

Disease/Syndrome(s)

Arthritis, Septic *on page 18*

Joint Replacement, Early Infection *on page 32*

Meningitis, Pediatric (>2 months of age) *on page 35*

Pneumonia, Community-Acquired *on page 45*

Organism(s)

Borrelia burgdorferi *on page 84*

Haemophilus ducreyi *on page 156*

Neisseria gonorrhoeae *on page 215*

Streptococcus pneumoniae, Drug-Resistant *on page 270*

Pregnancy Risk Factor B

Contraindications Hypersensitivity to ceftriaxone sodium, any component, or cephalosporins; **do not use in hyperbilirubinemic neonates**, particularly those who are premature since ceftriaxone is reported to displace bilirubin from albumin binding sites

Warnings/Precautions Modify dosage in patients with severe renal impairment, prolonged use may result in superinfection; use with caution in patients with a history of penicillin allergy, especially IgE-mediated reactions (eg, anaphylaxis, urticaria); may cause antibiotic-associated colitis or colitis secondary to *C. difficile*

Adverse Reactions

1% to 10%:

Dermatologic: Rash (1.7%)

Gastrointestinal: Diarrhea (2.7%)

Hematologic: Eosinophilia (6%), thrombocytosis (5.1%), leukopenia (2.1%)

Hepatic: Elevated transaminases (3.1% to 3.3%)

Local: Pain, induration at injection site (1%)

Renal: Increased BUN (1.2%)

<1%: Phlebitis, pruritus, fever, chills, anemia, hemolytic anemia, neutropenia, lymphopenia, thrombocytopenia, prolonged PT, nausea, vomiting, dysgeusia, increased alkaline phosphatase, increased bilirubin, increased creatinine, urinary casts, headache, dizziness, candidiasis, vaginitis, diaphoresis, flushing

Other reactions with cephalosporins include anaphylaxis, paresthesia, Stevens-Johnson syndrome, toxic epidermal necrolysis, erythema multiforme, angioedema, pseudomembranous colitis, hemolytic anemia, encephalopathy, asterixis, neuromuscular excitability, seizures, serum-sickness reactions, renal dysfunction, interstitial nephritis, toxic nephropathy, cholestasis, aplastic anemia, hemolytic anemia, pancytopenia, agranulocytosis, colitis, hemorrhage, superinfection

Overdosage/Toxicology

Symptoms of overdose include neuromuscular hypersensitivity, convulsions especially with renal insufficiency; many beta-lactam antibiotics have the potential to cause neuromuscular hyperirritability or seizures

Hemodialysis may be helpful to aid in the removal of the drug from the blood, otherwise most treatment is supportive or symptom directed

Drug Interactions

Increased effect:

Aminoglycosides may result in synergistic antibacterial activity

High-dose probenecid decreases clearance

Increased toxicity: Aminoglycosides increase nephrotoxic potential

Stability Reconstituted solution (100 mg/mL) is stable for 3 days at room temperature and 3 days when refrigerated; for I.V. infusion in NS or D_5W solution is stable for 3 days at room temperature, 10 days when refrigerated, or 26 weeks when frozen; after freezing, thawed solution is stable for 3 days at room temperature or 10 days when refrigerated

Mechanism of Action Inhibits bacterial cell wall synthesis by binding to one or more of the penicillin-binding proteins (PBPs) which in turn inhibits the final transpeptidation step of peptidoglycan synthesis in bacterial cell walls, thus inhibiting cell wall biosynthesis. Bacteria eventually lyse due to ongoing activity of cell wall autolytic enzymes (autolysins and murein hydrolases) while cell wall assembly is arrested.

Pharmacodynamics/Kinetics

Absorption: I.M.: Well absorbed

Distribution: Widely distributed throughout the body including gallbladder, lungs, bone, bile, CSF (diffuses into the CSF at higher concentrations when the meninges are inflamed); crosses placenta, reaches amniotic fluid and milk

Protein binding: 85% to 95%

Half-life: Normal renal and hepatic function: 5-9 hours

Neonates: Postnatal:

1-4 days: 16 hours

9-30 days: 9 hours

Time to peak serum concentration: I.M.: Within 1-2 hours

Elimination: Excreted unchanged in urine (33% to 65%) by glomerular filtration and in feces

Usual Dosage I.M., I.V.:

Neonates:

Postnatal age ≤7 days: 50 mg/kg/day given every 24 hours

Postnatal age >7 days:

≤2000 g: 50 mg/kg/day given every 24 hours

>2000 g: 50-75 mg/kg/day given every 24 hours

Gonococcal prophylaxis: 25-50 mg/kg as a single dose (dose not to exceed 125 mg)

Gonococcal infection: 25-50 mg/kg/day (maximum dose: 125 mg) given every 24 hours for 10-14 days

Infants and Children: 50-75 mg/kg/day in 1-2 divided doses every 12-24 hours; maximum: 2 g/24 hours

Meningitis: 100 mg/kg/day divided every 12-24 hours, up to a maximum of 4 g/ 24 hours; loading dose of 75 mg/kg/dose may be given at start of therapy

Otitis media: Single I.M. injection

Uncomplicated gonococcal infections, sexual assault, and STD prophylaxis: I.M.: 125 mg as a single dose plus doxycycline

Complicated gonococcal infections:

Infants: I.M., I.V.: 25-50 mg/kg/day in a single dose (maximum: 125 mg/ dose); treat for 7 days for disseminated infection and 7-14 days for documented meningitis

<45 kg: 50 mg/kg/day once daily; maximum: 1 g/day; for ophthalmia, peritonitis, arthritis, or bacteremia: 50-100 mg/kg/day divided every 12-24 hours; maximum: 2 g/day for meningitis or endocarditis

>45 kg: 1 g/day once daily for disseminated gonococcal infections; 1-2 g dose every 12 hours for meningitis or endocarditis

Acute epididymitis: I.M.: 250 mg in a single dose

Adults: 1-2 g every 12-24 hours (depending on the type and severity of infection); maximum dose: 2 g every 12 hours for treatment of meningitis

Uncomplicated gonorrhea: I.M.: 250 mg as a single dose

Surgical prophylaxis: 1 g 30 minutes to 2 hours before surgery

Dosing adjustment in renal or hepatic impairment: No change necessary

Hemodialysis: Not dialyzable (0% to 5%); administer dose postdialysis

Peritoneal dialysis: Administer 750 mg every 12 hours

Monitoring Parameters Observe for signs and symptoms of anaphylaxis

Test Interactions Positive direct Coombs', false-positive urinary glucose test using cupric sulfate (Benedict's solution, Clinitest®, Fehling's solution), false-positive serum or urine creatinine with Jaffé reaction

Nursing Implications For I.M. injection, the maximum concentration is 250 mg/ mL; ceftriaxone can be diluted with 1:1 water and 1% lidocaine for I.M. administration. Do not admix with aminoglycosides in same bottle/bag.

Additional Information Sodium content of 1 g: 60 mg (2.6 mEq)

(Continued)

Ceftriaxone *(Continued)*

Dosage Forms
Infusion, as sodium, premixed (frozen): 1 g in $D_{3.8}W$ (50 mL); 2 g in $D_{2.4}W$ (50 mL)

Powder for injection, as sodium: 250 mg, 500 mg, 1 g, 2 g, 10 g

Selected Readings
Donowitz GR and Mandell GL, "Beta-Lactam Antibiotics," *N Engl J Med*, 1988, 318(7):419-26 and 318(8):490-500.

Klein NC and Cunha BA, "Third-Generation Cephalosporins," *Med Clin North Am*, 1995, 79(4):705-19.

Marshall WF and Blair JE, "The Cephalosporins," *Mayo Clin Proc*, 1999, 74(2):187-95.

Schaad UB, Suter S, Gianella-Borradori A, et al, "A Comparison of Ceftriaxone and Cefuroxime for the Treatment of Bacterial Meningitis in Children," *N Engl J Med*, 1990, 322(3):141-7.

Ceftriaxone Sodium *see Ceftriaxone on page 655*

Cefuroxime *(se fyoor OKS eem)*

Related Information
Antimicrobial Activity Against Selected Organisms *on page 983*

U.S. Brand Names Ceftin® Oral; Kefurox® Injection; Zinacef® Injection

Synonyms Cefuroxime Axetil; Cefuroxime Sodium

Generic Available No

Use Treatment of infections caused by staphylococci, group B streptococci, *H. influenzae* (type A and B), *E. coli*, *Enterobacter*, *Salmonella*, and *Klebsiella*; treatment of susceptible infections of the lower respiratory tract, otitis media, urinary tract, skin and soft tissue, bone and joint, sepsis, and gonorrhea

Pregnancy Risk Factor B

Contraindications Hypersensitivity to cefuroxime, any component, or cephalosporins

Warnings/Precautions Modify dosage in patients with severe renal impairment, prolonged use may result in superinfection; use with caution in patients with a history of penicillin allergy, especially IgE-mediated reactions (eg, anaphylaxis, urticaria); may cause antibiotic-associated colitis or colitis secondary to *C. difficile*

Adverse Reactions
1% to 10%:
Hematologic: Eosinophilia (7%), decreased hemoglobin and hematocrit (10%)
Hepatic: Increased transaminases (4%), increased alkaline phosphatase (2%)
Local: Thrombophlebitis (1.7%)
<1%: Anaphylaxis, erythema multiforme, toxic epidermal necrolysis, Stevens-Johnson syndrome, interstitial nephritis, dizziness, fever, headache, rash, nausea, vomiting, diarrhea, stomach cramps, GI bleeding, colitis, neutropenia, leukopenia, increased creatinine, increased BUN, pain at injection site, vaginitis, seizures, angioedema, pseudomembranous colitis

Other reactions with cephalosporins include toxic nephropathy, cholestasis, agranulocytosis, colitis, pancytopenia, aplastic anemia, hemolytic anemia, hemorrhage, prolonged PT, encephalopathy, asterixis, neuromuscular excitability, serum-sickness reactions, superinfection

Overdosage/Toxicology
After acute overdose, most agents cause only nausea, vomiting, and diarrhea, although neuromuscular hypersensitivity and seizures are possible, especially in patients with renal insufficiency; many beta-lactam antibiotics have the potential to cause neuromuscular hyperirritability or seizures

Hemodialysis may be helpful to aid in the removal of the drug from the blood but not usually indicated, otherwise most treatment is supportive or symptom directed following GI decontamination

Drug Interactions
Increased effect: High-dose probenecid decreases clearance
Increased toxicity: Aminoglycosides increase nephrotoxic potential

Stability Reconstituted solution is stable for 24 hours at room temperature and 48 hours when refrigerated; I.V. infusion in NS or D_5W solution is stable for 24 hours at room temperature, 7 days when refrigerated, or 26 weeks when frozen; after freezing, thawed solution is stable for 24 hours at room temperature or 21 days when refrigerated

Mechanism of Action Inhibits bacterial cell wall synthesis by binding to one or more of the penicillin-binding proteins (PBPs) which in turn inhibits the final transpeptidation step of peptidoglycan synthesis in bacterial cell walls, thus inhibiting cell wall biosynthesis. Bacteria eventually lyse due to ongoing activity of cell wall autolytic enzymes (autolysins and murein hydrolases) while cell wall assembly is arrested.

Pharmacodynamics/Kinetics

Absorption: Oral (cefuroxime axetil): Increased when given with or shortly after food or infant formula (37% to 52%)

Distribution: Widely distributed to body tissues and fluids; crosses blood-brain barrier; therapeutic concentrations achieved in CSF even when meninges are not inflamed; crosses placenta and reaches breast milk

Protein binding: 33% to 50%

Bioavailability, axetil: Oral: 37% to 52%

Half-life:

Neonates:

≤3 days: 5.1-5.8 hours

6-14 days: 2-4.2 hours

3-4 weeks: 1-1.5 hours

Adults: 1-2 hours (prolonged in renal impairment)

Time to peak serum concentration: I.M.: Within 15-60 minutes

Elimination: Primarily excreted 66% to 100% as unchanged drug in urine by both glomerular filtration and tubular secretion

Usual Dosage

Children:

Pharyngitis, tonsillitis: Oral:

Suspension: 20 mg/kg/day (maximum: 500 mg/day) in 2 divided doses

Tablet: 125 mg every 12 hours

Acute otitis media, impetigo: Oral:

Suspension: 30 mg/kg/day (maximum: 1 g/day) in 2 divided doses

Tablet: 250 mg every 12 hours

I.M., I.V.: 75-150 mg/kg/day divided every 8 hours; maximum dose: 6 g/day

Meningitis: Not recommended (doses of 200-240 mg/kg/day divided every 6-8 hours have been used); maximum dose: 9 g/day

Adults:

Oral: 250-500 mg twice daily; uncomplicated urinary tract infection: 125-250 mg every 12 hours

I.M., I.V.: 750 mg to 1.5 g/dose every 8 hours or 100-150 mg/kg/day in divided doses every 6-8 hours; maximum: 6 g/24 hours

Dosing adjustment in renal impairment:

Cl_{cr} 10-20 mL/minute: Administer every 12 hours

Cl_{cr} <10 mL/minute: Administer every 24 hours

Hemodialysis: Dialyzable (25%)

Note: Cefuroxime axetil film-coated tablets and oral suspension are not bioequivalent and are not substitutable on a mg/mg basis

Continuous arteriovenous or venovenous hemodiafiltration (CAVH) effects: Dose as for Cl_{cr} 10-20 mL/minute

Monitoring Parameters Observe for signs and symptoms of anaphylaxis during first dose; with prolonged therapy, monitor renal, hepatic, and hematologic function periodically

Test Interactions Positive direct Coombs', false-positive urinary glucose test using cupric sulfate (Benedict's solution, Clinitest®, Fehling's solution), false-positive serum or urine creatinine with Jaffé reaction

Patient Information Report prolonged diarrhea; entire course of medication (10-14 days) should be taken to ensure eradication of organism; may interfere with oral contraceptives; females should report symptoms of vaginitis

Nursing Implications Do not admix with aminoglycosides in same bottle/bag; obtain specimens for culture and sensitivity prior to the first dose

Additional Information Sodium content of 1 g: 54.2 mg (2.4 mEq)

Dosage Forms

Infusion, as sodium, premixed (frozen) (Zinacef®): 750 mg (50 mL); 1.5 g (50 mL)

Powder for injection, as sodium: 750 mg, 1.5 g, 7.5 g

Powder for injection, as sodium (Kefurox®, Zinacef®): 750 mg, 1.5 g, 7.5 g

Powder for oral suspension, as axetil (tutti-frutti flavor) (Ceftin®): 125 mg/5 mL (50 mL, 100 mL, 200 mL)

Tablet, as axetil (Ceftin®): 125 mg, 250 mg, 500 mg

(Continued)

Cefuroxime *(Continued)*

Selected Readings

"Antimicrobial Prophylaxis in Surgery," *Med Lett Drugs Ther*, 1993, 35(906):91-4.

Donowitz GR and Mandell GL, "Beta-Lactam Antibiotics," *N Engl J Med*, 1988, 318(7):419-26 and 318(8):490-500.

Gentry LO, Zeluff BJ, and Cooley DA, "Antibiotic Prophylaxis in Open-Heart Surgery: A Comparison of Cefamandole, Cefuroxime, and Cefazolin," *Ann Thorac Surg*, 1988, 46(2):167-71.

Marshall WF and Blair JE, "The Cephalosporins," *Mayo Clin Proc*, 1999, 74(2):187-95.

Perry CM and Brogden RN, "Cefuroxime Axetil. A Review of Its Antibacterial Activity, Pharmacokinetic Properties and Therapeutic Efficacy," *Drugs*, 1996, 52(1):125-58.

Peterson CD, Lake KD, Arom KV, et al, "Antibiotic Prophylaxis in Open-Heart Surgery Patients: Comparison of Cefamandole and Cefuroxime," *Drug Intell Clin Pharm*, 1987, 21(9):728-32.

Cefuroxime Axetil *see* Cefuroxime *on page 658*

Cefuroxime Sodium *see* Cefuroxime *on page 658*

Cefzil® *see* Cefprozil *on page 649*

Cephalexin *(sef a LEKS in)*

Related Information

Antimicrobial Activity Against Selected Organisms *on page 983*

U.S. Brand Names Biocef; Keflex®; Keftab®

Canadian Brand Names Apo®-Cephalex; Novo-Lexin; Nu-Cephalex

Synonyms Cephalexin Hydrochloride; Cephalexin Monohydrate

Generic Available Yes

Use Treatment of susceptible bacterial infections, including those caused by group A beta-hemolytic *Streptococcus*, *Staphylococcus*, *Klebsiella pneumoniae*, *E. coli*, *Proteus mirabilis*, and *Shigella*; predominantly used for lower respiratory tract, urinary tract, skin and soft tissue, and bone and joint; prophylaxis against bacterial endocarditis in high-risk patients undergoing surgical or dental procedures who are allergic to penicillin

Pregnancy Risk Factor B

Contraindications Hypersensitivity to cephalexin, any component, or cephalosporins

Warnings/Precautions Modify dosage in patients with severe renal impairment, prolonged use may result in superinfection; use with caution in patients with a history of penicillin allergy, especially IgE-mediated reactions (eg, anaphylaxis, urticaria); may cause antibiotic-associated colitis or colitis secondary to *C. difficile*

Adverse Reactions

1% to 10%: Gastrointestinal: Diarrhea

<1%: Dizziness, fatigue, headache, rash, urticaria, angioedema, anaphylaxis, erythema multiforme, toxic epidermal necrolysis, Stevens-Johnson syndrome, serum-sickness reaction, nausea, vomiting, dyspepsia, gastritis, abdominal pain, pseudomembranous colitis, interstitial nephritis, agitation, hallucinations, confusion, arthralgia, eosinophilia, neutropenia, thrombocytopenia, anemia, increased transaminases, hepatitis, cholestasis

Other reactions with cephalosporins include anaphylaxis, vomiting, agranulocytosis, colitis, pancytopenia, aplastic anemia, hemolytic anemia, hemorrhage, prolonged PT, encephalopathy, asterixis, neuromuscular excitability, seizures, superinfection

Overdosage/Toxicology

After acute overdose, most agents cause only nausea, vomiting, and diarrhea, although neuromuscular hypersensitivity and seizures are possible, especially in patients with renal insufficiency; many beta-lactam antibiotics have the potential to cause neuromuscular hyperirritability or seizures

Hemodialysis may be helpful to aid in the removal of the drug from the blood but not usually indicated, otherwise most treatment is supportive or symptom directed following GI decontamination

Drug Interactions

Increased effect: High-dose probenecid decreases clearance

Increased toxicity: Aminoglycosides increase nephrotoxic potential

Stability Refrigerate suspension after reconstitution; discard after 14 days

Mechanism of Action Inhibits bacterial cell wall synthesis by binding to one or more of the penicillin-binding proteins (PBPs) which in turn inhibits the final transpeptidation step of peptidoglycan synthesis in bacterial cell walls, thus inhibiting cell wall biosynthesis. Bacteria eventually lyse due to ongoing activity of cell wall autolytic enzymes (autolysins and murein hydrolases) while cell wall assembly is arrested.

Pharmacodynamics/Kinetics

Absorption: Delayed in young children; may be decreased up to 50% in neonates

Distribution: Widely distributed into most body tissues and fluids, including gall-bladder, liver, kidneys, bone, sputum, bile, and pleural and synovial fluids; CSF penetration is poor; crosses placenta; appears in breast milk

Protein binding: 6% to 15%

Half-life:

Neonates: 5 hours

Children 3-12 months: 2.5 hours

Adults: 0.5-1.2 hours (prolonged with renal impairment)

Time to peak serum concentration: Oral: Within 1 hour

Elimination: 80% to 100% of dose excreted as unchanged drug in urine within 8 hours

Usual Dosage Oral:

Children: 25-50 mg/kg/day every 6 hours; severe infections: 50-100 mg/kg/day in divided doses every 6 hours; maximum: 3 g/24 hours

Adults: 250-1000 mg every 6 hours; maximum: 4 g/day

Prophylaxis of bacterial endocarditis: 2 g 1 hour prior to the procedure

Dosing adjustment in renal impairment: Adults:

Cl_{cr} 10-40 mL/minute: 250-500 mg every 8-12 hours

Cl_{cr} <10 mL/minute: 250 mg every 12-24 hours

Hemodialysis: Moderately dialyzable (20% to 50%)

Dietary Considerations Food: Peak antibiotic serum concentration is lowered and delayed, but total drug absorbed is not affected; take on an empty stomach. If GI distress, take with food.

Administration Administer on an empty stomach (ie, 1 hour prior to, or 2 hours after meals) to increase total absorption

Monitoring Parameters With prolonged therapy monitor renal, hepatic, and hematologic function periodically; monitor for signs of anaphylaxis during first dose

Test Interactions Positive direct Coombs', false-positive urinary glucose test using cupric sulfate (Benedict's solution, Clinitest®, Fehling's solution), false-positive serum or urine creatinine with Jaffé reaction, false-positive urinary proteins and steroids

Patient Information Report prolonged diarrhea; entire course of medication (10-14 days) should be taken to ensure eradication of organism; may interfere with oral contraceptives; females should report symptoms of vaginitis

Dosage Forms

Capsule, as monohydrate: 250 mg, 500 mg

Powder for oral suspension: 125 mg/5 mL (5 mL unit dose, 60 mL, 100 mL, 200 mL); 250 mg/5 mL (5 mL unit dose, 100 mL, 200 mL)

Suspension, oral, as monohydrate, pediatric: 100 mg/mL [5 mg/drop] (10 mL)

Tablet, as hydrochloride: 500 mg

Tablet, as monohydrate: 250 mg, 500 mg, 1 g

Selected Readings

Donowitz GR and Mandell GL, "Beta-Lactam Antibiotics," N Engl J Med, 1988, 318(7):419-26 and 318(8):490-500.

Marshall WF and Blair JE, "The Cephalosporins," Mayo Clin Proc, 1999, 74(2):187-95.

Smith GH, "Oral Cephalosporins in Perspective," DICP, 1990, 24(1):45-51.

Cephalexin Hydrochloride see Cephalexin on previous page

Cephalexin Monohydrate see Cephalexin on previous page

Cephalosporins, 1st Generation

Related Information

Antimicrobial Activity Against Selected Organisms on page 983

Refer to

Cefadroxil on page 629

Cefazolin on page 632

Cephalexin on page 660

Cephalothin on page 663

Cephapirin on page 664

Cephradine on page 666

(Continued)

Cephalosporins, 1st Generation *Continued)*

Drug of Choice or Alternative for

Disease/Syndrome(s)

Organism(s)

Cephalosporins, 2nd Generation

Related Information

Refer to

Drug of Choice or Alternative for

Disease/Syndrome(s)

Organism(s)

Cephalosporins, 3rd Generation

Related Information

Refer to

Drug of Choice or Alternative for

Disease/Syndrome(s)

Cephalothin (sef A loe thin)

Related Information
Antimicrobial Activity Against Selected Organisms *on page 983*

Canadian Brand Names Ceporacin®

Synonyms Cephalothin Sodium

Generic Available Yes

Use Treatment of infections when caused by susceptible strains in respiratory, genitourinary, gastrointestinal, skin and soft tissue, bone and joint infections; septicemia. Treatment of susceptible gram-positive bacilli and cocci (never enterococcus); some gram-negative bacilli including *E. coli*, *Proteus*, and *Klebsiella* may be susceptible.

Pregnancy Risk Factor B

Contraindications Hypersensitivity to cephalothin or cephalosporins

Warnings/Precautions Modify dosage in patients with severe renal impairment, prolonged use may result in superinfection; use with caution in patients with a history of penicillin allergy, especially IgE-mediated reactions (eg, anaphylaxis, urticaria); may cause antibiotic-associated colitis or colitis secondary to *C. difficile*

Adverse Reactions
1% to 10%: Gastrointestinal: Diarrhea, nausea, vomiting
<1%: Maculopapular and erythematous rash, dyspepsia, pseudomembranous colitis, bleeding, pain and induration at injection site

Other reactions with cephalosporins include anaphylaxis, erythema multiforme, toxic epidermal necrolysis, Stevens-Johnson syndrome, dizziness, fever, headache, CNS irritability, seizures, decreased hemoglobin, neutropenia, leukopenia, agranulocytosis, pancytopenia, aplastic anemia, hemolytic anemia, interstitial nephritis, toxic nephropathy, vaginitis, angioedema, cholestasis, hemorrhage, prolonged PT, serum-sickness reactions, superinfection

Overdosage/Toxicology
Symptoms of overdose include neuromuscular hypersensitivity, convulsions especially with renal insufficiency; many beta-lactam antibiotics have the potential to cause neuromuscular hyperirritability or seizures
Hemodialysis may be helpful to aid in the removal of the drug from the blood, otherwise most treatment is supportive or symptom directed

Stability Reconstituted solution is stable for 12-24 hours at room temperature and 96 hours when refrigerated; for I.V. infusion in NS or D_5W solution is stable for 24 hours at room temperature, 96 hours when refrigerated or 12 weeks when (Continued)

Cephalothin *(Continued)*

frozen; after freezing, thawed solution is stable for 24 hours at room temperature or 96 hours when refrigerated

Mechanism of Action Inhibits bacterial cell wall synthesis by binding to one or more of the penicillin-binding proteins (PBPs) which in turn inhibits the final transpeptidation step of peptidoglycan synthesis in bacterial cell walls, thus inhibiting cell wall biosynthesis. Bacteria eventually lyse due to ongoing activity of cell wall autolytic enzymes (autolysins and murein hydrolases) while cell wall assembly is arrested.

Pharmacodynamics/Kinetics

Distribution: Does not penetrate the CSF unless the meninges are inflamed; crosses the placenta; small amounts appear in breast milk

Protein binding: 65% to 80%

Metabolism: Partially deacetylated in the liver and kidney

Half-life: 30-60 minutes

Time to peak serum concentration: I.M.: Within 30 minutes

Elimination: 50% to 75% of a dose appearing as unchanged drug in urine

Usual Dosage I.M., I.V.:

Neonates:

Postnatal age <7 days:

<2000 g: 20 mg every 12 hours

>2000 g: 20 mg every 8 hours

Postnatal age >7 days:

<2000 g: 20 mg every 8 hours

>2000 g: 20 mg every 6 hours

Children: 75-125 mg/kg/day divided every 4-6 hours; maximum dose: 10 g in a 24-hour period

Adults: 500 mg to 2 g every 4-6 hours

Dosing interval in renal impairment:

Cl_{cr} 10-50 mL/minute: Administer every 6-8 hours

Cl_{cr} <10 mL/minute: Administer every 12 hours

Continuous arteriovenous or venovenous hemodiafiltration (CAVH) effects: Administer 1 g every 8 hours

Monitoring Parameters Observe for signs and symptoms of anaphylaxis during first dose

Test Interactions Positive direct Coombs', false-positive urinary glucose test using cupric sulfate (Benedict's solution, Clinitest®, Fehling's solution), false-positive serum or urine creatinine with Jaffé reaction, false-positive urinary proteins and steroids

Nursing Implications Do not admix with aminoglycosides in same bottle/bag

Additional Information Sodium content of 1 g: 64.4 mg (2.8 mEq)

Dosage Forms Powder for injection, as sodium: 1 g, 2 g

Selected Readings

Donowitz GR and Mandell GL, "Beta-Lactam Antibiotics," *N Engl J Med*, 1988, 318(7):419-26 and 318(8):490-500.

Marshall WF and Blair JE, "The Cephalosporins," *Mayo Clin Proc*, 1999, 74(2):187-95

Cephalothin Sodium *see Cephalothin on previous page*

Cephapirin *(sef a PYE rin)*

Related Information

Antimicrobial Activity Against Selected Organisms *on page 983*

U.S. Brand Names Cefadyl®

Synonyms Cephapirin Sodium

Generic Available No

Use Treatment of infections when caused by susceptible strains in respiratory, genitourinary, gastrointestinal, skin and soft tissue, bone and joint infections; septicemia. Treatment of susceptible gram-positive bacilli and cocci (never enterococcus); some gram-negative bacilli including *E. coli*, *Proteus*, and *Klebsiella* may be susceptible.

Pregnancy Risk Factor B

Contraindications Hypersensitivity to cephapirin sodium, any component, or cephalosporins

Warnings/Precautions Modify dosage in patients with severe renal impairment, prolonged use may result in superinfection; use with caution in patients with a history of penicillin allergy, especially IgE-mediated reactions (eg, anaphylaxis, urticaria); may cause antibiotic-associated colitis or colitis secondary to *C. difficile*

Adverse Reactions

1% to 10%: Gastrointestinal: Diarrhea

<1%: CNS irritation, seizures, fever, rash, urticaria, leukopenia, thrombocytopenia, increased transaminases

Other reactions with cephalosporins include anaphylaxis, erythema multiforme, toxic epidermal necrolysis, Stevens-Johnson syndrome, dizziness, fever, headache, encephalopathy, asterixis, neuromuscular excitability, seizures, nausea, vomiting, pseudomembranous colitis, decreased hemoglobin, agranulocytosis, pancytopenia, aplastic anemia, hemolytic anemia, interstitial nephritis, toxic nephropathy, pain at injection site, vaginitis, angioedema, cholestasis, hemorrhage, prolonged PT, serum-sickness reactions, superinfection

Overdosage/Toxicology

Symptoms of overdose include neuromuscular hypersensitivity, convulsions especially with renal insufficiency; many beta-lactam antibiotics have the potential to cause neuromuscular hyperirritability or seizures

Hemodialysis may be helpful to aid in the removal of the drug from the blood, otherwise most treatment is supportive or symptom directed

Drug Interactions

Increased effect: High-dose probenecid decreases clearance

Increased toxicity: Aminoglycosides increase nephrotoxic potential

Stability Reconstituted solution is stable for 24 hours at room temperature and 10 days when refrigerated; for I.V. infusion in NS or D_5W solution is stable for 24 hours at room temperature, 10 days when refrigerated or 14 days when frozen; after freezing, thawed solution is stable for 12 hours at room temperature or 10 days when refrigerated

Mechanism of Action Inhibits bacterial cell wall synthesis by binding to one or more of the penicillin-binding proteins (PBPs) which in turn inhibits the final transpeptidation step of peptidoglycan synthesis in bacterial cell walls, thus inhibiting cell wall biosynthesis. Bacteria eventually lyse due to ongoing activity of cell wall autolytic enzymes (autolysins and murein hydrolases) while cell wall assembly is arrested.

Pharmacodynamics/Kinetics

Distribution: Widely distributed into most body tissues and fluids including gallbladder, liver, kidneys, bone, sputum, bile, and pleural and synovial fluids; CSF penetration is poor; crosses the placenta and small amounts appear in breast milk

Protein binding: 22% to 25%

Metabolism: Partially in the liver, kidney, and plasma to metabolites (50% active)

Half-life: 36-60 minutes

Time to peak serum concentration: I.M.: Within 30 minutes

Elimination: 60% to 85% excreted as unchanged drug in urine

Usual Dosage I.M., I.V.:

Children: 10-20 mg/kg/dose every 6 hours up to 4 g/24 hours

Adults: 500 mg to 1 g every 6 hours up to 12 g/day

Perioperative prophylaxis: 1-2 g 30 minutes to 1 hour prior to surgery and every 6 hours as needed for 24 hours following

Dosing interval in renal impairment:

Cl_{cr} 10-50 mL/minute: Administer every 6-8 hours

Cl_{cr} <10 mL/minute: Administer every 12 hours

Continuous arteriovenous or venovenous hemodiafiltration (CAVH) effects: Administer 1 g every 8 hours

Monitoring Parameters Observe for signs and symptoms of anaphylaxis during first dose

Test Interactions Positive direct Coombs', false-positive urinary glucose test using cupric sulfate (Benedict's solution, Clinitest®, Fehling's solution), false-positive serum or urine creatinine with Jaffé reaction, false-positive urinary proteins and steroids

Nursing Implications Do not admix with aminoglycosides in same bottle/bag; obtain specimens for culture and sensitivity prior to administration of first dose

Additional Information Sodium content of 1 g: 55.2 mg (2.4 mEq)

Dosage Forms Powder for injection, as sodium: 500 mg, 1 g, 2 g, 4 g, 20 g

(Continued)

Cephapirin *(Continued)*

Selected Readings

Donowitz GR and Mandell GL, "Beta-Lactam Antibiotics," *N Engl J Med*, 1988, 318(7):419-26 and 318(8):490-500.

Marshall WF and Blair JE, "The Cephalosporins," *Mayo Clin Proc*, 1999, 74(2):187-95.

Cephapirin Sodium *see* Cephapirin *on page 664*

Cephradine *(SEF ra deen)*

Related Information

Antimicrobial Activity Against Selected Organisms *on page 983*

U.S. Brand Names Velosef®

Generic Available Yes

Use Treatment of infections when caused by susceptible strains in respiratory, genitourinary, gastrointestinal, skin and soft tissue, bone and joint infections. Treatment of susceptible gram-positive bacilli and cocci (never enterococcus); some gram-negative bacilli including *E. coli*, *Proteus*, and *Klebsiella* may be susceptible.

Pregnancy Risk Factor B

Contraindications Hypersensitivity to cephradine, any component, or cephalosporins

Warnings/Precautions Modify dosage in patients with severe renal impairment, prolonged use may result in superinfection; use with caution in patients with a history of penicillin allergy, especially IgE-mediated reactions (eg, anaphylaxis, urticaria); may cause antibiotic-associated colitis or colitis secondary to *C. difficile*

Adverse Reactions

1% to 10%: Gastrointestinal: Diarrhea

<1%: Rash, nausea, vomiting, pseudomembranous colitis, increased BUN, increased creatinine

Other reactions with cephalosporins include anaphylaxis, erythema multiforme, toxic epidermal necrolysis, Stevens-Johnson syndrome, dizziness, fever, headache, encephalopathy, asterixis, neuromuscular excitability, seizures, neutropenia, leukopenia, agranulocytosis, pancytopenia, aplastic anemia, hemolytic anemia, interstitial nephritis, toxic nephropathy, vaginitis, angioedema, cholestasis, hemorrhage, prolonged PT, serum-sickness reactions, superinfection

Overdosage/Toxicology

Symptoms of overdose include neuromuscular hypersensitivity, convulsions especially with renal insufficiency; many beta-lactam antibiotics have the potential to cause neuromuscular hyperirritability or seizures

Hemodialysis may be helpful to aid in the removal of the drug from the blood, otherwise most treatment is supportive or symptom directed

Drug Interactions

Increased effect: High-dose probenecid decreases clearance

Increased toxicity: Aminoglycosides increase nephrotoxic potential

Mechanism of Action Inhibits bacterial cell wall synthesis by binding to one or more of the penicillin-binding proteins (PBPs) which in turn inhibits the final transpeptidation step of peptidoglycan synthesis in bacterial cell walls, thus inhibiting cell wall biosynthesis. Bacteria eventually lyse due to ongoing activity of cell wall autolytic enzymes (autolysins and murein hydrolases) while cell wall assembly is arrested.

Pharmacodynamics/Kinetics

Absorption: Well absorbed

Distribution: Widely distributed into most body tissues and fluids including gallbladder, liver, kidneys, bone, sputum, bile, and pleural and synovial fluids; CSF penetration is poor; crosses the placenta and appears in breast milk

Protein binding: 18% to 20%

Half-life: 1-2 hours

Time to peak serum concentration: Oral: Within 1-2 hours

Elimination: ~80% to 90% unchanged drug is recovered in urine within 6 hours

Usual Dosage Oral:

Children ≥9 months: 25-50 mg/kg/day in divided doses every 6 hours

Adults: 250-500 mg every 6-12 hours

Dosing adjustment in renal impairment: Adults:

Cl$_{cr}$ 10-50 mL/minute: 250 mg every 6 hours

Cl$_{cr}$ <10 mL/minute: 125 mg every 6 hours

Monitoring Parameters Observe for signs and symptoms of anaphylaxis during first dose

Test Interactions Positive direct Coombs', false-positive urinary glucose test using cupric sulfate (Benedict's solution, Clinitest®, Fehling's solution), false-positive serum or urine creatinine with Jaffé reaction, false-positive urinary proteins and steroids

Patient Information Take until gone, do not miss doses; report diarrhea promptly; entire course of medication (10-14 days) should be taken to ensure eradication of organism; may interfere with oral contraceptives; females should report symptoms of vaginitis

Dosage Forms

Capsule: 250 mg, 500 mg

Powder for oral suspension: 125 mg/5 mL (5 mL, 100 mL, 200 mL); 250 mg/5 mL (5 mL, 100 mL, 200 mL)

Selected Readings

Donowitz GR and Mandell GL, "Beta-Lactam Antibiotics," *N Engl J Med*, 1988, 318(7):419-26 and 318(8):490-500.

Marshall WF and Blair JE, "The Cephalosporins," *Mayo Clin Proc*, 1999, 74(2):187-95.

Smith GH, "Oral Cephalosporins in Perspective," *DICP*, 1990, 24(1):45-51.

Ceporacin® *see* Cephalothin *on page 663*

Ceptaz™ *see* Ceftazidime *on page 651*

Certiva™ *see* Diphtheria, Tetanus Toxoids, and Acellular Pertussis Vaccine *on page 708*

Cetamide® Ophthalmic *see* Sulfacetamide Sodium *on page 927*

Cetapred® Ophthalmic *see* Sulfacetamide Sodium and Prednisolone *on page 928*

CFDN *see* Cefdinir *on page 633*

Chibroxin™ Ophthalmic *see* Norfloxacin *on page 844*

Chicken Pox Vaccine *see* Varicella Virus Vaccine *on page 970*

Chloramphenicol (klor am FEN i kole)

Related Information

Antimicrobial Activity Against Selected Organisms *on page 983*

U.S. Brand Names AK-Chlor® Ophthalmic; Chloromycetin®; Chloroptic® Ophthalmic

Canadian Brand Names Diochloram; Pentamycetin®; Sopamycetin

Generic Available Yes

Use Treatment of serious infections due to organisms resistant to other less toxic antibiotics or when its penetrability into the site of infection is clinically superior to other antibiotics to which the organism is sensitive; useful in infections caused by *Bacteroides*, *H. influenzae*, *Neisseria meningitidis*, *Salmonella*, and *Rickettsia*. Active against many vancomycin-resistant enterococci.

Drug of Choice or Alternative for

Disease/Syndrome(s)

Brain Abscess *on page 19*

Meningitis, Community-Acquired, Adult *on page 34*

Meningitis, Pediatric (>2 months of age) *on page 35*

Meningitis, Neonatal (<2 months of age) *on page 35*

Organism(s)

Bacillus anthracis *on page 73*

Bordetella pertussis *on page 81*

Burkholderia cepacia *on page 87*

Calymmatobacterium granulomatis *on page 89*

Coxiella burnetii *on page 115*

Ehrlichia Species *on page 130*

Enterococcus Species *on page 137*

Francisella tularensis *on page 148*

Haemophilus influenzae *on page 157*

Neisseria meningitidis *on page 217*

Rickettsia rickettsii *on page 243*

Salmonella Species *on page 245*

Streptococcus pneumoniae *on page 268*

(Continued)

Chloramphenicol *(Continued)*

Yersinia pestis on page 300

Pregnancy Risk Factor C

Contraindications Hypersensitivity to chloramphenicol or any component

Warnings/Precautions Use with caution in patients with impaired renal or hepatic function and in neonates; reduce dose with impaired liver function; use with care in patients with glucose 6-phosphate dehydrogenase deficiency. Serious and fatal blood dyscrasias have occurred after both short-term and prolonged therapy; should not be used when less potentially toxic agents are effective; prolonged use may result in superinfection.

Adverse Reactions <1%: Nightmares, headache, rash, diarrhea, stomatitis, enterocolitis, nausea, vomiting, bone marrow suppression, aplastic anemia, peripheral neuropathy, optic neuritis, gray syndrome

Three major toxicities associated with chloramphenicol include:

Aplastic anemia, an idiosyncratic reaction which can occur with any route of administration; usually occurs 3 weeks to 12 months after initial exposure to chloramphenicol

Bone marrow suppression is thought to be dose-related with serum concentrations >25 μg/mL and reversible once chloramphenicol is discontinued; anemia and neutropenia may occur during the first week of therapy

Gray syndrome is characterized by circulatory collapse, cyanosis, acidosis, abdominal distention, myocardial depression, coma, and death; reaction appears to be associated with serum levels ≥50 μg/mL; may result from drug accumulation in patients with impaired hepatic or renal function

Overdosage/Toxicology

Symptoms of overdose include anemia, metabolic acidosis, hypotension, hypothermia

Treatment is supportive following GI decontamination

Drug Interactions CYP2C9 enzyme inhibitor

Decreased effect: Phenobarbital and rifampin may decrease concentration of chloramphenicol

Increased toxicity: Chloramphenicol inhibits the metabolism of chlorpropamide, phenytoin, oral anticoagulants

Stability Refrigerate ophthalmic solution; constituted solutions remain stable for 30 days; use only clear solutions; frozen solutions remain stable for 6 months

Mechanism of Action Reversibly binds to 50S ribosomal subunits of susceptible organisms preventing amino acids from being transferred to growing peptide chains thus inhibiting protein synthesis

Pharmacodynamics/Kinetics

Distribution: Readily crosses placenta; appears in breast milk; distributes to most tissues and body fluids

Ratio of CSF to blood level (%):

Normal meninges: 66

Inflamed meninges: 66+

Protein binding: 60%

Metabolism: Extensive in the liver (90%) to inactive metabolites, principally by glucuronidation, chloramphenicol palmitate is hydrolyzed by lipases in the GI tract to the active base; chloramphenicol sodium succinate is hydrolyzed by esterases to active base

Half-life: (Prolonged with markedly reduced liver function or combined liver/kidney dysfunction):

Normal renal function: 1.6-3.3 hours

End stage renal disease: 3-7 hours

Cirrhosis: 10-12 hours

Neonates: Postnatal:

1-2 days: 24 hours

10-16 days: 10 hours

Elimination: 5% to 15% excreted as unchanged drug in the urine, 4% excreted in bile; in neonates, 6% to 80% may be excreted unchanged in urine

Usual Dosage

Meningitis: I.V.: Infants >30 days and Children: 50-100 mg/kg/day divided every 6 hours

Other infections: I.V.:

Infants >30 days and Children: 50-75 mg/kg/day divided every 6 hours; maximum daily dose: 4 g/day

Adults: 50-100 mg/kg/day in divided doses every 6 hours; maximum daily dose: 4 g/day

Ophthalmic: Children and Adults: Instill 1-2 drops or 1.25 cm (½" of ointment every 3-4 hours); increase interval between applications after 48 hours to 2-3 times/day

Otic solution: Instill 2-3 drops into ear 3 times/day

Topical: Gently rub into the affected area 1-4 times/day

Dosing adjustment/comments in hepatic impairment: Avoid use in severe liver impairment as increased toxicity may occur

Hemodialysis: Slightly dialyzable (5% to 20%) via hemo- and peritoneal dialysis; no supplemental doses needed in dialysis or continuous arteriovenous or veno-venous hemofiltration (CAVH/CAVHD)

Dietary Considerations Folic acid, iron salts, vitamin B_{12}: May decrease intestinal absorption of vitamin B_{12}; may have increased dietary need for riboflavin, pyridoxine, and vitamin B_{12}; monitor hematological status

Administration Do not administer I.M.

Monitoring Parameters CBC with reticulocyte and platelet counts, periodic liver and renal function tests, serum drug concentration

Reference Range

Therapeutic levels: 15-20 µg/mL; Toxic concentration: >40 µg/mL; Trough: 5-10 µg/mL

Timing of serum samples: Draw levels 1.5 hours and 3 hours after completion of I.V. or oral dose; trough levels may be preferred; should be drawn ≤1 hour prior to dose

Additional Information Sodium content of 1 g (injection): 51.8 mg (2.25 mEq)

Dosage Forms

Ointment, ophthalmic: 1% [10 mg/g] (3.5 g)

AK-Chlor®, Chloromycetin®, Chloroptic® S.O.P.: 1% [10 mg/g] (3.5 g)

Powder for injection, as sodium succinate: 1 g

Powder for ophthalmic solution (Chloromycetin®): 25 mg/vial (15 mL)

Solution: 0.5% [5 mg/mL] (7.5 mL, 15 mL)

Solution, ophthalmic (AK-Chlor®, Chloroptic®): 0.5% [5 mg/mL] (2.5 mL, 7.5 mL, 15 mL)

Solution, otic (Chloromycetin®): 0.5% (15 mL)

Selected Readings

Smilack JD, Wilson WR, and Cockerill FR 3d, "Tetracyclines, Chloramphenicol, Erythromycin, Clindamycin, and Metronidazole," *Mayo Clin Proc*, 1991, 66(12):1270-80.

Tunkel AR, Wispelwey B, and Scheld M, "Bacterial Meningitis: Recent Advances in Pathophysiology and Treatment," *Ann Intern Med*, 1990, 112(8):610-23.

Chloramphenicol and Prednisolone

(klor am FEN i kole & pred NIS oh lone)

Related Information

Chloramphenicol *on page 667*

U.S. Brand Names Chloroptic-P® Ophthalmic

Use Topical anti-infective and corticosteroid for treatment of ocular infections

Usual Dosage Ophthalmic: Instill 1-2 drops in eye(s) 2-4 times/day

Dosage Forms Ointment, ophthalmic: Chloramphenicol 1% and prednisolone 0.5% (3.5 g)

Chloramphenicol, Polymyxin B, and Hydrocortisone

(klor am FEN i kole, pol i MIKS in bee, & hye droe KOR ti sone)

Related Information

Chloramphenicol *on page 667*

Polymyxin B *on page 877*

Use Topical anti-infective and corticosteroid for treatment of ocular infections

Usual Dosage Apply ½" ribbon every 3-4 hours until improvement occurs

Dosage Forms Solution, ophthalmic: Chloramphenicol 1%, polymyxin B sulfate 10,000 units, and hydrocortisone acetate 0.5% per g (3.75 g)

Chlorhexidine Gluconate (klor HEKS i deen GLOO koe nate)

U.S. Brand Names BactoShield® Topical [OTC]; Betasept® [OTC]; Dyna-Hex® Topical [OTC]; Exidine® Scrub [OTC]; Hibiclens® Topical [OTC]; Hibistat® Topical [OTC]; Peridex® Oral Rinse; PerioGard®

Generic Available No

Use Skin cleanser for surgical scrub, cleanser for skin wounds, germicidal hand rinse, and as antibacterial dental rinse. Chlorhexidine is active against gram-positive and gram-negative organisms, facultative anaerobes, aerobes, and yeast.

Pregnancy Risk Factor B

Contraindications Known hypersensitivity to chlorhexidine gluconate

Warnings/Precautions Staining of oral surfaces, tooth restorations, and dorsum of tongue may occur; keep out of eyes and ears; for topical use only; there have been case reports of anaphylaxis following chlorhexidine disinfection

Adverse Reactions

>10%: Oral: Increase of tartar on teeth, changes in taste. Staining of oral surfaces (mucosa, teeth, dorsum of tongue) may be visible as soon as 1 week after therapy begins and is more pronounced when there is a heavy accumulation of unremoved plaque and when teeth fillings have rough surfaces. Stain does not have a clinically adverse effect but because removal may not be possible, patient with frontal restoration should be advised of the potential permanency of the stain.

1% to 10%: Gastrointestinal: Tongue irritation, oral irritation

<1%: Facial edema, nasal congestion, shortness of breath

Overdosage/Toxicology Symptoms of oral overdose include gastric distress, nausea, or signs of alcohol intoxication

Mechanism of Action The bactericidal effect of chlorhexidine is a result of the binding of this cationic molecule to negatively charged bacterial cell walls and extramicrobial complexes. At low concentrations, this causes an alteration of bacterial cell osmotic equilibrium and leakage of potassium and phosphorous resulting in a bacteriostatic effect. At high concentrations of chlorhexidine, the cytoplasmic contents of the bacterial cell precipitate and result in cell death.

Pharmacodynamics/Kinetics

Absorption: ~30% of chlorhexidine is retained in the oral cavity following rinsing and is slowly released into the oral fluids; chlorhexidine is poorly absorbed from the GI tract

Serum concentrations: Detectable levels are not present in the plasma 12 hours after administration

Elimination: Primarily through the feces (approximately 90%); <1% excreted in the urine

Usual Dosage Adults: Oral rinse (Peridex®):

Precede use of solution by flossing and brushing teeth; completely rinse toothpaste from mouth. Swish 15 mL undiluted oral rinse around in mouth for 30 seconds, then expectorate. Caution patient not to swallow the medicine. Avoid eating for 2-3 hours after treatment. (The cap on bottle of oral rinse is a measure for 15 mL.)

When used as a treatment of gingivitis, the regimen begins with oral prophylaxis. Patient treats mouth with 15 mL chlorhexidine, swishes for 30 seconds, then expectorates. This is repeated twice daily (morning and evening). Patient should have a re-evaluation followed by a dental prophylaxis every 6 months.

Cleanser:

Surgical scrub: Scrub 3 minutes and rinse thoroughly, wash for an additional 3 minutes

Hand wash: Wash for 15 seconds and rinse

Hand rinse: Rub 15 seconds and rinse

Patient Information

Oral rinse: Do not swallow, do not rinse after use; may cause reduced taste perception which is reversible; may cause discoloration of teeth

Topical administration is for external use only

Dosage Forms

Foam, topical, with isopropyl alcohol 4% (BactoShield®): 4% (180 mL)

Liquid, topical, with isopropyl alcohol 4%:

Dyna-Hex® Skin Cleanser: 2% (120 mL, 240 mL, 480 mL, 960 mL, 4000 mL); 4% (120 mL, 240 mL, 480 mL, 4000 mL)

BactoShield® 2: 2% (960 mL)
BactoShield®, Betasept®, Exidine® Skin Cleanser, Hibiclens® Skin Cleanser:
   4% (15 mL, 120 mL, 240 mL, 480 mL, 960 mL, 4000 mL)
Rinse:
   Oral (mint flavor) (Peridex®, PerioGard®): 0.12% with alcohol 11.6% (480 mL)
   Topical (Hibistat® Hand Rinse): 0.5% with isopropyl alcohol 70% (120 mL, 240
      mL)
Sponge/Brush (Hibiclens®): 4% with isopropyl alcohol 4% (22 mL)
Wipes (Hibistat®): 0.5% (50s)

Selected Readings
Emerson D and Pierce C, "A Case of a Single Ingestion of 4% Hibiclens®," *Vet Hum Toxicol*, 1988, 30(6):583.

Massano G, Ciocatto E, Rosabianca C, et al, "Striking Aminotransferase Rise After Chlorhexidine Self-Poisoning," *Lancet*, 1982, 1(8266):289.

Quinn MW and Bini RM, "Bradycardia Associated With Chlorhexidine Spray," *Arch Dis Child*, 1989, 64(6):892-3.

Yong D, Parker FC, and Foran SM, "Severe Allergic Reactions and Intra-Urethral Chlorhexidine Gluconate," *Med J Aust*, 1995, 162(5):257-8.

Chloromycetin® *see* Chloramphenicol *on page 667*

Chloroptic® Ophthalmic *see* Chloramphenicol *on page 667*

Chloroptic-P® Ophthalmic *see* Chloramphenicol and Prednisolone *on page 669*

Chloroquine and Primaquine (KLOR oh kwin & PRIM a kween)
Related Information
Chloroquine Phosphate *on next page*
Primaquine Phosphate *on page 882*
U.S. Brand Names Aralen® Phosphate With Primaquine Phosphate
Synonyms Primaquine and Chloroquine
Generic Available No
Use Prophylaxis of malaria, regardless of species, in all areas where the disease is endemic
Pregnancy Risk Factor C
Contraindications Retinal or visual field changes, known hypersensitivity to chloroquine or primaquine
Warnings/Precautions Use with caution in patients with psoriasis, porphyria, hepatic dysfunction, G-6-PD deficiency
Adverse Reactions
   1% to 10%: Gastrointestinal: Diarrhea, nausea
   <1%: Hypotension, EKG changes, fatigue, personality changes, headache, pruritus, hair bleaching, anorexia, vomiting, stomatitis, blood dyscrasias, retinopathy, blurred vision
Overdosage/Toxicology
   Symptoms of overdose include headache, visual changes, cardiovascular collapse, seizures, abdominal cramps, vomiting, cyanosis, methemoglobinemia, leukopenia, respiratory and cardiac arrest
   Following initial measures (immediate GI decontamination), treatment is supportive and symptomatic
Drug Interactions
   Decreased absorption if administered concomitantly with kaolin and magnesium trisilicate
   Increased toxicity/levels with cimetidine
Mechanism of Action Chloroquine concentrates within parasite acid vesicles and raises internal pH resulting in inhibition of parasite growth; may involve aggregates of ferriprotoporphyrin IX acting as chloroquine receptors causing membrane damage; may also interfere with nucleoprotein synthesis. Primaquine eliminates the primary tissue exoerythrocytic forms of *P. falciparum*; disrupts mitochondria and binds to DNA.
Pharmacodynamics/Kinetics
   Absorption: Oral: Both drugs are readily absorbed
   Distribution: Concentrated in liver, spleen, kidney, heart, and brain
   Protein binding: ~55%; binds strongly to melanin
   Metabolism: 25% of chloroquine is metabolized
   Elimination: Drug may remain in tissue for 3-5 days; up to 70% excreted unchanged
Usual Dosage Oral: Start at least 1 day before entering the endemic area; continue for 8 weeks after leaving the endemic area
   (Continued)

Chloroquine and Primaquine *(Continued)*

Children: For suggested weekly dosage (based on body weight), see table.

Adults: 1 tablet/week on the same day each week

Chloroquine and Primaquine

Weight		Chloroquine Base (mg)	Primaquine Base (mg)	Dose* (mL)
lb	kg			
10-15	4.5-6.8	20	3	2.5
16-25	7.3-11.4	40	6	5
26-35	11.8-15.9	60	9	7.5
36-45	16.4-20.5	80	12	10
46-55	20.9-25	100	15	12.5
56-100	25.4-45.4	150	22.5	½ tablet
100+	>45.4	300	45	1 tablet

*Dose based on liquid containing approximately 40 mg of chloroquine base and 6 mg primaquine base per 5 mL, prepared from chloroquine phosphate with primaquine phosphate tablets.

Monitoring Parameters Periodic CBC, examination for muscular weakness, and ophthalmologic examination in patients receiving prolonged therapy

Patient Information Take with meals; report any visual disturbances or difficulty in hearing or ringing in the ears; tablets are bitter tasting; may cause diarrhea, loss of appetite, nausea, stomach pain; notify physician if these become severe

Dosage Forms Tablet: Chloroquine phosphate 500 mg [base 300 mg] and primaquine phosphate 79 mg [base 45 mg]

Selected Readings

Panisko DM and Keystone JS, "Treatment of Malaria - 1990," *Drugs*, 1990, 39(2):160-89.
White NJ, "The Treatment of Malaria," *N Engl J Med*, 1996, 335(11):800-6.
Wyler DJ, "Malaria Chemoprophylaxis for the Traveler," *N Engl J Med*, 1993, 329(1):31-7.
Wyler DJ, "Malaria: Overview and Update," *Clin Infect Dis*, 1993, 16(4):449-56.

Chloroquine Phosphate (KLOR oh kwin FOS fate)

Related Information

Prevention of Malaria *on page 1057*

U.S. Brand Names Aralen® Phosphate

Generic Available Yes

Use Suppression or chemoprophylaxis of malaria; treatment of uncomplicated or mild-moderate malaria; extraintestinal amebiasis

Unlabeled use: Rheumatoid arthritis; discoid lupus erythematosus, scleroderma, pemphigus

Drug of Choice or Alternative for

Organism(s)

Plasmodium Species *on page 227*

Pregnancy Risk Factor C

Contraindications Retinal or visual field changes; patients with psoriasis; known hypersensitivity to chloroquine

Warnings/Precautions Use with caution in patients with liver disease, G-6-PD deficiency, alcoholism or in conjunction with hepatotoxic drugs, psoriasis, porphyria may be exacerbated; retinopathy (irreversible) has occurred with long or high-dose therapy; discontinue drug if any abnormality in the visual field or if muscular weakness develops during treatment

Adverse Reactions

>1%: Gastrointestinal: Nausea, diarrhea

<1%: Hypotension, EKG changes, fatigue, personality changes, headache, pruritus, hair bleaching, anorexia, vomiting, stomatitis, blood dyscrasias, retinopathy, blurred vision

Overdosage/Toxicology

Symptoms of overdose include headache, visual changes, cardiovascular collapse, seizures, abdominal cramps, vomiting, cyanosis, methemoglobinemia, leukopenia, respiratory and cardiac arrest

Following initial measures (immediate GI decontamination), treatment is supportive and symptomatic

Drug Interactions

Chloroquine and other 4-aminoquinolones may be decreased due to GI binding with kaolin or magnesium trisilicate

Increased effect: Cimetidine increases levels of chloroquine and probably other 4-aminoquinolones

Mechanism of Action Binds to and inhibits DNA and RNA polymerase; interferes with metabolism and hemoglobin utilization by parasites; inhibits prostaglandin effects; chloroquine concentrates within parasite acid vesicles and raises internal pH resulting in inhibition of parasite growth; may involve aggregates of ferriprotoporphyrin IX acting as chloroquine receptors causing membrane damage; may also interfere with nucleoprotein synthesis

Pharmacodynamics/Kinetics

Absorption: Oral: Rapid (~89%)

Distribution: Widely distributed in body tissues such as eyes, heart, kidneys, liver, and lungs where retention is prolonged; crosses the placenta; appears in breast milk

Metabolism: Partial hepatic metabolism occurs

Half-life: 3-5 days

Time to peak serum concentration: Within 1-2 hours

Elimination: ~70% excreted unchanged in urine; acidification of the urine increases elimination of drug; small amounts of drug may be present in urine months following discontinuation of therapy

Usual Dosage Oral (**dosage expressed in terms of mg of base**):

Suppression or prophylaxis of malaria:

Children: Administer 5 mg base/kg/week on the same day each week (not to exceed 300 mg base/dose); begin 1-2 weeks prior to exposure; continue for 4-6 weeks after leaving endemic area; if suppressive therapy is not begun prior to exposure, double the initial loading dose to 10 mg base/kg and administer in 2 divided doses 6 hours apart, followed by the usual dosage regimen

Adults: 300 mg/week (base) on the same day each week; begin 1-2 weeks prior to exposure; continue for 4-6 weeks after leaving endemic area; if suppressive therapy is not begun prior to exposure, double the initial loading dose to 600 mg base and administer in 2 divided doses 6 hours apart, followed by the usual dosage regimen

Acute attack:

Oral:

Children: 10 mg/kg on day 1, followed by 5 mg/kg 6 hours later and 5 mg/kg on days 2 and 3

Adults: 600 mg on day 1, followed by 300 mg 6 hours later, followed by 300 mg on days 2 and 3

I.M. (as hydrochloride):

Children: 5 mg/kg, repeat in 6 hours

Adults: Initial: 160-200 mg, repeat in 6 hours if needed; maximum: 800 mg first 24 hours; begin oral dosage as soon as possible and continue for 3 days until 1.5 g has been given

Extraintestinal amebiasis:

Children: Oral: 10 mg/kg once daily for 2-3 weeks (up to 300 mg base/day)

Adults:

Oral: 600 mg base/day for 2 days followed by 300 mg base/day for at least 2-3 weeks

I.M., as hydrochloride: 160-200 mg/day for 10 days; resume oral therapy as soon as possible

Dosing adjustment in renal impairment: Cl_{cr} <10 mL/minute: Administer 50% of dose

Hemodialysis: Minimally removed by hemodialysis

Monitoring Parameters Periodic CBC, examination for muscular weakness, and ophthalmologic examination in patients receiving prolonged therapy

Patient Information Take with meals; report any visual disturbances or difficulty in hearing or ringing in the ears; tablets are bitter tasting; may cause diarrhea, loss of appetite, nausea, stomach pain; notify physician if these become severe

(Continued)

Chloroquine Phosphate *(Continued)*

Dosage Forms
Injection: 50 mg [40 mg base]/mL (5 mL)
Tablet: 250 mg [150 mg base]; 500 mg [300 mg base]

Extemporaneous Preparations A 10 mg chloroquine base/mL suspension is made by pulverizing two Aralen® 500 mg phosphate = 300 mg base/tablet, levigating with sterile water, and adding by geometric proportion, a significant amount of the cherry syrup and levigating until a uniform mixture is obtained; qs ad to 60 mL with cherry syrup, stable for up to 4 weeks when stored in the refrigerator or at a temperature of 29°C

Mirochnick M, Barnett E, Clarke DF, et al, "Stability of Chloroquine in an Extemporaneously Prepared Suspension Stored at Three Temperatures," *Pediatr Infect Dis J*, 1994, 13(9):827-8.

Selected Readings
Panisko DM and Keystone JS, "Treatment of Malaria - 1990," *Drugs*, 1990, 39(2):160-89.
White NJ, "The Treatment of Malaria," *N Engl J Med*, 1996, 335(11):800-6.
Wyler DJ, "Malaria Chemoprophylaxis for the Traveler," *N Engl J Med*, 1993, 329(1):31-7.
Wyler DJ, "Malaria: Overview and Update," *Clin Infect Dis*, 1993, 16(4):449-56.

Chlortetracycline *(klor tet ra SYE kleen)*

U.S. Brand Names Aureomycin®

Synonyms Chlortetracycline Hydrochloride

Generic Available Yes

Use
Ophthalmic: Treatment of superficial ocular infections involving the conjunctiva or cornea due to strains of susceptible microorganisms
Topical: Treatment of superficial infections of the skin due to susceptible organisms, also infection prophylaxis in minor skin abrasions

Pregnancy Risk Factor D

Contraindications Hypersensitivity to tetracycline or any component; do not use topical formulation in eyes

Warnings/Precautions Prolonged use may cause superinfection; ophthalmic ointments may retard corneal epithelial healing

Adverse Reactions
1% to 10%: Dermatologic: Faint yellowing of skin
<1%: Edema, reddening of skin, photosensitivity, irritation

Mechanism of Action Inhibits bacterial protein synthesis by binding with the 30S and possibly the 50S ribosomal subunit(s) of susceptible bacteria; may also cause alterations in the cytoplasmic membrane; usually bacteriostatic, may be bactericidal

Usual Dosage
Ophthalmic:
Acute infections: Instill ½" (1.25 cm) every 3-4 hours until improvement
Mild to moderate infections: Instill ½" (1.25 cm) 2-3 times/day
Topical: Apply 1-4 times/day, cover with sterile bandage if needed

Patient Information
For ophthalmic use, tilt head back, place medication in conjunctival sac and close eye, apply light finger pressure on lacrimal sac following instillation
Topical is for external use only, contact physician if rash or irritation develops, may stain clothing

Nursing Implications Cleanse affected area of skin prior to application unless otherwise directed

Dosage Forms
Ointment, as hydrochloride:
Ophthalmic: 1% [10 mg/g] (3.5 g)
Topical: 3% (14.2 g, 30 g)

Chlortetracycline Hydrochloride *see* Chlortetracycline *on this page*

Cholera Vaccine *(KOL er a vak SEEN)*

Generic Available No

Use The World Health Organization no longer recommends cholera vaccination for travel to or from cholera-endemic areas. Some countries may still require evidence of a complete primary series or a booster dose given within 6 months of arrival. Vaccination should not be considered as an alternative to continued careful selection of foods and water. Ideally, cholera and yellow fever vaccines should be administered at least 3 weeks apart.

Pregnancy Risk Factor C

Contraindications Presence of any acute illness, history of severe systemic reaction, or allergic response following a prior dose of cholera vaccine

Warnings/Precautions There is no data on the safety of cholera vaccination during pregnancy. Use in pregnancy should reflect actual increased risk. Persons who have had severe local or systemic reactions to a previous dose should not be revaccinated. Have epinephrine (1:1000) available for immediate use.

Adverse Reactions All serious adverse reactions must be reported to the U.S. Department of Health and Human Services (DHHS) Vaccine Adverse Event Reporting System (VAERS) 1-800-822-7967.

>10%:

Central nervous system: Malaise, fever, headache

Local: Pain, edema, tenderness, erythema, and induration at injection site

Drug Interactions Decreased effect with yellow fever vaccine; data suggests that giving both vaccines within 3 weeks of each other may decrease the response to both

Stability Refrigerate, avoid freezing

Mechanism of Action Inactivated vaccine producing active immunization

Usual Dosage

Children:

6 months to 4 years: Two 0.2 mL doses I.M./S.C. 1 week to 1 month apart; booster doses (0.2 mL I.M./S.C.) every 6 months

5-10 years: Two 0.3 mL doses I.M./S.C. or two 0.2 mL intradermal doses 1 week to 1 month apart; booster doses (0.3 mL I.M./S.C. or 0.2 mL I.D.) every 6 months

Children ≥10 years and Adults: Two 0.5 mL doses given I.M./S.C. or two 0.2 mL doses I.D. 1 week to 1 month apart; booster doses (0.5 mL I.M. or S.C. or 0.2 mL I.D.) every 6 months

Administration Do not administer I.V.

Patient Information Local reactions can occur up to 7 days after injection

Nursing Implications Defer immunization in individuals with moderate or severe febrile illness

Additional Information Inactivated bacteria vaccine

Dosage Forms Injection: Suspension of killed *Vibrio cholerae* (Inaba and Ogawa types) 8 units of each serotype per mL (1.5 mL, 20 mL)

Ciclopirox (sye kloe PEER oks)

U.S. Brand Names Loprox®

Synonyms Ciclopirox Olamine

Generic Available No

Use Treatment of tinea pedis (athlete's foot), tinea cruris (jock itch), tinea corporis (ringworm), cutaneous candidiasis, and tinea versicolor (pityriasis)

Pregnancy Risk Factor B

Contraindications Known hypersensitivity to ciclopirox or any of its components; avoid occlusive wrappings or dressings

Warnings/Precautions For external use only; avoid contact with eyes

Adverse Reactions 1% to 10%:

Dermatologic: Pruritus

Local: Irritation, redness, burning, or pain

Mechanism of Action Inhibiting transport of essential elements in the fungal cell causing problems in synthesis of DNA, RNA, and protein

Pharmacodynamics/Kinetics

Absorption: <2% absorbed through intact skin

Distribution: To epidermis, corium (dermis), including hair, hair follicles, and sebaceous glands

Protein binding: 94% to 98%

Half-life: 1.7 hours

Elimination: Of the small amounts of systemically absorbed drug, majority excreted by the kidney with small amounts excreted in feces

Usual Dosage Children >10 years and Adults: Apply twice daily, gently massage into affected areas; if no improvement after 4 weeks of treatment, re-evaluate the diagnosis

(Continued)

Ciclopirox *(Continued)*

Patient Information Avoid contact with eyes; if sensitivity or irritation occurs, discontinue use

Dosage Forms

Cream, topical, as olamine: 1% (15 g, 30 g, 90 g)

Lotion, as olamine: 1% (30 mL, 60 mL)

Ciclopirox Olamine *see* Ciclopirox *on previous page*

Cidofovir (si DOF o veer)

U.S. Brand Names Vistide®

Generic Available No

Use Treatment of cytomegalovirus (CMV) retinitis in patients with acquired immunodeficiency syndrome (AIDS). **Note:** Should be administered with probenecid.

Drug of Choice or Alternative for

Organism(s)

Cytomegalovirus *on page 122*

Pregnancy Risk Factor C

Pregnancy/Breast-Feeding Implications

Clinical effect on the fetus: Although studies are inconclusive, adenocarcinomas have occurred in animal studies with cidofovir; use during pregnancy only if the potential benefit justifies the potential risk to the fetus

Breast-feeding/lactation: Excretion of cidofovir into breast milk is unknown

Contraindications Patients with hypersensitivity to cidofovir and in patients with a history of clinically severe hypersensitivity to probenecid or other sulfa-containing medications

Warnings/Precautions Dose-dependent nephrotoxicity requires dose adjustment or discontinuation if changes in renal function occur during therapy (eg, proteinuria, glycosuria, decreased serum phosphate, uric acid or bicarbonate, and elevated creatinine); avoid use in patients with creatinine >1.5 mg/dL; Cl_{cr} <55 mL/minute; use great caution with elderly patients; neutropenia and ocular hypotony have also occurred; safety and efficacy have not been established in children; administration must be accompanied by oral probenecid and intravenous saline prehydration; prepare admixtures in a class two laminar flow hood, wearing protective gear; dispose of cidofovir as directed

Adverse Reactions

>10%:

Central nervous system: Infection, chills, fever, headache, amnesia, anxiety, confusion, seizures, insomnia

Dermatologic: Alopecia, rash, acne, skin discoloration

Gastrointestinal: Nausea, vomiting, diarrhea, anorexia, abdominal pain, constipation, dyspepsia, gastritis

Hematologic: Thrombocytopenia, neutropenia, anemia

Neuromuscular & skeletal: Weakness, paresthesia

Ocular: Amblyopia, conjunctivitis, ocular hypotony

Renal: Tubular damage, proteinuria, increased creatinine

Respiratory: Asthma, bronchitis, coughing, dyspnea, pharyngitis

1% to 10%:

Cardiovascular: Hypotension, pallor, syncope, tachycardia

Central nervous system: Dizziness, hallucinations, depression, somnolence, malaise

Dermatologic: Pruritus, urticaria

Endocrine & metabolic: Hyperglycemia, hyperlipidemia, hypocalcemia, hypokalemia, dehydration

Gastrointestinal: Abnormal taste, stomatitis

Genitourinary: Glycosuria, urinary incontinence, urinary tract infections

Neuromuscular & skeletal: Skeletal pain

Ocular: Retinal detachment, iritis, uveitis, abnormal vision

Renal: Hematuria

Respiratory: Pneumonia, rhinitis, sinusitis

Miscellaneous: Diaphoresis, allergic reactions

Overdosage/Toxicology No reports of acute toxicity have been reported, however, hemodialysis and hydration may reduce drug plasma concentrations; probenecid may assist in decreasing active tubular secretion

Drug Interactions Increased effect/toxicity: Drugs with nephrotoxic potential (eg, amphotericin B, aminoglycosides, foscarnet, and I.V. pentamidine) should be avoided during cidofovir therapy

Stability Store admixtures under refrigeration for ≤24 hours

Mechanism of Action Cidofovir is converted to cidofovir diphosphate which is the active intracellular metabolite; cidofovir diphosphate suppresses CMV replication by selective inhibition of viral DNA synthesis. Incorporation of cidofovir into growing viral DNA chain results in reductions in the rate of viral DNA synthesis.

Pharmacodynamics/Kinetics The following pharmacokinetic data is based on a combination of cidofovir administered with probenecid:

Distribution: V_d: 0.54 L/kg; does not cross significantly into the CSF

Protein binding: <6%

Metabolism: Minimal; phosphorylation occurs intracellularly

Half-life, plasma: ~2.6 hours

Elimination: Renal tubular secretion and glomerular filtration

Usual Dosage

Induction: 5 mg/kg I.V. over 1 hour once weekly for 2 consecutive weeks

Maintenance: 5 mg/kg over 1 hour once every other week

Administer with probenecid - 2 g orally 3 hours prior to each cidofovir dose and 1 g at 2 and 8 hours after completion of the infusion (total: 4 g)

Hydrate with 1 L of 0.9% NS I.V. prior to cidofovir infusion; a second liter may be administered over a 1- to 3-hour period immediately following infusion, if tolerated

Dosing adjustment in renal impairment:

Cl_{cr} 41-55 mL/minute: 2 mg/kg

Cl_{cr} 30-40 mL/minute: 1.5 mg/kg

Cl_{cr} 20-29 mL/minute: 1 mg/kg

Cl_{cr} <19 mL/minute: 0.5 mg/kg

If the creatinine increases by 0.3-0.4 mg/dL, reduce the cidofovir dose to 3 mg/kg; discontinue therapy for increases ≥0.5 mg/dL or development of ≥3+ proteinuria

Monitoring Parameters Renal function (Cr, BUN, UAs), LFTs, WBCs, intraocular pressure and visual acuity

Patient Information Cidofovir is not a cure for CMV retinitis; regular follow-up ophthalmologic exams and careful monitoring of renal function are necessary; probenecid must be administered concurrently with cidofovir; report rash immediately to your physician; avoid use during pregnancy; use contraception during and for 3 months following treatment

Nursing Implications Administration of probenecid with a meal may decrease associated nausea; acetaminophen and antihistamines may ameliorate hypersensitivity reactions; dilute in 100 mL 0.9% saline; administer probenecid and I.V. saline before each infusion; allow the admixture to come to room temperature before administration

Dosage Forms Injection: 75 mg/mL (5 mL)

Selected Readings

Akler ME, Johnson DW, Burman WJ, et al, "Anterior Uveitis and Hypotony After Intravenous Cidofovir for the Treatment of Cytomegalovirus Retinitis," *Ophthalmology*, 1998, 105(4):651-7.

Alrabiah FA and Sacks SL, "New Antiherpesvirus Agents. Their Targets

Garcia CR, Torriani FJ, and Freeman WR, "Cidofovir in the Treatment of Cytomegalovirus (CMV) Retinitis," *Ocul Immunol Inflamm*, 1998, 6(3):195-203.

Hitchcock MJ, Jaffe HS, Martin JC, et al, "Cidofovir, a New Agent With Potent Anti-Herpes Virus Activity," *Antiviral Chem Chemother*, 1996, 7:115-27.

Lalezari JP, Holland GN, Kramer F, et al, "Randomized, Controlled Study of the Safety and Efficacy of Intravenous Cidofovir for the Treatment of Relapsing Cytomegalovirus Retinitis in Patients With AIDS," *J Acquir Immune Defic Syndr Hum Retrovirol*, 1998, 17(4):339-44.

Lea AP and Bryson HM, "Cidofovir," *Drugs*, 1996, 52(2):225-30.

Taskintuna I, Rahhal FM, Capparelli EV, et al, "Intravitreal and Plasma Cidofovir Concentrations After Intravitreal and Intravenous Administration in AIDS Patients With Cytomegalovirus Retinitis," *J Ocul Pharmacol Ther*, 1998, 14(2):147-51.

Whitley RJ, Jacobson MA, Friedberg DN, et al, "Guidelines for the Treatment of Cytomegalovirus Diseases in Patients With AIDS in the Era of Potent Antiretroviral Therapy: Recommendations of an International Panel. International AIDS Society-USA," *Arch Intern Med*, 1998, 158(9):957-69.

Ciloxan™ Ophthalmic see Ciprofloxacin on next page

Cinobac® Pulvules® see Cinoxacin on next page

Cinoxacin (sin OKS a sin)

U.S. Brand Names Cinobac® Pulvules®

Generic Available No

Use Treatment of urinary tract infections

Pregnancy Risk Factor B

Contraindications History of convulsive disorders, hypersensitivity to cinoxacin or any component or other quinolones

Warnings/Precautions CNS stimulation may occur (tremor, restlessness, confusion, and very rarely hallucinations or seizures). Use with caution in patients with known or suspected CNS disorders or renal impairment. Not recommended in children <18 years of age, ciprofloxacin (a related compound), has caused a transient arthropathy in children; prolonged use may result in superinfection; modify dosage in patients with renal impairment.

Adverse Reactions Generally well tolerated

1% to 10%:
  Central nervous system: Headache, dizziness
  Gastrointestinal: Heartburn, abdominal pain, GI bleeding, belching, flatulence, anorexia, nausea

<1%: Insomnia, confusion, seizures (rare), diarrhea, thrombocytopenia, photophobia, tinnitus

Overdosage/Toxicology
Symptoms of overdose include acute renal failure, seizures
GI decontamination and supportive care; not removed by peritoneal or hemodialysis

Drug Interactions
Decreased effect: Decreased urine levels with probenecid; decreased absorption with aluminum-, magnesium-, calcium-containing antacids
Increased serum levels: Probenecid

Mechanism of Action Inhibits microbial synthesis of DNA with resultant inhibition of protein synthesis

Pharmacodynamics/Kinetics
Absorption: Oral: Rapid and complete; food decreases peak levels by 30% but not total amount absorbed
Distribution: Crosses the placenta; concentrates in prostate tissue
Protein binding: 60% to 80%
Half-life: 1.5 hours, prolonged in renal impairment
Time to peak serum concentration: Oral: Within 2-3 hours
Elimination: ~60% excreted as unchanged drug in urine

Usual Dosage Children >12 years and Adults: Oral: 1 g/day in 2-4 doses for 7-14 days

Dosing interval in renal impairment:
Cl_{cr} 20-50 mL/minute: 250 mg twice daily
Cl_{cr} <20 mL/minute: 250 mg/day

Patient Information May be taken with food to minimize upset stomach; avoid antacid use; drink fluid liberally; may cause dizziness; use caution when driving or performing other tasks requiring alertness

Nursing Implications Hold antacids for 3-4 hours after giving

Dosage Forms Capsule: 250 mg, 500 mg

Cipro™ see Ciprofloxacin on page 678

Ciprofloxacin (sip roe FLOKS a sin)

Related Information
Antimicrobial Activity Against Selected Organisms on page 983
Tuberculosis Guidelines on page 1114

U.S. Brand Names Ciloxan™ Ophthalmic; Cipro™; Cipro™ I.V.

Synonyms Ciprofloxacin Hydrochloride

Generic Available No

Use Treatment of documented or suspected infections of the lower respiratory tract, sinuses, skin and skin structure, bone/joints, and urinary tract including prostatitis due to susceptible bacterial strains; especially indicated for pseudomonal infections and those due to multidrug-resistant gram-negative organisms, chronic bacterial prostatitis, infectious diarrhea, complicated gramnegative and anaerobic intra-abdominal infections (with metronidazole) due to *E. coli* (enteropathic strains), *B. fragilis*, *P. mirabilis*, *K. pneumoniae*, *P. aeruginosa*,

Campylobacter jejuni or *Shigella*; approved for acute sinusitis caused by *H. influenzae* or *M. catarrhalis*; also used to treat typhoid fever due to *Salmonella typhi* (although eradication of the chronic typhoid carrier state has not been proven), osteomyelitis when parenteral therapy is not feasible, and sexually transmitted diseases such as uncomplicated cervical and urethral gonorrhea due to *Neisseria gonorrhoeae*; used ophthalmologically for superficial ocular infections (corneal ulcers, conjunctivitis) due to susceptible strains

Drug of Choice or Alternative for

Disease/Syndrome(s)

Cholangitis, Acute *on page 21*
Otitis Externa, Severe (Malignant) *on page 40*
Pelvic Inflammatory Disease *on page 41*

Organism(s)

Burkholderia cepacia on page 87
Haemophilus ducreyi on page 156
Legionella pneumophila on page 185
Mycobacterium avium-intracellulare on page 201
Neisseria gonorrhoeae on page 215
Pseudomonas aeruginosa on page 235
Rickettsia rickettsii on page 243
Salmonella Species on page 245
Shigella Species on page 251

Pregnancy Risk Factor C

Contraindications Hypersensitivity to ciprofloxacin, any component or other quinolones

Warnings/Precautions Not recommended in children <18 years of age; has caused transient arthropathy in children; CNS stimulation may occur (tremor, restlessness, confusion, and very rarely hallucinations or seizures); use with caution in patients with known or suspected CNS disorder; green discoloration of teeth in newborns has been reported; prolonged use may result in superinfection; may rarely cause inflamed or ruptured tendons (discontinue use immediately with signs of inflammation or tendon pain)

Adverse Reactions

1% to 10%:
Central nervous system: Headache, restlessness
Gastrointestinal: Nausea, diarrhea, vomiting, abdominal pain
Dermatologic: Rash
<1%: Dizziness, confusion, seizures, anemia, increased liver enzymes, tremor, arthralgia, ruptured tendons, acute renal failure

Overdosage/Toxicology

Symptoms of overdose include acute renal failure, seizures
GI decontamination and supportive care; not removed by peritoneal or hemodialysis

Drug Interactions CYP1A2 enzyme inhibitor

Decreased effect:

Enteral feedings may decrease plasma concentrations of ciprofloxacin probably by >30% inhibition of absorption. Ciprofloxacin should not be administered with enteral feedings. The feeding would need to be discontinued for 1-2 hours prior to and after ciprofloxacin administration. Nasogastric administration produces a greater loss of ciprofloxacin bioavailability than does nasoduodenal administration.

Aluminum/magnesium products, didanosine, and sucralfate may decrease absorption of ciprofloxacin by ≥90% if administered concurrently

RECOMMENDATION: Administer ciprofloxacin 2 hours before dose **or** administer ciprofloxacin at least 4 hours and preferably 6 hours after the dose of these agents **or** change to an H_2 antagonist or omeprazole

Calcium, iron, zinc, and multivitamins with minerals products may decrease absorption of ciprofloxacin significantly if administered concurrently

RECOMMENDATION: Administer ciprofloxacin 2 hours before dose **or** administer ciprofloxacin at least 2 hours after the dose of these agents

Increased toxicity:

Caffeine and theophylline → CNS stimulation when concurrent with ciprofloxacin

Cyclosporine may increase serum creatinine levels

Stability Refrigeration and room temperature: Prepared bags: 14 days; Premixed bags: Manufacturer expiration dating

(Continued)

Ciprofloxacin *(Continued)*

Mechanism of Action Inhibits DNA-gyrase in susceptible organisms; inhibits relaxation of supercoiled DNA and promotes breakage of double-stranded DNA

Pharmacodynamics/Kinetics

Absorption: Oral: Rapid from GI tract (~50% to 85%)

Distribution: Crosses the placenta; appears in breast milk; distributes widely throughout body; tissue concentrations often exceed serum concentrations especially in the kidneys, gallbladder, liver, lungs, gynecological tissue, and prostatic tissue; CSF concentrations reach 10% with noninflamed meninges and 14% to 37% with inflamed meninges

Protein binding: 16% to 43%

Metabolism: Partially metabolized in the liver

Half-life:

Children: 2.5 hours

Adults with normal renal function: 3-5 hours

Time to peak: Oral: T_{max}: 0.5-2 hours

Elimination: 30% to 50% excreted as unchanged drug in urine; 20% to 40% of dose excreted in feces primarily from biliary excretion

Usual Dosage

Children (see Warnings/Precautions):

Oral: 20-30 mg/kg/day in 2 divided doses; maximum: 1.5 g/day

Cystic fibrosis: 20-40 mg/kg/day divided every 12 hours

I.V.: 15-20 mg/kg/day divided every 12 hours

Cystic fibrosis: 15-30 mg/kg/day divided every 8-12 hours

Adults: Oral:

Urinary tract infection: 250-500 mg every 12 hours for 7-10 days, depending on severity of infection and susceptibility; (3 investigations (n=975) indicate the minimum effective dose for women with acute, uncomplicated urinary tract infection may be 100 mg twice daily for 3 days)

Lower respiratory tract, skin/skin structure infections: 500-750 mg twice daily for 7-14 days depending on severity and susceptibility

Bone/joint infections: 500-750 mg twice daily for 4-6 weeks, depending on severity and susceptibility

Infectious diarrhea: 500 mg every 12 hours for 5-7 days

Typhoid fever: 500 mg every 12 hours for 10 days

Urethral/cervical gonococcal infections: 250-500 mg as a single dose (CDC recommends concomitant doxycycline or azithromycin due to developing resistance; avoid use in Asian or Western Pacific travelers)

Disseminated gonococcal infection: 500 mg twice daily to complete 7 days of therapy (initial treatment with ceftriaxone 1 g I.M./I.V. daily for 24-48 hours after improvement begins)

Chancroid: 500 mg twice daily for 3 days

Mild to moderate sinusitis: 500 mg every 12 hours for 10 days

Adults: I.V.

Urinary tract infection: 200-400 mg every 12 hours for 7-10 days

Lower respiratory tract, skin/skin structure infection (mild to moderate): 400 mg every 12 hours for 7-14 days

Ophthalmic: Instill 1-2 drops in eye(s) every 2 hours while awake for 2 days and 1-2 drops every 4 hours while awake for the next 5 days

Dosing adjustment in renal impairment:

Cl_{cr} <30 mL/minute:

500 mg every 24 hours or

750 mg every 24 hours

Dialysis: Only small amounts of ciprofloxacin are removed by hemo- or peritoneal dialysis (<10%); usual dose: 250-500 mg every 24 hours following dialysis

Continuous arteriovenous or venovenous hemodiafiltration (CAVH) effects: Administer 200-400 mg I.V. every 12 hours

Dietary Considerations

Food: Decreases rate, but not extent, of absorption. Drug may cause GI upset; take without regard to meals (manufacturer prefers that drug is taken 2 hours after meals).

Dairy products, oral multivitamins, and mineral supplements: Absorption decreased by divalent and trivalent cations. These cations bind to and form insoluble complexes with quinolones. Avoid taking these substrates with ciprofloxacin. The manufacturer states that the usual dietary intake of calcium has not been shown to interfere with ciprofloxacin absorption.

Caffeine: Possible exaggerated or prolonged effects of caffeine. Ciprofloxacin reduces total body clearance of caffeine. Patients consuming regular large quantities of caffeinated beverages may need to restrict caffeine intake if excessive cardiac or CNS stimulation occurs.

Administration

Oral: May administer with food to minimize GI upset; avoid antacid use; drink plenty of fluids to maintain proper hydration and urine output

Parenteral: Administer by slow I.V. infusion over 60 minutes to reduce the risk of venous irritation (burning, pain, erythema, and swelling); final concentration for administration should not exceed 2 mg/mL

Monitoring Parameters Patients receiving concurrent ciprofloxacin, theophylline, or cyclosporine should have serum levels monitored

Reference Range Therapeutic: 2.6-3 µg/mL; Toxic: >5 µg/mL

Patient Information May be taken with food to minimize upset stomach; avoid antacids containing magnesium or aluminum, or products containing zinc or iron within 4 hours before or 2 hours after dosing; may cause dizziness or drowsiness; drink fluid liberally; consult your physician immediately if inflammation or tendon pain develop

Nursing Implications Hold antacids for 2 hours after giving

Dosage Forms

Infusion, as hydrochloride, in D_5W: 400 mg (200 mL)

Infusion, as hydrochloride, in NS or D_5W: 200 mg (100 mL)

Injection, as hydrochloride: 200 mg (20 mL); 400 mg (40 mL)

Solution, ophthalmic, as hydrochloride: 3.5 mg/mL (2.5 mL, 5 mL)

Suspension, oral, as hydrochloride: 250 mg/5 mL x 100 mL, 500 mg/5 mL x 100 mL

Tablet, as hydrochloride: 100 mg, 250 mg, 500 mg, 750 mg

Selected Readings

Davis R, Markham A, and Balfour JA, "Ciprofloxacin. An Updated Review of Its Pharmacology, Therapeutic Efficacy and Tolerability," *Drugs*, 1996, 51(6):1019-74.

Hooper DC and Wolfson JS, "Fluoroquinolone Antimicrobial Agents," *N Engl J Med*, 1991, 324(6):384-94.

Lomaestro BM and Bailie GR, "Quinolone-Cation Interactions: A Review," *DICP*, 1991, 25(11):1249-58.

Sanders CC, "Ciprofloxacin: *In Vitro* Activity, Mechanism of Action, and Resistance," *Rev Infect Dis*, 1988, 10(3):516-27.

Stein GE, "The 4-Quinolone Antibiotics: Past, Present, and Future," *Pharmacotherapy*, 1988, 8(6):301-14.

Walker RC and Wright AJ, "The Fluoroquinolones," *Mayo Clin Proc*, 1991, 66(12):1249-59.

Ciprofloxacin and Hydrocortisone

(sip roe FLOKS a sin & hye droe KOR ti sone)

Related Information

Ciprofloxacin *on page 678*

U.S. Brand Names Cipro® HC Otic

Use Treatment of acute otitis externa, sometimes known as "swimmer's ear"

Usual Dosage Children >1 year of age and Adults: Otic: The recommended dosage for all patients is 3 drops of the suspension in the affected ear twice daily for 7 days; twice-daily dosing schedule is more convenient for patients than that of existing treatments with hydrocortisone, which are typically administered three or four times a day; a twice-daily dosage schedule may be especially helpful for parents and caregivers of young children

Dosage Forms Suspension, otic: Ciprofloxacin hydrochloride 0.2% and hydrocortisone 1%

Ciprofloxacin Hydrochloride see Ciprofloxacin *on page 678*

Cipro® HC Otic see Ciprofloxacin and Hydrocortisone *on this page*

Cipro™ I.V. see Ciprofloxacin *on page 678*

Cla see Clarithromycin *on this page*

Claforan® see Cefotaxime *on page 642*

Clarithromycin (kla RITH roe mye sin)

Related Information

Antimicrobial Activity Against Selected Organisms *on page 983*

U.S. Brand Names Biaxin™

(Continued)

Clarithromycin *(Continued)*

Synonyms Cla

Generic Available No

Use In adults, for treatment of pharyngitis/tonsillitis, acute maxillary sinusitis, acute exacerbation of chronic bronchitis, pneumonia, uncomplicated skin/skin structure infections due to susceptible *S. pyogenes*, *S. pneumoniae*, *S. agalactiae*, viridans *Streptococcus*, *M. catarrhalis*, *C. trachomatis*, *Legionella* sp, *Mycoplasma pneumoniae*, *S. aureus*, *H. influenzae*; has activity against *M. avium* and *M. intracellulare* infection and is indicated for treatment of and prevention of disseminated mycobacterial infections due to *M. avium* complex disease (eg, patients with advanced HIV infection); indicated for the treatment of duodenal ulcer disease due to *H. pylori* in regimens with other drugs including amoxicillin and lansoprazole or omeprazole, ranitidine, bismuth citrate, bismuth subsalicylate, tetracycline and/or an H_2 antagonist (see index); also indicated for prophylaxis of bacterial endocarditis in patients who are allergic to penicillin and undergoing surgical or dental procedures

In children, for treatment of pharyngitis/tonsillitis, acute maxillary sinusitis, acute otitis media, uncomplicated skin/skin structure infections due to the above organisms; also for treatment of and prevention of disseminated mycobacterial infections due to *M. avium* complex disease (eg, patients with advanced HIV infection)

Exhibits the same spectrum of *in vitro* activity as erythromycin, but with significantly increased potency against those organisms

Drug of Choice or Alternative for

Disease/Syndrome(s)

Pneumonia, Community-Acquired *on page 45*

Sinusitis, Community-Acquired, Acute *on page 48*

Organism(s)

Legionella pneumophila on page 185

Moraxella catarrhalis on page 196

Mycobacterium avium-intracellulare on page 201

Mycoplasma pneumoniae on page 211

Ureaplasma urealyticum on page 292

Pregnancy Risk Factor C

Contraindications Hypersensitivity to clarithromycin, erythromycin, or any macrolide antibiotic; use with pimozide, astemizole, cisapride, terfenadine

Warnings/Precautions In presence of severe renal impairment with or without coexisting hepatic impairment, decreased dosage or prolonged dosing interval may be appropriate; antibiotic-associated colitis has been reported with use of clarithromycin; elderly patients have experienced increased incidents of adverse effects due to known age-related decreases in renal function

Adverse Reactions

1% to 10%:

Central nervous system: Headache

Gastrointestinal: Diarrhea, nausea, abnormal taste, dyspepsia, abdominal pain

<1%: Ventricular tachycardia; torsade de pointes; neutropenia; leukopenia; prolonged PT; increased AST, alkaline phosphatase, bilirubin, BUN, and serum creatinine; manic behavior; tremor; hypoglycemia

Overdosage/Toxicology

Symptoms of overdose include nausea, vomiting, diarrhea, prostration, reversible pancreatitis, hearing loss with or without tinnitus or vertigo

Treatment includes symptomatic and supportive care

Drug Interactions CYP3A3/4 enzyme substrate; CYP1A2 and 3A3/4 enzyme inhibitor

Increased levels:

Clarithromycin increases serum theophylline levels by as much as 20%

Significantly increases carbamazepine, cyclosporine, digoxin, ergot alkaloid, tacrolimus, omeprazole, and triazolam levels

Peak levels (but not AUC) of zidovudine are often increased; terfenadine and astemizole should be avoided with use of clarithromycin since plasma levels may be increased by more than 3 times; serious arrhythmias have occurred with cisapride and other drugs which inhibit cytochrome P-450 3A4 (eg, clarithromycin)

Fluconazole increases clarithromycin levels and AUC by ~25%; death has been reported with administration of pimozide and clarithromycin

Increases concentration of HMG-CoA reductase inhibitors (lovastatin and simvastatin)

Note: While other drug interactions (bromocriptine, disopyramide, lovastatin, phenytoin, and valproate) known to occur with erythromycin have not been reported in clinical trials with clarithromycin, concurrent use of these drugs should be monitored closely

Stability Reconstituted oral suspension should not be refrigerated because it might gel; microencapsulated particles of clarithromycin in suspension is stable for 14 days when stored at room temperature

Mechanism of Action Exerts its antibacterial action by binding to 50S ribosomal subunit resulting in inhibition of protein synthesis. The 14-OH metabolite of clarithromycin is twice as active as the parent compound against certain organisms.

Pharmacodynamics/Kinetics

Absorption: Highly stable in the presence of gastric acid (unlike erythromycin)

Distribution: Widely distributes into most body tissues with the exception of the CNS

Metabolism: Partially converted to the microbiologically active metabolite, 14-OH clarithromycin

Bioavailability: 50%; food delays but does not affect extent of bioavailability; T_{max}: 2-4 hours

Half-life: 5-7 hours

Elimination: Primarily renal excretion; clearance approximates normal GFR

Usual Dosage Safe use in children has not been established

Children ≥6 months: 15 mg/kg/day divided every 12 hours; dosages of 7.5 mg/kg twice daily up to 500 mg twice daily children with AIDS and disseminated MAC infection

Adults: Oral: Usual dose: 250-500 mg every 12 hours for 7-14 days

Upper respiratory tract: 250-500 mg every 12 hours for 10-14 days
Pharyngitis/tonsillitis: 250 mg every 12 hours for 10 days
Acute maxillary sinusitis: 500 mg every 12 hours for 14 days

Lower respiratory tract: 250-500 mg every 12 hours for 7-14 days
Acute exacerbation of chronic bronchitis due to:
M. catarrhalis and S. pneumoniae: 250 mg every 12 hours for 7-14 days
H. influenzae: 500 mg every 12 hours for 7-14 days
Pneumonia due to M. pneumoniae and S. pneumoniae: 250 mg every 12 hours for 7-14 days
Mycobacterial infection (prevention and treatment): 500 mg twice daily (use with other antimycobacterial drugs, eg, ethambutol, clofazimine, or rifampin)

Prophylaxis of bacterial endocarditis: 500 mg 1 hour prior to procedure

Uncomplicated skin and skin structure: 250 mg every 12 hours for 7-14 days

Helicobacter pylori: In combination regimen with bismuth subsalicylate, tetracycline, and an H_2-receptor antagonist; or in combination with omeprazole (and possibly metronidazole or amoxicillin) or ranitidine bismuth citrate (Tritec®) (and possibly tetracycline or amoxicillin or lansoprazole and amoxicillin): 250 mg twice daily to 500 mg 3 times/day (for first 2 weeks only of regimen with Tritec® or omeprazole)

Dosing adjustment in renal impairment: Adults: Oral:
Cl_{cr} <30 mL/minute: 500 mg loading dose, then 250 mg once or twice daily

Dosing adjustment in severe renal impairment: Decreased doses or prolonged dosing intervals are recommended

Patient Information May be taken with meals; finish all medication; do not skip doses; do not refrigerate oral suspension, more palatable when taken at room temperature

Dosage Forms

Granules for oral suspension: 125 mg/5 mL (50 mL, 100 mL); 250 mg/5 mL (50 mL, 100 mL)

Tablet, film coated: 250 mg, 500 mg

Selected Readings

Amsden GW, "Erythromycin, Clarithromycin, and Azithromycin: Are the Differences Real?" Clin Ther, 1996, 18(1):56-72.

(Continued)

LIVERPOOL JOHN MOORES UNIVERSITY
LEARNING SERVICES

Clarithromycin *(Continued)*

Barradell LB, Plosker GL, and McTavish D, "Clarithromycin. A Review of Its Pharmacological Properties and Therapeutic Use in *Mycobacterium avium-intracellulare* Complex Infection in Patients With Acquired Immune Deficiency Syndrome," *Drugs*, 1993, 46(2):289-312.

Goldman MP and Longworth DL, "The Role of Azithromycin and Clarithromycin in Clinical Practice," *Cleve Clin J Med*, 1993, 60(5):359-64.

Langtry HD and Brogden RN, "Clarithromycin. A Review of Its Efficacy in the Treatment of Respiratory Tract Infections in Immunocompetent Patients," *Drugs*, 1997, 53(6):973-1004.

Tartaglione TA, "Therapeutic Options for the Management and Prevention of *Mycobacterium avium* Complex Infection in Patients With the Acquired Immunodeficiency Syndrome," *Pharmacotherapy*, 1996, 16(2):171-82.

Zuckerman JM and Kaye KM, "The Newer Macrolides. Azithromycin and Clarithromycin," *Infect Dis Clin North Am*, 1995, 9(3):731-45.

Clavulin® *see* Amoxicillin and Clavulanate Potassium *on page 593*

Cleocin HCl® *see* Clindamycin *on this page*

Cleocin Pediatric® *see* Clindamycin *on this page*

Cleocin Phosphate® *see* Clindamycin *on this page*

Cleocin T® *see* Clindamycin *on this page*

Clinda-Derm® Topical Solution *see* Clindamycin *on this page*

Clindamycin (klin da MYE sin)

Related Information

Antimicrobial Activity Against Selected Organisms *on page 983*

U.S. Brand Names Cleocin HCl®; Cleocin Pediatric®; Cleocin Phosphate®; Cleocin T®; Clinda-Derm® Topical Solution; C/T/S® Topical Solution

Canadian Brand Names Dalacin® C [Hydrochloride]

Synonyms Clindamycin Hydrochloride; Clindamycin Phosphate

Generic Available Yes: Injection

Use Treatment against aerobic and anaerobic streptococci (except enterococci), most staphylococci, *Bacteroides* sp and *Actinomyces*; used topically in treatment of severe acne, vaginally for *Gardnerella vaginalis*, alternate treatment for toxoplasmosis; prophylaxis in the prevention of bacterial endocarditis in high-risk patients undergoing surgical or dental procedures in patients allergic to penicillin; may be useful in PCP

Drug of Choice or Alternative for

Disease/Syndrome(s)

Brain Abscess *on page 19*

Osteomyelitis, Diabetic Foot *on page 38*

Osteomyelitis, Healthy Adult *on page 39*

Osteomyelitis, Pediatric *on page 39*

Pelvic Inflammatory Disease *on page 41*

Pneumonia, Aspiration, Community-Acquired *on page 44*

Sinusitis, Community-Acquired, Chronic *on page 49*

Skin and Soft Tissue *on page 50*

Vaginosis, Bacterial *on page 54*

Organism(s)

Babesia microti on page 71

Bacteroides Species *on page 75*

Clostridium perfringens on page 105

Gardnerella vaginalis on page 151

Mycoplasma hominis and *Mycoplasma genitalium on page 210*

Staphylococcus aureus, Methicillin-Susceptible *on page 258*

Staphylococcus epidermidis, Methicillin-Susceptible *on page 263*

Streptococcus-Related Gram-Positive Cocci *on page 278*

Toxoplasma gondii on page 283

Pregnancy Risk Factor B

Contraindications Hypersensitivity to clindamycin or any component; previous pseudomembranous colitis, hepatic impairment

Warnings/Precautions Dosage adjustment may be necessary in patients with severe hepatic dysfunction; can cause severe and possibly fatal colitis; use with caution in patients with a history of pseudomembranous colitis; discontinue drug if significant diarrhea, abdominal cramps, or passage of blood and mucus occurs

Adverse Reactions

>10%: Gastrointestinal: Diarrhea

1% to 10%:

Dermatologic: Rashes

Gastrointestinal: Pseudomembranous colitis (more common with oral form), nausea, vomiting

<1%: Hypotension, urticaria, Stevens-Johnson syndrome, eosinophilia, neutropenia, granulocytopenia, thrombocytopenia, elevation of liver enzymes, thrombophlebitis, sterile abscess at I.M. injection site, polyarthritis, rare renal dysfunction

Overdosage/Toxicology

Symptoms of overdose include diarrhea, nausea, vomiting; following GI decontamination

Treatment is supportive

Drug Interactions CYP3A3/4 enzyme substrate

Increased duration of neuromuscular blockade from tubocurarine, pancuronium

Stability Do not refrigerate reconstituted oral solution because it will thicken; oral solution is stable for 2 weeks at room temperature following reconstitution; I.V. infusion solution in NS or D_5W solution is stable for 16 days at room temperature

Mechanism of Action Reversibly binds to 50S ribosomal subunits preventing peptide bond formation thus inhibiting bacterial protein synthesis; bacteriostatic or bactericidal depending on drug concentration, infection site, and organism

Pharmacodynamics/Kinetics

Absorption: ~10% of topically applied drug is absorbed systemically; 90% absorbed rapidly from GI tract following oral administration

Distribution: No significant levels are seen in CSF, even with inflamed meninges; crosses the placenta; distributes into breast milk; high concentrations in bone and urine

Metabolism: Hepatic

Half-life:

Neonates:

Premature: 8.7 hours

Full-term: 3.6 hours

Adults: 1.6-5.3 hours, average: 2-3 hours

Time to peak serum concentration:

Oral: Within 60 minutes

I.M.: Within 1-3 hours

Elimination: Most of drug eliminated by hepatic metabolism

Usual Dosage Avoid in neonates (contains benzyl alcohol)

Infants and Children:

Oral: 8-20 mg/kg/day as hydrochloride; 8-25 mg/kg/day as palmitate in 3-4 divided doses; minimum dose of palmitate: 37.5 mg 3 times/day

I.M., I.V.:

<1 month: 15-20 mg/kg/day

>1 month: 20-40 mg/kg/day in 3-4 divided doses

Children and Adults: Topical: Apply a thin film twice daily

Adults:

Oral: 150-450 mg/dose every 6-8 hours; maximum dose: 1.8 g/day

I.M., I.V.: 1.2-1.8 g/day in 2-4 divided doses; maximum dose: 4.8 g/day

Bacterial endocarditis prophylaxis: 600 mg 1 hour prior to the procedure

Pelvic inflammatory disease: I.V.: 900 mg every 8 hours with gentamicin 2 mg/kg, then 1.5 mg/kg every 8 hours; continue after discharge with doxycycline 100 mg twice daily or oral clindamycin 450 mg 5 times/day for 10-14 days

Pneumocystis carinii pneumonia:

Oral: 300-450 mg 4 times/day with primaquine

I.M., I.V.: 1200-2400 mg/day with pyrimethamine

I.V.: 600 mg 4 times/day with primaquine

Vaginal: One full applicator (100 mg) inserted intravaginally once daily before bedtime for 3 or 7 consecutive days

Dosing adjustment in hepatic impairment: Adjustment recommended in patients with severe hepatic disease

Administration Administer oral dosage form with a full glass of water to minimize esophageal ulceration

Monitoring Parameters Observe for changes in bowel frequency, monitor for colitis and resolution of symptoms; during prolonged therapy monitor CBC, liver and renal function tests periodically

Patient Information Report any severe diarrhea immediately and do not take antidiarrheal medication; take each oral dose with a full glass of water; finish all medication; do not skip doses; should not engage in sexual intercourse during (Continued)

Clindamycin *(Continued)*

treatment with vaginal product; avoid contact of topical gel/solution with eyes, abraded skin, or mucous membranes

Dosage Forms

Capsule, as hydrochloride: 75 mg, 150 mg, 300 mg

Cream, vaginal: 2% (40 g)

Gel, topical, as phosphate: 1% [10 mg/g] (7.5 g, 30 g)

Granules for oral solution, as palmitate: 75 mg/5 mL (100 mL)

Infusion, as phosphate, in D_5W: 300 mg (50 mL); 600 mg (50 mL)

Injection, as phosphate: 150 mg/mL (2 mL, 4 mL, 6 mL, 50 mL, 60 mL)

Lotion: 1% [10 mg/mL] (60 mL)

Pledgets: 1%

Solution, topical, as phosphate: 1% [10 mg/mL] (30 mL, 60 mL, 480 mL)

Selected Readings

Falagas ME and Gorbach SL, "Clindamycin and Metronidazole," *Med Clin North Am*, 1995, 79(4):845-67.

Smilack JD, Wilson WR, and Cockerill FR 3d, "Tetracyclines, Chloramphenicol, Erythromycin, Clindamycin, and Metronidazole," *Mayo Clin Proc*, 1991, 66(12):1270-80.

Clindamycin Hydrochloride *see* Clindamycin *on page 684*

Clindamycin Phosphate *see* Clindamycin *on page 684*

Clioquinol *(klye oh KWIN ole)*

U.S. Brand Names Vioform® [OTC]

Canadian Brand Names Clioquinol®

Synonyms Iodochlorhydroxyquin

Generic Available Yes: Cream

Use Topically in the treatment of tinea pedis, tinea cruris, and skin infections caused by dermatophytic fungi (ringworm)

Pregnancy Risk Factor C

Contraindications Not effective in the treatment of scalp or nail fungal infections; children <2 years of age, hypersensitivity to any component

Warnings/Precautions May irritate sensitized skin; topical application poses a potential risk of toxicity to infants and children; known to cause serious and irreversible optic atrophy and peripheral neuropathy with muscular weakness, sensory loss, spastic paraparesis, and blindness; use with caution in patients with iodine intolerance

Adverse Reactions 1% to 10%:

Dermatologic: Skin irritation, rash

Neuromuscular & skeletal: Peripheral neuropathy

Ocular: Optic atrophy

Mechanism of Action Chelates bacterial surface and trace metals needed for bacterial growth

Pharmacodynamics/Kinetics

Absorption: With an occlusive dressing, up to 40% of dose can be absorbed systemically during a 12-hour period; absorption is enhanced when applied under diapers

Half-life: 11-14 hours

Elimination: Conjugated and excreted in urine

Usual Dosage Children and Adults: Topical: Apply 2-3 times/day; do not use for longer than 7 days

Test Interactions Thyroid function tests (decreased ^{131}I uptake); false-positive ferric chloride test for phenylketonuria

Patient Information Cleanse affected area before application; can stain skin and fabrics; for external use only; avoid contact with eyes and mucous membranes

Nursing Implications Watch affected area for increased irritation

Dosage Forms

Cream: 3% (30 g)

Ointment, topical: 3% (30 g)

Selected Readings

American Academy of Pediatrics Committee on Drugs, "Clioquinol (Iodochlorhydroxyquin, Vioform®) and Iodoquinol (Diiodohydroxyquin): Blindness and Neuropathy," *Pediatrics*, 1990, 86(5):797-8.

Clioquinol® *see* Clioquinol *on this page*

Clioquinol and Hydrocortisone

(klye oh KWIN ole & hye droe KOR ti sone)

Related Information

Clioquinol *on previous page*

U.S. Brand Names Corque® Topical; Pedi-Cort V® Creme

Use Contact or atopic dermatitis; eczema; neurodermatitis; anogenital pruritus; mycotic dermatoses; moniliasis

Usual Dosage Apply in a thin film 3-4 times/day

Dosage Forms Cream: Clioquinol 3% and hydrocortisone 1% (20 g)

Clofazimine (kloe FA zi meen)

Related Information

Tuberculosis Guidelines *on page 1114*

U.S. Brand Names Lamprene®

Synonyms Clofazimine Palmitate

Generic Available No

Use Orphan drug: Treatment of dapsone-resistant leprosy; multibacillary dapsone-sensitive leprosy; erythema nodosum leprosum; *Mycobacterium avium-intracellulare* (MAI) infections

Drug of Choice or Alternative for Organism(s)

Mycobacterium avium-intracellulare on page 201

Pregnancy Risk Factor C

Contraindications Hypersensitivity to clofazimine or any component

Warnings/Precautions Use with caution in patients with GI problems; dosages >100 mg/day should be used for as short a duration as possible; skin discoloration may lead to depression

Adverse Reactions

>10%:

Dermatologic: Dry skin

Gastrointestinal: Abdominal pain, nausea, vomiting, diarrhea

Miscellaneous: Pink to brownish black discoloration of the skin and conjunctiva

1% to 10%:

Dermatologic: Rash, pruritus

Endocrine & metabolic: Elevated blood sugar

Gastrointestinal: Fecal discoloration

Genitourinary: Discoloration of urine

Ocular: Irritation of the eyes

Miscellaneous: Discoloration of sputum, sweat

<1%: Edema, vascular pain, dizziness, drowsiness, fatigue, headache, giddiness, taste disorder, fever, erythroderma, acneiform eruptions, monilial cheilosis, phototoxicity, hypokalemia, bowel obstruction, GI bleeding, anorexia, constipation, weight loss, eosinophilic enteritis, cystitis, eosinophilia, anemia, hepatitis, jaundice, enlarged liver, increased albumin, bilirubin, and AST, bone pain, neuralgia, diminished vision, lymphadenopathy

Overdosage/Toxicology Following GI decontamination, treatment is supportive

Drug Interactions Decreased effect with dapsone (unconfirmed)

Mechanism of Action Binds preferentially to mycobacterial DNA to inhibit mycobacterial growth; also has some anti-inflammatory activity through an unknown mechanism

Pharmacodynamics/Kinetics

Absorption: Oral: 45% to 70% absorbed slowly

Distribution: Remains in tissues for prolonged periods; appears in breast milk; highly lipophilic; deposited primarily in fatty tissue and cells of the reticuloendothelial system; taken up by macrophages throughout the body; also distributed to breast milk, mesenteric lymph nodes, adrenal glands, subcutaneous fat, liver, bile, gallbladder, spleen, small intestine, muscles, bones, and skin; does not appear to cross blood-brain barrier

Metabolism: Partially in the liver to two metabolites

Half-life:

Terminal: 8 days

Tissue: 70 days

Time to peak serum concentration: 1-6 hours with chronic therapy

(Continued)

Clofazimine *(Continued)*

Elimination: Mainly in feces; negligible amounts excreted unchanged in urine; small amounts excreted in sputum, saliva, and sweat

Usual Dosage Oral:

Children: Leprosy: 1 mg/kg/day every 24 hours in combination with dapsone and rifampin

Adults:

Dapsone-resistant leprosy: 100 mg/day in combination with one or more antileprosy drugs for 3 years; then alone 100 mg/day

Dapsone-sensitive multibacillary leprosy: 100 mg/day in combination with two or more antileprosy drugs for at least 2 years and continue until negative skin smears are obtained, then institute single drug therapy with appropriate agent

Erythema nodosum leprosum: 100-200 mg/day for up to 3 months or longer then taper dose to 100 mg/day when possible

Pyoderma gangrenosum: 300-400 mg/day for up to 12 months

Dosing adjustment in hepatic impairment: Should be considered in severe hepatic dysfunction

Patient Information Drug may cause a pink to brownish-black discoloration of the skin, conjunctiva, tears, sweat, urine, feces, and nasal secretions; although reversible, may take months to years to disappear after therapy is complete; take with meals

Dosage Forms Capsule, as palmitate: 50 mg

Selected Readings

"Drugs for AIDS and Associated Infections," *Med Lett Drugs Ther*, 1993, 35(904):79-86.

"Effect of Combined Therapy with Ansamycin, Clofazimine, Ethambutol, and Isoniazid for *Mycobacterium avium* Infection in Patients With AIDS," *J Infect Dis*, 1989, 159(4):784-7.

Hoy J, Mijch A, Sandland M, et al, "Quadruple-Drug Therapy for *Mycobacterium avium-intracellulare* Bacteremia in AIDS Patients," *J Infect Dis*, 1990, 161(4):801-5.

Kemper CA, Meng TC, Nussbaum J, et al, "Treatment of *Mycobacterium avium* Complex Bacteremia in AIDS With a Four-Drug Oral Regimen. Rifampin, Ethambutol, Clofazimine, and Ciprofloxacin" *Ann Intern Med*, 1992, 116(6):466-72.

Clofazimine Palmitate *see Clofazimine on previous page*

Clotrimazole *(kloe TRIM a zole)*

U.S. Brand Names Femizole-7® [OTC]; Fungoid® Solution; Gyne-Lotrimin® [OTC]; Lotrimin®; Lotrimin® AF Cream [OTC]; Lotrimin® AF Lotion [OTC]; Lotrimin® AF Solution [OTC]; Mycelex®; Mycelex®-7; Mycelex®-G

Generic Available No

Use Treatment of susceptible fungal infections, including oropharyngeal, candidiasis, dermatophytoses, superficial mycoses, and cutaneous candidiasis, as well as vulvovaginal candidiasis; limited data suggest that clotrimazole troches may be effective for prophylaxis against oropharyngeal candidiasis in neutropenic patients

Drug of Choice or Alternative for

Organism(s)

Malassezia furfur on page 192

Pregnancy Risk Factor B; C (oral)

Contraindications Hypersensitivity to clotrimazole or any component

Warnings/Precautions Clotrimazole should not be used for treatment of systemic fungal infection; safety and effectiveness of clotrimazole lozenges (troches) in children <3 years of age have not been established

Adverse Reactions

>10%: Hepatic: Abnormal LFTs (causal relationship between troches and elevated LFTs not clearly established)

1% to 10%:

Gastrointestinal: Nausea and vomiting may occur in patients on clotrimazole troches

Local: Mild burning, irritation, stinging to skin or vaginal area

Drug Interactions CYP3A3/4 and 3A5-7 inhibitor

Mechanism of Action Binds to phospholipids in the fungal cell membrane altering cell wall permeability resulting in loss of essential intracellular elements

Pharmacodynamics/Kinetics

Absorption: Topical: Negligible through intact skin

Time to peak serum concentration:
Oral topical administration: Salivary levels occur within 3 hours following 30 minutes of dissolution time in the mouth
Vaginal cream: High vaginal levels occur within 8-24 hours
Vaginal tablet: High vaginal levels occur within 1-2 days
Elimination: As metabolites via bile

Usual Dosage
Children >3 years and Adults:
Oral:
Prophylaxis: 10 mg troche dissolved 3 times/day for the duration of chemotherapy or until steroids are reduced to maintenance levels
Treatment: 10 mg troche dissolved slowly 5 times/day for 14 consecutive days
Topical: Apply twice daily; if no improvement occurs after 4 weeks of therapy, re-evaluate diagnosis
Children >12 years and Adults:
Vaginal:
Cream: Insert 1 applicatorful of 1% vaginal cream daily (preferably at bedtime) for 7 consecutive days
Tablet: Insert 100 mg/day for 7 days or 500 mg single dose
Topical: Apply to affected area twice daily (morning and evening) for 7 consecutive days

Monitoring Parameters Periodic liver function tests during oral therapy with clotrimazole lozenges

Patient Information May cause irritation to the skin; avoid contact with eyes; lozenge (troche) must be dissolved slowly in the mouth

Dosage Forms
Combination pack (Mycelex®-7): Vaginal tablet 100 mg (7's) and vaginal cream 1% (7 g)
Cream:
Topical (Lotrimin®, Lotrimin® AF, Mycelex®, Mycelex® OTC) : 1% (15 g, 30 g, 45 g, 90 g)
Vaginal (Femizole-7®, Gyne-Lotrimin®, Mycelex®-G): 1% (45 g, 90 g)
Lotion (Lotrimin®): 1% (30 mL)
Solution, topical (Fungoid®, Lotrimin®, Lotrimin® AF, Mycelex®, Mycelex® OTC): 1% (10 mL, 30 mL)
Tablet, vaginal (Gyne-Lotrimin®, Mycelex®-G): 100 mg (7s); 500 mg (1s)
Troche (Mycelex®): 10 mg
Twin pack (Mycelex®): Vaginal tablet 500 mg (1's) and vaginal cream 1% (7 g)

Cloxacillin (kloks a SIL in)
Related Information
Antimicrobial Activity Against Selected Organisms *on page 983*
U.S. Brand Names Cloxapen®; Tegopen®
Canadian Brand Names Apo®-Cloxi; Novo-Cloxin; Nu-Cloxi; Orbenin®; Taro-Cloxacillin®
Synonyms Cloxacillin Sodium
Generic Available Yes
Use Treatment of susceptible bacterial infections, notably penicillinase-producing staphylococci causing respiratory tract, skin and skin structure, bone and joint, urinary tract infections
Pregnancy Risk Factor B
Contraindications Hypersensitivity to cloxacillin or any component, or penicillins
Warnings/Precautions Monitor PT if patient concurrently on warfarin, elimination of drug is slow in renally impaired; use with caution in patients allergic to cephalosporins due to a low incidence of cross-hypersensitivity
Adverse Reactions
1% to 10%: Gastrointestinal: Nausea, diarrhea, abdominal pain
<1%: Fever, seizures with extremely high doses and/or renal failure, rash (maculopapular to exfoliative), vomiting, pseudomembranous colitis, vaginitis, eosinophilia, leukopenia, neutropenia, thrombocytopenia, agranulocytosis, anemia, hemolytic anemia, prolonged PT, hepatotoxicity, transient elevated LFTs, hematuria, interstitial nephritis, increased BUN/creatinine, serum sickness-like reactions, hypersensitivity
(Continued)

Cloxacillin *(Continued)*

Overdosage/Toxicology
Symptoms of penicillin overdose include neuromuscular hypersensitivity (agitation, hallucinations, asterixis, encephalopathy, confusion, and seizures) and electrolyte imbalance with potassium or sodium salts, especially in renal failure

Hemodialysis may be helpful to aid in the removal of the drug from the blood, otherwise most treatment is supportive or symptom directed

Drug Interactions
Decreased effect: Efficacy of oral contraceptives may be reduced

Increased effect: Disulfiram, probenecid may increase penicillin levels, increased effect of anticoagulants

Stability
Refrigerate oral solution after reconstitution; discard after 14 days; stable for 3 days at room temperature

Mechanism of Action
Inhibits bacterial cell wall synthesis by binding to one or more of the penicillin-binding proteins (PBPs) which in turn inhibits the final transpeptidation step of peptidoglycan synthesis in bacterial cell walls, thus inhibiting cell wall biosynthesis. Bacteria eventually lyse due to ongoing activity of cell wall autolytic enzymes (autolysins and murein hydrolases) while cell wall assembly is arrested.

Pharmacodynamics/Kinetics
Absorption: Oral: ~50%

Distribution: Crosses the placenta; appears in breast milk; distributed widely to most body fluids and bone; penetration into cells, into the eye, and across normal meninges is poor; inflammation increased amount that crosses the blood-brain barrier

Protein binding: 90% to 98%

Metabolism: Significant in the liver to active and inactive metabolites

Half-life: 0.5-1.5 hours (prolonged with renal impairment and in neonates)

Time to peak serum concentration: Oral: Within 0.5-2 hours

Elimination: In urine and through bile

Usual Dosage
Oral:

Children >1 month (<20 kg): 50-100 mg/kg/day in divided doses every 6 hours; up to a maximum of 4 g/day

Children (>20 kg) and Adults: 250-500 mg every 6 hours

Hemodialysis: Not dialyzable (0% to 5%)

Monitoring Parameters
Observe for signs and symptoms of anaphylaxis during first dose

Test Interactions
May interfere with urinary glucose tests using cupric sulfate (Benedict's solution, Clinitest®); may inactivate aminoglycosides *in vitro*; false-positive urine and serum proteins; false-positive in uric acid, urinary steroids

Patient Information
Take 1 hour before or 2 hours after meals; finish all medication; do not skip doses

Additional Information
Sodium content of 250 mg capsule: 13.8 mg (0.6 mEq); 5 mL of 125 mg/5 mL: 11 mg (0.48 mEq)

Dosage Forms
Capsule, as sodium: 250 mg, 500 mg

Powder for oral suspension, as sodium: 125 mg/5 mL (100 mL, 200 mL)

Selected Readings
Donowitz GR and Mandell GL, "Beta-Lactam Antibiotics," *N Engl J Med*, 1988, 318(7):419-26 and 318(8):490-500.

Wright AJ, "The Penicillins," *Mayo Clin Proc*, 1999, 74(3):290-307.

Cloxacillin Sodium *see* Cloxacillin *on previous page*

Cloxapen® *see* Cloxacillin *on previous page*

CMV-IGIV *see* Cytomegalovirus Immune Globulin (Intravenous-Human) *on page 697*

Colistimethate *(koe lis ti METH ate)*

U.S. Brand Names
Coly-Mycin® M Parenteral

Generic Available
No

Use
Treatment of infections due to sensitive strains of certain gram-negative bacilli which are resistant to other antibacterials or in patients allergic to other antibacterials

Not FDA approved: Used as inhalation in the prevention of *Pseudomonas aeruginosa* respiratory tract infections in immunocompromised patients, and used as inhalation adjunct agent for the treatment of *P. aeruginosa* infections in patients with cystic fibrosis and other seriously ill or chronically ill patients

Pregnancy Risk Factor B

Contraindications Hypersensitivity to colistimethate or any component

Warnings/Precautions Use with caution in patients with pre-existing renal disease

Adverse Reactions 1% to 10%:
Central nervous system: Slurring of speech, vertigo
Dermatologic: Urticaria
Gastrointestinal: GI upset
Renal: Nephrotoxicity
Respiratory: Respiratory arrest

Drug Interactions Other nephrotoxic drugs, neuromuscular blocking agents

Stability Freshly prepare any infusion and use for no longer than 24 hours

Mechanism of Action Hydrolyzed to colistin, which acts as a cationic detergent which damages the bacterial cytoplasmic membrane causing leaking of intracellular substances and cell death

Pharmacodynamics/Kinetics
Distribution: Widely distributed, except for CNS, synovial, pleural, and pericardial fluids
Half-life: 1.5-8 hours; may be as high as 2-3 days in anuric patients
Elimination: Excreted primarily unchanged in urine
Peak: About 2 hours

Usual Dosage Children and Adults:
I.M., I.V.: 2.5-5 mg/kg/day in 2-4 divided doses
Inhalation: 75 mg in 3 mL NS (4 mL total) via nebulizer twice daily

Dosing interval in renal impairment: Adults:
S_{cr} 0.7-1.2 mg/dL: 100-125 mg 2-4 times/day
S_{cr} 1.3-1.5 mg/dL: 75-115 mg twice daily
S_{cr} 1.6-2.5 mg/dL: 66-150 mg once or twice daily
S_{cr} 2.6-4 mg/dL: 100-150 mg every 36 hours

Dosage Forms Powder for injection, lyophilized: 150 mg

Selected Readings
Bauldoff GS, Nunley DR, Manzetti JD, et al, "Use of Aerosolized Colistin in Cystic Fibrosis Patients Awaiting Lung Transplantation," *Transplantation*, 1997, 64(5):748-52.
Conway SP, Pond MN, Watson A, et al, "Intravenous Colistin Sulphomethate in Acute Respiratory Exacerbations in Adult Patients With Cystic Fibrosis," *Thorax*, 1997, 52(11):987-93.
Jensen T, Pederson SS, Garne S, et al, "Colistin Inhalation Therapy in Cystic Fibrosis Patients with Chronic *Pseudomonas aeruginosa* Lung Infection," *J Antimicrob Chemother*, 1987, 19(6):831-8.
Zylberberg H, Vargaftig J, Barbieux C, et al, "Prolonged Efficiency of Secondary Prophylaxis with Colistin Aerosols for Respiratory Infection Due to *Pseudomonas aeruginosa* in Patients Infected With Human Immunodeficiency Virus," *Clin Infect Dis*, 1996, 23(3):641-3.

Colistin (koe LIS tin)

U.S. Brand Names Coly-Mycin® S Oral

Synonyms Polymyxin E

Generic Available No

Use Treatment of diarrhea in infants and children caused by susceptible organisms, especially *E. coli* and *Shigella*, however, other agents are preferred; treatment of superficial infections of external ear canal and of mastoidectomy and fenestration cavities

Pregnancy Risk Factor C

Contraindications Known hypersensitivity to colistin

Warnings/Precautions Use with caution in patients with impaired renal function; some systemic absorption may occur; potential for renal toxicity exists; prolonged use may lead to superinfection

Adverse Reactions <1%: Neuromuscular blockade, nephrotoxicity, respiratory arrest, nausea, vomiting, hypersensitivity reactions, superinfections

Stability Stable for 2 weeks when refrigerated, shake well; discard after 14 days

Mechanism of Action Polypeptide antibiotic that binds to and damages the bacterial cell membrane

Pharmacodynamics/Kinetics
Absorption: Oral: Slightly absorbed from GI tract (adults); unpredictable absorption occurs in infants, can lead to significant serum levels
(Continued)

Colistin *(Continued)*

Half-life: 2.8-4.8 hours, prolonged in renal insufficiency; with anuria: 48-72 hours
Elimination: ~65% to 75% excreted unchanged in urine

Usual Dosage Diarrhea: Children: Oral: 5-15 mg/kg/day in 3 divided doses given every 8 hours

Dosage Forms Powder for oral suspension: 25 mg/5 mL (60 mL)

Colistin, Neomycin, and Hydrocortisone

(koe LIS tin, nee oh MYE sin & hye droe KOR ti sone)

Related Information

Colistin *on previous page*
Neomycin *on page 833*

U.S. Brand Names Coly-Mycin® S Otic Drops; Cortisporin-TC® Otic

Use Treatment of superficial and susceptible bacterial infections of the external auditory canal; for treatment of susceptible bacterial infections of mastoidectomy and fenestration cavities

Usual Dosage

Children: 3 drops in affected ear 3-4 times/day
Adults: 4 drops in affected ear 3-4 times/day

Dosage Forms Suspension, otic:

Coly-Mycin® S Otic Drops: Colistin sulfate 0.3%, neomycin sulfate 0.47%, and hydrocortisone acetate 1% (5 mL, 10 mL)
Cortisporin-TC®: Colistin sulfate 0.3%, neomycin sulfate 0.33%, and hydrocortisone acetate 1% (5 mL, 10 mL)

Coly-Mycin® M Parenteral *see* Colistimethate *on page 690*

Coly-Mycin® S Oral *see* Colistin *on previous page*

Coly-Mycin® S Otic Drops *see* Colistin, Neomycin, and Hydrocortisone *on this page*

Combivir® *see* Zidovudine and Lamivudine *on page 979*

Compound S *see* Zidovudine *on page 977*

Comvax™ *see* Haemophilus b Conjugate and Hepatitis B Vaccine *on page 754*

Coptin® *see* Sulfadiazine *on page 929*

Corque® Topical *see* Clioquinol and Hydrocortisone *on page 687*

Cortatrigen® Otic *see* Neomycin, Polymyxin B, and Hydrocortisone *on page 836*

Cortisporin® Ophthalmic Ointment *see* Bacitracin, Neomycin, Polymyxin B, and Hydrocortisone *on page 620*

Cortisporin® Ophthalmic Suspension *see* Neomycin, Polymyxin B, and Hydrocortisone *on page 836*

Cortisporin® Otic *see* Neomycin, Polymyxin B, and Hydrocortisone *on page 836*

Cortisporin-TC® Otic *see* Colistin, Neomycin, and Hydrocortisone *on this page*

Cortisporin® Topical Cream *see* Neomycin, Polymyxin B, and Hydrocortisone *on page 836*

Cortisporin® Topical Ointment *see* Bacitracin, Neomycin, Polymyxin B, and Hydrocortisone *on page 620*

Cotrim® *see* Co-Trimoxazole *on this page*

Cotrim® DS *see* Co-Trimoxazole *on this page*

Co-Trimoxazole (koe trye MOKS a zole)

Related Information

Antimicrobial Activity Against Selected Organisms *on page 983*

U.S. Brand Names Bactrim™; Bactrim™ DS; Cotrim®; Cotrim® DS; Septra®; Septra® DS; Sulfamethoprim®; Sulfatrim®; Sulfatrim® DS; Uroplus® DS; Uroplus® SS

Canadian Brand Names Apo®-Sulfatrim; Novo-Trimel; Nu-Cotrimox; Pro-Trin®; Roubac®; Trisulfa®; Trisulfa-S®

Synonyms SMX-TMP; Sulfamethoxazole and Trimethoprim; TMP-SMX; Trimethoprim and Sulfamethoxazole

Generic Available Yes

Use

Oral treatment of urinary tract infections due to *E. coli, Klebsiella* and *Enterobacter* sp, *M. morganii, P. mirabilis* and *P. vulgaris*; acute otitis media in children and acute exacerbations of chronic bronchitis in adults due to suscep-tible strains of *H. influenzae* or *S. pneumoniae*; prophylaxis of *Pneumocystis carinii* pneumonitis (PCP), traveler's diarrhea due to enterotoxigenic *E. coli* or *Cyclospora*

I.V. treatment or severe or complicated infections when oral therapy is not feasible, for documented PCP, empiric treatment of PCP in immune compro-mised patients; treatment of documented or suspected shigellosis, typhoid fever, *Nocardia asteroides* infection, or other infections caused by susceptible bacteria

Unlabeled use: Cholera and *Salmonella*-type infections and nocardiosis; chronic prostatitis; as prophylaxis in neutropenic patients with *P. carinii* infec-tions, in leukemics, and in patients following renal transplantation, to decrease incidence of gram-negative rod infections

Drug of Choice or Alternative for

Disease/Syndrome(s)

Bronchitis *on page 20*
Otitis Media, Acute *on page 41*
Prostatitis *on page 47*
Sinusitis, Community-Acquired, Acute *on page 48*
Urinary Tract Infection, Perinephric Abscess *on page 52*
Urinary Tract Infection, Pyelonephritis *on page 53*
Urinary Tract Infection, Uncomplicated *on page 53*

Organism(s)

Aeromonas Species *on page 64*
Bartonella Species *on page 76*
Bordetella pertussis on page 81
Brucella Species *on page 85*
Burkholderia cepacia on page 87
Calymmatobacterium granulomatis on page 89
Cyclospora cayetanensis on page 120
Escherichia coli, Nonenterohemorrhagic *on page 147*
Haemophilus ducreyi on page 156
Haemophilus influenzae on page 157
Isospora belli on page 182
Listeria monocytogenes on page 189
Moraxella catarrhalis on page 196
Nocardia Species *on page 218*
Pneumocystis carinii on page 228
Providencia Species *on page 234*
Salmonella Species *on page 245*
Shigella Species *on page 251*
Staphylococcus aureus, Methicillin-Resistant *on page 256*
Staphylococcus epidermidis, Methicillin-Resistant *on page 261*
Staphylococcus saprophyticus on page 264
Stenotrophomonas maltophilia on page 265
Toxoplasma gondii on page 283
Vibrio cholerae on page 297

Pregnancy Risk Factor C

Pregnancy/Breast-Feeding Implications Do not use at term to avoid kernic-terus in the newborn and use during pregnancy only if risks outweigh the bene-fits since folic acid metabolism may be affected

Contraindications Hypersensitivity to any sulfa drug or any component; porphyria; megaloblastic anemia due to folate deficiency; infants <2 months of age; marked hepatic damage

Warnings/Precautions Use with caution in patients with G-6-PD deficiency, impaired renal or hepatic function; adjust dosage in patients with renal impair-ment; injection vehicle contains benzyl alcohol and sodium metabisulfite; fatali-ties associated with sulfonamides, although rare, have occurred due to severe reactions including Stevens-Johnson syndrome, toxic epidermal necrolysis, hepatic necrosis, agranulocytosis, aplastic anemia and other blood dyscrasias; discontinue use at first sign of rash; elderly patients and slow acetylators appear at greater risk for more severe adverse reactions; may cause hypoglycemia, particularly in malnourished patients or patients with renal or hepatic impairment; use with caution in patients with porphyria or thyroid dysfunction
(Continued)

Co-Trimoxazole (Continued)

Adverse Reactions

>10%:

Dermatologic: Allergic skin reactions including rashes and urticaria, photosensitivity

Gastrointestinal: Nausea, vomiting, anorexia

1% to 10%:

Dermatologic: Stevens-Johnson syndrome, toxic epidermal necrolysis (rare)

Hematologic: Blood dyscrasias

Hepatic: Hepatitis

<1%: Confusion, depression, hallucinations, seizures, fever, ataxia, kernicterus in neonates, erythema multiforme, stomatitis, diarrhea, pseudomembranous colitis, pancreatitis, thrombocytopenia, megaloblastic anemia, granulocytopenia, aplastic anemia, hemolysis (with G-6-PD deficiency), cholestatic jaundice, interstitial nephritis, serum sickness, pancytopenia, rhabdomyolysis

Overdosage/Toxicology

Symptoms of acute overdose include nausea, vomiting, GI distress, hematuria, crystalluria

Following GI decontamination, treatment is supportive; adequate fluid intake is essential; peritoneal dialysis is not effective and hemodialysis only moderately effective in removing co-trimoxazole

Drug Interactions CYP2C9 enzyme inhibitor

Decreased effect: Cyclosporines

Increased effect/toxicity: Phenytoin, cyclosporines (nephrotoxicity), methotrexate (displaced from binding sites), dapsone, sulfonylureas, and oral anticoagulants; may compete for renal secretion of methotrexate; digoxin concentrations increased

Stability Do not refrigerate injection; is less soluble in more alkaline pH; protect from light; do not use NS as a diluent; injection vehicle contains benzyl alcohol and sodium metabisulfite

Stability of parenteral admixture at room temperature (25°C):

5 mL/125 mL D_5W: 6 hours

5 mL/100 mL D_5W: 4 hours

5 mL/75 mL D_5W: 2 hours

Mechanism of Action Sulfamethoxazole interferes with bacterial folic acid synthesis and growth via inhibition of dihydrofolic acid formation from para-aminobenzoic acid; trimethoprim inhibits dihydrofolic acid reduction to tetrahydrofolate resulting in sequential inhibition of enzymes of the folic acid pathway

Pharmacodynamics/Kinetics

Absorption: Oral: 90% to 100%

Distribution: Crosses the placenta; distributes widely into body tissues, breast milk, and fluids including middle ear fluid, prostatic fluid, bile, aqueous humor, and CSF

Protein binding:

SMX: 68%

TMP: 68%

Metabolism:

SMX is N-acetylated and glucuronidated

TMP is metabolized to oxide and hydroxylated metabolites

Half-life:

SMX: 9 hours

TMP: 6-17 hours, both are prolonged in renal failure

Time to peak serum concentration: Within 1-4 hours

Elimination: In urine as metabolites and unchanged drug

Usual Dosage Dosage recommendations are based on the trimethoprim component

Children >2 months:

Mild to moderate infections: Oral, I.V.: 8 mg TMP/kg/day in divided doses every 12 hours

Serious infection/Pneumocystis: I.V.: 20 mg TMP/kg/day in divided doses every 6 hours

Urinary tract infection prophylaxis: Oral: 2 mg TMP/kg/dose daily

Prophylaxis of Pneumocystis: Oral, I.V.: 10 mg TMP/kg/day or 150 mg TMP/m^2/day in divided doses every 12 hours for 3 days/week; dose should not exceed 320 mg trimethoprim and 1600 mg sulfamethoxazole 3 days/week

Adults:

Urinary tract infection/chronic bronchitis: Oral: 1 double strength tablet every 12 hours for 10-14 days

Sepsis: I.V.: 15-20 mg TMP/kg/day divided every 6 hours

Pneumocystis carinii:

Prophylaxis: Oral: 1 double strength tablet daily or 3 times/week

Treatment: I.V., Oral: 15-20 mg TMP/kg/day in 3-4 divided doses

Dosing adjustment in renal impairment: Adults:

I.V.:

Cl_{cr} 15-30 mL/minute: Administer 2.5-5 mg/kg every 12 hours

Cl_{cr} <15 mL/minute: Administer 2.5-5 mg/kg every 24 hours

Oral:

Cl_{cr} 15-30 mL/minute: Administer 1 double strength tablet every 24 hours or 1 single strength tablet every 12 hours

Cl_{cr} <15 mL/minute: Not recommended

Administration Infuse over 60-90 minutes, must dilute well before giving; may be given less diluted in a central line; not for I.M. injection; maintain adequate fluid intake to prevent crystalluria

Test Interactions Increases creatinine (Jaffé alkaline picrate reaction); increased serum methotrexate by dihydrofolate reductase method

Patient Information Take oral medication with 8 oz of water on an empty stomach (1 hour before or 2 hours after meals) for best absorption; report any skin rashes immediately; finish all medication, do not skip doses

Nursing Implications Infuse over 60-90 minutes, must dilute well before giving; not for I.M. injection; maintain adequate fluid intake to prevent crystalluria

Dosage Forms The 5:1 ratio (SMX to TMP) remains constant in all dosage forms:

Injection: Sulfamethoxazole 80 mg and trimethoprim 16 mg per mL (5 mL, 10 mL, 20 mL, 30 mL, 50 mL)

Suspension, oral: Sulfamethoxazole 200 mg and trimethoprim 40 mg per 5 mL (20 mL, 100 mL, 150 mL, 200 mL, 480 mL)

Tablet: Sulfamethoxazole 400 mg and trimethoprim 80 mg

Tablet, double strength: Sulfamethoxazole 800 mg and trimethoprim 160 mg

Selected Readings

Cockerill FR and Edson RS, "Trimethoprim-Sulfamethoxazole," *Mayo Clin Proc*, 1991, 66(12):1260-9.

Fischl MA, Dickinson GM, and La Voie L, "Safety and Efficacy of Sulfamethoxazole and Trimethoprim Chemoprophylaxis for *Pneumocystis carinii* Pneumonia in AIDS," *JAMA*, 1988, 259(8):1185-9.

Hughes W, Leoung G, Kramer F, et al, "Comparison of Atovaquone (566C80) With Trimethoprim-Sulfamethoxazole to Treat *Pneumocystis carinii* Pneumonia in Patients With AIDS," *N Engl J Med*, 1993, 328(21):1521-7.

Lundstrom TS and Sobel JD, "Vancomycin, Trimethoprim-Sulfamethoxazole, and Rifampin," *Infect Dis Clin North Am*, 1995, 9(3):747-67.

Masur H, "Prevention and Treatment of *Pneumocystis* Pneumonia," *N Engl J Med*, 1992, 327(26):1853-60.

Sattler FR, Cowan R, Nielsen DM, et al, " Trimethoprim-Sulfamethoxazole Compared With Pentamidine for Treatment of *Pneumocystis carinii* Pneumonia in the Acquired Immunodeficiency Syndrome," *Ann Intern Med*, 1988, 109(4):280-7.

CP-99,219-27 *see* Trovafloxacin *on page 960*

Crixivan® *see* Indinavir *on page 773*

Crotamiton (kroe TAM i tonn)

U.S. Brand Names Eurax® Topical

Generic Available No

Use Treatment of scabies (*Sarcoptes scabiei*) and symptomatic treatment of pruritus

Drug of Choice or Alternative for

Organism(s)

Sarcoptes scabiei on page 247

Pregnancy Risk Factor C

Contraindications Hypersensitivity to crotamiton or other components; patients who manifest a primary irritation response to topical medications

Warnings/Precautions Avoid contact with face, eyes, mucous membranes, and urethral meatus; do not apply to acutely inflamed or raw skin; for external use only

(Continued)

Crotamiton *(Continued)*

Adverse Reactions <1%: Local irritation, pruritus, contact dermatitis, warm sensation

Overdosage/Toxicology

Symptoms of ingestion include burning sensation in mouth, irritation of the buccal, esophageal and gastric mucosa, nausea, vomiting and abdominal pain
There is no specific antidote; general measures to eliminate the drug and reduce its absorption, combined with symptomatic treatment, are recommended

Mechanism of Action Crotamiton has scabicidal activity against *Sarcoptes scabiei*; mechanism of action unknown

Usual Dosage Topical:

Scabicide: Children and Adults: Wash thoroughly and scrub away loose scales, then towel dry; apply a thin layer and massage drug onto skin of the entire body from the neck to the toes (with special attention to skin folds, creases, and interdigital spaces). Repeat application in 24 hours. Take a cleansing bath 48 hours after the final application. Treatment may be repeated after 7-10 days if live mites are still present.

Pruritus: Massage into affected areas until medication is completely absorbed; repeat as necessary

Patient Information For topical use only; all contaminated clothing and bed linen should be washed to avoid reinfestation

Nursing Implications Lotion: Shake well before using; avoid contact with face, eyes, mucous membranes, and urethral meatus

Dosage Forms

Cream: 10% (60 g)

Lotion: 10% (60 mL, 454 mL)

Selected Readings

Eichenfield LF, Honig PJ, "Blistering Disorders in Childhood," *Pediatr Clin North Am*, 1991, 38(4):959-76.

Hogan DJ, Schachner L, Tanglertsampan C, "Diagnosis and Treatment of Childhood Scabies and Pediculosis," *Pediatr Clin North Am*, 1991, 38(4):941-57.

Crystalline Penicillin *see* Penicillin G, Parenteral, Aqueous *on page 860*

Crystal Violet *see* Gentian Violet *on page 751*

Crysticillin® A.S. *see* Penicillin G Procaine *on page 862*

C/T/S® Topical Solution *see* Clindamycin *on page 684*

Cycloserine *(sye kloe SER een)*

Related Information

Tuberculosis Guidelines *on page 1114*

U.S. Brand Names Seromycin® Pulvules®

Generic Available No

Use Adjunctive treatment in pulmonary or extrapulmonary tuberculosis; has been studied for use in Gaucher's disease

Pregnancy Risk Factor C

Contraindications Known hypersensitivity to cycloserine

Warnings/Precautions Epilepsy, depression, severe anxiety, psychosis, severe renal insufficiency, chronic alcoholism

Adverse Reactions Percentage unknown: Cardiac arrhythmias, drowsiness, headache, dizziness, vertigo, seizures, confusion, psychosis, paresis, coma, rash, folate deficiency, elevated liver enzymes, tremor, vitamin B_{12} deficiency

Overdosage/Toxicology

Symptoms of overdose include confusion, agitation, CNS depression, psychosis, coma, seizures
Decontaminate with activated charcoal; can be hemodialyzed; management is supportive; administer 100-300 mg/day of pyridoxine to reduce neurotoxic effects; acute toxicity can occur with ingestions >1 g; chronic toxicity: >500 mg/day

Drug Interactions Increased toxicity: Alcohol, isoniazid, ethionamide increase toxicity of cycloserine; cycloserine inhibits the hepatic metabolism of phenytoin

Mechanism of Action Inhibits bacterial cell wall synthesis by competing with amino acid (D-alanine) for incorporation into the bacterial cell wall; bacteriostatic or bactericidal

Pharmacodynamics/Kinetics

Absorption: Oral: ~70% to 90% from the GI tract

Distribution: Crosses the placenta; appears in breast milk; distributed widely to most body fluids and tissues including CSF, breast milk, bile, sputum, lymph tissue, lungs, and ascitic, pleural, and synovial fluids

Half-life: 10 hours in patients with normal renal function

Metabolism: Extensive in liver

Time to peak serum concentration: Oral: Within 3-4 hours

Elimination: 60% to 70% of oral dose excreted unchanged in urine by glomerular filtration within 72 hours, small amounts excreted in feces, remainder is metabolized

Usual Dosage Some of the neurotoxic effects may be relieved or prevented by the concomitant administration of pyridoxine

Tuberculosis: Oral:

Children: 10-20 mg/kg/day in 2 divided doses up to 1000 mg/day for 18-24 months

Adults: Initial: 250 mg every 12 hours for 14 days, then administer 500 mg to 1 g/day in 2 divided doses for 18-24 months (maximum daily dose: 1 g)

Dosing interval in renal impairment:

Cl_{cr} 10-50 mL/minute: Administer every 24 hours

Cl_{cr} <10 mL/minute: Administer every 36-48 hours

Monitoring Parameters Periodic renal, hepatic, hematological tests, and plasma cycloserine concentrations

Reference Range Toxicity is greatly increased at levels >30 µg/mL

Patient Information May cause drowsiness; notify physician if skin rash, mental confusion, dizziness, headache, or tremors occur; do not skip doses; do not drink excessive amounts of alcoholic beverages

Dosage Forms Capsule: 250 mg

Selected Readings

Davidson PT and Le HQ, "Drug Treatment of Tuberculosis - 1992," *Drugs*, 1992, 43(5):651-73.

"Drugs for Tuberculosis," *Med Lett Drugs Ther*, 1993, 35(908):99-101.

Iseman MD, "Treatment of Multidrug-Resistant Tuberculosis," *N Engl J Med*, 1993, 329(11):784-91.

CytoGam™ see Cytomegalovirus Immune Globulin (Intravenous-Human) *on this page*

Cytomegalovirus Immune Globulin (Intravenous-Human)

(sye toe meg a low VYE rus i MYUN GLOB yoo lin in tra VEE nus HYU man)

U.S. Brand Names CytoGam™

Synonyms CMV-IGIV

Generic Available No

Use Attenuation of primary CMV disease associated with immunosuppressed recipients of kidney transplantation; especially indicated for CMV-negative recipients of CMV-positive donor; has been used as adjunct therapy in the treatment of CMV disease in immunocompromised patients

Pregnancy Risk Factor C

Contraindications Hypersensitivity to any component, patients with selective immunoglobulin A deficiency (increases potential for anaphylaxis), persons with IgA deficiency

Warnings/Precautions Studies indicate that product carries little or no risk for transmission of HIV; give with caution to patients with prior allergic reactions to human immunoglobulin preparations; do not perform skin testing

Adverse Reactions

1% to 10%:

Cardiovascular: Flushing of face

Gastrointestinal: Nausea, vomiting

Neuromuscular & skeletal: Muscle cramps, back pain

Respiratory: Wheezing

Miscellaneous: Diaphoresis

<1%: Tightness in the chest, dizziness, fever, headache, chills, aseptic meningitis syndrome, hypersensitivity reactions

Drug Interactions May inactivate live virus vaccines (eg, measles, mumps, rubella); if IGIV administration within 3 months of vaccination with live virus products, revaccinate

Stability Use reconstituted product within 6 hours; do not admix with other medications

(Continued)

Cytomegalovirus Immune Globulin (Intravenous-Human) *(Continued)*

Mechanism of Action CMV-IGIV is a preparation of immunoglobulin G derived from pooled healthy blood donors with a high titer of CMV antibodies; administration provides a passive source of antibodies against cytomegalovirus

Usual Dosage I.V.:

Dosing schedule:

Initial dose (within 72 hours after transplant): 150 mg/kg/dose

2, 4, 6, 8 weeks after transplant: 100 mg/kg/dose

12 and 16 weeks after transplant: 50 mg/kg/dose

Severe CMV pneumonia: Regimens of 400 mg/kg on days 1, 2, 7 or 8, followed by 200 mg/kg have been used

Administration rate: Administer at 15 mg/kg/hour initially, then increase to 30 mg/kg/hour after 30 minutes if no untoward reactions, then increase to 60 mg/kg/hour after another 30 minutes; volume not to exceed 75 mL/hour

Administration I.V. use only; administer as separate infusion; infuse beginning at 15 mg/kg/hour; may titrate up to 60 mg/kg/hour; do not administer faster than 75 mL/hour

Dosage Forms Powder for injection, lyophilized, detergent treated: 2500 mg ± 250 mg (50 mL)

Selected Readings

Levinson ML and Jacobson PA, "Treatment and Prophylaxis of Cytomegalovirus Disease," *Pharmacotherapy*, 1992, 12(4):300-18.

Reed EC, Bowden RA, Dandliker PS, et al, "Efficacy of Cytomegalovirus Immunoglobulin in Marrow Transplant Recipients With Cytomegalovirus Pneumonia," *J Infect Dis*, 1987, 156:641-5.

Reed EC, Bowden RA, Dandliker PS, et al, "Treatment of Cytomegalovirus Pneumonia With Ganciclovir and Intravenous Cytomegalovirus Immunoglobulin in Patients With Bone Marrow Transplants," *Ann Intern Med*, 1988, 109:783-8.

Snydman DR, "Cytomegalovirus Immunoglobulins in the Prevention and Treatment of Cytomegalovirus Disease," *Rev Infect Dis*, 1990, 12(Suppl 7):S839-48.

Cytovene® see Ganciclovir *on page 745*

d4T see Stavudine *on page 923*

Dalacin® C [Hydrochloride] see Clindamycin *on page 684*

Dapsone *(DAP sone)*

U.S. Brand Names Avlosulfon®

Synonyms Diaminodiphenylsulfone

Generic Available No

Use Treatment of leprosy and dermatitis herpetiformis (infections caused by *Mycobacterium leprae*)

Prophylaxis of toxoplasmosis in severely immunocompromised patients; alternative agent for *Pneumocystis carinii* pneumonia prophylaxis (given alone) and treatment (given with trimethoprim)

May be useful in relapsing polychondritis, prophylaxis of malaria, inflammatory bowel disorders, leishmaniasis, rheumatic/connective tissue disorders, brown recluse spider bites

Drug of Choice or Alternative for

Organism(s)

Pneumocystis carinii on page 228

Pregnancy Risk Factor C

Contraindications Hypersensitivity to dapsone or any component

Warnings/Precautions Use with caution in patients with severe anemia, G-6-PD, methemoglobin reductase or hemoglobin M deficiency; hypersensitivity to other sulfonamides; aplastic anemia, agranulocytosis and other severe blood dyscrasias have resulted in death; monitor carefully; treat severe anemia prior to therapy; serious dermatologic reactions (including toxic epidermal necrolysis) are rare but potential occurrences; sulfone reactions may also occur as potentially fatal hypersensitivity reactions; these, but not leprosy reactional states, require drug discontinuation; dapsone is carcinogenic in small animals

Adverse Reactions

1% to 10%: Hematologic: Hemolysis, methemoglobinemia

<1%: Reactional states (ie, abrupt changes in clinical activity occurring during any leprosy treatment; classified as reversal of erythema nodosum leprosum reactions), insomnia, headache, exfoliative dermatitis, photosensitivity,

nausea, vomiting, anemia, leukopenia, agranulocytosis, hepatitis, cholestatic jaundice, peripheral neuropathy (usually in nonleprosy patients), blurred vision, tinnitus, SLE

Overdosage/Toxicology

Symptoms of overdose include nausea, vomiting, confusion, hyperexcitability, seizures, cyanosis, hemolysis, methemoglobinemia, sulfhemoglobinemia, metabolic acidosis, hallucinations, hepatitis

Following decontamination, methylene blue 1-2 mg/kg I.V. is treatment of choice if MHb level is >15%; may repeat every 6-8 hours for 2-3 days if needed; if hemolysis is present, give I.V. fluids and alkalinize urine to prevent acute tubular necrosis

Drug Interactions CYP2C9, 2E1, and 3A3/4 enzyme substrate

Decreased effect/levels: Para-aminobenzoic acid, didanosine, and rifampin decrease dapsone effects

Increased toxicity: Folic acid antagonists may increase the risk of hematologic reactions of dapsone; probenecid decreases dapsone excretion; trimethoprim with dapsone may increase toxic effects of both drugs

Stability Protect from light

Mechanism of Action Competitive antagonists of para-aminobenzoic acid (PABA) and prevent normal bacterial utilization of PABA for the synthesis of folic acid

Pharmacodynamics/Kinetics

Absorption: Oral: Well absorbed

Distribution: V_d: 1.5 L/kg; throughout total body water and present in all tissues, especially liver and kidney

Metabolism: In the liver

Half-life, elimination: 30 hours (range: 10-50 hours)

Elimination: In urine

Usual Dosage Oral:

Leprosy:

Children: 1-2 mg/kg/24 hours, up to a maximum of 100 mg/day

Adults: 50-100 mg/day for 3-10 years

Dermatitis herpetiformis: Adults: Start at 50 mg/day, increase to 300 mg/day, or higher to achieve full control, reduce dosage to minimum level as soon as possible

Prophylaxis of *Pneumocystis carinii* pneumonia:

Children >1 month: 1 mg/kg/day; maximum: 100 mg

Adults: 100 mg/day

Treatment of *Pneumocystis carinii* pneumonia: Adults: 100 mg/day in combination with trimethoprim (15-20 mg/kg/day) for 21 days

Dosing in renal impairment: No specific guidelines are available

Monitoring Parameters Monitor patient for signs of jaundice and hemolysis; CBC weekly for first month, monthly for 6 months, and semiannually thereafter

Patient Information Frequent blood tests are required during early therapy; discontinue if rash develops and contact physician if persistent sore throat, fever, malaise, or fatigue occurs; may cause photosensitivity

Dosage Forms Tablet: 25 mg, 100 mg

Extemporaneous Preparations One report indicated that dapsone may not be well absorbed when administered to children as suspensions made from pulverized tablets

Mirochnick M, Clarke D, Brenn A, et al, "Low Serum Dapsone Concentrations in Children Receiving an Extemporaneously Prepared Oral Formulation," [Abstract Th B 365], APS-SPR, Baltimore, MD: 1992.

Jacobus Pharmaceutical Company (609) 921-7447 makes a 2 mg/mL proprietary liquid formulation available under an IND for the prophylaxis of *Pneumocystis carinii* pneumonia

Selected Readings
El-Sadr WM, Murphy RL, Yurik TM, et al, "Atovaquone Compared With Dapsone for the Prevention of *Pneumocystic carinii* in Patients With HIV Infection Who Cannot Tolerate Trimethoprim, Sulfonamides, or Both," *N Engl J Med*, 1998, 339(26):1889-95.

Medina I, Mills J, Leoung G, et al, "Oral Therapy for *Pneumocystis carinii* Pneumonia in the Acquired Immunodeficiency Syndrome. A Controlled Trial of Trimethoprim-Sulfamethoxazole Versus Trimethoprim-Dapsone," *N Engl J Med*, 1990, 323(12):776-82.

Daraprim® see Pyrimethamine on page 886
Daraprim® see Pyrimethamine on page 886

Daskil® see Terbinafine on page 936
Daskil® see Terbinafine on page 936

ddC *see* Zalcitabine *on page 974*

ddI *see* Didanosine *on page 704*

Deca-Durabolin® *see* Nandrolone *on page 829*

Declomycin® *see* Demeclocycline *on next page*

Dehydral™ *see* Methenamine *on page 814*

Delatest® Injection *see* Testosterone *on page 939*

Delatestryl® Injection *see* Testosterone *on page 939*

Delavirdine (de la VIR deen)

Related Information
HIV Therapeutic Information *on page 1008*

U.S. Brand Names Rescriptor®

Synonyms U-90152S

Use Treatment of HIV-1 infection in combination with at least two additional antiretroviral agents

Pregnancy Risk Factor C

Pregnancy/Breast-Feeding Implications
Clinical effects on the fetus: Administer during pregnancy only if benefits to mother outweigh risks to the fetus

Breast-feeding/lactation: HIV-infected mothers are discouraged from breast-feeding to decrease potential transmission of HIV

Contraindications Known hypersensitivity to delavirdine or any components

Warnings/Precautions Avoid use with terfenadine, astemizole, benzodiazepines, clarithromycin, dapsone, cisapride, rifabutin, rifampin; use with caution in patients with hepatic or renal dysfunction; due to rapid emergence of resistance, delavirdine should not be used as monotherapy; cross-resistance may be conferred to other non-nucleoside reverse transcriptase inhibitors, although potential for cross-resistance with protease inhibitors is low. Long-term effects of delavirdine are not known. Safety and efficacy have not been established in children. Rash, which occurs frequently, may require discontinuation of therapy; usually occurs within 1-3 weeks and lasts <2 weeks. Most patients may resume therapy following a treatment interruption.

Adverse Reactions >2%:
Central nervous system: Headache, fatigue
Dermatologic: Rash, pruritus
Gastrointestinal: Nausea, diarrhea, vomiting
Metabolic: Increased ALT and AST

Overdosage/Toxicology
Human reports of overdose with delavirdine are not available
GI decontamination and supportive measures are recommended, dialysis unlikely to be of benefit in removing drug since it is extensively metabolized by the liver and is highly protein bound

Drug Interactions CYP2D6 and 3A3/4 enzyme substrate; CYP2D6 and 3A3/4 enzyme inhibitor
Increased plasma concentrations of delavirdine: Clarithromycin, ketoconazole, fluoxetine
Decreased plasma concentrations of delavirdine: Carbamazepine, phenobarbital, phenytoin, rifabutin, rifampin, didanosine, saquinavir
Decreased absorption of delavirdine: Antacids, H_2-receptor antagonists, didanosine
Delavirdine increases plasma concentrations of: Indinavir, saquinavir, terfenadine, astemizole, clarithromycin, dapsone, rifabutin, ergot derivatives, alprazolam, midazolam, triazolam, dihydropyridines, cisapride, quinidine, warfarin
Delavirdine decreases plasma concentrations of: Didanosine

Mechanism of Action Delavirdine binds directly to reverse transcriptase, blocking RNA-dependent and DNA-dependent DNA polymerase activities

Pharmacodynamics/Kinetics
Absorption: Rapid; peak plasma concentrations at 1 hour
Distribution: Not reported
Metabolism: Hepatic; extensively metabolized by the cytochrome P-450 3A or possibly 2D6
Bioavailability: 85%; AUC may be higher in female patients
Protein binding: ~98%, primarily albumin
Half-life: 2-11 hours

Elimination: 44% in feces, 51% in urine, and <5% unchanged in urine; nonlinear kinetics exhibited. (Note: May reduce CYP3A activity and inhibit its own metabolism.)

Usual Dosage Adults: Oral: 400 mg 3 times/day

Dietary Considerations Delavirdine may be taken without regard to food

Administration Patients with achlorhydria should take the drug with an acidic beverage; antacids and delavirdine should be separated by 1 hour

Monitoring Parameters Liver function tests if administered with saquinavir

Patient Information Delavirdine is not a cure for HIV-1 nor has it been shown to reduce the risk of transmission; illnesses associated with HIV-1 infection may continue to be acquired at the same frequency. Stay under the care of a physician when using delavirdine; notify your physician if a rash occurs or symptoms of rash with fever, blistering, oral lesions, conjunctivitis, swelling, or muscle/joint pain.

Additional Information Potential compliance problems, frequency of administration and adverse effects should be discussed with patients before initiating therapy to help prevent the emergence of resistance.

Dosage Forms Tablet: 100 mg

Extemporaneous Preparations A dispersion of delavirdine may be prepared by adding 4 tablets to at least 3 oz of water; allow to stand for a few minutes and stir until uniform dispersion; drink immediately; rinse glass and mouth following ingestion to ensure total dose administered

Selected Readings
Havlir DV and Lange JM, "New Antiretrovirals and New Combinations," *AIDS*, 1998, 12(Suppl A):S165-74.

Demeclocycline (dem e kloe SYE kleen)

U.S. Brand Names Declomycin®

Synonyms Demeclocycline Hydrochloride; Demethylchlortetracycline

Generic Available No

Use Treatment of susceptible bacterial infections (acne, gonorrhea, pertussis and urinary tract infections) caused by both gram-negative and gram-positive organisms; used when penicillin is contraindicated (other agents are preferred); treatment of chronic syndrome of inappropriate secretion of antidiuretic hormone (SIADH)

Pregnancy Risk Factor D

Contraindications Hypersensitivity to demeclocycline, tetracyclines, or any component

Warnings/Precautions Do not administer to children <9 years of age; photosensitivity reactions occur frequently with this drug, avoid prolonged exposure to sunlight, do not use tanning equipment

Adverse Reactions

1% to 10%:
Dermatologic: Photosensitivity
Gastrointestinal: Nausea, diarrhea
<1%: Pericarditis, increased intracranial pressure, bulging fontanels in infants, dermatologic effects, pruritus, exfoliative dermatitis, diabetes insipidus syndrome, vomiting, esophagitis, anorexia, abdominal cramps, paresthesia, acute renal failure, azotemia, superinfections, anaphylaxis, pigmentation of nails

Overdosage/Toxicology
Symptoms of overdose include diabetes insipidus, nausea, anorexia, diarrhea
Following GI decontamination, treatment is supportive

Drug Interactions
Decreased effect with antacids (aluminum, calcium, zinc, or magnesium), bismuth salts, sodium bicarbonate, barbiturates, carbamazepine, hydantoins
Decreased effect of oral contraceptives
Increased effect of warfarin

Mechanism of Action Inhibits protein synthesis by binding with the 30S and possibly the 50S ribosomal subunit(s) of susceptible bacteria; may also cause alterations in the cytoplasmic membrane; inhibits the action of ADH in patients with chronic SIADH

Pharmacodynamics/Kinetics
Onset of action for diuresis in SIADH: Several days
(Continued)

Demeclocycline *(Continued)*

Absorption: ~50% to 80% from GI tract; food and dairy products reduce absorption

Protein binding: 41% to 50%

Metabolism: Small amounts metabolized in the liver to inactive metabolites; enterohepatically recycled

Half-life: Reduced renal function: 10-17 hours

Time to peak serum concentration: Oral: Within 3-6 hours

Elimination: As unchanged drug (42% to 50%) in urine

Usual Dosage Oral:

Children ≥8 years: 8-12 mg/kg/day divided every 6-12 hours

Adults: 150 mg 4 times/day or 300 mg twice daily

Uncomplicated gonorrhea (penicillin sensitive): 600 mg stat, 300 mg every 12 hours for 4 days (3 g total)

SIADH: 900-1200 mg/day or 13-15 mg/kg/day divided every 6-8 hours initially, then decrease to 600-900 mg/day

Dosing adjustment/comments in renal/hepatic impairment: Should be avoided in patients with renal/hepatic dysfunction

Administration Administer 1 hour before or 2 hours after food or milk with plenty of fluid

Monitoring Parameters CBC, renal and hepatic function

Test Interactions May interfere with tests for urinary glucose (false-negative urine glucose using Clinistix®, Tes-Tape®)

Patient Information Avoid prolonged exposure to sunlight or sunlamps; avoid taking antacids before tetracyclines

Dosage Forms

Capsule, as hydrochloride: 150 mg

Tablet, as hydrochloride: 150 mg, 300 mg

Selected Readings

Smilack JD, Wilson WR, and Cockerill FR 3d, "Tetracyclines, Chloramphenicol, Erythromycin, Clindamycin, and Metronidazole," *Mayo Clin Proc,* 1991, 66(12):1270-80.

Demeclocycline Hydrochloride *see* Demeclocycline *on previous page*

Demethylchlortetracycline *see* Demeclocycline *on previous page*

Denavir™ *see* Penciclovir *on page 857*

depAndro® Injection *see* Testosterone *on page 939*

Depotest® Injection *see* Testosterone *on page 939*

Depo®-Testosterone Injection *see* Testosterone *on page 939*

Dermazin™ *see* Silver Sulfadiazine *on page 919*

Devrom® [OTC] *see* Bismuth Subsalicylate *on page 622*

Dexacidin® *see* Neomycin, Polymyxin B, and Dexamethasone *on page 836*

Dexamethasone and Tobramycin *see* Tobramycin and Dexamethasone *on page 956*

Dexasporin® *see* Neomycin, Polymyxin B, and Dexamethasone *on page 836*

Dey-Drop® Ophthalmic Solution *see* Silver Nitrate *on page 918*

DFMO *see* Eflornithine *on page 719*

DHPG Sodium *see* Ganciclovir *on page 745*

Diaminodiphenylsulfone *see* Dapsone *on page 698*

Dicloxacillin *(dye kloks a SIL in)*

Related Information

Antimicrobial Activity Against Selected Organisms *on page 983*

U.S. Brand Names Dycill®; Dynapen®; Pathocil®

Synonyms Dicloxacillin Sodium

Generic Available Yes

Use Treatment of systemic infections such as pneumonia, skin and soft tissue infections, and osteomyelitis caused by penicillinase-producing staphylococci

Pregnancy Risk Factor B

Contraindications Known hypersensitivity to dicloxacillin, penicillin, or any components

Warnings/Precautions Monitor PT if patient concurrently on warfarin; elimination of drug is slow in neonates; use with caution in patients allergic to cephalosporins; bad taste of suspension may make compliance difficult

Adverse Reactions

1% to 10%: Gastrointestinal: Nausea, diarrhea, abdominal pain

<1%: Fever, seizures with extremely high doses and/or renal failure, rash (maculopapular to exfoliative), vomiting, pseudomembranous colitis, vaginitis, eosinophilia, leukopenia, neutropenia, thrombocytopenia, agranulocytosis, anemia, hemolytic anemia, prolonged PT, hepatotoxicity, transient elevated LFTs, hematuria, interstitial nephritis, increased BUN/creatinine, serum sickness-like reactions, hypersensitivity

Overdosage/Toxicology

Symptoms of penicillin overdose include neuromuscular hypersensitivity (agitation, hallucinations, asterixis, encephalopathy, confusion, and seizures) and electrolyte imbalance with potassium or sodium salts, especially in renal failure

Hemodialysis may be helpful to aid in the removal of the drug from the blood, otherwise most treatment is supportive or symptom directed

Drug Interactions

Decreased effect: Efficacy of oral contraceptives may be reduced; decreased effect of warfarin

Increased effect: Disulfiram, probenecid may increase penicillin levels

Stability Refrigerate suspension after reconstitution; discard after 14 days if refrigerated or 7 days if kept at room temperature; unit dose antibiotic oral syringes are stable for 48 hours

Mechanism of Action Inhibits bacterial cell wall synthesis by binding to one or more of the penicillin binding proteins (PBPs); which in turn inhibits the final transpeptidation step of peptidoglycan synthesis in bacterial cell walls, thus inhibiting cell wall biosynthesis. Bacteria eventually lyse due to ongoing activity of cell wall autolytic enzymes (autolysins and murein hydrolases) while cell wall assembly is arrested.

Pharmacodynamics/Kinetics

Absorption: 35% to 76% from GI tract; food decreases rate and extent of absorption

Distribution: Crosses the placenta; distributes into breast milk; distributed throughout body with highest concentrations in kidney and liver; CSF penetration is low

Protein binding: 96%

Half-life: 0.6-0.8 hours, slightly prolonged in patients with renal impairment

Time to peak serum concentration: Within 0.5-2 hours

Elimination: Prolonged in neonates; partially eliminated by the liver and excreted in bile, 56% to 70% is eliminated in urine as unchanged drug

Usual Dosage Oral:

Use in newborns not recommended

Children <40 kg: 12.5-25 mg/kg/day divided every 6 hours; doses of 50-100 mg/kg/day in divided doses every 6 hours have been used for therapy of osteomyelitis

Children >40 kg and Adults: 125-250 mg every 6 hours

Dosage adjustment in renal impairment: Not necessary

Hemodialysis: Not dialyzable (0% to 5%); supplemental dosage not necessary

Peritoneal dialysis: Supplemental dosage not necessary

Continuous arteriovenous or venovenous hemofiltration (CAVH/CAVHD): Supplemental dosage not necessary

Dietary Considerations Food: Decreases drug absorption rate; decreases drug serum concentration. Administer on an empty stomach 1 hour before or 2 hours after meals.

Monitoring Parameters Monitor prothrombin time if patient concurrently on warfarin; monitor for signs of anaphylaxis during first dose

Test Interactions False-positive urine and serum proteins; false-positive in uric acid, urinary steroids; may interfere with urinary glucose tests using cupric sulfate (Benedict's solution, Clinitest®); may inactivate aminoglycosides *in vitro*

Patient Information Take until all medication used; take 1 hour before or 2 hours after meals, do not skip doses

Additional Information

Sodium content of 250 mg capsule: 13 mg (0.6 mEq)

Sodium content of suspension 65 mg/5 mL: 27 mg (1.2 mEq)

Dosage Forms

Capsule, as sodium: 125 mg, 250 mg, 500 mg

(Continued)

Dicloxacillin *(Continued)*

Powder for oral suspension, as sodium: 62.5 mg/5 mL (80 mL, 100 mL, 200 mL)

Selected Readings

Donowitz GR and Mandell GL, "Beta-Lactam Antibiotics," *N Engl J Med*, 1988, 318(7):419-26 and 318(8):490-500.

Wright AJ, "The Penicillins," *Mayo Clin Proc*, 1999, 74(3):290-307.

Dicloxacillin Sodium *see* Dicloxacillin *on page 702*

Didanosine *(dye DAN oh seen)*

Related Information

HIV Therapeutic Information *on page 1008*

U.S. Brand Names Videx®

Synonyms ddI

Generic Available No

Use Treatment of HIV infection; always to be used in combination with at least two other antiretroviral agents

Drug of Choice or Alternative for

Organism(s)

Human Immunodeficiency Virus *on page 177*

Pregnancy Risk Factor B

Pregnancy/Breast-Feeding Implications

Clinical effects on the fetus: Administer during pregnancy only if benefits to mother outweigh risks to the fetus

Breast-feeding/lactation: HIV-infected mothers are discouraged from breast-feeding to decrease potential transmission of HIV

Contraindications Hypersensitivity to any component

Warnings/Precautions Peripheral neuropathy occurs in ~35% of patients receiving the drug. Pancreatitis (sometimes fatal) occurs in ~9%; risk factors for developing pancreatitis include a previous history of the condition, concurrent cytomegalovirus or *Mycobacterium avium-intracellulare* infection, and concomitant use of pentamidine or co-trimoxazole; discontinue didanosine if clinical signs of pancreatitis occur. Didanosine may cause retinal depigmentation in children receiving doses >300 mg/m^2/day. Patients should undergo retinal examination every 6-12 months. Lactic acidosis and severe hepatomegaly have occurred with antiretroviral nucleoside analogues. Use with caution in patients with decreased renal or hepatic function, phenylketonuria, sodium-restricted diets, or with edema, congestive heart failure or hyperuricemia; in high concentrations, didanosine is mutagenic.

Adverse Reactions

>10%:

Central nervous system: Anxiety, headache, irritability, insomnia, restlessness

Gastrointestinal: Abdominal pain, nausea, diarrhea

Neuromuscular & skeletal: Peripheral neuropathy

1% to 10%:

Central nervous system: Depression

Dermatologic: Rash, pruritus

Gastrointestinal: Pancreatitis (2% to 3%)

<1%: Seizures, anemia, granulocytopenia, leukopenia, thrombocytopenia, hepatitis, retinal depigmentation, renal impairment, hypersensitivity, lactic acidosis/hepatomegaly, alopecia, anaphylactoid reaction, diabetes mellitus, optic neuritis

Overdosage/Toxicology

Chronic overdose may cause pancreatitis, peripheral neuropathy, diarrhea, hyperuricemia, and hepatic impairment

There is no known antidote for didanosine overdose; treatment is asymptomatic

Drug Interactions Drugs whose absorption depends on the level of acidity in the stomach such as ketoconazole, itraconazole, and dapsone should be administered at least 2 hours prior to didanosine

Decreased effect: Didanosine may decrease absorption of quinolones or tetracyclines, didanosine should be held during PCP treatment with pentamidine; didanosine may decrease levels of indinavir

Increased toxicity: Concomitant administration of other drugs which have the potential to cause peripheral neuropathy or pancreatitis may increase the risk of these toxicities

Stability Tablets should be stored in tightly closed bottles at 15°C to 30°C; undergoes rapid degradation when exposed to an acidic environment; tablets dispersed in water are stable for 1 hour at room temperature; reconstituted buffered solution is stable for 4 hours at room temperature; reconstituted pediatric solution is stable for 30 days if refrigerated; unbuffered powder for oral solution must be reconstituted and mixed with an equal volume of antacid at time of preparation

Mechanism of Action Didanosine, a purine nucleoside analogue and the deamination product of dideoxyadenosine (ddA), inhibits HIV replication *in vitro* in both T cells and monocytes. Didanosine is converted within the cell to the mono-, di-, and triphosphates of ddA. These ddA triphosphates act as substrate and inhibitor of HIV reverse transcriptase substrate and inhibitor of HIV reverse transcriptase thereby blocking viral DNA synthesis and suppressing HIV replication.

Pharmacodynamics/Kinetics

Absorption: Subject to degradation by the acidic pH of the stomach; buffered to resist the acidic pH; as much as 50% reduction in the peak plasma concentration is observed in the presence of food

Distribution: V_d: 1.08 L/kg; children: 35.6 L/m^2

Protein binding: <5%

Metabolism: Has not been evaluated in man; studies conducted in dogs, shows didanosine extensively metabolized with allantoin, hypoxanthine, xanthine, and uric acid being the major metabolites found in the urine

Bioavailability: 42% (range: 2% to 89%)

Half-life:

Children and Adolescents: 0.8 hour

Adults:

Normal renal function: 1.5 hours; however, its active metabolite ddATP has an intracellular half-life >12 hours *in vitro*; this permits the drug to be dosed at 12-hour intervals; total body clearance averages 800 mL/minute

Impaired renal function: Half-life is increased, with values ranging from 2.5-5 hours

Elimination: ~55% of drug is eliminated unchanged in urine

Usual Dosage Oral (administer on an empty stomach):

Children: 180 mg/m^2/day divided every 12 hours **or** dosing is based on body surface area (m^2): See table.

Didanosine — Pediatric Dosing

Body Surface Area (m^2)	Dosing (Tablets) (mg bid)
≤0.4	25
0.5-0.7	50
0.8-1	75
1.1-1.4	100

Adults: Dosing is based on patient weight: See table on next page.

Note: Children >1 year and Adults should receive 2 tablets per dose and children <1 year should receive 1 tablet per dose for adequate buffering and absorption; tablets should be chewed; didanosine has also been used as 300 mg once daily
(Continued)

Didanosine *(Continued)*

Didanosine — Adult Dosing

Patient Weight (kg)	Dosing (Tablets) (mg bid)
35-49	125
50-74	200
≥75	300

Recommended Dose (mg) of Didanosine by Body Weight

Creatinine Clearance (mL/min)	≥60 kg		<60 kg		Interval (hours)
	Tablet[a]	Solution[b]	Tablet[a]	Solution[b]	
≥60	200	250	125	167	12
30-59	100	100	75	100	12
10-29	150	167	100	100	24
<10	100	100	75	100	24

[a] Chewable/dispersible buffered tablet; 2 tablets must be taken with each dose; different strengths of tablets may be combined to yield the recommended dose.

[b] Buffered powder for oral solution

Dosing adjustment in renal impairment:
Hemodialysis: Removed by hemodialysis (40% to 60%)

Dosing adjustment in hepatic impairment: Should be considered

Monitoring Parameters Serum potassium, uric acid, creatinine; hemoglobin, CBC with neutrophil and platelet count, CD4 cells; viral load; liver function tests, amylase; weight gain; perform dilated retinal exam every 6 months

Patient Information Thoroughly chew tablets or manually crush or disperse 2 tablets in 1 oz of water prior to taking; for powder, open packet and pour contents into 4 oz of liquid; do not mix with fruit juice or other acid-containing liquid; stir until dissolved, drink immediately; do not take with meals

Nursing Implications Administer liquified powder immediately after dissolving; avoid creating dust if powder spilled, use wet mop or damp sponge

Additional Information Sodium content of buffered tablets: 264.5 mg (11.5 mEq)

Dosage Forms
Powder for oral solution:
Buffered (single dose packet): 100 mg, 167 mg, 250 mg, 375 mg
Pediatric: 2 g, 4 g
Tablet, buffered, chewable (mint flavor): 25 mg, 50 mg, 100 mg, 150 mg

Selected Readings
Hirsch MS and D'Aquila RT, "Therapy for Human Immunodeficiency Virus Infection," *N Engl J Med*, 1993, 328(23):1686-95.
Perry CM and Balfour JA, "Didanosine. An Update on Its Antiviral Activity, Pharmacokinetic Properties, and Therapeutic Efficacy in the Management of HIV Disease," *Drugs*, 1996, 52(6):928-62.
Rathbun RC and Martin ES 3d, "Didanosine Therapy in Patients Intolerant of or Failing Zidovudine Therapy," *Ann Pharmacother*, 1992, 26(11):1347-51.
Sande MA, Carpenter CC, Cobbs CG, et al, "Antiretroviral Therapy for Adult HIV-Infected Patients," *JAMA*, 1993, 270(21):2583-9.

Dideoxycytidine *see* Zalcitabine *on page 974*

Diflucan® *see* Fluconazole *on page 732*

Diiodohydroxyquin *see* Iodoquinol *on page 781*

Diloxanide Furoate *(dye LOKS ah nide FYOOR oh ate)*
U.S. Brand Names Furamide®
Generic Available No
Use Treatment of amebiasis (asymptomatic cyst passers)
Drug of Choice or Alternative for
Organism(s)
Entamoeba histolytica on page 132
Additional Information Available from:
The Centers for Disease Control Drug and Immunobiologic Service
1600 Clifton Road

Building 1
Room 1259
Atlanta, GA 30333
Monday-Friday 8 AM to 4:30 PM
(404) 639-3670
Nonbusiness hours (emergencies only): (404) 639-3670

Selected Readings
"Drugs for Parasitic Infections," *Med Lett Drugs Ther*, 1998, 40(1017):1-12.

Dimethoxyphenyl Penicillin Sodium *see* Methicillin *on page 816*

Diochloram *see* Chloramphenicol *on page 667*

Diodoquin® *see* Iodoquinol *on page 781*

Diomycin *see* Erythromycin *on page 722*

Diphtheria and Tetanus Toxoid
(dif THEER ee a & TET a nus TOKS oyd)

Synonyms DT; Td; Tetanus and Diphtheria Toxoid

Generic Available Yes

Use Active immunity against diphtheria and tetanus when pertussis vaccine is contraindicated; tetanus prophylaxis in wound management
DT: Infants and children through 6 years of age
Td: Children and adults ≥7 years of age

Drug of Choice or Alternative for
Organism(s)
Corynebacterium diphtheriae on page 111

Pregnancy Risk Factor C

Pregnancy/Breast-Feeding Implications Clinical effects on the fetus: Td and T vaccines are not known to cause special problems for pregnant women or their unborn babies. While physicians do not usually recommend giving any drugs or vaccines to pregnant women, a pregnant women who needs Td vaccine should get it; wait until 2nd trimester if possible.

Contraindications Patients receiving immunosuppressive agents, prior anaphylactic, allergic, or systemic reactions; hypersensitivity to diphtheria and tetanus toxoid or any component; acute respiratory infection or other active infection

Warnings/Precautions History of a neurologic reaction or immediate hypersensitivity reaction following a previous dose. History of severe local reaction (Arthus-type) following previous dose (such individuals should not be given further routine or emergency doses of tetanus and diphtheria toxoids for 10 years). Do not confuse pediatric DT with adult diphtheria and tetanus toxoid (Td), absorbed (Td) is used in patients >7 years of age; primary immunization should be postponed until the second year of life due to possibility of CNS damage or convulsion; have epinephrine 1:1000 available.

Adverse Reactions Severe adverse reactions must be reported to the FDA
>10%: Central nervous system: Fretfulness, drowsiness
1% to 10%:
Central nervous system: Persistent crying
Gastrointestinal: Anorexia, vomiting
<1%: Tachycardia, hypotension, edema, convulsions (rarely), pain, redness, urticaria, pruritus, tenderness, Arthus-type hypersensitivity reactions, transient fever

Drug Interactions Decreased effect with immunosuppressive agents, immunoglobulins if given within 1 month (eg, concomitant administration with tetanus immune globulin decreased the immune response to Td)

Stability Refrigerate

Usual Dosage I.M.:
Infants and Children (DT):
6 weeks to 1 year: Three 0.5 mL doses at least 4 weeks apart; administer a reinforcing dose 6-12 months after the third injection
1-6 years: Two 0.5 mL doses at least 4 weeks apart; reinforcing dose 6-12 months after second injection; if final dose is given after seventh birthday, use adult preparation
4-6 years (booster immunization): 0.5 mL; not necessary if all 4 doses were given after fourth birthday - routinely administer booster doses at 10-year intervals with the adult preparation
(Continued)

Diphtheria and Tetanus Toxoid *(Continued)*

Children >7 years and Adults: Should receive Td; 2 primary doses of 0.5 mL each, given at an interval of 4-6 weeks; third (reinforcing) dose of 0.5 mL 6-12 months later; boosters every 10 years

Tetanus Prophylaxis in Wound Management

Number of Prior Tetanus Toxoid Doses	Clean, Minor Wounds		All Other Wounds	
	Td*	TIG†	Td*	TIG†
Unknown or <3	Yes	No	Yes	Yes
≥3‡	No#	No	No¶	No

*Adult tetanus and diphtheria toxoids; use pediatric preparations (DT or DTP) if the patient is <7 years old.

†Tetanus immune globulin.

‡If only three doses of fluid tetanus toxoid have been received, a fourth dose of toxoid, preferably an adsorbed toxoid, should be given.

#Yes, if >10 years since last dose.

¶Yes, if >5 years since last dose.

Adapted from Report of the Committee on Infectious Diseases, American Academy of Pediatrics, Elk Grove Village, IL: American Academy of Pediatrics, 1986.

Administration Administer only I.M.; do not inject the same site more than once

Patient Information DT, Td and T vaccines cause few problems (mild fever or soreness, swelling, and redness/knot at the injection site); these problems usually last 1-2 days, but this does not happen nearly as often as with DTP vaccine

Nursing Implications Shake well before giving

Additional Information Pediatric dosage form should only be used in patients ≤6 years of age. Federal law requires that the date of administration, the vaccine manufacturer, lot number of vaccine, and the administering person's name, title, and address be entered into the patient's permanent medical record.

Since protective tetanus and diphtheria antibodies decline with age, only 28% of persons >70 years of age in the U.S. are believed to be immune to tetanus, and most of the tetanus-induced deaths occur in people >60 years of age, it is advisable to offer Td especially to the elderly concurrent with their influenza and other immunization programs if history of vaccination is unclear; boosters should be given at 10-year intervals; earlier for wounds

Dosage Forms Injection:

Pediatric use:
Diphtheria 6.6 Lf units and tetanus 5 Lf units per 0.5 mL (5 mL)
Diphtheria 10 Lf units and tetanus 5 Lf units per 0.5 mL (0.5 mL, 5 mL)
Diphtheria 12.5 Lf units and tetanus 5 Lf units per 0.5 mL (5 mL)
Diphtheria 15 Lf units and tetanus 10 Lf units per 0.5 mL (5 mL)

Adult use:
Diphtheria 1.5 Lf units and tetanus 5 Lf units per 0.5 mL (0.5 mL, 5 mL)
Diphtheria 2 Lf units and tetanus 5 Lf units per 0.5 mL (5 mL)
Diphtheria 2 Lf units and tetanus 10 Lf units per 0.5 mL (5 mL)

Diphtheria CRM₁₉₇ Protein Conjugate *see Haemophilus b Conjugate Vaccine on page 756*

Diphtheria, Tetanus Toxoids, and Acellular Pertussis Vaccine

(dif THEER ee a, TET a nus TOKS oyds, & ay CEL yoo lar per TUS sis vak SEEN)

Related Information
Immunization Guidelines *on page 1041*

U.S. Brand Names Acel-Imune®; Certiva™; Infanrix™; TriHIBit®; Tripedia®

Synonyms DTaP

Use As fourth and fifth dose in primary immunization series against diphtheria, tetanus, and pertussis from age 15 months (Tripedia®) or 17 months (Acel-Imune®) through 7th birthday (recipients must have previously received 3 doses of whole-cell DTP (DTwP))

**Drug of Choice or Alternative for
Organism(s)**

Corynebacterium diphtheriae on page 111

Pregnancy Risk Factor C

Pregnancy/Breast-Feeding Implications Clinical effects on the fetus: Animal reproduction studies have not been conducted. It is not known whether the vaccine can cause fetal harm when administered to a pregnant woman or can affect reproductive capacity. Tripedia® vaccine is NOT recommended for use in a pregnant woman.

Contraindications Patients >7 years of age, patients with cancer, immunodeficiencies, an acute respiratory infection, or any other active infection; children with a history of neurologic disorders should not receive the pertussis or any component; history of any of the following effects from previous administration of pertussis vaccine precludes further use: >103°F fever (39.4°C), convulsions, focal neurologic signs, screaming episodes, shock, collapse, sleepiness or encephalopathy; known hypersensitivity to diphtheria and tetanus toxoids or pertussis vaccine; do not use for treatment of actual tetanus, diphtheria, or whooping cough infections

Warnings/Precautions DTaP should not be used in children <15 months of age and should not be used in children who have received fewer than 3 doses of DTP

Adverse Reactions All serious adverse reactions must be reported to the U.S. Department of Health and Human Services (DDHS) Vaccine Adverse Event Reporting System (VAERS) 1-800-822-7967.

<1%: Edema, convulsions, screaming episodes, malaise, sleepiness, focal neurological signs, shock, collapse, fever, chills, erythema, induration, rash, urticaria, tenderness, arthralgias

Drug Interactions Decreased effect with immunosuppressive agents, corticosteroids within 1 month

Stability Refrigerate at 2°C to 8°C (35°F to 46°F); do not freeze

Mechanism of Action Promotes active immunity to diphtheria, tetanus, and pertussis by inducing production of specific antibodies and antitoxins.

Usual Dosage Before administration, ensure that at least 3 doses of whole-cell DTP vaccine have been given. Give the fourth dose of DTaP at ~18 months of age, at least 6 months after the third DTwP. Give a fifth 0.5 mL dose at 4-6 years of age. Tetanus and diphtheria toxoids for adult use (Td) is the preferred agent for adults and older children.

Administration Administer only I.M. in anterolateral aspect of thigh or deltoid muscle of upper arm

Patient Information A nodule may be palpable at the injection site for a few weeks

Nursing Implications

Acetaminophen 10-15 mg/kg before and every 4 hours to 12-24 hours may reduce or prevent fever

Shake well before administering

The child's medical record should document that the small risk of postvaccination seizure and the benefits of the pertussis vaccination were discussed with the patient

Additional Information This preparation contains less endotoxin relative to DTP and, although immunogenic, it apparently is less reactogenic than DTP. Federal law requires that the date of administration, the vaccine manufacturer, lot number of vaccine, and the administering person's name, title, and address be entered into the patient's permanent medical record.

Dosage Forms Injection:

Acel-Imune®: Diphtheria 7.5 Lf units, tetanus 5 Lf units, and acellular pertussis vaccine 40 mcg per 0.5 mL (7.5 mL)

Tripedia®: Diphtheria 6.7 Lf units, tetanus 5 Lf units, and acellular pertussis vaccine 46.8 mcg per 0.5 mL (7.5 mL)

Infanrix™: Diphtheria 25 Lf units, tetanus 10 Lf units, and acellular pertussis vaccine 25 mcg per 0.5 mL (0.5 mL)

TriHIBit® vaccine [Tripedia® vaccine used to reconstitute ActHIB®]: 0.5 mL

Certiva™: Diphtheria 15 Lf units, tetanus 6 Lf, and acellular pertussis vaccine 40 mcg per 0.5 mL (7.5 mL)

Diphtheria, Tetanus Toxoids, and Whole-Cell Pertussis Vaccine, Adsorbed

(dif THEER ee a, TET a nus TOK soyds, & hole-sel per TUS is vak SEEN, ad SORBED)

Related Information

Immunization Guidelines *on page 1041*

U.S. Brand Names Tri-Immunol®

Synonyms DTP

Use Active immunization of infants and children through 6 years of age (between 2 months and the seventh birthday) against diphtheria, tetanus, and pertussis; recommended for primary immunization; start immunization if whooping cough or diphtheria is present in the community

For children who are severely immunocompromised or who are infected with HIV, DTP vaccine is indicated in the same schedule and dose as for immuno-competent children, including the use of acellular pertussis-containing vaccines (DTaP) as a booster. Although no specific studies with pertussis vaccine are available, if immunosuppressive therapy is to be discontinued shortly, it would be reasonable to defer immunization until at least 3 months after the patient last received therapy; otherwise, the patient should be vaccinated while still receiving therapy.

Pregnancy Risk Factor C

Contraindications

Known hypersensitivity to diphtheria and tetanus toxoids or pertussis vaccine, known hypersensitivity to thimerosal, thrombocytopenia

Patients >7 years of age history of any of the following effects from previous administration of pertussis vaccine precludes further use

Temperature of 105°F or higher **within 2 days** after getting DTP

Shock-collapse (becoming blue or pale, limp, and not responsive) **within 2 days** after getting DTP

Convulsion **within 3 days** after getting DTP

Crying that cannot be stopped which lasts for more than 3 hours at a time **within 2 days** after getting DTP

Warnings/Precautions Do not use DTP for treatment of actual tetanus, diphtheria, or whooping cough infections. The child's medical record should document that the small risk of past vaccination seizure and the benefits of the pertussis vaccination were discussed with the patient. If adverse reactions occurred with previous doses, immunization should be completed with diphtheria and tetanus toxoid absorbed (pediatric); have epinephrine 1:1000 available.

Adverse Reactions All serious adverse reactions must be reported to the U.S. Department of Health and Human Services (DHHS) Vaccine Adverse Event Reporting System (VAERS). Reporting forms and information about reporting requirements or completion of the form can be obtained from VAERS through a toll-free number 1-800-822-7967.

<1%: Convulsions, screaming episodes, malaise, sleepiness, focal neurological signs, shock, collapse, mild to moderate fever, chills, erythema, swelling induration, rash, urticaria, local tenderness, arthralgia

Drug Interactions Decreased effect: Immunosuppressive agents may result in aberrant responses to active immunization

Stability Refrigerate

Mechanism of Action Promotes active immunity to diphtheria, tetanus, and pertussis by inducing production of specific antibodies and antitoxins.

Usual Dosage For pediatric use only. Do not give to patients >7 years of age; primary immunization for children 2-6 years of age, ideally beginning at the age of 2-3 months

Primary immunization: Administer 0.5 mL I.M. on three occasions at 8-week intervals with a re-enforcing dose administered at 15-18 months of age

The booster doses are given when children are 4-6 years of age, 0.5 mL I.M. For booster doses thereafter, use the recommended dose of diphtheria and tetanus toxoids, adsorbed (adults) every 10 years; for patients not receiving immunization at usual times, consult authoritative source

Patient Information Most children have little or no problem from the DTP shot; many children will have fever or soreness, swelling, and redness where the shot was given. Usually these problems are mild and last 1-2 days. Some children will be cranky, drowsy, or not want to eat during this time.

Nursing Implications
Acetaminophen 10-15 mg/kg before and every 4 hours to 12-24 hours may reduce fever

Give vaccine only I.M.

The child's medical record should document that the small risk of past vaccination seizure and the benefits of the pertussis vaccination were discussed with the patient

Additional Information Inactivated/killed bacterial vaccine; federal law requires that the date of administration, the vaccine manufacturer, lot number of vaccine and the administering person's name, title and address be entered into the patient's permanent medical record

Dosage Forms Injection: 0.5 mL

Diphtheria, Tetanus Toxoids, Whole-Cell Pertussis, and *Haemophilus influenzae* Type b Conjugate Vaccines

(dif THEER ee a, TET a nus TOKS oyds, hole-sel per TUS sis, & hem OF fil us in floo EN za TIP bee KON joo gate vak SEEN)

U.S. Brand Names Tetramune®; Tripedia/ActHIB®

Synonyms DTwP-HIB

Use Active immunization of infants and children through 5 years of age (between 2 months and the sixth birthday) against diphtheria, tetanus, and pertussis and *Haemophilus* b disease when indications for immunization with DTP vaccine and HIB vaccine coincide

Drug of Choice or Alternative for
Organism(s)
Corynebacterium diphtheriae on page 111

Pregnancy Risk Factor C

Contraindications Children with any febrile illness or active infection, known hypersensitivity to *Haemophilus* b polysaccharide vaccine (thimerosal), children who are immunosuppressed or receiving immunosuppressive therapy; patients >7 years of age, patients with cancer, immunodeficiencies, an acute respiratory infection, or any other active infection; children with a history of neurologic disorders should not receive the pertussis any component; history of any of the following effects from previous administration of pertussis vaccine precludes further use: fever >103°F (39.4°C), convulsions, focal neurologic signs, screaming episodes, shock, collapse, sleepiness or encephalopathy; known hypersensitivity to diphtheria and tetanus toxoids or pertussis vaccine; do not use DTP for treatment of actual tetanus, diphtheria or whooping cough infections

Warnings/Precautions If adverse reactions occurred with previous doses, immunization should be completed with diphtheria and tetanus toxoid absorbed (pediatric); any febrile illness or active infection is reason for delaying use of *Haemophilus* b conjugate vaccine

Adverse Reactions
>10%:
Central nervous system: Fever, chills, irritability, restlessness, drowsiness
Local: Erythema, edema, induration, pain and warmth at injection site
1% to 10%:
Dermatologic: Rash
Gastrointestinal: Vomiting, diarrhea, loss of appetite
<1%: Convulsions, screaming episodes, malaise, sleepiness, focal neurological signs, shock, collapse, chills, urticaria, local tenderness, arthralgia, increased risk of *Haemophilus* b infections in the week after vaccination, rarely allergic or anaphylactic reactions

Drug Interactions Decreased effect: Immunosuppressive agents; may interfere with antigen detection tests

Stability Keep in refrigerator, may be frozen (not diluent) without affecting potency; unopened vials are stable for up to 24 hours at <70°C

Mechanism of Action Promotes active immunity to diphtheria, tetanus, pertussis, and *H. influenzae* by inducing production of specific antibodies and antitoxins.
(Continued)

Diphtheria, Tetanus Toxoids, Whole-Cell Pertussis, and *Haemophilus influenzae* Type b Conjugate Vaccines *(Continued)*

Usual Dosage The primary immunization for children 2 months to 5 years of age, ideally beginning at the age of 2-3 months or at 6-week check-up. Administer 0.5 mL I.M. on 3 occasions at ~2-month intervals, followed by a fourth 0.5 mL dose at ~15 months of age.

Administration Administer I.M. only

Patient Information A nodule may be palpable at the injection site for a few weeks

Nursing Implications

Acetaminophen 10-15 mg/kg before and every 4 hours to 12-24 hours may reduce or prevent fever

Shake well before administering

The child's medical record should document that the small risk of past vaccination seizure and the benefits of the pertussis vaccination were discussed with the patient

Additional Information Inactivated bacterial vaccine; federal law requires that the date of administration, the vaccine manufacturer, lot number of vaccine and the administering person's name, title, and address be entered into the patient's permanent medical record. **(Note:** Diphtheria and Tetanus Toxoids, and Acellular Pertussis and *Haemophilus influenzae* Type b Conjugate Vaccine is Tripedia/ActHIB®.)

Dosage Forms Injection: Diphtheria toxoid 12.5 Lf units, tetanus toxoid 5 Lf units, and whole-cell pertussis vaccine 4 units, and *Haemophilus influenzae* type b oligosaccharide 10 mcg per 0.5 mL (5 mL)

Diphtheria Toxoid Conjugate *see Haemophilus* b Conjugate Vaccine *on page 756*

Dirithromycin (dye RITH roe mye sin)

U.S. Brand Names Dynabac®

Generic Available No

Use Treatment of mild to moderate upper and lower respiratory tract infections due to *Moraxella catarrhalis*, *Streptococcus pneumoniae*, *Legionella pneumophila*, *Haemophilus influenzae*, or *Streptococcus pyogenes* (ie, acute exacerbation of chronic bronchitis, secondary bacterial infection of acute bronchitis, community-acquired pneumonia, pharyngitis/tonsillitis, and uncomplicated infections of the skin and skin structure due to *Staphylococcus aureus*)

Pregnancy Risk Factor C

Pregnancy/Breast-Feeding Implications

Clinical effects on the fetus: Animal studies indicate the use of dirithromycin during pregnancy should be avoided if possible

Breast-feeding/lactation: Use caution when administering to nursing women

Contraindications Hypersensitivity to any macrolide or component of dirithromycin; use with pimozide

Warnings/Precautions Contrary to potential serious consequences with other macrolides (eg, cardiac arrhythmias), the combination of terfenadine and dirithromycin has not shown alteration of terfenadine metabolism; however, caution should be taken during coadministration of dirithromycin and terfenadine; pseudomembranous colitis has been reported and should be considered in patients presenting with diarrhea subsequent to therapy with dirithromycin

Adverse Reactions

1% to 10%:

Central nervous system: Headache, dizziness, vertigo, insomnia

Dermatologic: Rash, pruritus, urticaria

Endocrine & metabolic: Hyperkalemia

Gastrointestinal: Abdominal pain, nausea, diarrhea, vomiting, dyspepsia, flatulence

Hematologic: Thrombocytosis, eosinophilia, segmented neutrophils

Neuromuscular & skeletal: Weakness, pain, increased CPK

Respiratory: Increased cough, dyspnea

<1%: Palpitations, vasodilation, syncope, edema, anxiety depression, somnolence, fever, malaise, dysmenorrhea, hypochloremia, hypophosphatemia,

dehydration, abnormal stools, anorexia, gastritis, constipation, abnormal taste, xerostomia, abdominal pain, mouth ulceration, polyuria, vaginitis, neutropenia, thrombocytopenia, decreased hemoglobin and hematocrit, increased bands and basophils, leukocytosis, monocytosis, increased ALT, AST, GGT, creatinine, phosphorus, uric acid, alkaline phosphatase, bilirubin, paresthesia, tremor, myalgia, amblyopia, tinnitus, epistaxis, hemoptysis, hyperventilation, hypoalbuminemia, flu-like syndrome, diaphoresis, thirst

Overdosage/Toxicology
Symptoms of overdose include nausea, vomiting, abdominal pain, diarrhea
Treatment is supportive; dialysis has not been found effective

Drug Interactions CYP3A3/4 enzyme inhibitor
Increased effect: Absorption of dirithromycin is slightly enhanced with concomitant antacids and H_2 antagonists; dirithromycin may, like erythromycin, increase the effect of alfentanil, anticoagulants, bromocriptine, carbamazepine, cyclosporine, digoxin, disopyramide, ergots, methylprednisolone, cisapride, astemizole

Increased toxicity: Avoid use with pimozide (due to risk of significant cardiotoxicity) and triazolam

Note: Interactions with nonsedating antihistamines (eg, terfenadine, astemizole), cisapride, and theophylline are not known to occur, however, caution is advised with coadministration.

Mechanism of Action After being converted during intestinal absorption to its active form, erythromycylamine, dirithromycin inhibits protein synthesis by binding to the 50S ribosomal subunits of susceptible microorganisms

Pharmacodynamics/Kinetics
Absorption: Rapidly absorbed and nonenzymatically hydrolyzed to erythromycylamine; T_{max}: 4 hours
Distribution: V_d: 800 L; rapidly and widely distributed (higher levels in tissues than plasma)
Protein binding: 14% to 30%
Metabolism: Hydrolyzed to erythromycylamine
Bioavailability: 10%
Half-life: 8 hours (range: 2-36 hours)
Elimination: Via bile (81% to 97% of dose)

Usual Dosage Adults: Oral: 500 mg once daily for 5-14 days (14 days required for treatment of community-acquired pneumonia due to *Legionella, Mycoplasma,* or *S. pneumoniae*; 10 days is recommended for treatment of *S. pyogenes* pharyngitis/tonsillitis)

Dosing adjustment in renal impairment: None necessary
Dosing adjustment in hepatic impairment: None needed in mild dysfunction; not studied in moderate to severe dysfunction

Administration Administer with food or within an hour following a meal
Monitoring Parameters Temperature, CBC
Patient Information Take with food or within an hour following a meal; do not cut, chew, or crush tablets; entire course of medication should be taken to ensure eradication of organism
Nursing Implications Do not crush tablets
Dosage Forms Tablet, enteric coated: 250 mg

Selected Readings
"Dirithromycin," *Med Lett Drugs Ther,* 1995, 37(962):109-10.
Sharma R and Cramer M, "Focus on Dirithromycin: A New Once Daily Macrolide Antibiotic," *Formulary,* 1995, 30:769-83.
Tartaglione TA, "Therapeutic Options for the Management and Prevention of *Mycobacterium avium* Complex Infection in Patients With the Acquired Immunodeficiency Syndrome," *Pharmacotherapy,* 1996, 16(2):171-82.
Wintermeyer SM, Abdel-Rahman SM, and Nahata MC, "Dirithromycin: A New Macrolide," *Ann Pharmacother,* 1996, 30(10):1141-9.

Doryx® *see Doxycycline on page 713*
Doxy® *see Doxycycline on page 713*
Doxychel® *see Doxycycline on page 713*
Doxycin *see Doxycycline on page 713*

Doxycycline (doks i SYE kleen)
U.S. Brand Names Atridox™; Bio-Tab® Oral; Doryx®; Doxy®; Doxychel®; Periostat™; Vibramycin®; Vibramycin® IV; Vibra-Tabs®
(Continued)

Doxycycline *(Continued)*

Canadian Brand Names Apo®-Doxy; Apo®-Doxy Tabs; Doxycin; Doxytec; Novo-Doxylin; Nu-Doxycycline

Synonyms Doxycycline Hyclate; Doxycycline Monohydrate

Generic Available Yes

Use Principally in the treatment of infections caused by susceptible *Rickettsia*, *Chlamydia*, and *Mycoplasma* along with uncommon susceptible gram-negative and gram-positive organisms; alternative to mefloquine for malaria prophylaxis; treatment for syphilis in penicillin-allergic patients; often active against vancomycin-resistant enterococci; used for community-acquired pneumonia and other common infections due to susceptible organisms; sclerosing agent for pleural effusions

Drug of Choice or Alternative for

Disease/Syndrome(s)

Bronchitis *on page 20*
Pelvic Inflammatory Disease *on page 41*
Pneumonia, Community-Acquired *on page 45*
Urethritis, Nongonococcal *on page 51*

Organism(s)

Actinomyces Species *on page 61*
Bartonella Species *on page 76*
Borrelia burgdorferi on page 84
Brucella Species *on page 85*
Campylobacter jejuni on page 90
Chlamydia pneumoniae on page 95
Chlamydia psittaci on page 97
Chlamydia trachomatis on page 99
Coxiella burnetii on page 115
Ehrlichia Species *on page 130*
Enterococcus Species *on page 137*
Leptospira interrogans on page 186
Mycoplasma pneumoniae on page 211
Neisseria gonorrhoeae on page 215
Rickettsia rickettsii on page 243
Staphylococcus aureus, Methicillin-Resistant *on page 256*
Stenotrophomonas maltophilia on page 265
Treponema pallidum on page 285
Ureaplasma urealyticum on page 292
Vibrio cholerae on page 297
Yersinia pestis on page 300

Pregnancy Risk Factor D

Contraindications Hypersensitivity to doxycycline, tetracycline or any component; children <8 years of age; severe hepatic dysfunction

Warnings/Precautions Use of tetracyclines during tooth development may cause permanent discoloration of the teeth and enamel hypoplasia; prolonged use may result in superinfection; photosensitivity reaction may occur with this drug; avoid prolonged exposure to sunlight or tanning equipment. Do not administer to children ≤8 years of age.

Adverse Reactions

>10%: Miscellaneous: Discoloration of teeth in children

1% to 10%: Gastrointestinal: Esophagitis

<1%: Increased intracranial pressure, bulging fontanels in infants, rash, photosensitivity, nausea, diarrhea, neutropenia, eosinophilia, hepatotoxicity, phlebitis

Overdosage/Toxicology

Symptoms of overdose include nausea, anorexia, diarrhea

Following GI decontamination, supportive care only; fluid support may be required for hypotension

Drug Interactions CYP3A3/4 enzyme substrate

Decreased effect with antacids containing aluminum, calcium, or magnesium

Iron and bismuth subsalicylate may decrease doxycycline bioavailability

Barbiturates, phenytoin, and carbamazepine decrease doxycycline's half-life

Increased effect of warfarin

Stability Tetracyclines form toxic products when outdated or when exposed to light, heat, or humidity; reconstituted solution is stable for 72 hours (refrigerated);

for I.V. infusion in NS or D_5W solution, complete infusion should be completed within 12 hours; discard remaining solution

Mechanism of Action Inhibits protein synthesis by binding with the 30S and possibly the 50S ribosomal subunit(s) of susceptible bacteria; may also cause alterations in the cytoplasmic membrane

Pharmacodynamics/Kinetics

Absorption: Almost completely from the GI tract; absorption can be reduced by food or milk by 20%

Distribution: Widely distributed into body tissues and fluids including synovial, pleural, prostatic, seminal fluids, and bronchial secretions; saliva, aqueous humor, and CSF penetration is poor; readily crosses placenta and appears in breast milk

Protein binding: 90%

Metabolism: Not metabolized in the liver, instead is partially inactivated in the GI tract by chelate formation

Half-life: 12-15 hours (usually increases to 22-24 hours with multiple dosing)
End stage renal disease: 18-25 hours

Time to peak serum concentration: Within 1.5-4 hours

Elimination: In urine (23%) and feces (30%)

Usual Dosage Oral, I.V.:

Children ≥8 years (<45 kg): 2-5 mg/kg/day in 1-2 divided doses, not to exceed 200 mg/day

Children >8 years (>45 kg) and Adults: 100-200 mg/day in 1-2 divided doses

Acute gonococcal infection: 200 mg immediately, then 100 mg at bedtime on the first day followed by 100 mg twice daily for 3 days **or** 300 mg immediately followed by 300 mg in 1 hour

Primary and secondary syphilis: 300 mg/day in divided doses for ≥10 days

Uncomplicated chlamydial infections: 100 mg twice daily for ≥7 days

Endometritis, salpingitis, parametritis, or peritonitis: 100 mg I.V. twice daily with cefoxitin 2 g every 6 hours for 4 days and for ≥48 hours after patient improves; then continue with oral therapy 100 mg twice daily to complete a 10- to 14-day course of therapy

Sclerosing agent for pleural effusion injection: 500 mg as a single dose in 30-50 mL of NS or SWI

Dosing adjustment in renal impairment: Cl_{cr} <10 mL/minute: 100 mg every 24 hours

Dialysis: Not dialyzable; 0% to 5% by hemo- and peritoneal methods or by continuous arteriovenous or venovenous hemofiltration (CAVH/CAVHD); no supplemental dosage necessary

Administration Infuse I.V. doxycycline over 1 hour; may administer with meals to decrease GI upset

Test Interactions False-negative urine glucose using Clinistix®, Tes-Tape®

Patient Information Avoid unnecessary exposure to sunlight; finish all medication; do not skip doses

Nursing Implications Avoid extravasation

Dosage Forms

Capsule, as hyclate:
Doxychel®, Vibramycin®: 50 mg
Doxy®, Doxychel®, Vibramycin®: 100 mg

Capsule, as monohydrate (Monodox®): 50 mg, 100 mg

Capsule, coated pellets, as hyclate (Doryx®): 100 mg

Powder for injection, as hyclate (Doxy®, Doxychel®, Vibramycin® IV): 100 mg, 200 mg

Powder for oral suspension, as monohydrate (raspberry flavor) (Vibramycin®): 25 mg/5 mL (60 mL)

Syrup, as calcium (raspberry-apple flavor) (Vibramycin®): 50 mg/5 mL (30 mL, 473 mL)

Tablet, as hyclate
Doxychel®: 50 mg
Bio-Tab®, Doxychel®, Vibra-Tabs®: 100 mg

Selected Readings
Joshi N and Miller DQ, "Doxycycline Revisited," *Arch Int Med*, 1997, 157(13):1421-8.
Smilack JD, Wilson WR, and Cockerill FR 3d, "Tetracyclines, Chloramphenicol, Erythromycin, Clindamycin, and Metronidazole," *Mayo Clin Proc*, 1991, 66(12):1270-80.
US Department of Health and Human Services, "1993 Sexually Transmitted Diseases Treatment Guidelines," *MMWR Morb Mortal Wkly Rep*, 1993, 42(RR-14).
Wyler DJ, "Malaria: Overview and Update," *Clin Infect Dis*, 1993, 16(4):449-56.

Doxycycline Hyclate *see Doxycycline on page 713*

Doxycycline Monohydrate *see Doxycycline on page 713*

Doxytec *see Doxycycline on page 713*

Dronabinol (droe NAB i nol)

U.S. Brand Names Marinol®

Synonyms Tetrahydrocannabinol; THC

Generic Available Yes

Use Treatment of "AIDS-wasting" syndrome; used when conventional antiemetics fail to relieve the nausea and vomiting associated with cancer chemotherapy

Restrictions C-II

Pregnancy Risk Factor B

Contraindications Use only for cancer chemotherapy-induced nausea; should not be used in patients with a history of schizophrenia or in patients with known hypersensitivity to dronabinol or any component

Warnings/Precautions Use with caution in patients with heart disease, hepatic disease, or seizure disorders; reduce dosage in patients with severe hepatic impairment

Adverse Reactions

>10%: Central nervous system: Drowsiness, dizziness, detachment, anxiety, difficulty concentrating, mood change

1% to 10%:

Cardiovascular: Orthostatic hypotension, tachycardia

Central nervous system: Ataxia, depression, headache, vertigo, hallucinations, memory lapse

Gastrointestinal: Xerostomia

Neuromuscular & skeletal: Paresthesia, weakness

<1%: Syncope, nightmares, speech difficulties, diarrhea, myalgia, tinnitus, diaphoresis

Overdosage/Toxicology Symptoms of overdose include tachycardia, hypertension, and hypotension

Drug Interactions Increased toxicity (drowsiness) with alcohol, barbiturates, benzodiazepines

Stability Store in a cool place

Mechanism of Action Not well defined, probably inhibits the vomiting center in the medulla oblongata

Pharmacodynamics/Kinetics

Absorption: Oral: Erratic

Protein binding: 97% to 99%

Metabolism: Extensive first-pass metabolism; metabolized in the liver to several metabolites, some of which are active

Half-life: 19-24 hours

Time to peak serum concentration: Within 2-3 hours

Elimination: In feces and urine

Usual Dosage Oral:

Children: NCI protocol recommends 5 mg/m^2 starting 6-8 hours before chemotherapy and every 4-6 hours after to be continued for 12 hours after chemotherapy is discontinued

Adults: 5 mg/m^2 1-3 hours before chemotherapy, then administer 5 mg/m^2/dose every 2-4 hours after chemotherapy for a total of 4-6 doses/day; dose may be increased up to a maximum of 15 mg/m^2/dose if needed (dosage may be increased by 2.5 mg/m^2 increments)

AIDS wasting: Initial: 2.5 mg twice daily (before lunch and dinner); titrate up to a maximum of 20 mg/day

Dietary Considerations Alcohol: Additive CNS effect, avoid use

Monitoring Parameters CNS effects, heart rate, blood pressure

Reference Range Antinauseant effects: 5-10 ng/mL

Test Interactions Decreases FSH, LH, growth hormone, testosterone

Patient Information Avoid activities such as driving which require motor coordination, avoid alcohol and other CNS depressants; may impair coordination and judgment

Nursing Implications Raise bed rails, institute safety measures, assist with ambulation

Dosage Forms Capsule: 2.5 mg, 5 mg, 10 mg

Selected Readings
Lane M, Smith FE, Sullivan RA, et al, "Dronabinol and Prochlorperazine Alone and in Combination as Antiemetic Agents for Cancer Chemotherapy," *Am J Clin Oncol*, 1990, 13(6):480-4.

Drotic® Otic *see* Neomycin, Polymyxin B, and Hydrocortisone *on page 836*

Dr Scholl's Athlete's Foot [OTC] *see* Tolnaftate *on page 956*

Dr Scholl's Maximum Strength Tritin [OTC] *see* Tolnaftate *on page 956*

DT *see* Diphtheria and Tetanus Toxoid *on page 707*

DTaP *see* Diphtheria, Tetanus Toxoids, and Acellular Pertussis Vaccine *on page 708*

DTP *see* Diphtheria, Tetanus Toxoids, and Whole-Cell Pertussis Vaccine, Adsorbed *on page 710*

DTwP-HIB *see* Diphtheria, Tetanus Toxoids, Whole-Cell Pertussis, and *Haemophilus influenzae* Type b Conjugate Vaccines *on page 711*

Durabolin® *see* Nandrolone *on page 829*

Duratest® Injection *see* Testosterone *on page 939*

Durathate® Injection *see* Testosterone *on page 939*

Duricef® *see* Cefadroxil *on page 629*

Dycill® *see* Dicloxacillin *on page 702*

Dynabac® *see* Dirithromycin *on page 712*

Dynacin® Oral *see* Minocycline *on page 823*

Dyna-Hex® Topical [OTC] *see* Chlorhexidine Gluconate *on page 670*

Dynapen® *see* Dicloxacillin *on page 702*

Ear-Eze® Otic *see* Neomycin, Polymyxin B, and Hydrocortisone *on page 836*

E-Base® *see* Erythromycin *on page 722*

Econazole (e KONE a zole)

U.S. Brand Names Spectazole™ Topical

Canadian Brand Names Ecostatin®

Synonyms Econazole Nitrate

Generic Available No

Use Topical treatment of tinea pedis (athlete's foot), tinea cruris (jock itch), tinea corporis (ringworm), tinea versicolor, and cutaneous candidiasis

Pregnancy Risk Factor C

Pregnancy/Breast-Feeding Implications Clinical effect on the fetus: Do not use during the 1st trimester of pregnancy, unless essential to a patient's welfare; use during the 2nd and 3rd trimesters only if clearly needed

Contraindications Known hypersensitivity to econazole or any component

Warnings/Precautions Discontinue drug if sensitivity or chemical irritation occurs; not for ophthalmic or intravaginal use

Adverse Reactions 1% to 10%:
Dermatologic: Pruritus, erythema
Local: Burning, stinging

Mechanism of Action Alters fungal cell wall membrane permeability; may interfere with RNA and protein synthesis, and lipid metabolism

Pharmacodynamics/Kinetics
Absorption: Topical: <10%
Metabolism: In the liver to >20 metabolites
Elimination: <1% of applied dose recovered in urine or feces

Usual Dosage Children and Adults: Topical:
Tinea pedis, tinea cruris, tinea corporis, tinea versicolor: Apply sufficient amount to cover affected areas once daily
Cutaneous candidiasis: Apply sufficient quantity twice daily (morning and evening)
Duration of treatment: Candidal infections and tinea cruris, versicolor, and corporis should be treated for 2 weeks and tinea pedis for 1 month; occasionally, longer treatment periods may be required

Patient Information For external use only; avoid eye contact; if condition worsens or persists, or irritation occurs, notify physician

Dosage Forms Cream, as nitrate: 1% (15 g, 30 g, 85 g)

Econazole Nitrate *see* Econazole *on this page*

Ecostatin® see Econazole on previous page

E.E.S.® see Erythromycin on page 722

Efavirenz (e FAV e renz)

Related Information

HIV Therapeutic Information on page 1008

U.S. Brand Names Sustiva™

Use Treatment of HIV-1 infections in combination with at least two other antiretroviral agents. Also has some activity against hepatitis B virus and herpes viruses.

Pregnancy Risk Factor C

Pregnancy/Breast-Feeding Implications Teratogenic effects have been observed in Primates receiving efavirenz. Pregnancy should be avoided. Women of childbearing potential should undergo pregnancy testing prior to initiation of efavirenz. Barrier contraception should be used in combination with other (hormonal) methods of contraception.

Contraindications Clinically significant hypersensitivity to any component of the formulation

Warnings/Precautions Do not use as single-agent therapy; avoid pregnancy; women of childbearing potential should undergo pregnancy testing prior to initiation of therapy; do not administer with other agents metabolized by cytochrome P-450 isoenzyme 3A4 including astemizole, cisapride, midazolam, triazolam or ergot alkaloids (potential for life-threatening adverse effects); history of mental illness/drug abuse (predisposition to psychological reactions); may cause depression and/or other psychiatric symptoms including impaired concentration, dizziness or drowsiness (avoid potentially hazardous tasks such as driving or operating machinery if these effects are noted); discontinue if severe rash (involving blistering, desquamation, mucosal involvement or fever) develops. Caution in patients with known or suspected hepatitis B or C infection (monitoring of liver function is recommended); hepatic impairment. Persistent elevations of serum transaminases >5 times the upper limit of normal should prompt evaluation - benefit of continued therapy should be weighed against possible risk of hepatotoxicity. Children are more susceptible to development of rash - prophylactic antihistamines may be used

Adverse Reactions

2% to 10%:

Central nervous system: Dizziness (2% to 10%), inability to concentrate (0% to 9%), insomnia (0% to 7%), headache (5% to 6%) abnormal dreams (0% to 4%), somnolence (0% to 3%), depression (0% to 2%), anorexia (0% to 5%), nervousness (0% to 2%), fatigue (2% to 7%), hypoesthesia (1% to 2%)

Dermatologic: Rash (5% to 20%), pruritus (0% to 2%)

Gastrointestinal: Nausea (0% to 12%), vomiting (0% to 7%), diarrhea (2% to 12%), dyspepsia (0% to 4%), abdominal pain (0% to 3%)

Hepatic: Increased transaminases (2% to 3%)

Miscellaneous: Increased sweating (0% to 2%)

<2%: Edema (peripheral), syncope, flushing, palpitations, tachycardia, fever, pain, malaise, ataxia, depression, seizures, hallucinations, psychosis, depersonalization, amnesia, anxiety, apathy, emotional lability, agitation, confusion, euphoria, impaired coordination, migraine, speech disorder, vertigo, alopecia, eczema, folliculitis, skin exfoliation, urticaria, increased cholesterol and triglycerides, hot flashes, pancreatitis, dry mouth, taste disturbance, flatulence, renal calculus, hematuria, hepatitis, thrombophlebitis, asthenia, neuralgia, paresthesia, peripheral neuropathy, tremor, arthralgia, myalgia, abnormal vision, diplopia, tinnitus, asthma, alcohol intolerance, allergic reaction, parosmia

Pediatric patients: Rash (40%), diarrhea (39%), fever (26%), cough (25%), nausea/vomiting (16%), central nervous system reactions (9%)

Overdosage/Toxicology

Increased central nervous system symptoms and involuntary muscle contractions have been reported in accidental overdose

Treatment is supportive, activated charcoal may enhance elimination; dialysis is unlikely to remove drug

Drug Interactions

Increased effect: CYP3A4, 2C9, 2C19 inhibitor; CYP3A4 inducer; coadministration with medications metabolized by these enzymes may lead to increased concentration-related effects. Astemizole, cisapride, midazolam, triazolam and ergot alkaloids may result in life-threatening toxicities. The AUC of nelfinavir is increased (20%); AUC of both ritonavir and efavirenz are increased by 20% during concurrent therapy. The AUC of ethinyl estradiol is increased 37% by efavirenz (clinical significance unknown). May increase effect of warfarin.

Decreased effect: Other inducers of this enzyme (including phenobarbital, rifampin and rifabutin) may decrease serum concentrations of efavirenz. Concentrations of indinavir may be reduced; dosage increase to 1000 mg 3 times/day is recommended. Concentrations of saquinavir may be decreased (use as sole protease inhibitor is not recommended). Plasma concentrations of clarithromycin are decreased (clinical significance unknown). May decrease effect of warfarin.

Stability Store below 25°C (77°F)

Mechanism of Action As a non-nucleoside reverse transcriptase inhibitor, efavirenz has activity against HIV-1 by binding to reverse transcriptase. It consequently blocks the RNA-dependent and DNA-dependent DNA polymerase activities including HIV-1 replication. It does not require intracellular phosphorylation for antiviral activity.

Pharmacodynamics/Kinetics
Absorption: Increased 50% by fatty meals
Distribution: Highly protein bound (>99%) primarily to albumin; CSF concentrations exceed free fraction in serum
Metabolism: Hepatic
Half-life: Single dose: 52-76 hours; after multiple doses: 40-55 hours
Time to peak concentration: 3-8 hours
Elimination: 14% to 34% in urine (as metabolites) and 16% to 41% in feces (primarily as efavirenz)

Usual Dosage Oral: Dosing at bedtime is recommended to limit central nervous system effects; should not be used as single-agent therapy

Children: Dosage is based on body weight
10 kg to <15 kg: 200 mg once daily
15 kg to <20 kg: 250 mg once daily
20 kg to <25 kg: 300 mg once daily
25 kg to <32.5 kg: 350 mg once daily
32.5 kg to <40 kg: 400 mg once daily
≥40 kg: 600 mg once daily
Adults: 600 mg once daily

Dosing adjustment in renal impairment: None recommended
Dosing comments in hepatic impairment: Limited clinical experience, use with caution

Dietary Considerations May be taken with or without food. Avoid high-fat meals when taking this medication. High-fat meals increase the absorption of efavirenz.

Monitoring Parameters Serum transaminases (discontinuation of treatment should be considered for persistent elevations greater than five times the upper limit of normal), cholesterol, triglycerides, signs and symptoms of infection

Test Interactions False-positive test for cannabinoids have been reported when the CEDIA DAU Multilevel THC assay is used. False-positive results with other assays for cannabinoids have not been observed.

Patient Information Take efavirenz exactly as prescribed; report all side effects to your physician; do not alter dose or discontinue without consulting physician; may cause dizziness, drowsiness, impaired concentration, delusions or depression; taking at bedtime may minimize these effects; caution in performing potentially hazardous tasks such as operating machinery or driving; do not get pregnant; avoid high-fat meals

Dosage Forms Capsule: 50 mg, 100 mg, 200 mg

Selected Readings
"Three New Drugs for HIV Infection," *Med Lett Drugs Ther*, 1998, 40(1041):114-6.

Eflornithine (ee FLOR ni theen)

U.S. Brand Names Ornidyl®
Synonyms DFMO; Eflornithine Hydrochloride
Generic Available No
Use Treatment of meningoencephalitic stage of *Trypanosoma brucei gambiense* infection (sleeping sickness)
(Continued)

Eflornithine *(Continued)*

Pregnancy Risk Factor C

Contraindications Hypersensitivity to eflornithine or any component

Warnings/Precautions Must be diluted before use; frequent monitoring for myelosuppression should be done; use with caution in patients with a history of seizures and in patients with renal impairment; serial audiograms should be obtained; due to the potential for relapse, patients should be followed up for at least 24 months

Adverse Reactions

>10%: Hematologic (reversible): Anemia (55%), leukopenia (37%), thrombocytopenia (14%)

1% to 10%:

Central nervous system: Seizures (may be due to the disease) (8%), dizziness

Dermatologic: Alopecia

Gastrointestinal: Vomiting, diarrhea

Hematologic: Eosinophilia

Otic: Hearing impairment

<1%: Facial edema, headache, abdominal pain, anorexia, weakness

Overdosage/Toxicology No known antidote; treatment is supportive; in mice and rats, CNS depression, seizures, death have occurred

Stability Must be diluted before use and used within 24 hours of preparation

Mechanism of Action Eflornithine exerts antitumor and antiprotozoal effects through specific, irreversible ("suicide") inhibition of the enzyme ornithine decarboxylase (ODC). ODC is the rate-limiting enzyme in the biosynthesis of putrescine, spermine, and spermidine, the major polyamines in nucleated cells. Polyamines are necessary for the synthesis of DNA, RNA, and proteins and are, therefore, necessary for cell growth and differentiation. Although many microorganisms and higher plants are able to produce polyamines from alternate biochemical pathways, all mammalian cells depend on ornithine decarboxylase to produce polyamines. Eflornithine inhibits ODC and rapidly depletes animal cells of putrescine and spermidine; the concentration of spermine remains the same or may even increase. Rapidly dividing cells appear to most susceptible to the effects of eflornithine.

Pharmacodynamics/Kinetics

Absorption: Well absorbed from GI tract

Bioavailability: 54% to 58%

Half-life: 3-3.5 hours

Elimination: Mainly excreted unchanged in urine via glomerular filtration

Usual Dosage Adults: I.V. infusion: 100 mg/kg/dose given every 6 hours (over at least 45 minutes) for 14 days

Dosing adjustment in renal impairment: Dose should be adjusted although no specific guidelines are available

Monitoring Parameters CBC with platelet counts

Patient Information Report any persistent or unusual fever, sore throat, fatigue, bleeding, or bruising; frequent blood tests are needed during therapy

Dosage Forms Injection, as hydrochloride: 200 mg/mL (100 mL)

Selected Readings

"Drugs for Parasitic Infections," *Med Lett Drugs Ther*, 1998, 40(1017):1-12.

Eflornithine Hydrochloride *see* Eflornithine *on previous page*

Elimite™ Cream *see* Permethrin *on page 868*

E-Mycin® *see* Erythromycin *on page 722*

Endantadine® *see* Amantadine *on page 586*

End Lice® Liquid [OTC] *see* Pyrethrins *on page 885*

Engerix-B® *see* Hepatitis B Vaccine *on page 761*

Enhanced-potency Inactivated Poliovirus Vaccine *see* Poliovirus Vaccine, Inactivated *on page 875*

Enoxacin *(en OKS a sin)*

U.S. Brand Names Penetrex™

Generic Available No

Use Treatment of complicated and uncomplicated urinary tract infections caused by susceptible gram-negative and gram-positive bacteria and uncomplicated urethral or cervical gonorrhea due to *N. gonorrhoeae*

Drug of Choice or Alternative for
Organism(s)
  Neisseria gonorrhoeae on page 215
Pregnancy Risk Factor C
Contraindications Hypersensitivity to enoxacin, any component, or other quinolones
Warnings/Precautions Use with caution in patients with a history of convulsions or epilepsy, renal dysfunction, psychosis, elevated intracranial pressure, prepubertal children, and pregnancy; nalidixic acid and ciprofloxacin (related compounds) have been associated with erosions of the cartilage in weight-bearing joints and other signs of arthropathy in immature animals and children; similar precautions are advised for enoxacin although no data is available; has rarely caused ruptured tendons (discontinue immediately with signs of inflammation or tendon pain)

Adverse Reactions
  1% to 10%:
    Central nervous system: Dizziness (<3%), headache (<2%), vertigo (3%)
    Gastrointestinal: Nausea (2.9%), vomiting (6% to 9%), abdominal pain (1% to 2%), diarrhea (1% to 2%)
  <1%: Palpitations, syncope, edema, restlessness, confusion, seizures, fatigue, drowsiness, depression, insomnia, confusion, chills, fever, rash, photosensitivity, pruritus, exfoliative dermatitis, hypo/hyperkalemia, GI bleeding, dyspepsia, xerostomia, constipation, flatulence, anorexia, vaginitis, anemia, leukopenia, eosinophilia, leukocytosis, increased liver enzymes, tremor, arthralgia, ruptured tendons, paresthesias, visual disturbances, increased serum BUN and creatinine, acute renal failure, proteinuria

Overdosage/Toxicology
  Symptoms of overdose include acute renal failure, seizures
  GI decontamination and supportive care; diazepam for seizures; not removed by peritoneal or hemodialysis

Drug Interactions CYP1A2 enzyme inhibitor
  Decreased effect of enoxacin with antacids (magnesium, aluminum), iron and zinc salts, sucralfate, bismuth salts, antineoplastics
  Increased toxicity/levels of warfarin, cyclosporine, digoxin, caffeine, and theophylline with enoxacin
  Increased levels of enoxacin with cimetidine, probenecid

Mechanism of Action Inhibits DNA-gyrase in susceptible organisms; inhibits relaxation of supercoiled DNA and promotes breakage of double-stranded DNA

Pharmacodynamics/Kinetics
  Absorption: 98%
  Distribution: Penetrates well into tissues and body secretions
  Half-life: 3-6 hours (average)
  Elimination: Primarily in urine, however, significant drug concentrations are achieved in feces

Usual Dosage Adults: Oral:
  Complicated urinary tract infection: 400 mg twice daily for 14 days
  Cystitis: 200 mg twice daily for 7 days
  Uncomplicated gonorrhea: 400 mg as single dose
  Dosing adjustment in renal impairment: Cl_{cr} <50 mL/minute: Administer 50% of dose

Patient Information May be taken with food to minimize upset stomach; avoid antacid use; drink fluids liberally

Dosage Forms Tablet: 200 mg, 400 mg

Selected Readings
  Hooper DC and Wolfson JS, "Fluoroquinolone Antimicrobial Agents," *N Engl J Med*, 1991, 324(6):384-94.
  Lomaestro BM and Bailie GR, "Quinolone-Cation Interactions: A Review," *DICP*, 1991, 25(11):1249-58.
  Patel SS and Spencer CM, "Enoxacin: A Reappraisal of Its Clinical Efficacy in the Treatment of Genitourinary Tract Infections," *Drugs*, 1996, 51(1):137-60.
  Stein GE, "The 4-Quinolone Antibiotics: Past, Present, and Future," *Pharmacotherapy*, 1988, 8(6):301-14.
  Walker RC and Wright AJ, "The Fluoroquinolones," *Mayo Clin Proc*, 1991, 66(12):1249-59.

Epivir® *see Lamivudine on page 793*

Epivir® HBV *see Lamivudine on page 793*

Eramycin® *see Erythromycin on next page*

Erybid™ see Erythromycin on this page
Eryc® see Erythromycin on this page
EryPed® see Erythromycin on this page
Ery-Tab® see Erythromycin on this page
Erythro-Base® see Erythromycin on this page
Erythrocin® see Erythromycin on this page

Erythromycin (er ith roe MYE sin)
Related Information
Antimicrobial Activity Against Selected Organisms on page 983

U.S. Brand Names E-Base®; E.E.S.®; E-Mycin®; Eramycin®; Eryc®; EryPed®; Ery-Tab®; Erythrocin®; Ilosone®; PCE®

Canadian Brand Names Apo®-Erythro E-C; Diomycin; Erybid™; Erythro-Base®; Novo-Rythro Encap; PMS-Erythromycin

Synonyms Erythromycin Base; Erythromycin Estolate; Erythromycin Ethylsuccinate; Erythromycin Gluceptate; Erythromycin Lactobionate; Erythromycin Stearate

Generic Available Yes

Use Treatment of susceptible bacterial infections including *S. pyogenes*, some *S. pneumoniae*, some *S. aureus*, *M. pneumoniae*, *Legionella pneumophila*, diphtheria, pertussis, chancroid, *Chlamydia*, erythrasma, *N. gonorrhoeae*, *E. histolytica*, syphilis and nongonococcal urethritis, and *Campylobacter* gastroenteritis; used in conjunction with neomycin for decontaminating the bowel; also used in the treatment of gastroparesis

Drug of Choice or Alternative for
Disease/Syndrome(s)
Impetigo on page 32
Pharyngitis on page 43
Pneumonia, Community-Acquired on page 45
Urethritis, Nongonococcal on page 51

Organism(s)
Bartonella Species on page 76
Bordetella pertussis on page 81
Calymmatobacterium granulomatis on page 89
Campylobacter jejuni on page 90
Chlamydia pneumoniae on page 95
Chlamydia psittaci on page 97
Chlamydia trachomatis on page 99
Corynebacterium diphtheriae on page 111
Corynebacterium Species, Other Than *C. jeikeium* on page 113
Haemophilus ducreyi on page 156
Legionella pneumophila on page 185
Mycoplasma pneumoniae on page 211
Rhodococcus Species on page 242
Streptococcus agalactiae on page 266
Streptococcus pneumoniae on page 268
Streptococcus pyogenes on page 274
Ureaplasma urealyticum on page 292

Pregnancy Risk Factor B

Contraindications Hepatic impairment, known hypersensitivity to erythromycin or its components; pre-existing liver disease (erythromycin estolate); concomitant use with pimozide, terfenadine, astemizole, or cisapride

Warnings/Precautions Hepatic impairment with or without jaundice has occurred, it may be accompanied by malaise, nausea, vomiting, abdominal colic, and fever; discontinue use if these occur; avoid using erythromycin lactobionate in neonates since formulations may contain benzyl alcohol which is associated with toxicity in neonates; observe for superinfections

Adverse Reactions
>10%: Gastrointestinal: Abdominal pain, cramping, nausea, vomiting
1% to 10%:
Gastrointestinal: Oral candidiasis
Hepatic: Cholestatic jaundice
Local: Phlebitis at the injection site
Miscellaneous: Hypersensitivity reactions

<1%: Ventricular arrhythmias, fever, rash, hypertrophic pyloric stenosis, diarrhea, pseudomembranous colitis, eosinophilia, cholestatic jaundice (most common with estolate), thrombophlebitis, allergic reactions

Overdosage/Toxicology

Symptoms of overdose include nausea, vomiting, and diarrhea

General and supportive care only

Drug Interactions CYP3A3/4 enzyme substrate; CYP1A2 and 3A3/4 enzyme inhibitor

Increased toxicity:

Erythromycin decreases clearance of carbamazepine, cyclosporine, and triazolam, alfentanil, bromocriptine, digoxin (~10% of patients), disopyramide, ergot alkaloids, methylprednisolone; may decrease clearance of protease inhibitors

Erythromycin may decrease theophylline clearance and increase theophylline's half-life by up to 60% (patients on high-dose theophylline and erythromycin or who have received erythromycin for >5 days may be at higher risk)

Decreases metabolism of terfenadine, cisapride, and astemizole resulting in an increase in Q-T interval and potential heart failure

Inhibits felodipine (and other dihydropyridine calcium antagonist) metabolism in the liver resulting in a twofold increase in levels and consequent toxicity

Death has been reported by potentiation of pimozide's cardiotoxicity when given concurrently with erythromycin

May potentiate anticoagulant effect of warfarin and decrease metabolism of vinblastine

Concurrent use of erythromycin and lovastatin and simvastatin may result in significantly increased levels and rhabdomyolysis

Stability

Erythromycin lactobionate should be reconstituted with sterile water for injection without preservatives to avoid gel formation; the reconstituted solution is stable for 2 weeks when refrigerated for 24 hours at room temperature

Erythromycin I.V. infusion solution is stable at pH 6-8. Stability of lactobionate is pH dependent; I.V. form has the longest stability in 0.9% sodium chloride (NS) and should be prepared in this base solution whenever possible. Do not use D_5W as a diluent unless sodium bicarbonate is added to solution. If I.V. must be prepared in D_5W, 0.5 mL of the 8.4% sodium bicarbonate solution should be added per each 100 mL of D_5W.

Stability of parenteral admixture at room temperature (25°C) and at refrigeration temperature (4°C): 24 hours

Standard diluent: 500 mg/250 mL D_5W/NS; 750 mg/250 mL D_5W/NS; 1 g/250 mL D_5W/NS

Refrigerate oral suspension

Mechanism of Action Inhibits RNA-dependent protein synthesis at the chain elongation step; binds to the 50S ribosomal subunit resulting in blockage of transpeptidation

Pharmacodynamics/Kinetics

Absorption: Variable but better with salt forms than with base form; 18% to 45% absorbed orally, ethylsuccinate may be better absorbed with food

Distribution: Crosses the placenta; appears in breast milk

Relative diffusion of antimicrobial agents from blood into cerebrospinal fluid (CSF): Minimal even with inflammation

Ratio of CSF to blood level (%):

Normal meninges: 1-12

Inflamed meninges: 7-25

Protein binding: 75% to 90%

Metabolism: In the liver by demethylation

Half-life: 1.5-2 hours (peak)

End stage renal disease: 5-6 hours

Time to peak serum concentration: 4 hours for the base, 30 minutes to 2.5 hours for the ethylsuccinate; delayed in the presence of food; due to differences in absorption

Elimination: 2% to 15% excreted as unchanged drug in urine and major excretion in feces (via bile)

(Continued)

Erythromycin *(Continued)*

Usual Dosage

Infants and Children (Note: 400 mg ethylsuccinate = 250 mg base, stearate, or estolate salts):

Oral: 30-50 mg/kg/day divided every 6-8 hours; may double doses in severe infections

Preop bowel preparation: 20 mg/kg erythromycin base at 1, 2, and 11 PM on the day before surgery combined with mechanical cleansing of the large intestine and oral neomycin

I.V.: Lactobionate: 20-40 mg/kg/day divided every 6 hours

Adults:

Oral:

Base: 250-500 mg every 6-12 hours

Ethylsuccinate: 400-800 mg every 6-12 hours

Preop bowel preparation: Oral: 1 g erythromycin base at 1, 2, and 11 PM on the day before surgery combined with mechanical cleansing of the large intestine and oral neomycin

I.V.: Lactobionate: 15-20 mg/kg/day divided every 6 hours or 500 mg to 1 g every 6 hours, or given as a continuous infusion over 24 hours (maximum: 4 g/24 hours)

Children and Adults: Ophthalmic: Instill ½" (1.25 cm) 2-8 times/day depending on the severity of the infection

Dialysis: Slightly dialyzable (5% to 20%); no supplemental dosage necessary in hemo or peritoneal dialysis or in continuous arteriovenous or venovenous hemofiltration (CAVH/CAVHD)

Erythromycin has been used as a prokinetic agent to improve gastric emptying time and intestinal motility. In adults, 200 mg was infused I.V. initially followed by 250 mg orally 3 times/day 30 minutes before meals. In children, erythromycin 3 mg/kg I.V. has been infused over 60 minutes initially followed by 20 mg/kg/day orally in 3-4 divided doses before meals or before meals and at bedtime

Dietary Considerations Food: Increased drug absorption with meals. Drug may cause GI upset; may take with food.

Administration Can administer with food to decrease GI upset

Test Interactions False-positive urinary catecholamines

Patient Information Refrigerate after reconstitution, take until gone, do not skip doses; chewable tablets should not be swallowed whole; report to physician if persistent diarrhea occurs; discard any unused portion after 10 days; absorption of estolate, ethylsuccinate, and base in a delayed release form are unaffected by food; take stearate salt and nondelayed release base preparations 2 hours before or after meals

Nursing Implications Some formulations may contain benzyl alcohol as a preservative; use with extreme care in neonates; do not crush enteric coated drug product; GI upset, including diarrhea, is common; I.V. infusion may be very irritating to the vein; if phlebitis/pain occurs with used dilution, consider diluting further (eg, 1:5) and administer over ≥20-60 minutes, if fluid status of the patient will tolerate, or consider administering in larger available vein

Additional Information Due to differences in absorption, 400 mg erythromycin ethylsuccinate produces the same serum levels as 250 mg erythromycin base, stearate, or estolate. Do not use D_5W as a diluent unless sodium bicarbonate is added to solution; infuse over 30 minutes.

Sodium content of oral suspension (ethylsuccinate) 200 mg/5 mL: 29 mg (1.3 mEq)

Sodium content of base Filmtab® 250 mg: 70 mg (3 mEq)

Dosage Forms

Erythromycin base:

Capsule, delayed release: 250 mg

Capsule, delayed release, enteric coated pellets (Eryc®): 250 mg

Ointment, ophthalmic: 0.55 (3.5 g)

Tablet, delayed release: 333 mg

Tablet, enteric coated (E-Mycin®, Ery-Tab®, E-Base®): 250 mg, 333 mg, 500 mg

Tablet, film coated: 250 mg, 500 mg

Tablet, polymer coated particles (PCE®): 333 mg, 500 mg

Erythromycin estolate:
  Capsule (Ilosone® Pulvules®): 250 mg
  Suspension, oral (Ilosone®): 125 mg/5 mL (480 mL); 250 mg/5 mL (480 mL)
  Tablet (Ilosone®): 500 mg
Erythromycin ethylsuccinate:
  Granules for oral suspension (EryPed®): 400 mg/5 mL (60 mL, 100 mL, 200 mL)
  Powder for oral suspension (E.E.S.®): 200 mg/5 mL (100 mL, 200 mL)
  Suspension, oral (E.E.S.®, EryPed®): 200 mg/5 mL (5 mL, 100 mL, 200 mL, 480 mL); 400 mg/5 mL (5 mL, 60 mL, 100 mL, 200 mL, 480 mL)
  Suspension, oral [drops] (EryPed®): 100 mg/2.5 mL (50 mL)
  Tablet (E.E.S.®): 400 mg
  Tablet, chewable (EryPed®): 200 mg
Erythromycin gluceptate: Injection: 1000 mg (30 mL)
Erythromycin lactobionate: Powder for injection: 500 mg, 1000 mg
Erythromycin stearate: Tablet, film coated (Eramycin®, Erythrocin®): 250 mg, 500 mg

Selected Readings

Amsden GW, "Erythromycin, Clarithromycin, and Azithromycin: Are the Differences Real?" *Clin Ther*, 1996, 18(1):56-72.

Goldman MP and Longworth DL, "The Role of Azithromycin and Clarithromycin in Clinical Practice," *Cleve Clin J Med*, 1993, 60(5):359-64.

Smilack JD, Wilson WR, and Cockerill FR 3d, "Tetracyclines, Chloramphenicol, Erythromycin, Clindamycin, and Metronidazole," *Mayo Clin Proc*, 1991, 66(12):1270-80.

Tartaglione TA, "Therapeutic Options for the Management and Prevention of *Mycobacterium avium* Complex Infection in Patients With the Acquired Immunodeficiency Syndrome," *Pharmacotherapy*, 1996, 16(2):171-82.

Erythromycin and Benzoyl Peroxide

(er ith roe MYE sin & BEN zoe il per OKS ide)

Related Information

Erythromycin *on page 722*

U.S. Brand Names Benzamycin®

Use Topical control of acne vulgaris

Usual Dosage Apply twice daily, morning and evening

Dosage Forms Gel: Erythromycin 30 mg and benzoyl peroxide 50 mg per g

Erythromycin and Sulfisoxazole

(er ith roe MYE sin & sul fi SOKS a zole)

U.S. Brand Names Eryzole®; Pediazole®

Synonyms Sulfisoxazole and Erythromycin

Generic Available Yes

Use Treatment of susceptible bacterial infections of the upper and lower respiratory tract, otitis media in children caused by susceptible strains of *Haemophilus influenzae*, and many other infections in patients allergic to penicillin

Drug of Choice or Alternative for Disease/Syndrome(s)

Otitis Media, Acute *on page 41*

Pregnancy Risk Factor C

Contraindications Hepatic dysfunction, known hypersensitivity to erythromycin or sulfonamides; infants <2 months of age (sulfas compete with bilirubin for binding sites); patients with porphyria; concurrent use with pimozide, terfenadine, astemizole, or cisapride

Warnings/Precautions Use with caution in patients with impaired renal or hepatic function, G-6-PD deficiency (hemolysis may occur)

Adverse Reactions

>10%: Gastrointestinal: Abdominal pain, cramping, nausea, vomiting

1% to 10%:
  Gastrointestinal: Oral candidiasis
  Local: Phlebitis at the injection site
  Miscellaneous: Hypersensitivity reactions

<1%: Ventricular arrhythmias, fever, headache, rash, Stevens-Johnson syndrome, toxic epidermal necrolysis, hypertrophic pyloric stenosis, diarrhea, pseudomembranous colitis, crystalluria, eosinophilia, agranulocytosis, aplastic anemia, hepatic necrosis, cholestatic jaundice, thrombophlebitis, toxic nephrosis

(Continued)

Erythromycin and Sulfisoxazole *(Continued)*

Overdosage/Toxicology
Symptoms of overdose include nausea, vomiting, diarrhea, prostration, reversible pancreatitis, hearing loss with or without tinnitus or vertigo

General and supportive care only; keep patient well hydrated

Drug Interactions
Increased effect/toxicity/levels with erythromycin/sulfisoxazole on alfentanil, astemizole, terfenadine (resulting in potentially life-threatening prolonged Q-T interval), bromocriptine, carbamazepine, cyclosporine, digoxin, disopyramide, theophylline, triazolam, lovastatin/simvastatin, ergots, methylprednisolone, cisapride, pimozide, felodipine, phenytoin, barbiturate anesthetics, methotrexate, sulfonylureas, uricosuric agents, and warfarin; may inhibit metabolism of protease inhibitors

Increased toxicity of sulfonamides occurs with concurrent diuretics, indomethacin, methenamine, probenecid, and salicylates

Stability
Reconstituted suspension is stable for 14 days when refrigerated

Mechanism of Action
Erythromycin inhibits bacterial protein synthesis; sulfisoxazole competitively inhibits bacterial synthesis of folic acid from para-aminobenzoic acid

Pharmacodynamics/Kinetics
Erythromycin ethylsuccinate:
Absorption: Well absorbed from GI tract
Distribution: Crosses the placenta; appears in breast milk
Protein binding: 75% to 90%
Metabolism: In the liver
Half-life: 1-1.5 hours
Elimination: Unchanged drug is excreted and concentrated in bile

Sulfisoxazole acetyl: Hydrolyzed in the GI tract to sulfisoxazole which has the following characteristics:
Absorption: Readily absorbed
Distribution: Crosses the placenta; appears in breast milk
Protein binding: 85%
Half-life: 6 hours, prolonged in renal impairment
Elimination: 50% excreted in urine as unchanged drug

Usual Dosage
Oral (dosage recommendation is based on the product's erythromycin content):

Children ≥2 months: 50 mg/kg/day erythromycin and 150 mg/kg/day sulfisoxazole in divided doses every 6 hours; not to exceed 2 g erythromycin/day or 6 g sulfisoxazole/day for 10 days

Adults >45 kg: 400 mg erythromycin and 1200 mg sulfisoxazole every 6 hours

Dosing adjustment in renal impairment (sulfisoxazole must be adjusted in renal impairment):
Cl_{cr} 10-50 mL/minute: Administer every 8-12 hours
Cl_{cr} <10 mL/minute: Administer every 12-24 hours

Monitoring Parameters
CBC and periodic liver function test

Test Interactions
False-positive urinary protein

Patient Information
Maintain adequate fluid intake; avoid prolonged exposure to sunlight; discontinue if rash appears; take until gone, do not skip doses

Dosage Forms
Suspension, oral: Erythromycin ethylsuccinate 200 mg and sulfisoxazole acetyl 600 mg per 5 mL (100 mL, 150 mL, 200 mL, 250 mL)

Selected Readings
Rodriguez WJ, Schwartz RH, Sait T, et al, "Erythromycin-Sulfisoxazole vs Amoxicillin in the Treatment of Acute Otitis Media in Children," *Am J Dis Child*, 1985, 139(8):766-70.

Tartaglione TA, "Therapeutic Options for the Management and Prevention of *Mycobacterium avium* Complex Infection in Patients With the Acquired Immunodeficiency Syndrome," *Pharmacotherapy*, 1996, 16(2):171-82.

Erythromycin Base *see* Erythromycin *on page 722*

Erythromycin Estolate *see* Erythromycin *on page 722*

Erythromycin Ethylsuccinate *see* Erythromycin *on page 722*

Erythromycin Glucceptate *see* Erythromycin *on page 722*

Erythromycin Lactobionate *see* Erythromycin *on page 722*

Erythromycin Stearate *see* Erythromycin *on page 722*

Eryzole® *see* Erythromycin and Sulfisoxazole *on previous page*

Ethambutol (e THAM byoo tole)

Related Information
Tuberculosis Guidelines *on page 1114*

U.S. Brand Names Myambutol®

Canadian Brand Names Etibi®

Synonyms Ethambutol Hydrochloride

Generic Available No

Use Treatment of tuberculosis and other mycobacterial diseases in conjunction with other antituberculosis agents

Drug of Choice or Alternative for
Organism(s)
Mycobacterium avium-intracellulare on page 201
Mycobacterium bovis on page 203
Mycobacterium kansasii on page 204
Mycobacterium tuberculosis on page 207

Pregnancy Risk Factor B

Contraindications Hypersensitivity to ethambutol or any component; optic neuritis

Warnings/Precautions Use only in children whose visual acuity can accurately be determined and monitored (not recommended for use in children <13 years of age); dosage modification required in patients with renal insufficiency

Adverse Reactions
1% to 10%:
Central nervous system: Headache, confusion, disorientation
Endocrine & metabolic: Acute gout or hyperuricemia
Gastrointestinal: Abdominal pain, anorexia, nausea, vomiting
<1%: Malaise, mental confusion, fever, rash, pruritus, abnormal LFTs, peripheral neuritis, optic neuritis, anaphylaxis

Overdosage/Toxicology
Symptoms of overdose include decrease in visual acuity, anorexia, joint pain, numbness of the extremities
Following GI decontamination, treatment is supportive

Drug Interactions Decreased absorption with aluminum salts

Mechanism of Action Suppresses mycobacteria multiplication by interfering with RNA synthesis

Pharmacodynamics/Kinetics
Absorption: Oral: ~80%
Distribution: Well distributed throughout the body with high concentrations in kidneys, lungs, saliva, and red blood cells
Relative diffusion of antimicrobial agents from blood into CSF: Adequate with or without inflammation (exceeds usual MICs)
Ratio of CSF to blood level (%):
Normal meninges: 0
Inflamed meninges: 25
Protein binding: 20% to 30%
Metabolism: 20% metabolized by the liver to inactive metabolite
Half-life: 2.5-3.6 hours
End stage renal disease: 7-15 hours
Time to peak serum concentration: 2-4 hours
Elimination: ~50% excreted in the urine and 20% excreted in the feces as unchanged drug

Usual Dosage Oral:
Ethambutol is generally not recommended in children whose visual acuity cannot be monitored (<6 years of age). However, ethambutol should be considered for all children with organisms resistant to other drugs, when susceptibility to ethambutol has been demonstrated, or susceptibility is likely.
Note: A four-drug regimen (isoniazid, rifampin, pyrazinamide, and either streptomycin or ethambutol) is preferred for the initial, empiric treatment of TB. When the drug susceptibility results are available, the regimen should be altered as appropriate.

Children (>6 years) and Adults:
Daily therapy: 15-25 mg/kg/day (maximum: 2.5 g/day)
Directly observed therapy (DOT): Twice weekly: 50 mg/kg (maximum: 2.5 g)
DOT: 3 times/week: 25-30 mg/kg (maximum: 2.5 g)
(Continued)

Ethambutol (Continued)

Dosing interval in renal impairment:
Cl_{cr} 10-50 mL/minute: Administer every 24-36 hours
Cl_{cr} <10 mL/minute: Administer every 48 hours
Hemodialysis: Slightly dialyzable (5% to 20%); Administer dose postdialysis
Peritoneal dialysis: Dose for Cl_{cr} <10 mL/minute
Continuous arteriovenous or venovenous hemofiltration: Administer every 24-36 hours

Monitoring Parameters Periodic visual testing in patients receiving more than 15 mg/kg/day; periodic renal, hepatic, and hematopoietic tests

Patient Information Report any visual changes or rash to physician; may cause stomach upset, take with food; do not take within 2 hours of aluminum-containing antacids

Dosage Forms Tablet, as hydrochloride: 100 mg, 400 mg

Selected Readings
Davidson PT and Le HQ, "Drug Treatment of Tuberculosis - 1992," *Drugs*, 1992, 43(5):651-73.
"Drugs for Tuberculosis," *Med Lett Drugs Ther*, 1993, 35(908):99-101.
Havlir DV and Barnes PF, "Tuberculosis in Patients With Human Immunodeficiency Virus Infection," *N Engl J Med*, 1999, 340(5):367-73.
Iseman MD, "Treatment of Multidrug-Resistant Tuberculosis," *N Engl J Med*, 1993, 329(11):784-91.
"Prevention and Treatment of Tuberculosis Among Patients Infected With Human Immunodeficiency Virus: Principles of Therapy and Revised Recommendations. Centers for Disease Control and Prevention," *MMWR Morb Mortal Wkly Rep*, 1998, 47(RR-20):1-58.
Van Scoy RE and Wilkowske CJ, "Antituberculous Agents," *Mayo Clin Proc*, 1992, 67(2):179-87.

Ethambutol Hydrochloride *see Ethambutol on previous page*

Ethionamide (e thye on AM ide)

Related Information
Tuberculosis Guidelines *on page 1114*

U.S. Brand Names Trecator®-SC

Generic Available No

Use Treatment of tuberculosis and other mycobacterial diseases, in conjunction with other antituberculosis agents, when first-line agents have failed or resistance has been demonstrated

Pregnancy Risk Factor C

Contraindications Contraindicated in patients with severe hepatic impairment or in patients who are sensitive to the drug

Warnings/Precautions Use with caution in patients receiving cycloserine or isoniazid, in diabetics

Adverse Reactions
>10%: Gastrointestinal: Anorexia, nausea, vomiting
1% to 10%:
Cardiovascular: Postural hypotension
Central nervous system: Psychiatric disturbances, drowsiness
Gastrointestinal: Metallic taste, diarrhea
Hepatic: Hepatitis (5%), jaundice
Neuromuscular & skeletal: Weakness
<1%: Dizziness, seizures, headache, peripheral neuritis, rash, alopecia, hypothyroidism or goiter, hypoglycemia, gynecomastia, stomatitis, abdominal pain, thrombocytopenia, optic neuritis, blurred vision, olfactory disturbances

Overdosage/Toxicology
Symptoms of overdose include peripheral neuropathy, anorexia, joint pain
Following GI decontamination, treatment is supportive; pyridoxine may be given to prevent peripheral neuropathy

Mechanism of Action Inhibits peptide synthesis

Pharmacodynamics/Kinetics
Absorption: Rapid from GI tract (~80%)
Distribution: Crosses the placenta
Protein binding: 10%
Bioavailability: 80%
Half-life: 2-3 hours
Time to peak serum concentration: Oral: Within 3 hours
Elimination: As metabolites (active and inactive) and parent drug in urine

Usual Dosage Oral:
Children: 15-20 mg/kg/day in 2 divided doses, not to exceed 1 g/day
Adults: 500-1000 mg/day in 1-3 divided doses

Dosing adjustment in renal impairment: Cl_{cr} <50 mL/minute: Administer 50% of dose

Monitoring Parameters Initial and periodic serum ALT and AST

Patient Information Take with meals; notify physician of persistent or severe stomach upset, loss of appetite, or metallic taste; frequent blood tests are needed for monitoring; increase dietary intake of pyridoxine

Additional Information Neurotoxic effects may be relieved by the administration of pyridoxine

Dosage Forms Tablet, sugar coated: 250 mg

Selected Readings
Davidson PT and Le HQ, "Drug Treatment of Tuberculosis - 1992," *Drugs*, 1992, 43(5):651-73.
"Drugs for Tuberculosis," *Med Lett Drugs Ther*, 1993, 35(908):99-101.
Iseman MD, "Treatment of Multidrug-Resistant Tuberculosis," *N Engl J Med*, 1993, 329(11):784-91.

Ethoxynaphthamido Penicillin Sodium see Nafcillin on page 826

Etibi® see Ethambutol on page 727

Eurax® Topical see Crotamiton on page 695

Everone® Injection see Testosterone on page 939

Exelderm® see Sulconazole on page 926

Exidine® Scrub [OTC] see Chlorhexidine Gluconate on page 670

Exsel® see Selenium Sulfide on page 917

F_3T see Trifluridine on page 957

Famciclovir (fam SYE kloe veer)

U.S. Brand Names Famvir™

Use Management of acute herpes zoster (shingles) and recurrent episodes of genital herpes; treatment of recurrent herpes simplex in immunocompetent patients

Drug of Choice or Alternative for
Organism(s)
Herpes Simplex Virus on page 170
Varicella-Zoster Virus on page 294

Pregnancy Risk Factor B

Pregnancy/Breast-Feeding Implications
Clinical effects on the fetus: Use only if the benefit to the patient clearly exceeds the potential risk to the fetus
Breast-feeding/lactation: Due to potential for excretion of famciclovir in breast milk and for its associated tumorigenicity, discontinue nursing or discontinue the drug during lactation

Contraindications Hypersensitivity to famciclovir

Warnings/Precautions Has not been studied in immunocompromised patients or patients with ophthalmic or disseminated zoster; dosage adjustment is required in patients with renal insufficiency (Cl_{cr} <60 mL/minute) and in patients with noncompensated hepatic disease; safety and efficacy have not been established in children <18 years of age; animal studies indicated increases in incidence of carcinomas, mutagenic changes, and decreases in fertility with extremely large doses

Adverse Reactions
1% to 10%:
Central nervous system: Fatigue (4% to 6%), headache, fever (1% to 3%), dizziness (3% to 5%), somnolence (1% to 2%)
Dermatologic: Pruritus (1% to 4%)
Gastrointestinal: Diarrhea (4% to 8%), nausea, vomiting (1% to 5%), constipation (1% to 5%), anorexia (1% to 3%), abdominal pain (1% to 4%)
Neuromuscular & skeletal: Paresthesia (1% to 3%)
Respiratory: Sinusitis/pharyngitis (2%)
<1%: Rigors, arthralgia, upper respiratory infection

Overdosage/Toxicology Supportive and symptomatic care is recommended; hemodialysis may enhance elimination

Drug Interactions Increased effect/toxicity:
Cimetidine: Penciclovir AUC may increase due to impaired metabolism
Digoxin: C_{max} of digoxin increases by ~19%
Probenecid: Penciclovir serum levels significantly increase
Theophylline: Penciclovir AUC/C_{max} may increase and renal clearance decrease, although not clinically significant
(Continued)

Famciclovir (Continued)

Mechanism of Action After undergoing rapid biotransformation to the active compound, penciclovir, famciclovir is phosphorylated by viral thymidine kinase in HSV-1, HSV-2, and VZV-infected cells to a monophosphate form; this is then converted to penciclovir triphosphate and competes with deoxyguanosine triphosphate to inhibit HSV-2 polymerase (ie, herpes viral DNA synthesis/replication is selectively inhibited)

Pharmacodynamics/Kinetics

Absorption: Food decreases the maximum peak concentration and delays the time to peak; AUC remains the same

Distribution: V_{dss}: 0.98-1.08 L/kg

Protein binding: 20%

Metabolism: Rapidly deacetylated and oxidized to penciclovir (not by cytochrome P-450)

Bioavailability: 77%; T_{max}: 0.9 hours

Half-life: Penciclovir: 2-3 hours (10, 20, and 7 hours in HSV-1, HSV-2, and VZV-infected cells); linearly decreased with reductions in renal failure

Elimination: >90% of penciclovir is eliminated unchanged in urine; C_{max} and T_{max} are decreased and prolonged, respectively in patients with noncompensated hepatic impairment

Usual Dosage Adults: Oral:

Acute herpes zoster: 500 mg every 8 hours for 7 days

Recurrent herpes simplex in immunocompetent patients: 125 mg twice daily for 5 days

Genital herpes:

Recurrent episodes: 125 mg twice daily for 5 days

Prophylaxis: 250 mg twice daily

Dosing interval in renal impairment:

Cl_{cr} 40-59 mL/minute: Administer 500 mg every 12 hours

Cl_{cr} 20-39 mL/minute: Administer 500 mg every 24 hours

Cl_{cr} <20 mL/minute: Unknown

Patient Information Initiate therapy as soon as herpes zoster is diagnosed; may take medication with food or on an empty stomach

Additional Information Most effective if therapy is initiated within 72 hours of initial lesion

Dosage Forms Tablet: 125 mg, 250 mg, 500 mg

Selected Readings

Alrabiah FA and Sacks SL, "New Antiherpesvirus Agents. Their Targets and Therapeutic Potential," *Drugs*, 1996, 52(1):17-32.

Luber AD and Flaherty JF Jr, "Famciclovir for Treatment of Herpesvirus Infections," *Ann Pharmacother*, 1996, 30(9):978-85.

Perry CM and Wagstaff AJ, "Famciclovir. A Review of Its Pharmacological Properties and Therapeutic Efficacy in Herpesvirus Infections," *Drugs*, 1995, 50(2):396-415.

Sacks SL, "Genital Herpes Simplex Virus and Its Treatment Focus on Famciclovir," *Semin Dermatol*, 1996, 15(2 Suppl 1):32-6.

Tyring SK, "Efficacy of Famciclovir in the Treatment of Herpes Zoster," *Semin Dermatol*, 1996, 15(2 Suppl 1):27-31.

Famvir™ see Famciclovir *on previous page*

Fansidar® see Sulfadoxine and Pyrimethamine *on page 931*

5-FC see Flucytosine *on page 734*

Femizole-7® [OTC] see Clotrimazole *on page 688*

Femizol-M® [OTC] see Miconazole *on page 822*

Filgrastim (fil GRA stim)

U.S. Brand Names Neupogen® Injection

Synonyms G-CSF; Granulocyte Colony Stimulating Factor

Generic Available No

Use Decreases the period of neutropenia and the associated risk of infection in patients with nonmyeloid malignancies receiving myelosuppressive chemotherapeutic regimens associated with a significant incidence of severe neutropenia with fever; it has also been used in AIDS patients on zidovudine and in patients with noncancer chemotherapy-induced neutropenia

Pregnancy Risk Factor C

Contraindications Hypersensitivity to *E. coli* derived proteins or G-CSF

Warnings/Precautions Complete blood count and platelet count should be obtained prior to chemotherapy. Do not use G-CSF in the period 24 hours before to 24 hours after administration of cytotoxic chemotherapy because of the potential sensitivity of rapidly dividing myeloid cells to cytotoxic chemotherapy. Precaution should be exercised in the usage of G-CSF in any malignancy with myeloid characteristics. G-CSF can potentially act as a growth factor for any tumor type, particularly myeloid malignancies. Tumors of nonhematopoietic origin may have surface receptors for G-CSF.

Adverse Reactions As this drug is indicated for patients receiving chemotherapeutic regimens, many of the adverse reactions listed below occurred in equal numbers in the placebo arms of clinical trials secondary to the chemotherapeutic agents. Included in the adverse effects associated with filgrastim alone is medullary bone pain which has been reported in up to 24% of patients.

>10%:
    Central nervous system: Neutropenic fever, fever
    Dermatologic: Alopecia
    Gastrointestinal: Nausea, vomiting, diarrhea, mucositis
1% to 10%:
    Cardiovascular: Chest pain, fluid retention
    Central nervous system: Headache
    Dermatologic: Skin rash
    Gastrointestinal: Anorexia, stomatitis, constipation
    Hematologic: Leukocytosis
    Local: Pain at injection site
    Neuromuscular & skeletal: Weakness
    Respiratory: Dyspnea, cough, sore throat
<1%: Transient supraventricular arrhythmia, anaphylactic reaction, pericarditis, thrombophlebitis

Overdosage/Toxicology Signs and symptoms: Leukocytosis which was not associated with any clinical adverse effects; after discontinuing the drug there is a 50% decrease in circulating levels of neutrophils within 1-2 days, return to pretreatment levels within 1-7 days. No clinical adverse effects seen with high-dose producing ANC >10,000/mm^3

Stability Store at 2°C to 8°C (36°F to 46°F); do not expose to freezing or dry ice. Prior to administration, filgrastim may be allowed to be at room temperature for a maximum of 24 hours. It may be diluted in dextrose 5% in water to a concentration of ≥15 µg/mL for I.V. infusion administration. Minimum concentration is 15 µg/mL; concentrations <15 µg/mL require addition of albumin (1 mL of 5%) to the bag to prevent absorption. This diluted solution is stable for 7 days under refrigeration or at room temperature. **Filgrastim is incompatible with 0.9% sodium chloride (normal saline).**
Standard diluent: ≥375 µg/25 mL D$_5$W

Mechanism of Action Stimulates the production, maturation, and activation of neutrophils, G-CSF activates neutrophils to increase both their migration and cytotoxicity.

Pharmacodynamics/Kinetics
    Onset of action: Rapid elevation in neutrophil counts within the first 24 hours, reaching a plateau in 3-5 days
    Duration: ANC decreases by 50% within 2 days after discontinuing G-CSF; white counts return to the normal range in 4-7 days
    Absorption: S.C.: 100%; peak plasma levels can be maintained for up to 12 hours
    Distribution: V$_d$: 150 mL/kg; no evidence of drug accumulation over a 11- to 20-day period
    Metabolism: Systemic
    Bioavailability: Oral: Not bioavailable
    Half-life: 1.8-3.5 hours
    Time to peak serum concentration: S.C.: Within 2-6 hours

Usual Dosage Children and Adults:
    Initial dosing recommendations: 5 µg/kg/day administered S.C. or I.V. as a single daily infusion over 20-30 minutes

    Doses may be increased in increments of 5 µg/kg for each chemotherapy cycle, according to the duration and severity of the absolute neutrophil count (ANC) nadir. In phase III trials, efficacy was observed at doses of 4-6 µg/kg/day. (Continued)

Filgrastim *(Continued)*

Discontinue therapy if the ANC count is >10,000/mm^3 after the ANC nadir has occurred.

Length of therapy:

Bone marrow transplant patients: G-CSF should be administered daily for up to 30 days, until the ANC has reached 1000/mm^3 for 3 consecutive days following the expected chemotherapy-induced neutrophil nadir.

Chemotherapy-treated patients: G-CSF may be administered daily for up to 2 weeks until the ANC has reached 10,000/mm^3 following the expected chemotherapy-induced neutrophil nadir. Duration of therapy needed to attenuate chemotherapy-induced neutropenia may be dependent on the myelosuppressive potential of the chemotherapy regimen employed. Duration of therapy in clinical studies has ranged from 2 weeks to 3 years. Safety and efficacy of chronic administration have not been established.

Premature discontinuation of G-CSF therapy prior to the time of recovery from the expected neutrophil is generally not recommended. A transient increase in neutrophil counts is typically seen 1-2 days after initiation of therapy.

Administration May be administered undiluted by S.C. or by I.V. infusion over 15-60 minutes in D$_5$W; **incompatible** with sodium chloride solutions

Monitoring Parameters Complete blood cell count and platelet count should be obtained twice weekly. Leukocytosis (white blood cell counts of ≥100,000/mm^3) has been observed in ~2% of patients receiving G-CSF at doses above 5 µg/kg/day. Monitor platelets and hematocrit regularly. Monitor patients with pre-existing cardiac conditions closely as cardiac events (myocardial infarctions, arrhythmias) have been reported in premarketing clinical studies.

Reference Range No clinical benefit seen with ANC >10,000/mm^3

Patient Information Possible bone pain

Nursing Implications Do not mix with sodium chloride solutions

Additional Information Reimbursement hotline: 1-800-272-9376

Dosage Forms Injection, preservative free: 300 mcg/mL (1 mL, 1.6 mL)

Flagyl® Oral *see* Metronidazole *on page 817*

Flamazine® *see* Silver Sulfadiazine *on page 919*

Floxin® *see* Ofloxacin *on page 847*

Fluconazole *(floo KOE na zole)*

U.S. Brand Names Diflucan®

Generic Available No

Use Oral fluconazole should be used in persons able to tolerate oral medications; parenteral fluconazole should be reserved for patients who are both unable to take oral medications and are unable to tolerate amphotericin B (eg, due to hypersensitivity or renal insufficiency)

Indications for use in adult patients:

Oral or vaginal candidiasis unresponsive to nystatin or clotrimazole

Nonlife-threatening *Candida* infections (eg, cystitis, esophagitis)

Treatment of hepatosplenic candidiasis

Treatment of other *Candida* infections in persons unable to tolerate amphotericin B

Treatment of cryptococcal infections

Secondary prophylaxis for cryptococcal meningitis in persons with AIDS

Antifungal prophylaxis in allogeneic bone marrow transplant recipients

Drug of Choice or Alternative for Organism(s)

Blastomyces dermatitidis on page 78

Candida Species *on page 91*

Coccidioides immitis on page 109

Cryptococcus neoformans on page 117

Dematiaceous Fungi *on page 125*

Dermatophytes *on page 127*

Malassezia furfur on page 192

Prototheca Species *on page 233*

Pregnancy Risk Factor C

Contraindications Known hypersensitivity to fluconazole or other azoles; concomitant administration with terfenadine

Warnings/Precautions Should be used with caution in patients with renal and hepatic dysfunction or previous hepatotoxicity from other azole derivatives. Patients who develop abnormal liver function tests during fluconazole therapy should be monitored closely and discontinued if symptoms consistent with liver disease develop. **Should be used with caution in patients receiving cisapride or astemizole.**

Adverse Reactions
1% to 10%:
  Central nervous system: Headache
  Dermatologic: Rash
  Gastrointestinal: Nausea, vomiting, abdominal pain, diarrhea
<1%: Pallor, dizziness, hypokalemia, increased AST, ALT, or alkaline phosphatase

Overdosage/Toxicology
Symptoms of overdose include decreased lacrimation, salivation, respiration and motility, urinary incontinence, cyanosis
Treatment includes supportive measures, a 3-hour hemodialysis will remove 50%

Drug Interactions CYP2C9 enzyme inducer; CYP2C9, 2C18, and 2C19 enzyme inhibitor and CYP3A3/4 enzyme inhibitor (weak)
Decreased effect: Rifampin and cimetidine decrease concentrations of fluconazole; fluconazole may decrease the effect of oral contraceptives
Increased effect/toxicity:
  Coadministration with terfenadine or cisapride is contraindicated; use with caution with astemizole due to increased risk of significant cardiotoxicity
  Hydrochlorothiazide may decrease fluconazole clearance
  Fluconazole may also inhibit warfarin, phenytoin, cyclosporine, and theophylline, zidovudine, sulfonylureas, rifabutin, and warfarin clearance
  Nephrotoxicity of tacrolimus may be increased

Stability Parenteral admixture at room temperature (25°C): Manufacturer expiration dating; do not refrigerate
Standard diluent: 200 mg/100 mL NS (premixed); 400 mg/200 mL NS (premixed)

Mechanism of Action Interferes with cytochrome P-450 activity, decreasing ergosterol synthesis (principal sterol in fungal cell membrane) and inhibiting cell membrane formation

Pharmacodynamics/Kinetics
Distribution: Widely distributed throughout body with good penetration into CSF, eye, peritoneal fluid, sputum, skin, and urine; relative diffusion of antimicrobial agents from blood into CSF: Adequate with or without inflammation (exceeds usual MICs)
  Ratio of CSF to blood level (%):
    Normal meninges: 70-80
    Inflamed meninges: >70-80
Protein binding, plasma: 11% to 12%
Bioavailability: Oral: >90%
Half-life: 25-30 hours with normal renal function
Time to peak serum concentration: Oral: Within 2-4 hours
Elimination: 80% of a dose excreted unchanged in the urine

Usual Dosage The daily dose of fluconazole is the same for oral and I.V. administration

Fluconazole — Once Daily Dosing, Children

Indication	Day 1	Daily Therapy	Minimum Duration of Therapy
Oropharyngeal candidiasis	6 mg/kg	3 mg/kg	14 d
Esophageal candidiasis	6 mg/kg	3-12 mg/kg	21 d and for at least 2 wks following resolution of symptoms
Systemic candidiasis	—	6-12 mg/kg	28 d
Cryptococcal meningitis relapse	12 mg/kg 6 mg/kg	6-12 mg/kg 6 mg/kg	10-12 wk after CSF culture becomes negative

(Continued)

Fluconazole *(Continued)*

Neonates: First 2 weeks of life, especially premature neonates: Same dose as older children every 72 hours

Children: See table on previous page.

Adults: Oral, I.V.: See table for once daily dosing.

Fluconazole — Once Daily Dosing, Adults

Indication	Day 1	Daily Therapy	Minimum Duration of Therapy
Oropharyngeal candidiasis	200 mg	100 mg	14 d
Esophageal candidiasis	200 mg	100 mg	21 d
Systemic candidiasis	400 mg	200 mg	28 d
Cryptococcal meningitis acute	400 mg	200 mg	10-12 wk after CSF culture becomes negative
relapse	200 mg	200 mg	

Dosing adjustment/interval in renal impairment:

No adjustment for vaginal candidiasis single-dose therapy

For multiple dosing, administer usual load then adjust daily doses

Cl_{cr} 11-50 mL/minute: Administer 50% of recommended dose or administer every 48 hours

Hemodialysis: One dose after each dialysis

Continuous arteriovenous or venovenous hemodiafiltration (CAVH) effects: Dose as for Cl_{cr} 10-50 mL/minute

Administration Parenteral fluconazole must be administered by I.V. infusion over approximately 1-2 hours; do not exceed 200 mg/hour when giving I.V. infusion; maximum rate of infusion: 200 mg/hour

Monitoring Parameters Periodic liver function tests (AST, ALT, alkaline phosphatase), renal function tests, potassium

Patient Information May take with food; complete full course of therapy; contact physician or pharmacist if side effects develop; consider using an alternative method of contraception if taking concurrently with birth control pills

Dosage Forms

Injection: 2 mg/mL (100 mL, 200 mL)

Powder for oral suspension: 10 mg/mL (35 mL); 40 mg/mL (35 mL)

Tablet: 50 mg, 100 mg, 150 mg, 200 mg

Selected Readings

Amichai B and Grunwald MH, "Adverse Drug Reactions of the New Oral Antifungal Agents - Terbinafine, Fluconazole, and Itraconazole," *Int J Dermatol*, 1998, 37(6):410-5.

Como JA and Dismukes WE, "Oral Azole Drugs as Systemic Antifungal Therapy," *N Engl J Med*, 1993, 330(4):263-72.

Goa KL and Barradell LB, "Fluconazole. An Update of Its Pharmacodynamic and Pharmacokinetic Properties and Therapeutic Use in Major Superficial and Systemic Mycoses in Immunocompromised Patients," *Drugs*, 1995, 50(4):658-90.

Kauffman CA and Carver PL, "Antifungal Agents in the 1990s. Current Status and Future Developments," *Drugs*, 1997, 53(4):539-49.

Kowalsky SF and Dixon DM, "Fluconazole: A New Antifungal Agent," *Clin Pharm*, 1991, 10(3):179-94.

Lyman CA and Walsh TJ, "Systemically Administered Antifungal Agents. A Review of Their Clinical Pharmacology and Therapeutic Applications," *Drugs*, 1992, 44(1):9-35.

Perry CM, Whittington R, and McTavish D, "Fluconazole. An Update of Its Antimicrobial Activity, Pharmacokinetic Properties, and Therapeutic Use in Vaginal Candidiasis," *Drugs*, 1995, 49(6):984-1006.

Terrell CL, "Antifungal Agents. Part II. The Azoles," *Mayo Clin Proc*, 1999, 74(1):78-100.

Trepanier EF and Amsden GW, "Current Issues in Onchomycosis," *Ann Pharmacother*, 1998, 32(2):204-14.

Flucytosine *(floo SYE toe seen)*

U.S. Brand Names Ancobon®

Canadian Brand Names Ancotil®

Synonyms 5-FC; 5-Flurocytosine

Generic Available No

Use Adjunctive treatment of susceptible fungal infections (usually *Candida* or *Cryptococcus*); synergy with amphotericin B for selected fungal infections (*Cryptococcus* spp, *Candida* spp)

Drug of Choice or Alternative for
Disease/Syndrome(s)
Meningitis, Postsurgical *on page 36*
Organism(s)
Cryptococcus neoformans on page 117
Dematiaceous Fungi *on page 125*
Pregnancy Risk Factor C
Contraindications Hypersensitivity to flucytosine or any component
Warnings/Precautions Use with extreme caution in patients with renal impairment, bone marrow suppression, or in patients with AIDS; dosage modification required in patients with impaired renal function
Adverse Reactions
1% to 10%:
Dermatologic: Rash
Gastrointestinal: Abdominal pain, diarrhea, loss of appetite, nausea, vomiting
Hematologic: Anemia, leukopenia, thrombocytopenia
Hepatic: Hepatitis, jaundice
<1%: Cardiac arrest, confusion, hallucinations, dizziness, drowsiness, headache, parkinsonism, psychosis, ataxia, photosensitivity, temporary growth failure, hypoglycemia, hypokalemia, bone marrow suppression, elevated liver enzymes, paresthesia, hearing loss, respiratory arrest, anaphylaxis
Overdosage/Toxicology
Symptoms of overdose include nausea, vomiting, diarrhea, bone marrow suppression
Treatment is supportive
Drug Interactions Increased effect/toxicity with concurrent amphotericin administration; cytosine may inactivate flucytosine activity
Stability Protect from light
Mechanism of Action Penetrates fungal cells and is converted to fluorouracil which competes with uracil interfering with fungal RNA and protein synthesis
Pharmacodynamics/Kinetics
Absorption: Oral: 75% to 90%
Distribution: Into CSF, aqueous humor, joints, peritoneal fluid, and bronchial secretions
Metabolism: Minimal
Protein binding: 2% to 4%
Half-life: 3-8 hours
Anuria: May be as long as 200 hours
End stage renal disease: 75-200 hours
Time to peak serum concentration: Within 2-6 hours
Elimination: 75% to 90% excreted unchanged in the urine by glomerular filtration
Usual Dosage Children and Adults: Oral: 50-150 mg/kg/day in divided doses every 6 hours

Dosing interval in renal impairment: Use lower initial dose:
Cl_{cr} >50 mL/minute: Administer every 12 hours
Cl_{cr} 10-50 mL/minute: Administer every 16 hours
Cl_{cr} <10 mL/minute: Administer every 24 hours
Hemodialysis: Dialyzable (50% to 100%); administer dose posthemodialysis
Peritoneal dialysis: Adults: Administer 0.5-1 g every 24 hours
Continuous arteriovenous or venovenous hemodiafiltration (CAVH) effects: Dose as for Cl_{cr} 10-50 mL/minute
Monitoring Parameters Serum creatinine, BUN, alkaline phosphatase, AST, ALT, CBC; serum flucytosine concentrations
Reference Range
Therapeutic: 25-100 µg/mL (SI: 195-775 µmol/L); levels should not exceed 100-120 µg/mL to avoid toxic bone marrow depressive effects
Trough: Draw just prior to dose administration
Peak: Draw 2 hours after an oral dose administration
Test Interactions Flucytosine causes markedly false elevations in serum creatinine values when the Ektachem® analyzer is used
Patient Information Take capsules a few at a time with food over a 15-minute period to avoid nausea
Dosage Forms Capsule: 250 mg, 500 mg
Extemporaneous Preparations Flucytosine oral liquid has been prepared by using the contents of ten 500 mg capsules triturated in a mortar and pestle with a
(Continued)

Flucytosine *(Continued)*

small amount of distilled water; the mixture was transferred to a 500 mL volumetric flask; the mortar was rinsed several times with a small amount of distilled water and the fluid added to the flask; sufficient distilled water was added to make a total volume of 500 mL of a 10 mg/mL liquid; oral liquid was stable for 70 days when stored in glass or plastic prescription bottles at 4°C or for up to 14 days at room temperature.

Wintermeyer SM and Nahata MC, "Stability of Flucytosine in an Extemporaneously Compounded Oral Liquid," *Am J Health Syst Pharm*, 1996, 53:407-9.

Selected Readings
Lyman CA and Walsh TJ, "Systemically Administered Antifungal Agents. A Review of Their Clinical Pharmacology and Therapeutic Applications," *Drugs*, 1992, 44(1):9-35.

Patel R, "Antifungal Agents. Part I. Amphotericin B Preparations and Flucytosine," *Mayo Clin Proc*, 1998, 73(12):1205-25.

Flumadine® *see* Rimantadine *on page 908*

Fluogen® *see* Influenza Virus Vaccine *on page 775*

Fluoroquinolones
Refer to
Cinoxacin *on page 678*
Ciprofloxacin *on page 678*
Enoxacin *on page 720*
Grepafloxacin *on page 752*
Levofloxacin *on page 795*
Lomefloxacin *on page 798*
Nalidixic Acid *on page 829*
Norfloxacin *on page 844*
Ofloxacin *on page 847*
Sparfloxacin *on page 921*
Trovafloxacin *on page 960*

Drug of Choice or Alternative for
Disease/Syndrome(s)
Osteomyelitis, Healthy Adult *on page 39*
Prostatitis *on page 47*
Sinusitis, Community-Acquired, Acute *on page 48*
Urinary Tract Infection, Pyelonephritis *on page 53*

Organism(s)
Aeromonas Species *on page 64*
Alcaligenes Species *on page 65*
Bordetella bronchiseptica on page 80
Campylobacter jejuni on page 90
Chlamydia pneumoniae on page 95
Citrobacter Species *on page 102*
Enterobacter Species *on page 134*
Escherichia coli, Nonenterohemorrhagic *on page 147*
Haemophilus influenzae on page 157
Klebsiella Species *on page 183*
Legionella pneumophila on page 185
Moraxella catarrhalis on page 196
Mycoplasma hominis and *Mycoplasma genitalium on page 210*
Mycoplasma pneumoniae on page 211
Proteus Species *on page 232*
Pseudomonas aeruginosa on page 235
Serratia Species *on page 250*
Shigella Species *on page 251*
Staphylococcus saprophyticus on page 264
Stenotrophomonas maltophilia on page 265

Fluoxymesterone *(floo oks i MES te rone)*
U.S. Brand Names Halotestin®

Generic Available Yes

Use Treatment of "AIDS-wasting" syndrome; replacement of endogenous testicular hormone; in females, used as palliative treatment of breast cancer; stimulation of erythropoiesis, angioneurotic edema, postpartum breast engorgement

Restrictions C-III

Pregnancy Risk Factor X

Contraindications Serious cardiac disease, liver or kidney disease, hypersensitivity to fluoxymesterone or any component

Warnings/Precautions May accelerate bone maturation without producing compensatory gain in linear growth in children; in prepubertal children perform radiographic examination of the hand and wrist every 6 months to determine the rate of bone maturation and to assess the effect of treatment on the epiphyseal centers

Adverse Reactions

>10%:

Cardiovascular: Edema

Dermatologic: Acne

Endocrine & metabolic: Menstrual problems (amenorrhea), virilism, breast soreness

Genitourinary: Priapism

1% to 10%:

Cardiovascular: Edema

Dermatologic: Hirsutism (increase in pubic hair growth)

Gastrointestinal: GI irritation, nausea, vomiting

Genitourinary: Prostatic hypertrophy, prostatic carcinoma, impotence, testicular atrophy

Hepatic: Hepatic dysfunction

<1%: Hypercalcemia, leukopenia, polycythemia, hepatic necrosis, cholestatic hepatitis, hypersensitivity reactions, gynecomastia

Overdosage/Toxicology Symptoms of overdose include abnormal liver function tests, water retention

Drug Interactions

Decreased effect:

Fluphenazine effectiveness with anticholinergics

Barbiturate levels and decreased fluphenazine effectiveness when given together

Increased toxicity:

Anticoagulants: Fluoxymesterone may suppress clotting factors II, V, VII, and X; therefore, bleeding may occur in patients on anticoagulant therapy

Cyclosporine: May elevate cyclosporine serum levels

Insulin: May enhance hypoglycemic effect of insulin therapy

May decrease blood glucose concentrations and insulin requirements in patients with diabetes

With ethanol, effects of both drugs may increase

EPSEs and other CNS effects may increase when coadministered with lithium

May potentiate the effects of narcotics including respiratory depression

Stability Protect from light

Mechanism of Action Synthetic androgenic anabolic hormone responsible for the normal growth and development of male sex hormones and development of male sex organs and maintenance of secondary sex characteristics; synthetic testosterone derivative with significant androgen activity; stimulates RNA polymerase activity resulting in an increase in protein production; increases bone development

Pharmacodynamics/Kinetics

Absorption: Oral: Rapid

Protein binding: 98%

Metabolism: In the liver

Half-life: 10-100 minutes

Elimination: Enterohepatic circulation and urinary excretion (90%)

Halogenated derivative of testosterone with up to 5 times the activity of methyltestosterone

Usual Dosage Adults: Oral:

Male:

Hypogonadism: 5-20 mg/day

Delayed puberty: 2.5-20 mg/day for 4-6 months

Female:

Inoperable breast carcinoma: 10-40 mg/day in divided doses for 1-3 months

Breast engorgement: 2.5 mg after delivery, 5-10 mg/day in divided doses for 4-5 days

AIDS wasting: 10 mg twice daily

(Continued)

Fluoxymesterone *(Continued)*

Monitoring Parameters In prepubertal children, perform radiographic examination of the head and wrist every 6 months

Test Interactions Decreased levels of thyroxine-binding globulin; decreased total T_4 serum levels; increased resin uptake of T_3 and T_4

Patient Information Men should report overly frequent or persistent penile erections; women should report menstrual irregularities; all patients should report persistent GI distress, diarrhea, or jaundice

Dosage Forms Tablet: 2 mg, 5 mg, 10 mg

5-Flurocytosine *see* Flucytosine *on page 734*

Flushield® *see* Influenza Virus Vaccine *on page 775*

Fluviral® *see* Influenza Virus Vaccine *on page 775*

Fluviron® *see* Influenza Virus Vaccine *on page 775*

Fluzone® *see* Influenza Virus Vaccine *on page 775*

FML-S® Ophthalmic Suspension *see* Sulfacetamide Sodium and Fluorometholone *on page 928*

Fomivirsen *(foe MI vir sen)*

U.S. Brand Names Vitravene™

Synonyms Fomivirsen Sodium

Use Local treatment of cytomegalovirus (CMV) retinitis in patients with acquired immunodeficiency syndrome who are intolerant or insufficiently responsive to other treatments for CMV retinitis or when other treatments for CMV retinitis are contraindicated

Pregnancy Risk Factor C

Pregnancy/Breast-Feeding Implications Studies have not been conducted in pregnant women. Should be used in pregnancy only when potential benefit to the mother outweighs the potential risk to the fetus. Excretion in human milk is unknown. Use during breast-feeding is contraindicated - a decision to discontinue nursing or discontinue the drug is should be made.

Contraindications Hypersensitivity to fomivirsen or any component

Warnings/Precautions For ophthalmic use via intravitreal injection only. Uveitis occurs frequently, particularly during induction dosing. Do not use in patients who have received intravenous or intravitreal cidofovir within 2-4 weeks (risk of exaggerated inflammation is increased). Patients should be monitored for CMV disease in the contralateral eye and/or extraocular disease. Commonly increases intraocular pressure - monitoring is recommended.

Adverse Reactions

5% to 10%:

Central nervous system: Fever, headache

Gastrointestinal: Abdominal pain, diarrhea, nausea, vomiting

Hematologic: Anemia

Neuromuscular & skeletal: Asthenia

Ocular: Uveitis, abnormal vision, anterior chamber inflammation, blurred vision, cataract, conjunctival hemorrhage, decreased visual acuity, loss of color vision, eye pain, increased intraocular pressure, photophobia, retinal detachment, retinal edema, retinal hemorrhage, retinal pigment changes, vitreitis

Respiratory: Pneumonia, sinusitis

Miscellaneous: Systemic CMV, sepsis, infection

2% to 5%:

Cardiovascular: Chest pain

Central nervous system: Confusion, depression, dizziness, neuropathy, pain

Endocrine and metabolic: Dehydration

Gastrointestinal: Abnormal liver function, pancreatitis, anorexia, weight loss

Hematologic: Thrombocytopenia, lymphoma

Neuromuscular & skeletal: Back pain, cachexia

Ocular: Application site reaction, conjunctival hyperemia, conjunctivitis, corneal edema, decreased peripheral vision, eye irritation, keratic precipitates, optic neuritis, photopsia, retinal vascular disease, visual field defect, vitreous hemorrhage, vitreous opacity

Renal: Kidney failure

Respiratory: Bronchitis, dyspnea, cough

Miscellaneous: Allergic reaction, flu-like syndrome, diaphoresis (increased)

Drug Interactions Drug interactions between fomivirsen and other medications have not been conducted.

Stability Store between 2°C to 25°C (35°F to 77°F); protect from excessive heat or light

Mechanism of Action Inhibits synthesis of viral protein by binding to mRNA which blocks replication of cytomegalovirus through an antisense mechanism

Pharmacodynamics/Kinetics Pharmacokinetic studies have not been conducted in humans. In animal models, the drug is cleared from the eye after 7-10 days. It is metabolized by sequential nucleotide removal, with a small amount of the radioactivity from a dose appearing in the urine.

Usual Dosage Adults: Intravitreal injection: Induction: 330 mcg (0.05 mL) every other week for 2 doses, followed by maintenance dose of 330 mcg (0.05 mL) every 4 weeks

If progression occurs during maintenance, a repeat of the induction regimen may be attempted to establish resumed control. Unacceptable inflammation during therapy may be managed by temporary interruption, provided response has been established. Topical corticosteroids have been used to reduce inflammation.

Administration Administered by intravitreal injection following application of standard topical and/or local anesthetics and antibiotics.

Monitoring Parameters Immediately after injection, light perception and optic nerve head perfusion should be monitored. Anterior chamber paracentesis may be necessary if perfusion is not complete within 7-10 minutes after injection. Subsequent patient evaluation should include monitoring for contralateral CMV infection or extraocular CMV disease, and intraocular pressure prior to each injection.

Additional Information Because the mechanism of action of fomivirsen is different than other antiviral agents active against CMV, fomivirsen may be active against isolates resistant to ganciclovir, foscarnet, or cidofovir. The converse may also be true.

Dosage Forms Solution, for ocular injection: 6.6 mg/mL (0.25 mL)

Selected Readings
Leeds JM, Henry SP, Bistner S, et al, "Pharmacokinetics of an Antisense Oligonucleotide Injected Intravitreally in Monkeys," *Drug Metab Dispos*, 1998, 26(7):670-5.
Leeds JM, Henry SP, Truong L, et al, "Pharmacokinetics of a Potential Human Cytomegalovirus Therapeutic, a Phosphorothioate Oligonucleotide, After Intravitreal Injection in the Rabbit," *Drug Metab Dispos*, 1997, 25(8):921-6.

Fomivirsen Sodium *see* Fomivirsen *on previous page*

Formula Q® *see* Quinine *on page 890*

Fortaz® *see* Ceftazidime *on page 651*

Fortovase® *see* Saquinavir *on page 915*

Foscarnet (fos KAR net)

U.S. Brand Names Foscavir® Injection

Synonyms PFA; Phosphonoformate; Phosphonoformic Acid

Generic Available No

Use

Herpesvirus infections suspected to be caused by acyclovir-resistant (HSV, VZV) or ganciclovir-resistant (CMV) strains. This occurs almost exclusively in immunocompromised persons (eg, with advanced AIDS), who have received prolonged treatment for a herpesvirus infection.

CMV retinitis in persons with AIDS

Other CMV infections in persons unable to tolerate ganciclovir; may be given in combination with ganciclovir in patients who relapse after monotherapy with either drug

Drug of Choice or Alternative for

Organism(s)

Cytomegalovirus *on page 122*

Herpes Simplex Virus *on page 170*

Pregnancy Risk Factor C

Contraindications Hypersensitivity to foscarnet, Cl_{cr} <0.4 mL/minute/kg during therapy

Warnings/Precautions Renal impairment occurs to some degree in the majority of patients treated with foscarnet; renal impairment may occur at any time and is usually reversible within 1 week following dose adjustment or discontinuation of (Continued)

Foscarnet *(Continued)*

therapy, however, several patients have died with renal failure within 4 weeks of stopping foscarnet; therefore, renal function should be closely monitored. Foscarnet is deposited in teeth and bone of young, growing animals; it has adversely affected tooth enamel development in rats; safety and effectiveness in children have not been studied. Imbalance of serum electrolytes or minerals occurs in 6% to 18% of patients (hypocalcemia, low ionized calcium, hypo- or hyperphosphatemia, hypomagnesemia or hypokalemia).

Patients with a low ionized calcium may experience perioral tingling, numbness, paresthesias, tetany, and seizures. Seizures have been experienced by up to 10% of AIDS patients. Risk factors for seizures include a low baseline absolute neutrophil count (ANC), impaired baseline renal function and low total serum calcium. Some patients who have experienced seizures have died, while others have been able to continue or resume foscarnet treatment after their mineral or electrolyte abnormality has been corrected, their underlying disease state treated, or their dose decreased. Foscarnet has been shown to be mutagenic *in vitro* and in mice at very high doses. Information on the use of foscarnet is lacking in the elderly; dose adjustments and proper monitoring must be performed because of the decreased renal function common in older patients.

Adverse Reactions

>10%:
Central nervous system: Fever (65%), headache (26%), seizures (10%)
Gastrointestinal: Nausea (47%), diarrhea (30%), vomiting
Hematologic: Anemia (33%)
Renal: Abnormal renal function/decreased creatinine clearance (27%)

1% to 10%:
Central nervous system: Fatigue, malaise, dizziness, hypoesthesia, depression/confusion/anxiety (≥5%)
Dermatologic: Rash
Endocrine & metabolic: Electrolyte imbalance (especially potassium, calcium, magnesium, and phosphorus)
Gastrointestinal: Anorexia
Hematologic: Granulocytopenia, leukopenia (≥5%), thrombocytopenia, thrombosis
Local: Injection site pain
Neuromuscular & skeletal: Paresthesia, involuntary muscle contractions, rigors, neuropathy (peripheral), weakness
Ocular: Vision abnormalities
Respiratory: Coughing, dyspnea (≥5%)
Miscellaneous: Sepsis, diaphoresis (increased)

<1%: Cardiac failure, bradycardia, arrhythmias, cerebral edema, leg edema, peripheral edema, syncope, substernal chest pain, hypothermia, abnormal crying, malignant hyperpyrexia, vertigo, coma, speech disorders, gynecomastia, decreased gonadotropins, cholecystitis, cholelithiasis, hepatitis, hepatosplenomegaly, ascites, abnormal gait, dyskinesia, hypertonia, nystagmus, vocal cord paralysis

Overdosage/Toxicology

Symptoms of overdose include seizures, renal dysfunction, perioral or limb paresthesias, hypocalcemia
Treatment is supportive; I.V. calcium salts for hypocalcemia

Drug Interactions Increased toxicity: Pentamidine increases hypocalcemia; concurrent use with ciprofloxacin increases seizure potential; acute renal failure (reversible) has been reported with cyclosporin due most likely to toxic synergistic effect; other nephrotoxic drugs (amphotericin B, I.V. pentamidine, aminoglycosides, etc) should be avoided, if possible, to minimize additive renal risk with foscarnet

Stability

Foscarnet injection is a clear, colorless solution; it should be stored at room temperature and protected from temperatures >40°C and from freezing
Foscarnet should be diluted in D_5W or NS and transferred to PVC containers; stable for 24 hours at room temperature or refrigeration
For peripheral line administration, foscarnet **must** be diluted to 12 mg/mL with D_5W or NS
For central line administration, foscarnet may be administered undiluted

Incompatible with dextrose 30%, I.V. solutions containing calcium, magnesium, vancomycin, TPN

Mechanism of Action Pyrophosphate analogue which acts as a noncompetitive inhibitor of many viral RNA and DNA polymerases as well as HIV reverse transcriptase. Similar to ganciclovir, foscarnet is a virostatic agent. Foscarnet does not require activation by thymidine kinase.

Pharmacodynamics/Kinetics

Absorption: Oral: Poorly absorbed; I.V. therapy is needed for the treatment of viral infections in AIDS patients

Distribution: Up to 28% of cumulative I.V. dose may be deposited in bone

Metabolism: Biotransformation does not occur

Half-life: ~3 hours

Elimination: Up to 28% excreted unchanged in urine

Usual Dosage Adolescents and Adults: I.V.:

CMV retinitis:

Induction treatment: 60 mg/kg/dose every 8 hours **or** 100 mg/kg every 12 hours for 14-21 days

Maintenance therapy: 90-120 mg/kg/day as a single infusion

Acyclovir-resistant HSV induction treatment: 40 mg/kg/dose every 8-12 hours for 14-21 days

Dosage adjustment in renal impairment: See tables below and on next page

Hemodialysis:

Foscarnet is highly removed by hemodialysis (30% in 4 hours HD)

Doses of 50 mg/kg/dose posthemodialysis have been found to produce similar serum concentrations as doses of 90 mg/kg twice daily in patients with normal renal function

Doses of 60-90 mg/kg/dose loading dose (posthemodialysis) followed by 45 mg/kg/dose posthemodialysis (3 times/week) with the monitoring of weekly plasma concentrations to maintain peak plasma concentrations in the range of 400-800 μM has been recommended by some clinicians

Continuous arteriovenous or venovenous hemodiafiltration (CAVH) effects: Dose as for Cl_{cr} 10-50 mL/minute

Administration

Foscarnet is administered by intravenous infusion, using an infusion pump, at a rate not exceeding 1 mg/kg/minute

Undiluted (24 mg/mL) solution can be administered without further dilution when using a central venous catheter for infusion

For peripheral vein administration, the solution **must** be diluted to a final concentration **not to exceed** 12 mg/mL

The recommended dosage, frequency, and rate of infusion should not be exceeded

Patient Information Close monitoring is important and any symptom of electrolyte abnormalities should be reported immediately; maintain adequate fluid intake and hydration; regular ophthalmic examinations are necessary. Foscarnet is not a cure; disease progression may occur during or following treatment. Report any numbness in the extremities, paresthesias, or perioral tingling.

Nursing Implications Do not administer by rapid or bolus injection; follow administration guidelines carefully

Maintenance Dosing of Foscarnet in Patients with Abnormal Renal Function

Cl_{cr} (mL/min/kg)	CMV Equivalent to 90 mg/kg q24h	CMV Equivalent to 120 mg/kg q24h
<0.4	not recommended	not recommended
≥0.4-0.5	50 mg/kg every 48 hours	65 mg/kg every 48 hours
≥0.5-0.6	60 mg/kg every 48 hours	80 mg/kg every 48 hours
≥0.6-0.8	80 mg/kg every 48 hours	105 mg/kg every 48 hours
≥0.8-1.0	50 mg/kg every 24 hours	65 mg/kg every 24 hours
≥1-1.4	70 mg/kg every 24 hours	90 mg/kg every 24 hours
≥1.4	90 mg/kg every 24 hours	120 mg/kg every 24 hours

(Continued)

Foscarnet *(Continued)*

Dose Adjustment for Renal Impairment

The induction dose of foscarnet should be adjusted according to creatinine clearance as follows:

Creatinine Clearance (mL/min/kg)	Foscarnet Induction Dose (mg/kg q8h)
1.6	60
1.5	57
1.4	53
1.3	49
1.2	46
1.1	42
1	39
0.9	35
0.8	32
0.7	28
0.6	25
0.5	21
0.4	18

The maintenance dose of foscarnet should be adjusted according to creatinine clearance as follows:

Creatinine Clearance (mL/min/kg)	Foscarnet Maintenance Dose (mg/kg/day)
1.4	90-120
1.2-1.4	78-104
1-1.2	75-100
0.8-1	71-94
0.6-0.8	63-84
0.4-0.6	57-75

Additional Information Sodium loading with 500 mL of 0.9% sodium chloride solution before and after foscarnet infusion helps to minimize the risk of nephrotoxicity

Dosage Forms Injection: 24 mg/mL (250 mL, 500 mL)

Selected Readings

Chrisp P and Clissold SP, "Foscarnet. A Review of Its Antiviral Activity, Pharmacokinetic Properties and Therapeutic Use in Immunocompromised Patients With Cytomegalovirus Retinitis," *Drugs*, 1991, 41(1):104-29.

Deray G, Martinez F, Katlama C, et al, "Foscarnet Nephrotoxicity: Mechanism, Incidence and Prevention," *Am J Nephrol*, 1989, 9:316-21.

"Drugs for Non-HIV Viral Infections," *Med Lett Drugs Ther*, 1994, 36(919):27.

Jayaweera DT, "Minimising the Dosage-Limiting Toxicities of Foscarnet Induction Therapy," *Drug Saf*, 1997, 16(4):258-66.

Keating MR, "Antiviral Agents," *Mayo Clin Proc*, 1992, 67(2):160-78.

Whitley RJ, Jacobson MA, Friedberg DN, et al, "Guidelines for the Treatment of Cytomegalovirus Diseases in Patients With AIDS in the Era of Potent Antiretroviral Therapy: Recommendations of an International Panel. International AIDS Society-USA," *Arch Intern Med*, 1998, 158(9):957-69.

Foscavir® Injection *see* Foscarnet *on page 739*

Fosfomycin (fos foe MYE sin)

U.S. Brand Names Monurol™

Synonyms Fosfomycin Tromethamine

Use A single oral dose in the treatment of uncomplicated urinary tract infections in women due to susceptible strains of *E. coli* and *Enterococcus*; multiple doses have been investigated for complicated urinary tract infections in men; may have an advantage over other agents since it maintains high concentration in the urine for up to 48 hours

Pregnancy Risk Factor B

Pregnancy/Breast-Feeding Implications Breast-feeding/lactation: Milk concentration approximates 10% of plasma

Adverse Reactions

>1%:

Central nervous system: Headache

Dermatologic: Rash

Gastrointestinal: Diarrhea (2% to 8%), nausea, vomiting, epigastric discomfort, anorexia

<1%: Dizziness, drowsiness, fatigue, pruritus

Overdosage/Toxicology Symptomatic and supportive treatment is recommended in the event of an overdose.

Drug Interactions

Decreased effect: Antacids or calcium salts may cause precipitate formation and decrease fosfomycin absorption

Metoclopramide: Increased gastrointestinal motility may lower fosfomcyin tromethamine serum concentrations and urinary excretion. This drug interaction possibly could be extrapolated to other medications which increase gastrointestinal motility.

Mechanism of Action As a phosphoric acid derivative, fosfomycin inhibits bacterial wall synthesis (bactericidal) by inactivating the enzyme, pyruvyl transferase, which is critical in the synthesis of cell walls by bacteria; the tromethamine salt is preferable to the calcium salt due to its superior absorption

Pharmacodynamics/Kinetics

Absorption: Well absorbed

Distribution: V_d: 2 L/kg; high concentrations in urine; distributed well into other tissues, crosses maximally into CSF with inflamed meninges

Protein binding: Minimal (<3%)

Metabolism: None

Bioavailability: 34% to 58%

Half-life: 4-8 hours; prolonged in renal failure (50 hours with Cl_{cr} <10 mL/minute)

Time to peak serum concentration: 2 hours

Elimination: High urinary levels persist for >48 hours (100 mcg/mL); excreted unchanged

Usual Dosage Adults: Oral: Urinary tract infections:

Female: Single dose of 3 g in 4 oz of water

Male: 3 g once daily for 2-3 days for complicated urinary tract infections

Dosing adjustment in renal impairment: Decrease dose; 80% removed by dialysis, repeat dose after dialysis

Dosing adjustment in hepatic impairment: No dosage decrease needed

Administration Always mix with water before ingesting; do not administer in its dry form; pour contents of envelope into 90-120 mL of water (not hot), stir to dissolve and take immediately

Monitoring Parameters Signs and symptoms of urinary tract infection

Patient Information May be taken with or without food; avoid use of antacids or calcium salts within 4 hours before or 2 hours after taking fosfomycin; contact your physician if signs of allergy develop; if symptoms do not improve after 2-3 days, contact your healthcare provider

Additional Information Many gram-positive and gram-negative organisms such as *Staphylococcus*, pneumococci, *E. coli*, *Salmonella*, *Shigella*, *H. influenzae*, *Neisseria* spp, and some strains of *P. aeruginosa*, indole-negative *Proteus*, and *Providencia* are inhibited; *B. fragilis*, and anaerobic gram-negative cocci are resistant

Dosage Forms Powder, as tromethamine: 3 g, to be mixed in 4 oz of water

Selected Readings

Patel SS, Balfour JA, and Bryson HM, "Fosfomycin Tromethamine. A Review of Its Antibacterial Activity, Pharmacokinetic Properties, and Therapeutic Efficacy as a Single-Dose Oral Treatment for Acute Uncomplicated Lower Urinary Tract Infections," *Drugs*, 1997, 53(4):637-56.

Furanite® see Nitrofurantoin on page 842

Furazolidone (fyoor a ZOE li done)
U.S. Brand Names Furoxone®
Generic Available No
Use Treatment of bacterial or protozoal diarrhea and enteritis caused by susceptible organisms Giardia lamblia and Vibrio cholerae
Pregnancy Risk Factor C
Contraindications Known hypersensitivity to furazolidone; concurrent use of alcohol; patients <1 month of age because of the possibility of producing hemolytic anemia
Warnings/Precautions Use caution in patients with G-6-PD deficiency when administering large doses for prolonged periods; furazolidone inhibits monoamine oxidase
Adverse Reactions
>10%: Genitourinary: Discoloration of urine (dark yellow to brown)
1% to 10%:
Central nervous system: Headache
Gastrointestinal: Abdominal pain, diarrhea, nausea, vomiting
<1%: Orthostatic hypotension, fever, dizziness, drowsiness, malaise, rash, hypoglycemia, disulfiram-like reaction after alcohol ingestion, leukopenia, agranulocytosis, hemolysis in patients with G-6-PD deficiency, arthralgia
Overdosage/Toxicology
Symptoms of overdose include nausea, vomiting, serotonin crisis
Treatment is supportive care only; serotonin crisis may require dantrolene/bromocriptine
Drug Interactions
Increases toxicity of sympathomimetic amines, tricyclic antidepressants, MAO inhibitors, meperidine, anorexiants, dextromethorphan, fluoxetine, paroxetine, sertraline, trazodone
Increased effect/toxicity of levodopa
Disulfiram-like reaction with alcohol
Mechanism of Action Inhibits several vital enzymatic reactions causing antibacterial and antiprotozoal action
Pharmacodynamics/Kinetics
Absorption: Oral: Poor
Elimination: Oral: $\frac{1}{3}$ of dose is excreted in urine as active drug and metabolites
Usual Dosage Oral:
Children >1 month: 5-8 mg/kg/day in 4 divided doses for 7 days, not to exceed 400 mg/day or 8.8 mg/kg/day
Adults: 100 mg 4 times/day for 7 days
Dietary Considerations
Alcohol: Avoid use
Food: Marked elevation of blood pressure, hypertensive crisis, or hemorrhagic stroke may occur with foods high in amine content
Monitoring Parameters CBC
Test Interactions False-positive results for urine glucose with Clinitest®
Patient Information May discolor urine to a brown tint; avoid drinking alcohol during or for 4 days after therapy or eating tyramine-containing foods; consult with physician or pharmacist for a list of these foods. Do not take any prescription or nonprescription drugs without consulting the physician or pharmacist; if result not achieved at the end of treatment contact physician.
Dosage Forms
Liquid: 50 mg/15 mL (60 mL, 473 mL)
Tablet: 100 mg
Selected Readings
"Drugs for Parasitic Infections," Med Lett Drugs Ther, 1998, 40(1017):1-12.

Furoxone® see Furazolidone on this page
Gamimune® N see Immune Globulin, Intravenous on page 771
Gamma Benzene Hexachloride see Lindane on page 797
Gammabulin Immuno see Immune Globulin, Intramuscular on page 770
Gammagard® S/D see Immune Globulin, Intravenous on page 771
Gamma Globulin see Immune Globulin, Intramuscular on page 770
Gammar®-P I.V. see Immune Globulin, Intravenous on page 771

Gamulin® Rh *see* Rh₀(D) Immune Globulin *on page 896*

Ganciclovir (gan SYE kloe veer)

U.S. Brand Names Cytovene®; Vitrasert®
Synonyms DHPG Sodium; GCV Sodium; Nordeoxyguanosine
Generic Available No
Use

Parenteral: Treatment of CMV retinitis in immunocompromised individuals, including patients with acquired immunodeficiency syndrome; prophylaxis of CMV infection in transplant patients; may be given in combination with foscarnet in patients who relapse after monotherapy with either drug

Oral: Alternative to the I.V. formulation for maintenance treatment of CMV retinitis in immunocompromised patients, including patients with AIDS, in whom retinitis is stable following appropriate induction therapy and for whom the risk of more rapid progression is balanced by the benefit associated with avoiding daily I.V. infusions.

Implant: Treatment of CMV retinitis

Drug of Choice or Alternative for Organism(s)

Cytomegalovirus *on page 122*
Herpes Simplex Virus *on page 170*

Pregnancy Risk Factor C
Contraindications Absolute neutrophil count <500/mm³; platelet count <25,000/mm³; known hypersensitivity to ganciclovir or acyclovir
Warnings/Precautions Dosage adjustment or interruption of ganciclovir therapy may be necessary in patients with neutropenia and/or thrombocytopenia and patients with impaired renal function. Use with extreme caution in children since long-term safety has not been determined and due to ganciclovir's potential for long-term carcinogenic and adverse reproductive effects; ganciclovir may adversely affect spermatogenesis and fertility; due to its mutagenic potential, contraceptive precautions for female and male patients need to be followed during and for at least 90 days after therapy with the drug; take care to administer only into veins with good blood flow.

Adverse Reactions
>10%:
Central nervous system: Fever (38% to 48%)
Dermatologic: Rash (15% - oral, 10% - I.V.)
Gastrointestinal: Abdominal pain (17% to 19%), diarrhea (40%), nausea (25%), anorexia (15%), vomiting (13%)
Hematologic: Anemia (20% to 25%), leukopenia (30% to 40%)
1% to 10%:
Central nervous system: Confusion, neuropathy (8% to 9%), headache (4%)
Dermatologic: Pruritus (5%)
Hematologic: Thrombocytopenia (6%), neutropenia with ANC <500/mm³ (5% - oral, 14% - I.V.)
Neuromuscular & skeletal: Paresthesia (6% to 10%), weakness (6%)
Miscellaneous: Sepsis (4% - oral, 15% - I.V.)
<1%: Arrhythmia, hypertension, hypotension, edema, ataxia, dizziness, nervousness, psychosis, malaise, coma, seizures, alopecia, urticaria, eosinophilia, hemorrhage, increased LFTs, inflammation or pain at injection site, tremor, retinal detachment, visual loss, hyphema, uveitis (intravitreal implant) creatinine increased 2.5%, dyspnea, increased serum creatinine, azotemia

Overdosage/Toxicology
Symptoms of overdose include neutropenia, vomiting, hypersalivation, bloody diarrhea, cytopenia, testicular atrophy
Treatment is supportive; hemodialysis removes 50% of drug; hydration may be of some benefit

Drug Interactions
Decreased effect: Didanosine: A decrease in steady-state ganciclovir AUC may occur
Increased toxicity:
Immunosuppressive agents may increase cytotoxicity of ganciclovir
Imipenem/cilastatin may increase seizure potential
Zidovudine: Oral ganciclovir increased the AUC of zidovudine, although zidovudine decreases steady state levels of ganciclovir. Since both drugs have
(Continued)

Ganciclovir *(Continued)*

the potential to cause neutropenia and anemia, some patients may not tolerate concomitant therapy with these drugs at full dosage.

Probenecid: The renal clearance of ganciclovir is decreased in the presence of probenecid

Didanosine levels are increased with concurrent ganciclovir

Other nephrotoxic drugs (eg, amphotericin and cyclosporine) may have additive nephrotoxicity with ganciclovir

Stability

Preparation should take place in a vertical laminar flow hood with the same precautions as antineoplastic agents

Intact vials should be stored at room temperature and protected from temperatures >40°C

Reconstitute powder with sterile water **not** bacteriostatic water because parabens may cause precipitation

Reconstituted solution is stable for 12 hours at room temperature, however, conflicting data indicates that reconstituted solution is stable for 60 days under refrigeration (4°C)

Drug product should be reconstituted immediately before use and any unused portion should be discarded

Stability of parenteral admixture at room temperature (25°C) and at refrigeration temperature (4°C): 5 days

An in-line filter of 0.22-5 micron is recommended during the infusion of all ganciclovir solutions

Mechanism of Action Ganciclovir is phosphorylated to a substrate which competitively inhibits the binding of deoxyguanosine triphosphate to DNA polymerase resulting in inhibition of viral DNA synthesis

Pharmacodynamics/Kinetics

Absorption: Oral: Absolute bioavailability under fasting conditions: 5% and following food: 6% to 9%; following fatty meal: 28% to 31%

Distribution: V_d: 15.26 L/1.73 m^2; widely distributed to all tissues including CSF and ocular tissue; CSF concentration 24% to 67% of plasma concentration

Protein binding: 1% to 2%

Half-life: 1.7-5.8 hours; increases with impaired renal function

End stage renal disease: 5-28 hours

Elimination: Majority (80% to 99%) excreted as unchanged drug in the urine

Usual Dosage

CMV retinitis: Slow I.V. infusion (dosing is based on total body weight):

Children >3 months and Adults:

Induction therapy: 5 mg/kg/dose every 12 hours for 14-21 days followed by maintenance therapy

Maintenance therapy: 5 mg/kg/day as a single daily dose for 7 days/week or 6 mg/kg/day for 5 days/week

CMV retinitis: Oral: 1000 mg 3 times/day with food **or** 500 mg 6 times/day with food

Prevention of CMV disease in patients with advanced HIV infection and normal renal function: Oral: 1000 mg 3 times/day with food

Prevention of CMV disease in transplant patients: Same initial and maintenance dose as CMV retinitis except duration of initial course is 7-14 days, duration of maintenance therapy is dependent on clinical condition and degree of immunosuppression

Intravitreal implant: One implant for 5- to 8-month period; following depletion of ganciclovir, as evidenced by progression of retinitis, implant may be removed and replaced

Dosing adjustment in renal impairment:

I.V. (Induction):

Cl_{cr} 50-69 mL/minute: Administer 2.5 mg/kg/dose every 12 hours

Cl_{cr} 25-49 mL/minute: Administer 2.5 mg/kg/dose every 24 hours

Cl_{cr} 10-24 mL/minute: Administer 12.5 mg/kg/dose every 24 hours

Cl_{cr} <10 mL/minute: Administer 1.25 mg/kg/dose 3 times/week following hemodialysis

I.V. (Maintenance):

Cl_{cr} 50-69 mL/minute: Administer 2.5 mg/kg/dose every 24 hours

Cl_{cr} 25-49 mL/minute: Administer 1.25 mg/kg/dose every 24 hours

Cl_{cr} 10-24 mL/minute: Administer 0.625 mg/kg/dose every 24 hours

Cl_{cr} <10 mL/minute: Administer 0.625 mg/kg/dose 3 times/week following hemodialysis

Oral:

Cl_{cr} 50-69 mL/minute: Administer 1500 mg/day or 500 mg 3 times/day

Cl_{cr} 25-49 mL/minute: Administer 1000 mg/day or 500 mg twice daily

Cl_{cr} 10-24 mL/minute: Administer 500 mg/day

Cl_{cr} <10 mL/minute: Administer 500 mg 3 times/week following hemodialysis

Hemodialysis effects: Dialyzable (50%) following hemodialysis; administer dose postdialysis. During peritoneal dialysis, dose as for Cl_{cr} <10 mL/minute. During continuous arteriovenous or venovenous hemofiltration (CAVH/CAVHD), administer 2.5 mg/kg/dose every 24 hours.

Administration The same precautions utilized with antineoplastic agents should be followed with ganciclovir administration. Ganciclovir should not be administered by I.M., S.C., or rapid IVP administration; administer by slow I.V. infusion over at least 1 hour at a final concentration for administration not to exceed 10 mg/mL. **An IN-LINE filter of 0.22-5 micron is recommended during the infusion of all ganciclovir solutions.** Oral ganciclovir should be administered with food.

Monitoring Parameters CBC with differential and platelet count, serum creatinine, ophthalmologic exams

Patient Information Ganciclovir is not a cure for CMV retinitis; regular ophthalmologic examinations should be done; close monitoring of blood counts should be done while on therapy and dosage adjustments may need to be made; take with food to increase absorption

Nursing Implications Must be prepared in vertical flow hood; use chemotherapy precautions during administration; discard appropriately

Additional Information Sodium content of 500 mg vial: 46 mg

Dosage Forms

Capsule: 250 mg

Implant, intravitreal: 4.5 mg

Powder for injection, lyophilized: 500 mg (10 mL)

Selected Readings
Alrabiah FA and Sacks SL, "New Antiherpesvirus Agents. Their Targets and Therapeutic Potential," *Drugs*, 1996, 52(1):17-32.

"Drugs for Non-HIV Viral Infections," *Med Lett Drugs Ther*, 1994, 36(919):27.

Keating MR, "Antiviral Agents," *Mayo Clin Proc*, 1992, 67(2):160-78.

Matthews T and Boehme R, "Antiviral Activity and Mechanism of Action of Ganciclovir," *Rev Infect Dis*, 1988, 10(Suppl 3):S490-4.

Whitley RJ, Jacobson MA, Friedberg DN, et al, "Guidelines for the Treatment of Cytomegalovirus Diseases in Patients With AIDS in the Era of Potent Antiretroviral Therapy: Recommendations of an International Panel. International AIDS Society-USA," *Arch Intern Med*, 1998, 158(9):957-69.

Gantanol® *see* Sulfamethoxazole *on page 932*

Garamycin® *see* Gentamicin *on this page*

G-CSF *see* Filgrastim *on page 730*

GCV Sodium *see* Ganciclovir *on page 745*

Genapax® *see* Gentian Violet *on page 751*

Genaspor® [OTC] *see* Tolnaftate *on page 956*

Genoptic® Ophthalmic *see* Gentamicin *on this page*

Genoptic® S.O.P. Ophthalmic *see* Gentamicin *on this page*

Gentacidin® Ophthalmic *see* Gentamicin *on this page*

Gentafair® *see* Gentamicin *on this page*

Gentak® Ophthalmic *see* Gentamicin *on this page*

Gentamicin (jen ta MYE sin)

Related Information

Aminoglycoside Dosing and Monitoring *on page 1058*

U.S. Brand Names Garamycin®; Genoptic® Ophthalmic; Genoptic® S.O.P. Ophthalmic; Gentacidin® Ophthalmic; Gentafair®; Gentak® Ophthalmic; Gentrasul®; G-myticin® Topical; I-Gent®; Jenamicin® Injection; Ocumycin®

Synonyms Gentamicin Sulfate

Generic Available Yes

Use Treatment of susceptible bacterial infections, normally gram-negative organisms including *Pseudomonas*, *Proteus*, *Serratia*, and gram-positive *Staphylococcus*; treatment of bone infections, respiratory tract infections, skin and soft (Continued)

Gentamicin *(Continued)*

tissue infections, as well as abdominal and urinary tract infections, endocarditis, and septicemia; used topically to treat superficial infections of the skin or ophthalmic infections caused by susceptible bacteria; also for prevention of bacterial endocarditis prior to dental or surgical procedures

Drug of Choice or Alternative for
Disease/Syndrome(s)
Catheter Infection, Intravascular *on page 21*
Endocarditis, Acute, I.V. Drug Abuse *on page 26*
Endocarditis, Acute Native Valve *on page 26*
Endocarditis, Prosthetic Valve, Early *on page 27*
Endocarditis, Prosthetic Valve, Late *on page 28*
Endocarditis, Subacute Native Valve *on page 28*
Meningitis, Neonatal (<2 months of age) *on page 35*
Otitis Externa, Severe (Malignant) *on page 40*
Pelvic Inflammatory Disease *on page 41*
Pneumonia, Hospital-Acquired *on page 46*
Sinusitis, Hospital-Acquired *on page 49*
Urinary Tract Infection, Pyelonephritis *on page 53*
Organism(s)
Brucella Species *on page 85*
Calymmatobacterium granulomatis *on page 89*
Corynebacterium jeikeium *on page 113*
Enterococcus Species *on page 137*
Francisella tularensis *on page 148*
HACEK Group *on page 155*
Listeria monocytogenes *on page 189*
Staphylococcus aureus, Methicillin-Resistant *on page 256*
Staphylococcus epidermidis, Methicillin-Resistant *on page 261*
Streptococcus, Viridans Group *on page 279*
Yersinia pestis *on page 300*

Pregnancy Risk Factor C

Contraindications Hypersensitivity to gentamicin or other aminoglycosides

Warnings/Precautions Not intended for long-term therapy due to toxic hazards associated with extended administration; pre-existing renal insufficiency, vestibular or cochlear impairment, myasthenia gravis, hypocalcemia, conditions which depress neuromuscular transmission

Parenteral aminoglycosides have been associated with significant nephrotoxicity or ototoxicity; the ototoxicity may be directly proportional to the amount of drug given and the duration of treatment; tinnitus or vertigo are indications of vestibular injury and impending hearing loss; renal damage is usually reversible

Adverse Reactions
>10%:
  Central nervous system: Neurotoxicity (vertigo, ataxia)
  Neuromuscular & skeletal: Gait instability
  Otic: Ototoxicity (auditory), ototoxicity (vestibular)
  Renal: Nephrotoxicity, decreased creatinine clearance
1% to 10%:
  Cardiovascular: Edema
  Dermatologic: Skin itching, reddening of skin, rash
<1%: Drowsiness, headache, pseudomotor cerebri, photosensitivity, erythema, anorexia, nausea, vomiting, weight loss, increased salivation, enterocolitis, granulocytopenia, agranulocytosis, thrombocytopenia, elevated LFTs, burning, stinging, tremors, muscle cramps, weakness, dyspnea

Overdosage/Toxicology
Symptoms of overdose include ototoxicity, nephrotoxicity, and neuromuscular toxicity; serum level monitoring is recommended

The treatment of choice, following a single acute overdose, appears to be the maintenance of good urine output of at least 3 mL/kg/hour. Dialysis is of questionable value in the enhancement of aminoglycoside elimination. If required, hemodialysis is preferred over peritoneal dialysis in patients with normal renal function. Careful hydration may be all that is required to promote diuresis and therefore the enhancement of the drug's elimination. Chelation with penicillins is experimental.

Drug Interactions Increased toxicity:
    Penicillins, cephalosporins, amphotericin B, loop diuretics may increase nephrotoxic potential
    Neuromuscular blocking agents may increase neuromuscular blockade

Stability
    Gentamicin is a colorless to slightly yellow solution which should be stored between 2°C to 30°C, but refrigeration is not recommended
    I.V. infusion solutions mixed in NS or D_5W solution are stable for 24 hours at room temperature and refrigeration
    Premixed bag: Manufacturer expiration date
    Out of overwrap stability: 30 days

Mechanism of Action Interferes with bacterial protein synthesis by binding to 30S and 50S ribosomal subunits resulting in a defective bacterial cell membrane

Pharmacodynamics/Kinetics
    Absorption: Oral: Not absorbed
    Distribution: Crosses the placenta
    V_d: Increased by edema, ascites, fluid overload; decreased in patients with dehydration.
        Neonates: 0.4-0.6 L/kg
        Children: 0.3-0.35 L/kg
        Adults: 0.2-0.3 L/kg
    Relative diffusion of antimicrobial agents from blood into cerebrospinal fluid (CSF): Minimal even with inflammation
    Ratio of CSF to blood level (%):
        Normal meninges: Nil
        Inflamed meninges: 10-30
    Protein binding: <30%
    Half-life:
        Infants:
            <1 week: 3-11.5 hours
            1 week to 6 months: 3-3.5 hours
        Adults: 1.5-3 hours; end stage renal disease: 36-70 hours
    Time to peak serum concentration:
        I.M.: Within 30-90 minutes
        I.V.: 30 minutes after a 30-minute infusion
    Elimination: Clearance is directly related to renal function, eliminated almost completely by glomerular filtration of unchanged drug with excretion into the urine

Usual Dosage Individualization is critical because of the low therapeutic index
    Use of ideal body weight (IBW) for determining the mg/kg/dose appears to be more accurate than dosing on the basis of total body weight (TBW).
    In morbid obesity, dosage requirement may best be estimated using a dosing weight of IBW + 0.4 (TBW - IBW)
    Initial and periodic peak and trough plasma drug levels should be determined, particularly in critically ill patients with serious infections or in disease states known to significantly alter aminoglycoside pharmacokinetics (eg, cystic fibrosis, burns, or major surgery)

    Newborns: Intrathecal: 1 mg every day
    Infants >3 months: Intrathecal: 1-2 mg/day
    Infants and Children <5 years: I.M., I.V.: 2.5 mg/kg/dose every 8 hours*
        Cystic fibrosis: 2.5 mg/kg/dose every 6 hours
    Children >5 years: I.M., I.V.: 1.5-2.5 mg/kg/dose every 8 hours*
        Prevention of bacterial endocarditis: Dental, oral, upper respiratory procedures, GI/GU procedures: 2 mg/kg with ampicillin (50 mg/kg) 30 minutes prior to procedure
    *Some patients may require larger or more frequent doses (eg, every 6 hours) if serum levels document the need (ie, cystic fibrosis or febrile granulocytopenic patients)

    Adults: I.M., I.V.:
        Severe life-threatening infections: 2-2.5 mg/kg/dose
        Urinary tract infections: 1.5 mg/kg/dose
        Synergy (for gram-positive infections): 1 mg/kg/dose
        Prevention of bacterial endocarditis:
            Dental, oral, or upper respiratory procedures: 1.5 mg/kg not to exceed 80 mg with ampicillin (1-2 g) 30 minutes prior to procedure
(Continued)

Gentamicin *(Continued)*

GI/GU surgery: 1.5 mg/kg not to exceed 80 mg with ampicillin 2 g 30 minutes prior to procedure

Children and Adults:
Intrathecal: 4-8 mg/day
Ophthalmic:
Ointment: Instill ½" (1.25 cm) 2-3 times/day to every 3-4 hours
Solution: Instill 1-2 drops every 2-4 hours, up to 2 drops every hour for severe infections
Topical: Apply 3-4 times/day to affected area

Some clinicians suggest a daily dose of 4-7 mg/kg for all patients with normal renal function. This dose is at least as efficacious with similar, if not less, toxicity than conventional dosing. (See also Aminoglycoside Dosing and Monitoring *on page 1058*.)

Dosing interval in renal impairment:
Cl_{cr} ≥60 mL/minute: Administer every 8 hours
Cl_{cr} 40-60 mL/minute: Administer every 12 hours
Cl_{cr} 20-40 mL/minute: Administer every 24 hours
Cl_{cr} <20 mL/minute: Loading dose, then monitor levels
Hemodialysis: Dialyzable; removal by hemodialysis: 30% removal of aminoglycosides occurs during 4 hours of HD; administer dose after dialysis and follow levels
Removal by continuous ambulatory peritoneal dialysis (CAPD):
Administration via CAPD fluid:
Gram-negative infection: 4-8 mg/L (4-8 mcg/mL) of CAPD fluid
Gram-positive infection (ie, synergy): 3-4 mg/L (3-4 mcg/mL) of CAPD fluid
Administration via I.V., I.M. route during CAPD: Dose as for Cl_{cr} <10 mL/minute and follow levels
Removal via continuous arteriovenous or venovenous hemofiltration (CAVH/CAVHD): Dose as for Cl_{cr} 10-40 mL/minute and follow levels

Dosing adjustment/comments in hepatic disease: Monitor plasma concentrations

Dietary Considerations Calcium, magnesium, potassium: Renal wasting may cause hypocalcemia, hypomagnesemia, and/or hypokalemia

Monitoring Parameters Urinalysis, urine output, BUN, serum creatinine; hearing should be tested before, during, and after treatment; particularly in those at risk for ototoxicity or who will be receiving prolonged therapy (>2 weeks)

Reference Range
Timing of serum samples: Draw peak 30 minutes after 30-minute infusion has been completed or 1 hour after I.M. injection; draw trough immediately before next dose
Sample size: 0.5-2 mL blood (red top tube) or 0.1-1 mL serum (separated)
Therapeutic levels:
Peak:
Serious infections: 6-8 µg/mL (12-17 µmol/L)
Life-threatening infections: 8-10 µg/mL (17-21 µmol/L)
Urinary tract infections: 4-6 µg/mL
Synergy against gram-positive organisms: 3-5 µg/mL
Trough:
Serious infections: 0.5-1 µg/mL
Life-threatening infections: 1-2 µg/mL
Obtain drug levels after the third dose unless renal dysfunction/toxicity suspected

Test Interactions Penicillin may decrease aminoglycoside serum concentrations *in vitro*

Patient Information Report any dizziness or sensations of ringing or fullness in ears; do not touch ophthalmics to eye; use no other eye drops within 5-10 minutes of instilling ophthalmic

Nursing Implications Slower absorption and lower peak concentrations probably due to poor circulation in the atrophic muscle, may occur following I.M. injection in paralyzed patients (suggest I.V. route); aminoglycoside levels measured in blood taken from Silastic® central catheters can sometimes give falsely high readings (draw via separate lumen or peripheral site if possible, otherwise flush very well). Monitor serum creatinine and urine output; obtain drug levels after the third dose unless otherwise directed (eg, suspected toxicity or renal dysfunction). Peak levels are drawn 30 minutes after the end of a 30-minute infusion or 60 minutes following I.M. injection; trough levels are drawn within 30 minutes before the next dose; administer other antibiotic drugs at least 1 hour before or after gentamicin. Hearing should be tested before, during, and after treatment in patients at risk for ototoxicity.

Dosage Forms

Cream, topical, as sulfate (Garamycin®, G-myticin®): 0.1% (15 g)

Infusion, in D₅W, as sulfate: 60 mg, 80 mg, 100 mg

Infusion, in NS, as sulfate: 40 mg, 60 mg, 80 mg, 90 mg, 100 mg, 120 mg

Injection, as sulfate: 40 mg/mL (1 mL, 1.5 mL, 2 mL)

Pediatric, as sulfate: 10 mg/mL (2 mL)

Intrathecal, preservative free, as sulfate (Garamycin®): 2 mg/mL (2 mL)

Ointment, as sulfate:

Ophthalmic: 0.3% [3 mg/g] (3.5 g)

Garamycin®, Genoptic® S.O.P., Gentacidin®, Gentak®: 0.3% [3 mg/g] (3.5 g)

Topical (Garamycin®, G-myticin®): 0.1% (15 g)

Solution, ophthalmic, as sulfate: 0.3% (5 mL, 15 mL)

Garamycin®, Genoptic®, Gentacidin®, Gentak®: 0.3% (1 mL, 5 mL, 15 mL)

Selected Readings
Begg EJ and Barclay ML, "Aminoglycosides - 50 Years On," *Br J Clin Pharmacol*, 1995, 39(6):597-603.

Cunha BA, "Aminoglycosides: Current Role in Antimicrobial Therapy," *Pharmacotherapy*, 1988, 8(6):334-50.

Edson RS and Terrell CL, "The Aminoglycosides," *Mayo Clin Proc*, 1999, 74(5):519-28.

Gilbert DN, "Once-Daily Aminoglycoside Therapy," *Antimicrob Agents Chemother*, 1991, 35(3):399-405.

Hustinx WN, and Hoepelman IM, "Aminoglycoside Dosage Regimens. Is Once a Day Enough?" *Clin Pharmacokinet*, 1993, 25(6):427-32.

Iseman MD, "Treatment of Multidrug-Resistant Tuberculosis," *N Engl J Med*, 1993, 329(11):784-91.

Lortholary O, Tod M, Cohen Y, et al, "Aminoglycosides," *Med Clin North Am*, 1995, 79(4):761-87.

McCormack JP and Jewesson PJ, "A Critical Re-Evaluation of the "Therapeutic Range" of Aminoglycosides," *Clin Infect Dis*, 1992, 14(1):320-39.

Gentamicin Sulfate *see* Gentamicin *on page 747*

Gentian Violet (JEN shun VYE oh let)

U.S. Brand Names Genapax®

Synonyms Crystal Violet; Methylrosaniline Chloride

Generic Available Yes

Use Treatment of cutaneous or mucocutaneous infections caused by *Candida albicans* and other superficial skin infections

Pregnancy Risk Factor C

Contraindications Known hypersensitivity to gentian violet; ulcerated areas; patients with porphyria .

Warnings/Precautions Infants should be turned face down after application to minimize amount of drug swallowed; may result in tattooing of the skin when applied to granulation tissue; solution is for external use only; avoid contact with eyes

Adverse Reactions 1% to 10%:

Dermatologic: Irritation, vesicle formation, sensitivity reactions

Gastrointestinal: Esophagitis, ulceration of mucous membranes

Local: Burning

Respiratory: Laryngitis, tracheitis, laryngeal obstruction

Overdosage/Toxicology Signs and symptoms: Laryngeal obstruction

Mechanism of Action Topical antiseptic/germicide effective against some vegetative gram-positive bacteria, particularly *Staphylococcus* sp, and some yeast; it is much less effective against gram-negative bacteria and is ineffective against acid-fast bacteria

Usual Dosage

Children and Adults: Topical: Apply 0.5% to 2% locally with cotton to lesion 2-3 times/day for 3 days, do not swallow and avoid contact with eyes

Adults: Intravaginal: Insert one tampon for 3-4 hours once or twice daily for 12 days

Patient Information Drug stains skin and clothing purple; do not apply to an ulcerative lesion; may result in "tattooing" of the skin; when used for the treatment of vaginal candidiasis, coitus should be avoided; insert vaginal product (Continued)

Gentian Violet *(Continued)*

high into vagina. Use condoms or refrain from sexual intercourse to avoid reinfection.

Dosage Forms

Solution, topical: 1% (30 mL); 2% (30 mL)

Tampons: 5 mg (12s)

Gentrasul® *see* Gentamicin *on page 747*

Geocillin® *see* Carbenicillin *on page 626*

Geopen® *see* Carbenicillin *on page 626*

German Measles Vaccine *see* Rubella Virus Vaccine, Live *on page 914*

G-myticin® Topical *see* Gentamicin *on page 747*

Granulocyte Colony Stimulating Factor *see* Filgrastim *on page 730*

Grepafloxacin (grep a FLOX a sin)

U.S. Brand Names Raxar®

Synonyms OPC-17116

Use Treatment of acute bacterial exacerbations of chronic bronchitis caused by *Haemophilus influenzae*, *Streptococcus pneumoniae*, or *Moraxella catarrhalis*; community-acquired pneumonia caused by *Mycoplasma pneumoniae* or the organisms previously mentioned; uncomplicated gonorrhea caused by *Neisseria gonorrhoeae*, and nongonococcal cervicitis and urethritis caused by *Chlamydia trachomatis*

In vitro studies suggest similar or lesser activity against *Enterobacteriaceae* and *P. aeruginosa* but greater activity against gram-positive cocci, especially *S. pneumoniae*, and some anaerobes and *Chlamydia* spp.

Drug of Choice or Alternative for

Disease/Syndrome(s)

Pneumonia, Community-Acquired *on page 45*

Pregnancy Risk Factor C

Contraindications Previous hypersensitivity to grepafloxacin and other quinolone derivatives; in patients with hepatic failure; given concomitantly with class I and III antiarrhythmics or bepridil due to the potential risk of cardiac arrhythmias (including torsade de pointes); patients with Q-T$_c$ prolongation and use with drugs which prolong Q-T$_c$ interval

Warnings/Precautions Use caution in patients with cerebral arteriosclerosis or epilepsy, and in patients with GI disorders or hepatic or renal dysfunction; there is no data to support safety and efficacy in children <18 years of age

Adverse Reactions Percentage unknown: Syncope, headache, dizziness, fatigue, nausea, emesis due to medicinal taste, hepatotoxicity (ie, elevated serum transaminases), abdominal pain, diarrhea, hypersensitivity

Drug Interactions CYP1A2 enzyme substrate

Antacids decrease grepafloxacin levels by 60%; grepafloxacin decreases theophylline clearance by 50%; may inhibit the metabolism of other drugs metabolized by cytochrome P-450 enzymes; may have additive effect of Q-T$_c$ prolongation when administered with other agents that may prolong Q-T$_c$ interval

Mechanism of Action Inhibits DNA-gyrase in susceptible organisms; inhibits relaxation of supercoiled DNA and promotes breakage of double-stranded DNA

Pharmacodynamics/Kinetics

Absorption: Peak plasma levels at 2-3 hours

Distribution: V$_d$: 5 L/kg; high concentrations have been achieved in bile, gynecologic tissue, hair, blister fluid, lung and other tissue

Metabolism: Liver, unknown activity of metabolites

Bioavailability: 70%

Half-life: 15.7 hours

Elimination: Eliminated unchanged in urine (10%); the rest in bile, feces, and metabolites

Usual Dosage Oral:

Bronchitis: 400-600 mg/day for 10 days

Community-acquired pneumonia: 600 mg/day for 10 days

Nongonococcal urethritis or cervicitis: 400 mg/day for 7 days

Uncomplicated gonorrhea: 400 mg as a single dose

Monitoring Parameters CBC, signs/symptoms of infection, liver/renal function tests

Patient Information Call physician immediately if hallucinations, confusion, seizures, rash, itching, facial swelling, or shortness of breath develops

Dosage Forms Tablet, as hydrochloride: 200 mg

Selected Readings

"Grepafloxacin - A New Fluoroquinolone," *Med Lett Drugs Ther*, 1998, 40(1019):17-8.

Kozawa O, Uematsu T, Matsuno H, et al, "Comparative Study of Pharmacokinetics of Two New Fluoroquinolones, Belofloxacin and Grepafloxacin, in Elderly Subjects," *Antimicrob Agents Chemother*, 1996, 40(12):2824-8.

Wagstaff AJ and Balfour JA, "Grepafloxacin," *Drugs*, 1997, 53(5):817-24.

Grifulvin® V *see Griseofulvin on this page*

Grisactin-500® *see Griseofulvin on this page*

Grisactin® Ultra *see Griseofulvin on this page*

Griseofulvin (gri see oh FUL vin)

U.S. Brand Names Fulvicin® P/G; Fulvicin-U/F®; Grifulvin® V; Grisactin-500®; Grisactin® Ultra; Gris-PEG®

Canadian Brand Names Grisovin®-FP

Synonyms Griseofulvin Microsize; Griseofulvin Ultramicrosize

Generic Available No

Use Treatment of susceptible tinea infections of the skin, hair, and nails

Drug of Choice or Alternative for

Organism(s)

Dermatophytes *on page 127*

Pregnancy Risk Factor C

Contraindications Hypersensitivity to griseofulvin or any component; severe liver disease, porphyria (interferes with porphyrin metabolism)

Warnings/Precautions Safe use in children <2 years of age has not been established; during long-term therapy, periodic assessment of hepatic, renal, and hematopoietic functions should be performed; may cause fetal harm when administered to pregnant women; avoid exposure to intense sunlight to prevent photosensitivity reactions; hypersensitivity cross reaction between penicillins and griseofulvin is possible

Adverse Reactions

>10%: Dermatologic: Rash, urticaria

1% to 10%:

Central nervous system: Headache, fatigue, dizziness, insomnia, mental confusion

Dermatologic: Photosensitivity

Gastrointestinal: Nausea, vomiting, epigastric distress, diarrhea

Miscellaneous: Oral thrush

<1%: Angioneurotic edema, menstrual toxicity, GI bleeding, leukopenia, hepatotoxicity, proteinuria, nephrosis

Overdosage/Toxicology

Symptoms of overdose include lethargy, vertigo, blurred vision, nausea, vomiting, diarrhea

Following GI decontamination, treatment is supportive

Drug Interactions

Decreased effect:

Barbiturates may decrease levels of griseofulvin

Decreased warfarin, cyclosporine, and salicylate activity with griseofulvin

Griseofulvin decreases oral contraceptive effectiveness

Increased toxicity: With alcohol → tachycardia and flushing

Mechanism of Action Inhibits fungal cell mitosis at metaphase; binds to human keratin making it resistant to fungal invasion

Pharmacodynamics/Kinetics

Absorption: Ultramicrosize griseofulvin absorption is almost complete; absorption of microsize griseofulvin is variable (25% to 70% of an oral dose); absorption is enhanced by ingestion of a fatty meal (GI absorption of ultramicrosize is ~1.5 times that of microsize)

Distribution: Crosses the placenta

Metabolism: Extensive in the liver

Half-life: 9-22 hours

(Continued)

Griseofulvin (Continued)

Elimination: <1% excreted unchanged in urine; also excreted in feces and perspiration

Usual Dosage Oral:

Children >2 years:

Microsize: 10-15 mg/kg/day in single or divided doses

Ultramicrosize: 5.5-7.3 mg/kg/day in single or divided doses

Adults:

Microsize: 500 mg/day in single or divided doses for tinea corporis, cruris, capitis

Ultramicrosize: 330-375 mg/day in single or divided doses

Doses of 750-1000 mg (microsize) and 660-750 mg (ultramicrosize) have been used for infections more difficult to eradicate such as tinea unguium and tinea pedis

Duration of therapy depends on the site of infection:

Tinea corporis: 2-4 weeks

Tinea capitis: 4-6 weeks or longer

Tinea pedis: 4-8 weeks

Tinea unguium: 4-6 months

Monitoring Parameters Periodic renal, hepatic, and hematopoietic function tests

Test Interactions False-positive urinary VMA levels

Patient Information Avoid exposure to sunlight, take with fatty meal; if patient gets headache, it usually goes away with continued therapy; may cause dizziness, drowsiness, and impair judgment; do not take if pregnant; if you become pregnant, discontinue immediately

Dosage Forms

Microsize:

Capsule: 125 mg, 250 mg

Suspension, oral (Grifulvin® V): 125 mg/5 mL with alcohol 0.2% (120 mL)

Tablet:

Fulvicin-U/F®, Grifulvin® V: 250 mg

Fulvicin-U/F®, Grifulvin® V, Grisactin-500®: 500 mg

Ultramicrosize:

Tablet:

Fulvicin® P/G: 165 mg, 330 mg

Fulvicin® P/G, Grisactin® Ultra, Gris-PEG®: 125 mg, 250 mg

Grisactin® Ultra: 330 mg

Selected Readings

Trepanier EF and Amsden GW, "Current Issues in Onchomycosis," *Ann Pharmacother*, 1998, 32(2):204-14.

Griseofulvin Microsize see Griseofulvin on previous page

Griseofulvin Ultramicrosize see Griseofulvin on previous page

Grisovin®-FP see Griseofulvin on previous page

Gris-PEG® see Griseofulvin on previous page

Growth Hormone see Human Growth Hormone on page 764

G-well® see Lindane on page 797

Gyne-Lotrimin® [OTC] see Clotrimazole on page 688

Gyne-Sulf® see Sulfabenzamide, Sulfacetamide, and Sulfathiazole on page 927

Haemophilus b Conjugate and Hepatitis B Vaccine

(he MOF i lus bee KON joo gate & hep a TYE tis bee vak SEEN)

Related Information

Haemophilus b Conjugate Vaccine on page 756

Hepatitis B Vaccine on page 761

U.S. Brand Names Comvax™

Synonyms *Haemophilus* b (meningococcal protein conjugate) Conjugate Vaccine; Hib

Use

Immunization against invasive disease caused by *H. influenzae* type b and against infection caused by all known subtypes of hepatitis B virus in infants 8 weeks to 15 months of age born of HB$_s$Ag-negative mothers

Infants born of HB$_s$Ag-positive mothers or mothers of unknown HB$_s$Ag status should receive hepatitis B immune globulin and hepatitis B vaccine (Recombinant) at birth and should complete the hepatitis B vaccination series given according to a particular schedule

Pregnancy Risk Factor C

Contraindications Hypersensitivity to any component of the vaccine

Warnings/Precautions If used in persons with malignancies or those receiving immunosuppressive therapy or who are otherwise immunocompromised, the expected immune response may not be obtained.

Patients who develop symptoms suggestive of hypersensitivity after an injection should not receive further injections of the vaccine.

The decision to administer or delay vaccination because of current or recent febrile illness depends on the severity of symptoms and the etiology of the disease. Immunization should be delayed during the course of an acute febrile illness.

Adverse Reactions When administered during the same visit that DTP, OPV, IPV, Varicella Virus Vaccine, and M-M-R II vaccines are given, the rates of systemic reactions do not differ from those observed only when any of the vaccines are administered **All serious adverse reactions must be reported to the U.S. Department of Health and Human Services (DHHS) Vaccine Adverse Event Reporting System (VAERS) 1-800-822-7967.**

>10%: Central nervous system: Acute febrile reactions
1% to 10%:
  Central nervous system: Fever (up to 102.2°F), irritability, lethargy
  Gastrointestinal: Anorexia, diarrhea
  Local: Irritation at injection site
<1%: Convulsions, fever (>102.2°F), vomiting, allergic or anaphylactic reactions (difficulty in breathing, hives, itching, swelling of eyes, face, unusual tiredness or weakness)

Stability Store at 2°C to 8°C/36°F to 48°F

Mechanism of Action Hib conjugate vaccines use covalent binding of capsular polysaccharide of *Haemophilus influenzae* type b to OMPC carrier to produce an antigen which is postulated to convert a T-independent antigen into a T-dependent antigen to result in enhanced antibody response and on immunologic memory. Recombinant hepatitis B vaccine is a noninfectious subunit viral vaccine. The vaccine is derived from hepatitis B surface antigen (HB$_s$Ag) produced through recombinant DNA techniques from yeast cells. The portion of the hepatitis B gene which codes for HB$_s$Ag is cloned into yeast which is then cultured to produce hepatitis B vaccine.

Pharmacodynamics/Kinetics
  The seroconversion following one dose of Hib vaccine for children 18 months or 24 months of age or older is 75% to 90% respectively
  Onset of Hib serum antibody responses: 1-2 weeks after vaccination
  Duration: Hib Immunity appears to last 1.5 years
  Duration of action: Following all 3 doses of hepatitis B vaccine, immunity will last ~5-7 years

Usual Dosage Infants (>8 weeks of age): I.M.: 0.5 mL at 2, 4, and 12-15 months of age (total of 3 doses)

If the recommended schedule cannot be followed, the interval between the first two doses should be at least 2 months and the interval between the second and third dose should be as close as possible to 8-11 months.

Modified Schedule: Children who receive one dose of hepatitis B vaccine at or shortly after birth may receive Comvax™ on a schedule of 2, 4, and 12-15 months of age

Administration Administer 0.5 mL I.M. into anterolateral thigh [data suggests that injections given in the buttocks frequently are given into fatty tissue instead of into muscle to result in lower seroconversion rates]; **do not administer intravenously, intradermally, or subcutaneously**

Patient Information May use acetaminophen for postdose fever

Nursing Implications Defer immunization if infection or febrile illness present

Additional Information
  Inactivated bacterial vaccine and inactivated viral vaccine
  (Continued)

Haemophilus b Conjugate and Hepatitis B Vaccine
(Continued)

Federal law requires that the date of administration, the vaccine manufacturer, lot number of vaccine and the administering person's name, title and address be entered into the patient's permanent medical record

Dosage Forms Injection: 7.5 mcg *Haemophilus* b PRP and 5 mcg HB$_s$Ag/0.5 mL

Haemophilus b Conjugate Vaccine
(hem OF fi lus bee KON joo gate vak SEEN)

Related Information

Immunization Guidelines *on page 1041*

U.S. Brand Names ActHIB®; HibTITER®; OmniHIB™; PedvaxHIB™; ProHIBiT®; TriHIBIT™

Synonyms Diphtheria CRM$_{197}$ Protein Conjugate; Diphtheria Toxoid Conjugate; *Haemophilus* b Oligosaccharide Conjugate Vaccine; *Haemophilus* b Polysaccharide Vaccine; HbCV; Hib Polysaccharide Conjugate; PRP-D

Generic Available No

Use Routine immunization of children 2 months to 5 years of age against invasive disease caused by *H. influenzae*

Unimmunized children ≥5 years of age with a chronic illness known to be associated with increased risk of *Haemophilus influenzae* type b disease, specifically, persons with anatomic or functional asplenia or sickle cell anemia or those who have undergone splenectomy, should receive Hib vaccine.

Haemophilus b conjugate vaccines are not indicated for prevention of bronchitis or other infections due to *H. influenzae* in adults; adults with specific dysfunction or certain complement deficiencies who are at especially high risk of *H. influenzae* type b infection (HIV-infected adults); patients with Hodgkin's disease (vaccinated at least 2 weeks before the initiation of chemotherapy or 3 months after the end of chemotherapy)

Pregnancy Risk Factor C

Contraindications Children with any febrile illness or active infection, known hypersensitivity to *Haemophilus* b polysaccharide vaccine (thimerosal), children who are immunosuppressed or receiving immunosuppressive therapy

Warnings/Precautions Have epinephrine 1:1000 available; children in whom DTP or DT vaccination is deferred: The carrier proteins used in HbOC (but not PRP-OMP) are chemically and immunologically related to toxoids contained in DTP vaccine. Earlier or simultaneous vaccination with diphtheria or tetanus toxoids may be required to elicit an optimal anti-PRP antibody response to HbOC. In contrast, the immunogenicity of PRP-OMP is not affected by vaccination with DTP. In infants in whom DTP or DT vaccination is deferred, PRP-OMP may be advantageous for *Haemophilus influenzae* type b vaccination.

Children with immunologic impairment: Children with chronic illness associated with increased risk of *Haemophilus influenzae* type b disease may have impaired anti-PRP antibody responses to conjugate vaccination. Examples include those with HIV infection, immunoglobulin deficiency, anatomic or functional asplenia, and sickle cell disease, as well as recipients of bone marrow transplants and recipients of chemotherapy for malignancy. Some children with immunologic impairment may benefit from more doses of conjugate vaccine than normally indicated.

Adverse Reactions When administered during the same visit that DTP vaccine is given, the rates of systemic reactions do not differ from those observed only when DTP vaccine is administered. **All serious adverse reactions must be reported to the U.S. Department of Health and Human Services (DHHS) Vaccine Adverse Event Reporting System (VAERS) 1-800-822-7967.**

25%:
    Cardiovascular: Edema
    Dermatologic: Local erythema
    Local: Increased risk of *Haemophilus* b infections in the week after vaccination
    Miscellaneous: Warmth
>10%: Central nervous system: Acute febrile reactions
1% to 10%:
    Central nervous system: Fever (up to 102.2°F), irritability, lethargy
    Gastrointestinal: Anorexia, diarrhea

Local: Irritation at injection site

<1%: Edema of the eyes/face, convulsions, fever (>102.2°F), unusual fatigue, urticaria, itching, vomiting, weakness, dyspnea

Drug Interactions Decreased effect with immunosuppressive agents, immunoglobulins within 1 month may decrease antibody production

Stability Keep in refrigerator, may be frozen (not diluent) without affecting potency; reconstituted Hib-Imune® remains stable for only 8 hours, whereas HibVAX® remain stable for 30 days when refrigerated

Mechanism of Action Stimulates production of anticapsular antibodies and provides active immunity to *Haemophilus influenzae*

Pharmacodynamics/Kinetics

The seroconversion following one dose of Hib vaccine for children 18 months or 24 months of age or older is 75% to 90% respectively

Onset of serum antibody responses: 1-2 weeks after vaccination

Duration: Immunity appears to last 1.5 years

Usual Dosage Children: I.M.: 0.5 mL as a single dose should be administered according to one of the following "brand-specific" schedules; do not inject I.V.

Vaccination Schedule for *Haemophilus* b Conjugate Vaccines

Age at 1st Dose (mo)	HibTITER®		PedvaxHIB®		ProHIBiT®	
	Primary Series	Booster	Primary Series	Booster	Primary Series	Booster
2-6*	3 doses, 2 months apart	15 mo†	2 doses, 2 months apart	12 mo†		
7-11	2 doses, 2 months apart	15 mo†	2 doses, 2 months apart	15 mo†		
12-14	1 dose	15 mo†	1 dose	15 mo†		
15-60	1 dose	—	1 dose	—	1 dose	—

*It is not currently recommended that the various *Haemophilus* b conjugate vaccines be interchanged (ie, the same brand should be used throughout the entire vaccination series). If the health care provider does not know which vaccine was previously used, it is prudent that an infant, 2-6 months of age, be given a primary series of three doses.

†At least 2 months after previous dose.

Haemophilus influenzae Type b Conjugate Vaccines

Manufacturer	Abbreviation	Trade Name	Carrier Protein
Connaught Laboratories	PRP-D*	ProHiBit®	Diphtheria toxoid
Lederle Laboratories	HbOC	HibTITER®	CRM$_{197}$ (a nontoxic mutant diphtheria toxin)
Merck and Company	PRP-OMP	PedvaxHIB	OMP (an outer membrane protein complex of *Neisseria meningitidis*)
Pasteur Merieux Vaccines (Distributed by Connaught Laboratories, Inc, and SmithKline Beecham)	PRP-T**	ActHIB OmniHIB	Tetanus toxoid

* PRP-D is recommended by the American Academy of Pediatrics for only infants ≥12 months of age. HbOC, PRP-OMP, and PRP-T are recommended for infants beginning at approximately 2 months of age.

** PRP-T may be reconstituted with DTP, manufactured by Connaught Laboratories. Other licensed formulations of DTP have not been approved by the FDA for reconstitution and may not be used for this purpose.

Test Interactions May interfere with interpretation of antigen detection tests

Patient Information May use acetaminophen for postdose fever

(Continued)

Haemophilus b Conjugate Vaccine *(Continued)*

Nursing Implications Defer immunization if infection or febrile illness present. Do not administer I.V.

Additional Information Federal law requires that the date of administration, the vaccine manufacturer, lot number of vaccine, and the administering person's name, title, and address be entered into the patient's permanent medical record

Dosage Forms Injection:

ActHIB®, HibTITER®, OmniHIB™: Capsular oligosaccharide 10 mcg and diphtheria CRM$_{197}$ protein ~25 mcg per 0.5 mL (0.5 mL, 2.5 mL, 5 mL)

PedvaxHIB™: Purified capsular polysaccharide 15 mcg and *Neisseria meningitidis* OMPC 250 mcg per dose (0.5 mL)

ProHIBiT®: Purified capsular polysaccharide 25 mcg and conjugated diphtheria toxoid protein 18 mcg per dose (0.5 mL, 2.5 mL, 5 mL)

TriHIBit™ vaccine [Tripedia® vaccine used to reconstitute ActHIB®]: 0.5 mL

Haemophilus b (meningococcal protein conjugate) Conjugate Vaccine *see Haemophilus* b Conjugate and Hepatitis B Vaccine *on page 754*

Haemophilus b Oligosaccharide Conjugate Vaccine *see Haemophilus* b Conjugate Vaccine *on page 756*

Haemophilus b Polysaccharide Vaccine *see Haemophilus* b Conjugate Vaccine *on page 756*

Halfan® *see* Halofantrine *on this page*

Halofantrine (ha loe FAN trin)

U.S. Brand Names Halfan®

Use Treatment of mild to moderate acute malaria caused by susceptible strains of *Plasmodium falciparum* and *Plasmodium vivax*

Drug of Choice or Alternative for Organism(s)

Plasmodium Species *on page 227*

Pregnancy Risk Factor X

Contraindications Pregnancy

Warnings/Precautions Monitor closely for decreased hematocrit and hemoglobin, patients with chronic liver disease

Adverse Reactions

>10%: Dermatologic: Pruritus

1% to 10%:

Cardiovascular: Edema

Central nervous system: Malaise, headache

Gastrointestinal: Nausea, vomiting

Hematologic: Leukocytosis

Hepatic: Elevated LFTs

Local: Tenderness

Neuromuscular & skeletal: Myalgia

Respiratory: Cough

Miscellaneous: Lymphadenopathy

<1%: Sterile abscesses, anaphylactic shock, tachycardia, urticaria, asthma, hypotension, hypoglycemia

Mechanism of Action Similar to mefloquine; destruction of asexual blood forms, possible inhibition of proton pump

Pharmacodynamics/Kinetics

Mean time to parasite clearance: 40-84 hours

Absorption: Erratic and variable; serum levels are proportional to dose up to 1000 mg; doses greater than this should be divided; may be increased 60% with high fat meals

Distribution: V_d: 570 L/kg; widely distributed in most tissues

Metabolism: To active metabolite in liver

Half-life: 23 hours; metabolite: 82 hours; may be increased in active disease

Elimination: Essentially unchanged in urine

Usual Dosage Oral:

Children <40 kg: 8 mg/kg every 6 hours for 3 doses; repeat in 1 week

Adults: 500 mg every 6 hours for 3 doses; repeat in 1 week

Monitoring Parameters Closely for jaundice, other signs of hepatotoxicity; CBC, LFTs, parasite counts

Test Interactions Increased serum transaminases, bilirubin

Patient Information Take with food, avoid high fat meals; notify physician of persistent nausea, vomiting, abdominal pain, light stools, dark urine

Additional Information Not available in the United States

Dosage Forms
Suspension: 100 mg/5 mL
Tablet: 250 mg

Selected Readings
White NJ, "The Treatment of Malaria," *N Engl J Med*, 1996, 335(11):800-6.

Haloprogin (ha loe PROE jin)

U.S. Brand Names Halotex®

Generic Available No

Use Topical treatment of tinea pedis (athlete's foot), tinea cruris (jock itch), tinea corporis (ringworm), tinea manuum caused by *Trichophyton rubrum*, *Trichophyton tonsurans*, *Trichophyton mentagrophytes*, *Microsporum canis*, or *Epidermophyton floccosum*. Topical treatment of *Malassezia furfur*.

Pregnancy Risk Factor B

Contraindications Hypersensitivity to haloprogin or any component

Warnings/Precautions Safety and efficacy have not been established in children

Adverse Reactions <1%: Pruritus, folliculitis, vesicle formation, erythema, irritation, burning sensation

Mechanism of Action Interferes with fungal DNA replication to inhibit yeast cell respiration and disrupt its cell membrane

Pharmacodynamics/Kinetics
Absorption: Poorly through the skin (~11%)
Metabolism: To trichlorophenol
Elimination: In urine, 75% as unchanged drug

Usual Dosage Topical: Children and Adults: Apply liberally twice daily for 2-3 weeks; intertriginous areas may require up to 4 weeks of treatment

Patient Information Avoid contact with eyes; for external use only; improvement should occur within 4 weeks; discontinue use if sensitization or irritation occur

Dosage Forms
Cream: 1% (15 g, 30 g)
Solution, topical: 1% with alcohol 75% (10 mL, 30 mL)

Halotestin® see Fluoxymesterone on page 736

Halotex® see Haloprogin on this page

Havrix® see Hepatitis A Vaccine on this page

HbCV see Haemophilus b Conjugate Vaccine on page 756

HBIG see Hepatitis B Immune Globulin on next page

H-BIG® see Hepatitis B Immune Globulin on next page

HDCV see Rabies Virus Vaccine on page 893

Head & Shoulders® Intensive Treatment [OTC] see Selenium Sulfide on page 917

Helidac™ see Bismuth Subsalicylate, Metronidazole, and Tetracycline on page 623

Hepatitis A Immunization see page 1055

Hepatitis A Vaccine (hep a TYE tis aye vak SEEN)

Related Information
Hepatitis A Immunization on page 1055

U.S. Brand Names Havrix®; VAQTA®

Use For populations desiring protection against hepatitis A or for populations at high risk of exposure to hepatitis A virus (travelers to developing countries, household and sexual contacts of persons infected with hepatitis A), child day care employees, patients with chronic liver disease, illicit drug users, male homosexuals, institutional workers (eg, institutions for the mentally and physically handicapped persons, prisons, etc), and healthcare workers who may be exposed to hepatitis A virus (eg, laboratory employees); protection lasts for approximately 15 years

Drug of Choice or Alternative for Organism(s)
Hepatitis A Virus on page 161

Pregnancy Risk Factor C

(Continued)

Hepatitis A Vaccine *(Continued)*

Contraindications Hypersensitivity to any component of hepatitis A vaccine

Warnings/Precautions Use caution in patients with serious active infection, cardiovascular disease, or pulmonary disorders; treatment for anaphylactic reactions should be immediately available

Adverse Reactions All serious adverse reactions must be reported to the U.S. Department of Health and Human Services (DHHS) Vaccine Adverse Event Reporting System (VAERS) 1-800-822-7967.

Percentage unknown: Fatigue, fever (rare), transient liver function test abnormalities

>10%:

Central nervous system: Headache

Local: Pain, tenderness, and warmth

1% to 10%:

Gastrointestinal: Abdominal pain (1.2%)

Local: Cutaneous reactions at the injection site (soreness, edema, and redness)

Respiratory: Pharyngitis (1.2%)

Drug Interactions No interference of immunogenicity was reported when mixed with hepatitis B vaccine

Mechanism of Action As an inactivated virus vaccine, hepatitis A vaccine offers active immunization against hepatitis A virus infection at an effective immune response rate in up to 99% of subjects

Pharmacodynamics/Kinetics

Onset of action (protection): 3 weeks after a single dose

Duration: Neutralizing antibodies have persisted for >3 years; unconfirmed evidence indicates that antibody levels may persist for 5-10 years

Usual Dosage I.M.:

Havrix®:

Children 2-18 years: 720 ELISA units (administered as 2 injections of 360 ELISA units [0.5 mL]) 15-30 days prior to travel with a booster 6-12 months following primary immunization; the deltoid muscle should be used for I.M. injection

Adults: 1440 ELISA units(1 mL) 15-30 days prior to travel with a booster 6-12 months following primary immunization; injection should be in the deltoid

VAQTA®:

Children 2-17 years: 25 units (0.5 mL) with 25 units (0.5 mL) booster to be given 6-18 months after primary immunization

Adults: 50 units (1 mL) with 50 units (1 mL) booster to be given 6 months after primary immunization

Administration Inject I.M. into the deltoid muscle, if possible

Monitoring Parameters Liver function tests

Reference Range Seroconversion for Havrix®: Antibody >20 milli-international units/mL

Additional Information Some investigators suggest simultaneous or sequential administration of inactivated hepatitis A vaccine and immune globulin for postexposure protection, especially for travelers requiring rapid immunization, although a slight decrease in vaccine immunogenicity may be observed with this technique

Dosage Forms

Injection: 360 ELISA units/0.5 mL (0.5 mL); 1440 ELISA units/mL (1 mL)

Injection, pediatric: 720 ELISA units/0.5 mL (0.5 mL)

Injection (VAQTA®): 50 units/mL (1 mL)

Selected Readings

Bancroft WH, "Hepatitis A Vaccine," *N Engl J Med*, 1992, 327(7):453-7.

Koff RS, "Hepatitis A," *Lancet*, 1998, 351(9116):1643-9.

Lemon SM, "Inactivated Hepatitis A Vaccines," *JAMA*, 1994, 271(17):1363-4.

Niu MT, Salive M, Krueger C, et al, "Two-Year Review of Hepatitis A Vaccine Safety: Data From the Vaccine Adverse Event Reporting System (VAERS)," *Clin Infect Dis*, 1998, 26(6):1475-6.

Hepatitis B Immune Globulin

(hep a TYE tis bee i MYUN GLOB yoo lin)

Related Information

Postexposure Prophylaxis for Hepatitis B *on page 1054*

U.S. Brand Names H-BIG®; Hep-B Gammagee®; HyperHep®

Synonyms HBIG

Generic Available No

Use Provide prophylactic passive immunity to hepatitis B infection to those individuals exposed; newborns of mothers known to be hepatitis B surface antigen positive; hepatitis B immune globulin is not indicated for treatment of active hepatitis B infections and is ineffective in the treatment of chronic active hepatitis B infection

Drug of Choice or Alternative for

Organism(s)

Hepatitis B Virus *on page 162*

Pregnancy Risk Factor C

Contraindications Hypersensitivity to hepatitis B immune globulin or any component; allergies to gamma globulin or anti-immunoglobulin antibodies; allergies to thimerosal; IgA deficiency; I.M. injections in patients with thrombocytopenia or coagulation disorders

Adverse Reactions

1% to 10%:

Central nervous system: Dizziness, malaise

Dermatologic: Urticaria, angioedema, rash, erythema

Local: Pain and tenderness at injection site

Neuromuscular & skeletal: Arthralgia

<1%: Anaphylaxis

Drug Interactions Interferes with immune response of live virus vaccines

Stability Refrigerate at 2°C to 8°C (36°F to 46°F); do not freeze

Mechanism of Action Hepatitis B immune globulin (HBIG) is a nonpyrogenic sterile solution containing 10% to 18% protein of which at least 80% is monomeric immunoglobulin G (IgG). HBIG differs from immune globulin in the amount of anti-HBs. Immune globulin is prepared from plasma that is not preselected for anti-HBs content. HBIG is prepared from plasma preselected for high titer anti-HBs. In the U.S., HBIG has an anti-HBs high titer >1:100,000 by IRA. There is no evidence that the causative agent of AIDS is transmitted by HBIG.

Pharmacodynamics/Kinetics

Absorption: Slow

Time to peak serum concentration: 1-6 days

Usual Dosage I.M.:

Newborns: Hepatitis B: 0.5 mL as soon after birth as possible (within 12 hours); may repeat at 3 months in order for a higher rate of prevention of the carrier state to be achieved; at this time an active vaccination program with the vaccine may begin

Adults: Postexposure prophylaxis: 0.06 mL/kg as soon as possible after exposure (ie, within 24 hours of needlestick, ocular, or mucosal exposure or within 14 days of sexual exposure); usual dose: 3-5 mL; repeat at 28-30 days after exposure

Note: HBIG may be administered at the same time (but at a different site) or up to 1 month preceding hepatitis B vaccination without impairing the active immune response

Administration I.M. injection only in gluteal or deltoid region; to prevent injury from injection, care should be taken when giving to patients with thrombocytopenia or bleeding disorders

Additional Information Has been administered intravenously in hepatitis B-positive liver transplant patients

Dosage Forms Injection:

H-BIG®: 4 mL, 5 mL

HyperHep®: 0.5 mL, 1 mL, 5 mL

Hepatitis B Inactivated Virus Vaccine (plasma derived) *see* Hepatitis B Vaccine *on this page*

Hepatitis B Inactivated Virus Vaccine (recombinant DNA) *see* Hepatitis B Vaccine *on this page*

Hepatitis B Vaccine (hep a TYE tis bee vak SEEN)

Related Information

Immunization Guidelines *on page 1041*

U.S. Brand Names Engerix-B®; Recombivax HB®

Synonyms Hepatitis B Inactivated Virus Vaccine (plasma derived); Hepatitis B Inactivated Virus Vaccine (recombinant DNA)

(Continued)

Hepatitis B Vaccine *(Continued)*

Generic Available No

Use Immunization against infection caused by all known subtypes of hepatitis B virus, in individuals considered at high risk of potential exposure to hepatitis B virus or HBsAg-positive materials; see chart.

Pre-exposure Prophylaxis for Hepatitis B

Health care workers*
Special patient groups
Hemodialysis patients†
Recipients of certain blood products‡
Lifestyle factors
Homosexual and bisexual men
Intravenous drug abusers
Heterosexually active persons with multiple sexual partners or recently
acquired sexually transmitted diseases
Environmental factors
Household and sexual contacts of HBV carriers
Prison inmates
Clients and staff of institutions for the mentally retarded
Residents, immigrants and refugees from areas with endemic HBV infection
International travelers at increased risk of acquiring HBV infection

*The risk of hepatitis B virus (HBV) infection for health care workers varies both between hospitals and within hospitals. Hepatitis B vaccination is recommended for all health care workers with blood exposure.

†Hemodialysis patients often respond poorly to hepatitis B vaccination. Patients with chronic renal disease should be vaccinated as early as possible, ideally before they require hemodialysis. In addition, their anti-HBs levels should be monitored at 6- to 12-month intervals to assess the need for revaccination.

‡Patients with hemophilia should be immunized subcutaneously, not intramuscularly.

Pregnancy Risk Factor C

Contraindications Hypersensitivity to yeast, hypersensitivity to hepatitis B vaccine or any component

Adverse Reactions All serious adverse reactions must be reported to the U.S. Department of Health and Human Services (DHHS) Vaccine Adverse Event Reporting System (VAERS) 1-800-822-7967.

>10%:
  Central nervous system: Fever, malaise, fatigue (14%), headache
  Local: Mild local tenderness (22%), local inflammatory reaction
1% to 10%:
  Gastrointestinal: Nausea, vomiting
  Respiratory: Pharyngitis
<1%: Tachycardia, hypotension, sensation of warmth, flushing, lightheadedness, chills, somnolence, insomnia, irritability, agitation, pruritus, rash, erythema, urticaria, GI disturbances, constipation, abdominal cramps, dyspepsia, anorexia, dysuria, arthralgia, myalgia, stiffness in back/neck/arm or shoulder, earache, rhinitis, cough, epistaxis, diaphoresis

Drug Interactions Decreased effect: Immunosuppressive agents

Stability Refrigerate, do not freeze

Mechanism of Action Recombinant hepatitis B vaccine is a noninfectious subunit viral vaccine. The vaccine is derived from hepatitis B surface antigen (HBsAg) produced through recombinant DNA techniques from yeast cells. The portion of the hepatitis B gene which codes for HBsAg is cloned into yeast which is then cultured to produce hepatitis B vaccine.

Pharmacodynamics/Kinetics Duration of action: Following all 3 doses of hepatitis B vaccine, immunity will last approximately 5-7 years

Usual Dosage See tables on next page.

Immunization Regimen of Three I.M. Hepatitis B Vaccine Doses

Age	Initial		1 mo		6 mo	
	Recom-bivax HB® (mL)	Engerix-B® (mL)	Recom-bivax HB® (mL)	Engerix-B® (mL)	Recom-bivax HB® (mL)	Engerix-B® (mL)
Birth* to 10 y	0.25	0.5	0.25	0.5	0.25	0.5
11-19 y	0.5	1	0.5	1	0.5	1
≥20 y	1	1	1	1	1	1
Dialysis or immunocom-promised patients		2†		2†		2†

*Infants born of HBsAg-negative mothers.
†Two 1 mL doses given at different sites.

Recommended Dosage for Infants Born to HBsAg-Positive Mothers

Treatment	Birth	Within 7 d	1 mo	6 mo
Engerix-B® (pediatric dose 10 mcg/0.5 mL)	*	0.5 mL*	0.5 mL	0.5 mL
Recombivax HB® (pediatric dose 5 mcg/0.5 mL)	*	0.5 mL*	0.5 mL	0.5 mL
Hepatitis B immune globulin	0.5 mL	—	—	—

*The first dose may be given at birth at the same time as HBIG, but give in the opposite anterolateral thigh. This may better ensure vaccine absorption.

Administration I.M. injection only; in adults, the deltoid muscle is the preferred site; the anterolateral thigh is the recommended site in infants and young children

Patient Information Must complete full course of injections for adequate immunization

Nursing Implications Rare chance of anaphylactoid reaction; have epinephrine available

Additional Information Inactivated virus vaccine; federal law requires that the date of administration, the vaccine manufacturer, lot number of vaccine, and the administering person's name, title and address be entered into the patient's permanent medical record

Dosage Forms Injection:
Recombinant DNA (Engerix-B®)
Pediatric formulation: Hepatitis B surface antigen 10 mcg/0.5 mL (0.5 mL)
Adult formulation: Hepatitis B surface antigen 20 mcg/mL (1 mL)
Recombinant DNA (Recombivax HB®):
Pediatric formulation: Hepatitis B surface antigen 2.5 mg/0.5 mL (0.5 mL/3 mL)
Adolescent/high-risk infant formulation: Hepatitis B surface antigen 5 mcg/0.5 mL (0.5 mL)
Adult formulation: Hepatitis B surface antigen 10 mcg/mL (1 mL, 3 mL)
Dialysis formulation, recombinant DNA: Hepatitis B surface antigen 40 mcg/mL (1 mL)

Hep-B Gammagee® see Hepatitis B Immune Globulin on page 760

Hexachlorocyclohexane see Lindane on page 797

Hexamethylenetetramine see Methenamine on page 814

Hexit® see Lindane on page 797

Hib see Haemophilus b Conjugate and Hepatitis B Vaccine on page 754

Hibiclens® Topical [OTC] see Chlorhexidine Gluconate on page 670

Hibistat® Topical [OTC] see Chlorhexidine Gluconate on page 670

Hib Polysaccharide Conjugate see Haemophilus b Conjugate Vaccine on page 756

HibTITER® see Haemophilus b Conjugate Vaccine on page 756

Hip-Rex™ see Methenamine on page 814

Hiprex® see Methenamine on page 814

Histerone® Injection see Testosterone on page 939

Hivid® see Zalcitabine on page 974

HIV Therapeutic Information see page 1008

Human Diploid Cell Cultures Rabies Vaccine *see* Rabies Virus Vaccine *on page 893*

Human Diploid Cell Cultures Rabies Vaccine (Intradermal use) *see* Rabies Virus Vaccine *on page 893*

Human Growth Hormone (HYU man grothe HOR mone)

U.S. Brand Names Serostim® Injection

Synonyms Growth Hormone; Somatrem; Somatropin

Generic Available No

Use Serostim® is indicated for the treatment of AIDS wasting or cachexia. Continued use of this agent should be re-evaluated if patients do not begin to respond within 2 weeks. There are at least 7 other human growth hormone products used for long-term treatment of growth failure from lack of adequate endogenous growth hormone secretion or treatment of children who have growth failure associated with chronic renal insufficiency up until the time of renal transplantation.

Pregnancy Risk Factor B

Contraindications Closed epiphyses, known hypersensitivity to drug; progression of any underlying intracranial lesion or actively growing intracranial tumor

Warnings/Precautions Use with caution in patients with diabetes; when administering to newborns, reconstitute with sterile water for injection

Adverse Reactions Many Serostim® adverse reactions in HIV patients had similar rates as placebo

1% to 10%: Endocrine & metabolic: Hypothyroidism

<1%: Rash, itching, hypoglycemia, pain at injection site, increased skin turgor, musculoskeletal discomfort, carpal tunnel, pancreatitis

Overdosage/Toxicology Symptoms include hypoglycemia, hyperglycemia, acromegaly

Stability Serostim®: Store at room temperature, once reconstituted, solutions should be refrigerated and used within 24 hours

Mechanism of Action Serostim® is an anabolic and anticatabolic agent which interacts with myocytes, hepatocytes, lymphocytes, and hematopoietic cell receptors. In patients with AIDS wasting, Serostim® increases lean body mass, decreases body fat with subsequent weight gain.

Pharmacodynamics/Kinetics

Absorption: I.M.: Well absorbed

Distribution: V_d: 12 L

Metabolism: Cleared in kidney

Bioavailability: 70% to 90% after S.C. administration

Half-life: 4.3 hours

Usual Dosage Not indicated for children

S.C.: Administer daily at bedtime; see table for dosing recommendations

Weight Range	Dose*
>55 kg	6 mg/day
45-55 kg	5 mg/day
35-45 kg	4 mg/day

*Based on an approximate daily dosage of 0.1 mg/kg.

Administration Do not shake; administer S.C. or I.M.; refer to product labeling; when administering to newborns, reconstitute with sterile water for injection

Monitoring Parameters Growth curve, periodic thyroid function tests, bone age (annually), periodical urine testing for glucose, somatomedin C levels

Patient Information Rotate injection sites

Nursing Implications Watch for glucose intolerance

Dosage Forms Injection: Serostim®: 4 mg ~12 units; 5 mg ~15 units (5 mL); 6 mg ~18 units (5 mL); each vial is reconstituted with 1 mL sterile water for injection

Selected Readings

Howrie DL, "Growth Hormone for the Treatment of Growth Failure in Children," *Clin Pharm*, 1987, 6(4):283-91.

Humatin® *see* Paromomycin *on page 856*

Hybolin™ Decanoate *see* Nandrolone *on page 829*

Hybolin™ Improved *see* Nandrolone *on page 829*

Hydroxychloroquine (hye droks ee KLOR oh kwin)

U.S. Brand Names Plaquenil®

Synonyms Hydroxychloroquine Sulfate

Generic Available No

Use Suppresses and treats acute attacks of malaria; treatment of systemic lupus erythematosus and rheumatoid arthritis

Pregnancy Risk Factor C

Contraindications Retinal or visual field changes attributable to 4-aminoquinolines; hypersensitivity to hydroxychloroquine, 4-aminoquinoline derivatives, or any component

Warnings/Precautions Use with caution in patients with hepatic disease, G-6-PD deficiency, psoriasis, and porphyria; long-term use in children is not recommended; perform baseline and periodic (6 months) ophthalmologic examinations; test periodically for muscle weakness

Adverse Reactions

>10%:

Central nervous system: Headache

Dermatologic: Itching

Gastrointestinal: Diarrhea, loss of appetite, nausea, stomach cramps, vomiting

Ocular: Ciliary muscle dysfunction

1% to 10%:

Central nervous system: Dizziness, lightheadedness, nervousness, restlessness

Dermatologic: Bleaching of hair, rash, discoloration of skin (black-blue)

Ocular: Ocular toxicity, keratopathy, retinopathy

<1%: Emotional changes, seizures, agranulocytosis, aplastic anemia, neutropenia, thrombocytopenia, neuromyopathy, ototoxicity

Overdosage/Toxicology

Symptoms of overdose include headache, drowsiness, visual changes, cardiovascular collapse, and seizures followed by respiratory and cardiac arrest

Treatment is symptomatic; activated charcoal will bind the drug following GI decontamination; urinary alkalinization will enhance renal elimination

Drug Interactions

Chloroquine and other 4-aminoquinolones may be decreased due to GI binding with kaolin or magnesium trisilicate

Increased effect: Cimetidine increases levels of chloroquine and probably other 4-aminoquinolones

Mechanism of Action Interferes with digestive vacuole function within sensitive malarial parasites by increasing the pH and interfering with lysosomal degradation of hemoglobin; inhibits locomotion of neutrophils and chemotaxis of eosinophils; impairs complement-dependent antigen-antibody reactions

Pharmacodynamics/Kinetics

Absorption: Oral: Complete

Protein binding: 55%

Metabolism: In the liver

Half-life: 32-50 days

Elimination: Metabolites and unchanged drug slowly excreted in urine, may be enhanced by urinary acidification

Usual Dosage Note: Hydroxychloroquine sulfate 200 mg is equivalent to 155 mg hydroxychloroquine base and 250 mg chloroquine phosphate. Oral:

Children:

Chemoprophylaxis of malaria: 5 mg/kg (base) once weekly; should not exceed the recommended adult dose; begin 2 weeks before exposure; continue for 4-6 weeks after leaving endemic area; if suppressive therapy is not begun prior to the exposure, double the initial dose and give in 2 doses, 6 hours apart

Acute attack: 10 mg/kg (base) initial dose; followed by 5 mg/kg at 6, 24, and 48 hours

JRA or SLE: 3-5 mg/kg/day divided 1-2 times/day; avoid exceeding 7 mg/kg/day

Adults:

Chemoprophylaxis of malaria: 310 mg base/week on same day each week; begin 2 weeks before exposure; continue for 4-6 weeks after leaving

(Continued)

Hydroxychloroquine *(Continued)*

endemic area; if suppressive therapy is not begun prior to the exposure, double the initial dose and give in 2 doses, 6 hours apart

Acute attack: 620 mg first dose day 1; 310 mg in 6 hours day 1; 310 mg in 1 dose day 2; and 310 mg in 1 dose on day 3

Rheumatoid arthritis: 310-465 mg/day to start taken with food or milk; increase dose until optimum response level is reached; usually after 4-12 weeks dose should be reduced by $1/2$ and a maintenance dose of 155-310 mg/day given

Lupus erythematosus: 310 mg every day or twice daily for several weeks depending on response; 155-310 mg/day for prolonged maintenance therapy

Administration Administer with food or milk

Monitoring Parameters Ophthalmologic exam, CBC

Patient Information Take with food or milk; complete full course of therapy; wear sunglasses in bright sunlight; notify physician if blurring or other vision changes, ringing in the ears, or hearing loss occurs

Nursing Implications Periodic blood counts and eye examinations are recommended when patient is on chronic therapy

Dosage Forms Tablet, as sulfate: 200 mg [base 155 mg]

Extemporaneous Preparations A 25 mg/mL hydroxychloroquine sulfate suspension is made by removing the coating off of fifteen 200 mg hydroxychloroquine sulfate tablets with a towel moistened with alcohol; tablets are ground to a fine powder and levigated to a paste with 15 mL of Ora-Plus® suspending agent; add an additional 45 mL of suspending agent and levigate until a uniform mixture is obtained; qs ad to 120 mL with sterile water for irrigation; a 30 day expiration date is recommended, although stability testing has not been performed

Pesko LJ, "Compounding: Hydroxychloroquine," *Am Druggist*, 1993, 207:57.

Selected Readings
"Drugs for Parasitic Infections," *Med Lett Drugs Ther*, 1998, 40(1017):1-12.
Panisko DM and Keystone JS, "Treatment of Malaria - 1990," *Drugs*, 1990, 39(2):160-89.
White NJ, "The Treatment of Malaria," *N Engl J Med*, 1996, 335(11):800-6.

Hydroxychloroquine Sulfate *see* Hydroxychloroquine *on previous page*

Hyperab® *see* Rabies Immune Globulin (Human) *on page 892*

HyperHep® *see* Hepatitis B Immune Globulin *on page 760*

Hyper-Tet® *see* Tetanus Immune Globulin (Human) *on page 941*

HypRho®-D *see* Rh₀(D) Immune Globulin *on page 896*

HypRho®-D Mini-Dose *see* Rh₀(D) Immune Globulin *on page 896*

IFLrA *see* Interferon Alfa-2a *on page 776*

IFN *see* Interferon Alfa-2a *on page 776*

IFN-alpha 2 *see* Interferon Alfa-2b *on page 778*

IG *see* Immune Globulin, Intramuscular *on page 770*

I-Gent® *see* Gentamicin *on page 747*

IGIM *see* Immune Globulin, Intramuscular *on page 770*

Ilosone® *see* Erythromycin *on page 722*

Imipemide *see* Imipenem and Cilastatin *on this page*

Imipenem and Cilastatin *(i mi PEN em & sye la STAT in)*

Related Information
Antimicrobial Activity Against Selected Organisms *on page 983*

U.S. Brand Names Primaxin®

Synonyms Imipemide

Generic Available No

Use Treatment of respiratory tract, urinary tract, intra-abdominal, gynecologic, bone and joint, skin structure, and polymicrobic infections as well as bacterial septicemia and endocarditis. Antibacterial activity includes resistant gram-negative bacilli (*Pseudomonas aeruginosa* and *Enterobacter* sp), gram-positive bacteria (methicillin-sensitive *Staphylococcus aureus* and *Streptococcus* sp) and anaerobes.

Drug of Choice or Alternative for
Disease/Syndrome(s)
Fever, Neutropenic *on page 30*
Osteomyelitis, Diabetic Foot *on page 38*
Peritonitis, Spontaneous Bacterial *on page 43*

Organism(s)

Pregnancy Risk Factor C

Contraindications Hypersensitivity to imipenem/cilastatin or any component

Warnings/Precautions Dosage adjustment required in patients with impaired renal function; safety and efficacy in children <12 years of age have not yet been established; prolonged use may result in superinfection; use with caution in patients with a history of seizures or hypersensitivity to beta-lactams; elderly patients often require lower doses

Adverse Reactions

1% to 10%:

Gastrointestinal: Nausea (1% to 2%), diarrhea (1% to 2%), vomiting (1% to 2%)

Local: Phlebitis (3%)

<1%: Hypotension, palpitations, seizures, rash, pseudomembranous colitis, neutropenia (including agranulocytosis), eosinophilia, anemia, positive Coombs' test, thrombocytopenia, prolonged PT, increased LFTs, pain at injection site, increased BUN/creatine, abnormal urinalysis

Overdosage/Toxicology

Symptoms of overdose include neuromuscular hypersensitivity, seizures

Hemodialysis may be helpful to aid in the removal of the drug from the blood; otherwise most treatment is supportive or symptom directed

Drug Interactions Increased toxicity: Beta-lactam antibiotics, probenecid may increase toxic potential

Stability

Imipenem/cilastatin powder for injection should be stored at <30°C

Reconstituted solutions are stable 10 hours at room temperature and 48 hours at refrigeration (4°C) with NS

If reconstituted with 5% or 10% dextrose injection, 5% dextrose and sodium bicarbonate, 5% dextrose and 0.9% sodium chloride, is stable for 4 hours at room temperature and 24 hours when refrigerated

Imipenem/cilastatin is most stable at a pH of 6.5-7.5; imipenem is inactivated at acidic or alkaline pH

Standard diluent: 500 mg/100 mL NS; 1 g/250 mL NS

Comments: All IVPB should be prepared fresh; do not use dextrose as a diluent due to limited stability

Mechanism of Action Inhibits bacterial cell wall synthesis by binding to one or more of the penicillin binding proteins (PBPs); which in turn inhibits the final transpeptidation step of peptidoglycan synthesis in bacterial cell walls, thus inhibiting cell wall biosynthesis. Bacteria eventually lyse due to ongoing activity of cell wall autolytic enzymes (autolysins and murein hydrolases) while cell wall assembly is arrested. Cilastatin prevents renal metabolism of imipenem by competitive inhibition of dehydropeptidase along the brush border of the renal tubules.

Pharmacodynamics/Kinetics

Absorption: I.M.: Imipenem: 60% to 75%; cilastatin: 95% to 100%

Distribution: Imipenem appears in breast milk; crosses the placenta; distributed rapidly and widely to most tissues and fluids including sputum, pleural fluid, peritoneal fluid, interstitial fluid, bile, aqueous humor, reproductive organs, and bone; highest concentrations in pleural fluid, interstitial fluid, peritoneal fluid, and reproductive organs; low concentrations in cerebrospinal fluid

(Continued)

Imipenem and Cilastatin *(Continued)*

Metabolism: Imipenem is metabolized in the kidney by dehydropeptidase, this activity is blocked by cilastatin; cilastatin is partially metabolized in the kidneys

Half-life: Both: 60 minutes, extended with renal insufficiency

Elimination: Both: ~70% excreted unchanged in urine

Usual Dosage Dosing based on imipenem component:

Children: I.V.:

3 months to 3 years: 25 mg/kg every 6 hours; maximum: 2 g/day

≥3 years: 15 mg/kg/every 6 hours

Adults: I.V.:

Mild to moderate infection: 250-500 mg every 6-8 hours

Severe infections with only **moderately susceptible** organisms: 1 g every 6-8 hours

Mild to moderate infection **only**: I.M.: 500-750 mg every 12 hours (**Note:** 750 mg is recommended for intra-abdominal and more severe respiratory, dermatologic, or gynecologic infections; total daily I.M. dosages >1500 mg are not recommended; deep I.M. injection should be carefully made into a large muscle mass only)

Dosing adjustment in renal impairment: See table.

Imipenem/Cilastatin

Creatinine Clearance mL/min/1.73 m²	Frequency	Dose (mg)
30-70	q8h	500
20-30	q12h	500
5-20	q12h	250

Hemodialysis: Imipenem (**not cilastatin**) is moderately dialyzable (20% to 50%); administer dose postdialysis

Peritoneal dialysis: Dose as for Cl_{cr} <10 mL/minute

Continuous arteriovenous or venovenous hemofiltration (CAVH/CAVHD): Dose as for Cl_{cr} 20-30 mL/minute; monitor for seizure activity; imipenem is well removed by CAVH but cilastatin is not; removes 20 mg of imipenem per liter of filtrate per day

Administration Not for direct infusion; vial contents must be transferred to 100 mL of infusion solution; final concentration should not exceed 5 mg/mL; infuse each 250-500 mg dose over 20-30 minutes; infuse each 1 g dose over 40-60 minutes; watch for convulsions. If nausea and/or vomiting occur during administration, decrease the rate of I.V. infusion; do not mix with or physically add to other antibiotics; however, may administer concomitantly.

Monitoring Parameters Periodic renal, hepatic, and hematologic function tests; monitor for signs of anaphylaxis during first dose

Test Interactions Interferes with urinary glucose determination using Clinitest®

Additional Information Sodium content of 1 g injection:

I.M.: 64.4 mg (2.8 mEq)

I.V.: 73.6 mg (3.2 mEq)

Dosage Forms Powder for injection:

I.M.:

Imipenem 500 mg and cilastatin 500 mg

Imipenem 750 mg and cilastatin 750 mg

I.V.:

Imipenem 250 mg and cilastatin 250 mg

Imipenem 500 mg and cilastatin 500 mg

Selected Readings

Balfour JA, Bryson HM, and Brogden RN, "Imipenem/Cilastatin: An Update of Its Antibacterial Activity, Pharmacokinetics, and Therapeutic Efficacy in the Treatment of Serious Infections," *Drugs*, 1996, 51(1):99-136.

Barza M, "Imipenem: First of a New Class of Beta-Lactam Antibiotics," *Ann Intern Med*, 1985, 103(4):552-60.

Donowitz GR and Mandell GL, "Beta-Lactam Antibiotics," *N Engl J Med*, 1988, 318(7):419-26 and 318(8):490-500.

Hellinger WC and Brewer NS, "Carbapenems and Monobactams: Imipenem, Meropenem, and Aztreonam," *Mayo Clin Proc*, 1999, 74(4):420-34.

Imiquimod (i mi KWI mod)

U.S. Brand Names Aldara™

Use Treatment of external genital and perianal warts/condyloma acuminata in adults

Pregnancy Risk Factor B

Contraindications Hypersensitivity to imiquimod

Warnings/Precautions Imiquimod has not been evaluated for the treatment of urethral, intravaginal, cervical, rectal, or intra-anal human papilloma viral disease and is not recommended for these conditions. Topical imiquimod is not intended for ophthalmic use. Topical imiquimod administration is not recommended until genital/perianal tissue is healed from any previous drug or surgical treatment. Imiquimod has the potential to exacerbate inflammatory conditions of the skin.

Adverse Reactions

>10%: Local, mild/moderate: Erythema, itching, erosion, burning, excoriation/flaking, edema

1% to 10%:

Local, severe: Erythema, erosion, edema

Local, mild/moderate: Pain, induration, ulceration, scabbing, vesicles, soreness

Overdosage/Toxicology

Overdosage is unlikely because of minimal percutaneous absorption. Persistent topical overdosing of imiquimod could result in severe local skin reactions. The most clinically serious adverse event reported following multiple oral imiquimod doses of ≥200 mg was hypotension that resolved following oral or I.V. fluid administration.

Treat symptomatically

Stability Do not store at ≥30°C (86°F); avoid freezing

Mechanism of Action Mechanism of action is unknown; however, induces cytokines, including interferon-alpha and others

Pharmacodynamics/Kinetics

Absorption: Minimal

Elimination: Less than 0.9% of dose is excreted in urine and feces following topical administration

Usual Dosage

Adults: Topical: Apply 3 times/week prior to normal sleeping hours and leave on the skin for 6-10 hours. Following treatment period, remove cream by washing the treated area with mild soap and water. Examples of 3 times/week application schedules are: Monday, Wednesday, Friday; or Tuesday, Thursday, Saturday. Continue imiquimod treatment until there is total clearance of the genital/perianal warts for ≤16 weeks. A rest period of several days may be taken if required by the patient's discomfort or severity of the local skin reaction. Treatment may resume once the reaction subsides.

Nonocclusive dressings such as cotton gauze or cotton underwear may be used in the management of skin reactions. Handwashing before and after cream application is recommended. Imiquimod is packaged in single-use packets that contain sufficient cream to cover a wart area of up to 20 cm²; avoid use of excessive amounts of cream. Instruct patients to apply imiquimod to external or perianal warts. Apply a thin layer to the wart area and rub in until the cream is no longer visible. Do not occlude the application site.

Monitoring Parameters Reduction in wart size is indicative of a therapeutic response; patients should be monitored for signs and symptoms of hypersensitivity to imiquimod

Patient Information Imiquimod may weaken condoms and vaginal diaphragms; therefore, concurrent use is not recommended. This medication is for external use only; avoid contact with eyes. Do not occlude the treatment area with bandages or other covers or wraps. Avoid sexual (genital, anal, oral) contact while the cream is on the skin. Wash the treatment area with mild soap and water 6-10 hours following application of imiquimod.

Patients commonly experience local skin reactions such as erythema, erosion, excoriation/flaking, and edema at the site of application or surrounding areas. Most skin reactions are mild to moderate. Severe skin reactions can occur; promptly report severe reactions to physician. Uncircumcised males treating warts under the foreskin should retract the foreskin and clean the area daily.

Imiquimod is not a cure; new warts may develop during therapy.

(Continued)

Imiquimod *(Continued)*

Dosage Forms Cream, topical: 5% (250 mg single dose packets in boxes of 12)

Immune Globulin, Intramuscular

(i MYUN GLOB yoo lin, IN tra MUS kyoo ler)

Canadian Brand Names Gammabulin Immuno; Iveegam®

Synonyms Gamma Globulin; IG; IGIM; Immune Serum Globulin; ISG

Generic Available No

Use Household and sexual contacts of persons with hepatitis A, measles, varicella, and possibly rubella; travelers to high-risk areas outside tourist routes; staff, attendees, and parents of diapered attendees in day-care center outbreaks

For travelers, IG is not an alternative to careful selection of foods and water; immune globulin can interfere with the antibody response to parenterally administered live virus vaccines. Frequent travelers should be tested for hepatitis A antibody, immune hemolytic anemia, and neutropenia (with ITP, I.V. route is usually used).

Drug of Choice or Alternative for

Organism(s)

Hepatitis A Virus *on page 161*

Measles Virus *on page 193*

Pregnancy Risk Factor C

Contraindications Thrombocytopenia, hypersensitivity to immune globulin, thimerosal, IgA deficiency

Warnings/Precautions Skin testing should not be performed as local irritation can occur and be misinterpreted as a positive reaction; do not administer I.V.; IG should **not** be used to control outbreaks of measles; epidemiologic and laboratory data indicate current IMIG products do not have a discernible risk of transmitting HIV

Adverse Reactions

>10%: Local: Pain, tenderness, muscle stiffness at I.M. site

1% to 10%:

Cardiovascular: Flushing

Central nervous system: Chills

Gastrointestinal: Nausea

<1%: Lethargy, fever, urticaria, angioedema, erythema, vomiting, myalgia, hypersensitivity reactions

Drug Interactions Increased toxicity: Live virus, vaccines (measles, mumps, rubella); do not administer within 3 months after administration of these vaccines

Stability Keep in refrigerator; do not freeze

Mechanism of Action Provides passive immunity by increasing the antibody titer and antigen-antibody reaction potential

Pharmacodynamics/Kinetics

Duration of immune effect: Usually 3-4 weeks

Half-life: 23 days

Time to peak serum concentration: I.M.: Within 24-48 hours

Usual Dosage I.M.:

Hepatitis A:

Pre-exposure prophylaxis upon travel into endemic areas (hepatitis A vaccine preferred):

0.02 mL/kg for anticipated risk 1-3 months

0.06 mL/kg for anticipated risk >3 months

Repeat approximate dose every 4-6 months if exposure continues

Postexposure prophylaxis: 0.02 mL/kg given within 2 weeks of exposure

Measles:

Prophylaxis: 0.25 mL/kg/dose (maximum dose: 15 mL) given within 6 days of exposure followed by live attenuated measles vaccine in 3 months or at 15 months of age (whichever is later)

For patients with leukemia, lymphoma, immunodeficiency disorders, generalized malignancy, or receiving immunosuppressive therapy: 0.5 mL/kg (maximum dose: 15 mL)

Poliomyelitis: Prophylaxis: 0.3 mL/kg/dose as a single dose

Rubella: Prophylaxis: 0.55 mL/kg/dose within 72 hours of exposure

Varicella: Prophylaxis: 0.6-1.2 mL/kg (varicella zoster immune globulin preferred) within 72 hours of exposure

IgG deficiency: 1.3 mL/kg, then 0.66 mL/kg in 3-4 weeks

Hepatitis B: Prophylaxis: 0.06 mL/kg/dose (HBIG preferred)

Administration Intramuscular injection only

Test Interactions Skin tests should not be done

Nursing Implications Do not mix with other medications; skin testing should not be performed as local irritation can occur and be misinterpreted as a positive reaction

Dosage Forms Injection: I.M.: 165±15 mg (of protein)/mL (2 mL, 10 mL)

Selected Readings
ASHP Commission on Therapeutics, "ASHP Therapeutic Guidelines for Intravenous Immune Globulin," *Clin Pharm*, 1992, 11(2):117-36.
Berkman SA, Lee ML, and Gale RP, "Clinical Uses of Intravenous Immunoglobulins," *Ann Intern Med*, 1990, 112(4):278-92.

Immune Globulin, Intravenous

(i MYUN GLOB yoo lin, IN tra VEE nus)

U.S. Brand Names Gamimune® N; Gammagard® S/D; Gammar®-P I.V.; Polygam®; Polygam® S/D; Sandoglobulin®; Venoglobulin®-I; Venoglobulin®-S

Synonyms IVIG

Use Treatment of immunodeficiency sufficiency (hypogammaglobulinemia, agammaglobulinemia, IgG subclass deficiencies, severe combined immunodeficiency syndromes (SCIDS), Wiskott-Aldrich syndrome), idiopathic thrombocytopenic purpura; used in conjunction with appropriate anti-infective therapy to prevent or modify acute bacterial or viral infections in patients with iatrogenically-induced or disease-associated immunodepression; chronic lymphocytic leukemia (CLL) - chronic prophylaxis autoimmune neutropenia, bone marrow transplantation patients, autoimmune hemolytic anemia or neutropenia, refractory dermatomyositis/polymyositis, autoimmune diseases (myasthenia gravis, SLE, bullous pemphigoid, severe rheumatoid arthritis), Guillain-Barré syndrome; pediatric HIV infection to decrease frequency of serious bacterial infections

Pregnancy Risk Factor C

Contraindications Hypersensitivity to immune globulin or any component, IgA deficiency (except with the use of Gammagard®, Polygam®)

Warnings/Precautions Anaphylactic hypersensitivity reactions can occur, especially in IgA-deficient patients; studies indicate that the currently available products have no discernible risk of transmitting HIV or hepatitis B; aseptic meningitis may occur with high doses (≥2 g/kg)

Adverse Reactions
1% to 10%:
Cardiovascular: Flushing of the face, tachycardia
Central nervous system: Chills
Gastrointestinal: Nausea
Respiratory: Dyspnea
<1%: Hypotension, tightness in the chest, dizziness, fever, headache, diaphoresis, hypersensitivity reactions

Drug Interactions Increased toxicity: Live virus vaccines (measles, mumps, rubella); do not administer within 3 months after administration of these vaccines

Stability Stability and dilution is dependent upon the manufacturer and brand; do not mix with other drugs

Mechanism of Action Replacement therapy for primary and secondary immunodeficiencies; interference with F_c receptors on the cells of the reticuloendothelial system for autoimmune cytopenias and ITP; possible role of contained antiviral-type antibodies

Pharmacodynamics/Kinetics I.V. provides immediate antibody levels
Duration of immune effects: 3-4 weeks
Half-life: 21-24 days

Usual Dosage Children and Adults: I.V.:
Dosages should be based on ideal body weight and not actual body weight in morbidly obese patients; approved doses and regimens may vary between brands; check manufacturer guidelines
Primary immunodeficiency disorders: 200-400 mg/kg every 4 weeks or as per monitored serum IgG concentrations
Chronic lymphocytic leukemia (CLL): 400 mg/kg/dose every 3 weeks
Idiopathic thrombocytopenic purpura (ITP): Maintenance dose:
400 mg/kg/day for 2-5 consecutive days; or 1000 mg/kg every other day for 3 doses, if needed or
(Continued)

Intravenous Immune Globulin Product Comparison

	Gamimune® N	Gammagard® SD	Gammar®-IV	Polygam®	Sandoglobulin®	Venoglobulin®-I
FDA indication	Primary immunodeficiency, ITP	Primary immunodeficiency, ITP, CLL prophylaxis	Primary immunodeficiency	Primary immunodeficiency, ITP, CLL	Primary immunodeficiency, ITP	Primary immunodeficiency, ITP
Contraindication	IgA deficiency	None (caution with IgA deficiency)	IgA deficiency	None (caution with IgA deficiency)	IgA deficiency	IgA deficiency
IgA content	270 mcg/mL	0.92-1.6 mcg/mL	<20 mcg/mL	0.74±0.33 mcg/mL	720 mcg/mL	20-24 mcg/mL
Adverse reactions (%)	5.2	6	15	6	6	6
Plasma source	>2000 paid donors	4000-5000 paid donors	>8000 paid donors	50,000 voluntary donors	8000-15,000 voluntary donors	6000-9000 paid donors
Half-life	21 d	24 d	21-24 d	21-25 d	21-23 d	29 d
IgG subclass (%)						
IgG$_1$ (60-70)	60	67 (66.8)[1]	69	67	60.5 (55.3)[1]	62.3[2]
IgG$_2$ (19-31)	29.4	25 (25.4)	23	25	30.2 (35.7)	32.8
IgG$_3$ (5-8.4)	6.5	5 (7.4)	6	5	6.6 (6.3)	2.9
IgG$_4$ (0-7.4)	4.1	3 (0.3)	2	3	2.6 (2.6)	2
Monomers (%)	>95	>95	>98	>95	>92	>98
Gammaglobulin (%)	>98	>90	>98	>90	>96	>98
Storage	Refrigerate	Room temp	Room temp	Room temp	Room temp	Room temp
Recommendations for initial infusion rate	0.01-0.02 mL/kg/min	0.5 mL/kg/h	0.01-0.02 mL/kg/min	0.5 mL/kg/h	0.01-0.03 mL/kg/min	0.01-0.02 mL/kg/min
Maximum infusion rate	0.08 mL/kg/min	4 mL/kg/h	0.06 mL/kg/min	4 mL/kg/h	2.5 mL/kg/min	0.04 mL/kg/min
Maximum concentration for infusion (%)	10	5	5	10	12	10

[1]Skvaril F and Gardi A, "Differences Among Available Immunoglobulin Preparations for Intravenous Use," Pediatr Infect Dis J, 1988, 7:543-48.

[2]Roomer J, Morgenthaler JJ, Scherz R, et al, "Characterization of Various Immunoglobulin Preparations for Intravenous Application," Vox Sang, 1982, 42:62-73.

1000 mg/kg/day for 2 consecutive days; or up to 2000 mg/kg/day over 2-7 consecutive days

Chronic ITP: 400-2000 mg/kg/dose as needed to maintain appropriate platelet counts

Kawasaki disease:
400 mg/kg/day for 4 days within 10 days of onset of fever
800 mg/kg/day for 1-2 days within 10 days of onset of fever
2 g/kg for one dose only

Acquired immunodeficiency syndrome (patients must be symptomatic):
200-250 mg/kg/dose every 2 weeks
400-500 mg/kg/dose every month or every 4 weeks

Pediatric HIV: 400 mg/kg every 28 days

Autoimmune hemolytic anemia and neutropenia: 1000 mg/kg/dose for 2-3 days

Autoimmune diseases: 400 mg/kg/day for 4 days

Bone marrow transplant: 500 mg/kg beginning on days 7 and 2 pretransplant, then 500 mg/kg/week for 90 days post-transplant

Adjuvant to severe cytomegalovirus infections: 500 mg/kg/dose every other day for 7 doses

Severe systemic viral and bacterial infections: Children: 500-1000 mg/kg/week

Prevention of gastroenteritis: Infants and Children: Oral: 50 mg/kg/day divided every 6 hours

Guillain-Barré syndrome:
400 mg/kg/day for 4 days
1000 mg/kg/day for 2 days
2000 mg/kg/day for one day

Refractory dermatomyositis: 2 g/kg/dose every month x 3-4 doses

Refractory polymyositis: 1 g/kg/day x 2 days every month x 4 doses

Chronic inflammatory demyelinating polyneuropathy:
400 mg/kg/day for 5 doses once each month
800 mg/kg/day for 3 doses once each month
1000 mg/kg/day for 2 days once each month

Dosing adjustment/comments in renal impairment: Cl_{cr} <10 mL/minute: Avoid use

Administration I.V. use only; for initial treatment, a lower concentration and/or a slower rate of infusion should be used

Dosage Forms

Injection: Gamimune® N: 5% [50 mg/mL] (10 mL, 50 mL, 100 mL, 250 mL); 10% [100 mg/mL] (10 mL, 50 mL, 100 mL, 200 mL)

Powder for injection, lyophilized:
Gammar®-P I.V. (5% IgG and 3% albumin): 1 g, 2.5 g, 5 g, 10 g
Polygam®: 0.5 g, 2.5 g, 5 g, 10 g
Sandoglobulin®: 1 g, 3 g, 6 g, 12 g
Venoglobulin®-I: 0.5 g, 2.5 g, 5 g, 10 g
Detergent treated:
Gammagard® S/D: 2.5 g, 5 g, 10 g
Polygam® S/D: 2.5 g, 5 g, 10 g
Venoglobulin®-S: 5% [50 mg/mL] (50 mL, 100 mL, 200 mL); 10% [100 mg/mL] (50 mL, 100 mL, 200 mL)

Immune Serum Globulin *see* Immune Globulin, Intramuscular *on page 770*

Immunization Guidelines *see page 1041*

Imogam® *see* Rabies Immune Globulin (Human) *on page 892*

Imovax® Rabies I.D. Vaccine *see* Rabies Virus Vaccine *on page 893*

Imovax® Rabies Vaccine *see* Rabies Virus Vaccine *on page 893*

Indanyl Sodium *see* Carbenicillin *on page 626*

Indinavir *(in DIN a veer)*

Related Information
HIV Therapeutic Information *on page 1008*

U.S. Brand Names Crixivan®

Use Treatment of HIV infection when antiretroviral therapy is warranted; should always be used as part of a multidrug regimen (at least three antiretroviral agents)

Drug of Choice or Alternative for
Organism(s)
Human Immunodeficiency Virus *on page 177*
(Continued)

Indinavir *(Continued)*

Pregnancy Risk Factor C

Pregnancy/Breast-Feeding Implications
Clinical effects on the fetus: Administer during pregnancy only if benefits to mother outweigh risks to the fetus; hyperbilirubinemia may be exacerbated in neonates

Breast-feeding/lactation: HIV-infected mothers are discouraged from breast-feeding to decrease potential transmission of HIV

Contraindications Hypersensitivity to the drug or its components

Warnings/Precautions Because indinavir may cause nephrolithiasis the drug should be discontinued if signs and symptoms occur. Indinavir should not be administered concurrently with terfenadine, astemizole, cisapride, triazolam, and midazolam because of competition for metabolism of these drugs through the CYP3A4 system, and potential serious or life-threatening events. Patients with hepatic insufficiency due to cirrhosis should have dose reduction.

Adverse Reactions Protease inhibitors cause dyslipidemia which includes elevated cholesterol and triglycerides and a redistribution of body fat centrally to cause "protease paunch", buffalo hump, facial atrophy, and breast enlargement. These agents also cause hyperglycemia.

1% to 10%:
Central nervous system: Headache (5.6%), insomnia (3.1%)
Gastrointestinal: Mild elevation of indirect bilirubin (10%), abdominal pain (8.7%), nausea (11.7%), diarrhea/vomiting (4% to 5%), taste perversion (2.6%)
Neuromuscular & skeletal: Weakness (3.6%), flank pain (2.6%)
Renal: Kidney stones (2% to 3%)
<1%: Malaise, dizziness, somnolence, anorexia, xerostomia, decreased hemoglobin

Drug Interactions CYP3A3/4 enzyme substrate; CYP3A3/4 enzyme inhibitor
Decreased effect: Concurrent use of rifampin and rifabutin may decrease the effectiveness of indinavir (dosage increase of indinavir is recommended), dosage decreases of rifampin/rifabutin is recommended; the efficacy of protease inhibitors may be decreased when given with nevirapine
Increased toxicity: Gastric pH is lowered and absorption may be decreased when didanosine and indinavir are taken <1 hour apart; a reduction of dose is often required when coadministered with ketoconazole; terfenadine, astemizole, cisapride should be avoided with indinavir due to life-threatening cardiotoxicity; benzodiazepines with indinavir may result in prolonged sedation and respiratory depression

Stability Capsules are sensitive to moisture; medication should be stored and used in the original container and the desiccant should remain in the bottle

Mechanism of Action Indinavir is a human immunodeficiency virus protease inhibitor, binding to the protease activity site and inhibiting the activity of this enzyme. HIV protease is an enzyme required for the cleavage of viral polyprotein precursors into individual functional proteins found in infectious HIV. Inhibition prevents cleavage of these polyproteins resulting in the formation of immature noninfectious viral particles.

Pharmacodynamics/Kinetics
Absorption: Administration of indinavir with a high fat, high calorie diet resulted in a reduction in AUC and in maximum serum concentration (77% and 84% respectively). Administration with a lighter meal resulted in little or no change in these parameters.
Protein binding: 60% in the plasma
Metabolism: Highly metabolized by the cytochrome P-450 3A4 enzymes; seven metabolites of indinavir have been identified
Bioavailability: Oral: Good; T_{max}: 0.8 ± 0.3 hour
Half-life: 1.8 ± 0.4 hour
Elimination: In feces and urine

Usual Dosage Adults: Oral: 800 mg every 8 hours
Dosage adjustment in hepatic impairment: 600 mg every 8 hours with mild/medium impairment due to cirrhosis or with ketoconazole coadministration

Dietary Considerations Meals high in calories, fat, and protein result in a significant decrease in drug levels; grapefruit juice may decrease indinavir's AUC

Monitoring Parameters Monitor viral load, CD4 count, triglycerides, cholesterol, glucose

Patient Information Take with a full glass of water; any symptoms of kidney stones, including flank pain, dysuria, etc, indicates the drug should be discontinued and physician or pharmacist should be contacted. Drug should be administered on an empty stomach 1 hour before or 2 hours after a large meal. May take with a small, light meal. Indinavir should be stored and used in the original container.

Nursing Implications Administer around-the-clock to avoid significant fluctuation in serum levels; administer with plenty of water

Dosage Forms Capsule: 200 mg, 333 mg, 400 mg

Selected Readings

Deeks SG, Smith M, Holodniy M, et al, "HIV-1 Protease Inhibitors. A Review for Clinicians," *JAMA*, 1997, 277(2):145-53.

Kakuda TN, Struble KA, and Piscitelli SC, "Protease Inhibitors for the Treatment of Human Immunodeficiency Virus Infection," *Am J Health Syst Pharm*, 1998, 55(3):233-54.

Kaul DR, Cinti SK, Carver PL, et al, "HIV Protease Inhibitors: Advances in Therapy and Adverse Reactions, Including Metabolic Complications," *Pharmacotherapy*, 1999, 19(3):281-98.

McDonald CK and Kuritzkes DR, "Human Immunodeficiency Virus Type 1 Protease Inhibitors," *Arch Intern Med*, 1997, 157(9):951-9.

INF *see* Interferon Alfa-2b *on page 778*

Infanrix™ *see* Diphtheria, Tetanus Toxoids, and Acellular Pertussis Vaccine *on page 708*

Influenza Virus Vaccine (in floo EN za VYE rus vak SEEN)

Related Information
Immunization Guidelines *on page 1041*

U.S. Brand Names Fluogen®; Flushield®; Fluviron®; Fluzone®

Canadian Brand Names Fluviral®

Synonyms Influenza Virus Vaccine (inactivated whole-virus); Influenza Virus Vaccine (split-virus) Influenza Virus Vaccine (purified surface antigen)

Generic Available No

Use Provide active immunity to influenza virus strains contained in the vaccine; for high-risk persons, previous year vaccines should not be to prevent present year influenza

Groups at Increased Risk for Influenza-Related Complications:
- Persons ≥65 years of age
- Residents of nursing homes and other chronic-care facilities that house persons of any age with chronic medical conditions
- Adults and children with chronic disorders of the pulmonary or cardiovascular systems, including children with asthma
- Adults and children who have required regular medical follow-up or hospitalization during the preceding year because of chronic metabolic diseases (including diabetes mellitus), renal dysfunction, hemoglobinopathies, or immunosuppression (including immunosuppression caused by medications)

Children and teenagers (6 months to 18 years of age) who are receiving long-term aspirin therapy and therefore, may be at risk for developing Reye's syndrome after influenza

Pregnancy Risk Factor C

Contraindications Persons with allergy history to eggs or egg products, chicken, chicken feathers or chicken dander, hypersensitivity to thimerosal, influenza virus vaccine or any component, presence of acute respiratory disease or other active infections or illnesses, delay immunization in a patient with an active neurological disorder

Warnings/Precautions Although there is no evidence of maternal or fetal risk when vaccine is given in pregnancy, waiting until the 2nd or 3rd trimester to vaccinate the pregnant woman with a high-risk condition may be reasonable. Antigenic response may not be as great as expected in patients requiring immunosuppressive drug; hypersensitivity reactions may occur; because of potential for febrile reactions, risks and benefits must carefully be considered in patients with history of febrile convulsions; influenza vaccines from previous seasons must not be used; patients with sulfite sensitivity may be affected by this product. (Continued)

ιιιfluenza Virus Vaccine *(Continued)*

Adverse Reactions All serious adverse reactions must be reported to the U.S. Department of Health and Human Services (DHHS) Vaccine Adverse Event Reporting System (VAERS) 1-800-822-7967.

1% to 10%:
Central nervous system: Fever, malaise
Local: Tenderness, redness, or induration at the site of injection (<33%)
<1%: Guillain-Barré syndrome, fever, urticaria, angioedema, myalgia, asthma, anaphylactoid reactions (most likely to residual egg protein), allergic reactions

Drug Interactions
Decreased effect with immunosuppressive agents; some manufacturers and clinicians recommend that the flu vaccine not be administered with the DTP for the potential for increased febrile reactions (specifically whole-cell pertussis), and that one should wait at least 3 days. ACIP recommends that children at high risk for influenza may get the vaccine concomitantly with DTP
Increased effect/toxicity of theophylline and warfarin possible

Stability Refrigerate

Mechanism of Action Promotes immunity to influenza virus by inducing specific antibody production. Each year the formulation is standardized according to the U.S. Public Health Service. Preparations from previous seasons must not be used.

Usual Dosage I.M.:
Children:
6-35 months: 1-2 doses of 0.25 mL with ≥4 weeks between doses and the last dose administered before December
3-8 years: 1-2 doses of 0.5 mL (in anterolateral aspect of thigh) with ≥4 weeks between doses and the last dose administered before December
Children ≥9 years and Adults: 0.5 mL each year of appropriate vaccine for the year, one dose is all that is necessary; administer in late fall to allow maximum titers to develop by peak epidemic periods usually occurring in early December
Note: The split virus or purified surface antigen is recommended for children ≤12 years of age; if the child has received at least one dose of the 1978-79 or later vaccine, one dose is sufficient

Administration Inspect for particulate matter and discoloration prior to administration; for I.M. administration only

Additional Information Pharmacies will stock the formulations(s) standardized according to the USPHS requirements for the season. Influenza vaccines from previous seasons must not be used. Federal law requires that the date of administration, the vaccine manufacturer, lot number of vaccine, and the administering person's name, title and address be entered into the patient's permanent medical record.

Dosage Forms Injection:
Purified surface antigen (Flu-Imune®): 5 mL
Split-virus (Fluogen®, Fluzone®): 0.5 mL, 5 mL
Whole-virus (Fluzone®): 5 mL

Influenza Virus Vaccine (inactivated whole-virus) *see* Influenza Virus Vaccine *on previous page*

Influenza Virus Vaccine (split-virus) Influenza Virus Vaccine (purified surface antigen) *see* Influenza Virus Vaccine *on previous page*

INH *see* Isoniazid *on page 782*

α-2-interferon *see* Interferon Alfa-2b *on page 778*

Interferon Alfa-2a *(in ter FEER on AL fa-too aye)*

U.S. Brand Names Roferon-A®

Synonyms IFLrA; IFN; rIFN-A

Generic Available No

Use FDA approved: Patients >18 years of age: Hairy cell leukemia, AIDS-related Kaposi's sarcoma, chronic myelogenous leukemia (CML), Chronic Hepatitis C, adjuvant treatment to surgery for primary or recurrent malignant melanoma; multiple unlabeled uses; indications and dosage regimens are specific for a particular brand of interferon

Pregnancy Risk Factor C

Contraindications Hypersensitivity to alfa-2a interferon or any component of the product

Warnings/Precautions Use with caution in patients with seizure disorders, brain metastases, compromised CNS, multiple sclerosis, and patients with pre-existing cardiac disease, severe renal or hepatic impairment, or myelosuppression; safety and efficacy in children <18 years of age have not been established. Higher doses in the elderly or in malignancies other than hairy cell leukemia may result in severe obtundation.

Adverse Reactions

>10%:

Central nervous system: Dizziness, fatigue, malaise, fever (usually within 4-6 hours), chills

Dermatologic: Rash

Gastrointestinal: Xerostomia, nausea, vomiting, diarrhea, abdominal cramps, weight loss, metallic taste

Hematologic: Mildly myelosuppressive and well tolerated if used without adjunct antineoplastic agents; thrombocytosis has been reported, leukopenia (mainly neutropenia), anemia, thrombocytopenia, decreased hemoglobin, hematocrit, platelets

Neuromuscular & skeletal: Rigors, arthralgia

Miscellaneous: Flu-like syndrome, diaphoresis

1% to 10%:

Central nervous system: Headache, delirium, somnolence, neurotoxicity

Dermatologic: Alopecia, dry skin

Gastrointestinal: Anorexia, stomatitis

Hepatic: Hepatotoxicity

Neuromuscular & skeletal: Peripheral neuropathy, leg cramps

Ocular: Blurred vision

<1%: Tachycardia, arrhythmias, chest pain, hypotension, SVT, edema, confusion, sensory neuropathy, psychiatric effects, EEG abnormalities, depression, hypothyroidism, increased uric acid level, change in taste, increased hepatic transaminase, myalgia, visual disturbances, proteinuria, increased BUN/creatinine, coughing, dyspnea, nasal congestion, neutralizing antibodies, local sensitivity to injection

Usually patient can build up a tolerance to side effects

Overdosage/Toxicology

Symptoms of overdose include CNS depression, obtundation, flu-like symptoms, myelosuppression

Treatment is supportive

Drug Interactions

Increased effect:

Cimetidine: May augment the antitumor effects of interferon in melanoma

Theophylline: Clearance has been reported to be decreased in hepatitis patients receiving interferon

Increased toxicity: Vinblastine: Enhances interferon toxicity in several patients; increased incidence of paresthesia has also been noted

Stability Refrigerate (2°C to 8°C/36°F to 46°F); do not freeze; do not shake; after reconstitution, the solution is stable for 24 hours at room temperature and for 1 month when refrigerated

Pharmacodynamics/Kinetics

Absorption: Filtered and absorbed at the renal tubule

Distribution: The V_d of interferon is 31 L; but has been noted to be much greater (370-720 L) in leukemia patients receiving continuous infusion IFN; IFN does not penetrate the CSF

Metabolism: Majority of dose thought to be metabolized in the kidney

Bioavailability:

I.M.: 83%

S.C.: 90%

Half-life: Elimination:

I.M., I.V.: 2 hours after administration

S.C.: 3 hours

Time to peak serum concentration: I.M., S.C.: ~6-8 hours

Usual Dosage Refer to individual protocols

Infants and Children: Hemangiomas of infancy, pulmonary hemangiomatosis:

S.C.: 1-3 million units/m^2/day once daily

(Continued)

Interferon Alfa-2a *(Continued)*

Adults >18 years: I.M., S.C.:

Hairy cell leukemia:

Induction: 3 million units/day for 16-24 weeks.

Maintenance: 3 million units 3 times/week (may be treated for up to 20 consecutive weeks)

AIDS-related Kaposi's sarcoma:

Induction: 36 million units/day for 10-12 weeks

Maintenance: 36 million units 3 times/week (may begin with dose escalation from 3-9-18 million units each day over 3 consecutive days followed by 36 million units/day for the remainder of the 10-12 weeks of induction)

If severe adverse reactions occur, modify dosage (50% reduction) or temporarily discontinue therapy until adverse reactions abate

Administration S.C. administration is suggested for those who are at risk for bleeding or are thrombocytopenic; rotate S.C. injection site; patient should be well hydrated

Monitoring Parameters Baseline chest x-ray, EKG, CBC with differential, liver function tests, electrolytes, platelets, weight; patients with pre-existing cardiac abnormalities, or in advanced stages of cancer should have EKGs taken before and during treatment

Patient Information Do not change brands as changes in dosage may result; possible mental status changes may occur while on therapy; report to physician any persistent or severe sore throat, fever, fatigue, unusual bleeding, or bruising; do not operate heavy machinery while on therapy since changes in mental status may occur

Nursing Implications Do not freeze or shake solution; a flu-like syndrome (fever, chills) occurs in the majority of patients 2-6 hours after a dose; pretreatment with nonsteroidal anti-inflammatory drug (NSAID) or acetaminophen can decrease fever and its severity and alleviate headache

Dosage Forms

Injection: 3 million units/mL (1 mL); 6 million units/mL (3 mL); 9 million units/mL (0.9 mL, 3 mL); 36 million units/mL (1 mL)

Powder for injection: 6 million units/mL when reconstituted

Selected Readings

Barreca T, Corsini G, Franceschini R, et al, "Lichen Planus Induced by Interferon-Alpha-2a Therapy for Chronic Active Hepatitis C," *Eur J Gastroenterol Hepatol*, 1995, 7(4):367-8.

Fukumoto Y, Shigemitsu T, Kajii N, et al, "Abducent Nerve Paralysis During Interferon Alpha-2a Therapy in a Case of Chronic Active Hepatitis C," *Intern Med*, 1994, 33(10):637-40.

Haria M and Benfield P, "Interferon-Alpha-2a. A Review of Its Pharmacological Properties and Therapeutic Use in the Management of Viral Hepatitis," *Drugs*, 1995, 50(5):873-96.

Hoofnagle JH, "Alpha-Interferon Therapy of Chronic Hepatitis B, Current Status and Recommendations," *J Hepatol*, 1990, 11(Suppl 1):S100-7.

Morris DJ, "Adverse Effects and Drug Interactions of Clinical Importance With Antiviral Drugs," *Drug Saf*, 1994, 10(4):281-91.

Vial T and Descotes J, "Clinical Toxicity of the Interferons," *Drug Saf*, 1994, 10(2):115-50.

Interferon Alfa-2b (in ter FEER on AL fa too bee)

U.S. Brand Names Intron® A

Synonyms IFN-alpha 2; INF; α-2-interferon; rLFN-α2

Generic Available No

Use FDA approved: Patients >18 years of age: Hairy cell leukemia, condylomata acuminata, AIDS-related Kaposi's sarcoma, chronic hepatitis non-A, non-B(C), chronic hepatitis B; indications and dosage regimens are specific for a particular brand of interferon

Drug of Choice or Alternative for

Organism(s)

Hepatitis B Virus *on page 162*

Hepatitis C Virus *on page 164*

Pregnancy Risk Factor C

Contraindications Known hypersensitivity to interferon alfa-2b or any components, patients with pre-existing thyroid disease uncontrolled by medication, coagulation disorders, diabetics prone to DKA, pulmonary disease

Warnings/Precautions Use with caution in patients with seizure disorders, brain metastases, compromised CNS, multiple sclerosis, and patients with pre-existing cardiac disease, severe renal or hepatic impairment, or myelosuppression; safety and efficacy in children <18 years of age have not been established.

The U.S. Food and Drug Administration (FDA) currently recommends that procedures for proper handling and disposal of antineoplastic agents be considered. Higher doses in the elderly or in malignancies other than hairy cell leukemia may result in severe obtundation.

Adverse Reactions

>10%:
Central nervous system: Dizziness, tiredness
Dermatologic: Skin rash
Gastrointestinal: Diarrhea, xerostomia, metallic taste, anorexia, nausea, vomiting
Hematologic: Anemia, leukopenia, thrombocytopenia
Miscellaneous: Flu-like syndrome

1% to 10%:
Central nervous system: Neurotoxicity
Dermatologic: Dry skin, alopecia
Gastrointestinal: Stomatitis
Hepatic: Hepatotoxicity
Neuromuscular & skeletal: Leg cramps, peripheral neuropathy
Ocular: Blurred vision
Miscellaneous: Diaphoresis

<1%: Cardiotoxicity, hypothyroidism, weight loss, arrhythmias, hypotension, nasal congestion, edema, EEG abnormalities, confusion, sensory neuropathy, fever, headache, decreased hemoglobin, hematocrit, platelets, increased ALT and AST, myalgia, arthralgia, rigors, proteinuria, increased uric acid level, increased BUN/creatinine, coughing, chest pain, chills, neutralizing antibodies

Overdosage/Toxicology

Signs and symptoms include CNS depression, obtundation, flu-like symptoms, myelosuppression
Treatment is supportive

Drug Interactions

Increased effect: Cimetidine: May augment the antitumor effects of interferon in melanoma
Increased toxicity: Vinblastine: Enhances interferon toxicity in several patients; increased incidence of paresthesia has also been noted
Theophylline: Clearance has been reported to be decreased in hepatitis patients receiving interferon
Zidovudine: Increased myelosuppression

Stability

Store intact vials at refrigeration (2°C to 8°C); powder and premixed solutions are stable at 95°F to 113°F for 7 days
Reconstitute vials with diluent; solution is stable for 30 days under refrigeration (2°C to 8°C)
Standard I.M./S.C. dilution: Dose/syringe or dispense vial to floor
Solution is stable for 7 days at room temperature and 30 days under refrigeration (2°C to 8°C)

Mechanism of Action Alpha interferons are a family of proteins, produced by nucleated cells, that have antiviral, antiproliferative, and immune-regulating activity. There are 16 known subtypes of alpha interferons. Interferons interact with cells through high affinity cell surface receptors. Following activation, multiple effects can be detected including induction of gene transcription. Inhibits cellular growth, alters the state of cellular differentiation, interferes with oncogene expression, alters cell surface antigen expression, increases phagocytic activity of macrophages, and augments cytotoxicity of lymphocytes for target cells.

Pharmacodynamics/Kinetics

Absorption: Filtered and absorbed at the renal tubule
Distribution: V_d of interferon: 31 L; but has been noted to be much greater (370-720 L) in leukemia patients receiving continuous infusion IFN; IFN does not penetrate the CSF
Metabolism: Majority of dose thought to be metabolized in the kidney
Bioavailability:
I.M.: 83%
S.C.: 90%
Half-life: Elimination:
I.M., I.V.: 2 hours
(Continued)

Interferon Alfa-2b *(Continued)*

S.C.: 3 hours

Time to peak serum concentration: I.M., S.C.: ~6-8 hours

Usual Dosage Adults:

Hairy cell leukemia: I.M., S.C.: 2 million units/m² 3 times/week

AIDS-related Kaposi's sarcoma: I.M., S.C.: 30 million units/m² 3 times/week or 50 million units/m² I.V. 5 days/week every other week

Condylomata acuminata: Intralesionally: 1 million units/lesion 3 times/week for 3 weeks; not to exceed 5 million units per treatment (maximum: 5 lesions at one time)

Chronic hepatitis C: I.M., S.C.: 3 million units 3 times/week for approximately a 6-month course

Chronic hepatitis B: I.M., S.C.: 5 million IU/day or 10 million IU 3 times/week for 16 weeks; if severe adverse reactions occur, reduce dosage 50% or temporarily discontinue therapy until adverse reactions abate; when platelet/granulocyte count returns to normal, reinstitute therapy

Hemodialysis: Supplemental dose is not necessary

Peritoneal dialysis: Supplemental dose is not necessary

Monitoring Parameters Baseline chest x-ray, EKG, CBC with differential, liver function tests, electrolytes, thyroid function tests, platelets, weight; patients with pre-existing cardiac abnormalities, or in advanced stages of cancer should have EKGs taken before and during treatment

Patient Information Do not change brands of interferon as changes in dosage may result; do not operate heavy machinery while on therapy since changes in mental status may occur; report to physician any persistent or severe sore throat, fever, fatigue, unusual bleeding, or bruising

Nursing Implications Use acetaminophen to prevent or partially alleviate headache and fever; do not use 3, 5, 18, and 25 million unit strengths intralesionally, solutions are hypertonic; 50 million unit strength is not for use in condylomata, hairy cell leukemia, or chronic hepatitis.

Dosage Forms

Injection, albumin free: 3 million units (0.5 mL); 5 million units (0.5 mL); 10 million units (1 mL); 25 million units

Powder for injection, lyophilized: 18 million units, 50 million units

Selected Readings

Davis GL, Esteban-Mur R, Rustgi V, et al, "Interferon Alfa-2b Alone or in Combination With Ribavirin for the Treatment of Relapse of Chronic Hepatitis C," *N Engl J Med*, 1998, 339(21):1493-9.

"Drugs for Non-HIV Viral Infections," *Med Lett Drugs Ther*, 1994, 36(919):27.

McHutchison JG, Gordon SC, Schiff ER, et al, "Interferon Alfa-2b Alone or in Combination With Ribavirin as Initial Treatment for Chronic Hepatitis C," *N Engl J Med*, 1998, 339(21):1485-92.

Interferon Alfa-2b and Ribavirin Combination Pack

(in ter FEER on AL fa too bee & rye ba VYE rin com bi NAY shun pak)

Related Information

Interferon Alfa-2b *on page 778*

Ribavirin *on page 899*

U.S. Brand Names Rebetron™

Use The combination therapy of oral ribavirin with interferon alfa-2b, recombinant (Intron® A) injection is indicated for the treatment of chronic hepatitis C in patients with compensated liver disease who have relapsed after alpha interferon therapy.

Drug of Choice or Alternative for

Organism(s)

Hepatitis C Virus *on page 164*

Usual Dosage The recommended dosage of combination therapy is 3 million int. units of Intron® A injected subcutaneously 3 times/week and 1000-1200 mg of Rebetol® capsules administered orally in a divided daily (morning and evening) dose for 24 weeks; patients weighing 75 kg (165 pounds) or less should receive 1000 mg of Rebetol® daily (2 x 200 mg capsules in the morning and 3 x 200 mg capsules in the evening); while patients weighing more than 75 kg should receive 1200 mg of Rebetol® daily (3 x 200 mg capsules in the morning and 3 x 200 mg capsules in the evening)

Dosage Forms Combination package:

For patients ≤75 kg:

Each Rebetron™ combination package consists of:

A box containing 6 vials of Intron® A (3 million int. units in 0.5 mL per vial) and 6 syringes and alcohol swabs; two boxes containing 35 Rebetol® 200 mg capsules each for a total of 70 capsules (5 capsules per blister card)

One 18 million int. units multidose vial of Intron® A injection (22.8 million int. units per 3.8 mL; 3 million int. units/0.5 mL) and 6 syringes and alcohol swabs; two boxes containing 35 Rebetol® 200 mg capsules each for a total of 70 capsules (5 capsules per blister card)

One 18 million int. units Intron® A injection multidose pen (22.5 million int. units per 1.5 mL; 3 million int. units/0.2 mL) and 6 disposable needles and alcohol swabs; two boxes containing 35 Rebetol® 200 mg capsules each for a total of 70 capsules (5 capsules per blister card)

For patients >75 kg:

A box containing 6 vials of Intron® A injection (3 million int. units in 0.5 mL per vial) and 6 syringes and alcohol swabs; two boxes containing 42 Rebetol® 200 mg capsules each for a total of 84 capsules (6 capsules per blister card)

One 18 million int. units multidose vial of Intron® A injection (22.5 million int. units per 3.8 mL; 3 million int. units/0.5 mL) and 6 syringes and alcohol swabs; two boxes containing 42 Rebetol® 200 mg capsules each for a total of 84 capsules (6 capsules per blister card)

One 18 million int. units Intron® A injection multidose pen (22.5 million int. units per 1.5 mL; 3 million int. units/0.2 mL) and 6 disposable needles and alcohol swabs; two boxes containing 42 Rebetol® 200 mg capsules each for a total of 84 capsules (6 capsules per blister card)

For Rebetol® dose reduction:

A box containing 6 vials of Intron® A injection (3 million int. units in 0.5 mL per vial) and 6 syringes and alcohol swabs; one box containing 42 Rebetol® 200 mg capsules (6 capsules per blister card)

One 18 million int. units multidose vial of Intron® A injection (22.8 million int. units per 3.8 mL; 3 million int. units/0.5 mL) and 6 syringes and alcohol swabs; one box containing 42 Rebetol® 200 mg capsules (6 capsules per blister card)

One 18 million int. units Introl® A injection multidose pen (22.5 million int. units per 1.5 mL; 3 million int. units/0.2 mL) and 6 disposable needles and alcohol swabs; one box containing 42 Rebetol® 200 mg capsules (6 capsules per blister card)

Intron® A see Interferon Alfa-2b on page 778

Invirase® see Saquinavir on page 915

Iodochlorhydroxyquin see Clioquinol on page 686

Iodoquinol (eye oh doe KWIN ole)

U.S. Brand Names Yodoxin®

Canadian Brand Names Diodoquin®

Synonyms Diiodohydroxyquin

Generic Available No

Use Treatment of acute and chronic intestinal amebiasis; asymptomatic cyst passers; *Blastocystis hominis* infections; ineffective for amebic hepatitis or hepatic abscess

Drug of Choice or Alternative for

Organism(s)

Entamoeba histolytica on page 132

Pregnancy Risk Factor C

Contraindications Known hypersensitivity to iodine or iodoquinol; hepatic damage; pre-existing optic neuropathy

Warnings/Precautions Use with caution in patients with thyroid disease or neurological disorders

Adverse Reactions

>10%: Gastrointestinal: Diarrhea, nausea, vomiting, stomach pain

1% to 10%:

Central nervous system: Fever, chills, agitation, retrograde amnesia, headache

Dermatologic: Rash, urticaria

Endocrine & metabolic: Thyroid gland enlargement

(Continued)

Iodoquinol *(Continued)*

Neuromuscular & skeletal: Peripheral neuropathy, weakness
Ocular: Optic neuritis, optic atrophy, visual impairment
Miscellaneous: Itching of rectal area

Overdosage/Toxicology
Chronic overdose can result in vomiting, diarrhea, abdominal pain, metallic taste, paresthesias, paraplegia, and loss of vision; can lead to destruction of the long fibers of the spinal cord and optic nerve
Acute overdose: Delirium, stupor, coma, amnesia
Following GI decontamination, treatment is symptomatic

Mechanism of Action Contact amebicide that works in the lumen of the intestine by an unknown mechanism

Pharmacodynamics/Kinetics
Absorption: Oral: Poor and irregular
Metabolism: In the liver
Elimination: High percentage of dose excreted in feces

Usual Dosage Oral:
Children: 30-40 mg/kg/day (maximum: 650 mg/dose) in 3 divided doses for 20 days; not to exceed 1.95 g/day

Adults: 650 mg 3 times/day after meals for 20 days; not to exceed 1.95 g/day

Monitoring Parameters Ophthalmologic exam

Test Interactions May increase protein-bound serum iodine concentrations reflecting a decrease in ^{131}I uptake; false-positive ferric chloride test for phenylketonuria

Patient Information May take with food or milk to reduce stomach upset

Nursing Implications Tablets may be crushed and mixed with applesauce or chocolate syrup

Dosage Forms
Powder: 25 g
Tablet: 210 mg, 650 mg

Selected Readings
"Drugs for Parasitic Infections," *Med Lett Drugs Ther*, 1998, 40(1017):1-12.

Iodoquinol and Hydrocortisone

(eye oh doe KWIN ole & hye droe KOR ti sone)

Related Information
Iodoquinol *on previous page*

U.S. Brand Names Vytone® Topical

Use Treatment of eczema; infectious dermatitis; chronic eczematoid otitis externa; mycotic dermatoses

Usual Dosage Apply 3-4 times/day

Dosage Forms Cream: Iodoquinol 1% and hydrocortisone 1% (30 g)

IPOL™ *see* Poliovirus Vaccine, Inactivated *on page 875*

IPV *see* Poliovirus Vaccine, Inactivated *on page 875*

ISG *see* Immune Globulin, Intramuscular *on page 770*

Isoniazid (eye soe NYE a zid)

Related Information
Tuberculosis Guidelines *on page 1114*

U.S. Brand Names Laniazid®; Nydrazid®

Canadian Brand Names PMS-Isoniazid

Synonyms INH; Isonicotinic Acid Hydrazide

Generic Available Yes

Use Treatment of susceptible tuberculosis infections and prophylactically to those individuals exposed to tuberculosis

Drug of Choice or Alternative for
Organism(s)
Mycobacterium bovis *on page 203*
Mycobacterium kansasii *on page 204*
Mycobacterium tuberculosis *on page 207*

Pregnancy Risk Factor C

Contraindications Acute liver disease; hypersensitivity to isoniazid or any component; previous history of hepatic damage during isoniazid therapy

Warnings/Precautions Use with caution in patients with renal impairment and chronic liver disease. Severe and sometimes fatal hepatitis may occur or develop even after many months of treatment; patients must report any prodromal symptoms of hepatitis, such as fatigue, weakness, malaise, anorexia, nausea, or vomiting. Children with low milk and low meat intake should receive concomitant pyridoxine therapy. Periodic ophthalmic examinations are recommended even when usual symptoms do not occur; pyridoxine (10-50 mg/day) is recommended in individuals likely to develop peripheral neuropathies.

Adverse Reactions
>10%:
Gastrointestinal: Loss of appetite, nausea, vomiting, stomach pain
Hepatic: Mildly increased LFTs (10% to 20%)
Neuromuscular & skeletal: Weakness, peripheral neuropathy (dose-related incidence, 10% to 20% incidence with 10 mg/kg/day)
1% to 10%:
Central nervous system: Dizziness, slurred speech, lethargy
Hepatic: Progressive liver damage (increases with age; 2.3% in patients >50 years of age)
Neuromuscular & skeletal: Hyper-reflexia
<1%: Fever, seizures, mental depression, psychosis, rash, blood dyscrasias, arthralgia, blurred vision, loss of vision

Overdosage/Toxicology
Symptoms of overdose include nausea, vomiting, slurred speech, dizziness, blurred vision, hallucinations, stupor, coma, intractable seizures, onset of metabolic acidosis is 30 minutes to 3 hours. Because of the severe morbidity and high mortality rates with isoniazid overdose, patients who are asymptomatic after an overdose, should be monitored for 4-6 hours.
Pyridoxine has been shown to be effective in the treatment of intoxication, especially when seizures occur. Pyridoxine I.V. is administered on a milligram to milligram dose. If the amount of isoniazid ingested is unknown, 5 g of pyridoxine should be given over 3-5 minutes and may be followed by an additional 5 g in 30 minutes. Treatment is supportive; may require airway protection, ventilation; diazepam for seizures, sodium bicarbonate for acidosis; forced diuresis and hemodialysis can result in more rapid removal.

Drug Interactions CYP2E1 enzyme substrate; CYP2E1 enzyme inducer; and CYP1A2 enzyme inhibitor
Decreased effect of ketoconazole with isoniazid
Decreased effect/levels of isoniazid with aluminum salts
Increased toxicity/levels of oral anticoagulants, carbamazepine, cycloserine, meperidine, hydantoins, hepatically metabolized benzodiazepines with isoniazid; reaction with disulfiram occurs; enflurane with isoniazid may result in renal failure especially in rapid acetylators
Increased hepatic toxicity with alcohol or with rifampin and isoniazid

Stability Protect oral dosage forms from light

Mechanism of Action Unknown, but may include the inhibition of myocolic acid synthesis resulting in disruption of the bacterial cell wall

Pharmacodynamics/Kinetics
Absorption: Rapid and complete; rate can be slowed when orally administered with food
Distribution: Crosses the placenta; appears in breast milk; distributes into all body tissues and fluids including the CSF
Protein binding: 10% to 15%
Metabolism: By the liver with decay rate determined genetically by acetylation phenotype
Half-life:
Fast acetylators: 30-100 minutes
Slow acetylators: 2-5 hours; half-life may be prolonged in patients with impaired hepatic function or severe renal impairment
Time to peak serum concentration: Within 1-2 hours
Elimination: In urine (75% to 95%), feces, and saliva

Usual Dosage Recommendations often change due to resistant strains and newly developed information; consult *MMWR* for current CDC recommendations: Oral (injectable is available for patients who are unable to either take or absorb oral therapy):
Note: A four-drug regimen (isoniazid, rifampin, pyrazinamide, and either streptomycin or ethambutol) is preferred for the initial, empiric treatment of TB. When
(Continued)

Isoniazid *(Continued)*

the drug susceptibility results are available, the regimen should be altered as appropriate.

Infants and Children:

Prophylaxis: 10 mg/kg/day in 1-2 divided doses (maximum: 300 mg/day) 6 months in patients who do not have HIV infection and 12 months in patients who have HIV infection

Treatment:

Daily therapy: 10-20 mg/kg/day in 1-2 divided doses (maximum: 300 mg/day)

Directly observed therapy (DOT): Twice weekly therapy: 20-40 mg/kg (maximum: 900 mg/day); 3 times/week therapy: 20-40 mg/kg (maximum: 900 mg)

Adults:

Prophylaxis: 300 mg/day for 6 months in patients who do not have HIV infection and 12 months in patients who have HIV infection

Treatment:

Daily therapy: 5 mg/kg/day given daily (usual dose: 300 mg/day); 10 mg/kg/day in 1-2 divided doses in patients with disseminated disease

Directly observed therapy (DOT): Twice weekly therapy: 15 mg/kg (maximum: 900 mg); 3 times/week therapy: 15 mg/kg (maximum: 900 mg)

Note: Concomitant administration of 6-50 mg/day pyridoxine is recommended in malnourished patients or those prone to neuropathy (eg, alcoholics, diabetics)

Hemodialysis: Dialyzable (50% to 100%)
Administer dose postdialysis

Peritoneal dialysis effects: Dose for Cl_{cr} <10 mL/minute

Continuous arteriovenous or venovenous hemofiltration (CAVH/CAVHD): Dose for Cl_{cr} <10 mL/minute

Dosing adjustment in hepatic impairment: Dose should be reduced in severe hepatic disease

Monitoring Parameters Periodic liver function tests; monitoring for prodromal signs of hepatitis

Reference Range Therapeutic: 1-7 µg/mL (SI: 7-51 µmol/L); Toxic: 20-710 µg/mL (SI: 146-5176 µmol/L)

Test Interactions False-positive urinary glucose with Clinitest®

Patient Information Report any prodromal symptoms of hepatitis (fatigue, weakness, nausea, vomiting, dark urine, or yellowing of eyes) or any burning, tingling, or numbness in the extremities

Dosage Forms
Injection: 100 mg/mL (10 mL)
Syrup (orange flavor): 50 mg/5 mL (473 mL)
Tablet: 50 mg, 100 mg, 300 mg

Extemporaneous Preparations A 10 mg/mL oral suspension was stable for 21 days when refrigerated when compounded as follows:

Triturate ten 10 mg tablets in a mortar, reduce to a fine powder, then add 10 mL of purified water U.S.P. to make a paste; then transfer to a graduate and qs to 100 mL with sorbitol (do not use sugar-based solutions)

Shake well before using and keep in refrigerator

Nahata MC and Hipple TF, *Pediatric Drug Formulations*, 3rd ed, Cincinnati, OH: Harvey Whitney Books Co, 1997.

Selected Readings
Davidson PT and Le HQ, "Drug Treatment of Tuberculosis - 1992," *Drugs*, 1992, 43(5):651-73.
Havlir DV and Barnes PF, "Tuberculosis in Patients With Human Immunodeficiency Virus Infection," *N Engl J Med*, 1999, 340(5):367-73.
"Drugs for Tuberculosis," *Med Lett Drugs Ther*, 1993, 35(908):99-101.
Iseman MD, "Treatment of Multidrug-Resistant Tuberculosis," *N Engl J Med*, 1993, 329(11):784-91.
"Prevention and Treatment of Tuberculosis Among Patients Infected With Human Immunodeficiency Virus: Principles of Therapy and Revised Recommendations. Centers for Disease Control and Prevention," *MMWR Morb Mortal Wkly Rep*, 1998, 47(RR-20):1-58.
Van Scoy RE and Wilkowske CJ, "Antituberculosis Agents," *Mayo Clin Proc*, 1992, 67(2):179-87.

Isonicotinic Acid Hydrazide *see* Isoniazid *on page 782*

Isopto® Cetamide® Ophthalmic *see* Sulfacetamide Sodium *on page 927*

Isopto® Cetapred® Ophthalmic *see* Sulfacetamide Sodium and Prednisolone *on page 928*

Itraconazole (i tra KOE na zole)

U.S. Brand Names Sporanox®

Generic Available No

Use Treatment of susceptible fungal infections in immunocompromised and immunocompetent patients including blastomycosis and histoplasmosis; also indicated for aspergillosis, and onychomycosis of the toenail; treatment of onychomycosis of the fingernail without concomitant toenail infection via a pulse-type dosing regimen; has activity against *Aspergillus*, *Candida*, *Coccidioides*, *Cryptococcus*, *Sporothrix*, tinea unguium

Oral solution (not capsules) is marketed for oral and esophageal candidiasis

Useful in superficial mycoses including dermatophytoses (eg, tinea capitis), pityriasis versicolor, sebopsoriasis, vaginal and chronic mucocutaneous candidiases; systemic mycoses including candidiasis, meningeal and disseminated cryptococcal infections, paracoccidioidomycosis, coccidioidomycoses; miscellaneous mycoses such as sporotrichosis, chromomycosis, leishmaniasis, fungal keratitis, alternariosis, zygomycosis

Intravenous solution is indicated in the treatment of blastomycosis, histoplasmosis (nonmeningeal), and aspergillosis (in patients intolerant or refractory to amphotericin B therapy)

Drug of Choice or Alternative for

Organism(s)

Aspergillus Species *on page 70*
Blastomyces dermatitidis on page 78
Candida Species *on page 91*
Coccidioides immitis on page 109
Cryptococcus neoformans on page 117
Dematiaceous Fungi *on page 125*
Dermatophytes *on page 127*
Histoplasma capsulatum on page 173
Malassezia furfur on page 192
Penicillium marneffei on page 226

Pregnancy Risk Factor C

Contraindications Known hypersensitivity to other azoles; concomitant administration with astemizole, cisapride, lovastatin, midazolam, simvastatin, or triazolam

Warnings/Precautions Rare cases of serious cardiovascular adverse event, including death, ventricular tachycardia and torsade de pointes have been observed due to increased terfenadine and cisapride concentrations induced by itraconazole; patients who develop abnormal liver function tests during itraconazole therapy should be monitored and therapy discontinued if symptoms of liver disease develop

Adverse Reactions Listed incidences are for higher doses appropriate for systemic fungal infections

>10%: Gastrointestinal: Nausea (10.6%)

1% to 10%:

Cardiovascular: Edema (3.5%), hypertension (3.2%)
Central nervous system: Headache (4%), fatigue (2% to 3%), malaise (1.2%), fever (2.5%)
Dermatologic: Rash (8.6%)
Endocrine & metabolic: Decreased libido (1.2%), hypertriglyceridemia
Gastrointestinal: Abdominal pain (1.5%), vomiting (5%), diarrhea (3%)
Hepatic: Abnormal liver function (2.7%), hepatitis

<1%: Dizziness, somnolence, pruritus, hypokalemia, anorexia, impotence, albuminuria, adrenal suppression, gynecomastia

Overdosage/Toxicology

Overdoses are well tolerated

Following decontamination, if possible, supportive measures only are required; dialysis is not effective

Drug Interactions CYP3A3/4 enzyme inhibitor

Decreased effect:

Decreased serum levels with carbamazepine, didanosine, isoniazid, phenobarbital, phenytoin, rifabutin, and rifampin; may cause a decreased effect of oral contraceptives; alternative birth control is recommended

(Continued)

Itraconazole (Continued)

Decreased/undetectable serum levels with rifampin - **should not be administered concomitantly with rifampin**

Absorption requires gastric acidity; therefore, antacids, H$_2$ antagonists (cimetidine and ranitidine), omeprazole, and sucralfate significantly reduce bioavailability resulting in treatment failures and should not be administered concomitantly; amphotericin B or fluconazole should be used instead

Increased toxicity:

May increase cyclosporine or tacrolimus levels (by 50%) when high doses are used

Itraconazole increases serum levels of lovastatin (possibly 20-fold) and other HMG-CoA inhibitors due to inhibition of CYP3A4

May increase phenytoin serum concentration

May inhibit warfarins metabolism

May increase digoxin serum levels

May increase busulfan, cisapride, terfenadine, and vinca alkaloid levels - **concomitant administration is not recommended** due to increased risk of cardiotoxicity

Itraconazole may increase astemizole levels resulting in prolonged Q-T intervals - **concomitant administration is contraindicated**

May increase amlodipine, benzodiazepine, buspirone, corticosteroids, and oral hypoglycemics levels; use with caution in patients prescribed medications eliminated by P-450 3A4 metabolism

Stability Dilute with 0.9% sodium chloride only; do not dilute in dextrose or lactated Ringer's; may be stored refrigerated or at room temperature for 48 hours; use dedicated infusion line; do not mix with any other medication

Mechanism of Action Interferes with cytochrome P-450 activity, decreasing ergosterol synthesis (principal sterol in fungal cell membrane) and inhibiting cell membrane formation

Pharmacodynamics/Kinetics

Absorption: Requires gastric acidity; capsule better absorbed with food, solution better absorbed on empty stomach

Distribution: Apparent volume averaged 796±185 L or 10 L/kg; highly lipophilic and tissue concentrations are higher than plasma concentrations. The highest itraconazole concentrations are achieved in adipose, omentum, endometrium, cervical and vaginal mucus, and skin/nails. Aqueous fluids, such as cerebrospinal fluid and urine, contain negligible amounts of itraconazole; steady-state concentrations are achieved in 13 days with multiple administration of itraconazole 100-400 mg/day.

Protein binding: 99.9% bound to plasma proteins; metabolite hydroxy-itraconazole is 99.5% bound to plasma proteins

Metabolism: Extensive by the liver into >30 metabolites including hydroxy-itraconazole which is the major metabolite and appears to have in vitro antifungal activity. The main metabolic pathway is oxidation; may undergo saturation metabolism with multiple dosing

Bioavailability: Increased from 40% fasting to 100% postprandial; absolute oral bioavailability: 55%; hypochlorhydria has been reported in HIV-infected patients; therefore, oral absorption in these patients may be decreased

Half-life: Oral: After single 200 mg dose: 21±5 hours; 64 hours at steady-state; I.V.: steady-state: 35 hours

Elimination: ~3% to 18% excreted in feces; ~0.03% of parent drug excreted renally and 40% of dose excreted as inactive metabolites in urine

Usual Dosage Oral: Capsule: To facilitate absorption, administer itraconazole capsules after meals. Solution: Should be taken on an empty stomach. Absorption of both products is significantly increased when taken with a cola beverage.

Children: Efficacy and safety have not been established; a small number of patients 3-16 years of age have been treated with 100 mg/day for systemic fungal infections with no serious adverse effects reported

Adults:

Blastomycosis/histoplasmosis: 200 mg once daily, if no obvious improvement or there is evidence of progressive fungal disease, increase the dose in 100 mg increments to a maximum of 400 mg/day; doses >200 mg/day are given in 2 divided doses; length of therapy varies from 1 day to >6 months depending on the condition and mycological response

Aspergillosis: 200-400 mg/day

Onychomycosis: 200 mg once daily for 12 consecutive weeks

Life-threatening infections: Loading dose: 200 mg 3 times/day (600 mg/day) should be given for the first 3 days of therapy

Oropharyngeal and esophageal candidiasis: Oral solution: 100-200 mg once daily

I.V.: 200 mg twice daily for 4 doses, followed by 200 mg daily

Dosing adjustment in renal impairment: Not necessary; itraconazole infection is not recommended in patients with Cl$_{cr}$ <30 mL/minute

Hemodialysis: Not dialyzable

Dosing adjustment in hepatic impairment: May be necessary, but specific guidelines are not available

Dietary Considerations Food increases absorption of capsule and decreases absorption of the solution

Administration

Oral: Doses >200 mg/day are given in 2 divided doses; do not administer with antacids.

I.V.: Infuse over 1 hour

Patient Information Take capsule with food; take solution on an empty stomach; report any signs and symptoms that may suggest liver dysfunction so that the appropriate laboratory testing can be done; signs and symptoms may include unusual fatigue, anorexia, nausea and/or vomiting, jaundice, dark urine, or pale stool

Dosage Forms

Capsule: 100 mg

Injection kit: 10 mg/mL - 25 mL ampul, one 50 mL (100 mL capacity) bag 0.9% sodium chloride, one filtered infusion set

Solution, oral: 100 mg/10 mL (150 mL)

Selected Readings

Amichai B and Grunwald MH, "Adverse Drug Reactions of the New Oral Antifungal Agents - Terbinafine, Fluconazole, and Itraconazole," *Int J Dermatol*, 1998, 37(6):410-5.

Cleary JD, Taylor JW, and Chapman SW, "Itraconazole in Antifungal Therapy," *Ann Pharmacother*, 1992, 26(4):502-9.

Grant SM and Clissold SP, "Itraconazole. A Review of Its Pharmacodynamic and Pharmacokinetic Properties, and Therapeutic Use in Superficial and Systemic Mycoses," *Drugs*, 1989, 37(3):310-44.

Haria M, Bryson HM, and Goa KL, "Itraconazole: A Reappraisal of Its Pharmacological Properties and Therapeutic Use in the Management of Superficial Fungal Infections," *Drugs*, 1996, 51(4):585-620.

Jennings TS and Hardin TC, "Treatment of Aspergillosis With Itraconazole," *Ann Pharmacother*, 1993, 27(10):1206-11.

Kauffman CA and Carver PL, "Antifungal Agents in the 1990s. Current Status and Future Developments," *Drugs*, 1997, 53(4):539-49.

Lyman CA and Walsh TJ, "Systemically Administered Antifungal Agents. A Review of Their Clinical Pharmacology and Therapeutic Applications," *Drugs*, 1992, 44(1):9-35.

Terrell CL, "Antifungal Agents. Part II. The Azoles," *Mayo Clin Proc*, 1999, 74(1):78-100.

Trepanier EF and Amsden GW, "Current Issues in Onchomycosis," *Ann Pharmacother*, 1998, 32(2):204-14.

Iveegam® *see* Immune Globulin, Intramuscular *on page 770*

Ivermectin (eye ver MEK tin)

U.S. Brand Names Mectizan®; Stromectol®

Generic Available No

Use Treatment of the following infections: Strongyloidiasis of the intestinal tract due the nematode parasite *Strongyloides stercoralis*. Onchocerciasis due to the nematode parasite *Onchocerca volvulus*. Ivermectin is only active against the immature form of *Onchocerca volvulus*, and the intestinal forms of *Strongyloides stercoralis*. Ivermectin has been used for other parasitic infections including *Ascaris lumbricoides*, bancroftian filariasis, *Brugia malayi*, scabies, *Enterobius vermicularis*, *Mansonella ozzardi*, *Trichuris trichiura*

Drug of Choice or Alternative for

Organism(s)

Strongyloides stercoralis on page 281

Pregnancy Risk Factor C

Contraindications Hypersensitivity to Ivermectin or any component

Warnings/Precautions Data have shown that antihelmintic drugs like Ivermectin may cause cutaneous and/or systemic reactions (Mazzoti reaction) of (Continued)

Ivermectin *(Continued)*

varying severity including ophthalmological reactions in patients with onchocerciasis. These reactions are probably due to allergic and inflammatory responses to the death of microfilariae. Patients with hyper-reactive onchodermatitis may be more likely than others to experience severe adverse reactions, especially edema and aggravation of the onchodermatitis. Repeated treatment may be required in immunocompromised patients (eg, HIV); control of extraintestinal strongyloidiasis may necessitate suppressive (once monthly) therapy.

Adverse Reactions

Percentage unknown: Transient tachycardia, peripheral and facial edema, hypotension, mild EKG changes, dizziness, headache, somnolence, vertigo, insomnia, hyperthermia, pruritus, rash, urticaria, diarrhea, nausea, abdominal pain, vomiting, leukopenia, eosinophilia, increased ALT and AST, weakness, myalgia, tremor, limbitis, punctate opacity, mild conjunctivitis, blurred vision

Mazzotti reaction (with onchocerciasis): Pruritus, edema, rash, fever, lymphadenopathy, ocular damage

Overdosage/Toxicology

Accidental intoxication with, or significant exposure to unknown quantities of veterinary formulations of Ivermectin in humans, either by ingestion, inhalation, injection, or exposure to body surfaces, has resulted in the following adverse effects: rash, edema, headache, dizziness, asthenia, nausea, vomiting, and diarrhea; other adverse effects that have been reported include seizure and ataxia

Treatment is supportive; usual methods for decontamination are recommended

Mechanism of Action Ivermectin is a semisynthetic antihelminthic agent; it binds selectively and with strong affinity to glutamate-gated chloride ion channels which occur in invertebrate nerve and muscle cells. This leads to increased permeability of cell membranes to chloride ions then hyperpolarization of the nerve or muscle cell, and death of the parasite.

Pharmacodynamics/Kinetics

Peak response: 3-6 months

Absorption: Well absorbed

Distribution: Does not cross the blood-brain barrier

Half life: 16-35 hours

Metabolism: Hepatic, >97%

Elimination: <1% excreted in urine, the remainder in feces

Usual Dosage Oral:

Children ≥5 years: 150 mcg/kg as a single dose; treatment for onchocerciasis may need to be repeated every 3-12 months until the adult worms die

Adults:

Strongyloidiasis: 200 mcg/kg as a single dose; follow-up stool examinations

Onchocerciasis: 150 mcg/kg as a single dose; retreatment may be required every 3-12 months until the adult worms die

Monitoring Parameters Skin and eye microfilarial counts, periodic ophthalmologic exams

Patient Information If infected with strongyloidiasis, repeated stool examinations are required to document clearance of the organisms; repeated follow-up and retreatment is usually required in the treatment of onchocerciasis

Nursing Implications Ensure that patients take Ivermectin with water

Additional Information Available from:

The Centers for Disease Control Drug and Immunobiologic Service
1600 Clifton Road
Building 1
Room 1259
Atlanta, GA 30333
Monday-Friday 8 AM to 4:30 PM
(404) 639-3670
Nonbusiness hours (emergencies only): (404) 639-2888

Dosage Forms Tablet: 6 mg

Selected Readings

de Silva N, Guyatt H, and Bundy D, "Anthelmintics. A Comparative Review of Their Clinical Pharmacology," *Drugs*, 1997, 53(5):769-88.

"Drugs for Parasitic Infections," *Med Lett Drugs Ther*, 1998, 40(1017):1-12.

IVIG *see* Immune Globulin, Intravenous *on page 771*

Jaa Amp® Trihydrate *see* Ampicillin *on page 604*

Japanese Encephalitis Virus Vaccine, Inactivated
(jap a NEESE en sef a LYE tis VYE rus vak SEEN, in ak ti VAY ted)

U.S. Brand Names JE-VAX®

Use Active immunization against Japanese encephalitis for persons 1 year of age and older who plan to spend 1 month or more in endemic areas in Asia, especially persons traveling during the transmission season or visiting rural areas; consider vaccination for shorter trips to epidemic areas or extensive outdoor activities in rural endemic areas; elderly (>55 years of age) individuals should be considered for vaccination, since they have increased risk of developing symptomatic illness after infection; **those planning travel to or residence in endemic areas should consult the Travel Advisory Service (Central Campus) for specific advice**

Pregnancy Risk Factor C

Contraindications Serious adverse reaction (generalized urticaria or angioedema) to a prior dose of this vaccine; proven or suspected hypersensitivity to proteins or rodent or neural origin; hypersensitivity to thimerosal (used as a preservative). *CDC recommends that the following should not generally receive the vaccine, unless benefit to the individual clearly outweighs the risk:*

- those acutely ill or with active infections
- persons with heart, kidney, or liver disorders
- persons with generalized malignancies such as leukemia or lymphoma
- persons with a history of multiple allergies or hypersensitivity to components of the vaccine
- pregnant women, unless there is a very high risk of Japanese encephalitis during the woman's stay in Asia

Warnings/Precautions Severe adverse reactions manifesting as generalized urticaria or angioedema may occur within minutes following vaccination, or up to 17 days later; most reactions occur within 10 days, with the majority within 48 hours; observe vaccinees for 30 minutes after vaccination; warn them of the possibility of delayed generalized urticaria and to remain where medical care is readily available for 10 days following any dose of the vaccine; because of the potential for severe adverse reactions, Japanese encephalitis vaccine is **not** recommended for all persons traveling to or residing in Asia; safety and efficacy in infants <1 year of age have not been established; therefore, immunization of infants should be deferred whenever possible; it is not known whether the vaccine is excreted in breast milk

Adverse Reactions Report allergic or unusual adverse reactions to the Vaccine Adverse Event Reporting System (VAERS) 1-800-822-7967.

Percentage unknown: Commonly tenderness, redness, and swelling at injection site; systemic side effects include fever, headache, malaise, rash, chills, dizziness, myalgia, nausea, vomiting, abdominal pain, urticaria, itching with or without accompanying rash, and hypotension; rarely, anaphylactic reaction, encephalitis, encephalopathy, seizure, peripheral neuropathy, erythema multiforme, erythema nodosum, angioedema, dyspnea, and joint swelling

Drug Interactions Simultaneous administration of DTP vaccine and Japanese encephalitis vaccine does not compromise the immunogenicity of either vaccine; data on administration with other vaccines, chloroquine, or mefloquine are lacking

Stability Refrigerate, discard 8 hours after reconstitution

Usual Dosage U.S. recommended primary immunization schedule:

Children >3 years and Adults: S.C.: Three 1 mL doses given on days 0, 7, and 30. Give third dose on day 14 when time does not permit waiting; 2 doses a week apart produce immunity in about 80% of vaccines; the longest regimen yields highest titers after 6 months.

Children 1-3 years: S.C.: Three 0.5 mL doses given on days 0, 7, and 30; abbreviated schedules should be used only when necessary due to time constraints

Booster dose: Give after 2 years, or according to current recommendation

Note: Travel should not commence for at least 10 days after the last dose of vaccine, to allow adequate antibody formation and recognition of any delayed adverse reaction

(Continued)

Japanese Encephalitis Virus Vaccine, Inactivated
(Continued)

Advise concurrent use of other means to reduce the risk of mosquito exposure when possible, including bed nets, insect repellents, protective clothing, avoidance of travel in endemic areas, and avoidance of outdoor activity during twilight and evening periods

Patient Information Adverse reactions may occur shortly after vaccination or up to 17 days (usually within 10 days) after vaccination

Additional Information Japanese encephalitis vaccine is currently available only from the Centers for Disease Control. Contact Centers for Disease Control at (404) 639-6370 (Mon-Fri) or (404) 639-2888 (nights, weekends, or holidays).

Dosage Forms Powder for injection, lyophilized: 1 mL, 10 mL

Jenamicin® Injection *see Gentamicin on page 747*

JE-VAX® *see Japanese Encephalitis Virus Vaccine, Inactivated on previous page*

Kanamycin (kan a MYE sin)
Related Information
Tuberculosis Guidelines *on page 1114*
U.S. Brand Names Kantrex®
Synonyms Kanamycin Sulfate
Generic Available Yes
Use

Oral: Preoperative bowel preparation in the prophylaxis of infections and adjunctive treatment of hepatic coma (oral kanamycin is not indicated in the treatment of systemic infections); treatment of susceptible bacterial infection including gram-negative aerobes, gram-positive *Bacillus* as well as some mycobacteria

Parenteral: Rarely used in antibiotic irrigations during surgery

Pregnancy Risk Factor D

Contraindications Hypersensitivity to kanamycin or any component or other aminoglycosides

Warnings/Precautions Use with caution in patients with pre-existing renal insufficiency, vestibular or cochlear impairment, myasthenia gravis, conditions which depress neuromuscular transmission

Parenteral aminoglycosides are associated with nephrotoxicity or ototoxicity; the ototoxicity may be proportional to the amount of drug given and the duration of treatment; tinnitus or vertigo are indications of vestibular injury and impending hearing loss; renal damage is usually reversible

Adverse Reactions Percentage unknown: Edema, neurotoxicity, drowsiness, headache, pseudomotor cerebri, skin itching, redness, rash, photosensitivity, erythema, nausea, vomiting, diarrhea (most common with oral form), malabsorption syndrome with prolonged and high-dose therapy of hepatic coma; anorexia, weight loss, increased salivation, enterocolitis, granulocytopenia, agranulocytosis, thrombocytopenia, burning, stinging, weakness, tremors, muscle cramps, ototoxicity (auditory), ototoxicity (vestibular), nephrotoxicity, dyspnea

Overdosage/Toxicology

Symptoms of overdose include ototoxicity, nephrotoxicity, and neuromuscular toxicity

The treatment of choice following a single acute overdose appears to be the maintenance of good urine output of at least 3 mL/kg/hour. Dialysis is of questionable value in the enhancement of aminoglycoside elimination. If required, hemodialysis is preferred over peritoneal dialysis in patients with normal renal function. Careful hydration may be all that is required to promote diuresis and, therefore, the enhancement of the drug's elimination.

Drug Interactions

Increased toxicity:

Penicillins, cephalosporins, amphotericin B, diuretics may increase nephrotoxicity; polypeptide antibiotics may increase risk of respiratory paralysis and renal dysfunction

Neuromuscular blocking agents with oral kanamycin may increase neuromuscular blockade; a small increase in warfarin's effect may occur due to decreased absorption of vitamin K

Decreased toxicity: Methotrexate with kanamycin (oral) may be less well absorbed as may digoxin (minor) and vitamin A

Stability Darkening of vials does not indicate loss of potency

Mechanism of Action Interferes with protein synthesis in bacterial cell by binding to ribosomal subunit

Pharmacodynamics/Kinetics

Absorption: Oral: Not absorbed following administration

Relative diffusion of antimicrobial agents from blood into cerebrospinal fluid (CSF): Good only with inflammation (exceeds usual MICs)

Ratio of CSF to blood level (%):

Normal meninges: Nil

Inflamed meninges: 43

Half-life: 2-4 hours, increases in anuria to 80 hours

End stage renal disease: 40-96 hours

Time to peak serum concentration: I.M.: 1-2 hours

Elimination: Entirely in the kidney, principally by glomerular filtration

Usual Dosage

Children: Infections: I.M., I.V.: 15 mg/kg/day in divided doses every 8-12 hours

Adults:

Infections: I.M., I.V.: 5-7.5 mg/kg/dose in divided doses every 8-12 hours (<15 mg/kg/day)

Preoperative intestinal antisepsis: Oral: 1 g every 4-6 hours for 36-72 hours

Hepatic coma: Oral: 8-12 g/day in divided doses

Intraperitoneal: After contamination in surgery: 500 mg diluted in 20 mL distilled water; other irrigations: 0.25% solutions

Aerosol: 250 mg 2-4 times/day (250 mg diluted with 3 mL of NS and nebulized)

Dosing adjustment/interval in renal impairment:

Cl_{cr} 50-80 mL/minute: Administer 60% to 90% of dose or administer every 8-12 hours

Cl_{cr} 10-50 mL/minute: Administer 30% to 70% of dose or administer every 12 hours

Cl_{cr} <10 mL/minute: Administer 20% to 30% of dose or administer every 24-48 hours

Hemodialysis: Dialyzable (50% to 100%)

Administration Adults: Dilute to 100-200 mL and infuse over 30 minutes; give I.M. deeply in gluteal muscle

Monitoring Parameters Serum creatinine and BUN every 2-3 days; peak and trough concentrations; hearing

Reference Range Therapeutic: Peak: 25-35 µg/mL; Trough: 4-8 µg/mL; Toxic: Peak: >35 µg/mL; Trough: >10 µg/mL

Patient Information Report any dizziness or sensations of ringing or fullness in ears

Dosage Forms

Capsule, as sulfate: 500 mg

Injection, as sulfate:

Pediatric: 75 mg (2 mL)

Adults: 500 mg (2 mL); 1 g (3 mL)

Selected Readings

Begg EJ and Barclay ML, "Aminoglycosides - 50 Years On," *Br J Clin Pharmacol*, 1995, 39(6):597-603.

Cunha BA, "Aminoglycosides: Current Role in Antimicrobial Therapy," *Pharmacotherapy*, 1988, 8(6):334-50.

"Drugs for Tuberculosis," *Med Lett Drugs Ther*, 1993, 35(908):99-101.

Iseman MD, "Treatment of Multidrug-Resistant Tuberculosis," *N Engl J Med*, 1993, 329(11):784-91.

Kanamycin Sulfate *see Kanamycin on previous page*

Kantrex® *see Kanamycin on previous page*

Keflex® *see Cephalexin on page 660*

Keftab® *see Cephalexin on page 660*

Kefurox® Injection *see Cefuroxime on page 658*

Kefzol® *see Cefazolin on page 632*

Ketoconazole (kee toe KOE na zole)

U.S. Brand Names Nizoral®

Generic Available No

(Continued)

Ketoconazole *(Continued)*

Use Treatment of susceptible fungal infections, including candidiasis, oral thrush, blastomycosis, histoplasmosis, paracoccidioidomycosis, coccidioidomycosis, chromomycosis, candiduria, chronic mucocutaneous candidiasis, as well as, certain recalcitrant cutaneous dermatophytoses; used topically for treatment of tinea corporis, tinea cruris, tinea versicolor, and cutaneous candidiasis, seborrheic dermatitis

Drug of Choice or Alternative for
Organism(s)

Pregnancy Risk Factor C

Contraindications Hypersensitivity to ketoconazole or any component; CNS fungal infections (due to poor CNS penetration); coadministration with terfenadine, astemizole, or cisapride is contraindicated due to risk of potentially fatal cardiac arrhythmias

Warnings/Precautions Rare cases of serious cardiovascular adverse event, including death, ventricular tachycardia and torsade de pointes have been observed due to increased terfenadine concentrations induced by ketoconazole. Use with caution in patients with impaired hepatic function; has been associated with hepatotoxicity, including some fatalities; perform periodic liver function tests; high doses of ketoconazole may depress adrenocortical function.

Adverse Reactions
Oral:
  1% to 10%:
    Dermatologic: Pruritus (1.5%)
    Gastrointestinal: Nausea/vomiting (3% to 10%), abdominal pain (1.2%)
  <1%: Headache, dizziness, somnolence, fever, chills, bulging fontanelles, depression, gynecomastia, diarrhea, impotence, thrombocytopenia, leukopenia, hemolytic anemia, hepatotoxicity, photophobia
Cream: Severe irritation, pruritus, stinging (~5%)
Shampoo: Increases in normal hair loss, irritation (<1%), abnormal hair texture, scalp pustules, mild dryness of skin, itching, oiliness/dryness of hair

Overdosage/Toxicology
Symptoms of overdose include dizziness, headache, nausea, vomiting, diarrhea; overdoses are well tolerated
Treatment includes supportive measures and gastric decontamination

Drug Interactions CYP3A3/4 enzyme substrate; CYP1A2, 3A3/4, and 3A5-7 enzyme inhibitor
Decreased effect:
  Decreased ketoconazole serum levels with isoniazid and phenytoin; decreased/undetectable serum levels with rifampin - **should not be administered concomitantly with rifampin;** theophylline and oral hypoglycemic serum levels may be decreased
  Absorption requires gastric acidity; therefore, antacids, H$_2$ antagonists (cimetidine and ranitidine), omeprazole, and sucralfate significantly reduce bioavailability resulting in treatment failures; should not be administered concomitantly
Increased toxicity:
  May increase cyclosporine levels (by 50%) when high doses are used
  Inhibits warfarin metabolism resulting in increased anticoagulant effect
  Increases corticosteroid bioavailability and decreases steroid clearance
  Increases phenytoin, digoxin, terfenadine, astemizole, and cisapride concentrations; **concomitant administration with astemizole or cisapride is contraindicated;** may significantly increase levels and toxicity of lovastatin and simvastatin due to CYP3A4 inhibition; a disulfiram-type reaction may occur with concomitant ethanol

Mechanism of Action Alters the permeability of the cell wall by blocking fungal cytochrome P-450; inhibits biosynthesis of triglycerides and phospholipids by fungi; inhibits several fungal enzymes that results in a build-up of toxic concentrations of hydrogen peroxide

Pharmacodynamics/Kinetics

Absorption: Oral: Rapid (~75%); no detectable absorption following use of the shampoo

Distribution: Well distributed to inflamed joint fluid, saliva, bile, urine, breast milk, sebum, cerumen, feces, tendons, skin and soft tissues, and testes; crosses blood-brain barrier poorly; only negligible amounts reach CSF

Protein binding: 93% to 96%

Metabolism: Partially in the liver by enzymes to inactive compounds

Bioavailability: Decreases as pH of the gastric contents increases

Half-life, biphasic:

Initial: 2 hours

Terminal: 8 hours

Time to peak serum concentration: 1-2 hours

Elimination: Primarily in feces (57%) with smaller amounts excreted in urine (13%)

Usual Dosage

Oral:

Children ≥2 years: 3.3-6.6 mg/kg/day as a single dose for 1-2 weeks for candidiasis, for at least 4 weeks in recalcitrant dermatophyte infections, and for up to 6 months for other systemic mycoses

Adults: 200-400 mg/day as a single daily dose for durations as stated above

Shampoo: Apply twice weekly for 4 weeks with at least 3 days between each shampoo

Topical: Rub gently into the affected area once daily to twice daily

Dosing adjustment in hepatic impairment: Dose reductions should be considered in patients with severe liver disease

Hemodialysis: Not dialyzable (0% to 5%)

Monitoring Parameters Liver function tests

Patient Information Cream is for topical application to the skin only; avoid contact with the eye; avoid taking antacids at the same time as ketoconazole; may take with food; may cause drowsiness, impair judgment or coordination. Notify physician of unusual fatigue, anorexia, vomiting, dark urine, or pale stools.

Nursing Implications Administer 2 hours prior to antacids to prevent decreased absorption due to the high pH of gastric contents

Dosage Forms

Cream: 2% (15 g, 30 g, 60 g)

Shampoo: 2% (120 mL)

Tablet: 200 mg

Extemporaneous Preparations A 20 mg/mL suspension may be made by pulverizing twelve 200 mg ketoconazole tablets to a fine powder; add 40 mL Ora-Plus® in small portions with thorough mixing; incorporate Ora-Sweet® to make a final volume of 120 mL and mix thoroughly; refrigerate (no stability information is available)

Allen LV, "Ketoconazole Oral Suspension," *US Pharm*, 1993, 18(2):98-9, 101.

Selected Readings

Como JA and Dismukes WE, "Oral Azole Drugs as Systemic Antifungal Therapy," *N Engl J Med*, 1993, 330(4):263-72.

Lyman CA and Walsh TJ, "Systemically Administered Antifungal Agents. A Review of Their Clinical Pharmacology and Therapeutic Applications," *Drugs*, 1992, 44(1):9-35.

Terrell CL, "Antifungal Agents. Part II. The Azoles," *Mayo Clin Proc*, 1999, 74(1):78-100.

KI *see* Potassium Iodide *on page 879*

Klaron® Lotion *see* Sulfacetamide Sodium *on page 927*

Kwell® *see* Lindane *on page 797*

Kwellada™ *see* Lindane *on page 797*

L-AmB *see* Amphotericin B, Liposomal *on page 602*

Lamisil® *see* Terbinafine *on page 936*

Lamivudine (la MI vyoo deen)

Related Information

HIV Therapeutic Information *on page 1008*

U.S. Brand Names Epivir®; Epivir® HBV

Synonyms 3TC

(Continued)

Lamivudine *(Continued)*

Use Treatment of HIV infection when antiretroviral therapy is warranted; should always be used as part of a multidrug regimen (at least three antiretroviral agents); indicated for the treatment of chronic hepatitis B associated with evidence of hepatitis B viral replication and active liver inflammation

Drug of Choice or Alternative for Organism(s)

Hepatitis B Virus *on page 162*

Human Immunodeficiency Virus *on page 177*

Pregnancy Risk Factor C

Pregnancy/Breast-Feeding Implications

Clinical effects on the fetus: Use only if the potential benefits outweigh the risks. Combination therapy with zidovudine and lamivudine is currently being investigated to decrease the maternal/fetal transmission of HIV.

Breast-feeding/lactation: HIV-infected mothers are discouraged from breast-feeding to decrease postnatal transmission of HIV

Contraindications Hypersensitivity to lamivudine or any component

Warnings/Precautions A decreased dosage is recommended in patients with renal dysfunction since AUC, C_{max}, and half-life increased with diminishing renal function; use with extreme caution in children with history of pancreatitis or risk factors for development of pancreatitis. Do not use as monotherapy in treatment of HIV.

Adverse Reactions

>10%:

Central nervous system: Headache, insomnia, malaise, fatigue, pain

Gastrointestinal: Nausea, diarrhea, vomiting

Neuromuscular & skeletal: Peripheral neuropathy, paresthesia

Respiratory: Nasal signs and symptoms, cough

1% to 10%:

Central nervous system: Dizziness, depression, fever, chills

Dermatologic: Rashes

Gastrointestinal: Anorexia, abdominal pain, dyspepsia, elevated amylase

Hematologic: Neutropenia, anemia

Hepatic: Increased AST, ALT

Neuromuscular & skeletal: Myalgia, arthralgia

<1%: Pancreatitis, thrombocytopenia, hyperbilirubinemia

Overdosage/Toxicology

Very limited information is available although there have been no clinical signs or symptoms noted and hematologic tests remained normal in overdose

No antidote is available; unknown dialyzability

Drug Interactions Increased effect: Zidovudine concentrations increase (~39%) with coadministration with lamivudine; trimethoprim/sulfamethoxazole increases lamivudine's AUC and decreases its renal clearance by 44% and 29%, respectively; although the AUC was not significantly affected, absorption of lamivudine was slowed and C_{max} was 40% lower when administered to patients in the fed versus the fasted state

Stability Store solution at 2°C to 25°C tightly closed

Mechanism of Action After lamivudine is triphosphorylated, the principle mode of action is inhibition of HIV reverse transcription via viral DNA chain termination; inhibits RNA- and DNA-dependent DNA polymerase activities of reverse transcriptase. The monophosphate form of lamivudine is incorporated into the viral DNA by hepatitis B virus polymerase, resulting in DNA chain termination.

Pharmacodynamics/Kinetics

Absorption: Oral: Rapid

Distribution: V_d: 1.3 L/kg

Protein binding, plasma: <36%

Metabolism: 5.6% metabolized to trans-sulfoxide metabolite

Bioavailability: Absolute; Cp_{max} decreased with food although AUC not significantly affected

Children: 66%

Adults: 87%

Half-life:

Children: 2 hours

Adults: 5-7 hours

Elimination: Most eliminated unchanged in urine

Usual Dosage Oral: Use with at least two other antiretroviral agents when treating HIV

Children 3 months to 12 years: 4 mg/kg twice daily (maximum: 150 mg twice daily)

Adolescents 12-16 years and Adults: 150 mg twice daily

Prevention of HIV following needlesticks: 150 mg twice daily (with zidovudine and a protease inhibitor)

Adults <50 kg: 2 mg/kg twice daily

Treatment of hepatitis B: 100 mg/day

Dosing interval in renal impairment in patients >16 years for HIV:
Cl_{cr} 30-49 mL/minute: Administer 150 mg once daily
Cl_{cr} 15-29 mL/minute: Administer 150 mg first dose, then 100 mg once daily
Cl_{cr} 5-14 mL/minute: Administer 150 mg first dose, then 50 mg once daily
Cl_{cr} <5 mL/minute: Administer 50 mg first dose, then 25 mg once daily

Dosing interval in renal impairment in patients with hepatitis B:
Cl_{cr} 30-49: Administer 100 mg first dose then 50 mg once daily
Cl_{cr} 15-29: Administer 100 mg first dose then 25 mg once daily
Cl_{cr} 5-14: Administer 35 mg first dose then 15 mg once daily
Cl_{cr} <5: Administer 35 mg first dose then 10 mg once daily

Dialysis: No data available

Monitoring Parameters Amylase, bilirubin, liver enzymes, hematologic parameters, viral load, and CD4 count; signs and symptoms of pancreatitis

Patient Information Patients may still experience illnesses associated with HIV infection; lamivudine is not a cure for HIV infection nor has it been shown to reduce the risk of transmission to others; long-term effects are unknown; take exactly as prescribed; children should be monitored for symptoms of pancreatitis

Additional Information Lamivudine has been well studied in the treatment of chronic hepatitis B infection. Potential compliance problems, frequency of administration and adverse effects should be discussed with patients before initiating therapy to help prevent the emergence of resistance.

Dosage Forms

Solution, oral: 5 mg/mL (240 mL); 10 mg/mL (240 mL)

Tablet: 100 mg, 150 mg

Selected Readings

Dienstag JL, Perrillo, RP, Schiff, ER, et al, "A Preliminary Trial of Lamivudine for Chronic Hepatitis B Infection," *N Engl J Med*, 1995, 333(25):1657-61.

Eron JJ, Benoit SL, Jemsek J, et al, "Treatment with Lamivudine, Zidovudine, or Both in HIV-Positive Patients with 200 to 500 CD4+ Cells per Cubic Millimeter," *N Engl J Med*, 1995, 333(25):1662-9.

Lai CL, Chien RN, Leung NW, et al, "A One-Year Trial of Lamivudine for Chronic Hepatitis B," *N Engl J Med*, 1998, 339(2):61-8.

Perry CM and Faulds D, "Lamivudine. A Review of Its Antiviral Activity, Pharmacokinetic Properties and Therapeutic Efficacy in the Management of HIV Infection," *Drugs*, 1997, 53(4):657-80.

Lamprene® *see* Clofazimine *on page 687*

Laniazid® *see* Isoniazid *on page 782*

Lariam® *see* Mefloquine *on page 809*

LazerSporin-C® Otic *see* Neomycin, Polymyxin B, and Hydrocortisone *on page 836*

Levaquin™ *see* Levofloxacin *on this page*

Levofloxacin (lee voe FLOKS a sin)

U.S. Brand Names Levaquin™

Use Acute maxillary sinusitis due to *S. pneumoniae*, *H. influenzae*, or *M. catarrhalis*; treatment of uncomplicated urinary tract infection due to *E. coli*, *K. pneumoniae*, or *S. saprophyticus*; used for acute bacterial exacerbation of chronic bronchitis and community-acquired pneumonia due to *S. aureus*, *S. pneumoniae*, *H. influenzae*, *H. parainfluenzae*, or *M. catarrhalis*, *C. pneumoniae*, *L. pneumophila*, or *M. pneumoniae*; may be used for uncomplicated skin and skin structure infection (due to *S. aureus* or *S. pyogenes*) and complicated urinary tract infection due to gram-negative *Enterobacter* sp, including acute pyelonephritis (caused by *E. coli*)

Drug of Choice or Alternative for

Disease/Syndrome(s)

Pneumonia, Community-Acquired *on page 45*

Pregnancy Risk Factor C

(Continued)

Levofloxacin *(Continued)*

Pregnancy/Breast-Feeding Implications

Clinical effects on the fetus: Avoid use in pregnant women unless the benefit justifies the potential risk to the fetus

Breast-feeding/lactation: Quinolones are known to distribute well into breast milk; consequently, use during lactation should be avoided, if possible

Contraindications Hypersensitivity to levofloxacin, any component, or other quinolones; pregnancy, lactation

Warnings/Precautions Not recommended in children <18 years of age; other quinolones have caused transient arthropathy in children; CNS stimulation may occur (tremor, restlessness, confusion, and very rarely hallucinations or seizures); use with caution in patients with known or suspected CNS disorders or renal dysfunction; prolonged use may result in superinfection; if an allergic reaction (itching, urticaria, dyspnea, pharyngeal or facial edema, loss of consciousness, tingling, cardiovascular collapse) occurs, discontinue the drug immediately; use caution to avoid possible photosensitivity reactions during and for several days following fluoroquinolone therapy; pseudomembranous colitis may occur and should be considered in patients who present with diarrhea

Adverse Reactions >1%:

Central nervous system: Dizziness, headache, insomnia

Dermatologic: Rash

Gastrointestinal: Nausea, vomiting

Hematologic: Leukopenia, thrombocytopenia

Hepatic: Increased transaminases

Neuromuscular & skeletal: Tremor, arthralgia

Overdosage/Toxicology

Symptoms of overdose include acute renal failure, seizures

Treatment should include GI decontamination and supportive care; not removed by peritoneal or hemodialysis

Drug Interactions CYP1A2 enzyme inhibitor (minor)

Decreased effect: Decreased absorption with antacids containing aluminum, magnesium, and/or calcium (by up to 98% if given at the same time); phenytoin serum levels may be reduced by quinolones; antineoplastic agents may also decrease serum levels of fluoroquinolones

Increased toxicity/serum levels: Quinolones may cause increased levels of digoxin, caffeine, warfarin, cyclosporine. Cimetidine and probenecid increase quinolone levels; an increased incidence of seizures may occur with foscarnet.

Stability Stable for 72 hours when diluted to 5 mg/mL in a compatible I.V. fluid and stored at room temperature; stable for 14 days when stored at room temperature; stable for 6 months when frozen, do not refreeze; do not thaw in microwave or by bath immersion; **incompatible** with mannitol and sodium bicarbonate

Mechanism of Action As the S (-) enantiomer of the fluoroquinolone, ofloxacin, levofloxacin, inhibits DNA-gyrase in susceptible organisms thereby inhibits relaxation of supercoiled DNA and promotes breakage of DNA strands. DNA gyrase (topoisomerase II), is an essential bacterial enzyme that maintains the superhelical structure of DNA and is required for DNA replication and transcription, DNA repair, recombination, and transposition.

Pharmacodynamics/Kinetics

Absorption: Well absorbed

Distribution: V_d: 1.25 L/kg; CSF concentrations ~15% of serum levels; high concentrations are achieved in prostate and gynecological tissues, sinus, breast milk, and saliva

Protein binding: 50%

Metabolism: Hepatic, minimal

Half-life: 6 hours

Bioavailability: 100%

Time to peak serum concentration: 1 hour

Elimination: Most excreted unchanged in urine

Usual Dosage Adults: Oral, I.V. (infuse I.V. solution over 60 minutes):

Acute bacterial exacerbation of chronic bronchitis: 500 mg every 24 hours for at least 7 days

Community-acquired pneumonia: 500 mg every 24 hours for 7-14 days

Acute maxillary sinusitis: 500 mg every 24 hours for 10-14 days

Uncomplicated skin infections: 500 mg every 24 hours for 7-10 days

Uncomplicated urinary tract infections: 250 mg once daily for 3 days

Complicated urinary tract infections include acute pyelonephritis: 250 mg every 24 hours for 10 days

Dosing adjustment in renal impairment:
Cl$_{cr}$ 20-49 mL/minute: Administer 250 mg every 24 hours (initial: 500 mg)
Cl$_{cr}$ 10-19 mL/minute: Administer 250 mg every 48 hours (initial: 500 mg for most infections; 250 mg for renal infections)
Hemodialysis/CAPD: 250 mg every 48 hours (initial: 500 mg)

Monitoring Parameters Evaluation of organ system functions (renal, hepatic, ophthalmologic, and hematopoietic) is recommended periodically during therapy; the possibility of crystalluria should be assessed; WBC and signs of infection

Patient Information May be taken with or without food; drink plenty of fluids; avoid exposure to direct sunlight during therapy and for several days following; do not take antacids within 4 hours before or 2 hours after dosing; contact your physician immediately if signs of allergy occur; do not discontinue therapy until your course has been completed; take a missed dose as soon as possible, unless it is almost time for your next dose.

Nursing Implications Infuse I.V. solutions over 60 minutes

Dosage Forms
Infusion, in D$_5$W: 5 mg/mL (50 mL, 100 mL)
Injection: 25 mg/mL (20 mL)
Tablet: 250 mg, 500 mg

Selected Readings
Ernst ME, Ernst EJ, and Klepser ME, "Levofloxacin and Trovafloxacin: The Next Generation of Fluoroquinolones?" *Am J Health Syst Pharm*, 1997, 54(22):2569-84.

Hoogkamp-Korstanje JA, "*In vitro* Activities of Ciprofloxacin, Levofloxacin, Lomefloxacin, Ofloxacin, Pefloxacin, Sparfloxacin, and Trovafloxacin Against Gram-Positive and Gram-Negative Pathogens From Respiratory Tract Infections," *J Antimicrob Chemother*, 1997, 40(3):427-31.

Martin SJ, Meyer JM, Chuck SK, et al, "Levofloxacin and Sparfloxacin: New Quinolone Antibiotics," *Ann Pharmacother*, 1998, 32(3):320-36.

North DS, Fish DN, and Redington JJ, "Levofloxacin, A Second-Generation Fluoroquinolone," *Pharmacotherapy*, 1998, 18(5):915-35.

Pfaller MA and Jones RN, "Comparative Antistreptococcal Activity of Two Newer Fluoroquinolones, Levofloxacin and Sparfloxacin," *Diagn Microbiol Infect Dis*, 1997, 29(3):199-201.

"Sparfloxacin and Levofloxacin," *Med Lett Drugs Ther*, 1997, 39(999):41-3.

Lice-Enz® Shampoo [OTC] *see* Pyrethrins *on page 885*

Lindane (LIN dane)

U.S. Brand Names G-well®; Kwell®; Scabene®

Canadian Brand Names Hexit®; Kwellada™; PMS-Lindane

Synonyms Benzene Hexachloride; Gamma Benzene Hexachloride; Hexachlorocyclohexane

Generic Available Yes

Use Treatment of scabies (*Sarcoptes scabiei*), *Pediculus capitis* (head lice), and *Pediculus pubis* (crab lice); FDA recommends reserving lindane as a second-line agent or with inadequate response to other therapies

Drug of Choice or Alternative for
Organism(s)
Lice *on page 188*
Sarcoptes scabiei on page 247

Pregnancy Risk Factor B

Pregnancy/Breast-Feeding Implications Clinical effects on the fetus: There are no well controlled studies in pregnant women; treat no more than twice during a pregnancy

Contraindications Hypersensitivity to lindane or any component; premature neonates; acutely inflamed skin or raw, weeping surfaces

Warnings/Precautions Not considered a drug of first choice; use with caution in infants and small children, and patients with a history of seizures; avoid contact with face, eyes, mucous membranes, and urethral meatus. Because of the potential for systemic absorption and CNS side effects, lindane should be used with caution; consider permethrin or crotamiton agent first.

Adverse Reactions <1%: Cardiac arrhythmia, dizziness, restlessness, headache, ataxia, eczematous eruptions, contact dermatitis, skin and adipose tissue may act as repositories, nausea, vomiting, aplastic anemia, hepatitis, burning and stinging, hematuria, pulmonary edema
(Continued)

Lindane *(Continued)*

Overdosage/Toxicology

Symptoms of overdose include vomiting, restlessness, ataxia, seizures, arrhythmias, pulmonary edema, hematuria, hepatitis. Absorbed through skin and mucous membranes and GI tract, has occasionally caused serious CNS, hepatic and renal toxicity when used excessively for prolonged periods, or when accidental ingestion has occurred.

If ingested, perform gastric lavage and general supportive measures; diazepam 0.01 mg/kg can be used to control seizures.

Drug Interactions Increased toxicity: Oil-based hair dressing may increase toxic potential

Mechanism of Action Directly absorbed by parasites and ova through the exoskeleton; stimulates the nervous system resulting in seizures and death of parasitic arthropods

Pharmacodynamics/Kinetics

Absorption: Systemic absorption of up to 13% may occur

Distribution: Stored in body fat and accumulates in brain; skin and adipose tissue may act as repositories

Metabolism: By the liver

Half-life: Children: 17-22 hours

Time to peak serum concentration: Topical: Children: 6 hours

Elimination: In urine and feces

Usual Dosage Children and Adults: Topical:

Scabies: Apply a thin layer of lotion or cream and massage it on skin from the neck to the toes (head to toe in infants). For adults, bathe and remove the drug after 8-12 hours; for children, wash off 6-8 hours after application (for infants, wash off 6 hours after application); repeat treatment in 7 days if lice or nits are still present

Pediculosis, capitis and pubis: 15-30 mL of shampoo is applied and lathered for 4-5 minutes; rinse hair thoroughly and comb with a fine tooth comb to remove nits; repeat treatment in 7 days if lice or nits are still present

Administration Drug should not be administered orally, for topical use only; apply to dry, cool skin

Patient Information Topical use only, do not apply to face, avoid getting in eyes; do **not** apply lotion immediately after a hot, soapy bath. Clothing and bedding should be washed in hot water or by dry cleaning to kill the scabies mite. Combs and brushes may be washed with lindane shampoo then thoroughly rinsed with water. Notify physician if condition worsens; treat sexual contact simultaneously.

Dosage Forms

Cream: 1% (60 g, 454 g)

Lotion: 1% (60 mL, 473 mL, 4000 mL)

Shampoo: 1% (60 mL, 473 mL, 4000 mL)

Selected Readings

Liu LX and Weller PF, "Antiparasitic Drugs," *N Engl J Med*, 1996, 334(18):1178-84.

Linezolid *(li NE zoh lid)*

Synonyms PNU-100766

Use Investigational use: Has been studied in the treatment of a variety of infections caused by *Enterococcus faecium* and *E. faecalis* including vancomycin-resistant strains. Also has activity against many streptococcal species and many upper respiratory tract pathogens.

Contraindications Hypersensitivity to linezolid

Pharmacodynamics/Kinetics

Distribution: V_d: 40-50 L

Protein binding: 31%

Metabolism: Three metabolites

Bioavailability: Oral: 100%

Half-life: 5-7 hours

Elimination: Urinary excretion, 20% to 30% unchanged

Additional Information Product information not available at the time of this writing.

Lomefloxacin *(loe me FLOKS a sin)*

Related Information

Antimicrobial Activity Against Selected Organisms *on page 983*

U.S. Brand Names Maxaquin®

Synonyms Lomefloxacin Hydrochloride

Use Lower respiratory infections, acute bacterial exacerbation of chronic bronchitis, skin infections, sexually transmitted diseases, and urinary tract infections caused by *E. coli, K. pneumoniae, P. mirabilis, P. aeruginosa*; also has gram-positive activity including *S. pneumoniae* and some staphylococci

Pregnancy Risk Factor C

Contraindications Hypersensitivity to lomefloxacin or other members of the quinolone group such as nalidixic acid, oxolinic acid, cinoxacin, norfloxacin, and ciprofloxacin; avoid use in children <18 years of age due to association of other quinolones with transient arthropathies

Warnings/Precautions Use with caution in patients with epilepsy or other CNS diseases which could predispose them to seizures

Adverse Reactions

1% to 10%:

Central nervous system: Headache, dizziness

Dermatologic: Photosensitivity

Gastrointestinal: Nausea

<1%: Flushing, chest pain, hypotension, hypertension, edema, syncope, tachycardia, bradycardia, arrhythmia, extrasystoles, cyanosis, cardiac failure, angina pectoris, myocardial infarction, facial edema, fatigue, malaise, chills, convulsions, vertigo, coma, purpura, rash, gout, hypoglycemia, abdominal pain, vomiting, flatulence, constipation, xerostomia, discoloration of tongue, abnormal taste, urinary disorders, dysuria, thrombocytopenia, increased fibrinolysis, back pain, hyperkinesia, tremor, paresthesias, leg cramps, myalgia, weakness, earache, hematuria, anuria, dyspnea, cough, epistaxis, diaphoresis (increased), allergic reaction, flu-like symptoms, decreased heat tolerance, thirst

Overdosage/Toxicology

Symptoms of overdose include acute renal failure, seizures

GI decontamination and supportive care; diazepam for seizures; not removed by peritoneal or hemodialysis

Drug Interactions

Decreased effect: Decreased absorption with antacids containing aluminum, magnesium, and/or calcium (by up to 98% if given at the same time)

Increased toxicity/serum levels: Quinolones cause increased levels of caffeine, warfarin, cyclosporine, and theophylline; cimetidine, probenecid increase quinolone levels

Mechanism of Action Inhibits DNA-gyrase in susceptible organisms thereby inhibits relaxation of supercoiled DNA and promotes breakage of DNA strands. DNA gyrase (topoisomerase II), is an essential bacterial enzyme that maintains the superhelical structure of DNA and is required for DNA replication and transcription, DNA repair, recombination, and transposition.

Pharmacodynamics/Kinetics

Absorption: Well absorbed

Distribution: V_d: 2.4-3.5 L/kg; distributed well into bronchus, prostatic tissue, and urine

Protein binding: 20%

Half-life, elimination: 5-7.5 hours

Elimination: Primarily unchanged in urine

Usual Dosage

Lower respiratory and urinary tract infections (UTI): Adults: Oral: 400 mg once daily for 10-14 days

Urinary tract infection (UTI) due to susceptible organisms:

Uncomplicated cystitis caused by *Escherichia coli*: Adult female: Oral: 400 mg once daily for 3 successive days

Uncomplicated cystitis caused by *Klebsiella pneumoniae, Proteus mirabilis*, or *Staphylococcus saprophyticus*: Adult female: 400 mg once daily for 10 successive days

Complicated UTI caused by *Escherichia coli, Klebsiella pneumoniae, Proteus mirabilis*, or *Pseudomonas aeruginosa*: Adults: Oral: 400 mg once daily for 14 successive days

Surgical prophylaxis: 400 mg 2-6 hours before surgery

Uncomplicated gonorrhea: 400 mg as a single dose

No dosage adjustment is needed for elderly patients with normal renal function

(Continued)

Lomefloxacin *(Continued)*

Dosing adjustment in renal impairment:
Cl_{cr} 11-39 mL/minute: Loading dose: 400 mg; then 200 mg every day
Hemodialysis: Same as above

Dietary Considerations May be taken without regard to meals

Dosage Forms Tablet, as hydrochloride: 400 mg

Selected Readings

Hooper DC and Wolfson JS, "Fluoroquinolone Antimicrobial Agents," *N Engl J Med*, 1991, 324(6):384-94.

Lomaestro BM and Bailie GR, "Quinolone-Cation Interactions: A Review," *DICP*, 1991, 25(11):1249-58.

Stein GE, "The 4-Quinolone Antibiotics: Past, Present, and Future," *Pharmacotherapy*, 1988, 8(6):301-14.

Walker RC and Wright AJ, "The Fluoroquinolones," *Mayo Clin Proc*, 1991, 66(12):1249-59.

Lomefloxacin Hydrochloride *see Lomefloxacin on page 798*

Loprox® *see Ciclopirox on page 675*

Lorabid™ *see Loracarbef on this page*

Loracarbef *(lor a KAR bef)*

Related Information
Antimicrobial Activity Against Selected Organisms *on page 983*

U.S. Brand Names Lorabid™

Generic Available No

Use Infections caused by susceptible organisms involving the respiratory tract, acute otitis media, sinusitis, skin and skin structure, bone and joint, and urinary tract and gynecologic

Pregnancy Risk Factor B

Contraindications Patients with a history of hypersensitivity to loracarbef or cephalosporins

Warnings/Precautions Modify dosage in patients with severe renal impairment; prolonged use may result in superinfection; use with caution in patients with a previous history of hypersensitivity to other beta-lactam antibiotics (eg, penicillins, cephalosporins)

Adverse Reactions
1% to 10%
Central nervous system: Headache (3.2%)
Gastrointestinal: Diarrhea (3.6%), nausea (2.5%)
Respiratory: Rhinitis (1.6%)
<1%: Rash, vomiting, somnolence

Other reactions with cephalosporins include anaphylaxis, erythema multiforme, toxic epidermal necrolysis, Stevens-Johnson syndrome, dizziness, fever, headache, encephalopathy, asterixis, neuromuscular excitability, seizures, nausea, vomiting, pseudomembranous colitis, decreased hemoglobin, agranulocytosis, pancytopenia, aplastic anemia, hemolytic anemia, thrombocytopenia, interstitial nephritis, toxic nephropathy, pain at injection site, vaginitis, angioedema, cholestasis, transaminase elevation, hemorrhage, prolonged PT, serum-sickness reactions, and superinfection

Overdosage/Toxicology
Symptoms of overdose include abdominal discomfort, diarrhea
Supportive care only

Drug Interactions
Increased effect: Probenecid may decrease cephalosporin elimination
Increased toxicity: Furosemide, aminoglycosides may be a possible additive to nephrotoxicity

Stability Suspension may be kept at room temperature for 14 days

Mechanism of Action Inhibits bacterial cell wall synthesis by binding to one or more of the penicillin binding proteins (PBPs); inhibits the final transpeptidation step of peptidoglycan synthesis in bacterial cell walls, thus inhibiting cell wall biosynthesis. It is thought that beta-lactam antibiotics inactivate transpeptidase via acylation of the enzyme with cleavage of the CO-N bond of the beta-lactam ring. Upon exposure to beta-lactam antibiotics, bacteria eventually lyse due to ongoing activity of cell wall autolytic enzymes (autolysins and murein hydrolases) while cell wall assembly is arrested.

Pharmacodynamics/Kinetics
Absorption: Oral: Rapid

Half-life, elimination: ~1 hour
Time to peak serum concentration: Oral: Within 1 hour
Elimination: Plasma clearance: ~200-300 mL/minute

Usual Dosage Oral:
Children:
Acute otitis media: 15 mg/kg twice daily for 10 days
Pharyngitis and impetigo: 7.5-15 mg/kg twice daily for 10 days
Adults:
Uncomplicated urinary tract infections: 200 mg once daily for 7 days
Skin and soft tissue: 200-400 mg every 12-24 hours
Uncomplicated pyelonephritis: 400 mg every 12 hours for 14 days
Upper/lower respiratory tract infection: 200-400 mg every 12-24 hours for 7-14 days

Dosing comments in renal impairment:
Cl_{cr} 10-49 mL/minute: 50% of usual dose at usual interval or usual dose given half as often
Cl_{cr} <10 mL/minute: Administer usual dose every 3-5 days
Hemodialysis: Doses should be administered after dialysis sessions

Patient Information Take on an empty stomach at least 1 hour before or 2 hours after meals; finish all medication

Dosage Forms
Capsule: 200 mg, 400 mg
Suspension, oral: 100 mg/5 mL (50 mL, 100 mL); 200 mg/5 mL (50 mL, 100 mL)

Selected Readings
Force RW and Nahata MC, "Loracarbef: A New Orally Administered Carbacephem Antibiotic," *Ann Pharmacother*, 1993, 27(3):321-9.
Marshall WF and Blair JE, "The Cephalosporins," *Mayo Clin Proc*, 1999, 74(2):187-95.
Schatz BS, Karavokiros KT, Taeubel MA, et al, "Comparison of Cefprozil, Cefpodoxime Proxetil, Loracarbef, Cefixime, and Ceftibuten," *Ann Pharmacother*, 1996, 30(3):258-68.

Lotrimin® *see* Clotrimazole *on page 688*

Lotrimin® AF Cream [OTC] *see* Clotrimazole *on page 688*

Lotrimin® AF Lotion [OTC] *see* Clotrimazole *on page 688*

Lotrimin® AF Powder [OTC] *see* Miconazole *on page 822*

Lotrimin® AF Solution [OTC] *see* Clotrimazole *on page 688*

Lotrimin® AF Spray Liquid [OTC] *see* Miconazole *on page 822*

Lotrimin® AF Spray Powder [OTC] *see* Miconazole *on page 822*

Lugol's Solution *see* Potassium Iodide *on page 879*

Lyme Disease Vaccine (LIME dee seas vak SEEN)

Related Information
Lyme Disease Vaccine Guidelines *on page 1053*

U.S. Brand Names LYMErix®

Synonyms Lyme Disease Vaccine (Recombinant OspA)

Use Active immunization against Lyme disease in individuals between 15-70 years of age. Individuals most at risk are those who live, work, or travel to *B. burgdorfi*-infected, tick-infested, grassy/wooded areas.

Drug of Choice or Alternative for
Organism(s)
Borrelia burgdorferi on page 84

Pregnancy Risk Factor C

Pregnancy/Breast-Feeding Implications It is not known whether Lyme disease vaccine is excreted in human milk. Because many drugs are excreted in milk, caution should be exercised when the vaccine is given to nursing mothers. Healthcare professionals are encouraged to register pregnant women who receive the vaccine with the SKB vaccination pregnancy registry (1-800-366-8900, ext 5231).

Contraindications Known hypersensitivity to any component of the vaccine. Vaccination should be postponed during acute moderate to severe febrile illness (minor illness is generally not a contraindication). Safety and efficacy in patients <15 years of age have not been established.

Warnings/Precautions Do not administer to patients with treatment-resistant Lyme arthritis. Will not prevent disease in patients with prior infection and offers no protection against other tick-borne diseases. Immunosuppressed patients or those receiving immunosuppressive therapy (vaccine may not be effective) - (Continued)

Lyme Disease Vaccine *(Continued)*

defer vaccination until 3 months after therapy. Avoid in patients receiving anticoagulant therapy (due to intramuscular injection). The physician should take all known precautions for prevention of allergic or other reactions. Administer with caution to patients with known or suspected latex allergy (applies only to the LYMErix Tip-Lok™ syringe, vaccine vial does not contain natural rubber). Duration of immunity has not been established.

Adverse Reactions (Limited to overall self-reported events occurring within 30 days following a dose)

>10%: Local: Injection site pain (21.9%)

1% to 10%:

Central nervous system: Headache (5.6%), fatigue (3.9%), fever (2.6%), chills (2%), dizziness (1%)

Dermatologic: Rash (1.4%)

Gastrointestinal: Nausea (1.1%)

Neuromuscular & skeletal: Arthralgia (6.8%), myalgia (4.8%), muscle aches (2.8%), back pain (1.9%), stiffness (1%)

Respiratory: Upper respiratory tract infection (4.4%), sinusitis (3.2%), pharyngitis (2.5%), rhinitis (2.4%), cough (1.5%), bronchitis (1.1%)

Miscellaneous: Viral infection (2.8%), flu-like syndrome (2.5%)

Solicited adverse event rates were higher than unsolicited event rates (above). These included local reactions of soreness (93.5%), redness (41.8%), and swelling (29.9%). In addition, general systemic symptoms included fatigue (40.8%), headache (38.6%), arthralgia (25.6%), rash (11.7%), and fever (3.5%)

Patients with a history of Lyme disease were noted to experience a higher frequency of early musculoskeletal reactions. Other differences in the observed rate of adverse reactions were not significantly different between vaccine and placebo recipients.

Drug Interactions No data available

Stability Store between 2°C and 8°C (36°F and 46°F).

Mechanism of Action Lyme disease vaccine is a recombinant, noninfectious lipoprotein (OspA) derived from the outer surface of *Borrelia burgdorferi*, the causative agent of Lyme disease. Vaccination stimulates production of antibodies directed against this organism, including antibodies against the LA-2 epitope, which have bactericidal activity. Since OspA expression is down-regulated after inoculation into the human host, at least part of the vaccine's efficacy may be related to neutralization of bacteria within the midgut of the tick vector, preventing transmission to the human host.

Usual Dosage Adults: I.M.: Vaccination with 3 doses of 30 mcg (0.5 mL), administered at 0, 1, and 12 months, is recommended for optimal protection

Administration Intramuscular injection into the deltoid region is recommended. Do not administer intravenously, intradermally, or subcutaneously. The vaccine should be used as supplied without dilution. Shake well before withdrawal and use.

Test Interactions Vaccination will result in a positive *B. burgdorferi* IgG via ELISA (Western blot testing is recommended)

Patient Information Vaccination consists of a series of three injections over 12 months. Failure to complete the sequence may result in suboptimal protection. The vaccine may not provide 100% protection against Lyme disease, nor does it protect against other tick-borne disease. Individuals at risk should continue to use standard protective measures.

Dosage Forms Injection:

Vial: 30 mcg/0.5 mL

Prefilled syringe (Tip-Lok™): 30 mcg/0.5 mL

Selected Readings

Sigal LH, Zahradnik JM, Lavin P, et al, "A Vaccine Consisting of Recombinant *Borrelia burgdorferi* Outer-Surface Protein A to Prevent Lyme Disease," *N Engl J Med*, 1998, 339(4):216-22.

Steere AC, Sikand VK, Meurice F, et al, "Vaccination Against Lyme Disease With Recombinant *Borrelia burgdorferi* Outer-Surface Lipoprotein A With Adjuvant," *N Engl J Med*, 1998, 339(4):209-15.

Wormser GP, "Lyme Disease Vaccine," *Infection*, 1996, 24(2):203-7.

Lyme Disease Vaccine Guidelines *see page 1053*

Lyme Disease Vaccine (Recombinant OspA) *see* Lyme Disease Vaccine *on previous page*

Macrolides

Refer to

Azithromycin *on page 613*

Clarithromycin *on page 681*

Dirithromycin *on page 712*

Erythromycin *on page 722*

Erythromycin and Sulfisoxazole *on page 725*

Troleandomycin *on page 960*

Drug of Choice or Alternative for

Disease/Syndrome(s)

Sinusitis, Community-Acquired, Acute *on page 48*

Sinusitis, Community-Acquired, Chronic *on page 49*

Sinusitis, Hospital-Acquired *on page 49*

Organism(s)

Mycoplasma hominis and *Mycoplasma genitalium* on page 210

Streptococcus pneumoniae on page 268

Mafenide (MA fe nide)

U.S. Brand Names Sulfamylon® Topical

Synonyms Mafenide Acetate

Generic Available No

Use Adjunct in the treatment of second and third degree burns to prevent septicemia caused by susceptible organisms such as *Pseudomonas aeruginosa*; prevention of graft loss of meshed autografts on excised burn wounds

Pregnancy Risk Factor C

Contraindications Hypersensitivity to mafenide, sulfites, or any component

Warnings/Precautions Use with caution in patients with renal impairment and in patients with G-6-PD deficiency; prolonged use may result in superinfection

Adverse Reactions

>10%:

Central nervous system: Pain

Local: Burning sensation, excoriation

1% to 10%:

Cardiovascular: Facial edema

Dermatologic: Rash

Miscellaneous: Dyspnea

<1%: Erythema, hyperchloremia, metabolic acidosis, bone marrow suppression, hemolytic anemia, bleeding, porphyria, hyperventilation, tachypnea, hypersensitivity

Mechanism of Action Interferes with bacterial folic acid synthesis through competitive inhibition of para-aminobenzoic acid

Pharmacodynamics/Kinetics

Absorption: Diffuses through devascularized areas and is rapidly absorbed from burned surface

Metabolism: To para-carboxybenzene sulfonamide which is a carbonic anhydrase inhibitor

Time to peak serum concentration: Topical: 2-4 hours

Elimination: In urine as metabolites

Usual Dosage Children and Adults: Topical: Apply once or twice daily with a sterile gloved hand; apply to a thickness of approximately 16 mm; the burned area should be covered with cream at all times

Monitoring Parameters Acid base balance

Patient Information Discontinue and call physician immediately if rash, blisters, or swelling appear while using cream; discontinue if condition persists or worsens while using this product; for external use only

Dosage Forms Cream, topical, as acetate: 85 mg/g (56.7 g, 113.4 g, 411 g)

Malathion (mal a THYE on)

U.S. Brand Names Ovide™

Generic Available No

Use Treatment of head lice and their ova

Drug of Choice or Alternative for
Organism(s)
Lice *on page 188*

Pregnancy Risk Factor B

Contraindications Known hypersensitivity to malathion

Usual Dosage Sprinkle Ovide™ lotion on dry hair and rub gently until the scalp is thoroughly moistened; pay special attention to the back of the head and neck. Allow to dry naturally - use no heat and leave uncovered. After 8-12 hours, the hair should be washed with a nonmedicated shampoo; rinse and use a fine-toothed comb to remove dead lice and eggs. If required, repeat with second application in 7-9 days. Further treatment is generally not necessary. Other family members should be evaluated to determine if infested and if so, receive treatment.

Patient Information Topical use only

Dosage Forms Lotion: 0.5% (59 mL)

Selected Readings
"Drugs for Parasitic Infections," *Med Lett Drugs Ther,* 1998, 40(1017):1-12.

Mandelamine® *see* Methenamine *on page 814*

Mandol® *see* Cefamandole *on page 630*

Mantoux *see* Tuberculin Tests *on page 962*

Marcillin® *see* Ampicillin *on page 604*

Marinol® *see* Dronabinol *on page 716*

Maxaquin® *see* Lomefloxacin *on page 798*

Maximum Strength Desenex® Antifungal Cream [OTC] *see* Miconazole *on page 822*

Maxipime® *see* Cefepime *on page 634*

Maxitrol® *see* Neomycin, Polymyxin B, and Dexamethasone *on page 836*

Measles and Rubella Vaccines, Combined

(MEE zels & roo BEL a vak SEENS, kom BINED)

Related Information
Immunization Guidelines *on page 1041*

U.S. Brand Names M-R-VAX® II

Synonyms Rubella and Measles Vaccines, Combined

Generic Available No

Use Simultaneous immunization against measles and rubella

Note: Trivalent measles - mumps - rubella (MMR) vaccine is the preferred immunizing agent for most children and many adults. Adults born before 1957 are generally considered to be immune and need not be revaccinated.

Pregnancy Risk Factor C

Contraindications Immune deficiency condition, pregnancy

Warnings/Precautions Immunocompromised persons, history of anaphylactic reaction following receipt of neomycin

Adverse Reactions All serious adverse reactions must be reported to the U.S. Department of Health and Human Services (DHHS) Vaccine Adverse Event Reporting System (VAERS) 1-800-822-7967.

>10%:
Cardiovascular: Edema
Central nervous system: Fever (<100°F)
Local: Burning or stinging, induration
1% to 10%:
Central nervous system: Fever (100°F to 103°F usually between 5th and 12th days postvaccination)
Dermatologic: Rash (rarely generalized)
<1%: Fatigue, convulsions, encephalitis, confusion, severe headache, fever (>103°F, prolonged), palsies, Guillain-Barré syndrome, ataxia, urticaria,

itching, reddening of skin (especially around ears and eyes), erythema multiforme, vomiting, sore throat, diarrhea, thrombocytopenic purpura, diplopia, stiff neck, dyspnea, cough, rhinitis, lymphadenopathy, coryza, allergic reactions

Drug Interactions Whole blood, interferon immune globulin, radiation therapy, and immunosuppressive drugs (eg, corticosteroids) may result in insufficient response to immunization. DTP, OPV, MMR, Hib, and hepatitis B may be given concurrently; other virus vaccine administration should be separated by ≥1 month from measles.

Stability Refrigerate prior to use, use as soon as possible; discard if not used within 8 hours of reconstitution

Mechanism of Action Promotes active immunity to measles and rubella by inducing specific antibodies including measles-specific IgG and IgM and rubella hemagglutination-inhibiting antibodies.

Usual Dosage Children at 15 months and Adults: S.C.: Inject 0.5 mL into outer aspect of upper arm; no routine booster for rubella

Administration Not for I.V. administration

Test Interactions May temporarily depress tuberculin skin test sensitivity and reduce the seroconversion.

Patient Information Parents should monitor children closely for fever 5-11 days after vaccination; females should not become pregnant within 3 months of vaccination

Additional Information Federal law requires that the date of administration, the vaccine manufacturer, lot number of vaccine, and the administering person's name, title and address be entered into the patient's permanent medical record

Adults born before 1957 are generally considered to be immune to measles; all born in or after 1957 without documentation of live vaccine on or after first birthday, physician-diagnosed measles, or laboratory evidence of immunity should be vaccinated with two doses separated by or less than 1 month. For those previously vaccinated with one dose of measles vaccine, revaccination is indicated for students entering institutions of higher learning, for healthcare workers at time of employment, and for travelers to endemic areas. Guidelines for rubella vaccination are the same with the exception of birth year. All adults should be vaccinated against rubella. A booster dose of rubella vaccine is not necessary. Women who are pregnant when vaccinated or become pregnant within 3 months of vaccination should be consulted on the risks to the fetus; although the risks appear negligible. MMR is the vaccine of choice if recipients are likely to be susceptible to mumps as well as measles and rubella.

Dosage Forms Injection: 1000 TCID$_{50}$ each of live attenuated measles virus vaccine and live rubella virus vaccine

Measles, Mumps, and Rubella Vaccines, Combined
(MEE zels, mumpz & roo BEL a vak SEENS, kom BINED)

Related Information
Immunization Guidelines on page 1041

U.S. Brand Names M-M-R® II

Synonyms MMR; Mumps, Measles and Rubella Vaccines, Combined; Rubella, Measles and Mumps Vaccines, Combined

Generic Available No

Use Measles, mumps, and rubella prophylaxis

Pregnancy Risk Factor C

Pregnancy/Breast-Feeding Implications Clinical effects on the fetus: It is not known whether the drug can cause fetal harm or affect reproduction capacity (contracting natural measles during pregnancy can increase fetal risk)

Contraindications Blood dyscrasias, cancers affecting the bone marrow or lymphatic systems, known hypersensitivity to measles, mumps and rubella vaccine, known hypersensitivity to neomycin, acute infections, and respiratory illness, pregnancy; known hypersensitivity to eggs, chicken or chicken feathers, severely immunocompromised persons

Warnings/Precautions
Females should not become pregnant within 3 months of vaccination
MMR vaccine should not be given within 3 months of immune globulin or whole blood
Have epinephrine available during and after administration
(Continued)

Measles, Mumps, and Rubella Vaccines, Combined
(Continued)

MMR vaccine should not be administered to severely immunocompromised persons with the exception of asymptomatic children with HIV (ACIP and AAP recommendation)

Severely immunocompromised patients and symptomatic HIV-infected patients who are exposed to measles should receive immune globulin, regardless of prior vaccination status

The immunogenicity of measles virus vaccine is decreased if vaccine is administered <6 months after immune globulin

Adverse Reactions All serious adverse reactions must be reported to the U.S. Department of Health and Human Services (DHHS) Vaccine Adverse Event Reporting System (VAERS) 1-800-822-7967.

>10%:
  Cardiovascular: Edema
  Central nervous system: Fever (<100°F)
  Local: Burning or stinging, induration
1% to 10%:
  Central nervous system: Fever (100°F to 103°F usually between 5th and 12th days postvaccination)
  Dermatologic: Rash (rarely generalized)
<1%: Fatigue, convulsions, encephalitis, confusion, severe headache, fever (>103°F, prolonged), palsies, Guillain-Barré syndrome, ataxia, urticaria, itching, reddening of skin (especially around ears and eyes), erythema multiforme, vomiting, sore throat, diarrhea, thrombocytopenic purpura, diplopia, stiff neck, dyspnea, cough, rhinitis, lymphadenopathy, coryza, allergic reactions

Drug Interactions Decreased effect when immune globulin is given within 3 months and with concurrent use of corticosteroids and other immunosuppressant agents; decreased effect with concurrent infection, immunoglobulin in 3 months, other live vaccines with the exception of attenuated measles, rubella, or polio

Stability Refrigerate, protect from light prior to reconstitution; use as soon as possible; discard 8 hours after reconstitution

Mechanism of Action Promotes active immunity to measles, mumps, and rubella by inducing specific antibodies including measles-specific IgG and IgM and rubella hemagglutination-inhibiting antibodies.

Usual Dosage

Infants <12 months of age: If there is risk of exposure to measles, single-antigen measles vaccine should be administered at 6-11 months of age with a second dose (of MMR) at >12 months of age

Administer S.C. in outer aspect of the upper arm to children ≥15 months of age: 0.5 mL at 15 months of age and then repeated at 4-6 years* of age

In some areas, MMR vaccine may be given at 12 months

*Many experts recommend that this dose of MMR be given at entry to middle school or junior high school

Administration Not for I.V. administration

Test Interactions Temporary suppression of TB skin test reactivity with onset approximately 3 days after administration

Patient Information Pregnancy should be avoided for 3 months following vaccination

Nursing Implications Not for I.V. administration

Additional Information Federal law requires that the date of administration, the vaccine manufacturer, lot number of vaccine, and the administering person's name, title and address be entered into the patient's permanent medical record

Adults born before 1957 are generally considered to be immune to measles and mumps; all born in or after 1957 without documentation of live vaccine on or after first birthday, physician-diagnosed measles or mumps, or laboratory evidence of immunity should be vaccinated with two doses separated by no less than 1 month; for those previously vaccinated with one dose of measles vaccine, revaccination is indicated for students entering institutions of higher learning, health care workers at time of employment, and for travelers to endemic areas. Guidelines for rubella vaccination are the same with the exception of birth year; all adults should be vaccinated against rubella. Booster doses of mumps and rubella are not necessary; women who are pregnant when vaccinated or become pregnant within 3 months should be counseled on the risks to the fetus; although the risks appear negligible.

Dosage Forms Injection: 1000 TCID$_{50}$ each of measles virus vaccine and rubella virus vaccine, 5000 TCID$_{50}$ mumps virus vaccine

Measles Virus Vaccine, Live, Attenuated

(MEE zels VYE rus vak SEEN, live, a ten YOO ated)

Related Information

Immunization Guidelines *on page 1041*

U.S. Brand Names Attenuvax®

Synonyms More Attenuated Enders Strain; Rubeola Vaccine

Generic Available No

Use Adults born before 1957 are generally considered to be immune. All those born in or after 1957 without documentation of live vaccine on or after first birthday, physician-diagnosed measles, or laboratory evidence of immunity should be vaccinated, ideally with two doses of vaccine separated by no less than 1 month. For those previously vaccinated with one dose of measles vaccine, revaccination is recommended for students entering colleges and other institutions of higher education, for healthcare workers at the time of employment, and for international travelers who visit endemic areas.

MMR is the vaccine of choice if recipients are likely to be susceptible to rubella and/or mumps as well as to measles. Persons vaccinated between 1963 and 1967 with a killed measles vaccine, followed by live vaccine within 3 months, or with a vaccine of unknown type should be revaccinated with live measles virus vaccine.

Pregnancy Risk Factor C

Contraindications Pregnant females, known anaphylactoid reaction to eggs, known hypersensitivity to neomycin, acute respiratory infections, activated tuberculosis, immunosuppressed patients

Warnings/Precautions Avoid use in immunocompromised patients; defer administration in presence of acute respiratory or other active infections or inactive, untreated tuberculosis; avoid pregnancy for 3 months following vaccination; history of febrile seizures, hypersensitivity reactions may occur

Adverse Reactions All serious adverse reactions must be reported to the U.S. Department of Health and Human Services (DHHS) Vaccine Adverse Event Reporting System (VAERS) 1-800-822-7967.

>10%:

Cardiovascular: Edema

Central nervous system: Fever (<100°F)

Local: Burning or stinging, induration

1% to 10%:

Central nervous system: Fever (100°F to 103°F usually between 5th and 12th days postvaccination)

Dermatologic: Rash (rarely generalized)

<1%: Fatigue, convulsions, encephalitis, confusion, severe headache, fever (>103°F, prolonged), palsies, Guillain-Barré syndrome, ataxia, urticaria, itching, reddening of skin (especially around ears and eyes), erythema multiforme, vomiting, sore throat, diarrhea, thrombocytopenic purpura, diplopia, stiff neck, dyspnea, cough, rhinitis, lymphadenopathy, coryza, allergic reactions

Drug Interactions Whole blood, interferon immune globulin, radiation therapy, and immunosuppressive drugs (eg, corticosteroids) may result in insufficient response to immunization. DTP, OPV, MMR, Hib, and hepatitis B may be given concurrently; other virus vaccine administration should be separated by ≥1 month from measles.

Stability Refrigerate at 2°C to 8°C (36°F to 46°F); discard if left at room temperature for over 8 hours; protect from light

Mechanism of Action Promotes active immunity to measles virus by inducing specific measles IgG and IgM antibodies.

Usual Dosage Children ≥15 months and Adults: S.C.: 0.5 mL in outer aspect of the upper arm, no routine boosters

Administration Vaccine should not be given I.V.; S.C. injection preferred

Test Interactions May temporarily depress tuberculin skin test sensitivity

(Continued)

Measles Virus Vaccine, Live, Attenuated *(Continued)*

Patient Information Parents should monitor children closely for fever for 5-11 days after vaccination; females should not become pregnant within 3 months of vaccination

Additional Information Federal law requires that the date of administration, the vaccine manufacturer, lot number of vaccine, and the administering person's name, title and address be entered into the patient's permanent medical record

Dosage Forms Injection: 1000 $TCID_{50}$ per dose

Mebendazole *(me BEN da zole)*

U.S. Brand Names Vermox®

Generic Available No

Use Treatment of pinworms (*Enterobius vermicularis*), whipworms (*Trichuris trichiura*), roundworms (*Ascaris lumbricoides*), and hookworms (*Ancylostoma duodenale*)

Drug of Choice or Alternative for
Organism(s)
  Ancylostoma duodenale on page 66
  Ascaris on page 69
  Enterobius vermicularis on page 136
  Trichinella spiralis on page 289

Pregnancy Risk Factor C

Contraindications Hypersensitivity to mebendazole or any component

Warnings/Precautions Pregnancy and children <2 years of age are relative contraindications since safety has not been established; not effective for hydatid disease

Adverse Reactions
  1% to 10%: Gastrointestinal: Abdominal pain, diarrhea, nausea, vomiting
  <1%: Fever, dizziness, headache, rash, itching, alopecia (with high doses), neutropenia (sore throat, unusual fatigue), unusual weakness, angioedema, seizures

Overdosage/Toxicology
  Symptoms of overdose include abdominal pain, altered mental status
  Treatment should include GI decontamination and supportive care

Drug Interactions Decreased effect: Anticonvulsants such as carbamazepine and phenytoin may increase metabolism of mebendazole

Mechanism of Action Selectively and irreversibly blocks glucose uptake and other nutrients in susceptible adult intestine-dwelling helminths

Pharmacodynamics/Kinetics
  Absorption: Only 2% to 10%
  Distribution: Distributed to serum, cyst fluid, liver, omental fat, and pelvic, pulmonary, and hepatic cysts; highest concentrations found in liver; relatively high concentrations also found in muscle-encysted *Trichinella spiralis* larvae; crosses placenta
  Protein binding: High, 95%
  Metabolism: Extensive in the liver
  Half-life: 1-11.5 hours
  Time to peak serum concentration: Within 2-4 hours
  Elimination: Primarily excreted in feces with 5% to 10% eliminated in urine

Usual Dosage Children and Adults: Oral:
  Pinworms: 100 mg as a single dose; may need to repeat after 2 weeks; treatment should include family members in close contact with patient
  Whipworms, roundworms, hookworms: One tablet twice daily, morning and evening on 3 consecutive days; if patient is not cured within 3-4 weeks, a second course of treatment may be administered
  Capillariasis: 200 mg twice daily for 20 days

  Dosing adjustment in hepatic impairment: Dosage reduction may be necessary in patients with liver dysfunction
  Hemodialysis: Not dialyzable (0% to 5%)

Monitoring Parameters Check for helminth ova in feces within 3-4 weeks following the initial therapy

Patient Information Tablets may be chewed, swallowed whole, or crushed and mixed with food; hygienic precautions should be taken to prevent reinfection such as wearing shoes and washing hands

Dosage Forms Tablet, chewable: 100 mg

Selected Readings
de Silva N, Guyatt H, and Bundy D, "Anthelmintics. A Comparative Review of Their Clinical Pharmacology," *Drugs*, 1997, 53(5):769-88.
"Drugs for Parasitic Infections," *Med Lett Drugs Ther*, 1998, 40(1017):1-12.

Meclan® *see Meclocycline on this page*

Meclocycline (me kloe SYE kleen)
U.S. Brand Names Meclan®
Synonyms Meclocycline Sulfosalicylate
Generic Available No
Use Topical treatment of inflammatory acne vulgaris
Pregnancy Risk Factor B
Contraindications Known hypersensitivity to tetracyclines or any component
Warnings/Precautions Use with caution in patients allergic to formaldehyde; for external use only
Adverse Reactions
>10%: Topical: Follicular staining, yellowing of the skin, burning/stinging feeling
1% to 10%: Topical: Pain, redness, skin irritation, dermatitis
Mechanism of Action Inhibits bacterial protein synthesis by binding with the 30S and possibly the 50S ribosomal subunit(s) of susceptible bacteria; may also cause alterations in the cytoplasmic membrane
Pharmacodynamics/Kinetics Absorption: Topical: Very little
Usual Dosage Children >11 years and Adults: Topical: Apply generously to affected areas twice daily
Monitoring Parameters Periodic assessment of hematologic and hepatic function
Patient Information Apply generously until skin is wet; avoid contact with eyes, nose, and mouth; stinging may occur with application, but soon stops; if skin is discolored yellow, washing will remove the color
Dosage Forms Cream, topical, as sulfosalicylate: 1% (20 g, 45 g)

Meclocycline Sulfosalicylate *see Meclocycline on this page*

Mectizan® *see Ivermectin on page 787*

Medi-Quick® Topical Ointment [OTC] *see Bacitracin, Neomycin, and Polymyxin B on page 619*

Mefloquine (ME floe kwin)
Related Information
Prevention of Malaria *on page 1057*
U.S. Brand Names Lariam®
Synonyms Mefloquine Hydrochloride
Generic Available No
Use Treatment of acute malarial infections and prevention of malaria
Drug of Choice or Alternative for
Organism(s)
Plasmodium Species *on page 227*
Pregnancy Risk Factor C
Contraindications Hypersensitivity to any component
Warnings/Precautions Caution is warranted with lactation; discontinue if unexplained neuropsychiatric disturbances occur, caution in epilepsy patients or in patients with significant cardiac disease. If mefloquine is to be used for a prolonged period, periodic evaluations including liver function tests and ophthalmic examinations should be performed. (Retinal abnormalities have not been observed with mefloquine in humans; however, it has with long-term administration to rats.) In cases of life-threatening, serious, or overwhelming malaria infections due to *Plasmodium falciparum*, patients should be treated with intravenous antimalarial drug. Mefloquine may be given orally to complete the course. Caution should be exercised with regard to driving, piloting airplanes, and operating machines since dizziness, disturbed sense of balance; neuropsychiatric reactions have been reported with mefloquine.
Adverse Reactions
1% to 10%:
Central nervous system: Difficulty concentrating, headache, insomnia, lightheadedness, vertigo
(Continued)

Mefloquine *(Continued)*

Gastrointestinal: Vomiting (3%), diarrhea, stomach pain, nausea

Ocular: Visual disturbances

Otic: Tinnitus

<1%: Bradycardia, extrasystoles, syncope, anxiety, dizziness, confusion, seizures, hallucinations, mental depression, psychosis

Overdosage/Toxicology

Symptoms of overdose include vomiting, diarrhea; cardiotoxic

Following GI contamination supportive care only

Drug Interactions

Decreased effect of valproic acid

Increased toxicity of beta-blockers; chloroquine, quinine, and quinidine (hold treatment until at least 12 hours after these later drugs)

Mechanism of Action Mefloquine is a quinoline-methanol compound structurally similar to quinine; mefloquine's effectiveness in the treatment and prophylaxis of malaria is due to the destruction of the asexual blood forms of the malarial pathogens that affect humans, *Plasmodium falciparum, P. vivax, P. malariae, P. ovale*

Pharmacodynamics/Kinetics

Absorption: Oral: Well absorbed

Distribution: V_d: 19 L/kg; concentrates in erythrocytes; appears in breast milk; distributed to blood, urine, CSF, and tissues; concentrates in erythrocytes

Protein binding: 98%

Half-life: 21-22 days

Elimination: ~1.5% to 9% of dose excreted unchanged in urine

Usual Dosage Oral:

Children: Malaria prophylaxis:

15-19 kg: 1/4 tablet

20-30 kg: 1/2 tablet

31-45 kg: 3/4 tablet

>45 kg: 1 tablet

Administer weekly starting 1 week before travel, continuing weekly during travel and for 4 weeks after leaving endemic area

Adults:

Treatment of mild to moderate malaria infection: 5 tablets (1250 mg) as a single dose with at least 8 oz of water

Malaria prophylaxis: 1 tablet (250 mg) weekly starting 1 week before travel, continuing weekly during travel and for 4 weeks after leaving endemic area

Monitoring Parameters LFTS; ocular examination

Patient Information Begin therapy before trip and continue after; do not take drug on empty stomach; take with food and at least 8 oz of water; women of childbearing age should use reliable contraception during prophylaxis treatment and for 2 months after the last dose; be aware of signs and symptoms of malaria when traveling to an endemic area. Caution should be exercised with regard to driving, piloting airplanes, and operating machines since dizziness, disturbed sense of balance, or neuropsychiatric reactions have been reported with mefloquine.

Dosage Forms Tablet, as hydrochloride: 250 mg

Selected Readings

Panisko DM and Keystone JS, "Treatment of Malaria - 1990," *Drugs,* 1990, 39(2):160-89.

White NJ, "The Treatment of Malaria," *N Engl J Med,* 1996, 335(11):800-6.

Wyler DJ, "Malaria Chemoprophylaxis for the Traveler," *N Engl J Med,* 1993, 329(1):31-7.

Mefloquine Hydrochloride *see* Mefloquine *on previous page*

Mefoxin® *see* Cefoxitin *on page 646*

Megace® *see* Megestrol Acetate *on this page*

Megacillin® **Susp** *see* Penicillin G Benzathine, Parenteral *on page 859*

Megestrol Acetate *(me JES trole AS e tate)*

U.S. Brand Names Megace®

Generic Available Yes

Use Treatment of "AIDS-wasting" syndrome; palliative treatment of breast and endometrial carcinomas, appetite stimulation, and promotion of weight gain in cachexia

Pregnancy Risk Factor X

Contraindications Hypersensitivity to megestrol or any component

Warnings/Precautions The U.S. Food and Drug Administration (FDA) currently recommends that procedures for proper handling and disposal of antineoplastic agents be considered. Use during the first few months of pregnancy is not recommended. Use with caution in patients with a history of thrombophlebitis. Elderly females may have vaginal bleeding or discharge and need to be forewarned of this side effect and inconvenience.

Adverse Reactions

>10%:
  Cardiovascular: Edema
  Endocrine & metabolic: Breakthrough bleeding and amenorrhea, spotting, changes in menstrual flow
  Neuromuscular & skeletal: Weakness

1% to 10%:
  Central nervous system: Insomnia, depression, fever, headache
  Dermatologic: Allergic rash with or without pruritus, melasma or chloasma, rash, and rarely alopecia
  Endocrine & metabolic: Changes in cervical erosion and secretions, increased breast tenderness, amenorrhea, changes in vaginal bleeding pattern, edema, fluid retention, hyperglycemia
  Gastrointestinal: Weight gain (not attributed to edema or fluid retention), nausea, vomiting, stomach cramps
  Hepatic: Cholestatic jaundice, hepatotoxicity
  Local: Thrombophlebitis
  Neuromuscular & skeletal: Carpal tunnel syndrome
  Respiratory: Hyperpnea

Overdosage/Toxicology Toxicity is unlikely following simple exposures of excessive doses

Mechanism of Action A synthetic progestin with antiestrogenic properties which disrupt the estrogen receptor cycle. Megace® interferes with the normal estrogen cycle and results in a lower LH titer. May also have a direct effect on the endometrium. Megestrol is an antineoplastic progestin thought to act through an antileutenizing effect mediated via the pituitary.

Pharmacodynamics/Kinetics

Onset of action: At least 2 months of continuous therapy is necessary
Absorption: Oral: Well absorbed
Metabolism: Completely metabolized in the liver to free steroids and glucuronide conjugates
Time to peak serum concentration: Oral: Within 1-3 hours
Half-life, elimination: 15-20 hours
Elimination: In urine as steroid metabolites and inactive compound, some in feces and bile

Usual Dosage Adults: Oral (refer to individual protocols):

Female:
  Breast carcinoma: 40 mg 4 times/day
  Endometrial: 40-320 mg/day in divided doses; use for 2 months to determine efficacy; maximum doses used have been up to 800 mg/day
  Uterine bleeding: 40 mg 2-4 times/day
AIDS wasting: HIV-related cachexia: Initial dose: 800 mg/day; daily doses of 400 and 800 mg/day were found to be clinically effective

Monitoring Parameters Monitor for tumor response; observe for signs of thromboembolic phenomena; monitor for thromboembolism

Test Interactions Altered thyroid and liver function tests

Patient Information Exposure to megestrol during the first 4 months of pregnancy may pose risks to the fetus; notify physician if sudden loss of vision, double vision, migraine headache occur, or if pain in calves with warmth and tenderness develops; may cause photosensitivity, wear protective clothing or sunscreen

Dosage Forms

Suspension, oral: 40 mg/mL with alcohol 0.06% (236.6 mL)
Tablet: 20 mg, 40 mg

Selected Readings

Jeffrey LP, Chairman, National Study Commission on Cytotoxic Exposure. Position Statement. "The Handling of Cytotoxic Agents by Women Who Are Pregnant, Attempting to Conceive, or Breast-Feeding," January 12, 1987.

Meningococcal Polysaccharide Vaccine, Groups A, C, Y, and W-135

(me NIN joe kok al pol i SAK a ride vak SEEN, groops aye, see, why, & dubl yoo won thur tee fyve)

Related Information

Immunization Guidelines *on page 1041*

U.S. Brand Names Menomune®-A/C/Y/W-135

Generic Available No

Use

Immunization of persons 2 years of age and above in epidemic or endemic areas as might be determined in a population delineated by neighborhood, school, dormitory, or other reasonable boundary. The prevalent serogroup in such a situation should match a serogroup in the vaccine. Individuals at particular high-risk include persons with terminal component complement deficiencies and those with anatomic or functional asplenia.

Travelers visiting areas of a country that are recognized as having hyperendemic or epidemic meningococcal disease

Vaccinations should be considered for household or institutional contacts of persons with meningococcal disease as an adjunct to appropriate antibiotic chemoprophylaxis as well as medical and laboratory personnel at risk of exposure to meningococcal disease

Pregnancy Risk Factor C

Contraindications Children <2 years of age

Warnings/Precautions Patients who undergo splenectomy secondary to trauma or nonlymphoid tumors respond well; however, those asplenic patients with lymphoid tumors who receive either chemotherapy or irradiation respond poorly; pregnancy, unless there is substantial risk of infection.

Adverse Reactions All serious adverse reactions must be reported to the U.S. Department of Health and Human Services (DHHS) Vaccine Adverse Event Reporting System (VAERS) 1-800-822-7967.

>10%:

Central nervous system: Pain (17.5% to 24%)

Dermatologic: Erythema (0.8% to 31.7%), induration (4.8% to 8.3%)

Local: Tenderness (24% to 29%)

1% to 10%: Central nervous system: Headache (1.2% to 4.1%), malaise (≤2.6%), fever (0.4% to 3.1%), chills (≤1.7%)

Drug Interactions Decreased effect with administration of immunoglobulin within 1 month

Stability Discard remainder of vaccine within 5 days after reconstitution; store reconstituted vaccine in refrigerator

Mechanism of Action Induces the formation of bactericidal antibodies to meningococcal antigens; the presence of these antibodies is strongly correlated with immunity to meningococcal disease caused by *Neisseria meningitidis* groups A, C, Y and W-135.

Pharmacodynamics/Kinetics

Onset: Antibody levels are achieved within 10-14 days after administration

Duration: Antibodies against group A and C polysaccharides decline markedly (to prevaccination levels) over the first 3 years following a single dose of vaccine, especially in children <4 years of age

Usual Dosage One dose S.C. (0.5 mL); the need for booster is unknown

Nursing Implications Epinephrine 1:1000 should be available to control allergic reaction

Dosage Forms Injection: 10 dose, 50 dose

Menomune®-A/C/Y/W-135 *see* Meningococcal Polysaccharide Vaccine, Groups A, C, Y, and W-135 *on this page*

Mentax® *see* Butenafine *on page 624*

Mepron™ *see* Atovaquone *on page 612*

Meronem® *see* Meropenem *on this page*

Meropenem (mer oh PEN em)

U.S. Brand Names Meronem®; Merrem® I.V.

Generic Available No

Use Intra-abdominal infections (complicated appendicitis and peritonitis) caused by viridans group streptococci, *E. coli*, *K. pneumoniae*, *P. aeruginosa*, *B. fragilis*, *B. thetaiotaomicron*, and *Peptostreptococcus* sp; also indicated for bacterial meningitis in pediatric patients >3 months of age caused by *S. pneumoniae*, *H. influenzae*, and *N. meningitidis*; meropenem has also been used to treat soft tissue infections, febrile neutropenia, and urinary tract infections

Drug of Choice or Alternative for

Disease/Syndrome(s)

Fever, Neutropenic *on page 30*
Meningitis, Pediatric (>2 months of age) *on page 35*
Osteomyelitis, Diabetic Foot *on page 38*
Peritonitis, Spontaneous Bacterial *on page 43*

Organism(s)

Acinetobacter Species *on page 58*
Alcaligenes Species *on page 65*
Bacteroides Species *on page 75*
Citrobacter Species *on page 102*
Clostridium perfringens on page 105
Enterobacter Species *on page 134*
Klebsiella Species *on page 183*
Proteus Species *on page 232*
Pseudomonas aeruginosa on page 235
Serratia Species *on page 250*

Pregnancy Risk Factor B

Pregnancy/Breast-Feeding Implications Although no teratogenic or infant harm has been found in studies, excretion in breast milk is not known and this drug should be used during pregnancy and lactation only if clearly indicated

Contraindications Patients with known hypersensitivity to meropenem, any component, or other carbapenems (eg, imipenem); patients who have experienced anaphylactic reactions to other beta-lactams

Warnings/Precautions Pseudomembranous colitis and hypersensitivity reactions have occurred and often require immediate drug discontinuation; thrombocytopenia has been reported in patients with significant renal dysfunction; seizures have occurred in patients with underlying neurologic disorders (less frequent than with Primaxin®); safety and efficacy have not been established for children <3 months of age; superinfection possible with long courses of therapy

Adverse Reactions

1% to 10%:
Central nervous system: Headache (2.8%)
Dermatologic: Rash, pruritus (1% to 2%)
Gastrointestinal: Diarrhea (5%), nausea/vomiting (4%), constipation (1.2%)
Local: Pain at injection site (3%), phlebitis, thrombophlebitis (1%)
Respiratory: Apnea (1.2%)

<1%: Hypotension, heart failure (MI and arrhythmias), tachycardia, hypertension, edema, seizures, insomnia, agitation, confusion, hallucinations, depression, seizures, fever, urticaria, anorexia, flatulence, ileus, oral moniliasis, glossitis, dysuria, RBCs in urine, cholestatic jaundice, hepatic failure, increase LFTs, anemia, hypo- and hypercytosis, bleeding events (epistaxis, melena, etc), paresthesia, whole body pain, renal failure, increased BUN/creatinine

Overdosage/Toxicology

No cases of acute overdosage are reported which have resulted in symptoms Supportive therapy recommended; meropenem and metabolite are removable by dialysis

Drug Interactions Increased effect: Probenecid competes with meropenem for active tubular secretion and inhibits the renal excretion of meropenem (half-life increased by 38%)

Stability Store at room temperature; when vials are reconstituted with NaCl/D₅W, they are stable for 2 hours/1 hour at room temperature or for 18 hours/8 hours when refrigerated; when diluted in minibags, they are stable for up to 24 hours refrigerated in NaCl and 6 hours in D₅W

Mechanism of Action Inhibits bacterial cell wall synthesis by binding to several of the penicillin-binding proteins, which in turn inhibit the final transpeptidation step of peptidoglycan synthesis in bacterial cell walls, thus inhibiting cell wall biosynthesis; bacteria eventually lyse due to ongoing activity of cell wall autolytic enzymes (autolysins and murein hydrolases) while cell wall assembly is arrested (Continued)

Meropenem *(Continued)*

Pharmacodynamics/Kinetics

Distribution: V_d: ~0.3 L/kg in adults (0.4-0.5 L/kg in children); penetrates well into most body fluids and tissues; CSF concentrations approximate those of the plasma

Protein binding: 2%

Metabolism: Hepatic; metabolizes to open beta-lactam form (inactive); not metabolized by same enzyme as imipenem which results in toxic metabolite

Half-life:

Normal renal function: 1-1.5 hours

Cl_{cr} 30-80 mL/minute: 1.9-3.3 hours

Cl_{cr} 2-30 mL/minute: 3.82-5.7 hours

Time to peak tissue concentration: 1 hour following infusion

Elimination: Renal, ~25% as the inactive metabolite

Usual Dosage I.V.:

Neonates:

Preterm: 20 mg/kg/dose every 12 hours (may be increased to 40 mg/kg/dose if treating a highly resistant organism such as *Pseudomonas aeruginosa*)

Full-term (<3 months of age): 20 mg/kg/dose every 8 hours (may be increased to 40 mg/kg/dose if treating a highly resistant organism such as *Pseudomonas aeruginosa*)

Children >3 months (<50 kg):

Intra-abdominal infections: 20 mg/kg every 8 hours (maximum dose: 1 g every 8 hours)

Meningitis: 40 mg/kg every 8 hours (maximum dose: 2 g every 8 hours)

Children >50 kg:

Intra-abdominal infections: 1 g every 8 hours

Meningitis: 2 g every 8 hours

Adults: 1 g every 8 hours

Dosing adjustment in renal impairment: Adults:

Cl_{cr} 26-50 mL/minute: Administer 1 g every 12 hours

Cl_{cr} 10-25 mL/minute: Administer 500 mg every 12 hours

Cl_{cr} <10 mL/minute: Administer 500 mg every 24 hours

Dialysis: Meropenem and its metabolites are readily dialyzable

Continuous arteriovenous or venovenous hemodiafiltration (CAVH) effects: Dose as for Cl_{cr} 10-50 mL/minute

Administration Administer I.V. infusion over 15-30 minutes; I.V. bolus injection over 3-5 minutes

Monitoring Parameters Monitor for signs of anaphylaxis during first dose

Additional Information 1 g of meropenem contains 90.2 mg of sodium as sodium carbonate (3.92 mEq)

Dosage Forms

Infusion: 500 mg (100 mL); 1 g (100 mL)

Infusion, ADD-vantage®: 500 mg (15 mL); 1 g (15 mL)

Injection: 25 mg/mL (20 mL); 33.3 mg/mL (30 mL)

Selected Readings

Fish DN and Singletary TJ, "Meropenem, A New Carbapenem Antibiotic," *Pharmacotherapy*, 1997, 17(4):644-69.

Hellinger WC and Brewer NS, "Carbapenems and Monobactams: Imipenem, Meropenem, and Aztreonam," *Mayo Clin Proc*, 1999, 74(4):420-34.

Wiseman LR, Wagstaff AJ, Brogden RN, et al, "Meropenem. A Review of Its Antibacterial Activity, Pharmacokinetic Properties, and Clinical Efficacy," *Drugs*, 1995, 50(1):73-101.

Merrem® I.V. *see* Meropenem *on page 812*

Meruvax® II *see* Rubella Virus Vaccine, Live *on page 914*

Mestatin® *see* Nystatin *on page 845*

Methenamine *(meth EN a meen)*

U.S. Brand Names Hiprex®; Mandelamine®; Urex®

Canadian Brand Names Dehydral™; Hip-Rex™; Urasal®

Synonyms Hexamethylenetetramine; Methenamine Hippurate; Methenamine Mandelate

Generic Available Yes

Use Prophylaxis or suppression of recurrent urinary tract infections; urinary tract discomfort secondary to hypermotility

Pregnancy Risk Factor C

Contraindications Severe dehydration, renal insufficiency, hepatic insufficiency in patients receiving hippurate salt, hypersensitivity to methenamine or any component; patients receiving sulfonamides

Warnings/Precautions Use with caution in patients with hepatic disease, gout, and the elderly; doses of 8 g/day for 3-4 weeks may cause bladder irritation, some products may contain tartrazine; methenamine should not be used to treat infections outside of the lower urinary tract. Use care to maintain an acid pH of the urine, especially when treating infections due to urea splitting organisms (eg, *Proteus* and strains of *Pseudomonas*); reversible increases in LFTs have occurred during therapy especially in patients with hepatic dysfunction.

Adverse Reactions
1% to 10%:
Dermatologic: Rash (3.5%)
Gastrointestinal: Nausea, dyspepsia (3.5%)
Genitourinary: Dysuria (3.5%)
<1%: Bladder irritation, crystalluria (especially with large doses), increased AST and ALT (reversible, rare)

Overdosage/Toxicology Well tolerated; treatment includes GI decontamination, if possible, and supportive care

Drug Interactions
Decreased effect: Sodium bicarbonate and acetazolamide will decrease effect secondary to alkalinization of urine
Increased toxicity: Sulfonamides (may precipitate)

Stability Protect from excessive heat

Mechanism of Action Methenamine is hydrolyzed to formaldehyde and ammonia in acidic urine; formaldehyde has nonspecific bactericidal action

Pharmacodynamics/Kinetics
Absorption: Readily absorbed from GI tract
Metabolism: 10% to 30% of the drug will be hydrolyzed by gastric juices unless it is protected by an enteric coating; ~10% to 25% is metabolized in the liver
Half-life: 3-6 hours
Elimination: Occurs via glomerular filtration and tubular secretion with ~70% to 90% of dose excreted unchanged in urine within 24 hours

Usual Dosage Oral:
Children:
<6 years: 0.25 g/30 lb 4 times/day
6-12 years:
Hippurate: 25-50 mg/kg/day divided every 12 hours or 0.5-1 g twice daily
Mandelate: 50-75 mg/kg/day divided every 6 hours or 0.5 g 4 times/day
Children >12 years and Adults:
Hippurate: 1 g twice daily
Mandelate: 1 g 4 times/day after meals and at bedtime

Dosing adjustment/comments in renal impairment: Cl_{cr} <50 mL/minute: Avoid use

Monitoring Parameters Urinalysis, periodic liver function tests in patients

Test Interactions Increases catecholamines and VMA (U); decreases HIAA (U)

Patient Information Take with food to minimize GI upset; take with ascorbic acid to acidify urine; drink sufficient fluids to ensure adequate urine flow. Avoid excessive intake of alkalinizing foods (citrus fruits and milk products) or medication (bicarbonate, acetazolamide); notify physician if skin rash, painful urination or excessive abdominal pain occur.

Nursing Implications Urine should be acidic (pH <5.5) for maximum effect

Additional Information Should not be used to treat infections outside of the lower urinary tract; methenamine has little, if any, role in the treatment or prevention of infections in patients with indwelling urinary (Foley) catheters; furthermore, in noncatheterized patients, more effective antibiotics are available for the prevention or treatment of urinary tract infections; the influence of decreased renal function on the pharmacologic effects of methenamine results are unknown

Dosage Forms
Suspension, oral: 0.5 g/5 mL (480 mL)
Tablet, as hippurate (Hiprex®, Urex®): 1 g (Hiprex® contains tartrazine dye)
Tablet, as mandelate, enteric coated: 500 mg, 1 g

Methenamine Hippurate *see Methenamine on previous page*

Methenamine Mandelate *see* Methenamine *on page 814*

Methicillin (meth i SIL in)
Related Information
Antimicrobial Activity Against Selected Organisms *on page 983*
U.S. Brand Names Staphcillin®
Synonyms Dimethoxyphenyl Penicillin Sodium; Methicillin Sodium; Sodium Methicillin
Generic Available No
Use Treatment of susceptible bacterial infections such as osteomyelitis, septicemia, endocarditis, and CNS infections due to penicillinase-producing strains of *Staphylococcus*; other antistaphylococcal penicillins are usually preferred
Pregnancy Risk Factor B
Contraindications Known hypersensitivity to methicillin or any penicillin
Warnings/Precautions Elimination rate will be slow in neonates; modify dosage in patients with renal impairment and in the elderly; use with caution in patients with cephalosporin hypersensitivity
Adverse Reactions
1% to 10%:
Dermatologic: Rash
Renal: Acute interstitial nephritis
<1%: Fever, rash, hemorrhagic cystitis, eosinophilia, anemia, leukopenia, neutropenia, thrombocytopenia, phlebitis, serum sickness-like reactions
Overdosage/Toxicology
Symptoms of penicillin overdose include neuromuscular hypersensitivity (agitation, hallucinations, asterixis, encephalopathy, confusion, and seizures) and electrolyte imbalance with potassium or sodium salts, especially in renal failure
Hemodialysis may be helpful to aid in the removal of the drug from the blood, otherwise most treatment is supportive or symptom directed
Drug Interactions
Decreased effect: Efficacy of oral contraceptives may be reduced
Increased effect: Disulfiram, probenecid may increase penicillin levels, increased effect of anticoagulants
Stability Reconstituted solution is stable for 24 hours at room temperature and 4 days when refrigerated; discard solutions if it has a distinctive hydrogen sulfide odor and/or color turns to a deep orange; **incompatible** with aminoglycosides and tetracyclines
Mechanism of Action Inhibits bacterial cell wall synthesis by binding to one or more of the penicillin binding proteins (PBPs); which in turn inhibits the final transpeptidation step of peptidoglycan synthesis in bacterial cell walls, thus inhibiting cell wall biosynthesis. Bacteria eventually lyse due to ongoing activity of cell wall autolytic enzymes (autolysins and murein hydrolases) while cell wall assembly is arrested.
Pharmacodynamics/Kinetics
Distribution: Crosses the placenta; distributes into milk
Protein binding: 40%
Metabolism: Only partially
Half-life (with normal renal function):
Neonates:
<2 weeks: 2-3.9 hours
>2 weeks: 0.9-3.3 hours
Children 2-16 years: 0.8 hour
Adults: 0.4-0.5 hour
Time to peak serum concentration:
I.M.: 0.5-1 hour
I.V. infusion: Within 5 minutes
Elimination: ~60% to 70% of dose eliminated unchanged in urine within 4 hours by tubular secretion and glomerular filtration
Usual Dosage I.M., I.V.:
Infants:
>7 days and >2000 g: 100 mg/kg/day in divided doses every 6 hours (for meningitis: 200 mg/kg/day)
>7 days and <2000 g: 75 mg/kg/day in divided doses every 8 hours (for meningitis: 150 mg/kg/day)

<7 days and >2000 g: Same as above

<7 days and <2000 g: 50 mg/kg/day in divided doses every 12 hours (for meningitis: 100 mg/kg/day)

Children: 100-300 mg/kg/day in divided doses every 4-6 hours

Adults: 4-12 g/day in divided doses every 4-6 hours

Dosing interval in renal impairment:

Cl_{cr} 10-50 mL/minute: Administer every 6-8 hours

Cl_{cr} <10 mL/minute: Administer every 8-12 hours

Hemodialysis: Not dialyzable (0% to 5%)

Administration Can be administered IVP at a rate not to exceed 200 mg/minute or intermittent infusion over 20-30 minutes; final concentration for administration should not exceed 20 mg/mL

Monitoring Parameters Observe for signs and symptoms of anaphylaxis during first dose

Test Interactions Interferes with tests for urinary and serum proteins, uric acid, urinary steroids; may cause false-positive Coombs' test; may inactivate aminoglycosides *in vitro*

Additional Information Sodium content of 1 g injection: 59.8-71.3 mg (2.6-3.1 mEq)

Dosage Forms Powder for injection, as sodium: 1 g, 4 g, 6 g, 10 g

Selected Readings

Donowitz GR and Mandell GL, "Beta-Lactam Antibiotics," *N Engl J Med*, 1988, 318(7):419-26 and 318(8):490-500.

Wright AJ, "The Penicillins," *Mayo Clin Proc*, 1999, 74(3):290-307.

Methicillin Sodium *see Methicillin on previous page*

Methylphenyl Isoxazolyl Penicillin *see Oxacillin on page 849*

Methylrosaniline Chloride *see Gentian Violet on page 751*

Metimyd® Ophthalmic *see Sulfacetamide Sodium and Prednisolone on page 928*

MetroGel® Topical *see Metronidazole on this page*

MetroGel®-Vaginal *see Metronidazole on this page*

Metro I.V.® Injection *see Metronidazole on this page*

Metronidazole (me troe NI da zole)

Related Information

Antimicrobial Activity Against Selected Organisms *on page 983*

U.S. Brand Names Flagyl® Oral; MetroGel® Topical; MetroGel®-Vaginal; Metro I.V.® Injection; Noritate® Cream; Protostat® Oral

Canadian Brand Names Apo®-Metronidazole; Novo-Nidazol

Synonyms Metronidazole Hydrochloride

Generic Available Yes

Use Treatment of susceptible anaerobic bacterial and protozoal infections in the following conditions: amebiasis, symptomatic and asymptomatic trichomoniasis; skin and skin structure infections; CNS infections; intra-abdominal infections; systemic anaerobic infections; topically for the treatment of acne rosacea; treatment of antibiotic-associated pseudomembranous colitis (AAPC), bacterial vaginosis; used in combination with other agents (eg, tetracycline, bismuth subsalicylate, and an H_2 antagonist) to treat duodenal ulcer disease due to *Helicobacter pylori*; also used in Crohn's disease and hepatic encephalopathy

Drug of Choice or Alternative for

Disease/Syndrome(s)

Brain Abscess *on page 19*

Cholangitis, Acute *on page 21*

Pelvic Inflammatory Disease *on page 41*

Vaginosis, Bacterial *on page 54*

Organism(s)

Bacteroides Species *on page 75*

Blastocystis hominis on page 78

Clostridium difficile on page 105

Clostridium perfringens on page 105

Clostridium tetani on page 107

Entamoeba histolytica on page 132

Gardnerella vaginalis on page 151

Giardia lamblia on page 153

(Continued)

Metronidazole *(Continued)*

Helicobacter pylori on page 160
Microsporidia *on page 195*
Mobiluncus Species *on page 196*
Trichomonas vaginalis on page 290

Pregnancy Risk Factor B

Contraindications Hypersensitivity to metronidazole or any component, 1st trimester of pregnancy since found to be carcinogenic in rats

Warnings/Precautions Use with caution in patients with liver impairment due to potential accumulation, blood dyscrasias; history of seizures, congestive heart failure, or other sodium-retaining states; reduce dosage in patients with severe liver impairment, CNS disease, and severe renal failure (Cl$_{cr}$ <10 mL/minute); if *H. pylori* is not eradicated in patients being treated with metronidazole in a regimen, it should be assumed that metronidazole-resistance has occurred and it should not again be used; seizures and neuropathies have been reported especially with increased doses and chronic treatment; if this occurs, discontinue therapy

Adverse Reactions

>10%:

Central nervous system: Dizziness, headache

Gastrointestinal (12%): Nausea, diarrhea, loss of appetite, vomiting

<1%: Ataxia, seizures, disulfiram-type reaction with alcohol, pancreatitis, xerostomia, metallic taste, furry tongue, vaginal candidiasis, leukopenia, thrombophlebitis, neuropathy, hypersensitivity, change in taste sensation, dark urine

Overdosage/Toxicology

Symptoms of overdose include nausea, vomiting, ataxia, seizures, peripheral neuropathy

Treatment is symptomatic and supportive

Drug Interactions CYP2C9 enzyme substrate; CYP2C9, 3A3/4, and 3A5-7 enzyme inhibitor

Decreased effect: Phenytoin, phenobarbital may decrease metronidazole half-life

Increased toxicity: Alcohol results in disulfiram-like reactions; metronidazole increases P-T prolongation with warfarin and increases lithium levels/toxicity; cimetidine may increase metronidazole levels

Stability

Metronidazole injection should be stored at 15°C to 30°C and protected from light

Product may be refrigerated but crystals may form; crystals redissolve on warming to room temperature

Prolonged exposure to light will cause a darkening of the product. However, short-term exposure to normal room light does not adversely affect metronidazole stability. Direct sunlight should be avoided.

Stability of parenteral admixture at room temperature (25°C): Out of overwrap stability: 30 days

Standard diluent: 500 mg/100 mL NS

Mechanism of Action Reduced to a product which interacts with DNA to cause a loss of helical DNA structure and strand breakage resulting in inhibition of protein synthesis and cell death in susceptible organisms

Pharmacodynamics/Kinetics

Absorption:

Oral: Well absorbed

Topical: Concentrations achieved systemically after application of 1 g topically are 10 times less than those obtained after a 250 mg oral dose

Distribution: To saliva, bile, seminal fluid, breast milk, bone, liver, and liver abscesses, lung and vaginal secretions; crosses placenta and blood-brain barrier; appears in breast milk; ratio of CSF to blood level: normal meninges: 16% to 43%, inflamed meninges: 100%

Protein binding: <20%

Metabolism: 30% to 60% in the liver

Half-life:

Neonates: 25-75 hours

Others: 6-8 hours, increases with hepatic impairment

End stage renal disease: 21 hours

Time to peak serum concentration: Within 1-2 hours

Elimination: Final excretion via the urine (20% to 40% as unchanged drug) and feces (6% to 15%)

Usual Dosage

Neonates: Anaerobic infections: Oral, I.V.:

0-4 weeks: <1200 g: 7.5 mg/kg/dose every 48 hours

Postnatal age <7 days:

1200-2000 g: 7.5 mg/kg/day every 24 hours

>2000 g: 15 mg/kg/day in divided doses every 12 hours

Postnatal age >7 days:

1200-2000 g: 15 mg/kg/day in divided doses every 12 hours

>2000 g: 30 mg/kg/day in divided doses every 12 hours

Infants and Children:

Amebiasis: Oral: 35-50 mg/kg/day in divided doses every 8 hours for 10 days

Trichomoniasis: Oral: 15-30 mg/kg/day in divided doses every 8 hours for 7 days

Anaerobic infections:

Oral: 15-35 mg/kg/day in divided doses every 8 hours

I.V.: 30 mg/kg/day in divided doses every 6 hours

Clostridium difficile (antibiotic-associated colitis): Oral: 20 mg/kg/day divided every 6 hours

Maximum dose: 2 g/day

Adults:

Amebiasis: Oral: 500-750 mg every 8 hours for 5-10 days

Trichomoniasis: Oral: 250 mg every 8 hours for 7 days or 2 g as a single dose

Anaerobic infections: Oral, I.V.: 500 mg every 6-8 hours, not to exceed 4 g/day

Antibiotic-associated pseudomembranous colitis: Oral: 250-500 mg 3-4 times/day for 10-14 days

H. pylori: 1 capsule with meals and at bedtime for 14 days in combination with other agents (eg, tetracycline, bismuth subsalicylate, and H_2 antagonist)

Vaginosis: 1 applicatorful (~37.5 mg metronidazole) intravaginally once or twice daily for 5 days; apply once in morning and evening if using twice daily, if daily, use at bedtime

Elderly: Use lower end of dosing recommendations for adults, do not administer as a single dose

Topical (acne rosacea therapy): Apply and rub a thin film twice daily, morning and evening, to entire affected areas after washing. Significant therapeutic results should be noticed within 3 weeks. Clinical studies have demonstrated continuing improvement through 9 weeks of therapy.

Dosing adjustment in renal impairment: Cl_{cr} <10 mL/minute: Administer every 12 hours

Hemodialysis: Extensively removed by hemodialysis and peritoneal dialysis (50% to 100%); administer dose posthemodialysis

Peritoneal dialysis: Dose as for Cl_{cr} <10 mL/minute

Continuous arteriovenous or venovenous hemofiltration (CAVH/CAVHD): Administer usual dose

Dosing adjustment/comments in hepatic disease: Unchanged in mild liver disease; reduce dosage in severe liver disease

Dietary Considerations

Alcohol: A disulfiram-like reaction characterized by flushing, headache, nausea, vomiting, sweating or tachycardia; patients should be warned to avoid alcohol during and 72 hours after therapy

Food: Peak antibiotic serum concentration lowered and delayed, but total drug absorbed not affected. Take on an empty stomach. Drug may cause GI upset; if GI upset occurs, take with food.

Test Interactions May interfere with AST, ALT, triglycerides, glucose, and LDH testing

Patient Information Urine may be discolored to a dark or reddish-brown; do not take alcohol for at least 24 hours after the last dose; avoid beverage alcohol or any topical products containing alcohol during therapy; may cause metallic taste; may be taken with food to minimize stomach upset; notify physician if numbness or tingling in extremities; avoid contact of the topical product with the eyes; cleanse areas to be treated well before application

Nursing Implications No Antabuse®-like reactions have been reported after **topical** application, although metronidazole can be detected in the blood; avoid contact between the drug and aluminum in the infusion set

Additional Information Sodium content of 500 mg (I.V.): 322 mg (14 mEq)

(Continued)

Metronidazole *(Continued)*

Dosage Forms

Capsule: 375 mg

Gel, topical: 0.75% [7.5 mg/mL] (30 g)

Gel, vaginal: 0.75% (5 g applicator delivering 37.5 mg; 70 g tube)

Injection, ready to use: 5 mg/mL (100 mL)

Powder for injection, as hydrochloride: 500 mg

Tablet: 250 mg, 500 mg

Extemporaneous Preparations

To prepare metronidazole suspension 50 mg/mL, pulverize ten 250 mg tablets; levigate with a small amount of distilled water; add 10 mL Cologel® and levigate; add sufficient quantity of cherry syrup to total 50 mL and levigate until a uniform mixture is obtained; stable for 30 days if refrigerated

Committee on Extemporaneous Formulations, ASHP Special Interest Group (SIG) on Pediatric Pharmacy Practice, *Handbook on Extemporaneous Formulations*, 1987.

Selected Readings

Falagas ME and Gorbach SL, "Clindamycin and Metronidazole," *Med Clin North Am*, 1995, 79(4):845-67.

Fekety R and Shah AB, "Diagnosis and Treatment of *Clostridium difficile* Colitis," *JAMA*, 1993, 269(1):71-5.

Freeman CD, Klutman NE, and Lamp KC, "Metronidazole. A Therapeutic Review and Update," *Drugs*, 1997, 54(5):679-708.

Kelly CP, Pothoulakis C, and LaMont JT, "*Clostridium difficile* Colitis," *N Engl J Med*, 1994, 330(4):257-62.

Smilack JD, Wilson WR, and Cockerill FR 3d, "Tetracyclines, Chloramphenicol, Erythromycin, Clindamycin, and Metronidazole," *Mayo Clin Proc*, 1991, 66(12):1270-80.

Metronidazole Hydrochloride *see* Metronidazole *on page 817*

Mezlin® *see* Mezlocillin *on this page*

Mezlocillin (mez loe SIL in)

Related Information

Antimicrobial Activity Against Selected Organisms *on page 983*

U.S. Brand Names Mezlin®

Synonyms Mezlocillin Sodium

Generic Available No

Use

Treatment of infections caused by susceptible gram-negative aerobic bacilli (*Klebsiella, Proteus, Escherichia coli, Enterobacter, Pseudomonas aeruginosa, Serratia*) involving the skin and skin structure, bone and joint, respiratory tract, urinary tract, gastrointestinal tract, as well as, septicemia

Drug of Choice or Alternative for Disease/Syndrome(s)

Cholangitis, Acute *on page 21*

Pregnancy Risk Factor B

Contraindications

Hypersensitivity to mezlocillin, any component, or penicillins

Warnings/Precautions

If bleeding occurs during therapy, mezlocillin should be discontinued; dosage modification required in patients with impaired renal function; use with caution in patients with renal impairment or biliary obstruction, or history of allergy to cephalosporins

Adverse Reactions

1% to 10%: Gastrointestinal: Nausea, diarrhea

<1%: Fever, seizures, dizziness, headache, rash, exfoliative dermatitis, hypokalemia, hypernatremia, vomiting, eosinophilia, leukopenia, neutropenia, thrombocytopenia, agranulocytosis, hemolytic anemia, prolonged bleeding time, positive direct Coombs' test, hepatotoxicity, increased liver enzymes, hematuria, increased BUN/serum creatinine, interstitial nephritis, serum sickness-like reactions

Overdosage/Toxicology

Symptoms of penicillin overdose include neuromuscular hypersensitivity (agitation, hallucinations, asterixis, encephalopathy, confusion, and seizures) and electrolyte imbalance with potassium or sodium salts, especially in renal failure

Hemodialysis may be helpful to aid in the removal of the drug from the blood, otherwise most treatment is supportive or symptom directed

Drug Interactions Aminoglycosides (synergy), probenecid (decreased clearance), vecuronium (increased duration of neuromuscular blockade), heparin (increased risk of bleeding); possible decrease in effectiveness of oral contraceptives; bacteriostatic action of tetracycline may impair bactericidal effects of the penicillins

Stability Reconstituted solution is stable for 48 hours at room temperature and 7 days when refrigerated; for I.V. infusion in NS or D_5W solution is stable for 48 hours at room temperature, 7 days when refrigerated or 28 days when frozen; after freezing, thawed solution is stable for 48 hours at room temperature or 7 days when refrigerated; if precipitation occurs under refrigeration, warm in water bath (37°C) for 20 minutes and shake well

Mechanism of Action Inhibits bacterial cell wall synthesis by binding to one or more of the penicillin binding proteins (PBPs); which in turn inhibits the final transpeptidation step of peptidoglycan synthesis in bacterial cell walls, thus inhibiting cell wall biosynthesis. Bacteria eventually lyse due to ongoing activity of cell wall autolytic enzymes (autolysins and murein hydrolases) while cell wall assembly is arrested.

Pharmacodynamics/Kinetics

Absorption: I.M.: 63%

Distribution: Into bile, heart, peritoneal fluid, sputum, bone; does not cross the blood-brain barrier well unless meninges are inflamed; crosses the placenta; distributes into breast milk at low concentrations

Protein binding: 30%

Metabolism: Minimal

Half-life: Dose dependent:

Neonates:

    <7 days: 3.7-4.4 hours

    >7 days: 2.5 hours

Children 2-19 years: 0.9 hour

Adults: 50-70 minutes, increased in renal impairment

Time to peak serum concentration:

  I.M.: 45-90 minutes after administration

  I.V. infusion: Within 5 minutes

Elimination: Principally as unchanged drug in urine, also excreted via bile

Usual Dosage I.M., I.V.:

Infants:

  ≤7 days, ≤2000 g: 75 mg/kg every 12 hours

  ≤7 days, >2000 g: Same as above

  >7 days, ≤2000 g: 75 mg/kg every 8 hours

  >7 days, >2000 g: 75 mg/kg every 6 hours

Children: 300 mg/kg/day divided every 4-6 hours; maximum: 24 g/day

Adults: Usual: 3-4 g every 4-6 hours

  Uncomplicated urinary tract infection: 1.5-2 g every 6 hours

  Serious infections: 200-300 mg/kg/day in 4-6 divided doses

Dosing interval in renal impairment:

  Cl_{cr} 10-30 mL/minute: Administer every 6-8 hours

  Cl_{cr} <10 mL/minute: Administer every 8 hours

  Hemodialysis: Moderately dialyzable (20% to 50%)

Dosing adjustment in hepatic impairment: Reduce dose by 50%

Administration Administer I.M. injections in large muscle mass, not more than 2 g/injection; I.M. injections given over 12-15 seconds will be less painful

Monitoring Parameters Observe for signs and symptoms of anaphylaxis during first dose

Test Interactions False-positive direct Coombs' test, false-positive urinary or serum protein, may inactivate aminoglycosides *in vitro*

Nursing Implications Administer at least 1 hour prior to aminoglycosides

Additional Information Minimum volume: 50 mL D_5W (concentration should not exceed 1 g/10 mL); sodium content of 1 g: 42.6 mg (1.85 mEq)

Dosage Forms Powder for injection, as sodium: 1 g, 2 g, 3 g, 4 g, 20 g

Selected Readings

Donowitz GR and Mandell GL, "Beta-Lactam Antibiotics," *N Engl J Med*, 1988, 318(7):419-26 and 318(8):490-500.

Wright AJ, "The Penicillins," *Mayo Clin Proc*, 1999, 74(3):290-307.

Mezlocillin Sodium *see* Mezlocillin *on previous page*

Micatin® Topical [OTC] *see* Miconazole *on next page*

Miconazole (mi KON a zole)

U.S. Brand Names Absorbine® Antifungal Foot Powder [OTC]; Breezee® Mist Antifungal [OTC]; Femizol-M® [OTC]; Fungoid® Creme; Fungoid® Tincture; Lotrimin® AF Powder [OTC]; Lotrimin® AF Spray Liquid [OTC]; Lotrimin® AF Spray Powder [OTC]; Maximum Strength Desenex® Antifungal Cream [OTC]; Micatin® Topical [OTC]; Monistat-Derm™ Topical; Monistat i.v.™ Injection; Monistat™ Vaginal; M-Zole® 7 Dual Pack [OTC]; Ony-Clear® Spray; Prescription Strength Desenex® Powder [OTC]; Zeasorb-AF® Powder [OTC]

Canadian Brand Names Monazole-7®

Synonyms Miconazole Nitrate

Generic Available No

Use

I.V.: Treatment of severe systemic fungal infections and fungal meningitis that are refractory to standard treatment

Topical: Treatment of vulvovaginal candidiasis and a variety of skin and mucous membrane fungal infections

Drug of Choice or Alternative for

Organism(s)

Malassezia furfur on page 192

Pregnancy Risk Factor C

Contraindications Hypersensitivity to miconazole, fluconazole, ketoconazole, polyoxyl 35 castor oil, or any component; concomitant administration with cisapride

Warnings/Precautions Administer I.V. with caution to patients with hepatic insufficiency; the safety of miconazole in patients <1 year of age has not been established; cardiorespiratory and anaphylaxis have occurred with excessively rapid administration

Adverse Reactions

>10%:

Central nervous system: Fever, chills (10%)

Dermatologic: Rash, itching, pruritus (21%)

Gastrointestinal: Anorexia, diarrhea, nausea (18%), vomiting (7%)

Local: Pain at injection site

1% to 10%: Dermatologic: Rash (9%)

<1%: Flushing of face or skin, drowsiness, anemia, thrombocytopenia

Overdosage/Toxicology

Symptoms of overdose include nausea, vomiting, drowsiness

Following GI decontamination, supportive care only

Drug Interactions CYP3A3/4 enzyme substrate; CYP2C enzyme inhibitor, CYP3A3/4 enzyme inhibitor (moderate), and CYP3A5-7 enzyme inhibitor

Warfarin (increased anticoagulant effect), oral sulfonylureas, amphotericin B (decreased antifungal effect of both agents), phenytoin (levels may be increased)

Increased risk of significant cardiotoxicity with concurrent administration of cisapride - concomitant administration is contraindicated (see interactions associated with ketoconazole)

Stability Protect from heat; darkening of solution indicates deterioration; stability of parenteral admixture at room temperature (25°C): 2 days

Mechanism of Action Inhibits biosynthesis of ergosterol, damaging the fungal cell wall membrane, which increases permeability causing leaking of nutrients

Pharmacodynamics/Kinetics

Absorption: Topical: Negligible

Distribution: Appears to be widely distributed to body tissues; penetrates well into inflamed joints, vitreous humor of eye, and peritoneal cavity, but poorly into saliva and sputum; crosses blood-brain barrier but only to a small extent

Protein binding: 91% to 93%

Metabolism: In the liver

Half-life, multiphasic:

Initial: 40 minutes

Secondary: 126 minutes

Terminal phase: 24 hours

Elimination: ~50% excreted in feces and <1% in urine as unchanged drug

Usual Dosage

Children:

<1 year: 15-30 mg/kg/day

1-12 years:
  I.V.: 20-40 mg/kg/day divided every 8 hours (do not exceed 15 mg/kg/dose)
  Topical: Apply twice daily for up to 1 month
Adults:
  Topical: Apply twice daily for up to 1 month
  I.T.: 20 mg every 1-2 days
  I.V.: Initial: 200 mg, then 0.6-3.6 g/day divided every 8 hours for up to 20 weeks
  Bladder candidal infections: 200 mg diluted solution instilled in the bladder
  Vaginal: Insert contents of 1 applicator of vaginal cream (100 mg) or 100 mg suppository at bedtime for 7 days, or 200 mg suppository at bedtime for 3 days

Hemodialysis: Not dialyzable (0% to 5%)

Administration Administer I.V. dose over 2 hours

Test Interactions Increases protein

Patient Information Avoid contact with the eyes; for vaginal product, insert high into vagina and complete full course of therapy; notify physician if itching or burning occur; refrain from intercourse to prevent reinfection

Nursing Implications Observe patient closely during first I.V. dose for allergic reactions

Additional Information
Miconazole: Monistat i.v.™
Miconazole nitrate: Micatin®, Monistat™, Monistat-Derm™

Dosage Forms
Cream:
  Topical, as nitrate: 2% (15 g, 30 g, 56.7 g, 85 g)
  Vaginal, as nitrate: 2% (45 g is equivalent to 7 doses)
Dual pack: Vaginal suppositories and external vulvar cream 2%
Injection: 1% [10 mg/mL] (20 mL)
Lotion, as nitrate: 2% (30 mL, 60 mL)
Powder, topical: 2% (45 g, 90 g, 113 g)
Spray, topical: 2% (105 mL)
Suppository, vaginal, as nitrate: 100 mg (7s); 200 mg (3s)
Tincture: 2% with alcohol (7.39 mL, 29.57 mL)

Miconazole Nitrate see Miconazole on previous page
MICRhoGAM™ see Rh₀(D) Immune Globulin on page 896
Microsulfon® see Sulfadiazine on page 929
Mini-Gamulin® Rh see Rh₀(D) Immune Globulin on page 896
Minocin® IV Injection see Minocycline on this page
Minocin® Oral see Minocycline on this page

Minocycline (mi noe SYE kleen)

U.S. Brand Names Dynacin® Oral; Minocin® IV Injection; Minocin® Oral
Canadian Brand Names Apo®-Minocycline; Syn-Minocycline
Synonyms Minocycline Hydrochloride
Generic Available Yes
Use Treatment of susceptible bacterial infections of both gram-negative and gram-positive organisms; acne, meningococcal carrier state
Drug of Choice or Alternative for
Organism(s)
  Burkholderia cepacia on page 87
  Nocardia Species on page 218
  Stenotrophomonas maltophilia on page 265
Pregnancy Risk Factor D
Contraindications Hypersensitivity to minocycline, other tetracyclines, or any component; children <8 years of age
Warnings/Precautions Should be avoided in renal insufficiency, children ≤8 years of age, pregnant and nursing women; photosensitivity reactions can occur with minocycline
Adverse Reactions
>10%: Miscellaneous: Discoloration of teeth in children
1% to 10%:
  Dermatologic: Photosensitivity
  Gastrointestinal: Nausea, diarrhea
(Continued)

Minocycline *(Continued)*

<1%: Pericarditis, increased intracranial pressure, bulging fontanels in infants, dermatologic effects, pruritus, exfoliative dermatitis, rash, pigmentation of nails, diabetes insipidus syndrome, vomiting, esophagitis, anorexia, abdominal cramps, paresthesia, acute renal failure, azotemia, superinfections, anaphylaxis

Overdosage/Toxicology

Symptoms of overdose include diabetes insipidus, nausea, anorexia, diarrhea

Following GI decontamination, supportive care only; fluid support may be required

Drug Interactions

Decreased effect with antacids (aluminum, calcium, zinc, or magnesium), bismuth salts, sodium bicarbonate, barbiturates, carbamazepine, hydantoins; decreased effect of oral contraceptives

Increased effect of warfarin

Mechanism of Action Inhibits bacterial protein synthesis by binding with the 30S and possibly the 50S ribosomal subunit(s) of susceptible bacteria; cell wall synthesis is not affected

Pharmacodynamics/Kinetics

Absorption: Well absorbed

Distribution: Crosses placenta; appears in breast milk; majority of a dose deposits for extended periods in fat

Protein binding: 70% to 75%

Half-life: 15 hours

Elimination: Eventually cleared renally

Usual Dosage

Children >8 years: Oral, I.V.: Initial: 4 mg/kg followed by 2 mg/kg/dose every 12 hours

Adults:

Infection: Oral, I.V.: 200 mg stat, 100 mg every 12 hours not to exceed 400 mg/24 hours

Acne: Oral: 50 mg 1-3 times/day

Hemodialysis: Not dialyzable (0% to 5%)

Administration Infuse I.V. minocycline over 1 hour

Patient Information Avoid unnecessary exposure to sunlight; do not take with antacids, iron products, or dairy products; finish all medication; do not skip doses; take 1 hour before or 2 hours after meals

Dosage Forms

Capsule:

As hydrochloride: 50 mg, 100 mg

As hydrochloride (Dynacin®, Vectrin®): 50 mg, 100 mg

Pellet-filled, as hydrochloride (Minocin®): 50 mg, 100 mg

Injection, as hydrochloride (Minocin® IV): 100 mg

Suspension, oral, as hydrochloride (Minocin®)50 mg/5 mL (60 mL)

Selected Readings

Smilack JD, Wilson WR, and Cockerill FR 3d, "Tetracyclines, Chloramphenicol, Erythromycin, Clindamycin, and Metronidazole," *Mayo Clin Proc*, 1991, 66(12):1270-80.

Mumps, Measles and Rubella Vaccines, Combined *see* Measles, Mumps, and Rubella Vaccines, Combined *on page 805*

Mumpsvax® *see* Mumps Virus Vaccine, Live *on this page*

Mumps Virus Vaccine, Live (mumpz VYE rus vak SEEN, live)

Related Information
Immunization Guidelines *on page 1041*

U.S. Brand Names Mumpsvax®

Generic Available No

Use Mumps prophylaxis by promoting active immunity

Note: Trivalent measles-mumps-rubella (MMR) vaccine is the preferred agent for most children and many adults; persons born prior to 1957 are generally considered immune and need not be vaccinated

Pregnancy Risk Factor C

Pregnancy/Breast-Feeding Implications Although mumps virus can infect the placenta and fetus, there is not good evidence that it causes congenital malformations

Warnings/Precautions Pregnancy, immunocompromised persons, history of anaphylactic reaction following egg ingestion or receipt of neomycin

Adverse Reactions All serious adverse reactions must be reported to the U.S. Department of Health and Human Services (DHHS) Vaccine Adverse Event Reporting System (VAERS) 1-800-822-7967.

>10%: Local: Burning or stinging at injection site
1% to 10%:
  Central nervous system: Fever (≤100°F)
  Dermatologic: Rash
  Endocrine & metabolic: Parotitis
<1%: Convulsions, confusion, severe or continuing headache, fever (>103°F), orchitis in postpubescent and adult males, thrombocytopenic purpura, anaphylactic reactions

Drug Interactions Whole blood, interferon immune globulin, radiation therapy, and immunosuppressive drugs (eg, corticosteroids) may result in insufficient response to immunization; may temporarily depress tuberculin skin test sensitivity and reduce the seroconversion. DTP, OPV, MMR, Hib, and hepatitis B may be given concurrently; other virus vaccine administration should be separated by ≥1 month.

Stability Refrigerate, protect from light, discard within 8 hours after reconstitution

Mechanism of Action Promotes active immunity to mumps virus by inducing specific antibodies.

Usual Dosage Children ≥15 months and Adults: 0.5 mL S.C. in outer aspect of the upper arm, no booster

Administration Reconstitute only with diluent provided; administer only S.C. on outer aspect of upper arm

Test Interactions Temporary suppression of tuberculosis skin test

Patient Information Pregnancy should be avoided for 3 months following vaccination; a little swelling of the glands in the cheeks and under the jaw may occur that lasts for a few days; this could happen from 1-2 weeks after getting the mumps vaccine; this happens rarely

Additional Information Federal law requires that the date of administration, the vaccine manufacturer, lot number of vaccine, and the administering person's name, title and address be entered into the patient's permanent medical record; all adults without documentation of live vaccine on or after the first birthday or physician-diagnosed mumps, or laboratory evidence or immunity (particularly males and young adults who work in or congregate in hospitals, colleges, and on military bases) should be vaccinated. It is reasonable to consider persons born before 1957 immune, but there is no contraindication to vaccination of older persons. Susceptible travelers should be vaccinated.

Dosage Forms Injection: Single dose

Mupirocin (myoo PEER oh sin)

U.S. Brand Names Bactroban®; Bactroban® Nasal

Synonyms Mupirocin Calcium; Pseudomonic Acid A

Generic Available No

(Continued)

Mupirocin *(Continued)*

Use Topical treatment of impetigo due to *Staphylococcus aureus*, beta-hemolytic *Streptococcus*, and *S. pyogenes*

Drug of Choice or Alternative for
Disease/Syndrome(s)
Impetigo *on page 32*

Pregnancy Risk Factor B

Contraindications Known hypersensitivity to mupirocin or polyethylene glycol

Warnings/Precautions Potentially toxic amounts of polyethylene glycol contained in the vehicle may be absorbed percutaneously in patients with extensive burns or open wounds; prolonged use may result in over growth of nonsusceptible organisms; for external use only; not for treatment of pressure sores

Adverse Reactions 1% to 10%:
Dermatologic: Pruritus, rash, erythema, dry skin
Local: Burning, stinging, tenderness, edema, pain

Stability Do not mix with Aquaphor®, coal tar solution, or salicylic acid

Mechanism of Action Binds to bacterial isoleucyl transfer-RNA synthetase resulting in the inhibition of protein and RNA synthesis

Pharmacodynamics/Kinetics
Absorption: Topical: Penetrates the outer layers of the skin; systemic absorption minimal through intact skin
Protein binding: 95%
Metabolism: Extensively to monic acid, principally in the liver and skin
Half-life: 17-36 minutes
Elimination: In urine

Usual Dosage
Topical: Children and Adults: Apply small amount to affected area 2-5 times/day for 5-14 days
Nasal: In adults (12 years of age and older), approximately one-half of the ointment from the single-use tube should be applied into one nostril and the other half into the other nostril twice daily for 5 days

Patient Information For topical use only; do not apply into the eye; discontinue if rash, itching, or irritation occurs; improvement should be seen in 5 days

Additional Information Not for treatment of pressure sores in elderly; contains polyethylene glycol vehicle

Dosage Forms Ointment, as calcium:
Intranasal: 2% (1 g single use tube)
Topical: 2% (15 g, 30 g)

Mupirocin Calcium *see Mupirocin on previous page*

Myambutol® *see Ethambutol on page 727*

Mycelex® *see Clotrimazole on page 688*

Mycelex®-7 *see Clotrimazole on page 688*

Mycelex®-G *see Clotrimazole on page 688*

Mycifradin® Sulfate Oral *see Neomycin on page 833*

Mycifradin® Sulfate Topical *see Neomycin on page 833*

Mycitracin® Topical [OTC] *see Bacitracin, Neomycin, and Polymyxin B on page 619*

Mycobutin® *see Rifabutin on page 900*

Mycogen II Topical *see Nystatin and Triamcinolone on page 846*

Mycolog®-II Topical *see Nystatin and Triamcinolone on page 846*

Myconel® Topical *see Nystatin and Triamcinolone on page 846*

Mycostatin® *see Nystatin on page 845*

Myco-Triacet® II *see Nystatin and Triamcinolone on page 846*

Mytrex® F Topical *see Nystatin and Triamcinolone on page 846*

M-Zole® 7 Dual Pack [OTC] *see Miconazole on page 822*

Nadopen-V® *see Penicillin V Potassium on page 865*

Nadostine® *see Nystatin on page 845*

Nafcil™ Injection *see Nafcillin on this page*

Nafcillin *(naf SIL in)*

Related Information
Antimicrobial Activity Against Selected Organisms *on page 983*

U.S. Brand Names Nafcil™ Injection; Nallpen® Injection; Unipen® Injection; Unipen® Oral

Synonyms Ethoxynaphthamido Penicillin Sodium; Nafcillin Sodium; Sodium Nafcillin

Generic Available Yes

Use Treatment of infections such as osteomyelitis, septicemia, endocarditis, and CNS infections caused by susceptible strains of staphylococcal species

Pregnancy Risk Factor B

Contraindications Hypersensitivity to nafcillin or any component or penicillins

Warnings/Precautions Extravasation of I.V. infusions should be avoided; modification of dosage is necessary in patients with both severe renal and hepatic impairment; elimination rate will be slow in neonates; use with caution in patients with cephalosporin hypersensitivity

Adverse Reactions Percentage unknown: Fever, pain, rash, nausea, diarrhea, neutropenia, thrombophlebitis; oxacillin (less likely to cause phlebitis) is often preferred in pediatric patients, acute interstitial nephritis, hypersensitivity reactions

Overdosage/Toxicology

Symptoms of penicillin overdose include neuromuscular hypersensitivity (agitation, hallucinations, asterixis, encephalopathy, confusion, and seizures) and electrolyte imbalance with potassium or sodium salts, especially in renal failure

Hemodialysis may be helpful to aid in the removal of the drug from the blood, otherwise most treatment is supportive or symptom directed

Drug Interactions

Decreased effect: Efficacy of oral contraceptives may be reduced; decreased effect of warfarin/anticoagulants

Increased effect: Disulfiram, probenecid may increase penicillin levels

Stability Refrigerate oral solution after reconstitution; discard after 7 days; reconstituted parenteral solution is stable for 3 days at room temperature and 7 days when refrigerated or 12 weeks when frozen; for I.V. infusion in NS or D_5W, solution is stable for 24 hours at room temperature and 96 hours when refrigerated

Mechanism of Action Interferes with bacterial cell wall synthesis during active multiplication, causing cell wall death and resultant bactericidal activity against susceptible bacteria

Pharmacodynamics/Kinetics

Absorption: Oral: Poor and erratic

Distribution: Widely distributed; CSF penetration is poor but enhanced by meningeal inflammation; crosses the placenta

Metabolism: Primarily in the liver; it undergoes enterohepatic circulation

Half-life:

Neonates:

<3 weeks: 2.2-5.5 hours

4-9 weeks: 1.2-2.3 hours

Children 3 months to 14 years: 0.75-1.9 hours

Adults: 30 minutes to 1.5 hours, with normal renal and hepatic function

Time to peak serum concentration:

Oral: Within 2 hours

I.M.: Within 30-60 minutes

Elimination: Primarily eliminated in bile, 10% to 30% in urine as unchanged drug; undergoes enterohepatic recycling

Usual Dosage

Neonates:

<2000 g, <7 days: 50 mg/kg/day divided every 12 hours

<2000 g, >7 days: 75 mg/kg/day divided every 8 hours

>2000 g, <7 days: 50 mg/kg/day divided every 8 hours

>2000 g, >7 days: 75 mg/kg/day divided every 6 hours

Children:

Oral: 25-50 mg/kg/day in 4 divided doses

I.M.: 25 mg/kg twice daily

I.V.:

Mild to moderate infections: 50-100 mg/kg/day in divided doses every 6 hours

Severe infections: 100-200 mg/kg/day in divided doses every 4-6 hours

(Continued)

Nafcillin *(Continued)*

Maximum dose: 12 g/day
Adults:
Oral: 250-500 mg (up to 1 g) every 4-6 hours
I.M.: 500 mg every 4-6 hours
I.V.: 500-2000 mg every 4-6 hours

Dosing adjustment in renal impairment: Not necessary
Dialysis: Not dialyzable (0% to 5%) via hemodialysis; supplemental dosage not necessary with hemo- or peritoneal dialysis or continuous arteriovenous or venovenous hemofiltration (CAVH/CAVHD)

Monitoring Parameters Periodic CBC, urinalysis, BUN, serum creatinine, AST and ALT; observe for signs and symptoms of anaphylaxis during first dose

Test Interactions Positive direct Coombs' test, false-positive urinary and serum proteins, may inactivate aminoglycosides *in vitro*

Nursing Implications
Extravasation: Use cold packs
Hyaluronidase (Wydase®): Add 1 mL NS to 150 unit vial to make 150 units/mL of concentration; mix 0.1 mL of above with 0.9 mL NS in 1 mL syringe to make final concentration = 15 units/mL

Additional Information Sodium content of 1 g: 66.7 mg (2.9 mEq); other penicillinase-resistant penicillins (ie, dicloxacillin or cloxacillin) are preferred for oral therapy

Dosage Forms
Capsule, as sodium: 250 mg
Powder for injection, as sodium: 500 mg, 1 g, 2 g, 4 g, 10 g
Solution, as sodium: 250 mg/5 mL (100 mL)
Tablet, as sodium: 500 mg

Selected Readings
Donowitz GR and Mandell GL, "Beta-Lactam Antibiotics," *N Engl J Med*, 1988, 318(7):419-26 and 318(8):490-500.
Wright AJ, "The Penicillins," *Mayo Clin Proc*, 1999, 74(3):290-307.

Nafcillin Sodium *see* Nafcillin *on page 826*

Naftifine *(NAF ti feen)*

U.S. Brand Names Naftin®
Synonyms Naftifine Hydrochloride
Generic Available No
Use Topical treatment of tinea cruris (jock itch), tinea corporis (ringworm), and tinea pedis (athlete's foot)
Pregnancy Risk Factor B
Contraindications Hypersensitivity to any component
Warnings/Precautions For external use only
Adverse Reactions
>10%: Local: Burning, stinging
1% to 10%:
Dermatologic: Erythema, itching
Local: Dryness, irritation
Mechanism of Action Synthetic, broad-spectrum antifungal agent in the allylamine class; appears to have both fungistatic and fungicidal activity. Exhibits antifungal activity by selectively inhibiting the enzyme squalene epoxidase in a dose-dependent manner which results in the primary sterol, ergosterol, within the fungal membrane not being synthesized.
Pharmacodynamics/Kinetics
Absorption: Systemic, 6% for cream, ≤4% for gel
Half-life: 2-3 days
Elimination: Metabolites excreted in urine and feces
Usual Dosage Adults: Topical: Apply cream once daily and gel twice daily (morning and evening) for up to 4 weeks
Patient Information External use only; avoid eyes, mouth, and other mucous membranes; do not use occlusive dressings unless directed to do so; discontinue if irritation or sensitivity develops; wash hands after application
Dosage Forms
Cream, as hydrochloride: 1% (15 g, 30 g, 60 g)
Gel, topical, as hydrochloride: 1% (20 g, 40 g, 60 g)

Naftifine Hydrochloride *see Naftifine on previous page*
Naftin® *see Naftifine on previous page*

Nalidixic Acid (nal i DIKS ik AS id)

U.S. Brand Names NegGram®
Synonyms Nalidixinic Acid
Generic Available Yes
Use Treatment of urinary tract infections
Pregnancy Risk Factor B
Contraindications Hypersensitivity to nalidixic acid or any component; infants <3 months of age
Warnings/Precautions Use with caution in patients with impaired hepatic or renal function and prepubertal children; has been shown to cause cartilage degeneration in immature animals; may induce hemolysis in patients with G-6-PD deficiency

Adverse Reactions
>10%: Central nervous system: Dizziness, drowsiness, headache
1% to 10%: Gastrointestinal: Nausea, vomiting
<1%: Increased intracranial pressure, malaise, vertigo, confusion, toxic psychosis, convulsions, fever, chills, rash, urticaria, photosensitivity reactions, metabolic acidosis, leukopenia, thrombocytopenia, hepatotoxicity, visual disturbances

Overdosage/Toxicology
Symptoms of overdose include nausea, vomiting, toxic psychosis, convulsions, increased intracranial pressure, metabolic acidosis; severe overdose, intracranial hypertension, increased pressure, and seizures have occurred
After GI decontamination, treatment is symptomatic

Drug Interactions
Decreased effect with antacids
Increased effect of warfarin

Mechanism of Action Inhibits DNA polymerization in late stages of chromosomal replication

Pharmacodynamics/Kinetics
Distribution: Crosses the placenta; appears in breast milk; achieves significant antibacterial concentrations only in the urinary tract
Metabolism: Partly in the liver
Half-life: 6-7 hours; increases significantly with renal impairment
Time to peak serum concentration: Oral: Within 1-2 hours
Elimination: Excreted in urine as unchanged drug and 80% as metabolites; small amounts appear in feces

Usual Dosage Oral:
Children 3 months to 12 years: 55 mg/kg/day divided every 6 hours; suppressive therapy is 33 mg/kg/day divided every 6 hours

Adults: 1 g 4 times/day for 2 weeks; then suppressive therapy of 500 mg 4 times/day

Dosing comments in renal impairment: Cl_{cr} <50 mL/minute: Avoid use
Test Interactions False-positive urine glucose with Clinitest®, false increase in urinary VMA
Patient Information Avoid undue exposure to direct sunlight or use a sunscreen; take 1 hour before meals, but can take with food to decrease GI upset, finish all medication, do not skip doses; if persistent cough occurs, notify physician

Dosage Forms
Suspension, oral (raspberry flavor): 250 mg/5 mL (473 mL)
Tablet: 250 mg, 500 mg, 1 g

Nalidixinic Acid *see Nalidixic Acid on this page*
Nallpen® Injection *see Nafcillin on page 826*

Nandrolone (NAN droe lone)

U.S. Brand Names Androlone®; Androlone®-D; Deca-Durabolin®; Durabolin®; Hybolin™ Decanoate; Hybolin™ Improved; Neo-Durabolic
Synonyms Nandrolone Decanoate; Nandrolone Phenpropionate
Generic Available Yes
(Continued)

Nandrolone *(Continued)*

Use Treatment of "AIDS-wasting" syndrome; control of metastatic breast cancer; management of anemia of renal insufficiency

Restrictions C-III

Pregnancy Risk Factor X

Contraindications Carcinoma of breast or prostate, nephrosis, pregnancy and infants, hypersensitivity to any component

Warnings/Precautions Monitor diabetic patients carefully; anabolic steroids may cause peliosis hepatis, liver cell tumors, and blood lipid changes with increased risk of arteriosclerosis; use with caution in elderly patients, they may be at greater risk for prostatic hypertrophy; use with caution in patients with cardiac, renal, or hepatic disease or epilepsy

Adverse Reactions

Male:

Postpubertal:
>10%:
Dermatologic: Acne
Endocrine & metabolic: Gynecomastia
Genitourinary: Bladder irritability, priapism
1% to 10%:
Central nervous system: Insomnia, chills
Endocrine & metabolic: Decreased libido, hepatic dysfunction,
Gastrointestinal: Nausea, diarrhea
Genitourinary: Prostatic hypertrophy (elderly)
Hematologic: Iron deficiency anemia, suppression of clotting factors
<1%: Hepatic necrosis, hepatocellular carcinoma

Prepubertal:
>10%:
Dermatologic: Acne
Endocrine & metabolic: Virilism
1% to 10%:
Central nervous system: Chills, insomnia
Dermatologic: Hyperpigmentation
Gastrointestinal: Diarrhea, nausea
Hematologic: Iron deficiency anemia, suppression of clotting factors
<1%: Hepatocellular carcinoma, necrosis

Female:
>10%: Endocrine & metabolic: Virilism
1% to 10%:
Central nervous system: Chills, insomnia
Endocrine & metabolic: Hypercalcemia
Gastrointestinal: Nausea, diarrhea
Hematologic: Iron deficiency anemia, suppression of clotting factors
Hepatic: Hepatic dysfunction
<1%: Hepatic necrosis, hepatocellular carcinoma

Drug Interactions Increased toxicity: Oral anticoagulants, insulin, oral hypoglycemic agents, adrenal steroids, ACTH

Mechanism of Action Promotes tissue-building processes, increases production of erythropoietin, causes protein anabolism; increases hemoglobin and red blood cell volume

Pharmacodynamics/Kinetics
Metabolism: In the liver
Elimination: In urine

Usual Dosage Deep I.M. (into gluteal muscle):
Children 2-13 years: (decanoate): 25-50 mg every 3-4 weeks
Adults:
Male:
Breast cancer (phenpropionate): 50-100 mg/week
Anemia of renal insufficiency (decanoate): 100-200 mg/week
Female: 50-100 mg/week
Breast cancer (phenpropionate): 50-100 mg/week
Anemia of renal insufficiency (decanoate): 50-100 mg/week
AIDS wasting: 100 mg/week; up to 600 mg/week may be used

Administration Inject deeply I.M., preferably into the gluteal muscle

Test Interactions Altered glucose tolerance tests

Patient Information Virilization may occur in female patients; report menstrual irregularities; male patients report persistent penile erections; all patients should report persistent GI distress, diarrhea, dark urine, pale stools, yellow coloring of skin or sclera; diabetic patients should monitor glucose closely

Additional Information Both phenpropionate and decanoate are Injections in oil

Dosage Forms

Injection, as phenpropionate, in oil: 25 mg/mL (5 mL); 50 mg/mL (2 mL)

Injection, as decanoate, in oil: 50 mg/mL (1 mL, 2 mL); 100 mg/mL (1 mL, 2 mL); 200 mg/mL (1 mL)

Injection, repository, as decanoate: 50 mg/mL (2 mL); 100 mg/mL (2 mL); 200 mg/mL (2 mL)

Nandrolone Decanoate *see* Nandrolone *on page 829*

Nandrolone Phenpropionate *see* Nandrolone *on page 829*

Natacyn® Ophthalmic *see* Natamycin *on this page*

Natamycin (na ta MYE sin)

U.S. Brand Names Natacyn® Ophthalmic

Synonyms Pimaricin

Generic Available No

Use Treatment of blepharitis, conjunctivitis, and keratitis caused by susceptible fungi (*Aspergillus*, *Candida*), *Cephalosporium*, *Curvularia*, *Fusarium*, *Penicillium*, *Microsporum*, *Epidermophyton*, *Blastomyces dermatitidis*, *Coccidioides immitis*, *Cryptococcus neoformans*, *Histoplasma capsulatum*, *Sporothrix schenckii*, and *Trichomonas vaginalis*

Pregnancy Risk Factor C

Contraindications Known hypersensitivity to natamycin or any component

Warnings/Precautions Failure to improve (keratitis) after 7-10 days of administration suggests infection caused by a microorganism not susceptible to natamycin; inadequate as a single agent in fungal endophthalmitis

Adverse Reactions <1%: Blurred vision, photophobia, eye pain, eye irritation not present before therapy

Drug Interactions Increased toxicity: Topical corticosteroids (concomitant use contraindicated)

Stability Store at room temperature (8°C to 24°C/46°F to 75°F); protect from excessive heat and light; do not freeze

Mechanism of Action Increases cell membrane permeability in susceptible fungi

Pharmacodynamics/Kinetics

Absorption: Ophthalmic: <2% systemically absorbed

Distribution: Adheres to cornea and is retained in the conjunctival fornices

Usual Dosage Adults: Ophthalmic: Instill 1 drop in conjunctival sac every 1-2 hours, after 3-4 days reduce to 1 drop 6-8 times/day; usual course of therapy: 2-3 weeks

Patient Information Shake well before using, do not touch dropper to eye; notify physician if condition worsens or does not improve after 3-4 days

Dosage Forms Suspension, ophthalmic: 5% (15 mL)

Nebcin® Injection *see* Tobramycin *on page 953*

NebuPent™ Inhalation *see* Pentamidine *on page 866*

NegGram® *see* Nalidixic Acid *on page 829*

Nelfinavir (nel FIN a veer)

Related Information

HIV Therapeutic Information *on page 1008*

U.S. Brand Names Viracept®

Use In combination with other antiretroviral therapy in the treatment of HIV infection

Pregnancy Risk Factor B

Pregnancy/Breast-Feeding Implications Breast-feeding/lactation: Animal studies suggest that nelfinavir may be excreted in human milk; the CDC advises against breast-feeding by HIV-infected mothers to avoid postnatal transmission of the virus to the infant

(Continued)

Nelfinavir *(Continued)*

Contraindications Hypersensitivity to nelfinavir or product components; phenylketonuria; concurrent therapy with terfenadine, astemizole, cisapride, triazolam, or midazolam

Warnings/Precautions Avoid use of powder in phenylketonurics since contains phenylalanine; use extreme caution when administered to patients with hepatic insufficiency since nelfinavir is metabolized in the liver and excreted predominantly in the feces; avoid use, if possible, with terfenadine, astemizole, cisapride, triazolam, or midazolam. Concurrent use with some anticonvulsants may significantly limit nelfinavir's effectiveness.

Adverse Reactions Protease inhibitors cause dyslipidemia which includes elevated cholesterol and triglycerides and a redistribution of body fat centrally to cause "protease paunch," buffalo hump, facial atrophy, and breast enlargement. These agents also cause hyperglycemia.

>10%: Gastrointestinal: Diarrhea (19%)

1% to 10%:
Central nervous system: Decreased concentration
Dermatologic: Rash
Gastrointestinal: Nausea, flatulence, abdominal pain
Neuromuscular & skeletal: Weakness

<1%: Anxiety, depression, dizziness, emotional lability, hyperkinesia, insomnia, migraine, seizures, sleep disorder, somnolence, suicide ideation, fever, headache, malaise, dermatitis, pruritus, urticaria, increased LFTs, hyperlipemia, hyperuricemia, hypoglycemia, anorexia, dyspepsia, epigastric pain, mouth ulceration, GI bleeding, pancreatitis, vomiting, kidney calculus, sexual dysfunction, anemia, leukopenia, thrombocytopenia, hepatitis, arthralgia, arthritis, cramps, myalgia, myasthenia, myopathy, paresthesia, back pain, dyspnea, pharyngitis, rhinitis, sinusitis, diaphoresis, allergy

Overdosage/Toxicology No data available; however, unabsorbed drug should be removed via gastric lavage and activated charcoal; significant symptoms beyond gastrointestinal disturbances are likely following acute overdose; hemodialysis will not be effective due to high protein binding of nelfinavir

Drug Interactions CYP3A3/4 enzyme substrate; CYP3A3/4 enzyme inducer; CYP3A3/4 enzyme inhibitor

Increased effect:
Nelfinavir inhibits the metabolism of cisapride and astemizole and should, therefore, not be administered concurrently due to risk of life-threatening cardiac arrhythmias.
A 20% increase in rifabutin plasma AUC has been observed when coadministered with nelfinavir (decrease rifabutin's dose by 50%).
An increase in midazolam and triazolam serum levels may occur resulting in significant oversedation when administered with nelfinavir. These drugs should not be administered together.
Indinavir and ritonavir may increase nelfinavir plasma concentrations resulting in potential increases in side effects (the safety of these combinations have not been established).

Decreased effect:
Rifampin decreases nelfinavir's plasma AUC by ~82%; the two drugs should not be administered together.
Serum levels of the hormones in oral contraceptives may decrease significantly with administration of nelfinavir. Patients should use alternative methods of contraceptives during nelfinavir therapy.
Phenobarbital, phenytoin, and carbamazepine may decrease serum levels and consequently effectiveness of nelfinavir.
Nelfinavir's effectiveness may be decreased with concomitant nevirapine

Mechanism of Action Inhibits the HIV-1 protease; inhibition of the viral protease prevents cleavage of the gag-pol polyprotein resulting in the production of immature, noninfectious virus

Pharmacodynamics/Kinetics
Absorption: Food increases plasma concentration-time curve (AUC) by two- to threefold
Distribution: V_d: 2-7 L/kg
Metabolism: Via multiple cytochrome P-450 isoforms (eg, CYP3A); major metabolite has activity comparable to the parent drug

Protein binding: 98%

Half-life: 3.5-5 hours

Time to peak serum concentration: 2-4 hours

Elimination: 98% to 99% excreted in the feces (78% as metabolites and 22% as unchanged nelfinavir); 1% to 2% excreted in the urine

Usual Dosage Oral:

Children 2-13 years: 20-30 mg/kg 3 times/day with a meal or light snack; if tablets are unable to be taken, use oral powder in small amount of water, milk, formula, or dietary supplements; do not use acidic food/juice or store for >6 hours

Adults: 750 mg 3 times/day with meals

Dosing adjustment in renal impairment: No adjustment needed

Dosing adjustment in hepatic impairment: Use caution when administering to patients with hepatic impairment since eliminated predominantly by the liver

Monitoring Parameters LFTs, viral load, CD4 count, triglycerides, cholesterol, glucose

Patient Information Nelfinavir should be taken with food to increase its absorption; it is not a cure for HIV infection and the long-term effects of the drug are unknown at this time; the drug has not demonstrated a reduction in the risk of transmitting HIV to others. Take the drug as prescribed; if you miss a dose, take it as soon as possible and then return to your usual schedule (never double a dose, however). If tablets are unable to be taken, use oral powder in small amount of water, milk, formula, or dietary supplement; do not use acidic food/juice of store dilution for >6 hours. Use an alternative method of contraception from birth control pills during nelfinavir therapy.

Nursing Implications If diarrhea occurs, it may be treated with OTC antidiarrheals

Dosage Forms

Powder, oral: 50 mg/g (contains 11.2 mg phenylalanine)

Tablet: 250 mg

Selected Readings

Deeks SG, Smith M, Holodniy M, et al, "HIV-1 Protease Inhibitors. A Review for Clinicians," *JAMA*, 1997, 277(2):145-53.

Havlir DV and Lange JM, "New Antiretrovirals and New Combinations," *AIDS*, 1998, 12(Suppl A):S165-74.

Kakuda TN, Struble KA, and Piscitelli SC, "Protease Inhibitors for the Treatment of Human Immunodeficiency Virus Infection," *Am J Health Syst Pharm*, 1998, 55(3):233-54.

Kaul D, Cinti SK, Carver PL, et al, "HIV Protease Inhibitors: Advances in Therapy and Adverse Reactions, Including Metabolic Complications," *Pharmacotherapy*, 1999, 19(3):281-98.

McDonald CK and Kuritzkes DR, "Human Immunodeficiency Virus Type 1 Protease Inhibitors," *Arch Intern Med*, 1997, 157(9):951-9.

Perry CM and Benfield P, "Nelfinavir," *Drugs*, 1997, 54(1):81-7.

Neo-Cortef® *see* Neomycin and Hydrocortisone *on page 835*

NeoDecadron® Ophthalmic *see* Neomycin and Dexamethasone *on page 835*

NeoDecadron® Topical *see* Neomycin and Dexamethasone *on page 835*

Neo-Dexameth® Ophthalmic *see* Neomycin and Dexamethasone *on page 835*

Neo-Durabolic *see* Nandrolone *on page 829*

Neo-fradin® Oral *see* Neomycin *on this page*

Neomixin® Topical [OTC] *see* Bacitracin, Neomycin, and Polymyxin B *on page 619*

Neomycin (nee oh MYE sin)

U.S. Brand Names Mycifradin® Sulfate Oral; Mycifradin® Sulfate Topical; Neofradin® Oral; Neo-Tabs® Oral

Synonyms Neomycin Sulfate

Generic Available Yes

Use Orally to prepare GI tract for surgery; topically to treat minor skin infections; treat diarrhea caused by *E. coli*; adjunct in the treatment of hepatic encephalopathy

Drug of Choice or Alternative for

Disease/Syndrome(s)

Otitis Externa, Mild *on page 40*

Pregnancy Risk Factor C

Contraindications Hypersensitivity to neomycin or any component, or other aminoglycosides; patients with intestinal obstruction

(Continued)

Neomycin *(Continued)*

Warnings/Precautions Use with caution in patients with renal impairment, pre-existing hearing impairment, neuromuscular disorders; neomycin is more toxic than other aminoglycosides when given parenterally; **do not administer parenterally**; topical neomycin is a contact sensitizer with sensitivity occurring in 5% to 15% of patients treated with the drug; symptoms include itching, reddening, edema, and failure to heal; **do not use as peritoneal lavage** due to significant systemic adsorption of the drug

Adverse Reactions

1% to 10%:

Dermatologic: Dermatitis, rash, urticaria, erythema

Local: Burning

Ocular: Contact conjunctivitis

<1%: Nausea, vomiting, diarrhea, neuromuscular blockade, ototoxicity, nephrotoxicity

Overdosage/Toxicology

Symptoms of overdose (rare due to poor oral bioavailability) include ototoxicity, nephrotoxicity, and neuromuscular toxicity

The treatment of choice following a single acute overdose appears to be the maintenance of good urine output of at least 3 mL/kg/hour. Dialysis is of questionable value in the enhancement of aminoglycoside elimination. If required, hemodialysis is preferred over peritoneal dialysis in patients with normal renal function. Chelation with penicillin may be of benefit.

Drug Interactions

Decreased effect: May decrease GI absorption of digoxin and methotrexate

Increased effect: Synergistic effects with penicillins

Increased toxicity:

Oral neomycin may potentiate the effects of oral anticoagulants

Increased adverse effects with other neurotoxic, ototoxic, or nephrotoxic drugs

Stability Use reconstituted parenteral solutions within 7 days of mixing, when refrigerated

Mechanism of Action Interferes with bacterial protein synthesis by binding to 30S ribosomal subunits

Pharmacodynamics/Kinetics

Absorption: Oral, percutaneous: Poor (3%)

Distribution: V_d: 0.36 L/kg

Metabolism: Slight hepatic

Half-life: 3 hours (age and renal function dependent)

Time to peak serum concentration:

Oral: 1-4 hours

I.M.: Within 2 hours

Elimination: In urine (30% to 50% as unchanged drug); 97% of an oral dose eliminated unchanged in feces

Usual Dosage

Children: Oral:

Preoperative intestinal antisepsis: 90 mg/kg/day divided every 4 hours for 2 days; or 25 mg/kg at 1 PM, 2 PM, and 11 PM on the day preceding surgery as an adjunct to mechanical cleansing of the intestine and in combination with erythromycin base

Hepatic coma: 50-100 mg/kg/day in divided doses every 6-8 hours or 2.5-7 g/m²/day divided every 4-6 hours for 5-6 days not to exceed 12 g/day

Children and Adults: Topical: Apply ointment 1-4 times/day; topical solutions containing 0.1% to 1% neomycin have been used for irrigation

Adults: Oral:

Preoperative intestinal antisepsis: 1 g each hour for 4 doses then 1 g every 4 hours for 5 doses; or 1 g at 1 PM, 2 PM, and 11 PM on day preceding surgery as an adjunct to mechanical cleansing of the bowel and oral erythromycin; or 6 g/day divided every 4 hours for 2-3 days

Hepatic coma: 500-2000 mg every 6-8 hours or 4-12 g/day divided every 4-6 hours for 5-6 days

Chronic hepatic insufficiency: 4 g/day for an indefinite period

Hemodialysis: Dialyzable (50% to 100%)

Monitoring Parameters Renal function tests, audiometry in symptomatic patients

Patient Information Notify physician if redness, burning, itching, ringing in the ears, hearing impairment, or dizziness occurs of if condition does not improve in 3-4 days

Dosage Forms

Cream, as sulfate: 0.5% (15 g)

Injection, as sulfate: 500 mg

Ointment, topical, as sulfate: 0.5% (15 g, 30 g, 120 g)

Solution, oral, as sulfate: 125 mg/5 mL (480 mL)

Tablet, as sulfate: 500 mg [base 300 mg]

Selected Readings

Begg EJ and Barclay ML, "Aminoglycosides - 50 Years On," *Br J Clin Pharmacol*, 1995, 39(6):597-603.

Edson RS and Terrell CL, "The Aminoglycosides," *Mayo Clin Proc*, 1999, 74(5):519-28.

Neomycin and Dexamethasone

(nee oh MYE sin & deks a METH a sone)

Related Information

Neomycin *on page 833*

U.S. Brand Names AK-Neo-Dex® Ophthalmic; NeoDecadron® Ophthalmic; NeoDecadron® Topical; Neo-Dexameth® Ophthalmic

Use Treatment of steroid responsive inflammatory conditions of the palpebral and bulbar conjunctiva, lid, cornea, and anterior segment of the globe

Usual Dosage

Ophthalmic: Instill 1-2 drops in eye(s) every 3-4 hours

Topical: Apply thin coat 3-4 times/day until favorable response is observed, then reduce dose to one application/day

Dosage Forms

Cream: Neomycin sulfate 0.5% [5 mg/g] and dexamethasone 0.1% [1 mg/g] (15 g, 30 g)

Ointment, ophthalmic: Neomycin sulfate 0.35% [3.5 mg/g] and dexamethasone 0.05% [0.5 mg/g] (3.5 g)

Solution, ophthalmic: Neomycin sulfate 0.35% [3.5 mg/mL] and dexamethasone 0.1% [1 mg/mL] (5 mL)

Neomycin and Hydrocortisone

(nee oh MYE sin & hye droe KOR ti sone)

Related Information

Neomycin *on page 833*

U.S. Brand Names Neo-Cortef®

Use Treatment of susceptible topical bacterial infections with associated inflammation

Usual Dosage Topical: Apply to area in a thin film 2-4 times/day

Dosage Forms

Cream: Neomycin sulfate 0.5% and hydrocortisone 1% (20 g)

Ointment, topical: Neomycin sulfate 0.5% and hydrocortisone 0.5% (20 g); neomycin sulfate 0.5% and hydrocortisone 1% (20 g)

Solution, ophthalmic: Neomycin sulfate 0.5% and hydrocortisone 0.5% (5 mL)

Neomycin and Polymyxin B (nee oh MYE sin & pol i MIKS in bee)

Related Information

Neomycin *on page 833*

Polymyxin B *on page 877*

U.S. Brand Names Neosporin® Cream [OTC]; Neosporin® G.U. Irrigant

Synonyms Polymyxin B and Neomycin

Use Short-term as a continuous irrigant or rinse in the urinary bladder to prevent bacteriuria and gram-negative rod septicemia associated with the use of indwelling catheters; to help prevent infection in minor cuts, scrapes, and burns

Usual Dosage Children and Adults:

Bladder irrigation: **Not for injection;** add 1 mL irrigant to 1 liter isotonic saline solution and connect container to the inflow of lumen of 3-way catheter. Continuous irrigant or rinse in the urinary bladder for up to a maximum of 10 days with administration rate adjusted to patient's urine output; usually no more than 1 L of irrigant is used per day.

Topical: Apply cream 1-4 times/day to affected area

(Continued)

Neomycin and Polymyxin B *(Continued)*

Dosage Forms

Cream: Neomycin sulfate 3.5 mg and polymyxin B sulfate 10,000 units per g (0.94 g, 15 g)

Solution, irrigant: Neomycin sulfate 40 mg and polymyxin B sulfate 200,000 units per mL (1 mL, 20 mL)

Neomycin, Polymyxin B, and Dexamethasone

(nee oh MYE sin, pol i MIKS in bee, & deks a METH a sone)

Related Information

Neomycin *on page 833*

Polymyxin B *on page 877*

U.S. Brand Names AK-Trol®; Dexacidin®; Dexasporin®; Maxitrol®

Use Steroid-responsive inflammatory ocular conditions in which a corticosteroid is indicated and where bacterial infection or a risk of bacterial infection exists

Usual Dosage Children and Adults: Ophthalmic:

Ointment: Place a small amount (~½") in the affected eye 3-4 times/day or apply at bedtime as an adjunct with drops

Solution: Instill 1-2 drops into affected eye(s) every 3-4 hours; in severe disease, drops may be used hourly and tapered to discontinuation

Dosage Forms Ophthalmic:

Ointment: Neomycin sulfate 3.5 mg, polymyxin B sulfate 10,000 units and dexamethasone 0.1% per g (3.5 g, 5 g)

Suspension: Neomycin sulfate 3.5 mg, polymyxin B sulfate 10,000 units and dexamethasone 0.1% per mL (5 mL, 10 mL)

Neomycin, Polymyxin B, and Gramicidin

(nee oh MYE sin, pol i MIKS in bee, & gram i SYE din)

U.S. Brand Names AK-Spore® Ophthalmic Solution; Neosporin® Ophthalmic Solution; Ocutricin® Ophthalmic Solution

Generic Available Yes

Use Treatment of superficial ocular infection, infection prophylaxis in minor skin abrasions

Pregnancy Risk Factor C

Contraindications Hypersensitivity to neomycin, polymyxin B, gramicidin or any component

Warnings/Precautions Symptoms of neomycin sensitization include itching, reddening, edema, failure to heal; prolonged use may result in glaucoma, defects in visual acuity, posterior subcapsular cataract formation, and secondary ocular infections

Adverse Reactions 1% to 10%:

Cardiovascular: Edema

Dermatologic: Itching

Local: Reddening, failure to heal

Ocular: Low grade conjunctivitis

Mechanism of Action Interferes with bacterial protein synthesis by binding to 30S ribosomal subunits; binds to phospholipids, alters permeability, and damages the bacterial cytoplasmic membrane permitting leakage of intracellular constituents

Usual Dosage Children and Adults: Ophthalmic: Instill 1-2 drops 4-6 times/day or more frequently as required for severe infections

Patient Information Tilt head back, place medication in conjunctival sac, and close eyes; apply finger pressure on lacrimal sac for 1 minute following instillation

Dosage Forms Solution, ophthalmic: Neomycin sulfate 1.75 mg, polymyxin B sulfate 10,000 units, and gramicidin 0.025 mg per mL (2 mL, 10 mL)

Neomycin, Polymyxin B, and Hydrocortisone

(nee oh MYE sin, pol i MIKS in bee, & hye droe KOR ti sone)

Related Information

Neomycin *on page 833*

Polymyxin B *on page 877*

U.S. Brand Names AK-Spore® H.C. Ophthalmic Suspension; AK-Spore® H.C. Otic; Antibiotic® Otic; Bacticort® Otic; Cortatrigen® Otic; Cortisporin® Ophthalmic

Suspension; Cortisporin® Otic; Cortisporin® Topical Cream; Drotic® Otic; Ear-Eze® Otic; LazerSporin-C® Otic; Octicair® Otic; Otic-Care® Otic; OtiTricin® Otic; Otocort® Otic; Otomycin-HPN® Otic; Otosporin® Otic; PediOtic® Otic; UAD® Otic

Use Steroid-responsive inflammatory condition for which a corticosteroid is indicated and where bacterial infection or a risk of bacterial infection exists

Usual Dosage Duration of use should be limited to 10 days unless otherwise directed by the physician

Otic solution is used **only** for swimmer's ear (infections of external auditory canal)

Otic:

Children: Instill 3 drops into affected ear 3-4 times/day

Adults: Instill 4 drops 3-4 times/day; otic suspension is the preferred otic preparation

Children and Adults:

Ophthalmic: Drops: Instill 1-2 drops 2-4 times/day, or more frequently as required for severe infections; in acute infections, instill 1-2 drops every 15-30 minutes gradually reducing the frequency of administration as the infection is controlled

Topical: Apply a thin layer 1-4 times/day

Dosage Forms

Cream, topical: Neomycin sulfate 5 mg, polymyxin B sulfate 10,000 units, and hydrocortisone 10 mg per mL (7.5 g)

Solution, otic: Neomycin sulfate 5 mg, polymyxin B sulfate 10,000 units, and hydrocortisone 10 mg per mL (10 mL)

Suspension:

Ophthalmic: Neomycin sulfate 5 mg, polymyxin B sulfate 10,000 units, and hydrocortisone 10 mg per mL (7.5 mL)

Otic: Neomycin sulfate 5 mg, polymyxin B sulfate 10,000 units, and hydrocortisone 10 mg per mL (10 mL)

Neomycin, Polymyxin B, and Prednisolone

(nee oh MYE sin, pol i MIKS in bee, & pred NIS oh lone)

Related Information

Neomycin *on page 833*

Polymyxin B *on page 877*

U.S. Brand Names Poly-Pred® Ophthalmic Suspension

Use Steroid-responsive inflammatory ocular condition in which bacterial infection or a risk of bacterial ocular infection exists

Usual Dosage Children and Adults: Ophthalmic: Instill 1-2 drops every 3-4 hours; acute infections may require every 30-minute instillation initially with frequency of administration reduced as the infection is brought under control. To treat the lids: Instill 1-2 drops every 3-4 hours, close the eye and rub the excess on the lids and lid margins.

Dosage Forms Suspension, ophthalmic: Neomycin sulfate 0.35%, polymyxin B sulfate 10,000 units, and prednisolone acetate 0.5% per mL (5 mL, 10 mL)

Neomycin Sulfate *see Neomycin on page 833*

Neosporin® Cream [OTC] *see Neomycin and Polymyxin B on page 835*

Neosporin® G.U. Irrigant *see Neomycin and Polymyxin B on page 835*

Neosporin® Ophthalmic Ointment *see Bacitracin, Neomycin, and Polymyxin B on page 619*

Neosporin® Ophthalmic Solution *see Neomycin, Polymyxin B, and Gramicidin on previous page*

Neosporin® Topical Ointment [OTC] *see Bacitracin, Neomycin, and Polymyxin B on page 619*

Neo-Tabs® Oral *see Neomycin on page 833*

Neotopic *see Bacitracin, Neomycin, and Polymyxin B on page 619*

Neotricin HC® Ophthalmic Ointment *see Bacitracin, Neomycin, Polymyxin B, and Hydrocortisone on page 620*

Nephronex® *see Nitrofurantoin on page 842*

1-N-Ethyl Sisomicin *see Netilmicin on this page*

Netilmicin (ne til MYE sin)

Related Information

Aminoglycoside Dosing and Monitoring *on page 1058*

(Continued)

Netilmicin *(Continued)*

Antimicrobial Activity Against Selected Organisms *on page 983*

U.S. Brand Names Netromycin®

Canadian Brand Names Netromicina®

Synonyms 1-*N*-Ethyl Sisomicin

Generic Available No

Use Short-term treatment of serious or life-threatening infections including septicemia, peritonitis, intra-abdominal abscess, lower respiratory tract infections, urinary tract infections; skin, bone, and joint infections caused by susceptible organisms; active against *Pseudomonas aeruginosa*, *E. coli*, *Proteus*, *Klebsiella*, *Serratia*, *Enterobacter*, *Citrobacter*, and other gram-negative bacilli

Pregnancy Risk Factor D

Contraindications Known hypersensitivity to netilmicin (aminoglycosides, bisulfites)

Warnings/Precautions Use with caution in patients with pre-existing renal insufficiency, vestibular or cochlear impairment, myasthenia gravis, hypocalcemia, conditions which depress neuromuscular transmission. Parenteral aminoglycosides are associated with nephrotoxicity or ototoxicity; the ototoxicity may be proportional to the amount of drug given and the duration of treatment; tinnitus or vertigo are indications of vestibular injury and impending hearing loss; renal damage is usually reversible.

Adverse Reactions

>10%:
  Central nervous system: Neurotoxicity
  Otic: Ototoxicity (auditory), ototoxicity (vestibular)
  Renal: Nephrotoxicity, decreased creatinine clearance
1% to 10%: Dermatologic: Skin itching, redness, rash, swelling
<1%: Difficulty in breathing, drowsiness, weakness, headache, tremors, muscle cramps, pseudomotor cerebri, anorexia, nausea, vomiting, weight loss, increased salivation, enterocolitis, granulocytopenia, agranulocytosis, thrombocytopenia, photosensitivity, erythema, burning, stinging

Overdosage/Toxicology

Serum levels monitoring is recommended. Signs and symptoms of overdose include ototoxicity, nephrotoxicity, and neuromuscular toxicity.

Treatment of choice following a single acute overdose appears to be the maintenance of good urine output of at least 3 mL/kg/hour. Dialysis is of questionable value in the enhancement of aminoglycoside elimination. If required, hemodialysis is preferred over peritoneal dialysis in patients with normal renal function. Careful hydration may be all that is required to promote diuresis and therefore the enhancement of the drug's elimination. Chelation with penicillins is experimental.

Drug Interactions

Increased/prolonged effect of depolarizing and nondepolarizing neuromuscular blocking agents

Increased toxicity: Concurrent use of amphotericin, vancomycin, ethacrynic acid, furosemide and other nephrotoxic agents may increase nephrotoxicity

Mechanism of Action Interferes with protein synthesis in bacterial cell by binding to 30S ribosomal subunits

Pharmacodynamics/Kinetics

Absorption: I.M.: Well absorbed

Distribution: To extracellular fluid including serum, abscesses, ascitic, pericardial, pleural, synovial, lymphatic, and peritoneal fluids; high concentrations in urine; crosses placenta

Half-life: 2-3 hours (age and renal function dependent)

Time to peak serum concentration: I.M.: Within 30-60 minutes

Elimination: Excreted by glomerular filtration

Usual Dosage Individualization is critical because of the low therapeutic index. Use of ideal body weight (IBW) for determining the mg/kg/dose appears to be more accurate than dosing on the basis of total body weight (TBW). In morbid obesity, dosage requirement may best be estimated using a dosing weight of IBW + 0.4 (TBW - IBW). Peak and trough plasma drug levels should be determined, particularly in critically ill patients with serious infections or in disease states known to significantly alter aminoglycoside pharmacokinetics (eg, cystic fibrosis, burns, or major surgery).

I.M., I.V.:
Neonates <6 weeks: 2-3.25 mg/kg/dose every 12 hours
Children 6 weeks to 12 years: 1-2.5 mg/kg/dose every 8 hours
Children >12 years and Adults: 1.5-2 mg/kg/dose every 8-12 hours

Some clinicians suggest a daily dose of 4-7 mg/kg for all patients with normal renal function. This dose is at least as efficacious with similar, if not less, toxicity than conventional dosing. (See also Aminoglycoside Dosing and Monitoring *on page 1058*.)

Dosing adjustment in renal impairment: Initial dose:
All patients should receive a loading dose of at least 2 mg/kg (subsequent dosing should be base on serum concentrations)
Cl_{cr} ≥60 mL/minute: Administer every 8 hours
Cl_{cr} 40-60 mL/minute: Administer every 12 hours
Cl_{cr} 20-40 mL/minute: Administer every 24 hours
Continuous arteriovenous or venovenous hemodiafiltration (CAVH) effects:
Dose as for Cl_{cr} 10-40 mL/minute and follow levels

Reference Range Therapeutic: Peak: 4-10 µg/mL (SI: 8-21 µmol/L); Trough: <2 µg/mL (SI: 4 µmol/L); Toxic: Peak: >10 µg/mL (SI: >21 µmol/L); Trough: >2 µg/mL (SI: >4.2 µmol/L)

Test Interactions Penicillins may decrease aminoglycoside serum concentrations *in vitro*

Patient Information Report any dizziness or sensations of ringing or fullness in ears

Nursing Implications Peak levels are drawn 30 minutes after the end of a 30-minute infusion; trough levels are drawn within 30 minutes before the next dose; give other antibiotic drugs at least 1 hour before or after gentamicin, if possible.

Dosage Forms
Injection: 100 mg/mL (1.5 mL)
Injection:
Neonatal: 10 mg/mL (2 mL)
Pediatric: 25 mg/mL (2 mL)

Selected Readings
Begg EJ and Barclay ML, "Aminoglycosides - 50 Years On," *Br J Clin Pharmacol*, 1995, 39(6):597-603.
Blaser J, König C, Simmen HP, et al, "Monitoring Serum Concentrations for Once-Daily Netilmicin Dosing Regimens," *J Antimicrob Chemother*, 1994, 33(2):341-8.
Cunha BA, "Aminoglycosides: Current Role in Antimicrobial Therapy," *Pharmacotherapy*, 1988, 8(6):334-50.
Edson RS and Terrell CL, "The Aminoglycosides," *Mayo Clin Proc*, 1999, 74(5):519-28.
Lortholary O, Tod M, Cohen Y, et al, "Aminoglycosides," *Med Clin North Am*, 1995, 79(4):761-87.
McCormack JP and Jewesson PJ, "A Critical Reevaluation of the "Therapeutic Range" of Aminoglycosides," *Clin Infect Dis*, 1992, 14(1):320-39.
Rozdzinski E, Kern WV, Reichle A, et al, "Once-Daily Versus Trice-Daily Dosing of Netilmicin in Combination With β-lactam Antibiotics as Empirical Therapy for Febrile Neutropenic Patients," *J Antimicrob Chemother*, 1993, 31(4):585-98.

Netromicina® *see* Netilmicin *on page 837*

Netromycin® *see* Netilmicin *on page 837*

Neupogen® Injection *see* Filgrastim *on page 730*

Neutrexin® Injection *see* Trimetrexate Glucuronate *on page 958*

Nevirapine (ne VYE ra peen)
Related Information
HIV Therapeutic Information *on page 1008*

U.S. Brand Names Viramune®

Generic Available No

Use In combination therapy with other antiretroviral agents for the treatment of HIV-1 in adults

Drug of Choice or Alternative for
Organism(s)
Human Immunodeficiency Virus *on page 177*

Pregnancy Risk Factor C

Pregnancy/Breast-Feeding Implications
Clinical effects on the fetus: Administer nevirapine during pregnancy only if benefits to the mother outweigh the risk to the fetus
Breast-feeding/lactation: Avoid use during lactation, if possible
(Continued)

Nevirapine *(Continued)*

Contraindications Previous hypersensitivity to nevirapine or its components; concurrent use with oral contraceptives and protease inhibitors (indinavir, nelfinavir, ritonavir, saquinavir)

Warnings/Precautions Consider alteration of antiretroviral therapies if disease progression occurs while patients are receiving nevirapine. Resistant HIV virus emerges rapidly and uniformly when nevirapine is administered as monotherapy. Therefore, always administer in combination with at least one additional antiretroviral agent. Severe skin reactions (eg, Stevens-Johnson syndrome) have occurred, usually within 6 weeks. Therapy should be discontinued if any rash which develops does not resolve; although mild to moderate alterations in LFTs are not uncommon, however, severe hepatotoxic reactions may occur rarely, and if abnormalities reoccur after temporarily discontinuing therapy, treatment should be permanently halted. Safety and efficacy have not been established in children.

Adverse Reactions
>10%:
Central nervous system: Headache (11%), fever (8% to 11%)
Dermatologic: Rash (15% to 20%)
Gastrointestinal: Diarrhea (15% to 20%)
Hematologic: Neutropenia (10% to 11%)
1% to 10%:
Gastrointestinal: Ulcerative stomatitis (4%), nausea, abdominal pain (2%)
Hematologic: Anemia
Hepatic: Hepatitis, increased LFTs (2% to 4%)
Neuromuscular & skeletal: Peripheral neuropathy, paresthesia (2%), myalgia
<1%: Thrombocytopenia, Stevens-Johnson syndrome, hepatotoxicity, hepatic necrosis

Overdosage/Toxicology No toxicities have been reported with acute ingestions of large sums of tablets

Drug Interactions CYP3A3/4 enzyme substrate; CYP3A3/4 enzyme inducer; CYP3A3/4 enzyme inhibitor
Decreased effect: Rifampin and rifabutin may decrease nevirapine trough concentrations due to induction of CYP3A; since nevirapine may decrease concentrations of protease inhibitors, they should not be administered concomitantly or doses should be increased; nevirapine may decrease the effectiveness of oral contraceptives - suggest alternate method of birth control; decreased effect of ketoconazole
Increased effect/toxicity with cimetidine, macrolides, ketoconazole

Mechanism of Action As a non-nucleoside reverse transcriptase inhibitor, nevirapine has activity against HIV-1 by binding to reverse transcriptase. It consequently blocks the RNA-dependent and DNA-dependent DNA polymerase activities including HIV-1 replication. It does not require intracellular phosphorylation for antiviral activity.

Pharmacodynamics/Kinetics
Absorption: Oral: >90%
Distribution: V_d: 1.2-1.4 L/kg; widely distributed; distributes well into breast milk and crosses the placenta; CSF penetration approximates 50% of that found in the plasma
Protein binding, plasma: 50% to 60%
Metabolism: Extensively metabolized via cytochrome P-450 system (hydroxylation to inactive compounds); may undergo enterohepatic recycling
Half-life: Decreases over 2- to 4-week time with chronic dosing due to autoinduction (ie, half-life = 45 hours initially and decreases to 23 hours)
Time to peak serum concentration: 2-4 hours
Elimination: Renal elimination of metabolites; <3% of parent compound excreted in urine

Usual Dosage Adults: Oral:
Initial: 200 mg once daily for 14 days
Maintenance: 200 mg twice daily (in combination with an additional antiretroviral agent)

Monitoring Parameters Liver function tests periodically throughout therapy; observe for CNS side effects

Patient Information Report any right upper quadrant pain, jaundice, or rash to your physician immediately

Nursing Implications May be given with food, antacids, or didanosine; if a therapy is interrupted for >7 days, the dose should be decreased to the initial regimen and increased after 14 days

Additional Information Potential compliance problems, frequency of administration and adverse effects should be discussed with patients before initiating therapy to help prevent the emergence of resistance.

Dosage Forms

Suspension, oral: 50 mg/5 mL (240 mL)

Tablet: 200 mg

Selected Readings

D'Aquila RT, Hughes MD, Johnson VA, et al, "Nevirapine, Zidovudine, and Didanosine Compared With Zidovudine and Didanosine in Patients With HIV-1 Infection," *Ann Intern Med*, 1996, 124:1019-30.

Hammer SM, Kessler HA, and Saag MS, "Issues in Combination Antiretroviral Therapy: A Review," *J Acquired Immune Defic Syndr*, 1994, 7(Suppl 2):S24-37.

Havlir DV and Lange JM, "New Antiretrovirals and New Combinations," *AIDS*, 1998, 12(Suppl A):S165-74.

Weverling GJ, Lange JM, Jurriaans S, et al, "Alternative Multidrug Regimen Provides Improved Suppression of HIV-1 Replication Over Triple Therapy," *AIDS*, 1998, 12(11):F117-22.

N.G.T.® **Topical** *see* Nystatin and Triamcinolone *on page 846*

Niclocide® *see* Niclosamide *on this page*

Niclosamide (ni KLOE sa mide)

U.S. Brand Names Niclocide®

Generic Available No

Use Treatment of intestinal beef and fish tapeworm infections and dwarf tapeworm infections

Drug of Choice or Alternative for

Organism(s)

Cestodes *on page 94*

Pregnancy Risk Factor B

Contraindications Known hypersensitivity to niclosamide

Warnings/Precautions Affects cestodes of the intestine only; it is without effect in cysticercosis

Adverse Reactions

1% to 10%:

Central nervous system: Drowsiness, dizziness, headache

Gastrointestinal: Nausea, vomiting, loss of appetite, diarrhea

<1%: Rash, pruritus ani, oral irritation, fever, rectal bleeding, weakness, bad taste in mouth, diaphoresis, palpitations, constipation, alopecia, edema in the arm, backache

Overdosage/Toxicology

Signs and symptoms of overdose include nausea, vomiting, anorexia

In the event of an overdose, do not administer ipecac

Mechanism of Action Inhibits the synthesis of ATP through inhibition of oxidative phosphorylation in the mitochondria of cestodes

Pharmacodynamics/Kinetics

Absorption: Oral: Not significantly absorbed

Metabolism: Not appreciably metabolized by mammalian host, but may be metabolized in GI tract by the worm

Elimination: Excreted in feces

Usual Dosage Oral:

Beef and fish tapeworm:

Children:

11-34 kg: 1 g (2 tablets) as a single dose

>34 kg: 1.5 g (3 tablets) as a single dose

Adults: 2 g (4 tablets) in a single dose

May require a second course of treatment 7 days later

Dwarf tapeworm:

Children:

11-34 g: 1 g (2 tablets) chewed thoroughly in a single dose the first day, then 500 mg/day (1 tablet) for next 6 days

>34 g: 1.5 g (3 tablets) in a single dose the first day, then 1 g/day for 6 days

Adults: 2 g (4 tablets) in a single daily dose for 7 days

Monitoring Parameters Stool cultures

(Continued)

Niclosamide *(Continued)*

Patient Information Chew tablets thoroughly; tablets can be pulverized and mixed with water to form a paste for administration to children; can be taken with food; a mild laxative can be used for constipation

Nursing Implications Administer a laxative 2-3 hours after the niclosamide dose if treating *Taenia solium* infections to prevent the development of cysticercosis

Additional Information Not available in the U.S.

Dosage Forms Tablet, chewable (vanilla flavor): 500 mg

Selected Readings
"Drugs for Parasitic Infections," *Med Lett Drugs Ther*, 1998, 40(1017):1-12.

Nilstat® *see* Nystatin *on page 845*

Nitrofural *see* Nitrofurazone *on next page*

Nitrofurantoin *(nye troe fyoor AN toyn)*

Related Information

Antimicrobial Activity Against Selected Organisms *on page 983*

U.S. Brand Names Furadantin®; Furalan®; Furan®; Furanite®; Macrobid®; Macrodantin®

Canadian Brand Names Apo®-Nitrofurantoin; Nephronex®; Novo-Furan

Generic Available Yes: Tablet and suspension

Use Prevention and treatment of urinary tract infections caused by susceptible gram-negative and some gram-positive organisms; *Pseudomonas*, *Serratia*, and most species of *Proteus* are generally resistant to nitrofurantoin

Drug of Choice or Alternative for

Disease/Syndrome(s)

Urinary Tract Infection, Pyelonephritis *on page 53*

Organism(s)

Staphylococcus saprophyticus on page 264

Pregnancy Risk Factor B

Contraindications Hypersensitivity to nitrofurantoin or any component; renal impairment; infants <1 month (due to the possibility of hemolytic anemia)

Warnings/Precautions Use with caution in patients with G-6-PD deficiency, patients with anemia, vitamin B deficiency, diabetes mellitus or electrolyte abnormalities; therapeutic concentrations of nitrofurantoin are not attained in urine of patients with Cl_{cr} <40 mL/minute (elderly); use with caution if prolonged therapy is anticipated due to possible pulmonary toxicity; acute, subacute, or chronic (usually after 6 months of therapy) pulmonary reactions have been observed in patients treated with nitrofurantoin; if these occur, discontinue therapy; monitor closely for malaise, dyspnea, cough, fever, radiologic evidence of diffuse interstitial pneumonitis or fibrosis

Adverse Reactions Percentage unknown: Chest pains, chills, fever, fatigue, drowsiness, headache, dizziness, rash, itching, lupus-like syndrome, exfoliative dermatitis, stomach upset, diarrhea, loss of appetite/vomiting/nausea (most common), sore throat, hemolytic anemia, hepatitis, increased LFTs, weakness, paresthesia, numbness, arthralgia, cough, dyspnea, hypersensitivity, *C. difficile*-colitis

Overdosage/Toxicology

Symptoms of overdose include vomiting

Supportive care only

Drug Interactions

Decreased effect: Antacids, especially magnesium salts, decrease absorption of nitrofurantoin; nitrofurantoin may antagonize effects of norfloxacin

Increased toxicity: Probenecid (decreases renal excretion of nitrofurantoin); anticholinergic drugs increase absorption of nitrofurantoin

Mechanism of Action Inhibits several bacterial enzyme systems including acetyl coenzyme A interfering with metabolism and possibly cell wall synthesis

Pharmacodynamics/Kinetics

Absorption: Well absorbed from GI tract; the macrocrystalline form is absorbed more slowly due to slower dissolution, but causes less GI distress

Distribution: V_d: 0.8 L/kg; crosses the placenta; appears in breast milk

Protein binding: ~40%

Metabolism: 60% of drug metabolized by body tissues throughout the body, with exception of plasma, to inactive metabolites

Bioavailability: Increased by presence of food

Half-life: 20-60 minutes; prolonged with renal impairment

Elimination: As metabolites and unchanged drug (40%) in urine and small amounts in bile; renal excretion via glomerular filtration and tubular secretion

Usual Dosage Oral:

Children >1 month: 5-7 mg/kg/day in divided doses every 6 hours; maximum: 400 mg/day

Chronic therapy: 1-2 mg/kg/day in divided doses every 12-24 hours; maximum dose: 100 mg/day

Adults: 50-100 mg/dose every 6 hours

Macrocrystal/monohydrate: 100 mg twice daily

Prophylaxis or chronic therapy: 50-100 mg/dose at bedtime

Dosing adjustment in renal impairment: Cl_{cr} <50 mL/minute: Avoid use

Avoid use in hemo and peritoneal dialysis and continuous arteriovenous or venovenous hemofiltration (CAVH/CAVHD)

Dietary Considerations Alcohol: Avoid use

Administration Administer with meals to slow the rate of absorption and decrease adverse effects; suspension may be mixed with water, milk, fruit juice, or infant formula

Monitoring Parameters Signs of pulmonary reaction, signs of numbness or tingling of the extremities, periodic liver function tests

Test Interactions Causes false-positive urine glucose with Clinitest®

Patient Information Take with food or milk; may discolor urine to a dark yellow or brown color; notify physician if fever, chest pain, persistent, nonproductive cough, or difficulty breathing occurs; avoid alcohol

Additional Information Nitrofurantoin macrocrystal/monohydrate is Macrobid®

Dosage Forms

Capsule: 50 mg, 100 mg

Capsule:

Macrocrystal: 25 mg, 50 mg, 100 mg

Macrocrystal/monohydrate: 100 mg

Suspension, oral: 25 mg/5 mL (470 mL)

Nitrofurazone (nye troe FYOOR a zone)

U.S. Brand Names Furacin® Topical

Synonyms Nitrofural

Use Antibacterial agent in second and third degree burns and skin grafting

Pregnancy Risk Factor C

Contraindications Hypersensitivity to nitrofurazone or any component

Warnings/Precautions Use with caution in patients with renal impairment and patients with G-6-PD deficiency

Adverse Reactions Women should inform their physicians if signs or symptoms of any of the following occur thromboembolic or thrombotic disorders including sudden severe headache or vomiting, disturbance of vision or speech, loss of vision, numbness or weakness in an extremity, sharp or crushing chest pain, calf pain, shortness of breath, severe abdominal pain or mass, mental depression, or unusual bleeding. Notify physician if area under dermal patch becomes irritated or a rash develops.

Women should discontinue taking the medication if they suspect they are pregnant or become pregnant.

Drug Interactions Decreased effect: Sutilains decrease activity of nitrofurazone

Stability Avoid exposure to direct sunlight; excessive heat, strong fluorescent lighting, and alkaline materials

Mechanism of Action A broad antibacterial spectrum; it acts by inhibiting bacterial enzymes involved in carbohydrate metabolism; effective against a wide range of gram-negative and gram-positive organisms; bactericidal against most bacteria commonly causing surface infections including *Staphylococcus aureus, Streptococcus, Escherichia coli, Enterobacter cloacae, Clostridium perfringens, Aerobacter aerogenes*, and *Proteus* sp; not particularly active against most *Pseudomonas aeruginosa* strains and does not inhibit viruses or fungi. Topical preparations of nitrofurazone are readily soluble in blood, pus, and serum and are nonmacerating.

Usual Dosage Children and Adults: Topical: Apply once daily or every few days to lesion or place on gauze

(Continued)

Nitrofurazone *(Continued)*

Patient Information Notify physician if condition worsens or if irritation develops

Dosage Forms

Cream: 0.2% (28 g)

Ointment, soluble dressing, topical: 0.2% (28 g, 56 g, 454 g, 480 g)

Solution, topical: 0.2% (480 mL, 4000 mL)

Nix™ Creme Rinse *see Permethrin on page 868*

Nizoral® *see Ketoconazole on page 791*

Nordeoxyguanosine *see Ganciclovir on page 745*

Norfloxacin *(nor FLOKS a sin)*

Related Information

Antimicrobial Activity Against Selected Organisms *on page 983*

U.S. Brand Names Chibroxin™ Ophthalmic; Noroxin® Oral

Generic Available No

Use Uncomplicated urinary tract infections and cystitis caused by susceptible gram-negative and gram-positive bacteria; sexually transmitted disease (eg, uncomplicated urethral and cervical gonorrhea) caused by *N. gonorrhoeae*; prostatitis due to *E. coli*; ophthalmic solution for conjunctivitis

Drug of Choice or Alternative for

Organism(s)

Neisseria gonorrhoeae on page 215

Pregnancy Risk Factor C

Contraindications Known hypersensitivity to quinolones

Warnings/Precautions Not recommended in children <18 years of age; other quinolones have caused transient arthropathy in children; CNS stimulation may occur which may lead to tremor, restlessness, confusion, and very rarely to hallucinations or convulsive seizures; use with caution in patients with known or suspected CNS disorders; has rarely caused ruptured tendons (discontinue immediately with signs of inflammation or tendon pain)

Adverse Reactions

1% to 10%:

Central nervous system: Headache (2.7%), dizziness (1.8%), fatigue

Gastrointestinal: Nausea (2.8%)

<1%: Somnolence, depression, insomnia, fever, pruritus, hyperhidrosis, erythema, rash, abdominal pain, dyspepsia, constipation, flatulence, heartburn, xerostomia, diarrhea, vomiting, loose stools, anorexia, bitter taste, GI bleeding, increased liver enzymes, back pain, ruptured tendons, weakness, increased BUN/serum creatinine, acute renal failure

Overdosage/Toxicology

Symptoms of overdose include acute renal failure, seizures

Following GI decontamination, use supportive measures

Drug Interactions CYP1A2 and 3A3/4 enzyme inhibitor

Decreased effect: Decreased absorption with antacids containing aluminum, magnesium, and/or calcium (by up to 98% if given at the same time); decreased serum levels of fluoroquinolones by antineoplastics; nitrofurantoin may antagonize effects of norfloxacin; phenytoin serum levels may be decreased by fluoroquinolones

Increased toxicity/serum levels: Quinolones cause increased levels or toxicity of digoxin, caffeine, warfarin, cyclosporine, and possibly theophylline. Cimetidine and probenecid increase quinolone levels.

Mechanism of Action Norfloxacin is a DNA gyrase inhibitor. DNA gyrase is an essential bacterial enzyme that maintains the superhelical structure of DNA. DNA gyrase is required for DNA replication and transcription, DNA repair, recombination, and transposition; bactericidal.

Pharmacodynamics/Kinetics

Absorption: Oral: Rapid, up to 40%

Distribution: Crosses the placenta; small amounts appear in breast milk

Protein binding: 15%

Metabolism: In the liver

Half-life: 4.8 hours (can be higher with reduced glomerular filtration rates)

Time to peak serum concentration: Within 1-2 hours

Elimination: In urine and feces (30%)

Usual Dosage
Children >1 year and Adults: Ophthalmic: Instill 1-2 drops in affected eye(s) 4 times/day for up to 7 days

Adults: Oral:
Urinary tract infections: 400 mg twice daily for 3-21 days depending on severity of infection or organism sensitivity; maximum: 800 mg/day
Uncomplicated gonorrhea: 800 mg as a single dose (CDC recommends as an alternative regimen to ciprofloxacin or ofloxacin)
Prostatitis: 400 mg every 12 hours for 4 weeks

Dosing interval in renal impairment:
Cl_{cr} 10-30 mL/minute: Administer every 24 hours
Cl_{cr} <10 mL/minute: Do not use

Patient Information Tablets should be taken at least 1 hour before or at least 2 hours after a meal with a glass of water; patients receiving norfloxacin should be well hydrated; take all the medication, do not skip doses; do not take with antacids; contact your physician immediately with inflammation or tendon pain

Nursing Implications Hold antacids, sucralfate for 3-4 hours after giving

Dosage Forms
Solution, ophthalmic: 0.3% [3 mg/mL] (5 mL)
Tablet: 400 mg

Selected Readings
Hooper DC and Wolfson JS, "Fluoroquinolone Antimicrobial Agents," *N Engl J Med*, 1991, 324(6):384-94.

Lomaestro BM and Bailie GR, "Quinolone-Cation Interactions: A Review," *DICP*, 1991, 25(11):1249-58.

Stein GE, "The 4-Quinolone Antibiotics: Past, Present, and Future," *Pharmacotherapy*, 1988, 8(6):301-14.

Walker RC and Wright AJ, "The Fluoroquinolones," *Mayo Clin Proc*, 1991, 66(12):1249-59.

Noritate® Cream see Metronidazole on page 817

Noroxin® Oral see Norfloxacin on previous page

Nor-tet® Oral see Tetracycline on page 944

Norvir® see Ritonavir on page 909

Novacet® Topical see Sulfur and Sulfacetamide Sodium on page 936

Novamoxin® see Amoxicillin on page 592

Novo-AZT see Zidovudine on page 977

Novo-Cloxin see Cloxacillin on page 689

Novo-Doxylin see Doxycycline on page 713

Novo-Furan see Nitrofurantoin on page 842

Novo-Lexin see Cephalexin on page 660

Novo-Nidazol see Metronidazole on page 817

Novo-Pen-VK® see Penicillin V Potassium on page 865

Novo-Rythro Encap see Erythromycin on page 722

Novo-Soxazole see Sulfisoxazole on page 934

Novo-Tetra see Tetracycline on page 944

Novo-Trimel see Co-Trimoxazole on page 692

NP-27® [OTC] see Tolnaftate on page 956

Nu-Amoxi see Amoxicillin on page 592

Nu-Ampi Trihydrate see Ampicillin on page 604

Nu-Cephalex see Cephalexin on page 660

Nu-Cloxi see Cloxacillin on page 689

Nu-Cotrimox see Co-Trimoxazole on page 692

Nu-Doxycycline see Doxycycline on page 713

Nu-Pen-VK see Penicillin V Potassium on page 865

Nu-Tetra see Tetracycline on page 944

Nyaderm see Nystatin on this page

Nydrazid® see Isoniazid on page 782

Nystatin (nye STAT in)
U.S. Brand Names Mycostatin®; Nilstat®; Nystat-Rx®; Nystex®; O-V Staticin®
Canadian Brand Names Mestatin®; Nadostine®; Nyaderm; PMS-Nystatin
Generic Available Yes
(Continued)

Nystatin *(Continued)*

Use Treatment of susceptible cutaneous, mucocutaneous, and oral cavity fungal infections normally caused by the *Candida* species

Pregnancy Risk Factor B/C (oral)

Contraindications Hypersensitivity to nystatin or any component

Adverse Reactions

Percentage unknown: Contact dermatitis, Stevens-Johnson syndrome

1% to 10%: Gastrointestinal: Nausea, vomiting, diarrhea, stomach pain

<1%: Hypersensitivity reactions

Overdosage/Toxicology

Symptoms of overdose include nausea, vomiting, diarrhea

Treatment is supportive

Stability Keep vaginal inserts in refrigerator; protect from temperature extremes, moisture, and light

Mechanism of Action Binds to sterols in fungal cell membrane, changing the cell wall permeability allowing for leakage of cellular contents

Pharmacodynamics/Kinetics

Absorption: Not absorbed through mucous membranes or intact skin; poorly absorbed from the GI tract

Elimination: In feces as unchanged drug

Usual Dosage

Oral candidiasis:

Suspension (swish and swallow orally):

Premature infants: 100,000 units 4 times/day

Infants: 200,000 units 4 times/day or 100,000 units to each side of mouth 4 times/day

Children and Adults: 400,000-600,000 units 4 times/day

Troche: Children and Adults: 200,000-400,000 units 4-5 times/day

Powder for compounding: Children and Adults: 1/8 teaspoon (500,000 units) to equal approximately 1/2 cup of water; give 4 times/day

Mucocutaneous infections: Children and Adults: Topical: Apply 2-3 times/day to affected areas; very moist topical lesions are treated best with powder

Intestinal infections: Adults: Oral tablets: 500,000-1,000,000 units every 8 hours

Vaginal infections: Adults: Vaginal tablets: Insert 1 tablet/day at bedtime for 2 weeks

Patient Information The oral suspension should be swished about the mouth and retained in the mouth for as long as possible (several minutes) before swallowing. For neonates and infants, paint nystatin suspension into recesses of the mouth. Troches must be allowed to dissolve slowly and should not be chewed or swallowed whole. If topical irritation occurs, discontinue; for external use only; do not discontinue therapy even if symptoms are gone.

Dosage Forms

Cream: 100,000 units/g (15 g, 30 g)

Ointment, topical: 100,000 units/g (15 g, 30 g)

Powder, for preparation of oral suspension: 50 million units, 1 billion units, 2 billion units, 5 billion units

Powder, topical: 100,000 units/g (15 g)

Suspension, oral: 100,000 units/mL (5 mL, 60 mL, 480 mL)

Tablet:

Oral: 500,000 units

Vaginal: 100,000 units (15 and 30/box with applicator)

Troche: 200,000 units

Nystatin and Triamcinolone *(nye STAT in & trye am SIN oh lone)*

Related Information

Nystatin *on previous page*

U.S. Brand Names Mycogen II Topical; Mycolog®-II Topical; Myconel® Topical; Myco-Triacet® II; Mytrex® F Topical; N.G.T.® Topical; Tri-Statin® II Topical

Synonyms Triamcinolone and Nystatin

Use Treatment of cutaneous candidiasis

Usual Dosage Children and Adults: Topical: Apply sparingly 2-4 times/day

Dosage Forms

Cream: Nystatin 100,000 units and triamcinolone acetonide 0.1% (1.5 g, 15 g, 30 g, 60 g, 120 g)

Ointment, topical: Nystatin 100,000 units and triamcinolone acetonide 0.1% (15 g, 30 g, 60 g, 120 g)

Nystat-Rx® *see Nystatin on page 845*

Nystex® *see Nystatin on page 845*

Octicair® **Otic** *see Neomycin, Polymyxin B, and Hydrocortisone on page 836*

Ocuflox™ **Ophthalmic** *see Ofloxacin on this page*

Ocumycin® *see Gentamicin on page 747*

Ocusulf-10® **Ophthalmic** *see Sulfacetamide Sodium on page 927*

Ocutricin® **Ophthalmic Solution** *see Neomycin, Polymyxin B, and Gramicidin on page 836*

Ocutricin® **Topical Ointment** *see Bacitracin, Neomycin, and Polymyxin B on page 619*

Ofloxacin (oh FLOKS a sin)

Related Information
Antimicrobial Activity Against Selected Organisms *on page 983*
Tuberculosis Guidelines *on page 1114*

U.S. Brand Names Floxin®; Ocuflox™ Ophthalmic

Generic Available No

Use
Quinolone antibiotic for skin and skin structure, lower respiratory and urinary tract infections and sexually transmitted diseases. Active against many gram-positive and gram-negative aerobic bacteria.
Ophthalmic: Treatment of superficial ocular infections involving the conjunctiva or cornea due to strains of susceptible organisms

Drug of Choice or Alternative for
Disease/Syndrome(s)
Pelvic Inflammatory Disease *on page 41*
Organism(s)
Neisseria gonorrhoeae on page 215

Pregnancy Risk Factor C

Contraindications Hypersensitivity to ofloxacin or other members of the quinolone group such as nalidixic acid, oxolinic acid, cinoxacin, norfloxacin, and ciprofloxacin

Warnings/Precautions Use with caution in patients with epilepsy or other CNS diseases which could predispose seizures; use with caution in patients with renal impairment; failure to respond to an ophthalmic antibiotic after 2-3 days may indicate the presence of resistant organisms, or another causative agent; use caution with systemic preparation in children <18 years of age due to association of other quinolones with transient arthropathy; has rarely caused ruptured tendons (discontinue immediately with signs of inflammation or tendon pain)

Adverse Reactions
1% to 10%:
Cardiovascular: Chest pain (1% to 3%)
Central nervous system: Headache (1% to 9%), insomnia (3% to 7%), dizziness (1% to 5%), fatigue (1% to 3%), somnolence (1% to 3%), sleep disorders, nervousness (1% to 3%), pyrexia (1% to 3%), pain
Dermatologic: Rash/pruritus (1% to 3%)
Gastrointestinal: Diarrhea (1% to 4%), vomiting (1% to 3%), GI distress, cramps, abdominal cramps (1% to 3%), flatulence (1% to 3%), abnormal taste (1% to 3%), xerostomia (1% to 3%), decreased appetite, nausea (3% to 10%)
Genitourinary: Vaginitis (1% to 3%), external genital pruritus in women
Local: Pain at injection site
Ocular: Superinfection (ophthalmic), photophobia, lacrimation, dry eyes, stinging, visual disturbances (1% to 3%)
Miscellaneous: Trunk pain
<1%: Syncope, edema, hypertension, palpitations, vasodilation, anxiety, cognitive change, depression, dream abnormality, euphoria, hallucinations, vertigo, chills, malaise, extremity pain, weight loss, paresthesia, ruptured tendons, weakness, photophobia, photosensitivity, decreased hearing acuity, tinnitus, cough, thirst, vasculitis, Tourette's syndrome, hepatitis
(Continued)

Ofloxacin *(Continued)*

Overdosage/Toxicology
Symptoms of overdose include acute renal failure, seizures, nausea, vomiting
Treatment includes GI decontamination, if possible, and supportive care

Drug Interactions
Decreased effect: Decreased absorption with antacids containing aluminum, magnesium, and/or calcium (by up to 98% if given at the same time); fluoroquinolones may be decreased by antineoplastic agents

Increased toxicity/serum levels: Quinolones cause increased caffeine, warfarin, cyclosporine, procainamide, and possibly theophylline levels. Cimetidine and probenecid increase quinolone levels.

Mechanism of Action Ofloxacin is a DNA gyrase inhibitor. DNA gyrase is an essential bacterial enzyme that maintains the superhelical structure of DNA. DNA gyrase is required for DNA replication and transcription, DNA repair, recombination, and transposition; bactericidal

Pharmacodynamics/Kinetics
Absorption: Well absorbed; administration with food causes only minor alterations in absorption

Distribution: V_d: 2.4-3.5 L/kg

Protein binding: 20%

Half-life, elimination 5-7.5 hours

Elimination: Primarily unchanged in urine

Usual Dosage
Children >1 year and Adults: Ophthalmic: Instill 1-2 drops in affected eye(s) every 2-4 hours for the first 2 days, then use 4 times/day for an additional 5 days

Adults:

Lower respiratory tract infection: 400 mg every 12 hours for 10 days

Gonorrhea: 400 mg as a single dose

Cervicitis due to *C. trachomatis* and/or *N. gonorrhoeae*: 300 mg every 12 hours for 7 days

Skin/skin structure: 400 mg every 12 hours for 10 days

Urinary tract infection: 200-400 mg every 12 hours for 3-10 days

Prostatitis: 300 mg every 12 hours for 6 weeks

Dosing adjustment/interval in renal impairment: Adults: I.V., Oral:

Cl_{cr} 10-50 mL/minute: Administer 200-400 mg every 24 hours

Cl_{cr} <10 mL/minute: Administer 100-200 mg every 24 hours

Continuous arteriovenous or venovenous hemodiafiltration (CAVH) effects: Administer 300 mg every 24 hours

Patient Information Report any skin rash or other allergic reactions; avoid excessive sunlight; do not take with food; do not take within 2 hours of any products including antacids which contain zinc, magnesium, or aluminum; contact your physician immediately with signs of inflammation or tendon pain

Dosage Forms
Injection: 200 mg (50 mL); 400 mg (10 mL, 20 mL, 100 mL)

Solution, ophthalmic: 0.3% (5 mL)

Tablet: 200 mg, 300 mg, 400 mg

Selected Readings
Hooper DC and Wolfson JS, "Fluoroquinolone Antimicrobial Agents," *N Engl J Med*, 1991, 324(6):384-94.

Lomaestro BM and Bailie GR, "Quinolone-Cation Interactions: A Review," *DICP*, 1991, 25(11):1249-58.

Monk JP and Campoli-Richards DM, "Ofloxacin. A Review of Its Antibacterial Activity, Pharmacokinetic Properties and Therapeutic Use," *Drugs*, 1987, 33(4):346-91.

Stein GE, "The 4-Quinolone Antibiotics: Past, Present, and Future," *Pharmacotherapy*, 1988, 8(6):301-14.

US Department of Health and Human Services, "1993 Sexually Transmitted Diseases Treatment Guidelines," *MMWR Morb Mortal Wkly Rep*, 1993, 42(RR-14).

Walker RC and Wright AJ, "The Fluoroquinolones," *Mayo Clin Proc*, 1991, 66(12):1249-59.

Omnicef® *see Cefdinir on page 633*

OmniHIB™ *see Haemophilus b Conjugate Vaccine on page 756*

Omnipen® *see Ampicillin on page 604*

Omnipen®-N *see Ampicillin on page 604*

Ony-Clear® Spray *see Miconazole on page 822*

OPC-17116 *see Grepafloxacin on page 752*

Ophthalmics, Bacterial
Refer to

Ophthalmics, Viral
Refer to

Oxacillin (oks a SIL in)
Related Information
Antimicrobial Activity Against Selected Organisms *on page 983*
U.S. Brand Names Bactocill®; Prostaphlin®
Synonyms Methylphenyl Isoxazolyl Penicillin; Oxacillin Sodium
Generic Available Yes
Use Treatment of infections such as osteomyelitis, septicemia, endocarditis, and CNS infections caused by susceptible strains of *Staphylococcus*
Drug of Choice or Alternative for
Disease/Syndrome(s)
Arthritis, Septic *on page 18*
Pregnancy Risk Factor B
Contraindications Hypersensitivity to oxacillin or other penicillins or any component
Warnings/Precautions Elimination rate will be slow in neonates; modify dosage in patients with renal impairment and in the elderly; use with caution in patients with cephalosporin hypersensitivity
Adverse Reactions
1% to 10%: Gastrointestinal: Nausea, diarrhea
<1%: Fever, rash, vomiting, eosinophilia, leukopenia, neutropenia, thrombocytopenia, agranulocytosis, hepatotoxicity, increased AST, hematuria, acute interstitial nephritis, serum sickness-like reactions
Overdosage/Toxicology
Symptoms of penicillin overdose include neuromuscular hypersensitivity (agitation, hallucinations, asterixis, encephalopathy, confusion, and seizures) and
(Continued)

Oxacillin *(Continued)*

electrolyte imbalance with potassium or sodium salts, especially in renal failure

Hemodialysis may be helpful to aid in the removal of the drug from the blood, otherwise most treatment is supportive or symptom directed

Drug Interactions

Decreased effect: Efficacy of oral contraceptives may be reduced; effects of penicillins may be impaired by tetracycline

Increased effect: Disulfiram, probenecid may increase penicillin levels, increased effect of anticoagulants are possible with large I.V. doses

Stability Reconstituted parenteral solution is stable for 3 days at room temperature and 7 days when refrigerated; for I.V. infusion in NS or D_5W, solution is stable for 24 hours at room temperature

Mechanism of Action Inhibits bacterial cell wall synthesis by binding to one or more of the penicillin binding proteins (PBPs); which in turn inhibits the final transpeptidation step of peptidoglycan synthesis in bacterial cell walls, thus inhibiting cell wall biosynthesis. Bacteria eventually lyse due to ongoing activity of cell wall autolytic enzymes (autolysins and murein hydrolases) while cell wall assembly is arrested.

Pharmacodynamics/Kinetics

Absorption: Oral: 35% to 67%

Distribution: Into bile, synovial and pleural fluids, bronchial secretions; also distributes to peritoneal and pericardial fluids; crosses the placenta and appears in breast milk; penetrates the blood-brain barrier only when meninges are inflamed

Metabolism: In the liver to active metabolites

Half-life:

Children 1 week to 2 years: 0.9-1.8 hours

Adults: 23-60 minutes (prolonged with reduced renal function and in neonates)

Time to peak serum concentration:

Oral: Within 2 hours

I.M.: Within 30-60 minutes

Elimination: By kidneys and to small degree the bile as parent drug and metabolites

Usual Dosage

Neonates: I.M., I.V.:

Postnatal age <7 days:

<2000 g: 25 mg/kg/dose every 12 hours

>2000 g: 25 mg/kg/dose every 8 hours

Postnatal age >7 days:

<1200 g: 25 mg/kg/dose every 12 hours

1200-2000 g: 30 mg/kg/dose every 8 hours

>2000 g: 37.5 mg/kg/dose every 6 hours

Infants and Children:

Oral: 50-100 mg/kg/day divided every 6 hours

I.M., I.V.: 150-200 mg/kg/day in divided doses every 6 hours; maximum dose: 12 g/day

Adults:

Oral: 500-1000 mg every 4-6 hours for at least 5 days

I.M., I.V.: 250 mg to 2 g/dose every 4-6 hours

Dosing adjustment in renal impairment: Cl_{cr} <10 mL/minute: Use lower range of the usual dosage

Hemodialysis: Not dialyzable (0% to 5%)

Monitoring Parameters Observe for signs and symptoms of anaphylaxis during first dose

Test Interactions May interfere with urinary glucose tests using cupric sulfate (Benedict's solution, Clinitest®); may inactivate aminoglycosides *in vitro*; false-positive urinary and serum proteins

Patient Information Take orally on an empty stomach 1 hour before meals or 2 hours after meals; take all medication, do not skip doses

Additional Information Sodium content of 1 g: 64.4-71.3 mg (2.8-3.1 mEq)

Dosage Forms

Capsule, as sodium: 250 mg, 500 mg

Powder:
For injection, as sodium: 250 mg, 500 mg, 1 g, 2 g, 4 g, 10 g
For oral solution, as sodium: 250 mg/5 mL (100 mL)

Selected Readings
Donowitz GR and Mandell GL, "Beta-Lactam Antibiotics," *N Engl J Med*, 1988, 318(7):419-26 and 318(8):490-500.
Wright AJ, "The Penicillins," *Mayo Clin Proc*, 1999, 74(3):290-307.

Oxacillin Sodium *see* Oxacillin *on page 849*

Oxamniquine (oks AM ni kwin)
U.S. Brand Names Vansil™
Generic Available No
Use Treat all stages of *Schistosoma mansoni* infection
Drug of Choice or Alternative for
  Organism(s)
    Schistosoma mansoni on page 249
Pregnancy Risk Factor C
Warnings/Precautions Rare epileptiform convulsions have been observed within the first few hours of administration, especially in patients with a history of CNS pathology
Adverse Reactions
  >10%: Central nervous system: Dizziness, drowsiness, headache
  <10%:
    Central nervous system: Insomnia, malaise, hallucinations, behavior changes
    Gastrointestinal: GI effects, orange/red discoloration of urine
    Hepatic: Elevated LFTs
    Dermatologic: Rash, urticaria, pruritus
    Renal: Proteinuria
Drug Interactions May be synergistic with praziquantel
Mechanism of Action Not fully elucidated; causes worms to dislodge from their usual site of residence (mesenteric veins to the liver) by paralysis and contraction of musculature and subsequently phagocytized
Pharmacodynamics/Kinetics
  Absorption: Oral: Well absorbed
  Metabolism: Extensive in the GI tract via oxidation
  Half-life: 1-2.5 hours
  Time to peak: 1-3 hours
  Elimination: <2% unchanged in urine; up to 75% of metabolites excreted in urine
Usual Dosage Oral:
  Children <30 kg: 20 mg/kg in 2 divided doses of 10 mg/kg at 2- to 8-hour intervals

  Adults: 12-15 mg/kg as a single dose
Test Interactions May interfere with spectrometric or color reaction urinalysis
Patient Information Take with food
Additional Information Strains other than from the western hemisphere may require higher doses
Dosage Forms Capsule: 250 mg
Selected Readings
"Drugs for Parasitic Infections," *Med Lett Drugs Ther*, 1998, 40(1017):1-12.

Oxandrin® *see* Oxandrolone *on this page*

Oxandrolone (oks AN droe lone)
U.S. Brand Names Oxandrin®
Generic Available No
Use Treatment of "AIDS-wasting" syndrome; treatment of catabolic or tissue-depleting processes
Pregnancy Risk Factor X
Contraindications Severe renal or cardiac disease, benign prostatic hypertrophy with obstruction, undiagnosed genital bleeding, males with carcinoma of the breast or prostate
Warnings/Precautions May accelerate bone maturation without producing compensating gain in linear growth
(Continued)

Oxandrolone *(Continued)*

Adverse Reactions

Male:

Postpubertal:

>10%:
Dermatologic: Acne
Endocrine & metabolic: Gynecomastia
Genitourinary: Bladder irritability, priapism,

1% to 10%:
Central nervous system: Chills, insomnia
Endocrine & metabolic: Decreased libido
Gastrointestinal: Nausea, diarrhea
Genitourinary: Prostatic hypertrophy (geriatric)
Hematologic: Iron deficiency anemia, suppression of clotting factors
Hepatic: Hepatic dysfunction

<1%: Hepatic necrosis, hepatocellular carcinoma

Prepubertal:

>10%:
Dermatologic: Acne
Endocrine & metabolic: Virilism

1% to 10%:
Central nervous system: Chills, insomnia
Dermatologic: Hyperpigmentation
Gastrointestinal: Diarrhea, nausea
Hematologic: Iron deficiency anemia, suppression of clotting factors

<1%: Hepatic necrosis, hepatocellular carcinoma

Female:

>10%: Endocrine & metabolic: Virilism

1% to 10%:
Central nervous system: Chills, insomnia
Endocrine & metabolic: Hypercalcemia
Gastrointestinal: Nausea, diarrhea
Hematologic: Iron deficiency anemia, suppression of clotting factors
Hepatic: Hepatic dysfunction

<1%: Hepatic necrosis, hepatocellular carcinoma

Drug Interactions Oral anticoagulants, insulin requirements

Usual Dosage Adults: Oral:
AIDS wasting: 10 mg twice daily
Catabolic or tissue-depleting processes: 2.5 mg 2-4 times/day

Nursing Implications Perform radiographic examination of the hand and wrist every 6 months to determine the rate of bone maturation

Additional Information This medication is currently on the market as an "orphan drug." It is distributed by Gynex Pharmaceuticals, Inc to physicians who document their expertise in endocrinology and agree to participate in a study to gather data for the FDA.

Dosage Forms Tablet: 2.5 mg

Oxiconazole *(oks i KON a zole)*

U.S. Brand Names Oxistat®

Synonyms Oxiconazole Nitrate

Generic Available No

Use Treatment of tinea pedis (athlete's foot), tinea cruris (jock itch), and tinea corporis (ringworm)

Pregnancy Risk Factor B

Contraindications Hypersensitivity to this agent; not for ophthalmic use

Warnings/Precautions May cause irritation during therapy; if a sensitivity to oxiconazole occurs, therapy should be discontinued; avoid contact with eyes or vagina

Adverse Reactions 1% to 10%:
Dermatologic: Itching, erythema, dryness
Local: Transient burning, local irritation, stinging

Mechanism of Action The cytoplasmic membrane integrity of fungi is destroyed by oxiconazole which exerts a fungicidal activity through inhibition of ergosterol synthesis. Effective for treatment of tinea pedis, tinea cruris, and tinea corporis.

Active against *Trichophyton rubrum*, *Trichophyton mentagrophytes*, *Trichophyton violaceum*, *Microsporum canis*, *Microsporum audouini*, *Microsporum gypseum*, *Epidermophyton floccosum*, *Candida albicans*, and *Malassezia furfur*.

Pharmacodynamics/Kinetics
Absorption: In each layer of the dermis; very little is absorbed systemically after one topical dose
Distribution: To each layer of the dermis; excreted in breast milk
Elimination: <0.3% excreted in urine

Usual Dosage Children and Adults: Topical: Apply once to twice daily to affected areas for 2 weeks (tinea corporis/tinea cruris) to 1 month (tinea pedis)

Patient Information External use only; discontinue if sensitivity or chemical irritation occurs, contact physician if condition fails to improve in 3-4 days

Dosage Forms
Cream, as nitrate: 1% (15 g, 30 g, 60 g)
Lotion, as nitrate: 1% (30 mL)

Oxiconazole Nitrate *see* Oxiconazole *on previous page*

Oxistat® *see* Oxiconazole *on previous page*

Oxymetholone (oks i METH oh lone)
U.S. Brand Names Anadrol®
Canadian Brand Names Anapolon®
Generic Available No
Use Treatment of "AIDS-wasting" syndrome; anemias caused by the administration of myelotoxic drugs
Restrictions C-III
Pregnancy Risk Factor X
Contraindications Carcinoma of breast or prostate, nephrosis, pregnancy, hypersensitivity to any component
Warnings/Precautions Anabolic steroids may cause peliosis hepatis, liver cell tumors, and blood lipid changes with increased risk of arteriosclerosis; monitor diabetic patients carefully; use with caution in elderly patients, they may be at greater risk for prostatic hypertrophy; use with caution in patients with cardiac, renal, or hepatic disease or epilepsy

Adverse Reactions
Male:
Postpubertal:
>10%:
Dermatologic: Acne
Endocrine & metabolic: Gynecomastia
Genitourinary: Bladder irritability, priapism
1% to 10%:
Central nervous system: Insomnia, chills
Endocrine & metabolic: Decreased libido
Gastrointestinal: Nausea, diarrhea
Genitourinary: Prostatic hypertrophy (elderly)
Hematologic: Iron deficiency anemia, suppression of clotting factors
Hepatic: Hepatic dysfunction
<1%:
Hepatic: Hepatic necrosis, hepatocellular carcinoma
Prepubertal:
>10%:
Dermatologic: Acne
Endocrine & metabolic: Virilism
1% to 10%:
Central nervous system: Chills, insomnia
Dermatologic: Hyperpigmentation
Gastrointestinal: Diarrhea, nausea
Hematologic: Iron deficiency anemia, suppression of clotting factors
<1%: Hepatic: Hepatic necrosis, hepatocellular carcinoma

Female:
>10%: Endocrine & metabolic: Virilism
1% to 10%:
Central nervous system: Chills, insomnia
Endocrine & metabolic: Hypercalcemia
(Continued)

Oxymetholone *(Continued)*

Gastrointestinal: Nausea, diarrhea
Hematologic: Iron deficiency anemia, suppression of clotting factors
Hepatic: Hepatic dysfunction
<1%: Hepatic: Hepatic necrosis, hepatocellular carcinoma

Overdosage/Toxicology Abnormal liver function tests

Drug Interactions Increased toxicity: Increased oral anticoagulants, insulin requirements may be decreased

Mechanism of Action Stimulates receptors in organs and tissues to promote growth and development of male sex organs and maintains secondary sex characteristics in androgen-deficient males

Pharmacodynamics/Kinetics
Half-life: 9 hours
Elimination: Primarily in urine

Usual Dosage Adults:
AIDS wasting: 50 mg 3 times/day
Erythropoietic effects: Oral: 1-5 mg/kg/day in 1 daily dose; maximum: 100 mg/day; give for a minimum trial of 3-6 months because response may be delayed

Monitoring Parameters Liver function tests

Test Interactions Altered glucose tolerance tests, altered thyroid function tests, altered metyrapone tests

Dosage Forms Tablet: 50 mg

Oxytetracycline (oks i tet ra SYE kleen)

U.S. Brand Names Terramycin® I.M. Injection; Terramycin® Oral; Uri-Tet® Oral
Synonyms Oxytetracycline Hydrochloride
Generic Available Yes
Use Treatment of susceptible bacterial infections; both gram-positive and gram-negative, as well as, *Rickettsia* and *Mycoplasma* organisms
Pregnancy Risk Factor D
Contraindications Hypersensitivity to tetracycline or any component
Warnings/Precautions Avoid in children ≤8 years of age, pregnant and nursing women; photosensitivity can occur with oxytetracycline

Adverse Reactions
>10%: Miscellaneous: Discoloration of teeth and enamel hypoplasia (infants)
1% to 10%:
Dermatologic: Photosensitivity
Gastrointestinal: Nausea, diarrhea
<1%: Pericarditis, increased intracranial pressure, bulging fontanels in infants, pseudotumor cerebri, pruritus, exfoliative dermatitis, dermatologic effects, diabetes insipidus syndrome, vomiting, esophagitis, anorexia, abdominal cramps, antibiotic-associated pseudomembranous colitis, staphylococcal enterocolitis, hepatotoxicity, thrombophlebitis, paresthesia, renal damage, acute renal failure, azotemia, superinfections, anaphylaxis, pigmentation of nails, hypersensitivity reactions, candidal superinfection

Overdosage/Toxicology
Symptoms of overdose include nausea, anorexia, diarrhea
Following GI decontamination, supportive care only

Drug Interactions
Decreased effect with antacids containing aluminum, calcium or magnesium; iron and bismuth subsalicylate may decrease doxycycline bioavailability; barbiturates, phenytoin, and carbamazepine decrease doxycycline's half-life
Increased effect of warfarin

Mechanism of Action Inhibits bacterial protein synthesis by binding with the 30S and possibly the 50S ribosomal subunit(s) of susceptible bacteria, cell wall synthesis is not affected

Pharmacodynamics/Kinetics
Absorption:
Oral: Adequate (~75%)
I.M.: Poor
Distribution: Crosses the placenta
Metabolism: Small amounts in the liver
Half-life: 8.5-9.6 hours (increases with renal impairment)
Time to peak serum concentration: Within 2-4 hours

Elimination: In urine, while much higher amounts can be found in bile

Usual Dosage

Oral:

Children >8 years: 40-50 mg/kg/day in divided doses every 6 hours (maximum: 2 g/24 hours)

Adults: 250-500 mg/dose every 6-12 hours depending on severity of the infection

I.M.:

Children >8 years: 15-25 mg/kg/day (maximum: 250 mg/dose) in divided doses every 8-12 hours

Adults: 250 mg every 24 hours or 300 mg/day divided every 8-12 hours

Syphilis: 30-40 g in divided doses over 10-15 days

Gonorrhea: 1.5 g, then 500 mg every 6 hours for total of 9 g

Uncomplicated chlamydial infections: 500 mg every 6 hours for 7 days

Severe acne: 1 g/day then decrease to 125-500 mg/day

Dosing interval in renal impairment:

Cl_{cr} <10 mL/minute: Administer every 24 hours or avoid use if possible

Dosing adjustment/comments in hepatic impairment: Avoid use in patients with severe liver disease

Administration Injection for intramuscular use only; do not administer with antacids, iron products, or dairy products; administer 1 hour before or 2 hours after meals

Patient Information Avoid unnecessary exposure to sunlight; do not take with antacids, iron products, or dairy products; finish all medication; do not skip doses; take 1 hour before or 2 hours after meals

Dosage Forms

Capsule, as hydrochloride: 250 mg

Injection, as hydrochloride, with lidocaine 2%: 5% [50 mg/mL] (2 mL, 10 mL); 12.5% [125 mg/mL] (2 mL)

Oxytetracycline and Hydrocortisone
(oks i tet ra SYE kleen & hye droe KOR ti sone)

Related Information

Oxytetracycline *on previous page*

U.S. Brand Names Terra-Cortril® Ophthalmic Suspension

Use Treatment of susceptible ophthalmic bacterial infections with associated inflammation

Dosage Forms Suspension, ophthalmic: Oxytetracycline hydrochloride 0.5% and hydrocortisone 0.5% (5 mL)

Oxytetracycline and Polymyxin B
(oks i tet ra SYE kleen & pol i MIKS in bee)

Related Information

Oxytetracycline *on previous page*

Polymyxin B *on page 877*

U.S. Brand Names Terak® Ophthalmic Ointment; Terramycin® Ophthalmic Ointment; Terramycin® w/Polymyxin B Ophthalmic Ointment

Use Treatment of superficial ocular infections involving the conjunctiva and/or cornea

Usual Dosage Topical: Apply ½" of ointment onto the lower lid of affected eye 2-4 times/day

Dosage Forms

Ointment, ophthalmic/otic: Oxytetracycline hydrochloride 5 mg and polymyxin B 10,000 units per g (3.5 g)

Tablet, vaginal: Oxytetracycline hydrochloride 100 mg and polymyxin B 100,000 units (10s)

Oxytetracycline Hydrochloride *see* Oxytetracycline *on previous page*

Palivizumab (pah li VIZ u mab)

U.S. Brand Names Synagis®

Use Prevention of serious lower respiratory tract disease caused by respiratory syncytial virus (RSV) in pediatric patients at high risk of RSV disease; safety and efficacy were established in infants with bronchopulmonary dysplasia (BPD) and infants with a history of prematurity (≤35 weeks gestational age)

(Continued)

Palivizumab *(Continued)*

Pregnancy Risk Factor C

Pregnancy/Breast-Feeding Implications Animal reproduction studies have not been conducted; it is not known whether palivizumab can cause fetal harm when administered to a pregnant woman or could affect reproductive capacity

Contraindications Patients with a history of severe prior reaction to palivizumab or other components of the product

Warnings/Precautions Anaphylactoid reactions have not been observed following palivizumab administration; however, can occur after administration of proteins. Safety and efficacy of palivizumab have not been demonstrated in the treatment of established RSV disease.

Adverse Reactions The incidence of adverse events was similar between the palivizumab and placebo groups

>1%:
Central nervous system: Nervousness
Dermatologic: Fungal dermatitis, eczema, seborrhea
Gastrointestinal: Diarrhea, vomiting, gastroenteritis
Hematologic: Anemia
Hepatic: Increased ALT, liver function abnormality
Local: Injection site reaction
Ocular: Conjunctivitis
Respiratory: Cough, wheezing, bronchiolitis, pneumonia, bronchitis, asthma, croup, dyspnea, sinusitis, apnea
Miscellaneous: Oral moniliasis, failure to thrive, viral infection, flu syndrome

Overdosage/Toxicology No data from clinical studies are available

Drug Interactions No formal drug interaction studies have been conducted

Stability Store in refrigerator at a temperature between 2°C to 8°C (35.6°F to 46.4°F) in original container; do not freeze

Use aseptic technique when reconstituting; add 1 mL of sterile water for injection to a 100 mg vial; swirl vial gently for 30 seconds to avoid foaming. Do not shake vial. Allow to stand at room temperature for 20 minutes until the solution clarifies; solution should be administered with in 6 hours of reconstitution.

Mechanism of Action Exhibits neutralizing and fusion-inhibitory activity against RSV; these activities inhibit RSV replication in laboratory and clinical studies

Pharmacodynamics/Kinetics Half-life: ~18 days

Usual Dosage Children: I.M.: 15 mg/kg of body weight, monthly throughout RSV season (First dose administered prior to commencement of RSV season)

Administration Injection should (preferably) be in the anterolateral aspect of the thigh; gluteal muscle should not be used routinely; injection volume over 1 mL should be given as divided doses

Dose per month equals patient weight in cubagrams x 15 mg/kg divided by 100 mg/mL of palivizumab

Dosage Forms Injection, lyophilized: 100 mg

Selected Readings

Johnson S, Oliver C, Prince GA, et al, "Development of a Humanized Monoclonal Antibody (MEDI-493) With Potent *In Vitro* and *In Vivo* Activity Against Respiratory Syncytial Virus," *J Infect Dis,* 1997, 176(5):1215-24.

"Prevention of Respiratory Syncytial Virus Infections: Indications for the Use of Palivizumab and Update on the Use of RSV-IGIV. American Academy of Pediatrics Committee on Infectious Diseases and Committee of Fetus and Newborn," *Pediatrics,* 1998, 102(5):1211-6.

Simoes EA, Sondheimer HM, Top FH Jr, et al, "Respiratory Syncytial Virus Immune Globulin for Prophylaxis Against Respiratory Syncytial Virus Disease in Infants and Children With Congential Heart Disease. The Cardiac Study Group," *J Pediatr,* 1998, 133(4):492-9.

Subramanian KN, Weisman, LE, Rhodes T, et al, "Safety, Tolerance and Pharmacokinetics of a Humanized Monoclonal Antibody to Respiratory Syncytial Virus in Premature Infants With Bronchopulmonary Dysplasia. MEDI-493 Study Group," *Pediatr Infect Dis J,* 1998, 17(2):110-5.

Wandstrat TL, "Respiratory Syncytial Virus Immune Globulin Intravenous," *Ann Pharmacother,* 1997, 31(1):83-8.

Welliver RC, "Respiratory Syncytial Virus Immunoglobulin and Monoclonal Antibodies in the Prevention and Treatment of Respiratory Syncytial Virus Infection," *Semin Perinatol,* 1998, 22(1):87-95.

Panmycin® Oral *see* Tetracycline *on page 944*

Paromomycin *(par oh moe MYE sin)*

U.S. Brand Names Humatin®

Synonyms Paromomycin Sulfate

Generic Available No

Use Treatment of acute and chronic intestinal amebiasis; preoperatively to suppress intestinal flora; tapeworm infestations; has also been used in the treatment of *Cryptosporidium*

Drug of Choice or Alternative for

Organism(s)

Entamoeba histolytica on page 132

Pregnancy Risk Factor C

Contraindications Intestinal obstruction, renal failure, known hypersensitivity to paromomycin or components

Warnings/Precautions Use with caution in patients with impaired renal function or possible or proven ulcerative bowel lesions

Adverse Reactions

1% to 10%: Gastrointestinal: Diarrhea, abdominal cramps, nausea, vomiting, heartburn

<1%: Headache, vertigo, exanthema, rash, pruritus, steatorrhea, secondary enterocolitis, eosinophilia, ototoxicity

Overdosage/Toxicology

Symptoms of overdose include nausea, vomiting, diarrhea

Following GI decontamination, if possible; care is supportive and symptomatic

Drug Interactions

Decreased effect of digoxin, vitamin A, and methotrexate

Increased effect of oral anticoagulants, neuromuscular blockers, and polypeptide antibiotics

Mechanism of Action Acts directly on ameba; has antibacterial activity against normal and pathogenic organisms in the GI tract; interferes with bacterial protein synthesis by binding to 30S ribosomal subunits

Pharmacodynamics/Kinetics

Absorption: Not absorbed via oral route

Elimination: 100% unchanged in feces

Usual Dosage Oral:

Intestinal amebiasis: Children and Adults: 25-35 mg/kg/day in 3 divided doses for 5-10 days

Dientamoeba fragilis: Children and Adults: 25-30 mg/kg/day in 3 divided doses for 7 days

Cryptosporidium: Adults with AIDS: 1.5-2.25 g/day in 3-6 divided doses for 10-14 days (occasionally courses of up to 4-8 weeks may be needed)

Tapeworm (fish, dog, bovine, porcine):

Children: 11 mg/kg every 15 minutes for 4 doses

Adults: 1 g every 15 minutes for 4 doses

Hepatic coma: Adults: 4 g/day in 2-4 divided doses for 5-6 days

Dwarf tapeworm: Children and Adults: 45 mg/kg/dose every day for 5-7 days

Patient Information Take full course of therapy; do not skip doses; notify physician if ringing in ears, hearing loss, or dizziness occurs

Dosage Forms Capsule, as sulfate: 250 mg

Selected Readings

Danziger LH, Kanyok TP, and Novak RM, "Treatment of Cryptosporidial Diarrhea in an AIDS Patient With Paromomycin," *Ann Pharmacother*, 1993, 27(12):1460-2.

"Drugs for Parasitic Infections," *Med Lett Drugs Ther*, 1998, 40(1017):1-12.

Paromomycin Sulfate see Paromomycin *on previous page*

PAS see Aminosalicylate Sodium *on page 591*

Pathocil® see Dicloxacillin *on page 702*

PCE® see Erythromycin *on page 722*

Pediazole® see Erythromycin and Sulfisoxazole *on page 725*

Pedi-Cort V® Creme see Clioquinol and Hydrocortisone *on page 687*

PediOtic® Otic see Neomycin, Polymyxin B, and Hydrocortisone *on page 836*

PedvaxHIB™ see Haemophilus b Conjugate Vaccine *on page 756*

Penciclovir (pen SYE kloe veer)

U.S. Brand Names Denavir™

Generic Available No

Use Topical treatment of herpes simplex labialis (cold sores); potentially used for Epstein-Barr virus infections

Pregnancy Risk Factor B

(Continued)

Penciclovir *(Continued)*

Contraindications Previous and significant adverse reactions to famciclovir; hypersensitivity to the product or any of its components

Warnings/Precautions Penciclovir should only be used on herpes labialis on the lips and face; because no data are available, application to mucous membranes is not recommended. Avoid application in or near eyes since it may cause irritation. The effect of penciclovir has not been established in immunocompromised patients.

Adverse Reactions
Central nervous system: Headache (5.3%)
Dermatologic: Mild erythema (50%), local anesthesia (0.9%)

Mechanism of Action In cells infected with HSV-1 or HSV-2, viral thymidine kinase phosphorylates penciclovir to a monophosphate form which, in turn, is converted to penciclovir triphosphate by cellular kinases. Penciclovir triphosphate inhibits HSV polymerase competitively with deoxyguanosine triphosphate. Consequently, herpes viral DNA synthesis and, therefore, replication are selectively inhibited.

Pharmacodynamics/Kinetics Measurable penciclovir concentrations were not detected in plasma or urine of health male volunteers following single or repeat application of the 1% cream at a dose of 180 mg penciclovir daily (approximately 67 times the usual clinical dose)

Usual Dosage Apply cream at the first sign or symptom of cold sore (eg, tingling, swelling); apply every 2 hours during waking hours for 4 days

Monitoring Parameters Reduction in virus shedding, negative cultures for herpes virus; resolution of pain and healing of cold sore lesion

Patient Information Inform your physician if you experience significant burning, itching, stinging, or redness when using this medication

Additional Information Penciclovir is the active metabolite of the prodrug famciclovir. Penciclovir is an alternative to topical acyclovir for HSV-1 and HSV-2 infections. Neither drug will prevent recurring HSV attacks.

Dosage Forms Cream: 1% [10 mg/g] (2 g)

Selected Readings
Alrabiah FA and Sacks SL, "New Antiherpesvirus Agents. Their Targets and Therapeutic Potential," *Drugs*, 1996, 52(1):17-32.

Penetrex™ *see* Enoxacin *on page 720*
Penglobe® *see* Bacampicillin *on page 617*

Penicillin G Benzathine and Procaine Combined

(pen i SIL in jee BENZ a theen & PROE kane KOM bined)
U.S. Brand Names Bicillin® C-R; Bicillin® C-R 900/300
Synonyms Penicillin G Procaine and Benzathine Combined
Generic Available No
Use May be used in specific situations in the treatment of streptococcal infections
Pregnancy Risk Factor B
Contraindications Known hypersensitivity to penicillin or any component
Warnings/Precautions Use with caution in patients with impaired renal function, impaired cardiac function or seizure disorder

Overdosage/Toxicology
Many beta-lactam-containing antibiotics have the potential to cause neuromuscular hyperirritability or convulsive seizures
Hemodialysis may be helpful to aid in the removal of the drug from the blood, otherwise most treatment is supportive or symptom directed

Drug Interactions Probenecid, tetracyclines, methotrexate, aminoglycosides
Stability Store in the refrigerator
Mechanism of Action Inhibits bacterial cell wall synthesis by binding to one or more of the penicillin binding proteins (PBPs); which in turn inhibits the final transpeptidation step of peptidoglycan synthesis in bacterial cell walls, thus inhibiting cell wall biosynthesis. Bacteria eventually lyse due to ongoing activity of cell wall autolytic enzymes (autolysins and murein hydrolases) while cell wall assembly is arrested.

Usual Dosage I.M.:
Children:
<30 lb: 600,000 units in a single dose
30-60 lb: 900,000 units to 1.2 million units in a single dose

Children >60 lb and Adults: 2.4 million units in a single dose

Test Interactions May interfere with urinary glucose tests using cupric sulfate (Benedict's solution, Clinitest®); may inactivate aminoglycosides *in vitro*; positive direct Coombs' test, increased protein

Nursing Implications Administer by deep I.M. injection in the upper outer quadrant of the buttock

Dosage Forms

Injection:

300,000 units [150,000 units each of penicillin g benzathine and penicillin g procaine] (10 mL)

600,000 units [300,000 units each penicillin g benzathine and penicillin g procaine] (1 mL)

1,200,000 units [600,000 units each penicillin g benzathine and penicillin g procaine] (2 mL)

2,400,000 units [1,200,000 units each penicillin g benzathine and penicillin g procaine] (4 mL)

Injection: Penicillin g benzathine 900,000 units and penicillin g procaine 300,000 units per dose (2 mL)

Penicillin G Benzathine, Parenteral

(pen i SIL in jee BENZ a theen, pa Ren ter al)

U.S. Brand Names Bicillin® L-A; Permapen®

Canadian Brand Names Megacillin® Susp

Synonyms Benzathine Benzylpenicillin; Benzathine Penicillin G; Benzylpenicillin Benzathine

Generic Available No

Use Active against some gram-positive organisms, few gram-negative organisms such as *Neisseria gonorrhoeae*, and some anaerobes and spirochetes; used in the treatment of syphilis; used only for the treatment of mild to moderately severe infections caused by organisms susceptible to low concentrations of penicillin G or for prophylaxis of infections caused by these organisms

Drug of Choice or Alternative for

Organism(s)

Treponema pallidum on page 285

Pregnancy Risk Factor B

Contraindications Known hypersensitivity to penicillin or any component

Warnings/Precautions Use with caution in patients with impaired renal function, seizure disorder, or history of hypersensitivity to other beta-lactams; CDC and AAP do not currently recommend the use of penicillin G benzathine to treat congenital syphilis or neurosyphilis due to reported treatment failures and lack of published clinical data on its efficacy

Adverse Reactions

1% to 10%: Local: Pain

<1%: Convulsions, confusion, drowsiness, fever, rash, electrolyte imbalance, hemolytic anemia, positive Coombs' test, thrombophlebitis, myoclonus, acute interstitial nephritis, Jarisch-Herxheimer reaction, hypersensitivity reactions, anaphylaxis

Overdosage/Toxicology

Symptoms of penicillin overdose include neuromuscular hypersensitivity (agitation, hallucinations, asterixis, encephalopathy, confusion, and seizures) and electrolyte imbalance with potassium or sodium salts, especially in renal failure

Hemodialysis may be helpful to aid in the removal of the drug from the blood, otherwise most treatment is supportive or symptom directed

Drug Interactions

Decreased effect: Tetracyclines may decrease penicillin effectiveness; decreased oral contraceptive effect is possible

Increased effect:

Probenecid may increase penicillin levels

Aminoglycosides → synergistic efficacy; heparin and parenteral penicillins may result in increased bleeding

Stability Store in refrigerator

Mechanism of Action Interferes with bacterial cell wall synthesis during active multiplication, causing cell wall death and resultant bactericidal activity against susceptible bacteria

(Continued)

Penicillin G Benzathine, Parenteral *(Continued)*

Pharmacodynamics/Kinetics

Absorption: I.M.: Slow

Time to peak serum concentration: Within 12-24 hours; serum levels are usually detectable for 1-4 weeks depending on the dose; larger doses result in more sustained levels rather than higher levels

Usual Dosage I.M.: Administer undiluted injection; higher doses result in more sustained rather than higher levels. Use a penicillin G benzathine-penicillin G procaine combination to achieve early peak levels in acute infections.

Infants and Children:

Group A streptococcal upper respiratory infection: 25,000-50,000 units/kg as a single dose; maximum: 1.2 million units

Prophylaxis of recurrent rheumatic fever: 25,000-50,000 units/kg every 3-4 weeks; maximum: 1.2 million units/dose

Early syphilis: 50,000 units/kg as a single injection; maximum: 2.4 million units

Syphilis of more than 1-year duration: 50,000 units/kg every week for 3 doses; maximum: 2.4 million units/dose

Adults:

Group A streptococcal upper respiratory infection: 1.2 million units as a single dose

Prophylaxis of recurrent rheumatic fever: 1.2 million units every 3-4 weeks or 600,000 units twice monthly

Early syphilis: 2.4 million units as a single dose in 2 injection sites

Syphilis of more than 1-year duration: 2.4 million units in 2 injection sites once weekly for 3 doses

Not indicated as single drug therapy for neurosyphilis, but may be given 1 time/week for 3 weeks following I.V. treatment (refer to Penicillin G monograph for dosing)

Administration Administer by deep I.M. injection in the upper outer quadrant of the buttock do **not** administer I.V., intra-arterially, or S.C.; in children <2 years of age, I.M. injections should be made into the midlateral muscle of the thigh, not the gluteal region; when doses are repeated, rotate the injection site

Monitoring Parameters Observe for signs and symptoms of anaphylaxis during first dose

Test Interactions Positive direct Coombs' test, false-positive urinary and/or serum proteins, false-positive or -negative urinary glucose with Clinitest®

Patient Information Report any rash

Dosage Forms Injection: 300,000 units/mL (10 mL); 600,000 units/mL (1 mL, 2 mL, 4 mL)

Selected Readings

US Department of Health and Human Services, "1993 Sexually Transmitted Diseases Treatment Guidelines," *MMWR Morb Mortal Wkly Rep*, 1993, 42(RR-14).

Wright AJ, "The Penicillins," *Mayo Clin Proc*, 1999, 74(3):290-307.

Penicillin G, Parenteral, Aqueous

(pen i SIL in jee, pa REN ter al, AYE kwee us)

Related Information

Antimicrobial Activity Against Selected Organisms *on page 983*

U.S. Brand Names Pfizerpen®

Synonyms Benzylpenicillin Potassium; Benzylpenicillin Sodium; Crystalline Penicillin; Penicillin G Potassium; Penicillin G Sodium

Generic Available No

Use Active against some gram-positive organisms, generally not *Staphylococcus aureus*; some gram-negative organisms such as *Neisseria gonorrhoeae*, and some anaerobes and spirochetes

Drug of Choice or Alternative for

Disease/Syndrome(s)

Brain Abscess *on page 19*

Endocarditis, Subacute Native Valve *on page 28*

Meningitis, Community-Acquired, Adult *on page 34*

Pneumonia, Aspiration, Community-Acquired *on page 44*

Organism(s)

Actinomyces Species *on page 61*

Bacillus anthracis *on page 73*

Borrelia burgdorferi *on page 84*

Pregnancy Risk Factor B

Contraindications Known hypersensitivity to penicillin or any component

Warnings/Precautions Avoid intra-arterial administration or injection into or near major peripheral nerves or blood vessels since such injections may cause severe and/or permanent neurovascular damage; use with caution in patients with renal impairment (dosage reduction required), pre-existing seizure disorders, or with a history of hypersensitivity to cephalosporins

Adverse Reactions <1%: Convulsions, confusion, drowsiness, fever, rash, electrolyte imbalance, hemolytic anemia, positive Coombs' test, thrombophlebitis, myoclonus, acute interstitial nephritis, Jarisch-Herxheimer reaction, hypersensitivity reactions, anaphylaxis

Overdosage/Toxicology
Symptoms of penicillin overdose include neuromuscular hypersensitivity (agitation, hallucinations, asterixis, encephalopathy, confusion, and seizures) and electrolyte imbalance with potassium or sodium salts, especially in renal failure

Hemodialysis may be helpful to aid in the removal of the drug from the blood, otherwise most treatment is supportive or symptom directed

Drug Interactions
Decreased effect: Tetracyclines may decrease penicillin effectiveness; decreased oral contraceptive effect is possible
Increased effect:
Probenecid may increase penicillin levels
Aminoglycosides may result in synergistic efficacy; heparin and parenteral penicillins may result in increased bleeding

Stability
Penicillin G potassium is stable at room temperature
Reconstituted parenteral solution is stable for 7 days when refrigerated (2°C to 15°C)
Penicillin G potassium for I.V. infusion in NS or D_5W, solution is stable for 24 hours at room temperature
Incompatible with aminoglycosides; inactivated in acidic or alkaline solutions

Mechanism of Action Interferes with bacterial cell wall synthesis during active multiplication, causing cell wall death and resultant bactericidal activity against susceptible bacteria

Pharmacodynamics/Kinetics
Distribution: Crosses the placenta; appears in breast milk; penetration across the blood-brain barrier is poor, despite inflamed meninges
Relative diffusion of antimicrobial agents from blood into cerebrospinal fluid (CSF): Good only with inflammation (exceeds usual MICs)
Ratio of CSF to blood level (%):
Normal meninges: <1
Inflamed meninges: 3-5
Protein binding: 65%
Metabolism: In the liver (30%) to penicilloic acid
Half-life:
Neonates:
<6 days: 3.2-3.4 hours
(Continued)

Penicillin G, Parenteral, Aqueous *(Continued)*

7-13 days: 1.2-2.2 hours
>14 days: 0.9-1.9 hours
Children and adults with normal renal function: 20-50 minutes
End stage renal disease: 3.3-5.1 hours
Time to peak serum concentration:
I.M.: Within 30 minutes
I.V. Within 1 hour
Elimination: In urine

Usual Dosage I.M., I.V.:
Infants:
>7 days, >2000 g: 100,000 units/kg/day in divided doses every 6 hours
>7 days, <2000 g: 75,000 units/kg/day in divided doses every 8 hours
<7 days, >2000 g: 50,000 units/kg/day in divided doses every 8 hours
<7 days, <2000 g: 50,000 units/kg/day in divided doses every 12 hours
Infants and Children (sodium salt is preferred in children): 100,000-250,000 units/kg/day in divided doses every 4 hours
Severe infections: Up to 400,000 units/kg/day in divided doses every 4 hours; maximum dose: 24 million units/day
Adults: 2-24 million units/day in divided doses every 4 hours depending on sensitivity of the organism and severity of the infection
Congenital syphilis:
Newborns: 50,000 units/kg/day I.V. every 8-12 hours for 10-14 days
Infants: 50,000 units/kg every 4-6 hours for 10-14 days
Disseminated gonococcal infections or gonococcus ophthalmia (if organism proven sensitive): 100,000 units/kg/day in 2 equal doses (4 equal doses/day for infants >1 week)
Gonococcal meningitis: 150,000 units/kg in 2 equal doses (4 doses/day for infants >1 week)

Dosing interval in renal impairment:
Cl$_{cr}$ 30-50 mL/minute: Administer every 6 hours
Cl$_{cr}$ 10-30 mL/minute: Administer every 8 hours
Cl$_{cr}$ <10 mL/minute: Administer every 12 hours
Hemodialysis: Moderately dializable (20% to 50%)
Continuous arteriovenous or venovenous hemodiafiltration (CAVH) effects: Dose as for Cl$_{cr}$ 10-50 mL/minute

Administration Administer I.M. by deep injection in the upper outer quadrant of the buttock

Monitoring Parameters Observe for signs and symptoms of anaphylaxis during first dose

Test Interactions False-positive or -negative urinary glucose with Clinitest®, false-positive direct Coombs' test, false-positive urinary and/or serum proteins

Patient Information Report any rash or shortness of breath

Nursing Implications Dosage modification required in patients with renal insufficiency

Additional Information 1 million units is approximately equal to 625 mg
Penicillin G potassium: 1.7 mEq of potassium and 0.3 mEq of sodium per 1 million units of penicillin G
Penicillin G sodium: 2 mEq of sodium per 1 million units of penicillin G

Dosage Forms
Injection, as sodium: 5 million units
Injection:
Frozen premixed, as potassium: 1 million units, 2 million units, 3 million units
Powder, as potassium: 1 million units, 5 million units, 10 million units, 20 million units

Selected Readings
Donowitz GR and Mandell GL, "Beta-Lactam Antibiotics," *N Engl J Med*, 1988, 318(7):419-26 and 318(8):490-500.
Wright AJ, "The Penicillins," *Mayo Clin Proc*, 1999, 74(3):290-307.

Penicillin G Potassium *see* Penicillin G, Parenteral, Aqueous *on page 860*

Penicillin G Procaine *(pen i SIL in jee PROE kane)*
Related Information
Antimicrobial Activity Against Selected Organisms *on page 983*
U.S. Brand Names Crysticillin® A.S.; Wycillin®

Canadian Brand Names Ayercillin®

Synonyms APPG; Aqueous Procaine Penicillin G; Procaine Benzylpenicillin; Procaine Penicillin G

Generic Available Yes

Use Moderately severe infections due to *Treponema pallidum* and other penicillin G-sensitive microorganisms that are susceptible to low but prolonged serum penicillin concentrations

Drug of Choice or Alternative for

Disease/Syndrome(s)

Pharyngitis *on page 43*

Organism(s)

Corynebacterium diphtheriae on page 111

Treponema pallidum on page 285

Pregnancy Risk Factor B

Contraindications Known hypersensitivity to penicillin or any component; also contraindicated in patients hypersensitive to procaine

Warnings/Precautions May need to modify dosage in patients with severe renal impairment, seizure disorders, or history of hypersensitivity to cephalosporins; avoid I.V., intravascular, or intra-arterial administration of penicillin G procaine since severe and/or permanent neurovascular damage may occur

Adverse Reactions

>10%: Local: Pain at injection site

<1%: Myocardial depression, vasodilation, conduction disturbances, CNS stimulation, seizures, confusion, drowsiness, hemolytic anemia, positive Coombs' test, sterile abscess at injection site, myoclonus, interstitial nephritis, pseudo-anaphylactic reactions, Jarisch-Herxheimer reaction, hypersensitivity reactions

Overdosage/Toxicology

Symptoms of penicillin overdose include neuromuscular hypersensitivity (agitation, hallucinations, asterixis, encephalopathy, confusion, and seizures) and electrolyte imbalance with potassium or sodium salts, especially in renal failure

Hemodialysis may be helpful to aid in the removal of the drug from the blood, otherwise most treatment is supportive or symptom directed

Drug Interactions

Decreased effect: Tetracyclines may decrease penicillin effectiveness; decreased oral contraceptive effect is possible

Increased effect:

Probenecid may increase penicillin levels

Aminoglycosides may result in synergistic efficacy; heparin and parenteral penicillins may result in increased bleeding

Stability Store in refrigerator

Mechanism of Action Inhibits bacterial cell wall synthesis by binding to one or more of the penicillin binding proteins (PBPs); which in turn inhibits the final transpeptidation step of peptidoglycan synthesis in bacterial cell walls, thus inhibiting cell wall biosynthesis. Bacteria eventually lyse due to ongoing activity of cell wall autolytic enzymes (autolysins and murein hydrolases) while cell wall assembly is arrested.

Pharmacodynamics/Kinetics

Absorption: I.M.: Slowly absorbed

Distribution: Penetration across the blood-brain barrier is poor, despite inflamed meninges; appears in breast milk

Protein binding: 65%

Metabolism: ~30% of a dose is inactivated in the liver

Time to peak serum concentration: Within 1-4 hours; can persist within the therapeutic range for 15-24 hours

Elimination: Renal clearance is delayed in neonates, young infants, and patients with impaired renal function; 60% to 90% of the drug is excreted unchanged via renal tubular excretion

Usual Dosage I.M.:

Children: 25,000-50,000 units/kg/day in divided doses 1-2 times/day; not to exceed 4.8 million units/24 hours

Congenital syphilis: 50,000 units/kg/day for 10-14 days

Adults: 0.6-4.8 million units/day in divided doses every 12-24 hours

(Continued)

Penicillin G Procaine *(Continued)*

Endocarditis caused by susceptible viridans *Streptococcus* (when used in conjunction with an aminoglycoside): 1.2 million units every 6 hours for 2-4 weeks

Neurosyphilis: I.M.: 2-4 million units/day with 500 mg probenecid by mouth 4 times/day for 10-14 days; **penicillin G aqueous I.V. is the preferred agent**

Hemodialysis: Moderately dialyzable (20% to 50%)

Administration Procaine suspension for deep I.M. injection only; rotate the injection site; **do not administer I.V.**

Monitoring Parameters Periodic renal and hematologic function tests with prolonged therapy; fever, mental status, WBC count

Test Interactions Positive direct Coombs' test, false-positive urinary and/or serum proteins

Patient Information Notify physician if skin rash, itching, hives, or severe diarrhea occurs

Nursing Implications Renal and hematologic systems should be evaluated periodically during prolonged therapy; do not inject in gluteal muscle in children <2 years of age

Dosage Forms Injection, suspension: 300,000 units/mL (10 mL); 500,000 units/mL (1.2 mL); 600,000 units/mL (1 mL, 2 mL, 4 mL)

Selected Readings
Donowitz GR and Mandell GL, "Beta-Lactam Antibiotics," *N Engl J Med*, 1988, 318(7):419-26 and 318(8):490-500.
Wright AJ, "The Penicillins," *Mayo Clin Proc*, 1999, 74(3):290-307.

Penicillin G Procaine and Benzathine Combined *see* Penicillin G Benzathine and Procaine Combined *on page 858*

Penicillin G Sodium *see* Penicillin G, Parenteral, Aqueous *on page 860*

Penicillins, Extended Spectrum

Refer to
Mezlocillin *on page 820*
Piperacillin *on page 869*
Piperacillin and Tazobactam Sodium *on page 871*
Ticarcillin *on page 948*
Ticarcillin and Clavulanate Potassium *on page 950*

Drug of Choice or Alternative for
Disease/Syndrome(s)
Meningitis, Postsurgical *on page 36*
Meningitis, Post-traumatic *on page 37*
Otitis Externa, Severe (Malignant) *on page 40*
Pneumonia, Hospital-Acquired *on page 46*
Sepsis *on page 48*
Sinusitis, Hospital-Acquired *on page 49*

Organism(s)
Acinetobacter Species *on page 58*
Bordetella bronchiseptica *on page 80*
Burkholderia cepacia *on page 87*
Citrobacter Species *on page 102*
Enterobacter Species *on page 134*
Klebsiella Species *on page 183*
Proteus Species *on page 232*
Providencia Species *on page 234*
Pseudomonas aeruginosa *on page 235*
Serratia Species *on page 250*

Penicillins, Penicillinase-Resistant

Refer to
Cloxacillin *on page 689*
Dicloxacillin *on page 702*
Methicillin *on page 816*
Nafcillin *on page 826*
Oxacillin *on page 849*

Drug of Choice or Alternative for
Disease/Syndrome(s)
Catheter Infection, Intravascular *on page 21*
Endocarditis, Acute Native Valve *on page 26*

Organism(s)

Penicillin V Potassium (pen i SIL in vee poe TASS ee um)

Related Information
Antimicrobial Activity Against Selected Organisms *on page 983*

U.S. Brand Names Beepen-VK®; Betapen®-VK; Pen.Vee® K; Robicillin® VK; V-Cillin K®; Veetids®

Canadian Brand Names Apo®-Pen VK; Nadopen-V®; Novo-Pen-VK®; Nu-Pen-VK®; PVF® K

Synonyms Pen VK; Phenoxymethyl Penicillin

Generic Available Yes

Use Treatment of infections caused by susceptible organisms involving the respiratory tract, otitis media, sinusitis, skin, and urinary tract; prophylaxis in rheumatic fever

Drug of Choice or Alternative for
Disease/Syndrome(s)
Organism(s)

Pregnancy Risk Factor B

Contraindications Known hypersensitivity to penicillin or any component

Warnings/Precautions Use with caution in patients with severe renal impairment (modify dosage), history of seizures, or hypersensitivity to cephalosporins

Adverse Reactions
>10%: Gastrointestinal: Mild diarrhea, vomiting, nausea, oral candidiasis
<1%: Convulsions, fever, hemolytic anemia, positive Coombs' test, acute interstitial nephritis, hypersensitivity reactions, anaphylaxis

Overdosage/Toxicology
Symptoms of penicillin overdose include neuromuscular hypersensitivity (agitation, hallucinations, asterixis, encephalopathy, confusion, and seizures) and electrolyte imbalance with potassium or sodium salts, especially in renal failure
Hemodialysis may be helpful to aid in the removal of the drug from the blood, otherwise most treatment is supportive or symptom directed

Drug Interactions
Decreased effect: Tetracyclines may decrease penicillin effectiveness; decreased oral contraceptive effect is possible
Increased effect:
Probenecid may increase penicillin levels
Aminoglycosides may result in synergistic efficacy; heparin and parenteral penicillins may result in increased bleeding

Stability Refrigerate suspension after reconstitution; discard after 14 days

Mechanism of Action Inhibits bacterial cell wall synthesis by binding to one or more of the penicillin binding proteins (PBPs); which in turn inhibits the final transpeptidation step of peptidoglycan synthesis in bacterial cell walls, thus inhibiting cell wall biosynthesis. Bacteria eventually lyse due to ongoing activity of cell wall autolytic enzymes (autolysins and murein hydrolases) while cell wall assembly is arrested.

Pharmacodynamics/Kinetics
Absorption: Oral: 60% to 73% from GI tract
(Continued)

Penicillin V Potassium *(Continued)*

Distribution: Appears in breast milk

Plasma protein binding: 80%

Half-life: 0.5 hours; prolonged in patients with renal impairment

Time to peak serum concentration: Oral: Within 0.5-1 hour

Elimination: Penicillin V and its metabolites are excreted in urine mainly by tubular secretion

Usual Dosage Oral:

Systemic infections:

Children <12 years: 25-50 mg/kg/day in divided doses every 6-8 hours; maximum dose: 3 g/day

Children ≥12 years and Adults: 125-500 mg every 6-8 hours

Prophylaxis of pneumococcal infections:

Children <5 years: 125 mg twice daily

Children ≥5 years and Adults: 250 mg twice daily

Prophylaxis of recurrent rheumatic fever:

Children <5 years: 125 mg twice daily

Children ≥5 years and Adults: 250 mg twice daily

Dosing interval in renal impairment: Cl_{cr} <10 mL/minute: Administer 250 mg every 6 hours

Dietary Considerations Food: Decreases drug absorption rate; decreases drug serum concentration. Take on an empty stomach 1 hour before or 2 hours after meals.

Administration Administer on an empty stomach to increase oral absorption

Monitoring Parameters Periodic renal and hematologic function tests during prolonged therapy; monitor for signs of anaphylaxis during first dose

Test Interactions False-positive or -negative urinary glucose determination with Clinitest®, positive direct Coombs' test, false-positive urinary and/or serum proteins

Patient Information Take on an empty stomach 1 hour before or 2 hours after meals, take until gone, do not skip doses, report any rash or shortness of breath; shake liquid well before use

Additional Information 0.7 mEq of potassium per 250 mg penicillin V; 250 mg equals 400,000 units of penicillin

Dosage Forms 250 mg = 400,000 units

Powder for oral solution: 125 mg/5 mL (3 mL, 100 mL, 150 mL, 200 mL); 250 mg/5 mL (100 mL, 150 mL, 200 mL)

Tablet: 125 mg, 250 mg, 500 mg

Pentacarinat® Injection *see* Pentamidine *on this page*

Pentam-300® Injection *see* Pentamidine *on this page*

Pentamidine *(pen TAM i deen)*

U.S. Brand Names NebuPent™ Inhalation; Pentacarinat® Injection; Pentam-300® Injection

Synonyms Pentamidine Isethionate

Generic Available No

Use Treatment and prevention of pneumonia caused by *Pneumocystis carinii*; treatment of trypanosomiasis and visceral leishmaniasis

Drug of Choice or Alternative for

Organism(s)

Pneumocystis carinii on page 228

Pregnancy Risk Factor C

Contraindications Hypersensitivity to pentamidine isethionate or any component (inhalation and injection)

Warnings/Precautions Use with caution in patients with diabetes mellitus, renal or hepatic dysfunction; hypertension or hypotension; leukopenia, thrombocytopenia, asthma, hypo/hyperglycemia

Adverse Reactions Injection (I); Aerosol (A)

>10%:

Cardiovascular: Chest pain (A - 10% to 23%)

Central nervous system: Fatigue (A - 50% to 70%); dizziness (A - 31% to 47%)

Dermatologic: Rash (31% to 47%)

Endocrine & metabolic: Hyperkalemia

Gastrointestinal: Anorexia (A - 50% to 70%), nausea (A - 10% to 23%)

Local: Local reactions at injection site

Renal: Increased creatinine (I - 23%)

Respiratory: Wheezing (A - 10% to 23%), dyspnea (A - 50% to 70%), coughing (A - 31% to 47%), pharyngitis (10% to 23%)

1% to 10%:

Cardiovascular: Hypotension (I - 4%)

Central nervous system: Confusion/hallucinations (1% to 2%), headache (A - 1% to 5%)

Dermatologic: Rash (I - 3.3%)

Endocrine & metabolic: Hypoglycemia <25 mg/dL (I - 2.4%)

Gastrointestinal: Nausea/anorexia (I - 6%), diarrhea (A - 1% to 5%), vomiting

Hematologic: Severe leukopenia (I - 2.8%), thrombocytopenia <20,000/mm^3 (I - 1.7%), anemia (A - 1% to 5%)

Hepatic: Increased LFTs (I - 8.7%)

<1%: Hypotension <60 mm Hg systolic (I - 0.9%), tachycardia, arrhythmias, dizziness (I), fever, fatigue (I), hyperglycemia or hypoglycemia, hypocalcemia, pancreatitis, megaloblastic anemia, granulocytopenia, leukopenia, renal insufficiency, extrapulmonary pneumocystosis, irritation of the airway, pneumothorax, Jarisch-Herxheimer-like reaction, mild renal or hepatic injury

Overdosage/Toxicology

Symptoms of overdose include hypotension, hypoglycemia, cardiac arrhythmias

Treatment is supportive

Stability Do not refrigerate due to the possibility of crystallization; do not use NS as a diluent, NS is **incompatible** with pentamidine; reconstituted solutions (60-100 mg/mL) are stable for 48 hours at room temperature and do not require light protection; diluted solutions (1-2.5 mg/mL) in D_5W are stable for at least 24 hours at room temperature

Mechanism of Action Interferes with RNA/DNA, phospholipids and protein synthesis, through inhibition of oxidative phosphorylation and/or interference with incorporation of nucleotides and nucleic acids into RNA and DNA, in protozoa

Pharmacodynamics/Kinetics

Absorption: I.M.: Well absorbed

Distribution: Systemic accumulation of pentamidine does not appear to occur following inhalation therapy

Half-life, terminal: 6.4-9.4 hours; may be prolonged in patients with severe renal impairment

Elimination: 33% to 66% excreted in urine as unchanged drug

Usual Dosage

Children:

Treatment: I.M., I.V. (I.V. preferred): 4 mg/kg/day once daily for 10-14 days

Prevention:

I.M., I.V.: 4 mg/kg monthly or every 2 weeks

Inhalation (aerosolized pentamidine in children ≥5 years): 300 mg/dose given every 3-4 weeks via Respirgard® II inhaler (8 mg/kg dose has also been used in children <5 years)

Treatment of trypanosomiasis: I.V.: 4 mg/kg/day once daily for 10 days

Adults:

Treatment: I.M., I.V. (I.V. preferred): 4 mg/kg/day once daily for 14-21 days

Prevention: Inhalation: 300 mg every 4 weeks via Respirgard® II nebulizer

Dialysis: Not removed by hemo or peritoneal dialysis or continuous arteriovenous or venovenous hemofiltration (CAVH/CAVHD); supplemental dosage is not necessary

Dosing adjustment in renal impairment: Adults: I.V.:

Cl_{cr} 10-50 mL/minute: Administer 4 mg/kg every 24-36 hours

Cl_{cr} <10 mL/minute: Administer 4 mg/kg every 48 hours

Administration Infuse I.V. slowly over a period of at least 60 minutes or administer deep I.M.; patients receiving I.V. or I.M. pentamidine should be lying down and blood pressure should be monitored closely during administration of drug and several times thereafter until it is stable

Monitoring Parameters Liver function tests, renal function tests, blood glucose, serum potassium and calcium, EKG, blood pressure

(Continued)

Pentamidine *(Continued)*

Patient Information PCP pneumonia may still occur despite pentamidine use; notify physician of fever, shortness of breath, or coughing up blood; maintain adequate fluid intake

Nursing Implications Virtually indetectable amounts are transferred to health-care personnel during aerosol administration; **do not use NS as a diluent**

Dosage Forms

Inhalation, as isethionate: 300 mg

Powder for injection, as isethionate, lyophilized: 300 mg

Selected Readings

Goa KL and Campoli-Richards DM, "Pentamidine Isethionate. A Review of Its Antiprotozoal Activity, Pharmacokinetic Properties and Therapeutic Use in *Pneumocystis carinii* Pneumonia," *Drugs*, 1987, 33(3):242-58.

Masur H, "Prevention and Treatment of *Pneumocystis* Pneumonia," *N Engl J Med*, 1992, 327(26):1853-60.

Monk JP and Benfield P, "Inhaled Pentamidine. An Overview of Its Pharmacological Properties and a Review of Its Therapeutic Use in *Pneumocystis carinii* Pneumonia," *Drugs*, 1990, 39(5):741-56.

Sattler FR, Cowan R, Nielsen DM, et al, " Trimethoprim-Sulfamethoxazole Compared With Pentamidine for Treatment of *Pneumocystis carinii* Pneumonia in the Acquired Immunodeficiency Syndrome," *Ann Intern Med*, 1988, 109(4):280-7.

Pentamidine Isethionate *see* Pentamidine *on page 866*

Pentamycetin® *see* Chloramphenicol *on page 667*

Pen.Vee® K *see* Penicillin V Potassium *on page 865*

Pen VK *see* Penicillin V Potassium *on page 865*

Pepto-Bismol® [OTC] *see* Bismuth Subsalicylate *on page 622*

Peridex® Oral Rinse *see* Chlorhexidine Gluconate *on page 670*

PerioGard® *see* Chlorhexidine Gluconate *on page 670*

Periostat™ *see* Doxycycline *on page 713*

Permapen® *see* Penicillin G Benzathine, Parenteral *on page 859*

Permethrin *(per METH rin)*

U.S. Brand Names Elimite™ Cream; Nix™ Creme Rinse

Generic Available No

Use Single application treatment of infestation with *Pediculus humanus capitis* (head louse) and its nits or *Sarcoptes scabiei* (scabies); indicated for prophylactic use during epidemics of lice

Drug of Choice or Alternative for

Organism(s)

Lice *on page 188*

Sarcoptes scabiei on page 247

Pregnancy Risk Factor B

Contraindications Known hypersensitivity to pyrethyroid, pyrethrin, or chrysanthemums

Warnings/Precautions Treatment may temporarily exacerbate the symptoms of itching, redness, swelling; for external use only; use during pregnancy only if clearly needed

Adverse Reactions 1% to 10%:

Dermatologic: Pruritus, erythema, rash of the scalp

Local: Burning, stinging, tingling, numbness or scalp discomfort, edema

Mechanism of Action Inhibits sodium ion influx through nerve cell membrane channels in parasites resulting in delayed repolarization and thus paralysis and death of the pest

Pharmacodynamics/Kinetics

Absorption: Topical: Minimal (<2%)

Metabolism: In the liver by ester hydrolysis to inactive metabolites

Elimination: In urine

Usual Dosage Children >2 months and Adults: Topical:

Head lice: After hair has been washed with shampoo, rinsed with water, and towel dried, apply a sufficient volume of topical liquid to saturate the hair and scalp. Leave on hair for 10 minutes before rinsing off with water; remove remaining nits; may repeat in 1 week if lice or nits still present.

Scabies: Apply cream from head to toe; leave on for 8-14 hours before washing off with water; for infants, also apply on the hairline, neck, scalp, temple, and forehead; may reapply in 1 week if live mites appear

Permethrin 5% cream was shown to be safe and effective when applied to an infant <1 month of age with neonatal scabies; time of application was limited to 6 hours before rinsing with soap and water

Patient Information Avoid contact with eyes and mucous membranes during application; shake well before using; notify physician if irritation persists; clothing and bedding should be washed in hot water or dry cleaned to kill the scabies mite

Dosage Forms
Cream: 5% (60 g)
Liquid, topical: 1% (60 mL)

Selected Readings
"Drugs for Parasitic Infections," *Med Lett Drugs Ther*, 1998, 40(1017):1-12.
Liu LX and Weller PF, "Antiparasitic Drugs," *N Engl J Med*, 1996, 334(18):1178-84.

PFA *see Foscarnet on page 739*

Pfizerpen® *see Penicillin G, Parenteral, Aqueous on page 860*

Phenoxymethyl Penicillin *see Penicillin V Potassium on page 865*

Phosphonoformate *see Foscarnet on page 739*

Phosphonoformic Acid *see Foscarnet on page 739*

p-Hydroxyampicillin *see Amoxicillin on page 592*

Pima® *see Potassium Iodide on page 879*

Pimaricin *see Natamycin on page 831*

Pin-Rid® [OTC] *see Pyrantel Pamoate on page 883*

Pin-X® [OTC] *see Pyrantel Pamoate on page 883*

Piperacillin (pi PER a sil in)

Related Information
Antimicrobial Activity Against Selected Organisms *on page 983*

U.S. Brand Names Pipracil®

Synonyms Piperacillin Sodium

Generic Available No

Use Treatment of susceptible infections such as septicemia, acute and chronic respiratory tract infections, skin and soft tissue infections, and urinary tract infections due to susceptible strains of *Pseudomonas*, *Proteus*, and *Escherichia coli* and *Enterobacter*. Also active against some streptococci and some anaerobic bacteria.

Drug of Choice or Alternative for
Disease/Syndrome(s)
Cholangitis, Acute *on page 21*
Fever, Neutropenic *on page 30*
Organism(s)
Alcaligenes Species *on page 65*

Pregnancy Risk Factor B

Contraindications Hypersensitivity to piperacillin or any component or penicillins

Warnings/Precautions Dosage modification required in patients with impaired renal function; history of seizure activity; use with caution in patients with a history of beta-lactam allergy

Adverse Reactions Percentage unknown: Convulsions, confusion, drowsiness, fever, rash, electrolyte imbalance, hemolytic anemia, positive Coombs' test, abnormal platelet aggregation and prolonged PT (high doses), thrombophlebitis, myoclonus, acute interstitial nephritis, hypersensitivity reactions, anaphylaxis, Jarisch-Herxheimer reaction

Overdosage/Toxicology
Symptoms of penicillin overdose include neuromuscular hypersensitivity (agitation, hallucinations, asterixis, encephalopathy, confusion, and seizures) and electrolyte imbalance with potassium or sodium salts, especially in renal failure
Hemodialysis may be helpful to aid in the removal of the drug from the blood, otherwise most treatment is supportive or symptom directed

Drug Interactions
Decreased effect: Tetracyclines may decrease penicillin effectiveness; aminoglycosides → physical inactivation of aminoglycosides in the presence of high concentrations of piperacillin and potential toxicity in patients with mild-
(Continued)

Piperacillin *(Continued)*

moderate renal dysfunction; decreased efficacy of oral contraceptives is possible

Increased effect:

Probenecid may increase penicillin levels

Neuromuscular blockers may increase duration of blockade

Aminoglycosides → synergistic efficacy

Heparin with high-dose parenteral penicillins may result in increased risk of bleeding

Stability Reconstituted solution is stable (I.V. infusion) in NS or D_5W for 24 hours at room temperature, 7 days when refrigerated or 4 weeks when frozen; after freezing, thawed solution is stable for 24 hours at room temperature or 48 hours when refrigerated; 40 g bulk vial should **not** be frozen after reconstitution; **incompatible** with aminoglycosides

Mechanism of Action Inhibits bacterial cell wall synthesis by binding to one or more of the penicillin binding proteins (PBPs); which in turn inhibits the final transpeptidation step of peptidoglycan synthesis in bacterial cell walls, thus inhibiting cell wall biosynthesis. Bacteria eventually lyse due to ongoing activity of cell wall autolytic enzymes (autolysins and murein hydrolases) while cell wall assembly is arrested.

Pharmacodynamics/Kinetics

Absorption: I.M.: 70% to 80%

Distribution: Crosses the placenta; distributes into milk at low concentrations

Protein binding: 22%

Half-life: Dose-dependent; prolonged with moderately severe renal or hepatic impairment:

Neonates:

1-5 days: 3.6 hours

>6 days: 2.1-2.7 hours

Children:

1-6 months: 0.79 hour

6 months to 12 years: 0.39-0.5 hour

Adults: 36-80 minutes

Time to peak serum concentration: I.M.: Within 30-50 minutes

Elimination: Principally in urine and partially in feces (via bile)

Usual Dosage

Neonates: 100 mg/kg every 12 hours

Infants and Children: I.M., I.V.: 200-300 mg/kg/day in divided doses every 4-6 hours

Higher doses have been used in cystic fibrosis: 350-500 mg/kg/day in divided doses every 4-6 hours

Adults: I.M., I.V.:

Moderate infections (urinary tract infections): 2-3 g/dose every 6-12 hours; maximum: 2 g I.M./site

Serious infections: 3-4 g/dose every 4-6 hours; maximum: 24 g/24 hours

Uncomplicated gonorrhea: 2 g I.M. in a single dose accompanied by 1 g probenecid 30 minutes prior to injection

Dosing adjustment in renal impairment: Adults: I.V.:

Cl_{cr} 20-40 mL/minute: Administer 3-4 g every 8 hours

Cl_{cr} <20 mL/minute: Administer 3-4 g every 12 hours

Moderately dialyzable (20% to 50%)

Continuous arteriovenous or venovenous hemodiafiltration (CAVH) effects: Dose as for Cl_{cr} 10-50 mL/minute

Administration Administer at least 1 hour apart from aminoglycosides

Monitoring Parameters Observe for signs and symptoms for anaphylaxis during first dose

Test Interactions May interfere with urinary glucose tests using cupric sulfate (Benedict's solution, Clinitest®), may inactivate aminoglycosides *in vitro*, false-positive urinary and serum proteins, positive direct Coombs' test

Additional Information Sodium content of 1 g: 1.85 mEq

Dosage Forms Powder for injection, as sodium: 2 g, 3 g, 4 g, 40 g

Selected Readings

Donowitz GR and Mandell GL, "Beta-Lactam Antibiotics," *N Engl J Med*, 1988, 318(7):419-26 and 318(8):490-500.

Tan JS and File TM Jr, "Antipseudomonal Penicillins," *Med Clin North Am*, 1995, 79(4):679-93.

Wright AJ, "The Penicillins," *Mayo Clin Proc*, 1999, 74(3):290-307.

Piperacillin and Tazobactam Sodium
(pi PER a sil in & ta zoe BAK tam SOW dee um)

Related Information
Antimicrobial Activity Against Selected Organisms *on page 983*

U.S. Brand Names Zosyn™

Use Treatment of infections of lower respiratory tract, urinary tract, skin and skin structures, gynecologic, bone and joint infections, and septicemia caused by susceptible organisms. Tazobactam expands activity of piperacillin to include beta-lactamase producing strains of *S. aureus*, *H. influenzae*, *Bacteroides*, and other gram-negative bacteria.

Drug of Choice or Alternative for
Disease/Syndrome(s)
Cholangitis, Acute *on page 21*
Osteomyelitis, Diabetic Foot *on page 38*
Peritonitis, Spontaneous Bacterial *on page 43*
Pneumonia, Community-Acquired *on page 45*

Organism(s)
Bacteroides Species *on page 75*

Pregnancy Risk Factor B

Pregnancy/Breast-Feeding Implications Breast-feeding/lactation: Use by the breast-feeding mother may result in diarrhea, candidiasis, or allergic response in the infant

Contraindications Hypersensitivity to penicillins, beta-lactamase inhibitors, or any component

Warnings/Precautions Due to sodium load and to the adverse effects of high serum concentrations of penicillins, dosage modification is required in patients with impaired or underdeveloped renal function; use with caution in patients with seizures or in patients with history of beta-lactam allergy; safety and efficacy have not been established in children <12 years of age

Adverse Reactions
>10%: Gastrointestinal: Diarrhea (11.3%)

1% to 10%:
Cardiovascular: Hypertension (1.6%)
Central nervous system: Insomnia (6.7%), headache (7% to 8%), agitation (2%), fever (2.4%), dizziness (1.4%)
Dermatologic: Rash (4%), pruritus (3%)
Gastrointestinal: Constipation (7% to 8%), nausea (6.9%), vomiting/dyspepsia (3.3%)
Respiratory: Rhinitis/dyspnea (~1%)
Miscellaneous: Serum sickness-like reaction

<1%: Hypotension, edema, confusion, pseudomembranous colitis, bronchospasm

Several laboratory abnormalities have rarely been associated with piperacillin/tazobactam including reversible eosinophilia, and neutropenia (associated most often with prolonged therapy), positive direct Coombs' test, prolonged PT and PTT, transient elevations of LFTs, increased creatinine

Overdosage/Toxicology
Symptoms of penicillin overdose include neuromuscular hypersensitivity (agitation, hallucinations, asterixis, encephalopathy, confusion, and seizures) and electrolyte imbalance with potassium or sodium salts, especially in renal dysfunction

Hemodialysis may be helpful to aid in the removal of the drug from the blood, otherwise most treatment is supportive or symptom directed

Drug Interactions
Decreased effect: Tetracyclines may decrease penicillin effectiveness; aminoglycosides → physical inactivation of aminoglycosides in the presence of high concentrations of piperacillin and potential toxicity in patients with mild-moderate renal dysfunction; decreased efficacy of oral contraceptives is possible

Increased effect:
Probenecid may increase penicillin levels
Neuromuscular blockers may increase duration of blockade
Aminoglycosides → synergistic efficacy

(Continued)

Piperacillin and Tazobactam Sodium *(Continued)*

Heparin with high-dose parenteral penicillins may result in increased risk of bleeding

Stability Store at controlled room temperature; after reconstitution, solution is stable in NS or D_5W for 24 hours at room temperature and 7 days when refrigerated; use single dose vials immediately after reconstitution (discard unused portions after 24 hours at room temperature and 48 hours if refrigerated)

Mechanism of Action Inhibits bacterial cell wall synthesis by binding to one or more of the penicillin binding proteins (PBPs); which in turn inhibits the final transpeptidation step of peptidoglycan synthesis in bacterial cell walls, thus inhibiting cell wall biosynthesis. Bacteria eventually lyse due to ongoing activity of cell wall autolytic enzymes (autolysins and murein hydrolases) while cell wall assembly is arrested. Tazobactam inhibits many beta-lactamases, including staphylococcal penicillinase and Richmond and Sykes types II, III, IV, and V, including extended spectrum enzymes; it has only limited activity against class I beta-lactamases other than class Ic types.

Pharmacodynamics/Kinetics Both AUC and peak concentrations are dose proportional

Distribution: Distributes well into lungs, intestinal mucosa, skin, muscle, uterus, ovary, prostate, gallbladder, and bile; penetration into CSF is low in subject with noninflamed meninges

Metabolism:
  Piperacillin: 6% to 9%
  Tazobactam: ~26%

Protein binding:
  Piperacillin: ~26% to 33%
  Tazobactam: 31% to 32%

Half-life:
  Piperacillin: 1 hour
  Metabolite: 1-1.5 hours
  Tazobactam: 0.7-0.9 hour

Elimination: Both piperacillin and tazobactam are directly proportional to renal function

  Piperacillin: 50% to 70% eliminated unchanged in urine, 10% to 20% excreted in bile

  Tazobactam: Found in urine at 24 hours, with 26% as the inactive metabolite

Hemodialysis removes 30% to 40% of piperacillin and tazobactam; peritoneal dialysis removes 11% to 21% of tazobactam and 6% of piperacillin; hepatic impairment does not affect the kinetics of piperacillin or tazobactam significantly

Usual Dosage

Children <12 years: Not recommended due to lack of data

Children >12 years and Adults:

Severe infections: I.V.: Piperacillin/tazobactam 4/0.5 g every 8 hours or 3/0.375 g every 6 hours

Moderate infections: I.M.: Piperacillin/tazobactam 2/0.25 g every 6-8 hours; treatment should be continued for ≥7-10 days depending on severity of disease (Note: I.M. route not FDA-approved)

Dosing interval in renal impairment:
  Cl_{cr} 20-40 mL/minute: Administer 2/0.25 g every 6 hours
  Cl_{cr} <20 mL/minute: Administer 2/0.25 g every 8 hours

Hemodialysis: Administer 2/0.25 g every 8 hours with an additional dose of 0.75 g after each dialysis

Continuous arteriovenous or venovenous hemodiafiltration (CAVH) effects: Dose as for Cl_{cr} 10-50 mL/minute

Administration Administer by I.V. infusion over 30 minutes; reconstitute with 5 mL of diluent per 1 g of piperacillin and then further dilute; compatible diluents include NS, SW, dextran 6%, D_5W, D_5W with potassium chloride 40 mEq, bacteriostatic saline and water; not compatible with lactated Ringer's solution

Monitoring Parameters LFTs, creatinine, BUN, CBC with differential, serum electrolytes, urinalysis, PT, PTT; monitor for signs of anaphylaxis during first dose

Test Interactions Positive direct Coombs' test, ALT, AST, bilirubin, and LDH

Nursing Implications Discontinue primary infusion, if possible, during infusion and administer aminoglycosides separately from Zosyn™

Additional Information Sodium content of 1 g injection: 54 mg (2.35 mEq)

Dosage Forms Injection: Piperacillin sodium 2 g and tazobactam sodium 0.25 g; piperacillin sodium 3 g and tazobactam sodium 0.375 g; piperacillin sodium 4 g and tazobactam sodium 0.5 g (vials at an 8:1 ratio of piperacillin sodium/tazobactam sodium)

Selected Readings
"Piperacillin/Tazobactam," *Med Lett Drugs Ther*, 1994, 36(914):7-9.
Sanders WE Jr and Sanders CC, "Piperacillin/Tazobactam: A Critical Review of the Evolving Clinical Literature," *Clin Infect Dis*, 1996, 22(1):107-23.
Schoonover LL, Occhipinti DJ, Rodvold KA, et al, "Piperacillin/Tazobactam: A New Beta-Lactam/Beta-Lactamase Inhibitor Combination," *Ann Pharmacother*, 1995, 29(5):501-14.

Piperacillin Sodium *see Piperacillin on page 869*

Piperazine (PI per a zeen)

U.S. Brand Names Vermizine®

Synonyms Piperazine Citrate

Generic Available Yes

Use Treatment of pinworm and roundworm infections (used as an alternative to first-line agents, mebendazole, or pyrantel pamoate)

Pregnancy Risk Factor B

Contraindications Seizure disorders, liver or kidney impairment, hypersensitivity to piperazine or any component

Warnings/Precautions Use with caution in patients with anemia or malnutrition; avoid prolonged use especially in children

Adverse Reactions <1%: Dizziness, vertigo, weakness, seizures, EEG changes, headache, nausea, vomiting, diarrhea, hemolytic anemia, visual impairment, hypersensitivity reactions, bronchospasms

Drug Interactions Pyrantel pamoate (antagonistic mode of action)

Mechanism of Action Causes muscle paralysis of the roundworm by blocking the effects of acetylcholine at the neuromuscular junction

Pharmacodynamics/Kinetics
Absorption: Well absorbed from GI tract
Time to peak serum concentration: 1 hour
Elimination: Excreted in urine as metabolites and unchanged drug

Usual Dosage Oral:
Pinworms: Children and Adults: 65 mg/kg/day (not to exceed 2.5 g/day) as a single daily dose for 7 days; in severe infections, repeat course after a 1-week interval

Roundworms:
Children: 75 mg/kg/day as a single daily dose for 2 days; maximum: 3.5 g/day
Adults: 3.5 g/day for 2 days (in severe infections, repeat course, after a 1-week interval)

Monitoring Parameters Stool exam for worms and ova

Patient Information Take on empty stomach; if severe or persistent headache, loss of balance or coordination, dizziness, vomiting, diarrhea, or rash occurs, contact physician. If used for pinworm infections, all members of the family should be treated.

Dosage Forms
Syrup: 500 mg/5 mL (473 mL, 4000 mL)
Tablet: 250 mg

Selected Readings
"Drugs for Parasitic Infections," *Med Lett Drugs Ther*, 1998, 40(1017):1-12.

Piperazine Citrate *see Piperazine on this page*

Pipracil® *see Piperacillin on page 869*

Pitrex® *see Tolnaftate on page 956*

Plague Vaccine (plaig vak SEEN)

Generic Available No

Use Selected travelers to countries reporting cases for whom avoidance of rodents and fleas is impossible; all laboratory and field personnel working with *Yersinia pestis* organisms possibly resistant to antimicrobials; those engaged in *Yersinia pestis* aerosol experiments or in field operations in areas with enzootic plague where regular exposure to potentially infected wild rodents, rabbits, or their fleas cannot be prevented. Prophylactic antibiotics may be indicated
(Continued)

Plague Vaccine (Continued)

following definite exposure, whether or not the exposed persons have been vaccinated.

Pregnancy Risk Factor C

Contraindications Persons with known hypersensitivity to any of the vaccine constituents (see manufacturer's label); patients who have had severe local or systemic reactions to a previous dose; defer immunization in patients with a febrile illness until resolved

Warnings/Precautions Pregnancy, unless there is substantial and unavoidable risk of exposure; the expected immune response may not be obtained if plague vaccine is administered to immunosuppressed persons or patients receiving immunosuppressive therapy; be prepared with epinephrine injection (1:1000) in cases of anaphylaxis

Adverse Reactions All serious adverse reactions must be reported to the U.S. Department of Health and Human Services (DHHS) Vaccine Adverse Event Reporting System (VAERS) 1-800-822-7967.

>10%:
Dermatologic: Tenderness (20% to 80%)
1% to 10%:
Central nervous system: Malaise (10%), fever, headache (7% to 20%)
Dermatologic: Local erythema (4.5%)
Gastrointestinal: Nausea (3% to 13%),
<1%: Tachycardia, vomiting, sterile abscess

Drug Interactions Decreased effect with immunoglobulin, other live vaccine used within 1 month; accentuated side effects may occur if given on the same occasion as cholera vaccine or AKD or H-P typhoid vaccine

Mechanism of Action Promotes active immunity to plague in high-risk individuals.

Usual Dosage Three I.M. doses: First dose 1 mL, second dose (0.2 mL) 1 month later, third dose (0.2 mL) 5 months after the second dose; booster doses (0.2 mL) at 1- to 2-year intervals if exposure continues

Administration I.M. into deltoid muscle

Test Interactions Temporary suppression of tuberculosis skin test

Additional Information Federal law requires that the date of administration, the vaccine manufacturer, lot number of vaccine, and the administering person's name, title and address be entered into the patient's permanent medical record

Dosage Forms Injection: 2 mL, 20 mL

Plaquenil® see Hydroxychloroquine on page 765

PMS-Amantadine see Amantadine on page 586

PMS-Erythromycin see Erythromycin on page 722

PMS-Isoniazid see Isoniazid on page 782

PMS-Lindane see Lindane on page 797

PMS-Nystatin see Nystatin on page 845

PMS-Pyrazinamide see Pyrazinamide on page 884

Pneumococcal Polysaccharide Vaccine see Pneumococcal Polysaccharide Vaccine, Polyvalent on this page

Pneumococcal Polysaccharide Vaccine, Polyvalent

(noo moe KOK al pol i SAK a ride vak SEEN, pol i VAY lent)

Related Information

Immunization Guidelines on page 1041

U.S. Brand Names Pneumovax® 23; Pnu-Imune® 23

Synonyms Pneumococcal Polysaccharide Vaccine

Generic Available No

Use Children >2 years of age and adults who are at increased risk of pneumococcal disease and its complications because of underlying health conditions; older adults, including all those ≥65 years of age

Pregnancy Risk Factor C

Pregnancy/Breast-Feeding Implications The safety of vaccine in pregnant women has not been evaluated; it should not be given during pregnancy unless the risk of infection is high

Contraindications Active infections, Hodgkin's disease patients, <5 years of age, pregnancy, hypersensitivity to pneumococcal vaccine or any component;

<10 days prior to or during treatment with immunosuppressive drugs or radiation; (children <5 years of age do not respond satisfactorily to the capsular types of 23 capsular pneumococcal vaccine)

Warnings/Precautions Epinephrine injection (1:1000) must be immediately available in the case of anaphylaxis; use caution in individuals who have had episodes of pneumococcal infection within the preceding 3 years (pre-existing pneumococcal antibodies may result in increased reactions to vaccine); may cause relapse in patients with stable idiopathic thrombocytopenia purpura

Adverse Reactions All serious adverse reactions must be reported to the U.S. Department of Health and Human Services (DHHS) Vaccine Adverse Event Reporting System (VAERS) 1-800-822-7967.

>10%: Local: Induration and soreness at the injection site (~72%) (2-3 days)
<1%: Guillain-Barré syndrome, low-grade fever, erythema, rash, paresthesias, myalgia, arthralgia, anaphylaxis

Drug Interactions Decreased effect with immunosuppressive agents, immunoglobulin, other live vaccines within 1 month

Stability Refrigerate

Mechanism of Action Although there are more than 80 known pneumococcal capsular types, pneumococcal disease is mainly caused by only a few types of pneumococci. Pneumococcal vaccine contains capsular polysaccharides of 23 pneumococcal types which represent at least 98% of pneumococcal disease isolates in the United States and Europe. The pneumococcal vaccine with 23 pneumococcal capsular polysaccharide types became available in 1983. The 23 capsular pneumococcal vaccine contains purified capsular polysaccharides of pneumococcal types 1, 2, 3, 4, 5, 8, 9, 12, 14, 17, 19, 20, 22, 23, 26, 34, 43, 51, 56, 57, 67, 70 (American Classification). These are the main pneumococcal types associated with serious infections in the United States.

Usual Dosage Children >2 years and Adults: I.M., S.C.: 0.5 mL
Revaccination should be considered:
1. If ≥6 years since initial vaccination has elapsed, or
2. In patients who received 14-valent pneumococcal vaccine and are at highest risk (asplenic) for fatal infection or
3. At ≥6 years in patients with nephrotic syndrome, renal failure, or transplant recipients, or
4. 3-5 years in children with nephrotic syndrome, asplenia, or sickle cell disease

Administration Do not inject I.V., avoid intradermal, administer S.C. or I.M. (deltoid muscle or lateral midthigh)

Additional Information Federal law requires that the date of administration, the vaccine manufacturer, lot number of vaccine, and the administering person's name, title and address be entered into the patient's permanent medical record; inactivated bacteria vaccine

Dosage Forms Injection: 25 mcg each of 23 polysaccharide isolates/0.5 mL dose (0.5 mL, 1 mL, 5 mL)

Pneumovax® 23 *see* Pneumococcal Polysaccharide Vaccine, Polyvalent *on previous page*

PNU-100766 *see* Linezolid *on page 798*

Pnu-Imune® 23 *see* Pneumococcal Polysaccharide Vaccine, Polyvalent *on previous page*

Poliovirus Vaccine, Inactivated
(POE iee oh VYE rus vak SEEN, in ak ti VAY ted)
Related Information
Immunization Guidelines *on page 1041*
U.S. Brand Names IPOL™
Synonyms Enhanced-potency Inactivated Poliovirus Vaccine; IPV; Salk Vaccine
Generic Available No
Use Oral: Prevention of poliomyelitis for infants (6-12 weeks of age) and all unimmunized children and adolescents through 18 years of age for routine prophylaxis. Persons traveling to areas where wild poliovirus is epidemic or endemic, and certain health personnel.

Although a protective immune response to E-IPV cannot be assured in the immunocompromised individual, E-IPV is recommended because the vaccine is safe and some protection may result from its administration.
(Continued)

Poliovirus Vaccine, Inactivated *(Continued)*

Pregnancy Risk Factor C

Contraindications Hypersensitivity to any component including neomycin, streptomycin, or polymyxin B; defer vaccination for persons with acute febrile illness until recovery

Warnings/Precautions Although there is no convincing evidence documenting adverse effects of either OPV or E-IPV on the pregnant woman or developing fetus, it is prudent on theoretical grounds to avoid vaccinating pregnant women. However, if immediate protection against poliomyelitis is needed, OPV is recommended. OPV should not be given to immunocompromised individuals or to persons with known or possibly immunocompromised family members; E-IPV is recommended in such situations.

Adverse Reactions All serious adverse reactions must be reported to the U.S. Department of Health and Human Services (DHHS) Vaccine Adverse Event Reporting System (VAERS) 1-800-822-7967.

1% to 10%:
Central nervous system: Fever (>101.3°F)
Dermatologic: Rash
Local: Tenderness or pain at injection site
<1%: Fatigue, fussiness, sleepiness, crying, Guillain-Barré, reddening of skin, erythema, decreased appetite, weakness, dyspnea

Drug Interactions Decreased effect with immunosuppressive agents, immune globulin, other live vaccines within 1 month; may temporarily suppress tuberculin skin test sensitivity (4-6 weeks)

Mechanism of Action Immunization with poliovirus vaccine produces active immunity to the three types of polio virus.

Usual Dosage Subcutaneous: Adults: IPV is preferred for primary vaccination of adults, two doses S.C. 4-8 weeks apart, a third dose 6-12 months after the second. For adults with a completed primary series and for whom a booster is indicated, either OPV or E-IPV can be given. If immediate protection is needed, either OPV or E-IPV is recommended. Children at 6-12 weeks of age; second dose 6-8 weeks after first dose, and third dose 8-12 months after second dose
Booster: All children who have received primary immunization series, should receive a single follow-up dose and all children who have not should complete primary series
Children (older) and Adults (adolescents through 18 years of age): Two 0.5 mL doses 6-8 weeks apart and a third dose of 0.5 mL 6-12 months after second dose

Subcutaneous: **Enhanced-potency inactivated poliovirus vaccine (E-IPV) is preferred for primary vaccination of adults,** two doses S.C. 4-8 weeks apart, a third dose 6-12 months after the second. For adults with a completed primary series and for whom a booster is indicated, either OPV or E-IPV can be given. If immediate protection is needed, either OPV or E-IPV is recommended.

Nursing Implications Do not administer I.V.

Additional Information Federal law requires that the date of administration, the vaccine manufacturer, lot number of vaccine, and the administering person's name, title and address be entered into the patient's permanent medical record

Dosage Forms Injection, suspension (IPOL™): Three types of poliovirus (Types 1, 2 and 3) grown in monkey kidney cell cultures (0.5 mL)

Poliovirus Vaccine, Live, Trivalent, Oral

(POE lee oh VYE rus vak SEEN, live, try VAY lent, OR al)

Related Information

Immunization Guidelines *on page 1041*

U.S. Brand Names Orimune®

Synonyms OPV; Sabin Vaccine; TOPV

Generic Available No

Use Poliovirus immunization

Pregnancy Risk Factor C

Contraindications Persistent vomiting or diarrhea, patients allergic to sorbitol, streptomycin, or neomycin, known hypersensitivity to poliovirus vaccine

Warnings/Precautions The vaccine will not modify or prevent cases of existing or incubating poliomyelitis

Adverse Reactions All serious adverse reactions must be reported to the FDA.

Drug Interactions May temporarily suppress tuberculin skin test sensitivity (4-6 weeks), immunosuppressive agents, immune globulin

Stability Keep in freezer; vaccine must remain frozen to retain potency

Mechanism of Action Immunization with poliovirus vaccine produces active immunity to the three types of polio virus.

Usual Dosage Oral:

Infants: 0.5 mL dose at age 2 months, 4 months, and 18 months; optional dose may be given at 6 months in areas where poliomyelitis is endemic

Older Children, Adolescents, and Adults: Two 0.5 mL doses 8 weeks apart; third dose of 0.5 mL 6-12 months after second dose; a reinforcing dose of 0.5 mL should be given before entry to school, in children who received the third primary dose before their fourth birthday

Patient Information Because of the risk of vaccine-associated paralysis, unvaccinated family members and close personal contacts should be vaccinated prior to the child

Nursing Implications Reconstitute only with diluent provided; federal law requires that the date of administration, the vaccine manufacturer, lot number of vaccine, and the administering person's name, title and address be entered into the patient's permanent medical record

Dosage Forms Solution, oral: Mixture of type 1, 2, and 3 viruses in monkey kidney tissue (0.5 mL)

Polycillin® *see* Ampicillin *on page 604*

Polycillin-N® *see* Ampicillin *on page 604*

Polygam® *see* Immune Globulin, Intravenous *on page 771*

Polygam® S/D *see* Immune Globulin, Intravenous *on page 771*

Polymox® *see* Amoxicillin *on page 592*

Polymyxin B (pol i MIKS in bee)

Synonyms Polymyxin B Sulfate

Generic Available Yes

Use

Topical: Wound irrigation and bladder irrigation against *Pseudomonas aeruginosa*; used occasionally for gut decontamination

Parenteral use of polymyxin B has mainly been replaced by less toxic antibiotics; it is reserved for life-threatening infections caused by organisms resistant to the preferred drugs (eg, pseudomonal meningitis - intrathecal administration)

Drug of Choice or Alternative for

Disease/Syndrome(s)

Otitis Externa, Mild *on page 40*

Pregnancy Risk Factor B

Contraindications Concurrent use of neuromuscular blockers

Warnings/Precautions Use with caution in patients with impaired renal function, (modify dosage); polymyxin B-induced nephrotoxicity may be manifested by albuminuria, cellular casts, and azotemia. Discontinue therapy with decreasing urinary output and increasing BUN; neurotoxic reactions are usually associated with high serum levels, often in patients with renal dysfunction. Avoid concurrent or sequential use of other nephrotoxic and neurotoxic drugs (eg, aminoglycosides). The drug's neurotoxicity can result in respiratory paralysis from neuromuscular blockade, especially when the drug is given soon after anesthesia or muscle relaxants. Polymyxin B sulfate is most toxic when given parenterally; avoid parenteral use whenever possible.

Adverse Reactions <1%: Facial flushing, neurotoxicity (irritability, drowsiness, ataxia, perioral paresthesia, numbness of the extremities, and blurring of vision); drug fever, urticarial rash, hypocalcemia, hyponatremia, hypokalemia, hypochloremia, pain at injection site, neuromuscular blockade, weakness, nephrotoxicity, respiratory arrest, anaphylactoid reaction, meningeal irritation with intrathecal administration

Overdosage/Toxicology

Symptoms of overdose include respiratory paralysis, ototoxicity, nephrotoxicity
Supportive care is indicated as treatment; ventilatory support may be necessary

Drug Interactions Polymyxin may increase/prolong effect of neuromuscular blocking agents; aminoglycosides may increase polymyxin's risk of respiratory paralysis and renal dysfunction

(Continued)

Polymyxin B *(Continued)*

Stability Discard any unused solution after 72 hours. **Incompatible** with strong acids/alkalies, calcium, magnesium, cephalothin, cefazolin, chloramphenicol, heparin, penicillins.

Mechanism of Action Binds to phospholipids, alters permeability, and damages the bacterial cytoplasmic membrane permitting leakage of intracellular constituents

Pharmacodynamics/Kinetics

Absorption: Well absorbed from the peritoneum; minimal absorption from the GI tract (except in neonates) from mucous membranes or intact skin

Distribution: Minimal distribution into the CSF; crosses the placenta

Half-life: 4.5-6 hours, increased with reduced renal function

Time to peak serum concentration: I.M.: Within 2 hours

Elimination: Primarily as unchanged drug (>60%) in urine via glomerular filtration

Usual Dosage

Otic: 1-2 drops, 3-4 times/day; should be used sparingly to avoid accumulation of excess debris

Infants <2 years:
I.M.: Up to 40,000 units/kg/day divided every 6 hours (not routinely recommended due to pain at injection sites)
I.V.: Up to 40,000 units/kg/day by continuous I.V. infusion
Intrathecal: 20,000 units/day for 3-4 days, then 25,000 units every other day for at least 2 weeks after CSF cultures are negative and CSF (glucose) has returned to within normal limits

Children ≥2 years and Adults:
I.M.: 25,000-30,000 units/kg/day divided every 4-6 hours (not routinely recommended due to pain at injection sites)
I.V.: 15,000-25,000 units/kg/day divided every 12 hours or by continuous infusion
Intrathecal: 50,000 units/day for 3-4 days, then every other day for at least 2 weeks after CSF cultures are negative and CSF (glucose) has returned to within normal limits

Total daily dose should not exceed 2,000,000 units/day

Bladder irrigation: Continuous irrigant or rinse in the urinary bladder for up to 10 days using 20 mg (equal to 200,000 units) added to 1 L of normal saline; usually no more than 1 L of irrigant is used per day unless urine flow rate is high; administration rate is adjusted to patient's urine output

Topical irrigation or topical solution: 500,000 units/L of normal saline; topical irrigation should not exceed 2 million units/day in adults

Gut sterilization: Oral: 15,000-25,000 units/kg/day in divided doses every 6 hours

Clostridium difficile enteritis: Oral: 25,000 units every 6 hours for 10 days

Ophthalmic: A concentration of 0.1% to 0.25% is administered as 1-3 drops every hour, then increasing the interval as response indicates to 1-2 drops 4-6 times/day

Dosing adjustment/interval in renal impairment:

Cl_{cr} 20-50 mL/minute: Administer 75% to 100% of normal dose every 12 hours
Cl_{cr} 5-20 mL/minute: Administer 50% of normal dose every 12 hours
Cl_{cr} <5 mL/minute: Administer 15% of normal dose every 12 hours

Administration Dissolve 500,000 units in 300-500 mL D_5W for continuous I.V. drip; dissolve 500,000 units in 2 mL water for injection, saline, or 1% procaine solution for I.M. injection; dissolve 500,000 units in 10 mL physiologic solution for intrathecal administration

Monitoring Parameters Neurologic symptoms and signs of superinfection; renal function (decreasing urine output and increasing BUN may require discontinuance of therapy)

Reference Range Serum concentrations >5 µg/mL are toxic in adults

Patient Information Report any dizziness or sensations of ringing in the ear, loss of hearing, or any muscle weakness

Nursing Implications Parenteral use is indicated only in life-threatening infections caused by organisms not susceptible to other agents

Additional Information 1 mg = 10,000 units

Dosage Forms

Injection: 500,000 units (20 mL)

Solution, otic: 10,000 units of polymyxin B per mL in combination with hydrocortisone 0.5% solution (eg, Otobiotic®)

Suspension, otic: 10,000 units of polymixin B per mL in combination with hydrocortisone 1% and neomycin sulfate 0.5% (eg, PediOtic®)

Also available in a variety of other combination products for ophthalmic and otic use.

Polymyxin B and Hydrocortisone
(pol i MIKS in bee & hye droe KOR ti sone)
Related Information
Polymyxin B *on page 877*
U.S. Brand Names Otobiotic® Otic
Use Treatment of superficial bacterial infections of external ear canal
Usual Dosage Instill 4 drops 3-4 times/day
Dosage Forms Solution, otic: Polymyxin B sulfate 10,000 units and hydrocortisone 0.5% [5 mg/mL] per mL (10 mL, 15 mL)

Polymyxin B and Neomycin *see* Neomycin and Polymyxin B *on page 835*

Polymyxin B Sulfate *see* Polymyxin B *on page 877*

Polymyxin E *see* Colistin *on page 691*

Poly-Pred® Ophthalmic Suspension *see* Neomycin, Polymyxin B, and Prednisolone *on page 837*

Polysporin® Ophthalmic *see* Bacitracin and Polymyxin B *on page 619*

Polysporin® Topical *see* Bacitracin and Polymyxin B *on page 619*

Polytopic *see* Bacitracin and Polymyxin B *on page 619*

Polytrim® Ophthalmic *see* Trimethoprim and Polymyxin B *on page 958*

Postexposure Prophylaxis for Hepatitis B *see page 1054*

Potassium Iodide (poe TASS ee um EYE oh dide)
U.S. Brand Names Pima®; Potassium Iodide Enseals®; SSKI®; Thyro-Block®
Synonyms KI; Lugol's Solution; Strong Iodine Solution
Generic Available Yes
Use Used in the treatment of cutaneous sporotrichosis; facilitate bronchial drainage and cough; reduce thyroid vascularity prior to thyroidectomy and management of thyrotoxic crisis; block thyroidal uptake of radioactive isotopes of iodine in a radiation emergency
Drug of Choice or Alternative for
Organism(s)
Sporothrix schenckii *on page 253*
Pregnancy Risk Factor D
Contraindications Known hypersensitivity to iodine; hyperkalemia, pulmonary tuberculosis, pulmonary edema, bronchitis
Warnings/Precautions Prolonged use can lead to hypothyroidism; cystic fibrosis patients have an exaggerated response; can cause acne flare-ups, can cause dermatitis, some preparations may contain sodium bisulfite (allergy); use with caution in patients with a history of thyroid disease, patients with renal failure, or GI obstruction
Adverse Reactions 1% to 10%:
Central nervous system: Fever, headache
Dermatologic: Urticaria, acne, angioedema, cutaneous hemorrhage
Endocrine & metabolic: Goiter with hypothyroidism
Gastrointestinal: Metallic taste, GI upset, soreness of teeth and gums
Hematologic: Eosinophilia, hemorrhage (mucosal)
Neuromuscular & skeletal: Arthralgia
Respiratory: Rhinitis
Miscellaneous: Lymph node enlargement
Overdosage/Toxicology
Signs and symptoms: Angioedema, laryngeal edema in patients with hypersensitivity; muscle weakness, paralysis, peaked T waves, flattened P waves, prolongation of QRS complex, ventricular arrhythmias
Treatment: Removal of potassium can be accomplished by various means; removal through the GI tract with Kayexalate® administration; by way of the kidney through diuresis, mineralocorticoid administration or increased sodium intake; by hemodialysis or peritoneal dialysis; or by shifting potassium back into the cells by insulin and glucose infusion
(Continued)

Potassium Iodide *(Continued)*

Drug Interactions Increased effect/toxicity: Lithium → additive hypothyroid effect

Stability Store in tight, light-resistant containers at temperature <40°C; freezing should be avoided

Mechanism of Action Reduces viscosity of mucus by increasing respiratory tract secretions; inhibits secretion of thyroid hormone, fosters colloid accumulation in thyroid follicles

Pharmacodynamics/Kinetics

Onset of action: 24-48 hours

Peak effect: 10-15 days after continuous therapy

Elimination: In euthyroid patient, renal clearance rate is 2 times that of the thyroid

Usual Dosage Oral:

Sporotrichosis:

Oral: Initial:

Preschool: 50 mg/dose 3 times/day

Children: 250 mg/dose 3 times/day

Adults: 500 mg/dose 3 times/day

Oral increase 50 mg/dose daily

Maximum dose:

Preschool: 500 mg/dose 3 times/day

Children and Adults: 1-2 g/dose 3 times/day

Continue treatment for 4-6 weeks after lesions have completely healed

Adults: RDA: 130 mcg

Expectorant:

Children: 60-250 mg every 6-8 hours; maximum single dose: 500 mg

Adults: 300-650 mg 3-4 times/day

Preoperative thyroidectomy:

Children and Adults: 50-250 mg (1-5 drops SSKI®) 3 times/day **or** 0.1-0.3 mL (3-5 drops) of strong iodine (Lugol's solution) 3 times/day; give for 10 days before surgery

Thyrotoxic crisis:

Infants <1 year: 150-250 mg (3-5 drops SSKI®) 3 times/day

Children and Adults: 300-500 mg (6-10 drops SSKI®) 3 times/day or 1 mL strong iodine (Lugol's solution) 3 times/day

Graves' disease in neonates: 1 drop of strong iodine (Lugol's solution) 3 times/day

Monitoring Parameters Thyroid function tests

Patient Information Take after meals with food or milk or dilute with a large quantity of water, fruit juice, milk, or broth; discontinue use if stomach pain, skin rash, metallic taste, or nausea and vomiting occurs

Nursing Implications Must be diluted before administration of 240 mL of water, fruit juice, milk, or broth

Additional Information 10 drops of SSKI® = potassium iodide 500 mg

Dosage Forms

Solution, oral:

SSKI®: 1 g/mL (30 mL, 240 mL)

Lugol's Solution, strong iodine: Potassium iodide 100 mg and iodine 50 mg per mL (120 mL, 473 mL, 4000 mL)

Syrup: 325 mg/5 mL (473 mL, 4000 mL)

Tablet: 130 mg

Potassium Iodide Enseals® *see Potassium Iodide on page 879*

PPD *see Tuberculin Tests on page 962*

Praziquantel *(pray zi KWON tel)*

U.S. Brand Names Biltricide®

Generic Available No

Use All stages of schistosomiasis caused by all *Schistosoma* species pathogenic to humans; clonorchiasis and opisthorchiasis

Unlabeled use: Cysticercosis, flukes, and many intestinal tapeworms

Drug of Choice or Alternative for Organism(s)
Cestodes *on page 94*
Schistosoma mansoni on page 249

Pregnancy Risk Factor B

Contraindications Ocular cysticercosis, known hypersensitivity to praziquantel

Warnings/Precautions Use caution in patients with severe hepatic disease; patients with cerebral cysticercosis require hospitalization

Adverse Reactions
1% to 10%:
Central nervous system: Dizziness, drowsiness, headache, malaise
Gastrointestinal: Abdominal pain, loss of appetite, nausea, vomiting
Miscellaneous: Diaphoresis
<1%: CSF reaction syndrome in patients being treated for neurocysticercosis, fever, rash, urticaria, itching, diarrhea

Overdosage/Toxicology
Symptoms of overdose include dizziness, drowsiness, headache, liver function impairment
Treatment is supportive following GI decontamination; administer fast-acting laxative

Drug Interactions Hydantoins may decrease praziquantel levels causing treatment failures

Mechanism of Action Increases the cell permeability to calcium in schistosomes, causing strong contractions and paralysis of worm musculature leading to detachment of suckers from the blood vessel walls and to dislodgment

Pharmacodynamics/Kinetics
Absorption: Oral: ~80%; CSF concentration is 14% to 20% of plasma concentration
Distribution: CSF concentration is 14% to 20% of plasma concentration; appears in breast milk
Protein binding: ~80%
Metabolism: Extensive first-pass metabolism
Half-life:
Parent drug: 0.8-1.5 hours
Metabolites: 4.5 hours
Time to peak serum concentration: Within 1-3 hours
Elimination: Urinary excretion (99% as metabolites)

Usual Dosage Children >4 years and Adults: Oral:
Schistosomiasis: 20 mg/kg/dose 2-3 times/day for 1 day at 4- to 6-hour intervals
Flukes: 25 mg/kg/dose every 8 hours for 1-2 days
Cysticercosis: 50 mg/kg/day divided every 8 hours for 14 days
Tapeworms: 10-20 mg/kg as a single dose (25 mg/kg for *Hymenolepis nana*)
Clonorchiasis/opisthorchiasis: 3 doses of 25 mg/kg as a 1-day treatment

Patient Information Do not chew tablets due to bitter taste; take with food; caution should be used when performing tasks requiring mental alertness, may impair judgment and coordination

Nursing Implications Tablets can be halved or quartered

Dosage Forms Tablet, tri-scored: 600 mg

Selected Readings
de Silva N, Guyatt H, and Bundy D, "Anthelmintics. A Comparative Review of Their Clinical Pharmacology," *Drugs*, 1997, 53(5):769-88.
"Drugs for Parasitic Infections," *Med Lett Drugs Ther*, 1998, 40(1017):1-12.

Pred-G® Ophthalmic *see* Prednisolone and Gentamicin *on page 881*

Prednisolone and Gentamicin (pred NIS oh lone & jen ta MYE sin)

Related Information
Gentamicin *on page 747*

U.S. Brand Names Pred-G® Ophthalmic

Use Treatment of steroid responsive inflammatory conditions and superficial ocular infections due to strains of microorganisms susceptible to gentamicin such as *Staphylococcus*, *Streptococcus*, *E. coli*, *H. influenzae*, *Klebsiella*, *Neisseria*, *Pseudomonas*, *Proteus*, and *Serratia* species

Usual Dosage Children and Adults: Ophthalmic: 1 drop 2-4 times/day; during the initial 24-48 hours, the dosing frequency may be increased if necessary
(Continued)

Prednisolone and Gentamicin *(Continued)*

Dosage Forms

Ointment, ophthalmic: Prednisolone acetate 0.6% and gentamicin sulfate 0.3% (3.5 g)

Suspension, ophthalmic: Prednisolone acetate 1% and gentamicin sulfate 0.3% (2 mL, 5 mL, 10 mL)

Prescription Strength Desenex® [OTC] *see Miconazole on page 822*

Prevention of Malaria *see page 1057*

Preveon® *see Adefovir on page 584*

Priftin® *see Rifapentine on page 905*

Primaquine and Chloroquine *see Chloroquine and Primaquine on page 671*

Primaquine Phosphate (PRIM a kween FOS fate)

Synonyms Prymaccone

Generic Available No

Use Provides radical cure of *P. vivax* or *P. ovale* malaria after a clinical attack has been confirmed by blood smear or serologic titer and postexposure prophylaxis

Pregnancy Risk Factor C

Contraindications Acutely ill patients who have a tendency to develop granulocytopenia (rheumatoid arthritis, SLE); patients receiving other drugs capable of depressing the bone marrow (eg, quinacrine and primaquine)

Warnings/Precautions Use with caution in patients with G-6-PD deficiency, NADH methemoglobin reductase deficiency, acutely ill patients who have a tendency to develop granulocytopenia; patients receiving other drugs capable of depressing the bone marrow; do not exceed recommended dosage

Adverse Reactions

>10%:

Gastrointestinal: Abdominal pain, nausea, vomiting

Hematologic: Hemolytic anemia in G-6-PD deficiency

1% to 10%: Hematologic: Methemoglobinemia in NADH-methemoglobin reductase-deficient individuals

<1%: Arrhythmias, headache, pruritus, leukopenia, agranulocytosis, leukocytosis, interference with visual accommodation

Overdosage/Toxicology

Symptoms of acute overdose include abdominal cramps, vomiting, cyanosis, methemoglobinemia (possibly severe), leukopenia, acute hemolytic anemia (often significant), granulocytopenia; with chronic overdose, symptoms include ototoxicity and retinopathy

Following GI decontamination, treatment is supportive (fluids, anticonvulsants, blood transfusions, methylene blue if methemoglobinemia severe - 1-2 mg/kg over several minutes)

Drug Interactions Quinacrine may potentiate the toxicity of antimalarial compounds which are structurally related to primaquine

Mechanism of Action Eliminates the primary tissue exoerythrocytic forms of *P. falciparum*; disrupts mitochondria and binds to DNA

Pharmacodynamics/Kinetics

Absorption: Oral: Well absorbed

Metabolism: Liver metabolism to carboxyprimaquine, an active metabolite

Half-life: 3.7-9.6 hours

Time to peak serum concentration: Within 1-2 hours

Elimination: Only a small amount of unchanged drug excreted in urine

Usual Dosage Oral:

Children: 0.3 mg base/kg/day once daily for 14 days (not to exceed 15 mg/day) or 0.9 mg base/kg once weekly for 8 weeks not to exceed 45 mg base/week

Adults: 15 mg/day (base) once daily for 14 days or 45 mg base once weekly for 8 weeks

CDC treatment recommendations: Begin therapy during last 2 weeks of, or following a course of, suppression with chloroquine or a comparable drug

Monitoring Parameters Periodic CBC, visual color check of urine, glucose, electrolytes; if hemolysis suspected - CBC, haptoglobin, peripheral smear, urinalysis dipstick for occult blood

Patient Information Take with meals to decrease adverse GI effects; drug has a bitter taste; notify physician if a darkening of urine occurs or if shortness of breath, weakness or skin discoloration (chocolate cyanosis) occurs; complete full course of therapy

Dosage Forms Tablet: 26.3 mg [15 mg base]

Selected Readings

Panisko DM and Keystone JS, "Treatment of Malaria - 1990," *Drugs*, 1990, 39(2):160-89.
White NJ, "The Treatment of Malaria," *N Engl J Med*, 1996, 335(11):800-6.
Wyler DJ, "Malaria Chemoprophylaxis for the Traveler," *N Engl J Med*, 1993, 329(1):31-7.

Primaxin® *see* Imipenem and Cilastatin *on page 766*

Principen® *see* Ampicillin *on page 604*

Pristinamycin *see* Quinupristin/Dalfopristin *on page 891*

Pro-Amox® *see* Amoxicillin *on page 592*

Pro-Ampi® Trihydrate *see* Ampicillin *on page 604*

Procaine Benzylpenicillin *see* Penicillin G Procaine *on page 862*

Procaine Penicillin G *see* Penicillin G Procaine *on page 862*

ProHIBiT® *see* Haemophilus b Conjugate Vaccine *on page 756*

Proloprim® *see* Trimethoprim *on page 957*

Pronto® Shampoo [OTC] *see* Pyrethrins *on page 885*

Prostaphlin® *see* Oxacillin *on page 849*

Protease Inhibitors
Refer to
Amprenavir *on page 609*
Indinavir *on page 773*
Nelfinavir *on page 831*
Ritonavir *on page 909*
Saquinavir *on page 915*

Protostat® Oral *see* Metronidazole *on page 817*

Pro-Trin® *see* Co-Trimoxazole *on page 692*

PRP-D *see* Haemophilus b Conjugate Vaccine *on page 756*

Prymaccone *see* Primaquine Phosphate *on previous page*

Pseudomonic Acid A *see* Mupirocin *on page 825*

PVF® K *see* Penicillin V Potassium *on page 865*

Pyrantel Pamoate (pi RAN tel PAM oh ate)
U.S. Brand Names Antiminth® [OTC]; Pin-Rid® [OTC]; Pin-X® [OTC]; Reese's® Pinworm Medicine [OTC]

Generic Available No

Use Treatment of pinworms (*Enterobius vermicularis*), whipworms (*Trichuris trichiura*), roundworms (*Ascaris lumbricoides*), and hookworms (*Ancylostoma duodenale*)

Drug of Choice or Alternative for
Organism(s)
Ancylostoma duodenale *on page 66*
Ascaris *on page 69*
Enterobius vermicularis *on page 136*

Pregnancy Risk Factor C

Contraindications Known hypersensitivity to pyrantel pamoate

Warnings/Precautions Use with caution in patients with liver impairment, anemia, malnutrition, or pregnancy. Since pinworm infections are easily spread to others, treat all family members in close contact with the patient.

Adverse Reactions
1% to 10%: Gastrointestinal: Anorexia, nausea, vomiting, abdominal cramps, diarrhea
<1%: Dizziness, drowsiness, insomnia, headache, rash, elevated liver enzymes, tenesmus, weakness

Overdosage/Toxicology
Symptoms of overdose include anorexia, nausea, vomiting, cramps, diarrhea, ataxia
Treatment is supportive following GI decontamination

Drug Interactions Decreased effect with piperazine

Stability Protect from light

Mechanism of Action Causes the release of acetylcholine and inhibits cholinesterase; acts as a depolarizing neuromuscular blocker, paralyzing the helminths
(Continued)

Pyrantel Pamoate *(Continued)*

Pharmacodynamics/Kinetics

Absorption: Oral: Poor

Metabolism: Undergoes partial hepatic metabolism

Time to peak serum concentration: Within 1-3 hours

Elimination: In feces (50% as unchanged drug) and urine (7% as unchanged drug)

Usual Dosage Children and Adults (purgation is not required prior to use): Oral:

Roundworm, pinworm, or trichostrongyliasis: 11 mg/kg administered as a single dose; maximum dose: 1 g. **(Note:** For pinworm infection, dosage should be repeated in 2 weeks and all family members should be treated).

Hookworm: 11 mg/kg administered once daily for 3 days

Monitoring Parameters Stool for presence of eggs, worms, and occult blood, serum AST and ALT

Patient Information May mix drug with milk or fruit juice; strict hygiene is essential to prevent reinfection

Nursing Implications Shake well before pouring to assure accurate dosage; protect from light

Dosage Forms

Capsule: 180 mg

Liquid: 50 mg/mL (30 mL); 144 mg/mL (30 mL)

Suspension, oral (caramel-currant flavor): 50 mg/mL (60 mL)

Selected Readings

"Drugs for Parasitic Infections," *Med Lett Drugs Ther*, 1998, 40(1017):1-12.

Pyrazinamide *(peer a ZIN a mide)*

Related Information

Tuberculosis Guidelines *on page 1114*

Canadian Brand Names PMS-Pyrazinamide; Tebrazid

Synonyms Pyrazinoic Acid Amide

Generic Available No

Use Adjunctive treatment of tuberculosis in combination with other anti-tuberculosis agents

Drug of Choice or Alternative for

Organism(s)

Mycobacterium tuberculosis on page 207

Pregnancy Risk Factor C

Contraindications Severe hepatic damage; hypersensitivity to pyrazinamide or any component; acute gout

Warnings/Precautions Use with caution in patients with renal failure, chronic gout, diabetes mellitus, or porphyria

Adverse Reactions

1% to 10%:

Central nervous system: Malaise

Gastrointestinal: Nausea, vomiting, anorexia

Neuromuscular & skeletal: Arthralgia, myalgia

<1%: Fever, rash, itching, acne, photosensitivity, gout, dysuria, porphyria, thrombocytopenia, hepatotoxicity, interstitial nephritis

Overdosage/Toxicology

Symptoms of overdose include gout, gastric upset, hepatic damage (mild)

Treatment following GI decontamination is supportive

Mechanism of Action Converted to pyrazinoic acid in susceptible strains of *Mycobacterium* which lowers the pH of the environment; exact mechanism of action has not been elucidated

Pharmacodynamics/Kinetics Bacteriostatic or bactericidal depending on the drug's concentration at the site of infection

Absorption: Oral: Well absorbed

Distribution: Widely distributed into body tissues and fluids including the liver, lung, and CSF

Relative diffusion of antimicrobial agents from blood into cerebrospinal fluid (CSF): Adequate with or without inflammation (exceeds usual MICs)

Ratio of CSF to blood level (%): Inflamed meninges: 100

Protein binding: 50%

Metabolism: In the liver

Half-life: 9-10 hours
Time to peak serum concentration: Within 2 hours
Elimination: In urine (4% as unchanged drug)

Usual Dosage Oral (calculate dose on ideal body weight rather than total body weight): **Note:** A four-drug regimen (isoniazid, rifampin, pyrazinamide, and either streptomycin or ethambutol) is preferred for the initial, empiric treatment of TB. When the drug susceptibility results are available, the regimen should be altered as appropriate.

Children and Adults:
  Daily therapy: 15-30 mg/kg/day (maximum: 2 g/day)
  Directly observed therapy (DOT): Twice weekly: 50-70 mg/kg (maximum: 4 g)
  DOT: 3 times/week: 50-70 mg/kg (maximum: 3 g)
Elderly: Start with a lower daily dose (15 mg/kg) and increase as tolerated

Dosing adjustment in renal impairment: Cl$_{cr}$ <50 mL/minute: Avoid use or reduce dose to 12-20 mg/kg/day

Dosing adjustment in hepatic impairment: Reduce dose

Monitoring Parameters Periodic liver function tests, serum uric acid, sputum culture, chest x-ray 2-3 months into treatment and at completion

Test Interactions Reacts with Acetest® and Ketostix® to produce pinkish brown color

Patient Information Notify physician if fever, loss of appetite, malaise, nausea, vomiting, darkened urine, pale stools occur; do not stop taking without consulting a physician

Dosage Forms Tablet: 500 mg

Extemporaneous Preparations Pyrazinamide suspension can be compounded with simple syrup or 0.5% methylcellulose with simple syrup at a concentration of 100 mg/mL; the suspension is stable for 2 months at 4°C or 25°C when stored in glass or plastic bottles

To prepare pyrazinamide suspension in 0.5% methylcellulose with simple syrup: Crush 200 pyrazinamide 500 mg tablets and mix with a suspension containing 500 mL of 1% methylcellulose and 500 mL simple syrup. Add to this a suspension containing 140 crushed pyrazinamide tablets in 350 mL of 1% methylcellulose and 350 mL of simple syrup to make 1.7 L of suspension containing pyrazinamide 100 mg/mL in 0.5% methylcellulose with simple syrup.

Nahata MC, Morosco RS, and Peritre SP, "Stability of Pyrazinamide in Two Suspensions," *Am J Health Syst Pharm*, 1995, 52:1558-60.

Selected Readings
Davidson PT and Le HQ, "Drug Treatment of Tuberculosis - 1992," *Drugs*, 1992, 43(5):651-73.
"Drugs for Tuberculosis," *Med Lett Drugs Ther*, 1993, 35(908):99-101.
Havlir DV and Barnes PF, "Tuberculosis in Patients With Human Immunodeficiency Virus Infection," *N Engl J Med*, 1999, 340(5):367-73.
Iseman MD, "Treatment of Multidrug-Resistant Tuberculosis," *N Engl J Med*, 1993, 329(11):784-91.
"Prevention and Treatment of Tuberculosis Among Patients Infected With Human Immunodeficiency Virus: Principles of Therapy and Revised Recommendations. Centers for Disease Control and Prevention," *MMWR Morb Mortal Wkly Rep*, 1998, 47(RR-20):1-58.
Van Scoy RE and Wilkowske CJ, "Antituberculous Agents," *Mayo Clin Proc*, 1992, 67(2):179-87.

Pyrazinoic Acid Amide *see* Pyrazinamide *on previous page*

Pyrethrins (pye RE thrins)

U.S. Brand Names A-200™ Shampoo [OTC]; Barc® Liquid [OTC]; End Lice® Liquid [OTC]; Lice-Enz® Shampoo [OTC]; Pronto® Shampoo [OTC]; Pyrinex® Pediculicide Shampoo [OTC]; Pyrinyl II® Liquid [OTC]; Pyrinyl Plus® Shampoo [OTC]; R & C® Shampoo [OTC]; RID® Shampoo [OTC]; Tisit® Blue Gel [OTC]; Tisit® Liquid [OTC]; Tisit® Shampoo [OTC]; Triple X® Liquid [OTC]

Generic Available Yes

Use Treatment of *Pediculus humanus* infestations (head lice, body lice, pubic lice and their eggs)

Drug of Choice or Alternative for
  Organism(s)
    Lice *on page 188*

Pregnancy Risk Factor C

Contraindications Known hypersensitivity to pyrethrins, ragweed, or chrysanthemums

(Continued)

Pyrethrins *(Continued)*

Warnings/Precautions For external use only; do not use in eyelashes or eyebrows

Adverse Reactions 1% to 10%:
Dermatologic: Pruritus
Local: Burning, stinging, irritation with repeat use

Mechanism of Action Pyrethrins are derived from flowers that belong to the chrysanthemum family. The mechanism of action on the neuronal membranes of lice is similar to that of DDT. Piperonyl butoxide is usually added to pyrethrin to enhance the product's activity by decreasing the metabolism of pyrethrins in arthropods.

Pharmacodynamics/Kinetics
Onset of action: ~30 minutes
Absorption: Topical into the system is minimal
Metabolism: By ester hydrolysis and hydroxylation

Usual Dosage Application of pyrethrins: Topical:
Apply enough solution to completely wet infested area, including hair
Allow to remain on area for 10 minutes
Wash and rinse with large amounts of warm water
Use fine-toothed comb to remove lice and eggs from hair
Shampoo hair to restore body and luster
Treatment may be repeated if necessary once in a 24-hour period
Repeat treatment in 7-10 days to kill newly hatched lice

Patient Information For external use only; avoid touching eyes, mouth, or other mucous membranes; contact physician if irritation occurs or if condition does not improve in 2-3 days

Dosage Forms
Gel, topical: 0.3% (30 g)
Liquid, topical: 0.18% (60 mL); 0.2% (60 mL, 120 mL); 0.3% (60 mL, 118 mL, 120 mL, 177 mL, 237 mL, 240 mL)
Shampoo: 0.3% (59 mL, 60 mL, 118 mL, 120 mL, 240 mL); 0.33% (60 mL, 120 mL)

Selected Readings
"Drugs for Parasitic Infections," *Med Lett Drugs Ther*, 1998, 40(1017):1-12.
Liu LX and Weller PF, "Antiparasitic Drugs," *N Engl J Med*, 1996, 334(18):1178-84.

Pyrimethamine *(peer i METH a meen)*

U.S. Brand Names Daraprim®

Generic Available No

Use Prophylaxis of malaria due to susceptible strains of plasmodia; used in conjunction with quinine and sulfadiazine for the treatment of uncomplicated attacks of chloroquine-resistant *P. falciparum* malaria; used in conjunction with fast-acting schizonticide to initiate transmission control and suppression cure; synergistic combination with sulfonamide in treatment of toxoplasmosis

Drug of Choice or Alternative for
Disease/Syndrome(s)
Brain Abscess *on page 19*
Organism(s)
Toxoplasma gondii on page 283

Pregnancy Risk Factor C

Contraindications Megaloblastic anemia secondary to folate deficiency; known hypersensitivity to pyrimethamine, chloroguanide; resistant malaria

Warnings/Precautions When used for more than 3-4 days, it may be advisable to administer leucovorin to prevent hematological complications; monitor CBC and platelet counts every 2 weeks; use with caution in patients with impaired renal or hepatic function or with possible G-6-PD

Adverse Reactions
1% to 10%:
Gastrointestinal: Anorexia, abdominal cramps, vomiting
Hematologic: Megaloblastic anemia, leukopenia, thrombocytopenia, agranulocytosis
<1%: Insomnia, lightheadedness, fever, malaise, seizures, depression, rash, dermatitis, Stevens-Johnson syndrome, erythema multiforme, anaphylaxis, abnormal skin pigmentation, diarrhea, xerostomia, atrophic glossitis, pulmonary eosinophilia

Overdosage/Toxicology

Symptoms of overdose include megaloblastic anemia, leukopenia, thrombocytopenia, anorexia, CNS stimulation, seizures, nausea, vomiting, hematemesis

Following GI decontamination, leucovorin should be administered in a dosage of 5-15 mg/day I.M., I.V., or oral for 5-7 days or as required to reverse symptoms of folic acid deficiency; diazepam 0.1-0.25 mg/kg can be used to treat seizures

Drug Interactions

Decreased effect: Pyrimethamine effectiveness decreased by acid

Increased effect: Sulfonamides (synergy), methotrexate, TMP/SMX may increase the risk of bone marrow suppression; mild hepatotoxicity with lorazepam

Stability Pyrimethamine tablets may be crushed to prepare oral suspensions of the drug in water, cherry syrup, or sucrose-containing solutions at a concentration of 1 mg/mL; stable at room temperature for 5-7 days

Mechanism of Action Inhibits parasitic dihydrofolate reductase, resulting in inhibition of vital tetrahydrofolic acid synthesis

Pharmacodynamics/Kinetics

Absorption: Oral: Well absorbed

Distribution: Widely distributed ; mainly concentrated in blood cells, kidneys, lungs, liver, and spleen; crosses into CSF; crosses placenta; appears in breast milk

Metabolism: Hepatic

Half-life: 80-95 hours

Time to peak serum concentration: Within 1.5-8 hours

Elimination: 20% to 30% excreted unchanged in urine

Usual Dosage Oral:

Malaria chemoprophylaxis (for areas where chloroquine-resistant *P. falciparum* exists): Begin prophylaxis 2 weeks before entering endemic area:

Children: 0.5 mg/kg once weekly; not to exceed 25 mg/dose

or

Children:

<4 years: 6.25 mg once weekly

4-10 years: 12.5 mg once weekly

Children >10 years and Adults: 25 mg once weekly

Dosage should be continued for all age groups for at least 6-10 weeks after leaving endemic areas

Chloroquine-resistant *P. falciparum* malaria (when used in conjunction with quinine and sulfadiazine):

Children:

<10 kg: 6.25 mg/day once daily for 3 days

10-20 kg: 12.5 mg/day once daily for 3 days

20-40 kg: 25 mg/day once daily for 3 days

Adults: 25 mg twice daily for 3 days

Toxoplasmosis:

Infants for congenital toxoplasmosis: Oral: 1 mg/kg once daily for 6 months with sulfadiazine then every other month with sulfa, alternating with spiramycin.

Children: Loading dose: 2 mg/kg/day divided into 2 equal daily doses for 1-3 days (maximum: 100 mg/day) followed by 1 mg/kg/day divided into 2 doses for 4 weeks; maximum: 25 mg/day

With sulfadiazine or trisulfapyrimidines: 2 mg/kg/day divided every 12 hours for 3 days followed by 1 mg/kg/day once daily or divided twice daily for 4 weeks given with trisulfapyrimidines or sulfadiazine

Adults: 50-75 mg/day together with 1-4 g of a sulfonamide for 1-3 weeks depending on patient's tolerance and response, then reduce dose by 50% and continue for 4-5 weeks **or** 25-50 mg/day for 3-4 weeks

In HIV, life-long suppression is necessary to prevent relapse; leucovorin (5-10 mg/day) is given concurrently

Monitoring Parameters CBC, including platelet counts

Patient Information Take with meals to minimize vomiting; begin malaria prophylaxis at least 1-2 weeks prior to departure; discontinue at first sign of skin rash; notify physician if persistent fever, sore throat, bleeding or bruising occurs; regular blood work may be necessary in patients taking high doses

Dosage Forms Tablet: 25 mg

(Continued)

Pyrimethamine *(Continued)*

Extemporaneous Preparations Pyrimethamine tablets may be crushed to prepare oral suspensions of the drug in water, cherry syrup or sucrose-containing solutions at a concentration of 1 mg/mL; stable at room temperature for 5-7 days

McEvoy G, AHFS Drug Information 96. Bethesda, MD: American Society of Health-System Pharmacists, 1996.

Selected Readings

"Drugs for Parasitic Infections," *Med Lett Drugs Ther*, 1998, 40(1017):1-12.

Porter SB and Sande MA, "Toxoplasmosis of the Central Nervous System in the Acquired Immuno-deficiency Syndrome," *N Engl J Med*, 1992, 327(23):1643-8.

White NJ, "The Treatment of Malaria," *N Engl J Med*, 1996, 335(11):800-6.

Pyrinex® Pediculicide Shampoo [OTC] *see Pyrethrins on page 885*

Pyrinyl II® Liquid [OTC] *see Pyrethrins on page 885*

Pyrinyl Plus® Shampoo [OTC] *see Pyrethrins on page 885*

Quinaglute® Dura-Tabs® *see Quinidine on this page*

Quinalan® *see Quinidine on this page*

Quinidex® Extentabs® *see Quinidine on this page*

Quinidine (KWIN i deen)

U.S. Brand Names Cardioquin®; Quinaglute® Dura-Tabs®; Quinalan®; Quinidex® Extentabs®; Quinora®

Synonyms Quinidine Gluconate; Quinidine Polygalacturonate; Quinidine Sulfate

Generic Available Yes

Use Active against *Plasmodium falciparum* malaria (used as I.V.); prophylaxis after cardioversion of atrial fibrillation and/or flutter to maintain normal sinus rhythm; also used to prevent reoccurrence of paroxysmal supraventricular tachycardia, paroxysmal A-V junctional rhythm, paroxysmal ventricular tachycardia, paroxysmal atrial fibrillation, and atrial or ventricular premature contractions

Drug of Choice or Alternative for

Organism(s)

Plasmodium Species *on page 227*

Pregnancy Risk Factor C

Contraindications Patients with complete A-V block with an A-V junctional or idioventricular pacemaker; patients with intraventricular conduction defects (marked widening of QRS complex); patients with cardiac-glycoside induced A-V conduction disorders; hypersensitivity to the drug or cinchona derivatives

Warnings/Precautions Use with caution in patients with myocardial depression, sick sinus syndrome, incomplete A-V block, hepatic and/or renal insufficiency, myasthenia gravis; hemolysis may occur in patients with G-6-PD (glucose-6-phosphate dehydrogenase) deficiency; quinidine-induced hepatotoxicity, including granulomatous hepatitis can occur, increased serum AST and alkaline phosphatase concentrations, and jaundice may occur; use with caution in nursing women

Adverse Reactions

>10%: Gastrointestinal: Bitter taste, diarrhea, anorexia, nausea, vomiting, stomach cramping

1% to 10%:

Cardiovascular: Hypotension, syncope

Central nervous system: Lightheadedness, severe headache

Dermatologic: Rash

Ocular: Blurred vision

Otic: Tinnitus

Respiratory: Wheezing

<1%: Tachycardia, heart block, ventricular fibrillation, vascular collapse, confusion, delirium, fever, vertigo, angioedema, anemia, thrombocytopenic purpura, blood dyscrasias, impaired hearing, respiratory depression, pneumonitis, bronchospasm

Overdosage/Toxicology

Has a low toxic:therapeutic ratio and may easily produce fatal intoxication (acute toxic dose: 1 g in adults); symptoms of overdose include sinus bradycardia, sinus node arrest or asystole, P-R, QRS or Q-T interval prolongation, torsade de pointes (polymorphous ventricular tachycardia) and depressed myocardial contractility, which along with alpha-adrenergic or ganglionic blockade, may result in hypotension and pulmonary edema; other effects are anticholinergic (dry mouth, dilated pupils, and delirium) as well as seizures, coma and respiratory arrest

Treatment is primarily symptomatic and effects usually respond to conventional therapies (fluids, positioning, vasopressors, anticonvulsants, antiarrhythmics). **Note:** Do not use other type 1a or 1c antiarrhythmic agents to treat ventricular tachycardia; sodium bicarbonate may treat wide QRS intervals or hypotension; markedly impaired conduction or high degree A-V block, unresponsive to bicarbonate, indicates consideration of a pacemaker is needed.

Drug Interactions
Decreased serum concentrations with phenobarbital, phenytoin, and rifampin

Increased effect of nondepolarizing/depolarizing muscle relaxants and anticoagulants

Increased serum concentrations with verapamil, amiodarone, alkalinizing agents, diltiazem, and cimetidine

Increased plasma concentration of digoxin, closely monitor digoxin concentrations, digoxin dosage may need to be reduced (50%) when quinidine is initiated, new steady-state digoxin plasma concentrations occur in 5-7 days

Stability Do not use discolored parenteral solution

Mechanism of Action The drug probably interferes with *Plasmodium* DNA; depresses phase O of the action potential; decreased myocardial excitability and conduction velocity, and myocardial contractility by decreasing sodium influx during depolarization and potassium efflux in repolarization; also reduces calcium transport across cell membrane

Pharmacodynamics/Kinetics
Absorption: Well from GI tract

Distribution: All tissues except brain; concentrates in heart, liver, kidneys, and skeletal muscle; crosses the placenta and appears in breast milk

Metabolism: Extensively in the liver

Bioavailability: 80% (sulfate), 70% (gluconate)

Half-life:
Adults: 6-8 hours
Children: 2.5-6.7 hours
Increased half-life elderly, cirrhosis, and congestive heart failure

Elimination: Excretion in urine (15% to 25% as unchanged drug)

Usual Dosage Malaria:
Continuous infusion (preferred): Children and Adults: Loading dose: 10 mg/kg (in 250 mL NS) over 1-2 hours; then 20 µg/kg/minute for 72 hours or until patient can take orally, or until parasitemia is <1%
or
Intermittent infusion: Adults: Loading dose: 24 mg/kg (in 250 mL NS) over 4 hours, then 12 mg/kg every 8 hours (over 4 hours) until patient can take orally

Oral: Therapy with quinine is preferred over quinidine for treatment of malaria

Monitoring Parameters Complete blood counts, liver and renal function tests, should be routinely performed during long-term administration; monitor EKG during I.V. infusion; decrease infusion rate if Q-T interval is >0.6 seconds, if QRS increases to >25% of baseline, or if significant hypotension is present

Reference Range Therapeutic: 2-5 µg/mL (SI: 6.2-15.4 µmol/L). Patient dependent therapeutic response occurs at levels of 3-6 µg/mL (SI: 9.2-18.5 µmol/L). Optimal therapeutic level is method dependent

Patient Information Patients should notify their physician if rash, fever, unusual bleeding or bruising, ringing in the ears, or visual disturbances occur. Complete blood counts, liver and renal function tests should be routinely performed during long-term administration. Do not crush sustained release products.

Nursing Implications When injecting I.M., aspirate carefully to avoid injection into a vessel

Additional Information If serum concentration is >6 µg/mL, may reduce infusion rate

Dosage Forms
Injection, as gluconate (GENERIC): 80 mg/mL (10 mL)

Also comes in oral dosage forms for therapy of dysrhythmias

Selected Readings
Panisko DM and Keystone JS, "Treatment of Malaria - 1990," *Drugs*, 1990, 39(2):160-89.
Wyler DJ, "Malaria Chemoprophylaxis for the Traveler," *N Engl J Med*, 1993, 329(1):31-7.
Wyler DJ, "Malaria: Overview and Update," *Clin Infect Dis*, 1993, 16(4):449-56.

Quinidine Gluconate *see Quinidine on page 888*
Quinidine Polygalacturonate *see* Quinidine *on page 888*
Quinidine Sulfate *see Quinidine on page 888*

Quinine (KWYE nine)

U.S. Brand Names Formula Q®
Synonyms Quinine Sulfate
Generic Available Yes
Use In conjunction with other antimalarial agents, suppression or treatment of chloroquine-resistant *P. falciparum* malaria; has been used for treatment of *Babesia microti* infection in conjunction with clindamycin; prevention and treatment of nocturnal recumbency leg muscle cramps
Drug of Choice or Alternative for
    Organism(s)
      Babesia microti on page 71
Pregnancy Risk Factor X
Contraindications Tinnitus, optic neuritis, G-6-PD deficiency, hypersensitivity to quinine or any component, history of black water fever, and thrombocytopenia with quinine or quinidine
Warnings/Precautions Use with caution in patients with cardiac arrhythmias (quinine has quinidine-like activity) and in patients with myasthenia gravis
Adverse Reactions
    Percentage unknown: Cinchonism (risk of cinchonism is directly related to dose and duration of therapy): Severe headache, nausea, vomiting, diarrhea, blurred vision, tinnitus
    <1%: Flushing of the skin, anginal symptoms, fever, rash, pruritus, hypoglycemia, epigastric pain, hemolysis in G-6-PD deficiency, thrombocytopenia, hepatitis, nightblindness, diplopia, optic atrophy, impaired hearing, hypersensitivity reactions
Overdosage/Toxicology
    Symptoms of mild toxicity include nausea, vomiting, and cinchonism; severe intoxication may cause ataxia, obtundation, convulsions, coma, and respiratory arrest; with massive intoxication quinidine-like cardiotoxicity (hypotension, QRS and Q-T interval prolongation, A-V block, and ventricular arrhythmias) may be fatal; retinal toxicity occurs 9-10 hours after ingestion (blurred vision, impaired color perception, constriction of visual fields and blindness); other toxic effects include hypokalemia, hypoglycemia, hemolysis and congenital malformations when taken during pregnancy.
    Treatment includes symptomatic therapy with conventional agents (anticonvulsants, fluids, positioning, vasoconstrictors, antiarrhythmias). **Note:** Avoid type 1a and 1c antiarrhythmic drugs; treat cardiotoxicity with sodium bicarbonate; dialysis and hemoperfusion procedures are ineffective in enhancing elimination.
Drug Interactions CYP3A3/4 enzyme substrate; CYP3A3/4 enzyme inhibitor
    Decreased effect: Phenobarbital, phenytoin, aluminum salt antacids, and rifampin may decrease quinine serum concentrations
    Increased toxicity:
      To avoid risk of seizures and cardiac arrest, delay mefloquine dosing at least 12 hours after last dose of quinine
      Beta-blockers + quinine may increase bradycardia
      Quinine may enhance coumarin anticoagulants and potentiate nondepolarizing and depolarizing muscle relaxants
      Quinine may inhibit metabolism of astemizole resulting in toxic levels and potentially life-threatening cardiotoxicity
      Quinine may increase plasma concentration of digoxin by as much as twofold; closely monitor digoxin concentrations and decrease digoxin dose with initiation of quinine by one-half
      Verapamil, amiodarone, urinary alkalinizing agents, and cimetidine may increase quinine serum concentrations
Stability Protect from light
Mechanism of Action Depresses oxygen uptake and carbohydrate metabolism; intercalates into DNA, disrupting the parasite's replication and transcription; affects calcium distribution within muscle fibers and decreases the excitability of the motor end-plate region; cardiovascular effects similar to quinidine

Pharmacodynamics/Kinetics
Absorption: Oral: Readily absorbed mainly from the upper small intestine

Protein binding: 70% to 95%

Metabolism: Primarily in the liver

Half-life:

Children: 6-12 hours

Adults: 8-14 hours

Time to peak serum concentration: Within 1-3 hours

Elimination: In bile and saliva with <5% excreted unchanged in urine

Usual Dosage Oral:
Children:

Treatment of chloroquine-resistant malaria: 25-30 mg/kg/day in divided doses every 8 hours for 5-7 days in conjunction with another agent

Babesiosis: 25 mg/kg/day divided every 8 hours for 7 days

Adults:

Treatment of chloroquine-resistant malaria: 260-650 mg every 8 hours for 6-12 days in conjunction with another agent

Suppression of malaria: 325 mg twice daily and continued for 6 weeks after exposure

Babesiosis: 650 mg every 6-8 hours for 7 days

Leg cramps: 200-300 mg at bedtime

Dosing interval/adjustment in renal impairment:
Cl_{cr} 10-50 mL/minute: Administer every 8-12 hours or 75% of normal dose

Cl_{cr} <10 mL/minute: Administer every 24 hours or 30% to 50% of normal dose

Dialysis: Not removed

Peritoneal dialysis: Dose as for Cl_{cr} <10 mL/min

Continuous arteriovenous or venovenous hemodiafiltration (CAVH) effects: Dose for Cl_{cr} 10-50 mL/minute

Reference Range Toxic: >10 µg/mL

Test Interactions Positive direct Coombs' test, false elevation of urinary steroids and catecholamines

Patient Information Do not crush sustained release preparations. Avoid use of aluminum-containing antacids because of drug absorption problems; swallow dose whole to avoid bitter taste; may cause night blindness. Patients should notify their physician if rash, fever, unusual bleeding or bruising, ringing in the ears, visual disturbances, or syncope occur; seek emergency help if palpitations occur.

Dosage Forms
Capsule, as sulfate: 200 mg, 260 mg, 325 mg

Tablet, as sulfate: 260 mg

Selected Readings
Panisko DM and Keystone JS, "Treatment of Malaria - 1990," *Drugs*, 1990, 39(2):160-89.

White NJ, "The Treatment of Malaria," *N Engl J Med*, 1996, 335(11):800-6.

Wyler DJ, "Malaria Chemoprophylaxis for the Traveler," *N Engl J Med*, 1993, 329(1):31-7.

Wyler DJ, "Malaria: Overview and Update," *Clin Infect Dis*, 1993, 16(4):449-56.

Quinine Sulfate *see Quinine on previous page*

Quinora® *see Quinidine on page 888*

Quinsana Plus® [OTC] *see Tolnaftate on page 956*

Quinupristin/Dalfopristin (kwi NYOO pris tin/dal FOE pris tin)
U.S. Brand Names Synercid®

Synonyms Pristinamycin; RP59500

Use Investigational use: Has been studied in the treatment of a variety of infections caused by *Enterococcus faecium* (not *E. fecalis*) including vancomycin-resistant strains. May also be effective in the treatment of serious infections caused by *Staphylococcus* species including those resistant to methicillin.

Drug of Choice or Alternative for

Organism(s)

Enterococcus Species *on page 137*

Pregnancy Risk Factor Unknown

Contraindications Hypersensitivity to quinupristin, dalfopristin, or pristinamycin

Warnings/Precautions Use with caution in patients with hepatic or renal dysfunction. May cause pain and phlebitis when infused through a peripheral line.

(Continued)

Quinupristin/Dalfopristin *(Continued)*

Adverse Reactions Percentage unknown: Nausea, vomiting, diarrhea, increased LFTs, cutaneous reactions, infusion site reactions, myalgia, arthralgia

Drug Interactions May inhibit drugs metabolized through CYP3A4
Inhibits the metabolism of nifedipine and midazolam and inhibits terfenadine metabolism; also inhibits cyclosporine metabolism

Stability After reconstitution, stability is ~5 hours at room temperature and 54 hours if refrigerated at 2°C to 8°C.

Mechanism of Action Quinupristin/dalfopristin inhibits bacterial protein synthesis by binding to different sites on the 50S bacterial ribosomal subunit thereby inhibiting protein synthesis

Pharmacodynamics/Kinetics
Distribution: V_d:
Quinupristin: 1.4-1.6 L/kg
Dalfopristin: 0.6-1.9 L/kg
Protein binding:
Quinupristin: 55% to 78%
Dalfopristin: 11% to 26%
Metabolism: Extensively metabolized in the blood and liver
Half-life: Quinupristin/dalfopristin: 1.3-1.5 hours; each parent compound individually: ~1 hour
Elimination: Urinary excretion is mainly metabolites; less than 5% of the parent compounds appear unchanged in the urine; 75% of the drugs are excreted in the feces as metabolites

Usual Dosage I.V.: 7.5 mg/kg 2-3 times/day

Additional Information Product information not available at the time of this writing.

Selected Readings
Bryson HM and Spencer CM, "Quinupristin/Dalfopristin," *Drugs*, 1996, 52(3):406-15.
Chant C and Rybak MH, "Quinupristin/Dalfopristin (RP 59500): A New Streptogramin Antibiotic," *Ann Pharmacother*, 1995, 29(10):1022-7.
Griswold MW, Lomaestro BM, and Briceland LL, "Quinupristin-Dalfopristin (RP 59500): An Injectable Streptogramin Combination," *Am J Health Syst Pharm*, 1996, 53:2045-53.

Rabavert® *see Rabies Virus Vaccine* *on next page*

Rabies Immune Globulin (Human)
(RAY beez i MYUN GLOB yoo lin HYU man)

U.S. Brand Names Hyperab®; Imogam®

Synonyms RIG

Generic Available No

Use Part of postexposure prophylaxis of persons with rabies exposure who lack a history or pre-exposure or postexposure prophylaxis with rabies vaccine or a recently documented neutralizing antibody response to previous rabies vaccination; although it is preferable to administer RIG with the first dose of vaccine, it can be given up to 8 days after vaccination

Drug of Choice or Alternative for
Organism(s)
Rabies Virus *on page 237*

Pregnancy Risk Factor C

Contraindications Inadvertent I.V. administration; allergy to thimerosal or any component

Warnings/Precautions Use with caution in individuals with thrombocytopenia, bleeding disorders, or prior allergic reactions to immune globulins

Adverse Reactions
1% to 10%:
Central nervous system: Fever (mild)
Local: Soreness at injection site
<1%: Urticaria, angioedema, stiffness, soreness of muscles, anaphylactic shock

Drug Interactions Decreased effect: Live virus vaccines (eg, MMR, rabies) may have delayed or diminished antibody response with immune globulin administration; should not be administered within 3 months unless antibody titers dictate as appropriate

Stability Refrigerate

Mechanism of Action Rabies immune globulin is a solution of globulins dried from the plasma or serum of selected adult human donors who have been immunized with rabies vaccine and have developed high titers of rabies antibody. It generally contains 10% to 18% of protein of which not less than 80% is monomeric immunoglobulin G.

Usual Dosage Children and Adults: I.M.: 20 units/kg in a single dose (RIG should always be administered as part of rabies vaccine (HDCV)) regimen (as soon as possible after the first dose of vaccine, up to 8 days); infiltrate $^1/_2$ of the dose locally around the wound; administer the remainder I.M.

Note: Persons known to have an adequate titer or who have been completely immunized with rabies vaccine should not receive RIG, only booster doses of HDCV

Administration Intramuscular injection only; injection should be made into the deltoid muscle or anterolateral aspect of the thigh

Nursing Implications Severe adverse reactions can occur if patient receives RIG I.V.

Dosage Forms Injection: 150 units/mL (2 mL, 10 mL)

Selected Readings

"A New Rabies Vaccine," Med Lett Drugs Ther, 1998, 40(1029):64-5.

Dreesen DW and Hanlon CA, "Current Recommendations for the Prophylaxis and Treatment of Rabies," Drugs, 1998, 56(5):801-9.

Lang J and Plotkin SA, "Rabies Risk and Immunoprophylaxis in Children," Adv Pediatr Infect Dis, 1997, 13:219-55.

Strady A, Lang J, Lienard M, et al, "Antibody Persistence Following Pre-exposure Regimens of Cell-Culture Rabies Vaccines: 10-Year Follow-up and Proposal for a New Booster Policy," J Infect Dis, 1998, 177(5):1290-5.

Rabies Virus Vaccine (RAY beez VYE rus vak SEEN)

Related Information

Immunization Guidelines *on page 1041*

U.S. Brand Names Imovax® Rabies I.D. Vaccine; Imovax® Rabies Vaccine; Rabavert®

Synonyms HDCV; Human Diploid Cell Cultures Rabies Vaccine; Human Diploid Cell Cultures Rabies Vaccine (Intradermal use)

Generic Available No

Use Pre-exposure immunization: Vaccinate persons with greater than usual risk due occupation or avocation including veterinarians, rangers, animal handlers, certain laboratory workers, and persons living in or visiting countries for longer than 1 month where rabies is a constant threat.

Postexposure prophylaxis: If a bite from a carrier animal is unprovoked, if it is not captured and rabies is present in that species and area, administer rabies immune globulin (RIG) and the vaccine as indicated

The Food and Drug Administration has not approved the I.D. use of rabies vaccine for postexposure prophylaxis (only I.M.). The type of and schedule for postexposure prophylaxis depends upon the previous rabies vaccination status or the result of a previous or current serologic test for rabies antibody.

Drug of Choice or Alternative for

Organism(s)

Rabies Virus *on page 237*

Pregnancy Risk Factor C

Contraindications Developing febrile illness (during pre-exposure therapy only); allergy to neomycin, gentamicin, or amphotericin B; life-threatening allergic reactions to rabies vaccine or its components (however, carefully consider a patient's risk of rabies before continuing therapy)

Warnings/Precautions Report serious reactions to the State Health Department or the manufacturer/distributor, an immune complex reaction is possible 2-21 days following booster doses of HDCV; hypersensitivity reactions may be treated with antihistamines or epinephrine, if severe.

Use care to administer Imovax® rabies vaccine human and rabies vaccine adsorbed (RDA) only by I.M. route. Diploid cell (HDCV) (in the **deltoid only**) and Imovax® rabies I.D. vaccine by I.D. route only

Adverse Reactions Mild systemic reactions occur at an incidence of ~8% to 10% with RVA and 20% with HDCV. **All serious adverse reactions must be reported to the U.S. Department of Health and Human Services (DHHS) Vaccine Adverse Event Reporting System (VAERS) 1-800-822-7967.**
(Continued)

Rabies Virus Vaccine *(Continued)*

Cardiovascular: Edema

Central nervous system: Dizziness, malaise, encephalomyelitis, transverse myelitis, fever, pain, headache, neuroparalytic reactions

Dermatologic: Itching, erythema

Gastrointestinal: Nausea, abdominal pain

Local: Local discomfort, pain at injection site

Neuromuscular & skeletal: Myalgia

Note: Serum sickness reaction is much less frequent with RVA (<1%) vs the HDCV (6%)

Drug Interactions Decreased effect with immunosuppressive agents, corticosteroids, antimalarial drugs (ie, chloroquine); persons on these drugs should receive RIG (3 doses/1 mL each) by the I.M. route

Stability Refrigerate dried vaccine; HDCV can presumably tolerate 30 days at room temperature; reconstituted vaccine should be used immediately

Mechanism of Action Rabies vaccine is an inactivated virus vaccine which promotes immunity by inducing an active immune response. The production of specific antibodies requires about 7-10 days to develop. Rabies immune globulin or antirabies serum, equine (ARS) is given in conjunction with rabies vaccine to provide immune protection until an antibody response can occur.

Pharmacodynamics/Kinetics

Onset of effect: I.M.: Rabies antibody appears in the serum within 7-10 days

Peak effect: Within 30-60 days and persists for at least 1 year

Usual Dosage

Pre-exposure prophylaxis: 1 mL I.M. or 0.1 mL I.D. on days 0, 7, and 21 to 28. **Note:** Prolonging the interval between doses does not interfere with immunity achieved after the concluding dose of the basic series.

Postexposure prophylaxis: All postexposure treatment should begin with immediate cleansing of the wound with soap and water

Persons not previously immunized as above: Rabies immune globulin 20 units/kg body weight, half infiltrated at bite site if possible, remainder I.M.; and 5 doses of rabies vaccine, 1 mL I.M., one each on days 0, 3, 7, 14, 28

Persons who have previously received postexposure prophylaxis with rabies vaccine, received a recommended I.M. pre-exposure series of rabies vaccine or have a previously documented rabies antibody titer considered adequate: 1 mL of either vaccine I.M. only on days 0 and 3; do not administer RIG

Booster (for occupational or other continuing risk): 1 mL I.M. or 0.1 mL I.D. every 2-5 years or based on antibody titers

Administration HDCV may be given I.M. or I.D. (I.M. for postexposure prophylaxis); RVA may be given I.M. only; give I.M. injections in the deltoid muscle, not the gluteal, in adults and older children; for younger children, use the outer aspect of the thigh. I.D. injections are best given in the lateral aspect of the upper arm; travelers to endemic areas may receive the vaccine by the I.D. route if the 3-dose series can be completed >30 days before departure, otherwise give I.M.

Reference Range Antibody titers ≥115 as determined by rapid fluorescent-focus inhibition test are indicative of adequate response; collect titers on day 28 postexposure

Additional Information Federal law requires that the date of administration, the vaccine manufacturer, lot number of vaccine, and the administering person's name, title and address be entered into the patient's permanent medical record

Dosage Forms Injection:

Human diploid cell vaccine (HDCV): Rabies antigen 2.5 units/mL (1 mL)

Imovax® rabies I.D. vaccine: Rabies antigen 0.25 units/0.1 mL (1 mL)

Rabies vaccine (adsorbed): 1 mL

Selected Readings

"A New Rabies Vaccine," *Med Lett Drugs Ther*, 1998, 40(1029):64-5.

Dreesen DW and Hanlon CA, "Current Recommendations for the Prophylaxis and Treatment of Rabies," *Drugs*, 1998, 56(5):801-9.

Lang J and Plotkin SA, "Rabies Risk and Immunoprophylaxis in Children," *Adv Pediatr Infect Dis*, 1997, 13:219-55.

Strady A, Lang J, Lienard M, et al, "Antibody Persistence Following Preexposure Regimens of Cell-Culture Rabies Vaccines: 10-Year Follow-up and Proposal for a New Booster Policy," *J Infect Dis*, 1998, 177(5):1290-5.

Raxar® *see* Grepafloxacin *on page 752*

R & C® Shampoo [OTC] *see* Pyrethrins *on page 885*

Rebetol® *see* Ribavirin *on page 899*

Rebetron™ *see* Interferon Alfa-2b and Ribavirin Combination Pack *on page 780*

Recombivax HB® *see* Hepatitis B Vaccine *on page 761*

Reese's® **Pinworm Medicine [OTC]** *see* Pyrantel Pamoate *on page 883*

Rescriptor® *see* Delavirdine *on page 700*

RespiGam® *see* Respiratory Syncytial Virus Immune Globulin (Intravenous) *on this page*

Respiratory Syncytial Virus Immune Globulin (Intravenous)

(RES peer rah tor ee sin SISH al VYE rus i MYUN GLOB yoo lin in tra VEE nus)

U.S. Brand Names RespiGam®

Synonyms RSV-IGIV

Use Prevention of serious lower respiratory infection caused by respiratory syncytial virus (RSV) in children <24 months of age with bronchopulmonary dysplasia (BPD) or a history of premature birth (≤35 weeks gestation) (Palivizumab is now the preferred agent.)

Pregnancy Risk Factor C

Contraindications Selective IgA deficiency; history of severe prior reaction to any immunoglobulin preparation

Warnings/Precautions Use caution to avoid fluid overload in patients, particularly infants with bronchopulmonary dysplasia (BPD), when administering RSV-IGIV; hypersensitivity including anaphylaxis or angioneurotic edema may occur; keep epinephrine 1:1000 readily available during infusion; rare occurrences of aseptic meningitis syndrome have been associated with IGIV treatment, particularly with high doses; observe carefully for signs and symptoms of such and treat promptly

Adverse Reactions

1% to 10%:

Dermatologic: Rash (1%)

Cardiovascular: Tachycardia (1%), hypertension (1%), hypotension

Central nervous system: Fever (6%)

Endocrine & metabolic: Fluid overload (1%)

Gastrointestinal: Vomiting (2%), diarrhea (1%), gastroenteritis (1%)

Local: Injection site inflammation (1%)

Respiratory: Respiratory distress (2%), wheezing (2%), rales, hypoxia (1%), tachypnea (1%)

<1%: Edema, pallor, heart murmur, cyanosis, flushing, palpitations, chest tightness, dizziness, anxiety, eczema, pruritus, abdominal cramps, myalgia, arthralgia, cough, rhinorrhea, dyspnea

Overdosage/Toxicology

Likely symptoms of overdose include those associated with fluid overload

Treatment is supportive (eg, diuretics)

Drug Interactions

Decreased toxicity: Antibodies present in IVIG preparations may interfere with the immune response to live virus vaccines (eg, MMR); reimmunization is recommended if such vaccines are administered within 10 months following RSV-IVIG treatment; additionally, it is advised that booster doses of oral polio, DPT, and HIB be considered 3-4 months after the last dose of RSV-IVIG in order to ensure immunity

Stability Store between 2°C and 8°C; do not freeze or shake vial; avoid foaming; discard after single use since it is preservative free

Mechanism of Action RSV-IGIV is a sterile liquid immunoglobulin G containing neutralizing antibody to respiratory syncytial virus. It is effective in reducing the incidence and duration of RSV hospitalization and the severity of RSV illness in high risk infants.

Usual Dosage I.V.: 750 mg/kg/month according to the following infusion schedule:

1.5 mL/kg/hour for 15 minutes, then at 3 mL/kg/hour for the next 15 minutes if the clinical condition does not contraindicate a higher rate, and finally, administer at 6 mL/kg/hour until completion of dose

(Continued)

Respiratory Syncytial Virus Immune Globulin (Intravenous) *(Continued)*

Monitoring Parameters Monitor for symptoms of allergic reaction; check vital signs, cardiopulmonary status after each rate increase and thereafter at 30-minute intervals until 30 minutes following completion of the infusion

Nursing Implications Begin infusion within 6 hours and complete within 12 hours after entering vial. Observe for signs of intolerance during and after infusion; administer through an I.V. line using a constant infusion pump and through a separate I.V. line, if possible; begin infusion within 6 hours and complete within 12 hours after entering the vial; if needed, RSV-IGIV may be "piggy-backed" into dextrose with or without saline solutions, avoiding dilutions >2:1 with such line configurations. Filters are not necessary, but an in-line filter with a pore size >15 micrometers may be used.

Monitor vital signs frequently; adverse reactions may be related to the rate of administration; RSV-IGIV is made from human plasma and carries the possibility for transmission of blood-borne pathogenic agents

Additional Information Each vial contains 1-1.5 mEq sodium

Dosage Forms Injection: 2500 mg RSV immunoglobulin/50 mL vial

Selected Readings

American Academy of Pediatrics Committee on Infectious Diseases, Committee on Fetus and Newborn, "Respiratory Syncytial Virus Immune Globulin Intravenous: Indications for Use," *Pediatrics*, 1997, 99(4):645-50.

Ellenberg SS, Epstein JS, Fratantoni JC, et al, "A Trial of RSV Immune Globulin in Infants and Young Children: The FDA's View," *N Engl J Med*, 1994, 331(3):203-5.

Groothuis JR, Simoes EA, Levin MJ, et al, "Prophylactic Administration of Respiratory Syncytial Virus Immune Globulin to High-Risk Infants and Young Children. The Respiratory Syncytial Virus Immune Globulin Study Group," *N Engl J Med*, 1993, 329(21):1524-30.

Ottolini MG and Hemming VG, "Prevention and Treatment Recommendations for Respiratory Syncytial Virus Infection. Background and Clinical Experience 40 Years After Discovery," *Drugs*, 1997, 54(6):867-84.

"Prevention of Respiratory Syncytial Virus Infections: Indications for the Use of Palivizumab and Update on the Use of RSV-IGIV. American Academy of Pediatrics Committee on Infectious Diseases and Committee of Fetus and Newborn," *Pediatrics*, 1998, 102(5):1211-6.

Simoes EA, Sondheimer HM, Top FH Jr, et al, "Respiratory Syncytial Virus Immune Globulin for Prophylaxis Against Respiratory Syncytial Virus Disease in Infants and Children With Congential Heart Disease. The Cardiac Study Group," *J Pediatr*, 1998, 133(4):492-9.

Wandstrat TL, "Respiratory Syncytial Virus Immune Globulin Intravenous," *Ann Pharmacother*, 1997, 31(1):83-8.

Retrovir® *see* Zidovudine *on page 977*

Reverse Transcriptase Inhibitors
Refer to

Delavirdine *on page 700*
Didanosine *on page 704*
Lamivudine *on page 793*
Nevirapine *on page 839*
Stavudine *on page 923*
Zalcitabine *on page 974*
Zidovudine *on page 977*
Zidovudine and Lamivudine *on page 979*

Rh$_o$(D) Immune Globulin (ar aych oh (dee) i MYUN GLOB yoo lin)

U.S. Brand Names Gamulin® Rh; HypRho®-D; HypRho®-D Mini-Dose; MICRhoGAM™; Mini-Gamulin® Rh; RhoGAM™

Generic Available No

Use Prevention of isoimmunization in Rh-negative individuals exposed to Rh-positive blood during delivery of an Rh-positive infant, as a result of an abortion, following amniocentesis or abdominal trauma, or following a transfusion accident; prevention of hemolytic disease of the newborn if there is a subsequent pregnancy with an Rh-positive fetus

Pregnancy Risk Factor C

Contraindications Rh$_o$(D)-positive patient; known hypersensitivity to immune globulins or to thimerosal; transfusion of Rh$_o$(D)-positive blood in previous 3 months; prior sensitization to Rh$_o$(D)

Warnings/Precautions Use with caution in patients with thrombocytopenia or bleeding disorders, patients with IgA deficiency; do not inject I.V.; do not administer to neonates

Adverse Reactions <1%: Lethargy, splenomegaly, elevated bilirubin, pain at the injection site, myalgia, temperature elevation

Stability Reconstituted solution should be refrigerated and will remain stable for 30 days; solution that have been frozen should be discarded

Mechanism of Action Suppresses the immune response and antibody formation of Rh-negative individuals to Rh-positive red blood cells

Pharmacodynamics/Kinetics

Distribution: Appears in breast milk; however, not absorbed by the nursing infant

Half-life: 23-26 days

Usual Dosage Adults (administered I.M. to mothers **not** to infant) I.M.:

Obstetrical usage: 1 vial (300 mcg) prevents maternal sensitization if fetal packed red blood cell volume that has entered the circulation is <15 mL; if it is more, give additional vials. The number of vials = RBC volume of the calculated fetomaternal hemorrhage divided by 15 mL.

Postpartum prophylaxis: 300 mcg within 72 hours of delivery

Antepartum prophylaxis: 300 mcg at approximately 26-28 weeks gestation; followed by 300 mcg within 72 hours of delivery if infant is Rh-positive

Following miscarriage, abortion, or termination of ectopic pregnancy at up to 13 weeks of gestation: 50 mcg ideally within 3 hours, but may be given up to 72 hours after; if pregnancy has been terminated at 13 or more weeks of gestation, administer 300 mcg

Administration Administer I.M. in deltoid muscle; do **not** administer I.V.; the total volume can be given in divided doses at different sites at one time or may be divided and given at intervals, provided the total dosage is given within 72 hours of the fetomaternal hemorrhage or transfusion.

Patient Information Acetaminophen may be taken to ease minor discomfort after vaccination

Dosage Forms

Injection: Each package contains one single dose 300 mcg of Rh_o (D) immune globulin

Injection, microdose: Each package contains one single dose of microdose, 50 mcg of Rh_o (D) immune globulin

Selected Readings

Hartwell EA, "Use of Rh Immune Globulin: ASCP Practice Parameter. American Society of Clinical Pathologists," *Am J Clin Pathol*, 1998, 110(3):281-92.

"Rh_o(D) Immune Globulin I.V. for Prevention of Rh Isoimmunization and for Treatment of ITP," *Med Lett Drugs Ther*, 1996, 38(966):6-8.

Simpson KN, Coughlin CM, Eron J, et al, "Idiopathic Thrombocytopenia Purpura: Treatment Patterns and an Analysis of Cost Associated With Intravenous Immunoglobulin and Anti-D Therapy," *Semin Hematol*, 1998, 35(1 Suppl 1):58-64.

Ware RE and Zimmerman SA, "Anti-D: Mechanisms of Action," *Semin Hematol*, 1998, 35(1 Suppl 1):14-22.

Rh_o(D) Immune Globulin (Intravenous-Human)

(ar aych oh (dee) i MYUN GLOB yoo lin in tra VEE nus HYU man)

U.S. Brand Names WinRho SD®

Synonyms RholGIV

Use

Prevention of Rh isoimmunization in nonsensitized Rh_o(D) antigen-negative women within 72 hours after spontaneous or induced abortion, amniocentesis, chorionic villus sampling, ruptured tubal pregnancy, abdominal trauma, transplacental hemorrhage, or in the normal course of pregnancy unless the blood type of the fetus or father is known to be Rh_o(D) antigen-negative.

Suppression of Rh isoimmunization in Rh_o(D) antigen-negative female children and female adults in their childbearing years transfused with Rh_o(D) antigen-positive RBCs or blood components containing Rh_o(D) antigen-positive RBCs

Treatment of immune thrombocytopenic purpura (ITP) in nonsplenectomized Rh_o(D) antigen-positive patients

Pregnancy Risk Factor C

Contraindications Hypersensitivity to immune globulin or any component, IgA deficiency

Warnings/Precautions Anaphylactic hypersensitivity reactions can occur; studies indicate that there is no discernible risk of transmitting HIV or hepatitis B; do not administer by S.C. route; use only the I.V. route when treating ITP

(Continued)

Rh$_o$(D) Immune Globulin (Intravenous-Human)
(Continued)

Adverse Reactions 1% to 10%:

Central nervous system: Headache (2%), fever (1%), chills (<2%)

Hematologic: Hemolysis (hemoglobin decreased >2 g/dL in 5% to 10% of ITP patients)

Local: Slight edema and pain at the injection site

Overdosage/Toxicology

No symptoms are likely, however, high doses have been associated with a mild, transient hemolytic anemia

Treatment is supportive

Drug Interactions Increased toxicity: Live virus, vaccines (measles, mumps, rubella); do not administer within 3 months after administration of these vaccines

Stability Store at 2°C to 8°C; do not freeze; if not used immediately, store the product at room temperature for 4 hours; do not freeze the reconstituted product; use within 4 hours; discard unused portions

Mechanism of Action The Rh$_o$(D) antigen is responsible for most cases of Rh sensitization, which occurs when Rh-positive fetal RBCs enter the maternal circulation of an Rh-negative woman. Injection of anti-D globulin results in opsonization of the fetal RBCs, which are then phagocytized in the spleen, preventing immunization of the mother. Injection of anti-D into an Rh-positive patient with ITP coats the patient's own D-positive RBCs with antibody and, as they are cleared by the spleen, they saturate the capacity of the spleen to clear antibody-coated cells, sparing antibody-coated platelets. Other proposed mechanisms involve the generation of cytokines following the interaction between antibody-coated RBCs and macrophages.

Pharmacodynamics/Kinetics

Time to peak serum concentration: I.V.: 2 hours; I.M.: 5-10 days

Half-life: I.V.: 24 days; I.M.: 30 days

Usual Dosage

Prevention of Rh isoimmunization: I.V.: 1500 units (300 mcg) at 28 weeks gestation or immediately after amniocentesis if before 34 weeks gestation or after chorionic villus sampling; repeat this dose every 12 weeks during the pregnancy. Administer 600 units (120 mcg) at delivery (within 72 hours) and after invasive intrauterine procedures such as abortion, amniocentesis, or any other manipulation if at >34 weeks gestation. **Note:** If the Rh status of the baby is not known at 72 hours, administer Rh$_o$(D) immune globulin to the mother at 72 hours after delivery. If >72 hours have elapsed, do not withhold Rh$_o$(D) immune globulin, but administer as soon as possible, up to 28 days after delivery.

I.M.: Reconstitute vial with 1.25 mL and administer as above

Transfusion: Administer within 72 hours after exposure for treatment of incompatible blood transfusions or massive fetal hemorrhage as follows:

I.V.: 3000 units (600 mcg) every 8 hours until the total dose is administered (45 units [9 mcg] of Rh-positive blood/mL blood; 90 units [18 mcg] Rh-positive red cells/mL cells)

I.M.: 6000 units [1200 mcg] every 12 hours until the total dose is administered (60 units [12 mcg] of Rh-positive blood/mL blood; 120 units [24 mcg] Rh-positive red cells/mL cells)

Treatment of ITP: I.V.: Initial: 25-50 mcg/kg depending on the patient's hemoglobin concentration; maintenance: 25-60 mcg/kg depending on the clinical response

Administration The product should not be shaken when reconstituting or transporting; reconstitute the product shortly before use with NS, according to the manufacturer's guidelines; do not administer with other products

Nursing Implications Increasing the time of infusion from 1-3 minutes to 15-20 minutes may also help; pretreatment with acetaminophen, diphenhydramine, or prednisone can prevent the fever/chill reaction

Additional Information Rh$_o$(D) is IgA-depleted and is unlikely to cause an anaphylactic reaction in women with IgA deficiency and anti-IgA antibodies. Although immune globulins for I.M. use, manufactured in the U.S. have never been found to transmit any viral infection, Rh$_o$(D) is the only Rh$_o$(D) preparation treated with highly effective solvent detergent method of viral inactivation for hepatitis C, HIV, and hepatitis B; treatment of ITP in Rh-positive patients with an intact spleen appears to be about as effective as IVIG.

Dosage Forms Injection: 600 units [120 mcg], 1500 units [300 mcg] with 2.5 mL diluent

Selected Readings

Freiberg A and Mauger D, "Efficacy, Safety, and Dose Response of Intravenous Anti-D Immune Globulin (WinRho SDF) for the Treatment of Idiopathic Thrombocytopenic Purpura in Children," *Semin Hematol*, 1998, 35(1 Suppl 1):23-7.

Hartwell EA, "Use of Rh Immune Globulin: ASCP Practice Parameter. American Society of Clinical Pathologists," *Am J Clin Pathol*, 1998, 110(3):281-92.

Hong F, Ruiz R, Price H, et al, "Safety Profile of WinRho Anti-D," *Semin Hematol*, 1998, 35(1 Suppl 1):9-13.

Simpson KN, Coughlin CM, Eron J, et al, "Idiopathic Thrombocytopenia Purpura: Treatment Patterns and an Analysis of Cost Associated With Intravenous Immunoglobulin and Anti-D Therapy," *Semin Hematol*, 1998, 35(1 Suppl 1):58-64.

Ware RE and Zimmerman SA, "Anti-D: Mechanisms of Action," *Semin Hematol*, 1998, 35(1 Suppl 1):14-22.

RhoGAM™ *see* Rh$_o$(D) Immune Globulin *on page 896*

RholGIV *see* Rh$_o$(D) Immune Globulin (Intravenous-Human) *on page 897*

Ribavirin (rye ba VYE rin)

U.S. Brand Names Rebetol®; Virazole® Aerosol

Synonyms RTCA; Tribavirin

Generic Available No

Use Inhalation: Treatment of patients with respiratory syncytial virus (RSV) infections; may also be used in other viral infections including influenza A and B and adenovirus; specially indicated for treatment of severe lower respiratory tract RSV infections in patients with an underlying compromising condition (prematurity, bronchopulmonary dysplasia and other chronic lung conditions, congenital heart disease, immunodeficiency, immunosuppression), and recent transplant recipients

Oral capsules: The combination therapy of oral ribavirin with interferon alfa-2b, recombinant (Intron® A) injection is indicated for the treatment of chronic hepatitis C in patients with compensated liver disease who have relapsed after alpha interferon therapy.

Drug of Choice or Alternative for

Organism(s)

Respiratory Syncytial Virus *on page 239*

Pregnancy Risk Factor X

Contraindications Females of childbearing age; hypersensitivity to ribavirin; patients with autoimmune hepatitis

Warnings/Precautions Use with caution in patients requiring assisted ventilation because precipitation of the drug in the respiratory equipment may interfere with safe and effective patient ventilation; monitor carefully in patients with COPD and asthma for deterioration of respiratory function. Ribavirin is potentially mutagenic, tumor-promoting, and gonadotoxic. Anemia has been observed in patients receiving the interferon/ribavirin combination. Severe psychiatric events have also occurred including depression and suicidal behavior during combination therapy; avoid use in patients with a psychiatric history.

Adverse Reactions

Inhalation:

1% to 10%:

Central nervous system: Fatigue, headache, insomnia

Gastrointestinal: Nausea, anorexia

Hematologic: Anemia

<1%: Hypotension, cardiac arrest, digitalis toxicity, rash, skin irritation, conjunctivitis, mild bronchospasm, worsening of respiratory function, apnea

Note: Incidence of adverse effects in healthcare workers approximate 51% headache; 32% conjunctivitis; 10% to 20% rhinitis, nausea, rash, dizziness, pharyngitis, and lacrimation

Oral: (All adverse reactions are documented while receiving combination therapy with interferon alpha-2b)

>10%:

Cardiovascular: Chest pain

Central nervous system: Dizziness, headache, fatigue, fever, insomnia, irritability, depression, emotional lability, impaired concentration

Dermatologic: Alopecia, rash, pruritus

(Continued)

Ribavirin *(Continued)*

   Gastrointestinal: Nausea, anorexia, dyspepsia, vomiting
   Hematologic: Decreased hemoglobin and WBC
   Neuromuscular & skeletal: Myalgia, arthralgia, musculoskeletal pain, asternia, rigors
   Respiratory: Dyspnea, sinusitis
   Miscellaneous: Flu-like syndrome

   1% to 10%:
   Central nervous system: Nervousness
   Endocrine & metabolic: Thyroid function test abnormalities
   Gastrointestinal: Taste perversion

Drug Interactions Decreased effect of zidovudine

Stability Do not use any water containing an antimicrobial agent to reconstitute drug; reconstituted solution is stable for 24 hours at room temperature

Mechanism of Action Inhibits replication of RNA and DNA viruses; inhibits influenza virus RNA polymerase activity and inhibits the initiation and elongation of RNA fragments resulting in inhibition of viral protein synthesis

Pharmacodynamics/Kinetics

   Absorption: Absorbed systemically from the respiratory tract following nasal and oral inhalation; absorption is dependent upon respiratory factors and method of drug delivery; maximal absorption occurs with the use of the aerosol generator via an endotracheal tube; highest concentrations are found in the respiratory tract and erythrocytes

   Metabolism: Occurs intracellularly and may be necessary for drug action

   Half-life, plasma:
   Children: 6.5-11 hours
   Adults: 24 hours, much longer in the erythrocyte (16-40 days), which can be used as a marker for intracellular metabolism

   Time to peak serum concentration: Inhalation: Within 60-90 minutes

   Elimination: Hepatic metabolism is major route of elimination with 40% of the drug cleared renally as unchanged drug and metabolites

Usual Dosage Infants, Children, and Adults:

   Aerosol inhalation: Use with Viratek® small particle aerosol generator (SPAG-2) at a concentration of 20 mg/mL (6 g reconstituted with 300 mL of sterile water without preservatives)

   Aerosol only: 12-18 hours/day for 3 days, up to 7 days in length

Monitoring Parameters Respiratory function, CBC, reticulocyte count, I & O

Patient Information Do not use if pregnant.

Nursing Implications Keep accurate I & O record, discard solutions placed in the SPAG-2 unit at least every 24 hours and before adding additional fluid; healthcare workers who are pregnant or who may become pregnant should be advised of the potential risks of exposure and counseled about risk reduction strategies including alternate job responsibilities; ribavirin may adsorb to contact lenses

Dosage Forms

   Capsule: 200 mg; available only in Rebetron™ combination package
   Powder for aerosol: 6 g (100 mL)

Selected Readings

Davis GL, Esteban-Mur R, Rustgi V, et al, "Interferon Alfa-2b Alone or in Combination With Ribavirin for the Treatment of Relapse of Chronic Hepatitis C. International Hepatitis Interventional Therapy Group," *N Engl J Med*, 1998, 339(21):1493-9.

"Drugs for Non-HIV Viral Infections," *Med Lett Drugs Ther*, 1994, 36(919):27.

Keating MR, "Antiviral Agents," *Mayo Clin Proc*, 1992, 67(2):160-78.

McHutchison JG, Gordon SC, Schiff ER, et al, "Interferon Alfa-2b Alone or in Combination With Ribavirin as Initial Treatment for Chronic Hepatitis C. Hepatitis Interventional Therapy Group," *N Engl J Med*, 1998, 339(21):1485-92.

Ottolini MG and Hemming VG, "Prevention and Treatment Recommendations for Respiratory Syncytial Virus Infection. Background and Clinical Experience 40 Years After Discovery," *Drugs*, 1997, 54(6):867-84.

RID® Shampoo [OTC] *see* Pyrethrins *on page 885*

Rifabutin *(rif a BYOO tin)*

U.S. Brand Names Mycobutin®

Synonyms Ansamycin

Use Prevention of disseminated *Mycobacterium avium* complex (MAC) in patients with advanced HIV infection; also utilized in multiple drug regimens for treatment of MAC

Drug of Choice or Alternative for

Organism(s)

Mycobacterium avium-intracellulare on page 201

Pregnancy Risk Factor B

Contraindications Hypersensitivity to rifabutin or any other rifamycins; rifabutin is contraindicated in patients with a WBC <1000/mm^3 or a platelet count <50,000/mm^3; concurrent use with ritonavir

Warnings/Precautions Rifabutin as a single agent must not be administered to patients with active tuberculosis since its use may lead to the development of tuberculosis that is resistant to both rifabutin and rifampin; rifabutin should be discontinued in patients with AST >500 units/L or if total bilirubin is >3 mg/dL. Use with caution in patients with liver impairment; modification of dosage should be considered in patients with renal impairment.

Adverse Reactions

>10%:

Dermatologic: Rash (11%)

Genitourinary: Discolored urine (30%)

Hematologic: Neutropenia (25%), leukopenia (17%)

1% to 10%:

Central nervous system: Headache (3%)

Gastrointestinal: Nausea (6%), vomiting (1%), vomiting/nausea (3%), abdominal pain (4%), diarrhea (3%), anorexia (2%), flatulence (2%), eructation (3%)

Hematologic: Anemia, thrombocytopenia (5%)

Hepatic: Increased AST and ALT (7% to 9%)

Neuromuscular & skeletal: Myalgia

<1%: Chest pain, fever, insomnia, dyspepsia, taste perversion, uveitis

Overdosage/Toxicology

Symptoms of overdose include nausea, vomiting, hepatotoxicity, lethargy, CNS depression

Treatment is supportive; hemodialysis will remove rifabutin, its effect on outcome is unknown

Drug Interactions CYP3A3/4 enzyme inducer

Decreased plasma concentration (due to induction of liver enzymes) of verapamil, methadone, digoxin, cyclosporine, corticosteroids, oral anticoagulants, theophylline, barbiturates, chloramphenicol, ketoconazole, oral contraceptives, quinidine, halothane, protease inhibitors, non-nucleoside reverse transcriptase inhibitors, and perhaps clarithromycin

Increased concentration by indinavir; reduce to one-half standard dose when used with indinavir

Increased risk of rifabutin-induced hematologic and ocular toxicity (uveitis) with concurrent administration of drug that inhibits CYP450 enzymes such as protease inhibitors, erythromycin, clarithromycin, ketoconazole, and itraconazole

Mechanism of Action Inhibits DNA-dependent RNA polymerase at the beta subunit which prevents chain initiation

Pharmacodynamics/Kinetics

Absorption: Oral: Readily absorbed 53%

Distribution: V_d: 9.32 L/kg; distributes to body tissues including the lungs, liver, spleen, eyes, and kidneys

Protein binding: 85%

Metabolism: To active and inactive metabolites

Bioavailability: Absolute, 20% in HIV patients

Half life, terminal: 45 hours (range: 16-69 hours)

Peak serum level: Within 2-4 hours

Elimination: Renal and biliary clearance of unchanged drugs is 10%; 30% excreted in feces; 53% in urine as metabolites

Usual Dosage Oral:

Children: Efficacy and safety of rifabutin have not been established in children; a limited number of HIV-positive children with MAC have been given rifabutin for MAC prophylaxis; doses of 5 mg/kg once daily have been useful

(Continued)

Rifabutin *(Continued)*

Adults: 300 mg once daily; for patients who experience gastrointestinal upset, rifabutin can be administered 150 mg twice daily with food

Monitoring Parameters Periodic liver function tests, CBC with differential, platelet count

Patient Information May discolor urine, tears, sweat, or other body fluids to a red-orange color; take 1 hour before or 2 hours after a meal on an empty stomach; soft contact lenses may be permanently stained; report to physician any severe or persistent flu-like symptoms, nausea, vomiting, dark urine or pale stools, unusual bleeding or bruising, or any eye problems; can be taken with meals or sprinkled on applesauce

Dosage Forms Capsule: 150 mg

Selected Readings

Agins BD, Berman DS, Spicehandler D, et al, "Effect of Combined Therapy with Ansamycin, Clofazimine, Ethambutol, and Isoniazid for *Mycobacterium avium* Infection in Patients With AIDS," *J Infect Dis*, 1989, 159(4):784-7.

"Drugs for AIDS and Associated Infections," *Med Lett Drugs Ther*, 1993, 35(904):79-86.

Hoy J, Mijch A, Sandland M, et al, "Quadruple-Drug Therapy for *Mycobacterium avium-intracellulare* Bacteremia in AIDS Patients," *J Infect Dis*, 1990, 161(4):801-5.

Nightingale SD, Cameron DW, Gordin FM, et al, "Two Controlled Trials of Rifabutin Prophylaxis Against *Mycobacterium avium* Complex Infection in AIDS," *N Engl J Med*, 1993, 329(12):828-33.

Tseng AL and Walmsley SL, "Rifabutin-Associated Uveitis," *Ann Pharmacother*, 1995, 29(11):1149-55.

Rifadin® *see* Rifampin *on this page*

Rifadin® Injection *see* Rifampin *on this page*

Rifadin® Oral *see* Rifampin *on this page*

Rifamate® *see* Rifampin and Isoniazid *on page 905*

Rifampicin *see* Rifampin *on this page*

Rifampin *(RIF am pin)*

Related Information

Antimicrobial Activity Against Selected Organisms *on page 983*
Tuberculosis Guidelines *on page 1114*

U.S. Brand Names Rifadin® Injection; Rifadin® Oral; Rimactane® Oral

Canadian Brand Names Rifadin®; Rimactane®; Rofact™

Synonyms Rifampicin

Generic Available Yes

Use Management of active tuberculosis in combination with other agents; eliminate meningococci from asymptomatic carriers; prophylaxis of *Haemophilus influenzae* type b infection; used in combination with other anti-infectives in the treatment of staphylococcal infections

Drug of Choice or Alternative for

Organism(s)

Brucella Species *on page 85*
Legionella pneumophila *on page 185*
Mycobacterium bovis *on page 203*
Mycobacterium kansasii *on page 204*
Mycobacterium tuberculosis *on page 207*
Rhodococcus Species *on page 242*
Staphylococcus aureus, Methicillin-Resistant *on page 256*
Staphylococcus epidermidis, Methicillin-Resistant *on page 261*
Streptococcus pneumoniae, Drug-Resistant *on page 270*

Pregnancy Risk Factor C

Pregnancy/Breast-Feeding Implications Clinical effects on the fetus: Teratogenicity has occurred in rodents given may times the adult human dose

Contraindications Hypersensitivity to any rifamycins or any component

Warnings/Precautions Use with caution and modify dosage in patients with liver impairment; observe for hyperbilirubinemia; discontinue therapy if this in conjunction with clinical symptoms or any signs of significant hepatocellular damage develop; since rifampin has enzyme-inducing properties, porphyria exacerbation is possible; use with caution in patients with porphyria; do not use for meningococcal disease, only for short-term treatment of asymptomatic carrier states

Monitor for compliance and effects including hypersensitivity, decreased thrombocytopenia in patients on intermittent therapy; urine, feces, saliva, sweat, tears, and CSF may be discolored to red/orange; do not administer I.V. form via I.M. or S.C. routes; restart infusion at another site if extravasation occurs; remove soft contact lenses during therapy since permanent staining may occur; regimens of 600 mg once or twice weekly have been associated with a high incidence of adverse reactions including a flu-like syndrome

Adverse Reactions

Percentage unknown: Flushing, edema headache, drowsiness, dizziness, confusion, numbness, behavioral changes, pruritus, urticaria, pemphigoid reaction, eosinophilia, leukopenia, hemolysis, hemolytic anemia, thrombocytopenia (especially with high-dose therapy), hepatitis (rare), ataxia, myalgia, weakness, osteomalacia, visual changes, exudative conjunctivitis

1% to 10%:

Dermatologic: Rash (1% to 5%)

Gastrointestinal: (1% to 2%): Epigastric distress, anorexia, nausea, vomiting, diarrhea, cramps, pseudomembranous colitis, pancreatitis

Hepatic: Increased LFTs (up to 14%)

Overdosage/Toxicology

Symptoms of overdose include nausea, vomiting, hepatotoxicity

Treatment is supportive; lavage with activated charcoal is preferred to ipecac as emesis is frequently present with overdose; hemodialysis will remove rifampin, its effect on outcome is unknown

Drug Interactions CYP3A3/4 enzyme substrate; CYP1A2, 2C9, 3A3/4, and 3A5-7 enzyme inducer

Decreased effect: Rifampin induces liver enzymes which may decrease the plasma concentration of calcium channel blockers (verapamil, diltiazem, nifedipine), methadone, digitalis, cyclosporine, corticosteroids, oral anticoagulants, haloperidol, theophylline, barbiturates, chloramphenicol, imidazole antifungals, oral or systemic hormonal contraceptives, acetaminophen, benzodiazepines, hydantoins, sulfa drugs, enalapril, beta-blockers, chloramphenicol, clofibrate, dapsone, antiarrhythmics (disopyramide, mexiletine, quinidine, tocainide), diazepam, doxycycline, fluoroquinolones, levothyroxine, nortriptyline, progestins, tacrolimus, zidovudine, protease inhibitors, and non-nucleoside reverse transcriptase inhibitors.

Coadministration with INH or halothane may result in additive hepatotoxicity; probenecid and co-trimoxazole may increase rifampin levels while antacids may decrease its absorption

Stability Rifampin powder is reddish brown. Intact vials should be stored at room temperature and protected from excessive heat and light. Reconstituted vials are stable for 24 hours at room temperature

Stability of parenteral admixture at room temperature (25°C) is 4 hours for D_5W and 24 hours for NS

Mechanism of Action Inhibits bacterial RNA synthesis by binding to the beta subunit of DNA-dependent RNA polymerase, blocking RNA transcription

Pharmacodynamics/Kinetics

Absorption: Oral: Well absorbed

Time to peak serum concentration: Oral: 2-4 hours and persisting for up to 24 hours; food may delay or slightly reduce

Distribution: Crosses the blood-brain barrier well

Relative diffusion of antimicrobial agents from blood into cerebrospinal fluid (CSF): Adequate with or without inflammation (exceeds usual MICs)

Ratio of CSF to blood level (%):

Inflamed meninges: 25

Protein binding: 80%

Metabolism: Highly lipophilic; metabolized in the liver, undergoes enterohepatic recycling

Half-life: 3-4 hours, prolonged with hepatic impairment

End stage renal disease: 1.8-11 hours

Elimination: Undergoes enterohepatic recycling; principally excreted unchanged in the feces (60% to 65%) and urine (~30%); excreted unchanged: 15% to 30%; plasma rifampin concentrations are not significantly affected by hemodialysis or peritoneal dialysis

Usual Dosage Oral (I.V. infusion dose is the same as for the oral route):

Tuberculosis therapy:

Note: A four-drug regimen (isoniazid, rifampin, pyrazinamide, and either streptomycin or ethambutol) is preferred for the initial, empiric treatment of TB. (Continued)

Rifampin *(Continued)*

When the drug susceptibility results are available, the regimen should be altered as appropriate.

Infants and Children <12 years:

Daily therapy: 10-20 mg/kg/day usually as a single dose (maximum: 600 mg/day)

Directly observed therapy (DOT): Twice weekly: 10-20 mg/kg (maximum: 600 mg); 3 times/week: 10-20 mg/kg (maximum: 600 mg)

Adults:

Daily therapy: 10 mg/kg/day (maximum: 600 mg/day)

Directly observed therapy (DOT): Twice weekly: 10 mg/kg (maximum: 600 mg); 3 times/week: 10 mg/kg (maximum: 600 mg)

H. influenzae prophylaxis:

Infants and Children: 20 mg/kg/day every 24 hours for 4 days, not to exceed 600 mg/dose

Adults: 600 mg every 24 hours for 4 days

Meningococcal prophylaxis:

<1 month: 10 mg/kg/day in divided doses every 12 hours for 2 days

Infants and Children: 20 mg/kg/day in divided doses every 12 hours for 2 days

Adults: 600 mg every 12 hours for 2 days

Nasal carriers of *Staphylococcus aureus*:

Children: 15 mg/kg/day divided every 12 hours for 5-10 days in combination with other antibiotics

Adults: 600 mg/day for 5-10 days in combination with other antibiotics

Synergy for *Staphylococcus aureus* infections: Adults: 300-600 mg twice daily with other antibiotics

Dosing adjustment in hepatic impairment: Dose reductions may be necessary to reduce hepatotoxicity

Dietary Considerations Food: Rifampin is best taken on an empty stomach since food decreases the extent of absorption

Administration Administer on an empty stomach (ie, 1 hour prior to, or 2 hours after meals or antacids) to increase total absorption

Monitoring Parameters Periodic (baseline and every 2-4 weeks during therapy) monitoring of liver function (AST, ALT, bilirubin BSD), CBC; hepatic status and mental status, sputum culture, chest x-ray 2-3 months into treatment

Test Interactions Positive direct Coombs' test, rifampin inhibits standard assay's ability to measure serum folate and B$_{12}$, transient increase in LFTs and decreased biliary excretion of contrast media

Patient Information May discolor urine, tears, sweat, or other body fluids to a red-orange color; take 1 hour before or 2 hours after a meal on an empty stomach; soft contact lenses may be permanently stained; report to physician any severe or persistent flu-like symptoms, nausea, vomiting, dark urine or pale stools, or unusual bleeding or bruising; utilize an alternate form from oral/other systemic contraceptives during therapy; compliance and completion with course of therapy is very important; if you are a diabetic taking oral medications or if you regularly take oral anticoagulant therapy, your medication may need special and careful adjustment.

Dosage Forms

Capsule: 150 mg, 300 mg

Injection: 600 mg

Extemporaneous Preparations For pediatric and adult patients with difficulty swallowing or where lower doses are needed, the package insert lists an extemporaneous liquid suspension as follows:

Rifampin 1% w/v suspension (10 mg/mL) can be compounded using one of four syrups (Syrup NF, simple syrup, Syrpalta® syrup, or raspberry syrup)

Empty contents of four 300 mg capsules or eight 150 mg capsules onto a piece of weighing paper

If necessary, crush contents to produce a fine powder

Transfer powder blend to a 4 oz amber glass or plastic prescription bottle

Rinse paper and spatula with 20 mL of syrup and add the rinse to bottle; shake vigorously

Add 100 mL of syrup to the bottle and shake vigorously

This compounding procedure results in a 1% w/v suspension containing 10 mg rifampin/mL; stability studies indicate suspension is stable at room temperature (25°C ±3°C) or in refrigerator (2°C to 8°C) for 4 weeks; shake well prior to administration

Selected Readings

Davidson PT and Le HQ, "Drug Treatment of Tuberculosis - 1992," *Drugs*, 1992, 43(5):651-73.

"Drugs for Tuberculosis," *Med Lett Drugs Ther*, 1993, 35(908):99-101.

Havlir DV and Barnes PF, "Tuberculosis in Patients With Human Immunodeficiency Virus Infection," *N Engl J Med*, 1999, 340(5):367-73.

Iseman MD, "Treatment of Multidrug-Resistant Tuberculosis," *N Engl J Med*, 1993, 329(11):784-91.

Lundstrom TS and Sobel JD, "Vancomycin, Trimethoprim-Sulfamethoxazole, and Rifampin," *Infect Dis Clin North Am*, 1995, 9(3):747-67.

"Prevention and Treatment of Tuberculosis Among Patients Infected With Human Immunodeficiency Virus: Principles of Therapy and Revised Recommendations. Centers for Disease Control and Prevention," *MMWR Morb Mortal Wkly Rep*, 1998, 47(RR-20):1-58.

Van Scoy RE and Wilkowske CJ, "Antituberculosis Agents," *Mayo Clin Proc*, 1992, 67(2):179-87.

Vesely JJ, Pien FD, and Pien BC, "Rifampin, a Useful Drug for Nonmycobacterial Infections," *Pharmacotherapy*, 1998, 18(2):345-57.

Rifampin and Isoniazid (RIF am pin & eye soe NYE a zid)

Related Information

Isoniazid *on page 782*
Rifampin *on page 902*
Tuberculosis Guidelines *on page 1114*

U.S. Brand Names Rifamate®

Use Management of active tuberculosis

Drug of Choice or Alternative for Organism(s)

Mycobacterium tuberculosis on page 207

Usual Dosage Oral: 2 capsules/day

Dosage Forms Capsule: Rifampin 300 mg and isoniazid 150 mg

Rifampin, Isoniazid, and Pyrazinamide

(RIF am pin, eye soe NYE a zid, & peer a ZIN a mide)

Related Information

Isoniazid *on page 782*
Pyrazinamide *on page 884*
Rifampin *on page 902*
Tuberculosis Guidelines *on page 1114*

U.S. Brand Names Rifater®

Use Management of active tuberculosis

Dosage Forms Tablet: Rifampin 120 mg, isoniazid 50 mg, and pyrazinamide 300 mg

Rifapentine (RIF a pen teen)

U.S. Brand Names Priftin®

Use Treatment of pulmonary tuberculosis (indication is based on the 6-month follow-up treatment outcome observed in controlled clinical trial). Rifapentine must always be used in conjunction with at least one other antituberculosis drug to which the isolate is susceptible; it may also be necessary to add a third agent (either streptomycin or ethambutol) until susceptibility is known.

Pregnancy Risk Factor C

Pregnancy/Breast-Feeding Implications Has been shown to be teratogenic in rats and rabbits. Rat offspring showed cleft palates, right aortic arch, and delayed ossification and increased number of ribs. Rabbits displayed ovarian agenesis, pes varus, arhinia, microphthalmia, and irregularities of the ossified facial tissues. Rat studies also show decreased fetal weight, increased number of stillborns, and decreased gestational survival. No adequate well-controlled studies in pregnant women are available. Rifapentine should be used during pregnancy only if the potential benefits justifies the potential risk to the fetus.

Contraindications Patients with a history of hypersensitivity to rifapentine, rifampin, rifabutin, and any rifamycin analog

Warnings/Precautions Compliance with dosing regimen is absolutely necessary for successful drug therapy. patients with abnormal liver tests and/or liver disease should only be given rifapentine when absolutely necessary and under strict medical supervision. Monitoring of liver function tests should be carried out prior to therapy and then every 2-4 weeks during therapy if signs of liver disease

(Continued)

Rifapentine (Continued)

occur or worsen, rifapentine should be discontinued. Pseudomembranous colitis has been reported to occur with various antibiotics including other rifamycins. If this is suspected, rifapentine should be stopped and the patient treated with specific and supportive treatment. Experience in treating TB in HIV-infected patients is limited.

Rifapentine may produce a red-orange discoloration of body tissues/fluids including skin, teeth, tongue, urine, feces, saliva, sputum, tears, sweat, and cerebral spinal fluid. Contact lenses may become permanently stained. All patients treated with rifapentine should have baseline measurements of liver function tests and enzymes, bilirubin, and a complete blood count. patients should be seen monthly and specifically questioned regarding symptoms associated with adverse reactions. Routine laboratory monitoring in people with normal baseline measurements is generally not necessary.

Adverse Reactions

>10%: Endocrine & metabolic: Hyperuricemia (most likely due to pyrazinamide from initiation phase combination therapy)

1% to 10%:

Cardiovascular: Hypertension

Central nervous system: Headache, dizziness

Dermatologic: Rash, pruritus, acne

Gastrointestinal: Anorexia, nausea, vomiting, dyspepsia, diarrhea

Hematologic: Neutropenia, lymphopenia, anemia, leukopenia, thrombocytosis

Hepatic: Increased ALT, AST

Neuromuscular & skeletal: Arthralgia, pain

Renal: Pyuria, proteinuria, hematuria, urinary casts

Respiratory: Hemoptysis

<1%: Peripheral edema, aggressive reaction, fatigue, urticaria, skin discoloration, hyperkalemia, hypovolemia, increased alkaline phosphatase, increased LDH, constipation, esophagitis, gastritis, pancreatitis, thrombocytopenia, neutrophilia, leukocytosis, purpura, hematoma, bilirubinemia, hepatitis, gout, arthrosis

Overdosage/Toxicology There is no experience with treatment of acute overdose with rifapentine; experience with other rifamycins suggests that gastric lavage followed by activated charcoal may help adsorb any remaining drug from the GI tract. Hemodialysis or forced diuresis is not expected to enhance elimination of unchanged rifapentine in an overdose.

Drug Interactions CYP3A4 and 2C8/9 inducer. Rifapentine may increase the metabolism of coadministered drugs that are metabolized by these enzymes. Enzymes are induced within 4 days after the first dose and returned to baseline 14 days after discontinuation of rifapentine. The magnitude of enzyme induction is dose and frequency dependent. Rifampin has been shown to accelerate the metabolism and may reduce activity of the following drugs (therefore, rifapentine may also do the same): Phenytoin, disopyramide, mexiletine, quinidine, tocainide, chloramphenicol, clarithromycin, dapsone, doxycycline, fluoroquinolones, warfarin, fluconazole, itraconazole, ketoconazole, barbiturates, benzodiazepines, beta-blockers, diltiazem, nifedipine, verapamil, corticosteroids, cardiac glycoside preparations, clofibrate, oral or other systemic hormonal contraceptives, haloperidol, HIV protease inhibitors, sulfonylureas, cyclosporine, tacrolimus, levothyroxine, methadone, progestins, quinine, delavirdine, zidovudine, sildenafil, theophylline, amitriptyline, and nortriptyline.

Rifapentine should be used with extreme caution, if at all, in patients who are also taking protease inhibitors

Patients using oral or other systemic hormonal contraceptives should be advised to change to nonhormonal methods of birth control when receiving concomitant rifapentine.

Rifapentine metabolism is mediated by esterase activity, therefore, there is minimal potential for rifapentine metabolism to be affected by other drug therapy.

Stability Store at room temperature (15°C to 30°C; 59°F to 86°F); protect from excessive heat and humidity

Mechanism of Action Inhibits DNA-dependent RNA polymerase in susceptible strains of *Mycobacterium tuberculosis* (but not in mammalian cells). Rifapentine is bactericidal against both intracellular and extracellular MTB organisms. MTB resistant to other rifamycins including rifampin are likely to be resistant to rifapentine. Cross-resistance does not appear between rifapentine and other nonrifamycin antimycobacterial agents.

Pharmacodynamics/Kinetics

Absorption: Food increases AUC and C_{max} by 43% and 44% respectively.

Distribution: V_d: ~70.2 L

Metabolism: Hydrolyzed by an esterase and esterase enzyme to form the active metabolite 25-desacetyl rifapentine

Protein binding: Rifapentine and 25-desacetyl metabolite were 97.7% and 93.2% protein bound (mainly to albumin). Rifapentine and metabolite accumulate in human monocyte-derived macrophages with intracellular/extracellular ratios of 24:1 and 7:1 respectively.

Half-life: Rifapentine: 14-17 hours; 25-desacetyl rifapentine: 13 hours

Bioavailability: ~70%

Time to peak serum concentration: 5-6 hours

Elimination: Extent of renal excretion is unknown; excreted as parent drug and metabolite; 17% of administered dose is excreted via the kidneys

Usual Dosage

Children: No dosing information available

Adults: **Rifapentine should not be used alone**; initial phase should include a 3- to 4-drug regimen

Intensive phase of short-term therapy: 600 mg (four 150 mg tablets) given weekly (every 72 hours); following the intensive phase, treatment should continue with rifapentine 600 mg once weekly for 4 months in combination with INH or appropriate agent for susceptible organisms

Dosing adjustment in renal or hepatic impairment: Unknown

Dietary Considerations Food increases AUC and maximum serum concentration by 43% and 44% respectively as compared to fasting conditions

Monitoring Parameters Patients with pre-existing hepatic problems should have liver function tests monitored every 2-4 weeks during therapy

Test Interactions Rifampin has been shown to inhibit standard microbiological assays for serum folate and vitamin B_{12}; this should be considered for rifapentine; therefore, alternative assay methods should be considered.

Patient Information May produce a reddish coloration of urine, sweat, sputum, tears, and contact lenses may be permanently stained. oral or other systemic hormonal contraceptives may not be effective while taking rifapentine; alternative contraceptive measures should be used. Administration of rifapentine with food may decrease GI intolerance. Notify physician if experiencing fever, decreased appetite, malaise, nausea/vomiting, darkened urine, yellowish discoloration of skin or eyes, and pain or swelling of the joints. Adherence with the full course of therapy is essential; no doses of therapy should be missed.

Additional Information Rifapentine has only been studied in patients with tuberculosis receiving a 6-month short-course intensive regimen approval; outcomes have been based on 6-month follow-up treatment observed in clinical trial 008 as a surrogate for the 2-year follow-up generally accepted as evidence for efficacy in the treatment of pulmonary tuberculosis

Dosage Forms Tablet, film-coated: 150 mg

Selected Readings
Grosser J, Lounis N, Truffot-Pernot C, et al, "Once Weekly Rifapentine-Containing Regimens for Treatment of Tuberculosis in Mice," *Am J Respir Crit Care Med*, 1998, 157:1436-40.

Jarvis B and Lamb HM, "Rifapentine," *Drugs*, 1998, 56(4):607-16.

Keung AC, Eller MG, and Weir SJ, "Pharmacokinetics of Rifapentine in Patients With Varying Degrees of Hepatic Dysfunction," *J Clin Pharmacol*, 1998, 38:517-24.

Moghazeh SI, Pan X, Arain T, et al, "Comparative Antimycobacterial Activities of Rifampin, Rifapentine, and KRM-1648 Against a Collection of Rifampin-Resistant *Mycobacterium* Tuberculosis Isolates With Known rpoβ Mutations," *Antimicrob Agents Chemother*, 1996, 40:265-7.

Tam CM, Chan SL, Lam CW, et al, "Rifapentine and Isoniazid in the Continuation Phase of Treating Pulmonary Tuberculosis, Initial Report," *Am J Respir Crit Care Med*, 1998, 157:1726-33.

Rifater® *see* Rifampin, Isoniazid, and Pyrazinamide *on page 905*

rIFN-A *see* Interferon Alfa-2a *on page 776*

RIG *see* Rabies Immune Globulin (Human) *on page 892*

Rimactane® *see* Rifampin *on page 902*

Rimactane® Oral *see* Rifampin *on page 902*

Rimantadine (ri MAN ta deen)

U.S. Brand Names Flumadine®

Generic Available No

Use Prophylaxis (adults and children) and treatment (adults) of influenza A viral infection

Drug of Choice or Alternative for
Organism(s)
Influenza Virus *on page 181*

Pregnancy Risk Factor C

Pregnancy/Breast-Feeding Implications
Clinical effects on the fetus: Embryotoxic in high dose rat studies
Breast-feeding/lactation: Avoid use in nursing mothers due to potential adverse effect in infants; rimantadine is concentrated in milk

Contraindications Hypersensitivity to drugs of the adamantine class (rimantadine or amantadine)

Warnings/Precautions Use with caution in patients with liver disease, a history of recurrent and eczematoid dermatitis, uncontrolled psychosis or severe psychoneurosis, seizures in those receiving CNS stimulant drugs

Adverse Reactions 1% to 10%:
Cardiovascular: Orthostatic hypotension, edema
Central nervous system: Dizziness (1.9%), confusion, headache (1.4%), insomnia (2.1%), difficulty in concentrating, anxiety (1.3%), restlessness, irritability, hallucinations; incidence of CNS side effects may be less than that associated with amantadine
Gastrointestinal: Nausea (2.8%), vomiting (1.7%), xerostomia (1.5%), abdominal pain (1.4%), anorexia (1.6%)
Genitourinary: Urinary retention

Overdosage/Toxicology
Agitation, hallucinations, ventricular cardiac arrhythmias (torsade de pointes and PVCs), slurred speech, anticholinergic effects (dry mouth, urinary retention and mydriasis), ataxia, tremor, myoclonus, seizures and death have been reported with amantadine, a related drug
Treatment is symptomatic (do not use physostigmine); tachyarrhythmias may be treated with beta-blockers such as propranolol; dialysis is not recommended except possibly in renal failure

Drug Interactions
Acetaminophen: Reduction in AUC and peak concentration of rimantadine
Aspirin: Peak plasma and AUC concentrations of rimantadine are reduced
Cimetidine: Rimantadine clearance is decreased (~16%)

Mechanism of Action Blocks the uncoating of influenza A virus preventing penetration of virus into host and inhibiting viral growth

Pharmacodynamics/Kinetics
Absorption: Oral: Well absorbed
Metabolism: In the liver (hydroxylation and conjugation)
Half-life: 13-65 kg: 25 hours
Elimination: 25% as unchanged drug

Usual Dosage Oral:
Prophylaxis:
Children <10 years: 5 mg/kg give once daily
Children >10 years and Adults: 100 mg twice daily

Treatment: Adults: 100 mg twice daily

Dosing adjustment in renal impairment: Adults: Cl_{cr} <10 mL/minute: 100 mg every 24 hours
Elderly nursing home patients should receive 100 mg every 24 hours

Administration Initiation of rimantadine within 48 hours of the onset of influenza A illness halves the duration of illness and significantly reduces the duration of viral shedding and increased peripheral airways resistance; continue therapy for 5-7 days after symptoms begin

Monitoring Parameters Monitor for CNS or GI effects in elderly or patients with renal or hepatic impairment

Dosage Forms
Syrup: 50 mg/5 mL (60 mL, 240 mL, 480 mL)
Tablet: 100 mg

Selected Readings

Dolin R, Reichman RC, Madore HP, et al, "A Controlled Trial of Amantadine and Rimantadine in the Prophylaxis of Influenza A Infection," N Engl J Med, 1982, 307(10):580-4.

"Drugs for Non-HIV Viral Infections," Med Lett Drugs Ther, 1994, 36(919):27.

Keating MR, "Antiviral Agents," Mayo Clin Proc, 1992, 67(2):160-78.

Wintermeyer SM and Nahata MC, "Rimantadine: A Clinical Perspective," Ann Pharmacother, 1995, 29(3):299-310.

Ritonavir (rye TON a veer)

Related Information

HIV Therapeutic Information on page 1008

U.S. Brand Names Norvir®

Use In combination with other antiretroviral agents; treatment of HIV infection when therapy is warranted

Drug of Choice or Alternative for

Organism(s)

Human Immunodeficiency Virus on page 177

Pregnancy Risk Factor B

Pregnancy/Breast-Feeding Implications

Clinical effects on the fetus: Administer during pregnancy only if benefits to mother outweigh risks to the fetus

Breast-feeding/lactation: HIV-infected mothers are discouraged from breast-feeding to decrease postnatal transmission of HIV

Contraindicated Medications and Potential Alternatives*

Contraindicated Medications†			Potential Alternatives‡ (these alternatives may not be therapeutically equivalent)		
Drug Class	Generic Name	Brand Name	Generic Name	Brand Name	Exposed Patients
Analgesic	Meperidine	Demerol®	Acetaminophen	Tylenol®	N=135
	Piroxicam	Feldene®	Aspirin		N=43
	Propoxyphene	Darvon®	Oxycodone	Percodan®	N=23
Cardiovascular (antiarrhythmic)	Amiodarone Flecainide Propafenone Quinidine	Cordarone® Tambocor® Rythmol®	Very limited clinical experience		
Antimycobacterial	Rifabutin	Mycobutin®	Clarithromycin Ethambutol	Biaxin® Myambutol®	N=156§ N=66
Cardiovascular (calcium channel blocker)	Bepridil	Vascor®	Very limited clinical experience		
Cold and allergy (antihistamine)	Astemizole Terfenadine	Hismanal® Seldane®	Loratadine	Clarifin®	N=36
Ergot alkaloid (vasoconstrictor)	Dihydro-ergotamine Ergotamine	D.H.E. 45® various	Very limited clinical experience		
Gastrointestinal	Cisapride	Propulsid®	Very limited clinical experience		
Psychotropic (antidepressant)	Bupropion	Wellbutrin®	Desipramine	Norpramin®	¶
Psychotropic (neuroleptic)	Clozapine Pimozide	Clozaril® Orap™	Very limited clinical experience		
Psychotropic (sedative-hypnotic)	Alprazolam Clorazepate Diazepam Estazolam Flurazepam Midazolam Triazolam Zolpidem	Xanax® Tranxene® Valium® ProSom™ Dalmane® Versed® Halcion® Ambien®	Temazepam Lorazepam	Restoril® Ativan®	N=40 N=33

* During clinical trials, Norvir® was given to patients concomitantly taking a variety of medications. These medications were not evaluated in drug interaction studies. The number of Norvir®-treated patients exposed to each drug is provided in the last column.

† See Contraindications in the drug monograph.

‡ See Warnings/Precautions and Drug Interactions in the drug monograph.

§ Also evaluated in drug interaction study (N=22). See Results of Drug Interaction Studies table.

¶ No clinical experience with combination. Only evaluated in drug interaction study (N=14). See Results of Drug Interaction Studies table.

(Continued)

Ritonavir *(Continued)*

Contraindications Patients with known hypersensitivity to ritonavir or any ingredients; see contraindicated medications table on previous page

Warnings/Precautions Use caution in patients with hepatic insufficiency; safety and efficacy have not been established in children <16 years of age; use caution with benzodiazepines, antiarrhythmics (flecainide, encainide, bepridil, amiodarone, quinidine) and certain analgesics (meperidine, piroxicam, propoxyphene)

Results of Drug Interaction Studies

Co-administered Drug	Finding
Amiodarone	Increased risk of amiodarone toxicity, including cardiotoxicity
Astemizole	Increased risk of toxicity
Benzodiazepines	Increased risk of prolonged sedation and respiratory depression
Bepridil	Increased risk of bepridil toxicity, including cardiotoxicity
Bupropion	Increased risk of bupropion toxicity, including seizures
Cisapride	Increased risk of cardiotoxicity
Clarithromycin	77% increase in clarithromycin AUC; no dosage reduction is necessary in patients with normal renal function; for patients with Cl_{cr} from 30-60 mL/minute, decrease dose by 50%; for patients with Cl_{cr}<30 mL/minute, decrease dose by 75%
Clozapine	Increased risk of clozapine toxicity, including agranulocytosis, EKG changes, and seizures
Desipramine	145% increase in desipramine AUC; dosage reduction should be considered
Didanosine (ddL)	13% decrease in didanosine AUC; no dosage adjustment is necessary
Ethinyl estradiol	40% decrease in ethinyl estradiol AUC; increase ethinyl estradiol dose or substitute with another contraceptive
Flecainide	Increased risk of flecainide toxicity, including cardiotoxicity
Fluconazole	15% increase in ritonavir AUC
Meperidine	Increased risk of meperidine toxicity, including CNS side effects, seizures, and cardiac arrhythmias
Nevirapine	Efficacy of ritonavir may be decreased
Piroxicam	Increased risk of piroxicam
Propafenone	Increased risk of propafenone, including cardiotoxicity
Propoxyphene	Increased risk of propoxyphene toxicity, including respiratory depression
Quinidine	Increased risk of quinidine toxicity, including cardiotoxicity
Rifabutin	Efficacy of ritonavir may be decreased while the risk of rifabutin-induced hematologic toxicity may be increased
Saquinavir	Greater than 20-fold increase in saquinavir AUC
Sulfamethoxazole	20% decrease is sulfamethoxazole AUC; no dosage adjustment is necessary
Terfenadine	Increased risk of cardiotoxicity
Theophylline	43% decrease in theophylline AUC; increase in theophylline dose may be required
Zidovudine (AZT)	25% decrease in zidovudine AUC; no dosage adjustment is necessary
Zolpidem	Increased risk of prolonged sedation and respiratory depression

Adverse Reactions Protease inhibitors cause dyslipidemia which includes elevated cholesterol and triglycerides and a redistribution of body fat centrally to cause "protease paunch", buffalo hump, facial atrophy, and breast enlargement. These agents also cause hyperglycemia.

>10%:

Gastrointestinal: Diarrhea, nausea, vomiting, taste perversion
Endocrine & metabolic: Increased triglycerides
Hematologic: Anemia, leukopenia
Hepatic: Increased GGT

Neuromuscular & skeletal: Weakness

1% to 10%:

Cardiovascular: Vasodilation

Central nervous system: Fever, headache, malaise, dizziness, insomnia, somnolence, thinking abnormally

Dermatologic: Rash

Endocrine & metabolic: Hyperlipidemia, increased uric acid, glucose, potassium, calcium

Gastrointestinal: Abdominal pain, anorexia, constipation, dyspepsia, flatulence, local throat irritation

Hematologic: Neutropenia, eosinophilia, neutrophilia, leukocytosis, prolonged PT

Hepatic: Increased LFTs

Neuromuscular & skeletal: Increased CPK, myalgia, paresthesia

Respiratory: Pharyngitis

Miscellaneous: Diaphoresis

Overdosage/Toxicology Human experience is limited; there is no specific antidote for overdose with ritonavir. Dialysis is unlikely to be beneficial in significant removal of the drug. Charcoal or gastric lavage may be useful to remove unabsorbed drug.

Drug Interactions CYP1A2, 2A6, 2C9, 2C19, 2E1, and 3A3/4 enzyme substrate, CYP2D6 enzyme substrate (minor); CYP1A2 and 2D6 enzyme inducer; CYP2A6, 2C9, 1A2, 2C19, 2D6, 2E1, and 3A3/4 inhibitor

Ritonavir may significantly increase the AUC of the following drugs: Alfentanil, fentanyl, methadone, lidocaine, erythromycin, carbamazepine, nefazodone, sertraline, itraconazole, ketoconazole, miconazole, loratadine, quinine, amlodipine, diltiazem, felodipine, isradipine, nicardipine, nifedipine, nimodipine, nisoldipine, nitrendipine, verapamil, tamoxifen, bromocriptine, indinavir, fluvastatin, lovastatin, simvastatin, cyclosporine, tacrolimus, dexamethasone

Stability Store both capsules and oral solution in refrigerator (36°F to 46°F; 2°C to 80°C); may be left out at room temperature if used within 30 days

Mechanism of Action Ritonavir inhibits HIV protease and renders the enzyme incapable of processing of polyprotein precursor which leads to production of noninfectious immature HIV particles

Pharmacodynamics/Kinetics

Absorption: Variable, with or without food

Distribution: High concentrations are produced in serum and lymph nodes

Protein binding: 98% to 99%

Metabolism: Hepatic; 5 metabolites, low concentration of an active metabolite achieved in plasma (oxidative); see Drug Interactions

Half-life: 3-5 hours

Elimination: Renal clearance is negligible

Usual Dosage Oral:

Children: 250 mg/m² twice daily; titrate dose upward to 400 mg/m² twice daily (maximum: 600 mg twice daily)

Adults: 600 mg twice daily; dose escalation tends to avoid nausea that many patients experience upon initiation of full dosing. Escalate the dose as follows: 300 mg twice daily for 1 day, 400 mg twice daily for 2 days, 500 mg twice daily for 1 day, then 600 mg twice daily. Ritonavir may be better tolerated when used in combination with other antiretrovirals by initiating the drug alone and subsequently adding the second agent within 2 weeks.

If used in combination with saquinavir, dose is 400 mg twice daily

Dosing adjustment in renal impairment: None necessary

Dosing adjustment in hepatic impairment: Not determined; caution advised with severe impairment

Monitoring Parameters Triglycerides, cholesterol, LFTs, CPK, uric acid, glucose, basic HIV monitoring, viral load, and CD4 count

Patient Information Take with food, if possible; many drugs interact with ritonavir, consult with physician or pharmacist before adding any drug therapy including over-the-counter medications. Ritonavir is not a cure for HIV infection; long-term effects of ritonavir are unknown at this time. Taste of oral ritonavir solution may be enhanced by mixing with chocolate milk, Ensure®, or Advera®. Refrigeration is necessary for both capsules and solution.

(Continued)

Ritonavir *(Continued)*

Additional Information Potential compliance problems, frequency of administration and adverse effects should be discussed with patients before initiating therapy to help prevent the emergence of resistance.

Dosage Forms
Capsule: 100 mg
Solution, oral: 80 mg/mL (240 mL)

Selected Readings
Deeks SG, Smith M, Holodniy M, et al, "HIV-1 Protease Inhibitors. A Review for Clinicians," *JAMA*, 1997, 277(2):145-53.

Hsu A, Granneman GR, Cao G, et al, "Pharmacokinetic Interactions Between Two Human Immunodeficiency Virus Protease Inhibitors, Ritonavir and Saquinavir," *Clin Pharmacol Ther*, 1998, 63(4):453-64.

Kakuda TN, Struble KA, and Piscitelli SC, "Protease Inhibitors for the Treatment of Human Immunodeficiency Virus Infection," *Am J Health Syst Pharm*, 1998, 55(3):233-54.

Kaul DR, Cinti SK, Carver PL, et al, "HIV Protease Inhibitors: Advances in Therapy and Adverse Reactions, Including Metabolic Complications," *Pharmacotherapy*, 1999, 19(3):281-98.

Lea AP and Faulds D, "Ritonavir," *Drugs*, 1996, 52(4):541-6.

McDonald CK and Kuritzkes DR, "Human Immunodeficiency Virus Type 1 Protease Inhibitors," *Arch Intern Med*, 1997, 157(9):951-9.

rLFN-α2 *see Interferon Alfa-2b on page 778*

Robicillin® VK *see Penicillin V Potassium on page 865*

Rocephin® *see Ceftriaxone on page 655*

Rofact™ *see Rifampin on page 902*

Roferon-A® *see Interferon Alfa-2a on page 776*

RotaShield® *see Rotavirus Vaccine on this page*

Rotavirus Vaccine (RO ta vye rus vak SEEN)

U.S. Brand Names RotaShield®

Use Prevention of gastroenteritis caused by the rotavirus serotypes responsible for the majority of disease in infants and children in the U.S. (serotypes G 1, 2, 3, and 4)

Pregnancy Risk Factor C

Contraindications Known hypersensitivity to any component of the vaccine (due to the method of preparation, rotavirus vaccine may include small amounts of an aminoglycoside antibiotic, monosodium glutamate, and amphotericin B). Contraindicated in patients with ongoing diarrhea or vomiting.

Immunocompromised patients may shed virus for prolonged periods. RotaShield® is contraindicated in patients with known or suspected immune deficiency states, or in patients receiving therapy with agents which may compromise immune function (alkylating agents, antimetabolites, radiation, or high-dose systemic corticosteroids). Use of steroids when administered topically, via inhalation aerosol, or by intra-articular, tendon, or bursal injection does not contraindicate therapy. Although antibodies to rotavirus may be present in breast milk, there is no evidence that the efficacy of the rotavirus vaccine is diminished when administered to breast-fed infants.

Warnings/Precautions Vaccine administration may be delayed due to current or recent severe to moderate febrile illness. Minor illness with or without low-grade fever is not generally a contraindication. Do not administer parenterally. Do not administer to immunocompromised infants. Administer with caution to patients with possible latex allergy. Close association with immunosuppressed or other high-risk individuals should be avoided whenever possible for up to 4 weeks after administration. Data concerning administration to premature infants are insufficient to establish safety or efficacy. Prior to administration, the physician should take all known precautions for prevention of allergic or other reactions. A careful history for possible sensitivity should be taken and agents to control immediate allergic reactions, including epinephrine (1:1000), should be readily available.

Adverse Reactions
>10%: Central nervous system: Fever (>38°C to <39°C) (11% to 21%), decreased appetite (11% to 17%), irritability (36% to 41%), decreased activity (10% to 20%)

1% to 10%: Central nervous system: Fever (≥39°C) (1% to 2%)

The incidence of fever is greater when administered to infants >6 months of age. The highest incidence of adverse effects was associated with the first dose of the vaccine. By the third dose, there were no significant differences in the incidence of adverse effects between vaccine and placebo.

Drug Interactions No drug interactions have been reported. No data have been reported with respect to administration of orally or intravenously administered immune globulin-containing products.

Stability Store lyophilized vaccine at room temperature below 25°C. Lyophilized vaccine (and diluent) may be refrigerated. Reconstituted vaccine is stable for 60 minutes at room temperature and 4 hours under refrigeration.

Mechanism of Action The live virus vaccine stimulates production of IgG and IgA antibodies which cross-react with human serotypes. The four serotypes which cause the majority of infections in humans are neutralized by these antibodies.

Usual Dosage For oral administration only

Children: Three 2.5 mL doses are administered. The recommended schedule for immunization is at 2, 4, and 6 months of age. The first dose may be administered as early as 6 weeks of age, with subsequent doses at least 3 weeks apart. The third dose has been administered to infants up to 33 weeks of age with no increase in adverse reactions. Initiation of vaccination after the age of 6 months is not currently recommended due to an increased risk of fever. RotaShield® does not diminish the efficacy of OPV, DTP, or Hib when administered concurrently. Repeat dosing of vaccine is not recommended if an infant should regurgitate a dose.

Adults: Not approved for administration to adults

Administration Reconstitute lyophilized vaccine by adding diluent from Dispette®, then withdraw reconstituted solution back into Dispette® (may reuse cap to store until administration). Must be administered within 60 minutes of reconstitution if stored at room temperature, or within 4 hours of reconstitution if refrigerated. Place tip of Dispette® into the infant's mouth and slowly squeeze out contents.

Test Interactions A positive stool test for rotavirus may occur for at least one week after administration due to the presence of vaccine virus

Patient Information Parents must be instructed as to the importance of completing the vaccination sequence

Dosage Forms Powder, lyophilized, for oral solution: 2.5 mL diluent (Dispette®); specialized diluent contains citric acid and sodium bicarbonate

Selected Readings

Bernstein DI, Smith VE, Sherwood JR, et al, "Safety and Immunogenicity of Live, Attenuated Human Rotavirus Vaccine 89-12," *Vaccine*, 1998, 16(4):381-7.

Joensuu J, Koskenniemi E, Pang XL, et al, "Randomised Placebo-Controlled Trial of Rhesus-Human Reassortant Rotavirus Vaccine for Prevention of Severe Rotavirus Gastroenteritis," *Lancet*, 1997, 350(9086):1205-9.

Joensuu J, Koskenniemi E, and Vesikari T, "Prolonged Efficacy of Rhesus-Human Reassortant Rotavirus Vaccine," *Ped Inf Dis J*, 1998, 17(5):427-9.

Perez-Schael I, Guntinas MJ, Perez M, et al, "Efficacy of Rhesus Rotavirus Based Quadrivalent Vaccine in Infants and Young Children in Venezuela," *N Engl J Med*, 1997, 337(17):1181-7.

Tucker AW, Haddix AC, Bresee JS, et al, "Cost-Effectiveness Analysis of a Rotavirus Immunization Program for the United States," *JAMA*, 1998, 279(17):1371-6.

Vazquez J, Boher Y, Perez M, et al, "Immune Response to Three Doses of the Quadrivalent Rotavirus Vaccine: 1-Year Follow-up," *Vaccine*, 1998, 16(11-12):1179-83.

Ward RL, Dinsmore AM, Goldberg G, et al, "Shedding of Rotavirus After Administration of the Tetravalent Rhesus Rotavirus Vaccine," *Ped Inf Dis J*, 1998, 17(5):386-90.

Roubac® *see* Co-Trimoxazole *on page 692*

RP59500 *see* Quinupristin/Dalfopristin *on page 891*

RSV-IGIV *see* Respiratory Syncytial Virus Immune Globulin (Intravenous) *on page 895*

RTCA *see* Ribavirin *on page 899*

Rubella and Measles Vaccines, Combined *see* Measles and Rubella Vaccines, Combined *on page 804*

Rubella and Mumps Vaccines, Combined
(rue BEL a & mumpz vak SEENS, kom BINED)

U.S. Brand Names Biavax®II

Generic Available No

Use Promote active immunity to rubella and mumps by inducing production of antibodies

(Continued)

Rubella and Mumps Vaccines, Combined *(Continued)*

Note: Routine vaccination with trivalent MMR is recommended by ACIP as children enter kindergarten or first grade. AAP recommends a routine second vaccination as children enter into middle or junior high school.

Pregnancy Risk Factor C

Pregnancy/Breast-Feeding Implications Women who are pregnant when vaccinated or who become pregnant within 3 months of vaccination should be counseled on the theoretical risks to the fetus. The risk of rubella-associated malformations in these women is so small as to be negligible. MMR is the vaccine of choice if recipients are likely to be susceptible to measles or mumps as well as to rubella.

Contraindications Known hypersensitivity to neomycin, eggs; children <1 year, pregnant women, primary immunodeficient patients, patients receiving immunosuppressant drugs except corticosteroids

Warnings/Precautions Women planning on becoming pregnant in the next 3 months should not be vaccinated

Adverse Reactions All serious adverse reactions must be reported to the U.S. Department of Health and Human Services (DHHS) Vaccine Adverse Event Reporting System (VAERS) 1-800-822-7967.

>10%:
    Dermatologic: Local tenderness and erythema, urticaria, rash
    Neuromuscular & skeletal: Arthralgia
1% to 10%:
    Central nervous system: Malaise, moderate fever, headache
    Gastrointestinal: Sore throat
    Miscellaneous: Lymphadenopathy
<1%: High fever (>103°F), encephalitis, polyneuropathy, erythema multiforme, optic neuritis, hypersensitivity, allergic reactions to the vaccine

Drug Interactions Whole blood, interferon immune globulin, radiation therapy, and immunosuppressive drugs (eg, corticosteroids) may result in insufficient response to immunization; may temporarily depress tuberculin skin test sensitivity and reduce the seroconversion. DTP, OPV, MMR, Hib, and hepatitis B may be given concurrently; other virus vaccine administration should be separated by ≥1 month.

Stability Refrigerate, discard unused portion within 8 hours, protect from light

Usual Dosage Children >12 months (preferably at 15 months) and Adults: 1 vial (0.5 mL) in outer aspect of the upper arm; children vaccinated before 12 months of age should be revaccinated

Administration Administer S.C. only

Test Interactions Temporary suppression of TB skin test

Patient Information Patient may experience burning or stinging at the injection site; joint pain usually occurs 1-10 weeks after vaccination and persists 1-3 days

Nursing Implications Children immunized before 12 months of age should be reimmunized

Additional Information Federal law requires that the date of administration, the vaccine manufacturer, lot number of vaccine, and the administering person's name, title and address be entered into the patient's permanent medical record

Dosage Forms Injection (mixture of 2 viruses):
1. Wistar RA 27/3 strain of rubella virus
2. Jeryl Lynn (B level) mumps strain grown cell cultures of chick embryo

Rubella, Measles and Mumps Vaccines, Combined *see* Measles, Mumps, and Rubella Vaccines, Combined *on page 805*

Rubella Virus Vaccine, Live *(rue BEL a VYE rus vak SEEN, live)*

U.S. Brand Names Meruvax® II

Synonyms German Measles Vaccine

Generic Available No

Use Selective active immunization against rubella; vaccination is routinely recommended for persons from 12 months of age to puberty. All adults, both male and female, lacking documentation of live vaccine on or after first birthday, or laboratory evidence of immunity (particularly women of childbearing age and young adults who work in or congregate in hospitals, colleges, and on military bases) should be vaccinated. Susceptible travelers should be vaccinated.

Note: Trivalent measles - mumps - rubella (MMR) vaccine is the preferred immunizing agent for most children and many adults.

Pregnancy Risk Factor C

Pregnancy/Breast-Feeding Implications Women who are pregnant when vaccinated or who become pregnant within 3 months of vaccination should be counseled on the theoretical risks to the fetus. The risk of rubella-associated malformations in these women is so small as to be negligible. MMR is the vaccine of choice if recipients are likely to be susceptible to measles or mumps as well as to rubella.

Warnings/Precautions Pregnancy, immunocompromised persons, history of anaphylactic reaction following receipt of neomycin; do not administer with other live vaccines

Adverse Reactions All serious adverse reactions must be reported to the U.S. Department of Health and Human Services (DHHS) Vaccine Adverse Event Reporting System (VAERS) 1-800-822-7967.

>10%:
 Dermatologic: Local tenderness and erythema
 Neuromuscular & skeletal: Arthralgia
1% to 10%:
 Central nervous system: Malaise, moderate fever, headache
 Dermatologic: Rash, urticaria
 Gastrointestinal: Sore throat
 Miscellaneous: Lymphadenopathy
<1%: High fever (>103°F), encephalitis, polyneuropathy, erythema multiforme, optic neuritis, hypersensitivity, allergic reactions to the vaccine

Drug Interactions Whole blood, interferon immune globulin, radiation therapy, and immunosuppressive drugs (eg, corticosteroids) may result in insufficient response to immunization; may temporarily depress tuberculin skin test sensitivity and reduce the seroconversion. DTP, OPV, MMR, Hib, and hepatitis B may be given concurrently; other virus vaccine administration should be separated by ≥1 month from measles.

Stability Refrigerate, discard reconstituted vaccine after 8 hours; store at 2°C to 8°C (36°F to 46°F); ship vaccine at 10°C; may use dry ice, protect from light

Mechanism of Action Rubella vaccine is a live attenuated vaccine that contains the Wistar Institute RA 27/3 strain, which is adapted to and propagated in human diploid cell culture. Promotes active immunity by inducing rubella hemagglutination-inhibiting antibodies.

Pharmacodynamics/Kinetics Onset of effect: Antibodies to the vaccine are detectable within 2-4 weeks following immunization

Usual Dosage Children ≥12 months and Adults: S.C.: 0.5 mL in outer aspect of upper arm; children vaccinated before 12 months of age should be revaccinated

Test Interactions May depress tuberculin skin test sensitivity

Patient Information Patient may experience burning or stinging at the injection site; joint pain usually occurs 1-10 weeks after vaccination and persists 1-3 days

Nursing Implications Reconstituted vaccine should be used within 8 hours; S.C. injection only

Additional Information Live virus vaccine; federal law requires that the date of administration, the vaccine manufacturer, lot number of vaccine, and the administering person's name, title and address be entered into the patient's permanent record

Dosage Forms Injection, single dose: 1000 $TCID_{50}$ (Wistar RA 27/3 Strain)

Rubeola Vaccine see Measles Virus Vaccine, Live, Attenuated on page 807

Sabin Vaccine see Poliovirus Vaccine, Live, Trivalent, Oral on page 876

Salk Vaccine see Poliovirus Vaccine, Inactivated on page 875

Sandoglobulin® see Immune Globulin, Intravenous on page 771

Saquinavir (sa KWIN a veer)
Related Information
 HIV Therapeutic Information on page 1008
 U.S. Brand Names Fortovase®; Invirase®
 Synonyms Saquinavir Mesylate
 Use Treatment of HIV infection in selected patients; used in combination with at least two other antiretroviral agents
 (Continued)

Saquinavir *(Continued)*

Drug of Choice or Alternative for
Organism(s)
Human Immunodeficiency Virus *on page 177*

Pregnancy Risk Factor B

Pregnancy/Breast-Feeding Implications
Clinical effects on the fetus: Administer saquinavir during pregnancy only if benefits to the mother outweigh the risk to the fetus

Breast-feeding/lactation: HIV-infected mothers are discouraged from breast-feeding to decrease postnatal transmission of HIV

Contraindications Hypersensitivity to saquinavir or any components; exposure to direct sunlight without sunscreen or protective clothing; coadministration with terfenadine, cisapride, astemizole, triazolam, midazolam, or ergot derivatives

Warnings/Precautions The indication for saquinavir for the treatment of HIV infection is based on changes in surrogate markers. At present, there are no results from controlled clinical trials evaluating its effect on patient survival or the clinical progression of HIV infection (ie, occurrence of opportunistic infections or malignancies); use caution in patients with hepatic insufficiency; safety and efficacy have not been established in children <16 years of age; may exacerbate pre-existing hepatic dysfunction; use with caution in patients with hepatitis B or C and in cirrhosis

Adverse Reactions Protease inhibitors cause dyslipidemia which includes elevated cholesterol and triglycerides and a redistribution of body fat centrally to cause "protease paunch", buffalo hump, facial atrophy, and breast enlargement. These agents also cause hyperglycemia.

1% to 10%:

Dermatologic: Rash

Endocrine & metabolic: Hyperglycemia

Gastrointestinal: Diarrhea, abdominal discomfort, nausea, abdominal pain, buccal mucosa, ulceration

Neuromuscular & skeletal: Paresthesia, weakness, increased CPK

<1%: Headache, confusion, seizures, ataxia, pain, Stevens-Johnson syndrome, hypoglycemia, hyper- and hypokalemia, low serum amylase, upper quadrant abdominal pain, acute myeloblastic leukemia, hemolytic anemia, thrombocytopenia, jaundice, thrombophlebitis, ascites, bullous skin eruption, polyarthritis, portal hypertension, exacerbation of chronic liver disease, increased LFTs; altered AST, ALT, bilirubin, hemoglobin

Drug Interactions CYP3A3/4 enzyme substrate; CYP3A3/4 enzyme inhibitor

Decreased effect: Rifampin may decrease saquinavir's plasma levels and AUC by 40% to 80%; other enzyme inducers may induce saquinavir's metabolism (eg, phenobarbital, phenytoin, dexamethasone, carbamazepine); may decrease delavirdine concentrations

Increased effect: Ketoconazole significantly increases plasma levels and AUC of saquinavir; as a known, although not potent inhibitor of the cytochrome P-450 system, saquinavir may decrease the metabolism of terfenadine and astemizole, as well as cisapride, ergot derivatives, midazolam, and triazolam (and result in rare but serious effects including cardiac arrhythmias); other drugs which may have increased adverse effects if coadministered with saquinavir include calcium channel blockers, clindamycin, dapsone, and quinidine. Both clarithromycin and saquinavir levels/effects may be increased with coadministration. Delavirdine may increase concentration; ritonavir may increase AUC >17-fold; concurrent administration of nelfinavir results in increase in nelfinavir (18%) and saquinavir (mean: 392%).

Mechanism of Action As an inhibitor of HIV protease, saquinavir prevents the cleavage of viral polyprotein precursors which are needed to generate functional proteins in and maturation of HIV-infected cells

Pharmacodynamics/Kinetics
Absorption: Poor, increased with high fat meal. Fortovase® has improved absorption over Invirase®

Distribution: V_d: 700 L; does not distribute into CSF

Protein binding: ~98% bound to plasma proteins

Metabolism: Widely metabolized undergoing extensive first pass metabolism

Bioavailability: ~4% (Invirase®); 12% to 15% (Fortovase®)

Usual Dosage Adults: Oral:

Fortovase®: Six 200 mg capsules (1200 mg) 3 times/day within 2 hours after a meal in combination with a nucleoside analog

Invirase®: Three 200 mg capsules (600 mg) 3 times/day within 2 hours after a full meal in combination with a nucleoside analog

Dose of either Fortovase® or Invirase® in combination with ritonavir: 400 mg twice daily

Monitoring Parameters Monitor viral load, CD4 count, triglycerides, cholesterol, glucose

Patient Information Saquinavir is not a cure for HIV infection nor has it been found to reduce the transmission of HIV; opportunistic infections and other illnesses associated with AIDS may still occur; take saquinavir within 2 hours after a full meal; avoid direct sunlight when taking saquinavir

Nursing Implications Observe for signs of opportunistic infections and other illnesses associated with HIV; administer on a full stomach, if possible

Additional Information The indication for saquinavir for the treatment of HIV infection is based on changes in surrogate markers. At present, there are no results from controlled clinical trials evaluating the effect of regimens containing saquinavir on patient survival or the clinical progression of HIV infection, such as the occurrence of opportunistic infections or malignancies; in cell culture, saquinavir is additive to synergistic with AZT, ddC, and DDI without enhanced toxicity. According to the manufacturer, Invirase® will be phased out over time and completely replaced by Fortovase®. Potential compliance problems, frequency of administration and adverse effects should be discussed with patients before initiating therapy to help prevent the emergence of resistance.

Dosage Forms

Capsule (hard) as mesylate (Invirase®): 200 mg

Capsule (soft) (Fortovase®): 200 mg

Selected Readings

Deeks SG, Smith M, Holodniy M, et al, "HIV-1 Protease Inhibitors. A Review for Clinicians," *JAMA*, 1997, 277(2):145-53.

Hsu A, Granneman GR, Cao G, et al, "Pharmacokinetic Interactions Between Two Human Immuno-deficiency Virus Protease Inhibitors, Ritonavir and Saquinavir," *Clin Pharmacol Ther*, 1998, 63(4):453-64.

Kakuda TN, Struble KA, and Piscitelli SC, "Protease Inhibitors for the Treatment of Human Immuno-deficiency Virus Infection," *Am J Health Syst Pharm*, 1998, 55(3):233-54.

Kaul DR, Cinti SK, Carver PL, et al, "HIV Protease Inhibitors: Advances in Therapy and Adverse Reactions, Including Metabolic Complications," *Pharmacotherapy*, 1999, 19(3):281-98.

McDonald CK and Kuritzkes DR, "Human Immunodeficiency Virus Type 1 Protease Inhibitors," *Arch Intern Med*, 1997, 157(9):951-9.

Noble S and Faulds D, "Saquinavir: A Review of Its Pharmacology and Clinical Potential in the Management of HIV Infection," *Drugs*, 1996, 52(1):93-112.

Perry CM and Noble S, "Saquinavir Soft-Gel Capsule Formulation. A Review of Its Use in Patients With HIV Infection," *Drugs*, 1998, 55(3):461-86.

Vella S and Floridia M, "Saquinavir. Clinical Pharmacology and Efficacy," *Clin Pharmacokinet*, 1998, 34(3):189-201.

Saquinavir Mesylate see Saquinavir on page 915

Scabene® see Lindane on page 797

Sclavo-PPD Solution® see Tuberculin Tests on page 962

Sclavo Test-PPD® see Tuberculin Tests on page 962

Sebizon® Topical Lotion see Sulfacetamide Sodium on page 927

Selenium Sulfide (se LEE nee um SUL fide)

U.S. Brand Names Exsel®; Head & Shoulders® Intensive Treatment [OTC]; Selsun®; Selsun Blue® [OTC]; Selsun Gold® for Women [OTC]

Generic Available Yes

Use Treatment of itching and flaking of the scalp associated with dandruff, to control scalp seborrheic dermatitis; treatment of tinea versicolor

Drug of Choice or Alternative for

Organism(s)

Malassezia furfur on page 192

Pregnancy Risk Factor C

Contraindications Known hypersensitivity to selenium or any component

Warnings/Precautions Do not use on damaged skin to avoid any systemic toxicity; avoid topical use in very young children; safety of topical in infants has not been established

Adverse Reactions

>10%: Dermatologic: Unusual dryness or oiliness of scalp

(Continued)

Selenium Sulfide *(Continued)*

1% to 10%:
Central nervous system: Lethargy
Dermatologic: Alopecia or hair discoloration
Gastrointestinal: Vomiting following long-term use on damaged skin, abdominal pain, garlic breath
Local: Irritation
Neuromuscular & skeletal: Tremor
Miscellaneous: Diaphoresis

Overdosage/Toxicology Symptoms of overdose include nausea, vomiting, diarrhea

Mechanism of Action May block the enzymes involved in growth of epithelial tissue

Pharmacodynamics/Kinetics
Absorption: Topical: Not absorbed through intact skin, but can be absorbed through damaged skin
Elimination: Urine, feces, lungs, skin

Usual Dosage Topical:
Dandruff, seborrhea: Massage 5-10 mL into wet scalp, leave on scalp 2-3 minutes, rinse thoroughly, and repeat application; shampoo twice weekly for 2 weeks initially, then use once every 1-4 weeks as indicated depending upon control
Tinea versicolor: Apply the 2.5% lotion to affected area and lather with small amounts of water; leave on skin for 10 minutes, then rinse thoroughly; apply every day for 7 days

Patient Information Topical formulations are for external use only; notify physician if condition persists or worsens; avoid contact with eyes; thoroughly rinse after application

Dosage Forms
Lotion: 2.5% (120 mL)
Shampoo: 1% (120 mL, 210 mL, 240 mL, 330 mL); 2.5% (120 mL)

Selsun® *see* Selenium Sulfide *on previous page*

Selsun Blue® [OTC] *see* Selenium Sulfide *on previous page*

Selsun Gold® for Women [OTC] *see* Selenium Sulfide *on previous page*

Septa® Topical Ointment [OTC] *see* Bacitracin, Neomycin, and Polymyxin B *on page 619*

Septra® *see* Co-Trimoxazole *on page 692*

Septra® DS *see* Co-Trimoxazole *on page 692*

Seromycin® Pulvules® *see* Cycloserine *on page 696*

Serostim® Injection *see* Human Growth Hormone *on page 764*

Silvadene® *see* Silver Sulfadiazine *on next page*

Silver Nitrate *(SIL ver NYE trate)*

U.S. Brand Names Dey-Drop® Ophthalmic Solution

Synonyms $AgNO_3$

Generic Available Yes

Use Prevention of gonococcal ophthalmia neonatorum; cauterization of wounds and sluggish ulcers, removal of granulation tissue and warts; aseptic prophylaxis of burns

Pregnancy Risk Factor C

Contraindications Not for use on broken skin or cuts; hypersensitivity to silver nitrate or any component

Warnings/Precautions Do not use applicator sticks on the eyes; repeated applications of the ophthalmic solution into the eye can cause cauterization of the cornea and blindness

Adverse Reactions
>10%:
Dermatologic: Burning and skin irritation
Ocular: Chemical conjunctivitis
1% to 10%:
Dermatologic: Staining of the skin
Hematologic: Methemoglobinemia
Ocular: Cauterization of the cornea, blindness

Overdosage/Toxicology

Symptoms of overdose include pain and burning of mouth, salivation, vomiting, diarrhea, shock, coma, convulsions, death; blackening of skin and mucous membranes; absorbed nitrate can cause methemoglobinemia

Fatal dose is as low as 2 g

Administer sodium chloride in water (10 g/L) to cause precipitation of silver

Drug Interactions Decreased effect: Sulfacetamide preparations are incompatible

Stability Must be stored in a dry place; exposure to light causes silver to oxidize and turn brown, dipping in water causes oxidized film to readily dissolve

Mechanism of Action Free silver ions precipitate bacterial proteins by combining with chloride in tissue forming silver chloride; coagulates cellular protein to form an eschar; silver ions or salts or colloidal silver preparations can inhibit the growth of both gram-positive and gram-negative bacteria. This germicidal action is attributed to the precipitation of bacterial proteins by liberated silver ions. Silver nitrate coagulates cellular protein to form an eschar, and this mode of action is the postulated mechanism for control of benign hematuria, rhinitis, and recurrent pneumothorax.

Pharmacodynamics/Kinetics

Absorption: Because silver ions readily combine with protein, there is minimal GI and cutaneous absorption of the 0.5% and 1% preparations

Elimination: Although the highest amounts of silver noted on autopsy have been in the kidneys, excretion in urine is minimal

Usual Dosage

Neonates: Ophthalmic: Instill 2 drops immediately after birth (no later than 1 hour after delivery) into conjunctival sac of each eye as a single dose, allow to sit for ≥30 seconds; do not irrigate eyes following instillation of eye drops

Children and Adults:

Ointment: Apply in an apertured pad on affected area or lesion for approximately 5 days

Sticks: Apply to mucous membranes and other moist skin surfaces only on area to be treated 2-3 times/week for 2-3 weeks

Topical solution: Apply a cotton applicator dipped in solution on the affected area 2-3 times/week for 2-3 weeks

Monitoring Parameters With prolonged use, monitor methemoglobin levels

Patient Information Discontinue topical preparation if redness or irritation develop

Nursing Implications Silver nitrate solutions stain skin and utensils

Additional Information Applicators are **not** for ophthalmic use

Dosage Forms

Applicator, topical: 75% with potassium nitrate 25% (6")

Ointment, topical: 10% (30 g)

Solution:

Ophthalmic: 1% (wax ampuls)

Topical: 10% (30 mL); 25% (30 mL); 50% (30 mL)

Selected Readings

US Department of Health and Human Services, "1993 Sexually Transmitted Diseases Treatment Guidelines," *MMWR Morb Mortal Wkly Rep*, 1993, 42(RR-14).

Silver Sulfadiazine (SIL ver sul fa DYE a zeen)

U.S. Brand Names Silvadene®; SSD™; SSD AF®; Thermazene®

Canadian Brand Names Dermazin™; Flamazine®

Generic Available No

Use Prevention and treatment of infection in second and third degree burns

Pregnancy Risk Factor B

Contraindications Hypersensitivity to silver sulfadiazine or any component; premature infants or neonates <2 months of age because sulfonamides compete with bilirubin for protein binding sites which may displace bilirubin and cause kernicterus, pregnant women approaching or at term

Warnings/Precautions Use with caution in patients with G-6-PD deficiency, renal impairment, or history of allergy to other sulfonamides; sulfadiazine may accumulate in patients with impaired hepatic or renal function; fungal superinfection may occur; use of analgesic might be needed before application; systemic absorption is significant and adverse reactions may occur

(Continued)

Silver Sulfadiazine *(Continued)*

Adverse Reactions

1% to 10%:

Dermatologic: Itching, rash, erythema multiforme, discoloration of skin
Hematologic: Hemolytic anemia, leukopenia, agranulocytosis, aplastic anemia
Hepatic: Hepatitis
Renal: Interstitial nephritis
Miscellaneous: Allergic reactions may be related to sulfa component

<1%: Photosensitivity

Drug Interactions Decreased effect: Topical proteolytic enzymes are inactivated

Stability Silvadene® cream will occasionally darken either in the jar or after application to the skin. This color change results from a light catalyzed reaction which is a common characteristic of all silver salts. A similar analogy is the oxidation of silverware. The product of this color change reaction is silver oxide which ranges in color from gray to black. Silver oxide has rarely been associated with permanent skin discoloration. Additionally, the antimicrobial activity of the product is not substantially diminished because the color change reaction involves such a small amount of the active drug and is largely a surface phenomenon.

Mechanism of Action Acts upon the bacterial cell wall and cell membrane. Bactericidal for many gram-negative and gram-positive bacteria and is effective against yeast. Active against *Pseudomonas aeruginosa, Pseudomonas maltophilia, Enterobacter* species, *Klebsiella* species, *Serratia* species, *Escherichia coli, Proteus mirabilis, Morganella morganii, Providencia rettgeri, Proteus vulgaris, Providencia* species, *Citrobacter* species, *Acinetobacter calcoaceticus, Staphylococcus aureus, Staphylococcus epidermidis, Enterococcus* species, *Candida albicans, Corynebacterium diphtheriae,* and *Clostridium perfringens*

Pharmacodynamics/Kinetics

Absorption: Significant percutaneous absorption of silver sulfadiazine can occur especially when applied to extensive burns
Half-life: 10 hours and is prolonged in patients with renal insufficiency
Time to peak serum concentration: Within 3-11 days of continuous therapy
Elimination: ~50% excreted unchanged in urine

Usual Dosage Children and Adults: Topical: Apply once or twice daily with a sterile-gloved hand; apply to a thickness of $^1/_{16}$"; burned area should be covered with cream at all times

Monitoring Parameters Serum electrolytes, urinalysis, renal function tests, CBC in patients with extensive burns on long-term treatment

Patient Information For external use only; bathe daily to aid in debridement (if not contraindicated); apply liberally to burned areas; for external use only; notify physician if condition persists or worsens

Nursing Implications Evaluate the development of granulation

Additional Information Contains methylparaben and propylene glycol

Dosage Forms Cream, topical: 1% [10 mg/g] (20 g, 50 g, 85 g, 400 g, 1000 g)

Selected Readings

Kulick MI, Wong R, Okarma TB, et al, "Prospective Study of Side Effects Associated With the Use of Silver Sulfadiazine in Severely Burned Patients," *Ann Plast Surg,* 1985, 14(5):407-18.

Lockhart SP, Rushworth A, Azmy AA, et al, "Topical Silver Sulfadiazine: Side Effects and Urinary Excretion," *Burns Incl Therm Inj,* 1983, 10(1):9-12.

Smallpox Vaccine *(SMAL poks vak SEEN)*

Use There are no indications for the use of smallpox vaccine in the general civilian population. Laboratory workers involved with Orthopoxvirus or in the production and testing of smallpox vaccines should receive regular smallpox vaccinations. For advice on vaccine administration and contraindications, contact the Division of Immunization, CDC, Atlanta, GA 30333 (404-639-3356).

Pregnancy Risk Factor X

Somatropin *see* Human Growth Hormone *on page 764*
Sopamycetin *see* Chloramphenicol *on page 667*

Sparfloxacin (spar FLOKS a sin)
U.S. Brand Names Zagam®
Use Treatment of adults with community-acquired pneumonia caused by *C. pneumoniae, H. influenzae, H. parainfluenzae, M. catarrhalis, M. pneumoniae* or *S. pneumoniae*; also for treatment of acute bacterial exacerbations of chronic bronchitis caused by *C. pneumoniae, E. cloacae, H. influenzae, H. parainfluenzae, K. pneumoniae, M. catarrhalis, S. aureus,* or *S. pneumoniae*
Drug of Choice or Alternative for
Disease/Syndrome(s)
  Pneumonia, Community-Acquired *on page 45*
Pregnancy Risk Factor C
Pregnancy/Breast-Feeding Implications
  Clinical effects on the fetus: Avoid use in pregnant women unless the benefit justifies the potential risk to the fetus
  Breast-feeding/lactation: Quinolones are known to distribute well into breast milk; consequently use during lactation should be avoided if possible
Contraindications Hypersensitivity to sparfloxacin, any component, or other quinolones; a concurrent administration with drugs which increase the Q-T interval including: amiodarone, bepridil, bretylium, disopyramide, furosemide, procainamide, quinidine, sotalol, albuterol, astemizole, chloroquine, cisapride, halofantrine, phenothiazines, prednisone, terfenadine, and tricyclic antidepressants
Warnings/Precautions Not recommended in children <18 years of age, other quinolones have caused transient arthropathy in children; CNS stimulation may occur (tremor, restlessness, confusion, and very rarely hallucinations or seizures); use with caution in patients with known or suspected CNS disorder or renal dysfunction; prolonged use may result in superinfection; if an allergic reaction (itching, urticaria, dyspnea, pharyngeal or facial edema, loss of consciousness, tingling, cardiovascular collapse) occurs, discontinue the drug immediately; use caution to avoid possible photosensitivity reactions during and for several days following fluoroquinolone therapy; pseudomembranous colitis may occur and should be considered in patients who present with diarrhea
Adverse Reactions
  >1%:
    Central nervous system: Insomnia, agitation, sleep disorders, anxiety, delirium
    Gastrointestinal: Diarrhea, abdominal pain, vomiting
    Hematologic: Leukopenia, eosinophilia, anemia
    Hepatic: Increased LFTs
  <1%: Photosensitivity, rash, myalgia, arthralgia
Overdosage/Toxicology
  Symptoms of overdose include acute renal failure, seizures
  GI decontamination and supportive care; not removed by peritoneal or hemodialysis
Drug Interactions
  Decreased effect: Decreased absorption with antacids containing aluminum, magnesium, and/or calcium and by products containing zinc and iron salts when administered concurrently; phenytoin serum levels may be reduced by quinolones; antineoplastic agents may also decrease serum levels of fluoroquinolones
  Increased toxicity/serum levels: Quinolones cause increased levels of caffeine, warfarin, cyclosporine, and theophylline (although one study indicates that sparfloxacin may not affect theophylline metabolism), cimetidine and probenecid increase quinolone levels; an increased incidence of seizures may occur with foscarnet. Avoid use with drugs which increase Q-T interval as significant risk of cardiotoxicity may occur (see listing in Warnings/Precautions)
Mechanism of Action Inhibits DNA-gyrase in susceptible organisms; inhibits relaxation of supercoiled DNA and promotes breakage of double-stranded DNA
Pharmacodynamics/Kinetics
  Absorption: Oral absorption is unaffected by food or milk but can be reduced by approximately 50% by concurrent administration of aluminum- and magnesium-containing antacids
  Distribution: Widely distributed throughout the body
  (Continued)

Sparfloxacin *(Continued)*

Metabolism: Sparfloxacin is metabolized in the liver, but does not utilize the cytochrome P-450 system

Half-life: Mean terminal half life: 20 hours (range: 16-30 hours)

Elimination: Equally excreted in both the urine and feces; ~10% of an oral dose is excreted unchanged in the urine

Usual Dosage Adults: Oral:

Loading dose: 2 tablets (400 mg) on day 1

Maintenance: 1 tablet (200 mg)/day for 10 days total therapy (total 11 tablets)

Dosing adjustment in renal impairment: Cl_{cr} <50 mL/minute: Administer 400 mg on day 1, then 200 mg every 48 hours for a total of 9 days of therapy (total 6 tablets)

Monitoring Parameters Evaluation of organ system functions (renal, hepatic, ophthalmologic, and hematopoietic) is recommended periodically during therapy; the possibility of crystalluria should be assessed; WBC and signs and symptoms of infection

Patient Information May take with or without food; drink with plenty of fluids; avoid exposure to direct sunlight during therapy and for several days following; do not take antacids within 4 hours before or 2 hours after dosing; contact your physician immediately if signs of allergy occur; do not discontinue therapy until your course has been completed; take a missed dose as soon as possible, unless it is almost time for your next dose

Dosage Forms Tablet: 200 mg

Selected Readings

Goa KL, Bryson HM, and Markham A, "Sparfloxacin. A Review of Its Antibacterial Activity, Pharmacokinetic Properties, Clinical Efficacy, and Tolerability in Lower Respiratory Tract Infections," *Drugs*, 1997, 53(4):700-25.

Martin SJ, Meyer JM, Chuck SK, et al, "Levofloxacin and Sparfloxacin: New Quinolone Antibiotics," *Ann Pharmacother*, 1998, 32(3):320-36.

"Sparfloxacin and Levofloxacin," *Med Lett Drugs Ther*, 1997, 39(999):41-3.

Stein GE and Havlichek DH, "Sparfloxacin: Potential Clinical and Economic Impact in the Treatment of Respiratory Infections," *Pharmacotherapy*, 1997, 17(6):1139-47.

Zix JA, Geerdes-Fenge HF, Rau M, et al, "Pharmacokinetics of Sparfloxacin and Interaction With Cisapride and Sucralfate," *Antimicrob Agents Chemother*, 1997, 41(8):1668-72.

Spectam® *see* Spectinomycin *on this page*

Spectazole™ Topical *see* Econazole *on page 717*

Spectinomycin *(spek ti noe MYE sin)*

U.S. Brand Names Spectam®; Trobicin®

Synonyms Spectinomycin Hydrochloride

Generic Available No

Use Treatment of uncomplicated gonorrhea

Drug of Choice or Alternative for Organism(s)

Neisseria gonorrhoeae on page 215

Pregnancy Risk Factor B

Contraindications Hypersensitivity to spectinomycin or any component

Adverse Reactions <1%: Dizziness, headache, chills, urticaria, rash, pruritus, nausea, vomiting, pain at injection site

Overdosage/Toxicology Symptoms of overdose include paresthesia, dizziness, blurring of vision, ototoxicity, renal damage, nausea, sleeplessness, decrease in hemoglobin

Stability Use reconstituted solutions within 24 hours; reconstitute with supplied diluent only

Mechanism of Action A bacteriostatic antibiotic that selectively binds to the 30s subunits of ribosomes, and thereby inhibiting bacterial protein synthesis

Pharmacodynamics/Kinetics

Absorption: I.M.: Rapid and almost completely

Distribution: Concentrates in urine; does not distribute well into the saliva

Half-life: 1.7 hours

Elimination: Excreted almost entirely as unchanged drug in urine (70% to 100%)

Usual Dosage I.M.:

Children:

<45 kg: 40 mg/kg/dose 1 time (ceftriaxone preferred)

≥45 kg: See adult dose

Children >8 years who are allergic to PCNS/cephalosporins may be treated with oral tetracycline

Adults:

Uncomplicated urethral endocervical or rectal gonorrhea: 2 g deep I.M. or 4 g where antibiotic resistance is prevalent 1 time; 4 g (10 mL) dose should be given as two 5 mL injections, followed by doxycycline 100 mg twice daily for 7 days

Disseminated gonococcal infection: 2 g every 12 hours

Dosing adjustment in renal impairment: None necessary

Hemodialysis: 50% removed by hemodialysis

Administration For I.M. use only

Dosage Forms Powder for injection: 2 g, 4 g

Selected Readings

US Department of Health and Human Services, "1993 Sexually Transmitted Diseases Treatment Guidelines," *MMWR Morb Mortal Wkly Rep*, 1993, 42(RR-14).

Spectinomycin Hydrochloride *see* Spectinomycin *on previous page*

Spectrobid® *see* Bacampicillin *on page 617*

Sporanox® *see* Itraconazole *on page 785*

SSD™ *see* Silver Sulfadiazine *on page 919*

SSD AF® *see* Silver Sulfadiazine *on page 919*

SSKI® *see* Potassium Iodide *on page 879*

Staphcillin® *see* Methicillin *on page 816*

Stavudine (STAV yoo deen)

Related Information

HIV Therapeutic Information *on page 1008*

U.S. Brand Names Zerit®

Synonyms d4T

Use Treatment of adults with HIV infection in combination with other antiretroviral agents

Pregnancy Risk Factor C

Pregnancy/Breast-Feeding Implications

Clinical effects on the fetus: Administer during pregnancy only if benefits to mother outweigh risks to the fetus

Breast-feeding/lactation: HIV-infected mothers are discouraged from breast-feeding to decrease potential transmission of HIV

Contraindications Hypersensitivity to stavudine

Warnings/Precautions Use with caution in patients who demonstrate previous hypersensitivity to zidovudine, didanosine, zalcitabine, pre-existing bone marrow suppression, renal insufficiency, or peripheral neuropathy. Peripheral neuropathy may be the dose-limiting side effect. Zidovudine should not be used in combination with stavudine. Potentially fatal lactic acidosis and hepatomegaly have been reported. Use with caution in patients at risk of hepatic disease.

Adverse Reactions All adverse reactions reported below were similar to comparative agent, zidovudine, except for peripheral neuropathy, which was greater for stavudine.

>10%:

Central nervous system: Headache, chills, fever, malaise, insomnia, anxiety, depression, pain

Dermatologic: Rash

Gastrointestinal: Nausea, vomiting, diarrhea, pancreatitis, abdominal pain

Neuromuscular & skeletal: Peripheral neuropathy (15% to 21%)

1% to 10%:

Hematologic: Neutropenia, thrombocytopenia

Hepatic: Increased hepatic transaminases and bilirubin

Neuromuscular & skeletal: Myalgia, back pain, weakness

<1%: Lactic acidosis, hepatomegaly, hepatic failure, anemia, pancreatitis

Mechanism of Action Stavudine is a thymidine analog which interferes with HIV viral DNA dependent DNA polymerase resulting in inhibition of viral replication; nucleoside reverse transcriptase inhibitor

Pharmacodynamics/Kinetics

Distribution: V_d: 0.5 L/kg

Peak serum level: 1 hour after administration

Bioavailability: 86.4%

(Continued)

Stavudine *(Continued)*

Half-life: 1-1.6 hours
Elimination: Renal (40%)

Usual Dosage Oral:

Children: 2 mg/kg/day

Adults:

≥60 kg: 40 mg every 12 hours
<60 kg: 30 mg every 12 hours
Dose may be cut in half if symptoms of peripheral neuropathy occur

Dosing adjustment in renal impairment:

Cl_{cr} >50 mL/minute:

≥60 kg: 40 mg every 12 hours
<60 kg: 30 mg every 12 hours

Cl_{cr} 26-50 mL/minute:

≥60 kg: 20 mg every 12 hours
<60 kg: 15 mg every 12 hours

Hemodialysis:

≥60 kg: 20 mg every 24 hours
<60 kg: 15 mg every 24 hours

Monitoring Parameters Monitor liver function tests and signs and symptoms of peripheral neuropathy; monitor viral load and CD4 count

Patient Information Contact physician at first signs or symptoms of peripheral neuropathy

Additional Information Potential compliance problems, frequency of administration and adverse effects should be discussed with patients before initiating therapy to help prevent the emergence of resistance.

Dosage Forms

Capsule: 15 mg, 20 mg, 30 mg, 40 mg
Powder for oral solution: 1 mg/mL (200 mL)

Selected Readings

Dudley MN, Graham KK, Kaul S, et al, "Pharmacokinetics of Stavudine in Patients With AIDS and AIDS-Related Complex," *J Infect Dis*, 1992, 166(3):480-5.

Lea AP and Faulds D, "Stavudine: A Review of Its Pharmacodynamic and Pharmacokinetic Properties and Clinical Potential in HIV Infection," *Drugs*, 1996, 51(5):846-64.

Streptomycin *(strep toe MYE sin)*

Related Information

Antimicrobial Activity Against Selected Organisms *on page 983*
Tuberculosis Guidelines *on page 1114*

Generic Available Yes

Use Part of combination therapy of active tuberculosis; used in combination with other agents for treatment of streptococcal or enterococcal endocarditis, mycobacterial infections, plague, tularemia, and brucellosis

Drug of Choice or Alternative for

Organism(s)

Enterococcus Species *on page 137*
Francisella tularensis on page 148
Mycobacterium bovis on page 203
Mycobacterium tuberculosis on page 207
Yersinia pestis on page 300

Pregnancy Risk Factor D

Contraindications Hypersensitivity to streptomycin or any component

Warnings/Precautions Use with caution in patients with pre-existing vertigo, tinnitus, hearing loss, neuromuscular disorders, or renal impairment; modify dosage in patients with renal impairment; aminoglycosides are associated with significant nephrotoxicity or ototoxicity; the ototoxicity is directly proportional to the amount of drug given and the duration of treatment; tinnitus or vertigo are indications of vestibular injury and impending bilateral irreversible damage; renal damage is usually reversible

Adverse Reactions

1% to 10%:

Central nervous system: Neurotoxicity
Renal: Nephrotoxicity
Otic: Ototoxicity (auditory), ototoxicity (vestibular)

<1%: Skin rash, drug fever, headache, paresthesia, tremor, nausea, vomiting, eosinophilia, arthralgia, anemia, hypotension, difficulty in breathing, drowsiness, weakness

Overdosage/Toxicology

Symptoms of overdose include ototoxicity, nephrotoxicity, and neuromuscular toxicity

The treatment of choice following a single acute overdose appears to be the maintenance of good urine output of at least 3 mL/kg/hour. Dialysis is of questionable value in the enhancement of aminoglycoside elimination. If required, hemodialysis is preferred over peritoneal dialysis in patients with normal renal function. Careful hydration may be all that is required to promote diuresis and therefore the enhancement of the drug's elimination.

Drug Interactions

Increased/prolonged effect: Depolarizing and nondepolarizing neuromuscular blocking agents

Increased toxicity: Concurrent use of amphotericin may increase nephrotoxicity

Stability Depending upon manufacturer, reconstituted solution remains stable for 2-4 weeks when refrigerated; exposure to light causes darkening of solution without apparent loss of potency

Mechanism of Action Inhibits bacterial protein synthesis by binding directly to the 30S ribosomal subunits causing faulty peptide sequence to form in the protein chain

Pharmacodynamics/Kinetics

Absorption: I.M.: Absorbed well

Distribution: To extracellular fluid including serum, abscesses, ascitic, pericardial, pleural, synovial, lymphatic, and peritoneal fluids; crosses the placenta; small amounts appear in breast milk

Half-life:

Newborns: 4-10 hours

Adults: 2-4.7 hours and is prolonged with renal impairment

Elimination: Almost completely (90%) excreted as unchanged drug in urine, with small amounts (1%) excreted in bile, saliva, sweat, and tears

Usual Dosage

Children:

Daily therapy: 20-30 mg/kg/day (maximum: 1 g/day)

Directly observed therapy (DOT): Twice weekly: 25-30 mg/kg (maximum: 1.5 g)

DOT: 3 times/week: 25-30 mg/kg (maximum: 1 g)

Adults:

Daily therapy: 15 mg/kg/day (maximum: 1 g)

Directly observed therapy (DOT): Twice weekly: 25-30 mg/kg (maximum: 1.5 g)

DOT: 3 times/week: 25-30 mg/kg (maximum: 1 g)

Enterococcal endocarditis: 1 g every 12 hours for 2 weeks, 500 mg every 12 hours for 4 weeks in combination with penicillin

Streptococcal endocarditis: 1 g every 12 hours for 1 week, 500 mg every 12 hours for 1 week

Tularemia: 1-2 g/day in divided doses for 7-10 days or until patient is afebrile for 5-7 days

Plague: 2-4 g/day in divided doses until the patient is afebrile for at least 3 days

Elderly: 10 mg/kg/day, not to exceed 750 mg/day; dosing interval should be adjusted for renal function; some authors suggest not to give more than 5 days/week or give as 20-25 mg/kg/dose twice weekly

Dosing interval in renal impairment:

Cl_{cr} 10-50 mL/minute: Administer every 24-72 hours

Cl_{cr} <10 mL/minute: Administer every 72-96 hours

Removed by hemo and peritoneal dialysis: Administer dose postdialysis

Administration Inject deep I.M. into large muscle mass; may be administered I.V. over 30-60 minutes

Monitoring Parameters Hearing (audiogram), BUN, creatinine; serum concentration of the drug should be monitored in all patients; eighth cranial nerve damage is usually preceded by high-pitched tinnitus, roaring noises, sense of fullness in ears, or impaired hearing and may persist for weeks after drug is discontinued

(Continued)

Streptomycin *(Continued)*

Reference Range Therapeutic: Peak: 20-30 µg/mL; Trough: <5 µg/mL; Toxic: Peak: >50 µg/mL; Trough: >10 µg/mL

Test Interactions False-positive urine glucose with Benedict's solution or Clinitest®; penicillin may decrease aminoglycoside serum concentrations *in vitro*

Patient Information Report any unusual symptom of hearing loss, dizziness, roaring noises, or fullness in ears

Additional Information Due to the critical supply of streptomycin, the drug is being released on a per patient basis at no cost; patient specific information will be required to obtain the drug from Pfizer Inc. For more information, call 1-800-254-4445.

Dosage Forms Injection: 400 mg/mL (2.5 mL)

Selected Readings

Begg EJ and Barclay ML, "Aminoglycosides - 50 Years On," *Br J Clin Pharmacol*, 1995, 39(6):597-603.

Cunha BA, "Aminoglycosides: Current Role in Antimicrobial Therapy," *Pharmacotherapy*, 1988, 8(6):334-50.

Davidson PT and Le HQ, "Drug Treatment of Tuberculosis - 1992," *Drugs*, 1992, 43(5):651-73.

"Drugs for Tuberculosis," *Med Lett Drugs Ther*, 1993, 35(908):99-101.

Edson RS and Terrell CL, "The Aminoglycosides," *Mayo Clin Proc*, 1999, 74(5):519-28.

Havlir DV and Barnes PF, "Tuberculosis in Patients With Human Immunodeficiency Virus Infection," *N Engl J Med*, 1999, 340(5):367-73.

Iseman MD, "Treatment of Multidrug-Resistant Tuberculosis," *N Engl J Med*, 1993, 329(11):784-91.

Kim-Sing A, Kays MB, Vivien EJ, et al, "Intravenous Streptomycin Use in a Patient Infected With High-Level Gentamicin-Resistant *Streptococcus faecalis*," *Ann Pharmacother*, 1993, 27(6):712-4.

Morris JT and Cooper RH, "Intravenous Streptomycin: A Useful Route of Administration," *Clin Infect Dis*, 1994, 19(6):1150-1.

"Prevention and Treatment of Tuberculosis Among Patients Infected With Human Immunodeficiency Virus: Principles of Therapy and Revised Recommendations. Centers for Disease Control and Prevention," *MMWR Morb Mortal Wkly Rep*, 1998, 47(RR-20):1-58.

Van Scoy RE and Wilkowske CJ, "Antituberculous Agents," *Mayo Clin Proc*, 1992, 67(2):179-87.

Stromectol® *see Ivermectin on page 787*

Strong Iodine Solution *see Potassium Iodide on page 879*

Sulbactam and Ampicillin *see Ampicillin and Sulbactam on page 607*

Sulconazole *(sul KON a zole)*

U.S. Brand Names Exelderm®

Synonyms Sulconazole Nitrate

Generic Available No

Use Treatment of superficial fungal infections of the skin, including tinea cruris (jock itch), tinea corporis (ringworm), tinea versicolor, and possibly tinea pedis (athlete's foot - cream only)

Pregnancy Risk Factor C

Contraindications Known hypersensitivity to sulconazole

Warnings/Precautions Use with caution in nursing mothers; for external use only

Adverse Reactions 1% to 10%:

Dermatologic: Itching

Local: Burning, stinging, redness

Mechanism of Action Substituted imidazole derivative which inhibits metabolic reactions necessary for the synthesis of ergosterol, an essential membrane component. The end result is usually fungistatic; however, sulconazole may act as a fungicide in *Candida albicans* and parapsilosis during certain growth phases.

Pharmacodynamics/Kinetics

Absorption: Topical: About 8.7% absorbed percutaneously

Elimination: Mostly in urine

Usual Dosage Adults: Topical: Apply a small amount to the affected area and gently massage once or twice daily for 3 weeks (tinea cruris, tinea corporis, tinea versicolor) to 4 weeks (tinea pedis).

Patient Information For external use only; avoid contact with eyes; if burning or irritation develops, notify physician

Dosage Forms

Cream, as nitrate: 1% (15 g, 30 g, 60 g)

Solution, as nitrate, topical: 1% (30 mL)

Sulconazole Nitrate *see Sulconazole on this page*

Sulf-10® Ophthalmic *see* Sulfacetamide Sodium *on this page*

Sulfabenzamide, Sulfacetamide, and Sulfathiazole
(sul fa BENZ a mide, sul fa SEE ta mide & sul fa THYE a zole)

U.S. Brand Names Gyne-Sulf®; Sultrin™; Trysul®; Vagilia®; V.V.S.®

Synonyms Triple Sulfa

Generic Available Yes

Use Treatment of *Gardnerella vaginalis* vaginitis, although other agents are preferred

Pregnancy Risk Factor C

Contraindications Hypersensitivity to sulfabenzamide, sulfacetamide, sulfathiazole or any component

Warnings/Precautions If local irritation develops, discontinue therapy

Adverse Reactions
>10%: Local: Irritation, pruritus, urticaria
<1%: Allergic reactions, Stevens-Johnson syndrome

Mechanism of Action Interferes with microbial folic acid synthesis and growth via inhibition of para-aminobenzoic acid metabolism

Pharmacodynamics/Kinetics
Absorption: From the vagina is variable and unreliable
Metabolism: Primarily by acetylation
Elimination: Excreted by glomerular filtration into urine

Usual Dosage Adults:
Cream: Insert one applicatorful in vagina twice daily for 4-6 days; dosage may then be decreased to $1/2$ to $1/4$ of an applicatorful twice daily
Tablet: Insert one intravaginally twice daily for 10 days

Patient Information Complete full course of therapy; notify physician if burning, irritation, or signs of a systemic allergic reaction occur

Dosage Forms
Cream, vaginal: Sulfabenzamide 3.7%, sulfacetamide 2.86%, and sulfathiazole 3.42% (78 g with applicator, 90 g, 120 g)
Tablet, vaginal: Sulfabenzamide 184 mg, sulfacetamide 143.75 mg, and sulfathiazole 172.5 mg (20 tablets/box with vaginal applicator)

Sulfacetamide Sodium (sul fa SEE ta mide SOW dee um)

U.S. Brand Names AK-Sulf® Ophthalmic; Bleph®-10 Ophthalmic; Cetamide® Ophthalmic; Isopto® Cetamide® Ophthalmic; Klaron® Lotion; Ocusulf-10® Ophthalmic; Sebizon® Topical Lotion; Sodium Sulamyd® Ophthalmic; Sulf-10® Ophthalmic

Synonyms Sodium Sulfacetamide

Generic Available Yes

Use Treatment and prophylaxis of conjunctivitis due to susceptible organisms; corneal ulcers; adjunctive treatment with systemic sulfonamides for therapy of trachoma; topical application in scaling dermatosis (seborrheic); bacterial infections of the skin

Pregnancy Risk Factor C

Contraindications Hypersensitivity to sulfacetamide or any component, sulfonamides; infants <2 months of age

Warnings/Precautions Inactivated by purulent exudates containing PABA; use with caution in severe dry eye; ointment may retard corneal epithelial healing; sulfite in some products may cause hypersensitivity reactions; cross-sensitivity may occur with previous exposure to other sulfonamides given by other routes

Adverse Reactions
1% to 10%: Local: Irritation, stinging, burning
<1%: Headache, Stevens-Johnson syndrome, exfoliative dermatitis, toxic epidermal necrolysis, blurred vision, browache, hypersensitivity reactions

Drug Interactions Decreased effect: Silver, gentamicin (antagonism)

Stability Protect from light; discolored solution should not be used; **incompatible** with silver and zinc sulfate; sulfacetamide is inactivated by blood or purulent exudates

Mechanism of Action Interferes with bacterial growth by inhibiting bacterial folic acid synthesis through competitive antagonism of PABA

Pharmacodynamics/Kinetics
Half-life: 7-13 hours
Elimination: When absorbed, excreted primarily in urine as unchanged drug
(Continued)

Sulfacetamide Sodium *(Continued)*

Usual Dosage

Children >2 months and Adults: Ophthalmic:

Ointment: Apply to lower conjunctival sac 1-4 times/day and at bedtime

Solution: Instill 1-3 drops several times daily up to every 2-3 hours in lower conjunctival sac during waking hours and less frequently at night

Children >12 years and Adults: Topical:

Seborrheic dermatitis: Apply at bedtime and allow to remain overnight; in severe cases, may apply twice daily

Secondary cutaneous bacterial infections: Apply 2-4 times/day until infection clears

Monitoring Parameters Response to therapy

Patient Information Eye drops will burn upon instillation; wait at least 10 minutes before using another eye preparation; may sting eyes when first applied; do not touch container to eye, ointment will cause blurred vision; notify physician if condition does not improve in 3-4 days; may cause sensitivity to sunlight

Nursing Implications Assess whether patient can adequately instill drops or ointment

Dosage Forms

Lotion: 10% (59 mL, 85 mL)

Ointment, ophthalmic: 10% (3.5 g)

Solution, ophthalmic: 10% (1 mL, 2 mL, 2.5 mL, 5 mL, 15 mL); 15% (5 mL, 15 mL); 30% (15 mL)

Selected Readings

Lohr JA, Austin RD, Grossman M, et al, "Comparison of Three Topical Antimicrobials for Acute Bacterial Conjunctivitis," *Pediatr Infect Dis J,* 1988, 7(9):626-9.

Sulfacetamide Sodium and Fluorometholone

(sul fa SEE ta mide SOW dee um & flure oh METH oh lone)

Related Information

Sulfacetamide Sodium *on previous page*

U.S. Brand Names FML-S® Ophthalmic Suspension

Use Steroid-responsive inflammatory ocular conditions where infection is present or there is a risk of infection

Dosage Forms Suspension, ophthalmic: Sulfacetamide sodium 10% and fluoro-metholone 0.1% (5 mL, 10 mL)

Sulfacetamide Sodium and Phenylephrine

(sul fa SEE ta mide SOW dee um & fen il EF rin)

Related Information

Sulfacetamide Sodium *on previous page*

U.S. Brand Names Vasosulf® Ophthalmic

Use Treatment of conjunctivitis, corneal ulcer, and other superficial ocular infections due to susceptible microorganisms; adjunctive in systemic sulfonamide therapy

Usual Dosage Instill 1 or 2 drops into the lower conjunctival sac(s) every 2 or 3 hours during the day, less often at night

Dosage Forms Solution, ophthalmic: Sulfacetamide sodium 15% and phenyl-ephrine hydrochloride 0.125% (5 mL, 15 mL)

Sulfacetamide Sodium and Prednisolone

(sul fa SEE ta mide SOW dee um & pred NIS oh lone)

Related Information

Sulfacetamide Sodium *on previous page*

U.S. Brand Names AK-Cide® Ophthalmic; Blephamide® Ophthalmic; Cetapred® Ophthalmic; Isopto® Cetapred® Ophthalmic; Metimyd® Ophthalmic; Vasocidin® Ophthalmic

Use Steroid-responsive inflammatory ocular conditions where infection is present or there is a risk of infection; ophthalmic suspension may be used as an otic preparation

Usual Dosage Children >2 months and Adults: Ophthalmic:

Ointment: Apply to lower conjunctival sac 1-4 times/day

Solution: Instill 1-3 drops every 2-3 hours while awake

Dosage Forms

Ointment, ophthalmic:

AK-Cide®, Metimyd®, Vasocidin®: Sulfacetamide sodium 10% and predniso-lone acetate 0.5% (3.5 g)

Blephamide®: Sulfacetamide sodium 10% and prednisolone acetate 0.2% (3.5 g)

Cetapred®: Sulfacetamide sodium 10% and prednisolone acetate 0.25% (3.5 g)

Suspension, ophthalmic: Sulfacetamide sodium 10% and prednisolone sodium phosphate 0.25% (5 mL)

Suspension, ophthalmic:

AK-Cide®, Metimyd®: Sulfacetamide sodium 10% and prednisolone acetate 0.5% (5 mL)

Blephamide®: Sulfacetamide sodium 10% and prednisolone acetate 0.2% (2.5 mL, 5 mL, 10 mL)

Isopto® Cetapred®: Sulfacetamide sodium 10% and prednisolone acetate 0.25% (5 mL, 15 mL)

Vasocidin®: Sulfacetamide sodium 10% and prednisolone sodium phosphate: 0.25% (5 mL, 10 mL)

Sulfacet-R® Topical see Sulfur and Sulfacetamide Sodium on page 936

Sulfadiazine (sul fa DYE a zeen)

U.S. Brand Names Microsulfon®

Canadian Brand Names Coptin®

Generic Available Yes

Use Treatment of urinary tract infections and nocardiosis, rheumatic fever prophy-laxis; adjunctive treatment in toxoplasmosis; uncomplicated attack of malaria

Drug of Choice or Alternative for

Disease/Syndrome(s)

Brain Abscess on page 19

Organism(s)

Nocardia Species on page 218

Toxoplasma gondii on page 283

Pregnancy Risk Factor B (D at term)

Contraindications Porphyria, hypersensitivity to any sulfa drug or any compo-nent, pregnancy at term, children <2 months of age unless indicated for the treatment of congenital toxoplasmosis, sunscreens containing PABA, nursing mothers

Warnings/Precautions Use with caution in patients with impaired hepatic func-tion or impaired renal function, G-6-PD deficiency; dosage modification required in patients with renal impairment; fluid intake should be maintained ≥1500 mL/day, or administer sodium bicarbonate to keep urine alkaline; more likely to cause crystalluria because it is less soluble than other sulfonamides

Adverse Reactions

>10%:

Central nervous system: Fever, dizziness, headache

Dermatologic: Itching, rash, photosensitivity

Gastrointestinal: Anorexia, nausea, vomiting, diarrhea

1% to 10%:

Dermatologic: Lyell's syndrome, Stevens-Johnson syndrome

Hematologic: Granulocytopenia, leukopenia, thrombocytopenia, aplastic anemia, hemolytic anemia

Hepatic: Hepatitis

<1%: Thyroid function disturbance, crystalluria, jaundice, interstitial nephritis, acute nephropathy, hematuria, serum sickness-like reactions

Overdosage/Toxicology

Symptoms of overdose include drowsiness, dizziness, anorexia, abdominal pain, nausea, vomiting, hemolytic anemia, acidosis, jaundice, fever, agranulo-cytosis; doses of as little as 2-5 g/day may produce toxicity; the aniline radical is responsible for hematologic toxicity

High volume diuresis may aid in elimination and prevention of renal failure

Drug Interactions Decreased effect with PABA or PABA metabolites of drugs (eg, procaine, proparacaine, tetracaine, sunscreens); increased effect of oral anticoagulants and oral hypoglycemic agents

(Continued)

Sulfadiazine *(Continued)*

Stability Tablets may be crushed to prepare oral suspension of the drug in water or with a sucrose-containing solution; aqueous suspension with concentrations of 100 mg/mL should be stored in the refrigerator and used within 7 days

Mechanism of Action Interferes with bacterial growth by inhibiting bacterial folic acid synthesis through competitive antagonism of PABA

Pharmacodynamics/Kinetics

Absorption: Oral: Well absorbed

Distribution: Throughout body tissues and fluids including pleural, peritoneal, synovial, and ocular fluids; distributed throughout total body water; readily diffused into CSF; appears in breast milk

Metabolism: By N-acetylation

Half-life: 10 hours

Elimination: In urine as metabolites (15% to 40%) and as unchanged drug (43% to 60%)

Usual Dosage Oral:

Congenital toxoplasmosis:

Newborns and Children <2 months: 100 mg/kg/day divided every 6 hours in conjunction with pyrimethamine 1 mg/kg/day once daily and supplemental folinic acid 5 mg every 3 days for 6 months

Children >2 months: 25-50 mg/kg/dose 4 times/day

Toxoplasmosis:

Children >2 months: Loading dose: 75 mg/kg; maintenance dose: 120-150 mg/kg/day, maximum dose: 6 g/day; divided every 4-6 hours in conjunction with pyrimethamine 2 mg/kg/day divided every 12 hours for 3 days followed by 1 mg/kg/day once daily (maximum: 25 mg/day) with supplemental folinic acid

Adults: 2-4 g/day divided every 4-8 hours in conjunction with pyrimethamine 25 mg/day and with supplemental folinic acid

Prevention of recurrent attacks of rheumatic fever:

>30 kg: 1 g/day

<30 kg: 0.5 g/day

Patient Information Drink plenty of fluids; take on an empty stomach; avoid prolonged exposure to sunlight or wear protective clothing and sunscreen; notify physician if rash, difficulty breathing, severe or persistent fever, or sore throat occurs

Nursing Implications Maintain adequate hydration and monitor urine output

Dosage Forms Tablet: 500 mg

Selected Readings

Porter SB and Sande MA, "Toxoplasmosis of the Central Nervous System in the Acquired Immuno-deficiency Syndrome," *N Engl J Med*, 1992, 327(23):1643-8.

Sulfadiazine, Sulfamethazine, and Sulfamerazine

(sul fa DYE a zeen sul fa METH a zeen & sul fa MER a zeen)

Synonyms Multiple Sulfonamides; Trisulfapyrimidines

Generic Available No

Use Treatment of toxoplasmosis and other susceptible organisms, however, other agents are preferred

Pregnancy Risk Factor B (D at term)

Contraindications Porphyria, known hypersensitivity to any sulfa drug or any component

Mechanism of Action Interferes with microbial folic acid synthesis and growth via inhibition of para-aminobenzoic acid metabolism

Pharmacodynamics/Kinetics

Metabolism: By acetylation

Elimination: Excreted in urine via glomerular filtration

Usual Dosage Adults: Oral: 2-4 g to start, then 2-4 g/day in 3-6 divided doses

Test Interactions Increases cholesterol (S), protein, uric acid (S)

Patient Information Drink plenty of fluids

Dosage Forms Tablet: Sulfadiazine 167 mg, sulfamethazine 167 mg, and sulfamerazine 167 mg

Sulfadoxine and Pyrimethamine

(sul fa DOKS een & peer i METH a meen)

U.S. Brand Names Fansidar®

Generic Available No

Use Treatment of *Plasmodium falciparum* malaria in patients in whom chloroquine resistance is suspected; malaria prophylaxis for travelers to areas where chloroquine-resistant malaria is endemic

Drug of Choice or Alternative for

Organism(s)

Isospora belli on page 182

Plasmodium Species on page 227

Pregnancy Risk Factor C

Contraindications Known hypersensitivity to any sulfa drug, pyrimethamine, or any component; porphyria, megaloblastic anemia, severe renal insufficiency; children <2 months of age due to competition with bilirubin for protein binding sites

Warnings/Precautions Use with caution in patients with renal or hepatic impairment, patients with possible folate deficiency, and patients with seizure disorders, increased adverse reactions are seen in patients also receiving chloroquine; fatalities associated with sulfonamides, although rare, have occurred due to severe reactions including Stevens-Johnson syndrome, toxic epidermal necrolysis, hepatic necrosis, agranulocytosis, aplastic anemia and other blood dyscrasias; discontinue use at first sign of rash or any sign of adverse reaction; hemolysis occurs in patients with G-6-PD deficiency; leucovorin should be administered to reverse signs and symptoms of folic acid deficiency

Adverse Reactions

>10%:

Central nervous system: Ataxia, seizures, headache

Dermatologic: Photosensitivity

Gastrointestinal: Atrophic glossitis, vomiting, gastritis

Hematologic: Megaloblastic anemia, leukopenia, thrombocytopenia, pancytopenia

Neuromuscular & skeletal: Tremors

Miscellaneous: Hypersensitivity

1% to 10%:

Dermatologic: Stevens-Johnson syndrome

Hepatic: Hepatitis

<1%: Erythema multiforme, toxic epidermal necrolysis, rash, thyroid dysfunction, anorexia, glossitis, crystalluria, hepatic necrosis, respiratory failure

Overdosage/Toxicology

Symptoms of overdose include anorexia, vomiting, CNS stimulation including seizures, megaloblastic anemia, leukopenia, thrombocytopenia, crystalluria; leucovorin should be administered in a dosage of 3-9 mg/day for 3 days or as required to reverse symptoms of folic acid deficiency; doses of as little as 2-5 g/day may produce toxicity; the aniline radical is responsible for hematologic toxicity

High volume diuresis may aid in elimination and prevention of renal failure; diazepam can be used to control seizures

Drug Interactions

Decreased effect with PABA or PABA metabolites of local anesthetics

Increased toxicity with methotrexate, other sulfonamides, co-trimoxazole

Mechanism of Action Sulfadoxine interferes with bacterial folic acid synthesis and growth via competitive inhibition of para-aminobenzoic acid; pyrimethamine inhibits microbial dihydrofolate reductase, resulting in inhibition of tetrahydrofolic acid synthesis

Pharmacodynamics/Kinetics

Absorption: Oral: Well absorbed

Distribution:

Pyrimethamine: Widely distributed; mainly concentrated in blood cells, kidneys, lungs, liver, and spleen

Sulfadoxine: Well distributed like other sulfonamides

Metabolism:

Pyrimethamine: Hepatic

Sulfadoxine: None

(Continued)

Sulfadoxine and Pyrimethamine *(Continued)*

Half-life:
Pyrimethamine: 80-95 hours
Sulfadoxine: 5-8 days
Time to peak serum concentration: Within 2-8 hours
Elimination: Excreted in urine as parent compounds and several unidentified metabolites

Usual Dosage Children and Adults: Oral:
Treatment of acute attack of malaria: A single dose of the following number of Fansidar® tablets is used in sequence with quinine or alone:
2-11 months: $\frac{1}{4}$ tablet
1-3 years: $\frac{1}{2}$ tablet
4-8 years: 1 tablet
9-14 years: 2 tablets
>14 years: 2-3 tablets

Malaria prophylaxis:
The first dose of Fansidar® should be taken 1-2 days before departure to an endemic area (CDC recommends that therapy be initiated 1-2 weeks before such travel), administration should be continued during the stay and for 4-6 weeks after return. Dose = pyrimethamine 0.5 mg/kg/dose and sulfadoxine 10 mg/kg/dose up to a maximum of 25 mg pyrimethamine and 500 mg sulfadoxine/dose weekly.
2-11 months: $\frac{1}{8}$ tablet weekly **or** $\frac{1}{4}$ tablet once every 2 weeks
1-3 years: $\frac{1}{4}$ tablet once weekly **or** $\frac{1}{2}$ tablet once every 2 weeks
4-8 years: $\frac{1}{2}$ tablet once weekly **or** 1 tablet once every 2 weeks
9-14 years: $\frac{3}{4}$ tablet once weekly **or** $1\frac{1}{2}$ tablets once every 2 weeks
>14 years: 1 tablet once weekly **or** 2 tablets once every 2 weeks

Monitoring Parameters CBC, including platelet counts, and urinalysis should be performed periodically

Patient Information Begin prophylaxis at least 2 days before departure; drink plenty of fluids; avoid prolonged exposure to the sun; notify physician if rash, sore throat, pallor, or glossitis occurs

Dosage Forms Tablet: Sulfadoxine 500 mg and pyrimethamine 25 mg

Selected Readings
Panisko DM and Keystone JS, "Treatment of Malaria - 1990," *Drugs*, 1990, 39(2):160-89.
Wyler DJ, "Malaria Chemoprophylaxis for the Traveler," *N Engl J Med*, 1993, 329(1):31-7.
Wyler DJ, "Malaria: Overview and Update," *Clin Infect Dis*, 1993, 16(4):449-56.

Sulfamethoprim® *see Co-Trimoxazole on page 692*

Sulfamethoxazole *(sul fa meth OKS a zole)*

U.S. Brand Names Gantanol®; Urobak®
Canadian Brand Names Apo®-Sulfamethoxazole
Generic Available Yes: Tablet

Use Treatment of urinary tract infections, nocardiosis, toxoplasmosis, acute otitis media, and acute exacerbations of chronic bronchitis due to susceptible organisms

Pregnancy Risk Factor B (D at term)

Contraindications Porphyria, hypersensitivity to any sulfa drug or any component, pregnancy during 3rd trimester, children <2 months of age unless indicated for the treatment of congenital toxoplasmosis, sunscreens containing PABA

Warnings/Precautions Maintain adequate fluid intake to prevent crystalluria; use with caution in patients with renal or hepatic impairment, and patients with G-6-PD deficiency; should not be used for group A beta-hemolytic streptococcal infections

Adverse Reactions
>10%:
Central nervous system: Fever, dizziness, headache
Dermatologic: Itching, rash, photosensitivity
Gastrointestinal: Anorexia, nausea, vomiting, diarrhea
1% to 10%:
Dermatologic: Lyell's syndrome, Stevens-Johnson syndrome
Hematologic: Granulocytopenia, leukopenia, thrombocytopenia, aplastic anemia, hemolytic anemia
Hepatic: Hepatitis

<1%: Vasculitis, thyroid function disturbance, crystalluria, jaundice, hematuria, acute nephropathy, interstitial nephritis, serum sickness-like reactions

Overdosage/Toxicology
Symptoms of overdose include drowsiness, dizziness, anorexia, abdominal pain, nausea, vomiting, hemolytic anemia, acidosis, jaundice, fever, agranulocytosis; the aniline radical is responsible for hematologic toxicity
High volume diuresis may aid in elimination and prevention of renal failure

Drug Interactions
Decreased effect with PABA or PABA metabolites of drugs (ie, procaine, proparacaine, tetracaine); cyclosporine levels may be decreased
Increased effect/toxicity of oral anticoagulants, oral hypoglycemic agents, hydantoins, uricosuric agents, methotrexate when administered with sulfonamides
Increased toxicity of sulfonamides with diuretics, indomethacin, methenamine, probenecid, and salicylates

Stability Protect from light

Mechanism of Action Interferes with bacterial growth by inhibiting bacterial folic acid synthesis through competitive antagonism of PABA

Pharmacodynamics/Kinetics
Absorption: Oral: 90%
Distribution: Crosses the placenta; readily enters the CSF
Protein binding: 70%
Metabolism: Primarily in the liver, with 10% to 20% as the N-acetylated form in the plasma
Half-life: 9-12 hours, prolonged with renal impairment
Elimination: Unchanged drug (20%) and its metabolites are excreted in urine

Usual Dosage Oral:
Children >2 months: 50-60 mg/kg as single dose followed by 50-60 mg/kg/day divided every 12 hours; maximum: 3 g/24 hours or 75 mg/kg/day
Adults: Initial: 2 g, then 1 g 2-3 times/day; maximum: 3 g/24 hours

Dosing adjustment/interval in renal impairment:
Cl_{cr} 10-50 mL/minute: Administer every 12-24 hours
Cl_{cr} <10 mL/minute: Administer every 24 hours
Hemodialysis: Moderately dialyzable (20% to 50%)

Administration Administer around-the-clock to promote less variation in peak and trough serum levels

Monitoring Parameters Monitor urine output

Test Interactions May interfere with Jaffé alkaline picrate reaction assay for creatinine resulting in overestimations of ~10% in the range of normal values; decreased effect with PABA or PABA metabolites of drugs (ie, procaine, proparacaine, tetracaine)

Patient Information Drink plenty of fluids; avoid prolonged exposure to sunlight or wear protective clothing; avoid aspirin and vitamin C products, notify physician if rash, unusual bleeding, difficulty breathing, severe or persistent fever, or sore throat occurs

Nursing Implications Maintain adequate hydration

Dosage Forms
Suspension, oral (cherry flavor): 500 mg/5 mL (480 mL)
Tablet: 500 mg

Sulfamethoxazole and Phenazopyridine
(sul fa meth OKS a zole & fen az oh PEER i deen)

Related Information
Sulfamethoxazole on previous page

Use Treatment of urinary tract infections complicated with pain

Usual Dosage Oral: 4 tablets to start, then 2 tablets twice daily for up to 2 days, then switch to sulfamethoxazole only

Dosage Forms Tablet: Sulfamethoxazole 500 mg and phenazopyridine 100 mg

Sulfamethoxazole and Trimethoprim see Co-Trimoxazole on page 692

Sulfamylon® Topical see Mafenide on page 803

Sulfanilamide (sul fa NIL a mide)

U.S. Brand Names AVC™ Cream; AVC™ Suppository; Vagitrol®

Generic Available No

(Continued)

Sulfanilamide *(Continued)*

Use Treatment of vulvovaginitis caused by *Candida albicans*

Pregnancy Risk Factor C; kernicterus possible in nursing newborn, avoid breast-feeding if possible

Contraindications Hypersensitivity to sulfanilamide or any component

Warnings/Precautions Since sulfonamides may be absorbed from vaginal mucosa, the same precaution for oral sulfonamides apply (eg, blood dyscrasias); if a rash develops, terminate therapy immediately. Use vaginal applicators very cautiously after the 7th month of pregnancy.

Adverse Reactions Percentage unknown: Rarely, systemic reactions occur; increased discomfort, burning, allergic reactions, Stevens-Johnson syndrome (infrequent)

Mechanism of Action Interferes with microbial folic acid synthesis and growth via inhibition of para-aminiobenzoic acid metabolism; exerts a bacteriostatic action

Usual Dosage Adults: Female: Insert one applicatorful intravaginally once or twice daily continued through 1 complete menstrual cycle or insert one suppository intravaginally once or twice daily for 30 days

Patient Information Complete full course of therapy; notify physician if burning or irritation become severe or persist or if allergic symptoms occur; insert high into vagina; use of an applicator is not recommended during pregnancy; avoid sexual intercourse during treatment

Dosage Forms

Cream, vaginal (AVC™, Vagitrol®): 15% [150 mg/g] (120 g with applicator)
Suppository, vaginal (AVC™): 1.05 g (16s)

Sulfatrim® *see* Co-Trimoxazole *on page 692*

Sulfatrim® DS *see* Co-Trimoxazole *on page 692*

Sulfisoxazole *(sul fi SOKS a zole)*

Canadian Brand Names Novo-Soxazole; Sulfizole®

Synonyms Sulfisoxazole Acetyl; Sulphafurazole

Generic Available Yes

Use Treatment of urinary tract infections, otitis media, *Chlamydia*; nocardiosis; treatment of acute pelvic inflammatory disease in prepubertal children; often used in combination with trimethoprim

Drug of Choice or Alternative for Organism(s)

Nocardia Species *on page 218*

Pregnancy Risk Factor B (D at term)

Contraindications Hypersensitivity to any sulfa drug or any component, porphyria, pregnancy during 3rd trimester, infants <2 months of age (sulfas compete with bilirubin for protein binding sites), patients with urinary obstruction, sunscreens containing PABA

Warnings/Precautions Use with caution in patients with G-6-PD deficiency (hemolysis may occur), hepatic or renal impairment; dosage modification required in patients with renal impairment; risk of crystalluria should be considered in patients with impaired renal function

Adverse Reactions

>10%:

Central nervous system: Fever, dizziness, headache
Dermatologic: Itching, rash, photosensitivity
Gastrointestinal: Anorexia, nausea, vomiting, diarrhea

1% to 10%:

Dermatologic: Lyell's syndrome, Stevens-Johnson syndrome
Hematologic: Granulocytopenia, leukopenia, thrombocytopenia, aplastic anemia, hemolytic anemia
Hepatic: Hepatitis

<1%: Vasculitis, thyroid function disturbance, crystalluria, jaundice, hematuria, acute nephropathy, interstitial nephritis, serum sickness-like reactions

Overdosage/Toxicology

Symptoms of overdose include drowsiness, dizziness, anorexia, abdominal pain, nausea, vomiting, hemolytic anemia, acidosis, jaundice, fever, agranulocytosis; doses of as little as 2-5 g/day may produce toxicity; the aniline radical is responsible for hematologic toxicity

High volume diuresis may aid in elimination and prevention of renal failure

Drug Interactions

Decreased effect with PABA or PABA metabolites of drugs (ie, procaine, proparacaine, tetracaine); cyclosporine levels may be decreased

Increased effect/toxicity of oral anticoagulants, oral hypoglycemic agents, hydantoins, uricosuric agents, methotrexate when administered with sulfonamides

Increased toxicity of sulfonamides with diuretics, indomethacin, methenamine, probenecid, and salicylates

Stability Protect from light

Mechanism of Action Interferes with bacterial growth by inhibiting bacterial folic acid synthesis through competitive antagonism of PABA

Pharmacodynamics/Kinetics

Absorption: Sulfisoxazole acetyl is hydrolyzed in the GI tract to sulfisoxazole which is readily absorbed

Distribution: Crosses the placenta; excreted into breast milk

Ratio of CSF to blood level (%):

Normal meninges: 50-80

Inflamed meninges: 80+

Protein binding: 85% to 88%

Metabolized: In the liver by acetylation and glucuronide conjugation to inactive compounds

Half-life: 4-7 hours, prolonged with renal impairment

Elimination: Primarily in urine (95% within 24 hours), 40% to 60% as unchanged drug

Usual Dosage Not for use in patients <2 months of age:

Children >2 months: Oral: Initial: 75 mg/kg, followed by 120-150 mg/kg/day in divided doses every 4-6 hours; not to exceed 6 g/day

Pelvic inflammatory disease: 100 mg/kg/day in divided doses every 6 hours; used in combination with ceftriaxone

Chlamydia trachomatis: 100 mg/kg/day in divided doses every 6 hours

Adults: Oral: Initial: 2-4 g, then 4-8 g/day in divided doses every 4-6 hours

Pelvic inflammatory disease: 500 mg every 6 hours for 21 days; used in combination with ceftriaxone

Chlamydia trachomatis: 500 mg every 6 hours for 10 days

Dosing interval in renal impairment:

Cl_{cr} 10-50 mL/minute: Administer every 8-12 hours

Cl_{cr} <10 mL/minute: Administer every 12-24 hours

Hemodialysis: >50% removed by hemodialysis

Children and Adults: Ophthalmic:

Solution: Instill 1-2 drops to affected eye every 2-3 hours

Ointment: Apply small amount to affected eye 1-3 times/day and at bedtime

Monitoring Parameters CBC, urinalysis, renal function tests, temperature

Test Interactions False-positive protein in urine; false-positive urine glucose with Clinitest®

Patient Information Take with a glass of water on an empty stomach; avoid prolonged exposure to sunlight; report to physician any sore throat, mouth sores, rash, unusual bleeding, or fever; complete full course of therapy

Nursing Implications Maintain adequate fluid intake

Additional Information

Sulfisoxazole: Gantrisin® tablet

Sulfisoxazole acetyl: Gantrisin® pediatric syrup/suspension

Dosage Forms

Ointment, ophthalmic, as diolamine: 4% [40 mg/mL] (3.75 g)

Solution, ophthalmic, as diolamine: 4% [40 mg/mL] (15 mL)

Suspension, oral, pediatric, as acetyl (raspberry flavor): 500 mg/5 mL (480 mL)

Tablet: 500 mg

Sulfisoxazole Acetyl *see* Sulfisoxazole *on previous page*

Sulfisoxazole and Erythromycin *see* Erythromycin and Sulfisoxazole *on page 725*

Sulfisoxazole and Phenazopyridine
(sul fi SOKS a zole & fen az oh PEER i deen)

Related Information

Sulfisoxazole *on page 934*

U.S. Brand Names Azo-Sulfisoxazole

Use Treatment of urinary tract infections and nocardiosis

Usual Dosage Adults: Oral: 4-6 tablets to start, then 2 tablets 4 times/day for 2 days, then continue with sulfisoxazole only

Dosing adjustment/comments in renal impairment: Cl_{cr} <50 mL/minute: Avoid use of phenazopyridine

Dosage Forms Tablet: Sulfisoxazole 500 mg and phenazopyridine 50 mg

Sulfizole® *see* Sulfisoxazole *on page 934*

Sulfur and Sulfacetamide Sodium
(SUL fur & sul fa SEE ta mide SOW dee um)

Related Information

Sulfacetamide Sodium *on page 927*

U.S. Brand Names Novacet® Topical; Sulfacet-R® Topical

Use Aid in the treatment of acne vulgaris, acne rosacea and seborrheic dermatitis

Usual Dosage Topical: Apply in a thin film 1-3 times/day

Dosage Forms Lotion, topical: Sulfur colloid 5% and sulfacetamide sodium 10% (30 mL)

Sulphafurazole *see* Sulfisoxazole *on page 934*

Sultrin™ *see* Sulfabenzamide, Sulfacetamide, and Sulfathiazole *on page 927*

Sumycin® Oral *see* Tetracycline *on page 944*

Suprax® *see* Cefixime *on page 636*

Sustiva™ *see* Efavirenz *on page 718*

Symadine® *see* Amantadine *on page 586*

Symmetrel® *see* Amantadine *on page 586*

Synagis® *see* Palivizumab *on page 855*

Synercid® *see* Quinupristin/Dalfopristin *on page 891*

Syn-Minocycline *see* Minocycline *on page 823*

Tao® *see* Troleandomycin *on page 960*

Taro-Ampicillin® Trihydrate *see* Ampicillin *on page 604*

Taro-Cloxacillin® *see* Cloxacillin *on page 689*

TAT *see* Tetanus Antitoxin *on page 941*

Tazicef® *see* Ceftazidime *on page 651*

Tazidime® *see* Ceftazidime *on page 651*

3TC *see* Lamivudine *on page 793*

TCN *see* Tetracycline *on page 944*

Td *see* Diphtheria and Tetanus Toxoid *on page 707*

Tebrazid *see* Pyrazinamide *on page 884*

Tegopen® *see* Cloxacillin *on page 689*

Terak® Ophthalmic Ointment *see* Oxytetracycline and Polymyxin B *on page 855*

Terazol® *see* Terconazole *on page 938*

Terbinafine (TER bin a feen)

U.S. Brand Names Daskil®; Lamisil®

Synonyms Terbinafine Hydrochloride

Use Active against most strains of *Trichophyton mentagrophytes, Trichophyton rubrum*; may be effective for infections of *Microsporum gypseum* and *M. nanum, Trichophyton verrucosum, Epidermophyton floccosum, Candida albicans*, and *Scopulariopsis brevicaulis*

Oral: Onychomycosis of the toenail or fingernail due to susceptible dermatophytes

Topical: Antifungal for the treatment of tinea pedis (athlete's foot), tinea cruris (jock itch), and tinea corporis (ringworm)

Unlabeled use: Topical: Cutaneous candidiasis and pityriasis versicolor

Drug of Choice or Alternative for
Organism(s)
  Dermatophytes *on page 127*
Pregnancy Risk Factor B
Pregnancy/Breast-Feeding Implications
  Clinical effects on the fetus: Avoid use in pregnancy since treatment of onycho-
  mycosis is postponable
  Breast-feeding/lactation: Although minimal concentrations of terbinafine cross
  into breast milk after topical use, oral or topical treatment during lactation
  should be avoided
Contraindications Hypersensitivity to terbinafine, naftifine or any component;
  pre-existing liver or renal disease (≤50 mL/minute GFR)
Warnings/Precautions While rare, the following complications have been
  reported and may require discontinuation of therapy: Changes in the ocular lens
  and retina, pancytopenia, neutropenia, Stevens-Johnson syndrome, toxic
  epidermal necrolysis. Discontinue if symptoms or signs of hepatobiliary dysfunction or cholestatic hepatitis develop. If irritation/sensitivity develop with topical
  use, discontinue therapy.
Adverse Reactions
  1% to 10%:
    Oral:
      Central nervous system: Headache, dizziness, vertigo
      Dermatologic: Rash, pruritus, and alopecia with oral therapy;
      Gastrointestinal: Nausea, diarrhea, dyspepsia, abdominal pain, appetite
        decrease, taste disturbance
      Hematologic: Neutropenia, lymphocytopenia
      Hepatic: Cholestasis, jaundice, hepatitis, liver enzyme elevations
      Ocular: Visual disturbance
      Miscellaneous: Allergic reaction
    Topical:
      Dermatologic: Pruritus, contact dermatitis, dryness
      Local: Irritation, stinging
Drug Interactions
  Decreased effect: Cyclosporine clearance is increased (~15%) with concomi-
    tant terbinafine; rifampin increases terbinafine clearance (100%)
  Increased effect: Terbinafine clearance is decreased by cimetidine (33%) and
    terfenadine (16%); caffeine clearance is decreased by terfenadine (19%)
Stability Cream: Store at 5°C to 30°C/41°F to 86°F
Mechanism of Action Synthetic alkylamine derivative which inhibits squalene
  epoxidase, a key enzyme in sterol biosynthesis in fungi. This results in a defi-
  ciency in ergosterol within the fungal cell wall and results in fungal cell death.
Pharmacodynamics/Kinetics
  Absorption:
    Oral: >70%
    Topical: Limited (<5%)
  Distribution: V_d: 2000 L; distributed to sebum and skin predominantly
  Protein binding, plasma: >99%
  Metabolism: Hepatic; no active metabolites
  Bioavailability: Oral: 80% although undergoes first-pass metabolism (40%); does
    not involve significant (<5%) of total cytochrome P-450 capacity of liver; peak
    plasma levels occur at 1-2 hours
  Half-life: 22-26 hours; very slow release of drug from skin and adipose tissues
    occurs
  Elimination: ~75% of dose excreted in urine; 3.5% of a topically administered
    dose excreted in urine and feces
Usual Dosage Adults:
  Oral:
    Superficial mycoses: Fingernail: 250 mg/day for up to 6 weeks; toenail: 250
      mg/day for 12 weeks; doses may be given in two divided doses
    Systemic mycosis: 250-500 mg/day for up to 16 months
  Topical:
    Athlete's foot: Apply to affected area twice daily for at least 1 week, not to
      exceed 4 weeks
    Ringworm and jock itch: Apply to affected area once or twice daily for at least
      1 week, not to exceed 4 weeks
(Continued)

Terbinafine *(Continued)*

Dosing adjustment in renal impairment: Although specific guidelines are not available, dose reduction in significant renal insufficiency (GFR <50 mL/minute) is recommended

Monitoring Parameters CBC and LFTs at baseline and repeated if use is for >6 weeks

Patient Information Topical: Avoid contact with eyes, nose, or mouth during treatment with cream; nursing mothers should not use on breast tissue; advise physician if eyes or skin becomes yellow or if irritation, itching, or burning develops. Do not use occlusive dressings concurrent with therapy. Full clinical effect may require several months due to the time required for a new nail to grow.

Nursing Implications Patients should not be considered therapeutic failures until they have been symptom-free for 2-4 weeks off following a course of treatment; GI complaints usually subside with continued administration

Additional Information A meta-analysis of efficacy studies for toenail infections revealed that weighted average mycological cure rates for continuous therapy were 36.7% (griseofulvin), 54.7% (itraconazole), and 77% (terbinafine). Cure rate for 4-month pulse therapy for itraconazole and terbinafine were 73.3% and 80%. Additionally, the final outcome measure of final costs per cured infections for continuous therapy was significantly lower for terbinafine.

Dosage Forms
Cream: 1% (15 g, 30 g)
Tablet: 250 mg

Selected Readings

Abdel-Rahman SM and Nahata MC, "Oral Terbinafine: A New Antifungal Agent," *Ann Pharmacother,* 1997, 31(4):445-56.

Amichai B and Grunwald MH, "Adverse Drug Reactions of the New Oral Antifungal Agents - Terbinafine, Fluconazole, and Itraconazole," *Int J Dermatol,* 1998, 37(6):410-5.

Angello JT, et al, "A Cost/Efficacy Analysis of Oral Antifungals Indicated for the Treatment of Onychomycosis: Griseofulvin, Itraconazole, and Terbinafine," *Amer J Managed Care,* 1997, 3:443-50.

Dwyer CM, White MI, and Sinclair TS, "Cholestatic Jaundice Due to Terbinafine," *Br J Dermatol,* 1997, 136(6):976-7.

Gupta AK and Shear NH, "Terbinafine: An Update," *J Am Acad Dermatol,* 1997, 37(6):979-88.

Gupta AK, Sibbald RG, Knowles SR, et al, "Terbinafine Therapy May Be Associated With the Development of Psoriasis De Novo or Its Exacerbation: Four Case Reports and a Review of Drug Induced Psoriasis," *J Am Acad Dermatol,* 1997, 36(5 Part 2):858-62.

Jones TC, "Overview of the Use of Terbinafine in Children," *Br J Dermatol,* 1995, 132(5):683-9.

Trepanier EF and Amsden GW, "Current Issues in Onchomycosis," *Ann Pharmacother,* 1998, 32(2):204-14.

Terbinafine Hydrochloride *see* Terbinafine *on page 936*

Terconazole *(ter KONE a zole)*

U.S. Brand Names Terazol®

Synonyms Triaconazole

Generic Available No

Use Local treatment of vulvovaginal candidiasis

Pregnancy Risk Factor C

Contraindications Known hypersensitivity to terconazole or components of the vaginal cream or suppository

Warnings/Precautions Should be discontinued if sensitization or irritation occurs. Microbiological studies (KOH smear and/or cultures) should be repeated in patients not responding to terconazole in order to confirm the diagnosis and rule out other other pathogens.

Adverse Reactions 1% to 10%: Genitourinary: Vulvar/vaginal burning

Stability Room temperature (13°C to 30°C/59°F to 86°F)

Mechanism of Action Triazole ketal antifungal agent; involves inhibition of fungal cytochrome P-450. Specifically, terconazole inhibits cytochrome P-450-dependent 14-alpha-demethylase which results in accumulation of membrane disturbing 14-alpha-demethylsterols and ergosterol depletion.

Pharmacodynamics/Kinetics Absorption: Extent of systemic absorption after vaginal administration may be dependent on the presence of a uterus; 5% to 8% in women who had a hysterectomy versus 12% to 16% in nonhysterectomy women

Usual Dosage Adults: Female: Insert 1 applicatorful intravaginally at bedtime for 7 consecutive days

Patient Information Insert high into vagina; complete full course of therapy; contact physician if itching or burning occurs

Nursing Implications Watch for local irritation; assist patient in administration, if necessary; assess patient's ability to self-administer, may be difficult in patients with arthritis or limited range of motion

Dosage Forms
Cream, vaginal: 0.4% (45 g); 0.8% (20 g)
Suppository, vaginal: 80 mg (3s)

Selected Readings
Drug Facts and Comparisons, St Louis, MO: 1989, 528-9.

Terra-Cortril® Ophthalmic Suspension *see* Oxytetracycline and Hydrocortisone *on page 855*

Terramycin® I.M. Injection *see* Oxytetracycline *on page 854*

Terramycin® Ophthalmic Ointment *see* Oxytetracycline and Polymyxin B *on page 855*

Terramycin® Oral *see* Oxytetracycline *on page 854*

Terramycin® w/Polymyxin B Ophthalmic Ointment *see* Oxytetracycline and Polymyxin B *on page 855*

Tesamone® Injection *see* Testosterone *on this page*

Testoderm® Transdermal System *see* Testosterone *on this page*

Testopel® Pellet *see* Testosterone *on this page*

Testosterone (tes TOS ter one)

U.S. Brand Names Androderm® Transdermal System; Andro-L.A.® Injection; Andropository® Injection; Delatest® Injection; Delatestryl® Injection; depAndro® Injection; Depotest® Injection; Depo®-Testosterone Injection; Duratest® Injection; Durathate® Injection; Everone® Injection; Histerone® Injection; Tesamone® Injection; Testoderm® Transdermal System; Testopel® Pellet

Synonyms Aqueous Testosterone; Testosterone Cypionate; Testosterone Enanthate; Testosterone Propionate

Generic Available Yes

Use Treatment of "AIDS-wasting" syndrome; androgen replacement therapy in the treatment of delayed male puberty; postpartum breast pain and engorgement; inoperable breast cancer; male hypogonadism

Restrictions C-III

Pregnancy Risk Factor X

Contraindications Severe renal or cardiac disease, benign prostatic hypertrophy with obstruction, undiagnosed genital bleeding, males with carcinoma of the breast or prostate; hypersensitivity to testosterone or any component

Warnings/Precautions Perform radiographic examination of the hand and wrist every 6 months to determine the rate of bone maturation; may accelerate bone maturation without producing compensating gain in linear growth; has both androgenic and anabolic activity, the anabolic action may enhance hypoglycemia

Adverse Reactions
>10%:
Dermatologic: Acne
Endocrine & metabolic: Menstrual problems (amenorrhea), virilism, breast soreness
Genitourinary: Epididymitis, priapism, bladder irritability
1% to 10%:
Cardiovascular: Flushing, edema
Central nervous system: Excitation, aggressive behavior, sleeplessness, anxiety, mental depression, headache
Dermatologic: Hirsutism (increase in pubic hair growth)
Gastrointestinal: Nausea, vomiting, GI irritation
Genitourinary: Prostatic hypertrophy, prostatic carcinoma, impotence, testicular atrophy
Hepatic: Hepatic dysfunction
<1%: Gynecomastia, hypercalcemia, hypoglycemia, leukopenia, suppression of clotting factors, polycythemia, cholestatic hepatitis, hepatic necrosis, hypersensitivity reactions

Drug Interactions Cytochrome P-450 3A enzyme substrate
Increased toxicity: Effects of oral anticoagulants may be enhanced
(Continued)

Testosterone *(Continued)*

Mechanism of Action Principal endogenous androgen responsible for promoting the growth and development of the male sex organs and maintaining secondary sex characteristics in androgen-deficient males

Pharmacodynamics/Kinetics

Duration of effect: Based upon the route of administration and which testosterone ester is used; the cypionate and enanthate esters have the longest duration, up to 2-4 weeks after I.M. administration

Distribution: Crosses the placenta; appears in breast milk

Protein binding: 98% (to transcortin and albumin)

Metabolism: In the liver

Half-life: 10-100 minutes

Elimination: In urine (90%) and feces via bile (6%)

Usual Dosage

AIDS wasting: I.M.: 200-400 mg every 2 weeks

Delayed puberty: Males: Children: I.M.: 40-50 mg/m²/dose (cypionate or enanthate) monthly for 6 months

Initiation of pubertal growth: 40-50 mg/m²/dose (cypionate or enanthate) monthly until the growth rate falls to prepubertal levels (~5 cm/year)

During terminal growth phase: 100 mg/m²/dose (cypionate or enanthate) monthly until growth ceases

Maintenance virilizing dose: 100 mg/m²/dose (cypionate or enanthate) twice monthly or 50-400 mg/dose every 2-4 weeks

Inoperable breast cancer: Adults: I.M.: 200-400 mg every 2-4 weeks

Hypogonadism: Males: Adults:

I.M.:

Testosterone or testosterone propionate: 10-25 mg 2-3 times/week

Testosterone cypionate or enanthate: 50-400 mg every 2-4 weeks

Postpubertal cryptorchism: Testosterone or testosterone propionate: 10-25 mg 2-3 times/week

Topical: Initial: 6 mg/day system applied daily applied on scrotal skin. If scrotal area is inadequate, start with a 4 mg/day system. Transdermal system should be worn for 22-24 hours. Determine total serum testosterone after 3-4 weeks of daily application. If patients have not achieved desired results after 6-8 weeks of therapy, another form of testosterone replacement therapy should be considered.

Dosing adjustment/comments in hepatic disease: Reduce dose

Monitoring Parameters Periodic liver function tests, radiologic examination of wrist and hand every 6 months (when using in prepubertal children)

Reference Range Testosterone, urine: Male: 100-1500 ng/24 hours; Female: 100-500 ng/24 hours

Test Interactions May cause a decrease in creatinine and creatine excretion and an increase in the excretion of 17-ketosteroids, thyroid function tests

Patient Information Virilization may occur in female patients; report menstrual irregularities; male patients report persistent penile erections; all patients should report persistent GI distress, diarrhea, or jaundice

Nursing Implications Warm injection to room temperature and shaking vial will help redissolve crystals that have formed after storage; administer by deep I.M. injection into the upper outer quadrant of the gluteus maximus. Transdermal system should be applied on clean, dry, scrotal skin. Dry-shave scrotal hair for optimal skin contact. Do not use chemical depilatories.

Additional Information

Testosterone (aqueous): Andro®, Histerone®, Tesamone®

Testosterone cypionate: Andro-Cyp®, Andronate®, Depotest®, Depo®-Testosterone, Duratest®

Testosterone enanthate: Andro-L.A.®, Andropository®, Delatestryl®, Durathate®, Everone®, Testrin® P.A.

Testosterone propionate: Testex®

Dosage Forms

Injection:

Aqueous suspension: 25 mg/mL (10 mL, 30 mL); 50 mg/mL (10 mL, 30 mL); 100 mg/mL (10 mL, 30 mL)

In oil, as cypionate: 100 mg/mL (1 mL, 10 mL); 200 mg/mL (1 mL, 10 mL)

In oil, as enanthate: 100 mg/mL (5 mL, 10 mL); 200 mg/mL (5 mL, 10 mL)

In oil, as propionate: 50 mg/mL (10 mL, 30 mL); 100 mg/mL (10 mL, 30 mL)
Pellet: 75 mg (1 pellet per vial)
Transdermal system:
Androderm®: 2.5 mg/day; 5 mg/day
Testoderm®: 4 mg/day; 6 mg/day

Selected Readings
Borhan-Manesh F and Farnum JB, "Methyltestosterone-Induced Cholestasis. The Importance of Disproportionately Low Serum Alkaline Phosphatase Level," *Arch Intern Med*, 1989, 149(9):2127-9.

Cunningham GR, Cordero E, and Thornby JI, "Testosterone Replacement With Transdermal Therapeutic Systems. Physiological Serum Testosterone and Elevated Dihydrotestosterone Levels," *JAMA*, 1989, 261(17):2525-30.

Daigle RD, "Anabolic Steroids," *J Psychoactive Drugs*, 1990, 22(1):77-80.

Moller BB and Ekelund B, "Toxicity of Cyclosporine During Treatment With Androgens," *N Engl J Med*, 1985, 313(22):1416.

Ruch W and Jenny P, "Priapism Following Testosterone Administration for Delayed Male Puberty," *Am J Med*, 1989, 86(2):256.

Testosterone Cypionate *see* Testosterone *on page 939*

Testosterone Enanthate *see* Testosterone *on page 939*

Testosterone Propionate *see* Testosterone *on page 939*

Tetanus and Diphtheria Toxoid *see* Diphtheria and Tetanus Toxoid *on page 707*

Tetanus Antitoxin (TET a nus an tee TOKS in)
Synonyms TAT
Generic Available No
Use Tetanus prophylaxis or treatment of active tetanus only when tetanus immune globulin (TIG) is not available; tetanus immune globulin (Hyper-Tet®) is the preferred tetanus immunoglobulin for the treatment of active tetanus; may be given concomitantly with tetanus toxoid adsorbed when immediate treatment is required, but active immunization is desirable
Pregnancy Risk Factor D
Contraindications Patients sensitive to equine-derived preparations
Warnings/Precautions Tetanus antitoxin is not the same as tetanus immune globulin; sensitivity testing should be conducted in all individuals regardless of clinical history; have epinephrine 1:1000 available
Adverse Reactions Skin eruptions, erythema, urticaria, local pain, numbness, arthralgia, serum sickness may develop up to several weeks after injection in 10% of patients, anaphylaxis
Stability Refrigerate, do not freeze
Mechanism of Action Provides passive immunization; solution of concentrated globulins containing antitoxic antibodies obtained from horse serum after immunization against tetanus toxin
Usual Dosage
Prophylaxis: I.M., S.C.:
Children <30 kg: 1500 units
Children and Adults ≥30 kg: 3000-5000 units
Treatment: Children and Adults: Inject 10,000-40,000 units into wound; administer 40,000-100,000 units
Nursing Implications All patients should have sensitivity testing prior to starting therapy with tetanus antitoxin
Dosage Forms Injection, equine: Not less than 400 units/mL (12.5 mL, 50 mL)

Tetanus Immune Globulin (Human)
(TET a nus i MYUN GLOB yoo lin HYU man)
U.S. Brand Names Hyper-Tet®
Synonyms TIG
Generic Available No
Use Passive immunization against tetanus; tetanus immune globulin is preferred over tetanus antitoxin for treatment of active tetanus; part of the management of an unclean, nonminor wound in a person whose history of previous receipt of tetanus toxoid is unknown or who has received less than three doses of tetanus toxoid
Drug of Choice or Alternative for
Organism(s)
Clostridium tetani on page 107
(Continued)

Tetanus Immune Globulin (Human) *(Continued)*

Pregnancy Risk Factor C

Contraindications Hypersensitivity to tetanus immune globulin or any component; I.V. administration, patients with IgA deficiency

Warnings/Precautions Have epinephrine 1:1000 available for anaphylactic reactions

Adverse Reactions

>10%: Local: Pain, tenderness, erythema at injection site

1% to 10%:

Central nervous system: Fever (mild)

Dermatologic: Urticaria, angioedema

Neuromuscular & skeletal: Muscle stiffness

Miscellaneous: Anaphylaxis reaction

<1%: Sensitization to repeated injections

Drug Interactions Never administer tetanus toxoid and TIG in same syringe (toxoid will be neutralized); toxoid may be given at a separate site; concomitant administration with Td may decrease its immune response, especially in individuals with low prevaccination antibody titers

Stability Refrigerate

Mechanism of Action Passive immunity to tetanus

Pharmacodynamics/Kinetics Absorption: Well absorbed

Usual Dosage I.M.:

Prophylaxis of tetanus:

Children: 4 units/kg; some recommend administering 250 units to small children

Adults: 250 units

Treatment of tetanus:

Children: 500-3000 units; some should infiltrate locally around the wound

Adults: 3000-6000 units

Administration Do not administer I.V.; I.M. use only

Additional Information Tetanus immune globulin (TIG) must not contain <50 units/mL. Protein makes up 10% to 18% of TIG preparations. The great majority of this (≥90%) is IgG. TIG has almost no color or odor and it is a sterile, nonpyrogenic, concentrated preparation of immunoglobulins that has been derived from the plasma of adults hyperimmunized with tetanus toxoid. The pooled material from which the immunoglobulin is derived may be from fewer than 1000 donors. This plasma has been shown to be free of hepatitis B surface antigen.

Dosage Forms Injection: 250 units/mL

Tetanus Toxoid, Adsorbed *(TET a nus TOKS oyd, ad SORBED)*

Generic Available No

Use Selective induction of active immunity against tetanus in selected patients. **Note:** Tetanus and diphtheria toxoids for adult use (Td) is the preferred immunizing agent for most adults and for children after their seventh birthday. Young children should receive trivalent DTwP or DTaP (diphtheria/tetanus/pertussis - whole cell or acellular), as part of their childhood immunization program, unless pertussis is contraindicated, then TD is warranted.

Pregnancy Risk Factor C

Contraindications Hypersensitivity to tetanus toxoid or any component (may use the fluid tetanus toxoid to immunize the rare patient who is hypersensitive to aluminum adjuvant); avoid use with chloramphenicol or if neurological signs or symptoms occurred after prior administration; poliomyelitis outbreaks require deferral of immunizations; acute respiratory infections or other active infections may dictate deferral of administration of routine primary immunizing but not emergency doses

Warnings/Precautions Not equivalent to tetanus toxoid fluid; the tetanus toxoid adsorbed is the preferred toxoid for immunization and Td, TD or DTaP/DTwP are the preferred adsorbed forms; avoid injection into a blood vessel; have epinephrine (1:1000) available; not for use in treatment of tetanus infection nor for immediate prophylaxis of unimmunized individuals; immunosuppressive therapy or other immunodeficiencies may diminish antibody response, however it is recommended for routine immunization of symptomatic and asymptomatic HIV-infected patients; deferral of immunization until immunosuppression is discontinued or administration of an additional dose >1 month after treatment is recommended; allergic reactions may occur; epinephrine 1:1000 must be available; use in pediatrics should be deferred until >1 year of age when a history of a CNS disorder is present; elderly may not mount adequate antibody titers following immunization

Adverse Reactions
>10%: Local: Induration/redness at injection site
1% to 10%:
  Central nervous system: Chills, fever
  Local: Sterile abscess at injection site
  Miscellaneous: Allergic reaction
<1%: Fever (>103°F), malaise, neurological disturbances, blistering at injection site, Arthus-type hypersensitivity reactions

Drug Interactions Decreased response: If primary immunization is started in individuals receiving an immunosuppressive agent or corticosteroids, serologic testing may be needed to ensure adequate antibody response; concurrent use of TIG and tetanus toxoid may delay the development of active immunity by several days

Stability Refrigerate, do not freeze

Mechanism of Action Tetanus toxoid preparations contain the toxin produced by virulent tetanus bacilli (detoxified growth products of *Clostridium tetani*). The toxin has been modified by treatment with formaldehyde so that it has lost toxicity but still retains ability to act as antigen and produce active immunity; the aluminum salt, a mineral adjuvant, delays the rate of absorption and prolongs and enhances its properties; duration ~10 years.

Pharmacodynamics/Kinetics Duration of immunization following primary immunization: ~10 years

Usual Dosage Adults: I.M.:
Primary immunization: 0.5 mL; repeat 0.5 mL at 4-8 weeks after first dose and at 6-12 months after second dose
Routine booster doses are recommended only every 5-10 years

Administration Inject intramuscularly in the area of the vastus lateralis (midthigh laterally) or deltoid

Patient Information A nodule may be palpable at the injection site for a few weeks. DT, Td and T vaccines cause few problems; they may cause mild fever or soreness, swelling, and redness where the shot was given. These problems usually last 1-2 days, but this does not happen nearly as often as with DTP vaccine. Sometimes, adults who get these vaccines can have a lot of soreness and swelling where the shot was given.

Dosage Forms Injection, adsorbed:
Tetanus 5 Lf units per 0.5 mL dose (0.5 mL, 5 mL)
Tetanus 10 Lf units per 0.5 mL dose (0.5 mL, 5 mL)

Selected Readings
Bentley DW, "Vaccinations," *Clin Geriatr Med*, 1992, 8(4):745-60.
Gardner P and Schaffner W, "Immunization of Adults," *N Engl J Med*, 1993, 328(17):1252-8.

Tetanus Toxoid, Fluid (TET a nus TOKS oyd, FLOO id)

Synonyms Tetanus Toxoid Plain

Generic Available No

Use Detection of delayed hypersensitivity and assessment of cell-mediated immunity; active immunization against tetanus in the rare adult or child who is allergic to the aluminum adjuvant (a product containing adsorbed tetanus toxoid is preferred)

Pregnancy Risk Factor C

Contraindications Hypersensitivity to tetanus toxoid or any product components

Warnings/Precautions Epinephrine 1:1000 should be readily available; skin test responsiveness may be delayed or reduced in elderly patients

Adverse Reactions Percentage unknown: Very hypersensitive persons may develop a local reaction at the injection site; urticaria, anaphylactic reactions, shock and death are possible

Drug Interactions Increased effect: Cimetidine may augment delayed hypersensitivity responses to skin test antigens

Stability Refrigerate
(Continued)

Tetanus Toxoid, Fluid *(Continued)*

Mechanism of Action Tetanus toxoid preparations contain the toxin produced by virulent tetanus bacilli (detoxified growth products of *Clostridium tetani*). The toxin has been modified by treatment with formaldehyde so that is has lost toxicity but still retains ability to act as antigen and produce active immunity.

Usual Dosage

Anergy testing: Intradermal: 0.1 mL

Primary immunization (**Note:** Td, TD, DTaP/DTwP are recommended): Adults: Inject 3 doses of 0.5 mL I.M. or S.C. at 4- to 8-week intervals; administer fourth dose 6-12 months after third dose

Booster doses: I.M., S.C.: 0.5 mL every 10 years

Administration Must not be used I.V.; for skin testing, use 0.1 mL of 1:100 v/v or 0.02 mL of 1:10 v/v solution

Dosage Forms Injection, fluid:

Tetanus 4 Lf units per 0.5 mL dose (7.5 mL)

Tetanus 5 Lf units per 0.5 mL dose (0.5 mL, 7.5 mL)

Selected Readings

Gardner P and Schaffner W, "Immunization of Adults," *N Engl J Med*, 1993, 328(17):1252-8.

Tetanus Toxoid Plain *see* Tetanus Toxoid, Fluid *on previous page*

Tetracap® Oral *see* Tetracycline *on this page*

Tetracycline *(tet ra SYE kleen)*

U.S. Brand Names Achromycin® Ophthalmic; Achromycin® Topical; Nor-tet® Oral; Panmycin® Oral; Sumycin® Oral; Tetracap® Oral; Topicycline® Topical

Canadian Brand Names Apo®-Tetra; Novo-Tetra; Nu-Tetra

Synonyms TCN; Tetracycline Hydrochloride

Generic Available Yes

Use Treatment of susceptible bacterial infections of both gram-positive and gram-negative organisms; also infections due to *Mycoplasma*, *Chlamydia*, and *Rickettsia*; indicated for acne, exacerbations of chronic bronchitis, and treatment of gonorrhea and syphilis in patients that are allergic to penicillin; used concomitantly with metronidazole, bismuth subsalicylate and an H_2 antagonist for the treatment of duodenal ulcer disease induced by *H. pylori*

Drug of Choice or Alternative for

Disease/Syndrome(s)

Urethritis, Nongonococcal *on page 51*

Organism(s)

Bacillus anthracis on page 73

Bordetella pertussis on page 81

Calymmatobacterium granulomatis on page 89

Chlamydia pneumoniae on page 95

Chlamydia trachomatis on page 99

Coxiella burnetii on page 115

Ehrlichia Species *on page 130*

Francisella tularensis on page 148

Helicobacter pylori on page 160

Leptospira interrogans on page 186

Mycoplasma hominis and *Mycoplasma genitalium on page 210*

Mycoplasma pneumoniae on page 211

Rickettsia rickettsii on page 243

Ureaplasma urealyticum on page 292

Vibrio cholerae on page 297

Yersinia pestis on page 300

Pregnancy Risk Factor D; B (topical)

Pregnancy/Breast-Feeding Implications Breast-feeding/lactation: Excreted in breast milk; avoid use if possible in lactating mothers

Contraindications Hypersensitivity to tetracycline or any component; do not administer to children ≤8 years of age

Warnings/Precautions Use of tetracyclines during tooth development may cause permanent discoloration of the teeth and enamel, hypoplasia and retardation of skeletal development and bone growth with risk being the greatest for children <4 years and those receiving high doses; use with caution in patients with renal or hepatic impairment (eg, elderly) and in pregnancy; dosage modification required in patients with renal impairment since it may increase BUN as an antianabolic agent; pseudotumor cerebri has been reported with tetracycline use (usually resolves with discontinuation); outdated drug can cause nephropathy; superinfection possible; use protective measure to avoid photosensitivity

Adverse Reactions

>10%: Gastrointestinal: Discoloration of teeth and enamel hypoplasia (young children)

1% to 10%:
Dermatologic: Photosensitivity
Gastrointestinal: Nausea, diarrhea

<1%: Pericarditis, increased intracranial pressure, bulging fontanels in infants, pseudotumor cerebri, dermatologic effects, pruritus, pigmentation of nails, exfoliative dermatitis, diabetes insipidus syndrome, vomiting, esophagitis, anorexia, abdominal cramps, antibiotic-associated pseudomembranous colitis, staphylococcal enterocolitis, hepatotoxicity, thrombophlebitis, paresthesia, acute renal failure, azotemia, renal damage, superinfections, anaphylaxis, hypersensitivity reactions, candidal superinfection

Overdosage/Toxicology

Symptoms of overdose include nausea, anorexia, diarrhea
Following GI decontamination, supportive care only

Drug Interactions

Decreased effect: Calcium, magnesium or aluminum-containing antacids, oral contraceptives, iron, zinc, sodium bicarbonate, penicillins, cimetidine may decrease tetracycline absorption
Although no clinical evidence exists, may bind with bismuth or calcium carbonate, an excipient in bismuth subsalicylate, during treatment for *H. pylori*
Increased toxicity: Methoxyflurane anesthesia when concurrent with tetracycline may cause fatal nephrotoxicity; warfarin with tetracyclines may result in increased anticoagulation; tetracyclines may rarely increase digoxin serum levels

Stability Outdated tetracyclines have caused a Fanconi-like syndrome; protect oral dosage forms from light

Mechanism of Action Inhibits bacterial protein synthesis by binding with the 30S and possibly the 50S ribosomal subunit(s) of susceptible bacteria; may also cause alterations in the cytoplasmic membrane

Pharmacodynamics/Kinetics

Absorption: Oral: 75%
Distribution: Small amount appears in bile
Relative diffusion of antimicrobial agents from blood into cerebrospinal fluid (CSF): Good only with inflammation (exceeds usual MICs)
Ratio of CSF to blood level (%): Inflamed meninges: 25
Half-life:
Normal renal function: 8-11 hours
End stage renal disease: 57-108 hours
Elimination: Primary route is the kidney, with 60% of a dose excreted as unchanged drug in the urine; concentrated by liver in bile and feces in biologically active form

Usual Dosage

Children >8 years: Oral: 25-50 mg/kg/day in divided doses every 6 hours
Children >8 years and Adults:
Ophthalmic:
Ointment: Instill every 2-12 hours
Suspension: Instill 1-2 drops 2-4 times/day or more often as needed
Topical: Apply to affected areas 1-4 times/day
Adults: Oral: 250-500 mg/dose every 6 hours

Helicobacter pylori: Clinically effective treatment regimens include triple therapy with amoxicillin or tetracycline, metronidazole, and bismuth subsalicylate; amoxicillin, metronidazole, and H₂-receptor antagonist; or double therapy with amoxicillin and omeprazole. Adult dose: 850 mg 3 times/day to 500 mg 4 times/day

Dosing interval in renal impairment:

Cl_cr 50-80 mL/minute: Administer every 8-12 hours
Cl_cr 10-50 mL/minute: Administer every 12-24 hours
Cl_cr <10 mL/minute: Administer every 24 hours
(Continued)

Tetracycline *(Continued)*

Dialysis: Slightly dialyzable (5% to 20%) via hemo- and peritoneal dialysis nor via continuous arteriovenous or venovenous hemofiltration (CAVH/CAVHD); no supplemental dosage necessary

Dosing adjustment in hepatic impairment: Avoid use or maximum dose is 1 g/day

Dietary Considerations Food: Dairy products decrease effect of tetracycline

Administration Oral should be given on an empty stomach (ie, 1 hour prior to, or 2 hours after meals) to increase total absorption. Administer at least 1-2 hours prior to, or 4 hours after antacid because aluminum and magnesium cations may chelate with tetracycline and reduce its total absorption.

Monitoring Parameters Renal, hepatic, and hematologic function test, temperature, WBC, cultures and sensitivity, appetite, mental status

Test Interactions False-negative urine glucose with Clinistix®

Patient Information Take 1 hour before or 2 hours after meals with adequate amounts of fluid; avoid prolonged exposure to sunlight or sunlamps; avoid taking antacids, iron, or dairy products within 2 hours of taking tetracyclines; report persistent nausea, vomiting, yellow coloring of skin or eyes, dark urine, or pale stools; ophthalmic may cause transient burning or itching; topical is for external use only and may stain skin yellow

Additional Information

Tetracycline: Sumycin® syrup

Tetracycline hydrochloride: Nor-tet® capsule, Panmycin® capsule, Sumycin® capsule and tablet, Tetracyn® capsule

Dosage Forms

Capsule, as hydrochloride: 100 mg, 250 mg, 500 mg

Ointment:

Ophthalmic: 1% [10 mg/mL] (3.5 g)

Topical, as hydrochloride: 3% [30 mg/mL] (14.2 g, 30 g)

Solution, topical: 2.2 mg/mL (70 mL)

Suspension:

Ophthalmic: 1% [10 mg/mL] (0.5 mL, 1 mL, 4 mL)

Oral, as hydrochloride: 125 mg/5 mL (60 mL, 480 mL)

Tablet, as hydrochloride: 250 mg, 500 mg

Selected Readings

Smilack JD, Wilson WR, and Cockerill FR 3d, "Tetracyclines, Chloramphenicol, Erythromycin, Clindamycin, and Metronidazole," *Mayo Clin Proc*, 1991, 66(12):1270-80.

Tetracycline Hydrochloride *see* Tetracycline *on page 944*

Tetrahydrocannabinol *see* Dronabinol *on page 716*

Tetramune® *see* Diphtheria, Tetanus Toxoids, Whole-Cell Pertussis, and *Haemophilus influenzae* Type b Conjugate Vaccines *on page 711*

Thalidomide *(tha LI doe mide)*

U.S. Brand Names Thalomid®

Use Treatment of erythema nodosum leprosum

Orphan status: Crohn's disease

Investigational: Treatment or prevention of graft-versus-host reactions after bone marrow transplantation; in aphthous ulceration in HIV-positive patients; Langerhans cell histiocytosis, Behçet's syndrome; hypnotic agent; also may be effective in rheumatoid arthritis, discoid lupus, and erythema multiforme; useful in type 2 lepra reactions, but not type 1; can assist in healing mouth ulcers in AIDS patients

Pregnancy Risk Factor X

Pregnancy/Breast-Feeding Implications Embryotoxic with limb defects noted from the 27th to 40th gestational day of exposure; all cases of phocomelia occur from the 27th to 42nd gestational day; fetal cardiac, gastrointestinal, and genitourinary tract abnormalities have also been described

Contraindications Pregnancy or women in childbearing years, neuropathy (peripheral), thalidomide hypersensitivity

Warnings/Precautions Liver, hepatic, neurological disorders, constipation, congestive heart failure, hypertension

Adverse Reactions Percentage unknown: Tachycardia, sinus tachycardia, dizziness, headache, irritability, lethargy, fever, edema, alopecia, pruritus, amenorrhea, sexual dysfunction, nausea, vomiting, xerostomia, constipation, leukopenia, sensory neuropathy (peripheral) (after prolonged therapy due to neuronal degeneration), clonus, myoclonus

Mechanism of Action A derivative of glutethimide; mode of action for immunosuppression is unclear; inhibition of neutrophil chemotaxis and decreased monocyte phagocytosis may occur; may cause 50% to 80% reduction of tumor necrosis factor - alpha

Pharmacodynamics/Kinetics

Distribution: V_d: 120 L

Metabolism: Hepatic

Half-life: 8.7 hours

Peak plasma levels: 2-6 hours

Usual Dosage

Leprosy: Up to 400 mg/day; usual maintenance dose: 50-100 mg/day

Behçet's syndrome: 100-400 mg/day

Graft-vs-host reactions:

Children: 3 mg/kg 4 times/day

Adults: 100-1600 mg/day; usual initial dose: 200 mg 4 times/day for use up to 700 days

AIDS-related aphthous stomatitis: 200 mg twice daily for 5 days, then 200 mg/day for up to 8 weeks

Discoid lupus erythematosus: 100-400 mg/day; maintenance dose: 25-50 mg

Reference Range Therapeutic plasma thalidomide levels in graft-vs-host reactions are 5-8 µg/mL, although it has been suggested that lower plasma levels (0.5-1.5 µg/mL) may be therapeutic; peak serum thalidomide level after a 200 mg dose: 1.2 µg/mL

Additional Information Must be obtained via "STEPS Program" through Boston University

Selected Readings

Beckman DA and Brent RL, "Mechanism of Known Environmental Teratogens: Drugs and Chemicals," *Clin Perinatol*, 1986, 13(3):649-87.

Gunzler V, "Thalidomide in Human Immunodeficiency Virus (HIV) Patients. A Review of Safety Considerations," *Drug Saf*, 1992, 7(2):116-34.

Jacobson JM, Greenspan JS, Spritzler J, et al, "Thalidomide for the Treatment of Oral Aphthous Ulcers in Patients With Human Immunodeficiency Virus Infection. National Institute of Allergy and Infectious Diseases AIDS Clinical Trials Group," *N Engl J Med*, 1997, 336(21):1487-93.

Levien T, Baker DE, and Ballasiotes AA, "Reviews of Dexrazoxane and Thalidomide," *Hosp Pharm*, 1996, 31(5):487-8, 493-4, 499-500, 504, 508, 510.

Schuler U and Ehninger G, "Thalidomide: Rationale for Renewed Use in Immunological Disorders," *Drug Saf*, 1995, 12(6):364-9.

"Thalidomide," *Med Lett Drugs Ther*, 1998, 40(1038):103-4.

Thalomid® *see* Thalidomide *on previous page*

THC *see* Dronabinol *on page 716*

TheraCys® *see* BCG Vaccine *on page 620*

Thermazene® *see* Silver Sulfadiazine *on page 919*

Thiabendazole (thye a BEN da zole)

U.S. Brand Names Mintezol®

Synonyms Tiabendazole

Generic Available No

Use Treatment of strongyloidiasis, cutaneous larva migrans, visceral larva migrans, dracunculiasis, trichinosis, and mixed helminthic infections

Drug of Choice or Alternative for

Organism(s)

Ancylostoma duodenale *on page 66*

Strongyloides stercoralis *on page 281*

Trichinella spiralis *on page 289*

Pregnancy Risk Factor C

Contraindications Known hypersensitivity to thiabendazole

Warnings/Precautions Use with caution in patients with renal or hepatic impairment, malnutrition or anemia, or dehydration

Adverse Reactions

>10%:

Central nervous system: Seizures, hallucinations, delirium, dizziness, drowsiness, headache

Gastrointestinal: Anorexia, diarrhea, nausea, vomiting, drying of mucous membranes

(Continued)

Thiabendazole *(Continued)*

    Neuromuscular & skeletal: Numbness

    Otic: Tinnitus

    1% to 10%: Dermatologic: Rash, Stevens-Johnson syndrome

    <1%: Chills, malodor of urine, leukopenia, hepatotoxicity, blurred or yellow vision, nephrotoxicity, lymphadenopathy, hypersensitivity reactions

Overdosage/Toxicology

    Symptoms of overdose include altered mental status, visual problems

    Supportive care only following GI decontamination

Drug Interactions Increased levels of theophylline and other xanthines

Mechanism of Action Inhibits helminth-specific mitochondrial fumarate reductase

Pharmacodynamics/Kinetics

    Absorption: Rapid and well from GI tract

    Metabolism: Rapid

    Half-life: 1.2 hours

    Elimination: Excreted in feces (5%) and urine (87%), primarily as conjugated metabolites

Usual Dosage Purgation is not required prior to use; drinking of fruit juice aids in expulsion of worms by removing the mucous to which the intestinal tapeworms attach themselves.

    Children and Adults: Oral: 50 mg/kg/day divided every 12 hours (if >68 kg: 1.5 g/dose); maximum dose: 3 g/day

    Strongyloidiasis, ascariasis, uncinariasis, trichuriasis: For 2 consecutive days

    Cutaneous larva migrans: For 2-5 consecutive days

    Visceral larva migrans: For 5-7 consecutive days

    Trichinosis: For 2-4 consecutive days

    Dracunculosis: 50-75 mg/kg/day divided every 12 hours for 3 days

    Dosing comments in renal/hepatic impairment: Use with caution

Patient Information Take after meals, chew chewable tablet well; may decrease alertness, avoid driving or operating machinery; drinking of fruit juice aids in expulsion of worms by removing the mucous to which the intestinal tapeworms attach themselves

Dosage Forms

    Suspension, oral: 500 mg/5 mL (120 mL)

    Tablet, chewable (orange flavor): 500 mg

Selected Readings

    "Drugs for Parasitic Infections," *Med Lett Drugs Ther*, 1998, 40(1017):1-12.

Thyro-Block® *see* Potassium Iodide *on page 879*

Tiabendazole *see* Thiabendazole *on previous page*

Ticar® *see* Ticarcillin *on this page*

Ticarcillin *(tye kar SIL in)*

Related Information

    Antimicrobial Activity Against Selected Organisms *on page 983*

U.S. Brand Names Ticar®

Synonyms Ticarcillin Disodium

Generic Available No

Use Treatment of susceptible infections such as septicemia, acute and chronic respiratory tract infections, skin and soft tissue infections, and urinary tract infections due to susceptible strains of *Pseudomonas*, and other gram-negative bacteria

Pregnancy Risk Factor B

Contraindications Hypersensitivity to ticarcillin or any component or penicillins

Warnings/Precautions Due to sodium load and adverse effects (anemia, neuropsychological changes), use with caution and modify dosage in patients with renal impairment; serious and occasionally severe or fatal hypersensitivity (anaphylactoid) reactions have been reported in patients on penicillin therapy (especially with a history of beta-lactam hypersensitivity and/or a history of sensitivity to multiple allergens); use with caution in patients with seizures

Adverse Reactions Percentage unknown: Convulsions, confusion, drowsiness, fever, rash, electrolyte imbalance, hemolytic anemia, positive Coombs' test, eosinophilia, bleeding, thrombophlebitis, myoclonus, acute interstitial nephritis, hypersensitivity reactions, anaphylaxis, Jarisch-Herxheimer reaction

Overdosage/Toxicology

Symptoms of penicillin overdose include neuromuscular hypersensitivity (agitation, hallucinations, asterixis, encephalopathy, confusion, and seizures) and electrolyte imbalance with potassium or sodium salts, especially in renal failure

Hemodialysis may be helpful to aid in the removal of the drug from the blood, otherwise most treatment is supportive or symptom directed

Drug Interactions

Decreased effect:

Tetracyclines may decrease penicillin effectiveness

Aminoglycosides → physical inactivation of aminoglycosides in the presence of high concentrations of ticarcillin

Decreased effectiveness of oral contraceptives

Increased effect:

Probenecid may increase penicillin levels

Neuromuscular blockers may increase duration of blockade

Potential toxicity in patients with with mild-moderate renal dysfunction

Aminoglycosides → synergistic efficacy

Increased bleeding risk with large I.V. doses and anticoagulants

Stability Reconstituted solution is stable for 72 hours at room temperature and 14 days when refrigerated; for I.V. infusion in NS or D_5W solution is stable for 72 hours at room temperature, 14 days when refrigerated or 30 days when frozen; after freezing, thawed solution is stable for 72 hours at room temperature or 14 days when refrigerated; incompatible with aminoglycosides

Mechanism of Action Inhibits bacterial cell wall synthesis by binding to one or more of the penicillin binding proteins (PBPs); which in turn inhibits the final transpeptidation step of peptidoglycan synthesis in bacterial cell walls, thus inhibiting cell wall biosynthesis. Bacteria eventually lyse due to ongoing activity of cell wall autolytic enzymes (autolysins and murein hydrolases) while cell wall assembly is arrested.

Pharmacodynamics/Kinetics

Absorption: I.M.: 86%

Distribution: In blister fluid, lymph tissue, and gallbladder; crosses placenta; distributed into milk at low concentrations

Protein binding: 45% to 65%

Half-life:

Neonates:

<1 week: 3.5-5.6 hours

1-8 weeks: 1.3-2.2 hours

Children 5-13 years: 0.9 hour

Adults: 66-72 minutes, prolonged with renal impairment and/or hepatic impairment

Elimination: Almost entirely in urine as unchanged drug and its metabolites with small amounts excreted in feces (3.5%)

Usual Dosage Ticarcillin is generally given I.V., I.M. injection is only for the treatment of uncomplicated urinary tract infections and dose should not exceed 2 g/injection when administered I.M.

Neonates: I.M., I.V.:

Postnatal age <7 days:

<2000 g: 75 mg/kg/dose every 12 hours

>2000 g: 75 mg/kg/dose every 8 hours

Postnatal age >7 days:

<1200 g: 75 mg/kg/dose every 12 hours

1200-2000 g: 75 mg/kg/dose every 8 hours

>2000 g: 75 mg/kg/dose every 6 hours

Infants and Children:

Systemic infections: I.V.: 200-300 mg/kg/day in divided doses every 4-6 hours

Urinary tract infections: I.M., I.V.: 50-100 mg/kg/day in divided doses every 6-8 hours

Maximum dose: 24 g/day

Adults: I.M., I.V.: 1-4 g every 4-6 hours, usual dose: 3 g I.V. every 4-6 hours

(Continued)

Ticarcillin *(Continued)*

Dosing adjustment in renal impairment: Adults:

Cl_{cr} 30-60 mL/minute: 2 g every 4 hours or 3 g every 8 hours

Cl_{cr} 10-30 mL/minute: 2 g every 8 hours or 3 g every 12 hours

Cl_{cr} <10 mL/minute: 2 g every 12 hours

Moderately dialyzable (20% to 50%)

Continuous arteriovenous or venovenous hemodiafiltration (CAVH) effects: Dose as for Cl_{cr} 10-50 mL/minute

Administration Administer 1 hour apart from aminoglycosides

Monitoring Parameters Serum electrolytes, bleeding time, and periodic tests of renal, hepatic, and hematologic function; monitor for signs of anaphylaxis during first dose

Test Interactions May interfere with urinary glucose tests using cupric sulfate (Benedict's solution, Clinitest®); may inactivate aminoglycosides *in vitro*; false-positive urinary or serum protein

Nursing Implications Draw sample for culture and sensitivity before administering first dose, if possible

Additional Information Sodium content of 1 g: 119.6-149.5 mg (5.2-6.5 mEq)

Dosage Forms Powder for injection, as disodium: 1 g, 3 g, 6 g, 20 g, 30 g

Selected Readings

Donowitz GR and Mandell GL, "Beta-Lactam Antibiotics," *N Engl J Med*, 1988, 318(7):419-26 and 318(8):490-500.

Tan JS and File TM Jr, "Antipseudomonal Penicillins," *Med Clin North Am*, 1995, 79(4):679-93.

Wright AJ, "The Penicillins," *Mayo Clin Proc*, 1999, 74(3):290-307.

Ticarcillin and Clavulanate Potassium

(tye kar SIL in & klav yoo LAN ate poe TASS ee um)

Related Information

Antimicrobial Activity Against Selected Organisms *on page 983*

U.S. Brand Names Timentin®

Synonyms Ticarcillin and Clavulanic Acid

Generic Available No

Use Treatment of infections of lower respiratory tract, urinary tract, skin and skin structures, bone and joint, and septicemia caused by susceptible organisms. Clavulanate expands activity of ticarcillin to include beta-lactamase producing strains of *S. aureus*, *H. influenzae*, *Bacteroides* species, and some other gram-negative bacilli

Drug of Choice or Alternative for

Disease/Syndrome(s)

Cholangitis, Acute *on page 21*

Osteomyelitis, Diabetic Foot *on page 38*

Peritonitis, Spontaneous Bacterial *on page 43*

Pneumonia, Community-Acquired *on page 45*

Organism(s)

Bacteroides Species *on page 75*

Stenotrophomonas maltophilia on page 265

Pregnancy Risk Factor B

Contraindications Known hypersensitivity to ticarcillin, clavulanate, or any penicillin

Warnings/Precautions Not approved for use in children <12 years of age; use with caution and modify dosage in patients with renal impairment; use with caution in patients with a history of allergy to cephalosporins and in patients with CHF due to high sodium load

Adverse Reactions Percentage unknown: Convulsions, confusion, drowsiness, fever, rash, electrolyte imbalance, hemolytic anemia, positive Coombs' test, bleeding, thrombophlebitis, myoclonus, acute interstitial nephritis, hypersensitivity reactions, anaphylaxis, Jarisch-Herxheimer reaction

Overdosage/Toxicology

Symptoms of overdose include neuromuscular hypersensitivity, seizures; many beta-lactam containing antibiotics have the potential to cause neuromuscular hyperirritability or convulsive seizures

Hemodialysis may be helpful to aid in the removal of the drug from the blood, otherwise most treatment is supportive or symptom directed

Drug Interactions

Decreased effect:

Tetracyclines may decrease penicillin effectiveness

Aminoglycosides → physical inactivation of aminoglycosides in the presence of high concentrations of ticarcillin

Decreased effectiveness of oral contraceptives

Increased effect:

Probenecid may increase penicillin levels

Neuromuscular blockers may increase duration of blockade

Potential toxicity in patients with mild-moderate renal dysfunction

Aminoglycosides → synergistic efficacy

Increased bleeding risk with large I.V. doses and anticoagulants

Stability Reconstituted solution is stable for 6 hours at room temperature and 72 hours when refrigerated; for I.V. infusion in NS is stable for 24 hours at room temperature, 7 days when refrigerated or 30 days when frozen; after freezing, thawed solution is stable for 8 hours at room temperature; for I.V. infusion in D$_5$W solution is stable for 24 hours at room temperature, 3 days when refrigerated or 7 days when frozen; after freezing, thawed solution is stable for 8 hours at room temperature; darkening of drug indicates loss of potency of clavulanate potassium; incompatible with sodium bicarbonate, aminoglycosides

Mechanism of Action Inhibits bacterial cell wall synthesis by binding to one or more of the penicillin binding proteins (PBPs); which in turn inhibits the final transpeptidation step of peptidoglycan synthesis in bacterial cell walls, thus inhibiting cell wall biosynthesis. Bacteria eventually lyse due to ongoing activity of cell wall autolytic enzymes (autolysins and murein hydrolases) while cell wall assembly is arrested.

Pharmacodynamics/Kinetics

Distribution: Low concentrations of ticarcillin distribute into the CSF and increase when meninges are inflamed, otherwise widely distributed

Protein binding:

Ticarcillin: 45% to 65%

Clavulanic acid: 9% to 30% removed by hemodialysis

Metabolism: Clavulanic acid is metabolized in the liver

Half-life:

Clavulanate: 66-90 minutes

Ticarcillin: 66-72 minutes in patients with normal renal function; clavulanic acid does not affect the clearance of ticarcillin

Elimination: 45% excreted unchanged in urine, whereas 60% to 90% of ticarcillin excreted unchanged in urine

Usual Dosage I.V.:

Children and Adults <60 kg: 200-300 mg of ticarcillin component/kg/day in divided doses every 4-6 hours

Children >60 kg and Adults: 3.1 g (ticarcillin 3 g plus clavulanic acid 0.1 g) every 4-6 hours; maximum: 24 g/day

Urinary tract infections: 3.1 g every 6-8 hours

Dosing adjustment in renal impairment:

Cl$_{cr}$ 30-60 mL/minute: Administer 2 g every 4 hours or 3.1 g every 8 hours

Cl$_{cr}$ 10-30 mL/minute: Administer 2 g every 8 hours or 3.1 g every 12 hours

Cl$_{cr}$ <10 mL/minute: Administer 2 g every 12 hours

Moderately dialyzable (20% to 50%)

Continuous arteriovenous or venovenous hemodiafiltration (CAVH) effects: Dose as for Cl$_{cr}$ 10-50 mL/minute

Administration Infuse over 30 minutes; administer 1 hour apart from aminoglycosides

Monitoring Parameters Observe signs and symptoms of anaphylaxis during first dose

Test Interactions Positive Coombs' test, false-positive urinary proteins

Nursing Implications Draw sample for culture and sensitivity prior to first dose if possible

Additional Information Sodium content of 1 g: 4.75 mEq; potassium content of 1 g: 0.15 mEq

Dosage Forms

Infusion, premixed (frozen): Ticarcillin disodium 3 g and clavulanate potassium 0.1 g (100 mL)

(Continued)

LIVERPOOL JOHN MOORES UNIVERSITY
LEARNING SERVICES

Ticarcillin and Clavulanate Potassium *(Continued)*

Powder for injection: Ticarcillin disodium 3 g and clavulanate potassium 0.1 g (3.1 g, 31 g)

Selected Readings

Donowitz GR and Mandell GL, "Beta-Lactam Antibiotics," *N Engl J Med*, 1988, 318(7):419-26 and 318(8):490-500.

Itokazu GS and Danziger LH, "Ampicillin-Sulbactam and Ticarcillin-Clavulanic Acid: A Comparison of Their *In Vitro* Activity and Review of Their Clinical Efficacy," *Pharmacotherapy*, 1991, 11(5):382-414.

Wright AJ, "The Penicillins," *Mayo Clin Proc*, 1999, 74(3):290-307.

Tioconazole *(tye oh KONE a zole)*

U.S. Brand Names Vagistat-1® Vaginal [OTC]

Generic Available No

Use Local treatment of vulvovaginal candidiasis

Pregnancy Risk Factor C

Contraindications Known hypersensitivity to tioconazole

Warnings/Precautions Not effective when applied to the scalp; may interact with condoms and vaginal contraceptive diaphragms; avoid these products for 3 days following treatment

Adverse Reactions

1% to 10%: Genitourinary: Vulvar/vaginal burning

<1%: Vulvar itching, soreness, edema, or discharge; polyuria

Mechanism of Action A 1-substituted imidazole derivative with a broad antifungal spectrum against a wide variety of dermatophytes and yeasts, usually at a concentration ≤6.25 mg/L; has been demonstrated to be at least as active *in vitro* as other imidazole antifungals. *In vitro*, tioconazole has been demonstrated 2-8 times as potent as miconazole against common dermal pathogens including *Trichophyton mentagrophytes*, *T. rubrum*, *T. erinacei*, *T. tonsurans*, *Microsporum canis*, *Microsporum gypseum*, and *Candida albicans*. Both agents appear to be similarly effective against *Epidermophyton floccosum*.

Pharmacodynamics/Kinetics

Absorption: Intravaginal: Following application small amounts of drug are absorbed systemically (25%) within 2-8 hours; therapeutic levels persist for 3-5 days after single dose

Half-life: 21-24 hours

Elimination: Urine and feces in approximate equal amounts

Usual Dosage Adults: Vaginal: Insert 1 applicatorful in vagina, just prior to bedtime, as a single dose; therapy may extend to 7 days

Patient Information Insert high into vagina; contact physician if itching or burning continues; Vagistat-1® may interact with condoms and vaginal contraceptive diaphragms (ie, weaken latex); do not rely on these products for 3 days following treatment

Dosage Forms Cream, vaginal: 6.5% with applicator (4.6 g)

Tobramycin (toe bra MYE sin)

Related Information

Aminoglycoside Dosing and Monitoring *on page 1058*
Antimicrobial Activity Against Selected Organisms *on page 983*

U.S. Brand Names AKTob® Ophthalmic; Nebcin® Injection; TOBI™ Inhalation Solution; Tobrex® Ophthalmic

Synonyms Tobramycin Sulfate

Generic Available Yes

Use Treatment of documented or suspected infections caused by susceptible gram-negative bacilli including *Pseudomonas aeruginosa*; topically used to treat superficial ophthalmic infections caused by susceptible bacteria

Drug of Choice or Alternative for

Disease/Syndrome(s)

Meningitis, Postsurgical *on page 36*

Organism(s)

Burkholderia cepacia on page 87

Pregnancy Risk Factor C

Contraindications Hypersensitivity to tobramycin or other aminoglycosides or components

Warnings/Precautions Use with caution in patients with renal impairment; pre-existing auditory or vestibular impairment; and in patients with neuromuscular disorders; dosage modification required in patients with impaired renal function; aminoglycosides (I.M. & I.V.) are associated with significant nephrotoxicity or ototoxicity; the ototoxicity is directly proportional to the amount of drug given and the duration of treatment; tinnitus or vertigo are indications of vestibular injury; ototoxicity is often irreversible; renal damage is usually reversible

Adverse Reactions

1% to 10%:
Renal: Nephrotoxicity
Neuromuscular & skeletal: Neurotoxicity (neuromuscular blockade)
Otic: Ototoxicity (auditory), ototoxicity (vestibular)
<1%: Hypotension, drug fever, headache, drowsiness, rash, nausea, vomiting, eosinophilia, anemia, paresthesia, tremor, arthralgia, weakness, lacrimation, itching eyes, edema of the eyelid, keratitis, dyspnea

Overdosage/Toxicology

Symptoms of overdose include ototoxicity, nephrotoxicity, and neuromuscular toxicity

The treatment of choice following a single acute overdose appears to be the maintenance of good urine output of at least 3 mL/kg/hour. Dialysis is of questionable value in the enhancement of aminoglycoside elimination. If required, hemodialysis is preferred over peritoneal dialysis in patients with normal renal function. Careful hydration may be all that is required to promote diuresis and therefore the enhancement of the drug's elimination.

Drug Interactions

Increased effect: Extended spectrum penicillins (synergistic)
Increased toxicity:
Neuromuscular blockers increase neuromuscular blockade
Amphotericin B, cephalosporins, loop diuretics, and vancomycin may increase risk of nephrotoxicity

Stability

Tobramycin is stable at room temperature both as the clear, colorless solution and as the dry powder; reconstituted solutions remain stable for 24 hours at room temperature and 96 hours when refrigerated
Stability of parenteral admixture at room temperature (25°C) and at refrigeration temperature (4°C): 48 hours
Standard diluent: Dose/100 mL NS
Minimum volume: 50 mL NS
Incompatible with penicillins

Mechanism of Action Interferes with bacterial protein synthesis by binding to 30S and 50S ribosomal subunits resulting in a defective bacterial cell membrane

Pharmacodynamics/Kinetics

Absorption: I.M.: Rapid and complete
Time to peak serum concentration:
I.M.: Within 30-60 minutes
I.V.: Within 30 minutes

(Continued)

Tobramycin *(Continued)*

Distribution: To extracellular fluid including serum, abscesses, ascitic, pericardial, pleural, synovial, lymphatic, and peritoneal fluids; crosses the placenta; poor penetration into CSF, eye, bone, prostate

V_d: 0.2-0.3 L/kg; Pediatric patients: 0.2-0.7 L/kg

Protein binding: <30%

Half-life:

Neonates:

≤1200 g: 11 hours

>1200 g: 2-9 hours

Adults: 2-3 hours, directly dependent upon glomerular filtration rate

Adults with impaired renal function: 5-70 hours

Elimination: With normal renal function, about 90% to 95% of a dose is excreted in the urine within 24 hours

Usual Dosage Individualization is critical because of the low therapeutic index

Use of ideal body weight (IBW) for determining the mg/kg/dose appears to be more accurate than dosing on the basis of total body weight (TBW)

In morbid obesity, dosage requirement may best be estimated using a dosing weight of IBW + 0.4 (TBW - IBW)

Initial and periodic peak and trough plasma drug levels should be determined, particularly in critically ill patients with serious infections or in disease states known to significantly alter aminoglycoside pharmacokinetics (eg, cystic fibrosis, burns, or major surgery). Two to three serum level measurements should be obtained after the initial dose to measure the half-life in order to determine the frequency of subsequent doses.

Once daily dosing: Higher peak serum drug concentration to MIC ratios, demonstrated aminoglycoside postantibiotic effect, decreased renal cortex drug uptake, and improved cost-time efficiency are supportive reasons for the use of once daily dosing regimens for aminoglycosides. Current research indicates these regimens to be as effective for nonlife-threatening infections, with no higher incidence of nephrotoxicity, than those requiring multiple daily doses. Doses are determined by calculating the entire day's dose via usual multiple dose calculation techniques and administering this quantity as a single dose. Doses are then adjusted to maintain mean serum concentrations above the MIC(s) of the causative organism(s). (Example: 2.5-5 mg/kg as a single dose; expected Cp_{max}: 10-20 mcg/mL and Cp_{min}: <1 mcg/mL). Further research is needed for universal recommendation in all patient populations and gram-negative disease; exceptions may include those with known high clearance (eg, children, patients with cystic fibrosis, or burns who may require shorter dosage intervals) and patients with renal function impairment for whom longer than conventional dosage intervals are usually required.

Some clinicians suggest a daily dose of 4-7 mg/kg for all patients with normal renal function. This dose is at least as efficacious with similar, if not less, toxicity than conventional dosing. (See also Aminoglycoside Dosing and Monitoring *on page 1058*.)

Infants and Children <5 years: I.M., I.V.: 2.5 mg/kg/dose every 8 hours

Children >5 years: 1.5-2.5 mg/kg/dose every 8 hours

Note: Some patients may require larger or more frequent doses if serum levels document the need (ie, cystic fibrosis or febrile granulocytopenic patients).

Adults: I.M., I.V.:

Severe life-threatening infections: 2-2.5 mg/kg/dose

Urinary tract infection: 1.5 mg/kg/dose

Synergy (for gram-positive infections): 1 mg/kg/dose

Children and Adults: Ophthalmic: Instill 1-2 drops of solution every 4 hours; apply ointment 2-3 times/day; for severe infections apply ointment every 3-4 hours, or solution 2 drops every 30-60 minutes initially, then reduce to less frequent intervals

Inhalation:

Standard aerosolized tobramycin:

Children: 40-80 mg 2-3 times/day

Adults: 60-80 mg 3 times/day

High-dose regimen: Children ≥6 years and Adults: 300 mg every 12 hours (do not administer doses less than 6 hours apart); administer in repeated cycles of 28 days on drug followed by 28 days off drug

Dosing interval in renal impairment:
Cl_{cr} ≥60 mL/minute: Administer every 8 hours
Cl_{cr} 40-60 mL/minute: Administer every 12 hours
Cl_{cr} 20-40 mL/minute: Administer every 24 hours
Cl_{cr} 10-20 mL/minute: Administer every 48 hours
Cl_{cr} <10 mL/minute: Administer every 72 hours
Hemodialysis: Dialyzable; 30% removal of aminoglycosides occurs during 4 hours of HD - administer dose after dialysis and follow levels
Continuous arteriovenous or venovenous hemofiltration (CAVH/CAVHD): Dose as for Cl_{cr} of 10-40 mL/minute and follow levels
Administration in CAPD fluid:
Gram-negative infection: 4-8 mg/L (4-8 mcg/mL) of CAPD fluid
Gram-positive infection (ie, synergy): 3-4 mg/L (3-4 mcg/mL) of CAPD fluid
Administration IVPB/I.M.: Dose as for Cl_{cr} <10 mL/minute and follow levels

Dosing adjustment/comments in hepatic disease: Monitor plasma concentrations

Dietary Considerations Calcium, magnesium, potassium: Renal wasting may cause hypocalcemia, hypomagnesemia, and/or hypokalemia

Monitoring Parameters Urinalysis, urine output, BUN, serum creatinine, peak and trough plasma tobramycin levels; be alert to ototoxicity; hearing should be tested before and during treatment

Reference Range
Timing of serum samples: Draw peak 30 minutes after 30-minute infusion has been completed or 1 hour following I.M. injection or beginning of infusion; draw trough immediately before next dose
Therapeutic levels:
Peak:
Serious infections: 6-8 µg/mL (SI: 12-17 mg/L)
Life-threatening infections: 8-10 µg/mL (SI: 17-21 mg/L)
Urinary tract infections: 4-6 µg/mL (SI: 7-12 mg/L)
Synergy against gram-positive organisms: 3-5 µg/mL
Trough:
Serious infections: 0.5-1 µg/mL
Life-threatening infections: 1-2 µg/mL
Monitor serum creatinine and urine output; obtain drug levels after the third dose unless otherwise directed

Patient Information Report symptoms of superinfection; for eye drops - no other eye drops 5-10 minutes before or after tobramycin; report any dizziness or sensations of ringing or fullness in ears

Nursing Implications Eye solutions: Allow 5 minutes between application of "multiple-drop" therapy; obtain drug levels after the third dose; peak levels are drawn 30 minutes after the end of a 30-minute infusion or 1 hour after initiation of infusion or I.M. injection; the trough is drawn just before the next dose; administer penicillins or cephalosporins at least 1 hour apart from tobramycin

Dosage Forms
Injection, as sulfate (Nebcin®): 10 mg/mL (2 mL); 40 mg/mL (1.5 mL, 2 mL)
Ointment, ophthalmic (Tobrex®): 0.3% (3.5 g)
Powder for injection (Nebcin®): 40 mg/mL (1.2 g vials)
Solution, inhalation (TOBI™): 60 mg/mL (5 mL)
Solution, ophthalmic: 0.3% (5 mL)
AKTob®, Tobrex®: 0.3% (5 mL)

Selected Readings
Begg EJ and Barclay ML, "Aminoglycosides - 50 Years On," *Br J Clin Pharmacol*, 1995, 39(6):597-603.
Cunha BA, "Aminoglycosides: Current Role in Antimicrobial Therapy," *Pharmacotherapy*, 1988, 8(6):334-50.
Edson RS and Terrell CL, "The Aminoglycosides," *Mayo Clin Proc*, 1999, 74(5):519-28.
Gilbert DN, "Once-Daily Aminoglycoside Therapy," *Antimicrob Agents Chemother*, 1991, 35(3):399-405.
Hustinx WN, and Hoepelman IM, "Aminoglycoside Dosage Regimens. Is Once a Day Enough?" *Clin Pharmacokinet*, 1993, 25(6):427-32.
Lortholary O, Tod M, Cohen Y, et al, "Aminoglycosides," *Med Clin North Am*, 1995, 79(4):761-87.
McCormack JP and Jewesson PJ, "A Critical Reevaluation of the "Therapeutic Range" of Aminoglycosides," *Clin Infect Dis*, 1992, 14(1):320-39.

Tobramycin and Dexamethasone
(toe bra MYE sin & deks a METH a sone)

Related Information
Tobramycin *on page 953*

U.S. Brand Names TobraDex®

Synonyms Dexamethasone and Tobramycin

Use Treatment of external ocular infection caused by susceptible gram-negative bacteria and steroid responsive inflammatory conditions of the palpebral and bulbar conjunctiva, lid, cornea, and anterior segment of the globe

Usual Dosage Children and Adults: Ophthalmic: Instill 1-2 drops of solution every 4 hours; apply ointment 2-3 times/day; for severe infections apply ointment every 3-4 hours, or solution 2 drops every 30-60 minutes initially, then reduce to less frequent intervals

Dosage Forms
Ointment, ophthalmic: Tobramycin 0.3% and dexamethasone 0.1% (3.5 g)
Suspension, ophthalmic: Tobramycin 0.3% and dexamethasone 0.1% (2.5 mL, 5 mL)

Tobramycin Sulfate *see Tobramycin on page 953*

Tobrex® Ophthalmic *see Tobramycin on page 953*

Tolnaftate (tole NAF tate)

U.S. Brand Names Absorbine® Antifungal [OTC]; Absorbine® Jock Itch [OTC]; Absorbine Jr.® Antifungal [OTC]; Aftate® for Athlete's Foot [OTC]; Aftate® for Jock Itch [OTC]; Blis-To-Sol® [OTC]; Breezee® Mist Antifungal [OTC]; Dr Scholl's Athlete's Foot [OTC]; Dr Scholl's Maximum Strength Tritin [OTC]; Genaspor® [OTC]; NP-27® [OTC]; Quinsana Plus® [OTC]; Tinactin® [OTC]; Tinactin® for Jock Itch [OTC]; Ting® [OTC]; Zeasorb-AF® Powder [OTC]

Canadian Brand Names Pitrex®

Generic Available Yes

Use Treatment of tinea pedis, tinea cruris, tinea corporis, tinea manuum, tinea versicolor infections

Pregnancy Risk Factor C

Contraindications Known hypersensitivity to tolnaftate; nail and scalp infections

Warnings/Precautions Cream is not recommended for nail or scalp infections; keep from eyes; if no improvement within 4 weeks, treatment should be discontinued. Usually not effective alone for the treatment of infections involving hair follicles or nails.

Adverse Reactions 1% to 10%:
Dermatologic: Pruritus, contact dermatitis
Local: Irritation, stinging

Mechanism of Action Distorts the hyphae and stunts mycelial growth in susceptible fungi

Pharmacodynamics/Kinetics Onset of action: 24-72 hours

Usual Dosage Children and Adults: Topical: Wash and dry affected area; apply 1-3 drops of solution or a small amount of cream or powder and rub into the affected areas 2-3 times/day for 2-4 weeks

Patient Information Avoid contact with the eyes; apply to clean dry area; consult the physician if a skin irritation develops or if the skin infection worsens or does not improve after 10 days of therapy; does not stain skin or clothing

Nursing Implications Itching, burning, and soreness are usually relieved within 24-72 hours

Dosage Forms
Aerosol, topical:
Liquid: 1% (59.2 mL, 90 mL, 120 mL)
Powder: 1% (56.7 g, 100 g, 105 g, 150 g)
Cream: 1% (15 g, 30 g)
Gel, topical: 1% (15 g)
Powder, topical: 1% (45 g, 90 g)
Solution, topical: 1% (10 mL)

Topicycline® Topical *see Tetracycline on page 944*

TOPV *see Poliovirus Vaccine, Live, Trivalent, Oral on page 876*

Totacillin® *see Ampicillin on page 604*

Totacillin®-N *see Ampicillin on page 604*

Trecator®-SC *see Ethionamide on page 728*

Triacetyloleandomycin *see Troleandomycin on page 960*

Triaconazole *see Terconazole on page 938*

Triamcinolone and Nystatin *see Nystatin and Triamcinolone on page 846*

Tribavirin *see Ribavirin on page 899*

Trifluorothymidine *see Trifluridine on this page*

Trifluridine (trye FLURE i deen)

U.S. Brand Names Viroptic® Ophthalmic

Synonyms F_3T; Trifluorothymidine

Generic Available No

Use Treatment of primary keratoconjunctivitis and recurrent epithelial keratitis caused by herpes simplex virus types I and II

Pregnancy Risk Factor C

Contraindications Known hypersensitivity to trifluridine or any component

Warnings/Precautions Mild local irritation of conjunctival and cornea may occur when instilled but usually transient effects

Adverse Reactions

1% to 10%: Local: Burning, stinging

<1%: Hyperemia, palpebral edema, epithelial keratopathy, keratitis, stromal edema, increased intraocular pressure, hypersensitivity reactions

Stability Refrigerate at 2°C to 8°C (36°F to 46°F); storage at room temperature may result in a solution altered pH which could result in ocular discomfort upon administration and/or decreased potency

Mechanism of Action Interferes with viral replication by incorporating into viral DNA in place of thymidine, inhibiting thymidylate synthetase resulting in the formation of defective proteins

Pharmacodynamics/Kinetics Absorption: Ophthalmic instillation: Systemic absorption is negligible, while corneal penetration is adequate

Usual Dosage Adults: Instill 1 drop into affected eye every 2 hours while awake, to a maximum of 9 drops/day, until re-epithelialization of corneal ulcer occurs; then use 1 drop every 4 hours for another 7 days; do **not** exceed 21 days of treatment; if improvement has not taken place in 7-14 days, consider another form of therapy

Patient Information Notify physician if improvement is not seen after 7 days, condition worsens, or if irritation occurs; do not discontinue without notifying the physician, do not exceed recommended dosage

Dosage Forms Solution, ophthalmic: 1% (7.5 mL)

TriHIBit® *see Diphtheria, Tetanus Toxoids, and Acellular Pertussis Vaccine on page 708*

TriHIBIT™ *see Haemophilus b Conjugate Vaccine on page 756*

Tri-Immunol® *see Diphtheria, Tetanus Toxoids, and Whole-Cell Pertussis Vaccine, Adsorbed on page 710*

Trimethoprim (trye METH oh prim)

U.S. Brand Names Proloprim®; Trimpex®

Synonyms TMP

Generic Available Yes

Use Treatment of urinary tract infections due to susceptible strains of *E. coli, P. mirabilis, K. pneumoniae, Enterobacter* sp and coagulase-negative *Staphylococcus* including *S. saprophyticus*; acute otitis media in children; acute exacerbations of chronic bronchitis in adults; in combination with other agents for treatment of toxoplasmosis, *Pneumocystis carinii*; treatment of superficial ocular infections involving the conjunctiva and cornea

Drug of Choice or Alternative for

Organism(s)

Pneumocystis carinii on page 228

Pregnancy Risk Factor C

Contraindications Hypersensitivity to trimethoprim or any component, megaloblastic anemia due to folate deficiency

Warnings/Precautions Use with caution in patients with impaired renal or hepatic function or with possible folate deficiency

(Continued)

Trimethoprim *(Continued)*

Adverse Reactions
1% to 10%:
Dermatologic: Rash (3% to 7%), pruritus
Hematologic: Megaloblastic anemia (with chronic high doses)
<1%: Fever, exfoliative dermatitis, nausea, vomiting, epigastric distress, thrombocytopenia, neutropenia, leukopenia, cholestatic jaundice, increased LFTs, increased BUN/serum creatinine, hyperkalemia

Overdosage/Toxicology
Symptoms of acute toxicity includes: nausea, vomiting, confusion, dizziness; chronic overdose results in bone marrow suppression
Treatment of acute overdose is supportive following GI decontamination; treatment of chronic overdose is use of oral leucovorin 5-15 mg/day

Drug Interactions Increased effect/toxicity/levels of phenytoin; increased myelosuppression with methotrexate; may increase levels of digoxin

Mechanism of Action Inhibits folic acid reduction to tetrahydrofolate, and thereby inhibits microbial growth

Pharmacodynamics/Kinetics
Absorption: Oral: Readily and extensive
Protein binding: 42% to 46%
Metabolism: Partially in the liver
Half-life: 8-14 hours, prolonged with renal impairment
Time to peak serum concentration: Within 1-4 hours
Elimination: Significantly in urine (60% to 80% as unchanged drug)

Usual Dosage Oral:
Children: 4 mg/kg/day in divided doses every 12 hours
Adults: 100 mg every 12 hours or 200 mg every 24 hours; in the treatment of *Pneumocystis carinii* pneumonia; dose may be as high as 15-20 mg/kg/day in 3-4 divided doses

Dosing interval in renal impairment: Cl_{cr} 15-30 mL/minute: Administer 50 mg every 12 hours
Hemodialysis: Moderately dialyzable (20% to 50%)

Reference Range Therapeutic: Peak: 5-15 mg/L; Trough: 2-8 mg/L

Patient Information Take with milk or food; report any skin rash, persistent or severe fatigue, fever, sore throat, or unusual bleeding or bruising; complete full course of therapy

Dosage Forms Tablet: 100 mg, 200 mg

Trimethoprim and Polymyxin B
(trye METH oh prim & pol i MIKS in bee)

Related Information
Polymyxin B *on page 877*
Trimethoprim *on previous page*

U.S. Brand Names Polytrim® Ophthalmic

Use Treatment of surface ocular bacterial conjunctivitis and blepharoconjunctivitis

Usual Dosage Instill 1-2 drops in eye(s) every 4-6 hours

Dosage Forms Solution, ophthalmic: Trimethoprim sulfate 1 mg and polymyxin B sulfate 10,000 units per mL (10 mL)

Trimethoprim and Sulfamethoxazole *see* Co-Trimoxazole *on page 692*

Trimetrexate Glucuronate (tri me TREKS ate gloo KYOOR oh nate)

U.S. Brand Names Neutrexin® Injection

Use Alternative therapy for the treatment of moderate-to-severe *Pneumocystis carinii* pneumonia (PCP) in immunocompromised patients, including patients with acquired immunodeficiency syndrome (AIDS), who are intolerant of, or are refractory to, co-trimoxazole therapy or for whom co-trimoxazole and pentamidine are contraindicated. **Concurrent folinic acid (leucovorin) must always be administered.**

Pregnancy Risk Factor D

Contraindications Previous hypersensitivity to trimetrexate or methotrexate, severe existing myelosuppression

Warnings/Precautions Must be administered with concurrent leucovorin to avoid potentially serious or life-threatening toxicities; leucovorin therapy must extend for 72 hours past the last dose of trimetrexate; use with caution in patients with mild myelosuppression, severe hepatic or renal dysfunction, hypoproteinemia, hypoalbuminemia, or previous extensive myelosuppressive therapies

Adverse Reactions 1% to 10%:
Central nervous system: Seizures, fever
Dermatologic: Rash
Gastrointestinal: Stomatitis, nausea, vomiting
Hematologic: Neutropenia, thrombocytopenia, anemia
Hepatic: Increased LFTs
Neuromuscular & skeletal: Peripheral neuropathy
Renal: Increased serum creatinine
Miscellaneous: Flu-like illness, hypersensitivity reactions

Drug Interactions
Decreased effect of pneumococcal vaccine
Increased toxicity (infection rates) of yellow fever vaccine

Stability Reconstituted I.V. solution is stable for 24 hours at room temperature or 7 days when refrigerated; intact vials should be refrigerated at 2°C to 8°C

Mechanism of Action Exerts an antimicrobial effect through potent inhibition of the enzyme dihydrofolate reductase (DHFR)

Pharmacodynamics/Kinetics
Distribution: V_d: 0.62 L/kg
Metabolism: Extensive in the liver
Half-life: 15-17 hours

Usual Dosage Adults: I.V.: 45 mg/m^2 once daily over 60 minutes for 21 days; it is necessary to reduce the dose in patients with liver dysfunction, although no specific recommendations exist; concurrent folinic acid 20 mg/m^2 every 6 hours orally or I.V. for 24 days

Administration Reconstituted solution should be filtered (0.22 µM) prior to further dilution; final solution should be clear, hue will range from colorless to pale yellow; trimetrexate forms a precipitate instantly upon contact with chloride ion or leucovorin, therefore it should not be added to solutions containing sodium chloride or other anions; trimetrexate and leucovorin solutions **must** be administered separately; intravenous lines should be flushed with at least 10 mL of D$_5$W between trimetrexate and leucovorin

Monitoring Parameters Check and record patient's temperature daily; absolute neutrophil counts (ANC), platelet count, renal function tests (serum creatinine, BUN), hepatic function tests (ALT, AST, alkaline phosphatase)

Patient Information Report promptly any fever, rash, flu-like symptoms, numbness or tingling in the extremities, nausea, vomiting, abdominal pain, mouth sores, increased bruising or bleeding, black tarry stools

Nursing Implications Notify primary physician if there is fever ≥103°F, generalized rash, seizures, bleeding from any site, uncontrolled nausea/vomiting; laboratory abnormalities which warrant dose modification; any other clinical adverse event or laboratory abnormality occurring in therapy which is judged as serious for that patient or which causes unexplained effects or concern; initiate "Bleeding Precautions" for platelet counts ≤50,000/mm^3; initiate "Infection Control Measures" for absolute neutrophil counts (ANC) ≤1000/mm^3
Must administer folinic acid 20 mg/m^2 orally or I.V. every 6 hours for 24 days

Additional Information Not a vesicant; methotrexate derivative

Dosage Forms Powder for injection: 25 mg, 200 mg

Selected Readings
Fulton B, Wagstaff AJ, and McTavish D, "Trimetrexate. A Review of Its Pharmacodynamic and Pharmacokinetic Properties and Therapeutic Potential in the Treatment of *Pneumocystis carinii* Pneumonia," *Drugs*, 1995, 49(4):563-76.
Marshall JL and De Lap RJ, "Clinical Pharmacokinetics and Pharmacology of Trimetrexate," *Clin Pharmacokinet*, 1994, 26(3):190-200.
Masur H, "Prevention and Treatment of *Pneumocystis* Pneumonia," *N Engl J Med*, 1992, 327(26):1853-60.

Trimox® see Amoxicillin *on page 592*

Trimpex® see Trimethoprim *on page 957*

Tripedia® see Diphtheria, Tetanus Toxoids, and Acellular Pertussis Vaccine *on page 708*

Tripedia/ActHIB® see Diphtheria, Tetanus Toxoids, Whole-Cell Pertussis, and *Haemophilus influenzae* Type b Conjugate Vaccines *on page 711*

Triple Antibiotic® Topical see Bacitracin, Neomycin, and Polymyxin B *on page 619*

Triple Sulfa *see* Sulfabenzamide, Sulfacetamide, and Sulfathiazole *on page 927*

Triple X® **Liquid [OTC]** *see* Pyrethrins *on page 885*

Tri-Statin® **II Topical** *see* Nystatin and Triamcinolone *on page 846*

Trisulfa® *see* Co-Trimoxazole *on page 692*

Trisulfapyrimidines *see* Sulfadiazine, Sulfamethazine, and Sulfamerazine *on page 930*

Trisulfa-S® *see* Co-Trimoxazole *on page 692*

Trobicin® *see* Spectinomycin *on page 922*

Troleandomycin (troe lee an doe MYE sin)

U.S. Brand Names Tao®

Synonyms Triacetyloleandomycin

Generic Available No

Use Adjunct in the treatment of corticosteroid-dependent asthma due to its steroid-sparing properties; antibiotic with spectrum of activity similar to erythromycin

Pregnancy Risk Factor C

Contraindications Hypersensitivity to troleandomycin, other macrolides, or any component; concurrent use with cisapride

Warnings/Precautions Use with caution in patients with impaired hepatic function; chronic hepatitis may occur in patients with long or repetitive courses

Adverse Reactions
>10%: Gastrointestinal: Abdominal cramping and discomfort (dose-related)
1% to 10%:
   Dermatologic: Urticaria, rashes
   Gastrointestinal: Nausea, vomiting, diarrhea
<1%: Rectal burning, cholestatic jaundice

Overdosage/Toxicology
Symptoms of overdose include nausea, vomiting, diarrhea, hearing loss
Following GI decontamination, treatment is supportive

Drug Interactions CYP3A3/4 enzyme substrate; CYP3A3/4 and 3A5-7 enzyme inhibitor
Increased effect/toxicity/levels of carbamazepine, ergot alkaloids, methylprednisolone, oral contraceptives, theophylline, and triazolam; contraindicated with terfenadine, astemizole, cisapride, and pimozide due to decreased metabolism of this agent and resultant risk of cardiac arrhythmias and death

Mechanism of Action Decreases methylprednisolone clearance from a linear first order decline to a nonlinear decline in plasma concentration. Troleandomycin also has an undefined action independent of its effects on steroid elimination. Inhibits RNA-dependent protein synthesis at the chain elongation step; binds to the 50S ribosomal subunit resulting in blockage of transpeptidation.

Pharmacodynamics/Kinetics
Time to peak serum concentration: Within 2 hours
Elimination: 10% to 25% of dose excreted in urine as active drug; also excreted in feces via bile

Usual Dosage Oral:
Children 7-13 years: 25-40 mg/kg/day divided every 6 hours (125-250 mg every 6 hours)
   Adjunct in corticosteroid-dependent asthma: 14 mg/kg/day in divided doses every 6-12 hours not to exceed 250 mg every 6 hours; dose is tapered to once daily then alternate day dosing
Adults: 250-500 mg 4 times/day

Monitoring Parameters Hepatic function tests

Patient Information Complete full course of therapy; notify physician if persistent or severe abdominal pain, nausea, vomiting, jaundice, darkened urine, or fever occurs

Dosage Forms Capsule: 250 mg

Selected Readings
Tartaglione TA, "Therapeutic Options for the Management and Prevention of *Mycobacterium avium* Complex Infection in Patients With the Acquired Immunodeficiency Syndrome," *Pharmacotherapy,* 1996, 16(2):171-82.

Trovafloxacin (TROE va flox a sin)

U.S. Brand Names Trovan™

Synonyms Alatrovafloxacin Mesylate; CP-99,219-27

Use
Should be used only in life- or limb-threatening infections
Treatment of nosocomial pneumonia, community-acquired pneumonia, complicated intra-abdominal infections, gynecologic/pelvic infections, complicated skin and skin structure infections

Drug of Choice or Alternative for
Disease/Syndrome(s)
Peritonitis, Spontaneous Bacterial *on page 43*

Pregnancy Risk Factor C
Contraindications History of hypersensitivity to trovafloxacin, alatrofloxacin, quinolone antimicrobial agents or any other components of these products

Warnings/Precautions For use only in serious life- or limb-threatening infections. Initiation of therapy must occur in an inpatient healthcare facility. May alter GI flora resulting in pseudomembranous colitis due to *Clostridium difficile*; use with caution in patients with seizure disorders or severe cerebral atherosclerosis; discontinue if skin rash or pain, inflammation, or rupture of a tendon; photosensitivity; CNS stimulation may occur which may lead to tremor, restlessness, confusion, hallucinations, paranoia, depression, nightmares, insomnia, or lightheadedness. Hepatic reactions have resulted in death. Risk of hepatotoxicity is increased if therapy exceeds 14 days.

Adverse Reactions Note: Fatalities have occurred in patients developing hepatic necrosis

<10%:
Central nervous system: Dizziness, lightheadedness, headache
Dermatologic: Rash, pruritus
Gastrointestinal: Nausea, vomiting, diarrhea, abdominal pain
Genitourinary: Vaginitis
Hepatic: Increased LFTs
Local: Injection site reaction, pain, or inflammation

<1%: Anaphylaxis, hepatic necrosis, pancreatitis, Stevens-Johnson syndrome

Overdosage/Toxicology Empty the stomach by vomiting or gastric lavage. Observe carefully and give symptomatic and supportive treatment; maintain adequate hydration.

Drug Interactions Decreased effect of oral trovafloxacin:
Antacids containing magnesium or aluminum, sucralfate, citric acid buffered with sodium citrate, and metal cations: Administer oral trovafloxacin doses at least 2 hours before or 2 hours after

Morphine: Administer I.V. morphine at least 2 hours after oral trovafloxacin in the fasting state and at least 4 hours after oral trovafloxacin when taken with food

Stability Trovan™ I.V. should not be diluted with 0.9% sodium chloride injection, USP (normal saline), alone or in combination with other diluents. A precipitate may form under these conditions. In addition, Trovan™ I.V. should not be diluted with lactated Ringer's, USP.

Mechanism of Action Inhibits DNA-gyrase in susceptible organisms; inhibits relaxation of supercoiled DNA and promotes breakage of double-stranded DNA

Pharmacodynamics/Kinetics
Distribution: Concentration in most tissues greater than plasma or serum
Protein binding: 76%
Metabolism: Hepatic conjugation
Bioavailability: 88%
Half-life: 9-12 hours
Elimination: 50% excreted unchanged (43% feces, 6% urine)

Usual Dosage Adults:
Nosocomial pneumonia: I.V.: 300 mg single dose followed by 200 mg/day orally for a total duration of 10-14 days
Community-acquired pneumonia: Oral, I.V.: 200 mg/day for 7-14 days
Complicated intra-abdominal infections, including postsurgical infections/gynecologic and pelvic infections: I.V.: 300 mg as a single dose followed by 200 mg/day orally for a total duration of 7-14 days
Skin and skin structure infections, complicated, including diabetic foot infections: Oral, I.V.: 200 mg/day for 10-14 days
Dosage adjustment in renal impairment: No adjustment is necessary
Dosage adjustment for hemodialysis: None required; trovafloxacin not sufficiently removed by hemodialysis
(Continued)

Trovafloxacin *(Continued)*

Dosage adjustment in hepatic impairment:
Mild to moderate cirrhosis:
Initial dose for normal hepatic function: 300 mg I.V.; 200 mg I.V. or oral; 100 mg oral
Reduced dose: 200 mg I.V.; 100 mg I.V. or oral; 100 mg oral
Severe cirrhosis: No data available

Dietary Considerations Dairy products such as milk and yogurt reduce the absorption of oral trovafloxacin - avoid concurrent use. The bioavailability may also be decreased by enteral feedings.

Administration Administer IVPB over 60 minutes

Monitoring Parameters Periodic assessment of liver function tests should be considered

Patient Information Drink fluids liberally; do not take antacids containing magnesium or aluminum or products containing iron or zinc simultaneously or within 4 hours before or 2 hours after taking dose. May cause dizziness or lightheadedness; observe caution while driving or performing other tasks requiring alertness, coordination, or physical dexterity. CNS stimulation may occur (eg, tremor, restlessness, confusion). Avoid excessive sunlight/artificial ultraviolet light; discontinue drug if phototoxicity occurs. Avoid re-exposure to ultraviolet light. Reactions may recur up to several weeks after stopping therapy.

Dosage Forms
Injection, as mesylate (alatrofloxacin): 5 mg/mL (40 mL, 60 mL)
Tablet, as mesylate (trovafloxacin): 100 mg, 200 mg

Selected Readings
Ernst ME, Ernst EJ, and Klepser ME, "Levofloxacin and Trovafloxacin: The Next Generation of Fluoroquinolones?" *Am J Health Syst Pharm*, 1997, 54(22):2569-84.
Garey KW and Amsden GW, "Trovafloxacin: An Overview," *Pharmacotherapy*, 1999, 19(1):21-34.
Haria M and Lamb HA, "Trovafloxacin," *Drugs*, 1997, 54(3):435-45.
Hecht DW and Osmolski JR, "Comparison of Activities of Trovafloxacin (CP-99,219) and Five Other Agents Against 585 Anaerobes With Use of Three Media," *Clin Infect Dis*, 1996, 23(Suppl 1):S44-50.
"Trovafloxacin," *Med Lett Drugs Ther*, 1998, 40(1022):30-1.

Trovan™ *see* Trovafloxacin *on page 960*

Trysul® *see* Sulfabenzamide, Sulfacetamide, and Sulfathiazole *on page 927*

TST *see* Tuberculin Tests *on this page*

Tubasal® *see* Aminosalicylate Sodium *on page 591*

Tuberculin Purified Protein Derivative *see* Tuberculin Tests *on this page*

Tuberculin Skin Test *see* Tuberculin Tests *on this page*

Tuberculin Tests *(too BER kyoo lin tests)*

U.S. Brand Names Aplisol®; Aplitest®; Sclavo-PPD Solution®; Sclavo Test-PPD®; Tine Test PPD; Tubersol®

Synonyms Mantoux; PPD; Tine Test; TST; Tuberculin Purified Protein Derivative; Tuberculin Skin Test

Generic Available No

Use Skin test in diagnosis of tuberculosis, cell-mediated immunodeficiencies

Pregnancy Risk Factor C

Contraindications 250 TU strength should not be used for initial testing

Warnings/Precautions Do not administer I.V. or S.C.; epinephrine (1:1000) should be available to treat possible allergic reactions

Adverse Reactions 1% to 10%:
Dermatologic: Ulceration, vesiculation
Local: Pain at injection site
Miscellaneous: Necrosis

Drug Interactions Decreased effect: Reaction may be suppressed in patients receiving systemic corticosteroids, aminocaproic acid, or within 4-6 weeks following immunization with live or inactivated viral vaccines

Stability Refrigerate; Tubersol® opened vials are stable for up to 24 hours at <75°F

Mechanism of Action Tuberculosis results in individuals becoming sensitized to certain antigenic components of the *M. tuberculosis* organism. Culture extracts called tuberculins are contained in tuberculin skin test preparations. Upon intracutaneous injection of these culture extracts, a classic delayed (cellular) hypersensitivity reaction occurs. This reaction is characteristic of a delayed course (peak occurs >24 hours after injection, induration of the skin secondary to cell infiltration, and occasional vesiculation and necrosis). Delayed hypersensitivity reactions to tuberculin may indicate infection with a variety of nontuberculosis mycobacteria, or vaccination with the live attenuated mycobacterial strain of *M. bovis* vaccine, BCG, in addition to previous natural infection with *M. tuberculosis*.

Pharmacodynamics/Kinetics

Onset of action: Delayed hypersensitivity reactions to tuberculin usually occur within 5-6 hours following injection

Peak effect: Become maximal at 48-72 hours

Duration: Reactions subside over a few days

Usual Dosage Children and Adults: Intradermal: 0.1 mL about 4" below elbow; use ¼" to ½" or 26- or 27-gauge needle; significant reactions are ≥5 mm in diameter

Interpretation of induration of tuberculin skin test injections: Positive: ≥10 mm; inconclusive: 5-9 mm; negative: <5 mm

Interpretation of induration of Tine test injections: Positive: >2 mm and vesiculation present; inconclusive: <2 mm (give patient Mantoux test of 5 TU/0.1 mL - base decisions on results of Mantoux test); negative: <2 mm or erythema of any size (no need for retesting unless person is a contact of a patient with tuberculosis or there is clinical evidence suggestive of the disease)

Patient Information Return to physician for reaction interpretation at 48-72 hours

Nursing Implications Test dose: 0.1 mL intracutaneously; store in refrigerator; examine site at 48-72 hours after administration; whenever tuberculin is administered, a record should be made of the administration technique (Mantoux method, disposable multiple-puncture device), tuberculin used (OT or PPD), manufacturer and lot number of tuberculin used, date of administration, date of test reading, and the size of the reaction in millimeters (mm).

Dosage Forms Injection:

First test strength: 1 TU/0.1 mL (1 mL)

Intermediate test strength: 5 TU/0.1 mL (1 mL, 5 mL, 10 mL)

Second test strength: 250 TU/0.1 mL (1 mL)

Tine: 5 TU each test

Selected Readings

Dutt AK and Stead WW, "Tuberculosis," *Clin Geriatr Med*, 1992, 8(4):761-75.

Tuberculosis Guidelines *see page 1114*

Tubersol® *see* Tuberculin Tests *on previous page*

Typhim Vi® *see* Typhoid Vaccine *on this page*

Typhoid Vaccine (TYE foid vak SEEN)

U.S. Brand Names Typhim Vi®; Vivotif Berna™ Oral

Synonyms Typhoid Vaccine Live Oral Ty21a

Generic Available No

Use

Parenteral: Promotes active immunity to typhoid fever for patients intimately exposed to a typhoid carrier or foreign travel to a typhoid fever endemic area

Oral: For immunization of children >6 years of age and adults who expect intimate exposure of or household contact with typhoid fever, travelers to areas of world with risk of exposure to typhoid fever, and workers in microbiology laboratories with expected frequent contact with *S. typhi*

Typhoid vaccine: Live, attenuated Ty21a typhoid vaccine should not be administered to immunocompromised persons, including those known to be infected with HIV. Parenteral inactivated vaccine is a theoretically safer alternative for this group.

Pregnancy Risk Factor C

Contraindications Acute respiratory or other active infections, previous sensitivity to typhoid vaccine, congenital or acquired immunodeficient state, acute febrile illness, acute GI illness, other active infection, persistent diarrhea or vomiting

Warnings/Precautions Postpone use in presence of acute infection; use during pregnancy only when clearly needed, immune deficiency conditions; not all recipients of typhoid vaccine will be fully protected against typhoid fever. Travelers should take all necessary precautions to avoid contact or ingestion of potentially contaminated food or water sources. Unless a complete immunization schedule is followed, an optimum immune response may not be achieved. (Continued)

Typhoid Vaccine *(Continued)*

Adverse Reactions All serious adverse reactions must be reported to the U.S. Department of Health and Human Services (DHHS) Vaccine Adverse Event Reporting System (VAERS) 1-800-822-7967.

Oral:
1% to 10%:
Dermatologic: Rash
Gastrointestinal: Abdominal discomfort, stomach cramps, diarrhea, nausea, vomiting
<1%: Anaphylactic reaction

Injection:
>10%:
Central nervous system: Headache (9% to 30%), fever
Dermatologic: Erythema
Local: Tenderness, induration (6% to 40%)
Neuromuscular & skeletal: Myalgia (14% to 29%)
<1%: Hypotension

Drug Interactions Simultaneous administration with other vaccines which cause local or systemic adverse effects should be avoided

Decreased effect with concurrent use of sulfonamides or other antibiotics

Stability Refrigerate, do not freeze; potency is not harmed if mistakenly placed in freezer; however, remove from freezer as soon as possible and place in refrigerator; can still be used if exposed to temperature ≤80°F

Mechanism of Action Virulent strains of *Salmonella typhi* cause disease by penetrating the intestinal mucosa and entering the systemic circulation via the lymphatic vasculature. One possible mechanism of conferring immunity may be the provocation of a local immune response in the intestinal tract induced by oral ingesting of a live strain with subsequent aborted infection. The ability of *Salmonella typhi* to produce clinical disease (and to elicit an immune response) is dependent on the bacteria having a complete lipopolysaccharide. The live attenuate Ty21a strain lacks the enzyme UDP-4-galactose epimerase so that lipopolysaccharide is only synthesized under conditions that induce bacterial autolysis. Thus, the strain remains avirulent despite the production of sufficient lipopolysaccharide to evoke a protective immune response. Despite low levels of lipopolysaccharide synthesis, cells lyse before gaining a virulent phenotype due to the intracellular accumulation of metabolic intermediates.

Pharmacodynamics/Kinetics

Oral:
Onset of immunity to *Salmonella typhi*: Within about 1 week
Duration: ~5 years
Parenteral: Duration of immunity: ~3 years

Usual Dosage

S.C. (AKD and H-P):
Children 6 months to 10 years: 0.25 mL; repeat in ≥4 weeks (total immunization is 2 doses)
Children >10 years and Adults: 0.5 mL; repeat dose in ≥4 weeks (total immunization is 2 doses)
Booster: 0.25 mL every 3 years for children 6 months to 10 years and 0.5 mL every 3 years for children >10 years and adults; see Administration comments

Oral: Adults:
Primary immunization: 1 capsule on alternate days (day 1, 3, 5, and 7)
Booster immunization: Repeat full course of primary immunization every 5 years

Administration Only the H-P vaccine may be given intradermally and only for booster doses. The AKD vaccine may be given by jet injection; Typhim Vi® may be given I.M. and is indicated for children ≥2 years of age, give as a single 0.5 mL (25 mcg) injection in deltoid muscle

Patient Information Oral capsule should be taken 1 hour before a meal with cold or lukewarm drink, do not chew, swallow whole; systemic adverse effects may persist for 1-2 days. Take all 4 doses exactly as directed on alternate days to obtain a maximal response.

Nursing Implications The doses of vaccine are different between S.C. and intradermal; S.C. injection only should be used

Additional Information Inactivated bacteria vaccine; federal law requires that the date of administration, the vaccine manufacturer, lot number of vaccine, and the administering person's name, title and address be entered into the patient's permanent medical record

Dosage Forms

Capsule, enteric coated (Vivotif Berna™): Viable *S. typhi* Ty21a Colony-forming units 2-6 x 10⁹ and nonviable *S. typhi* Ty21a Colony-forming units 50 x 10⁹ with sucrose, ascorbic acid, amino acid mixture, lactose and magnesium stearate

Injection, suspension (H-P): Heat- and phenol-inactivated, killed Ty-2 strain of *S. typhi* organisms; provides 8 units/mL, ≤1 billion/mL and ≤35 mcg nitrogen/mL (5 mL, 10 mL)

Injection (Typhim Vi®): Purified Vi capsular polysaccharide 25 mcg/0.5 mL (0.5 mL)

Powder for suspension (AKD): 8 units/mL ≤1 billion/mL, acetone inactivated dried (50 doses)

Selected Readings

Gardner P and Schaffner W, "Immunization of Adults," *N Engl J Med*, 1993, 328(17):1252-8.

Valacyclovir (val ay SYE kloe veer)

U.S. Brand Names Valtrex®

Use Treatment of herpes zoster (shingles) in immunocompetent patients; episodic treatment or prophylaxis of recurrent genital herpes in immunocompetent patients; for first episode genital herpes

Drug of Choice or Alternative for

Organism(s)

Herpes Simplex Virus on page 170

Varicella-Zoster Virus on page 294

Pregnancy Risk Factor B

Pregnancy/Breast-Feeding Implications

Clinical effects on the fetus: Teratogenicity registry, thus far, has shown no increased rate of birth defects than that of the general population; however, the registry is small and use during pregnancy is only warranted if the potential benefit to the mother justifies the risk of the fetus

Breast-feeding/lactation: Avoid use in breast-feeding, if possible, since the drug distributes in high concentrations in breast milk

Contraindications Hypersensitivity to the drug or any component

Warnings/Precautions Thrombotic thrombocytopenic purpura/hemolytic uremic syndrome has occurred in immunocompromised patients; use caution and adjust the dose in elderly patients or those with renal insufficiency; safety and efficacy in children have not been established

Adverse Reactions

>10%:

Central nervous system: Headache (13% to 17%)

Gastrointestinal: Nausea (8% to 16%)

1% to 10%:

Central nervous system: Dizziness (2% to 4%)

(Continued)

Valacyclovir *(Continued)*

Dermatologic: Pruritus

Gastrointestinal: Diarrhea (4% to 5%), constipation (1% to 5%), abdominal pain (2% to 3%), anorexia (≤3%), vomiting (≤7%)

Neuromuscular & skeletal: Weakness (2% to 4%)

Miscellaneous: Photophobia

Overdosage/Toxicology

Symptoms of overdose include elevated serum creatinine, renal failure, and encephalitis, precipitation in renal tubules

Hemodialysis has resulted in up to 60% reduction in serum acyclovir levels after administration of acyclovir

Drug Interactions Decreased toxicity: Cimetidine and/or probenecid has decreased the rate but not the extent of valacyclovir conversion to acyclovir

Mechanism of Action Valacyclovir is rapidly and nearly completely converted to acyclovir by intestinal and hepatic metabolism. Acyclovir is converted to acyclovir monophosphate by virus-specific thymidine kinase then further converted to acyclovir triphosphate by other cellular enzymes. Acyclovir triphosphate inhibits DNA synthesis and viral replication by competing with deoxyguanosine triphosphate for viral DNA polymerase and being incorporated into viral DNA.

Pharmacodynamics/Kinetics

Distribution: Acyclovir: Widely distributed throughout the body including brain, kidney, lungs, liver, spleen, muscle, uterus, vagina, and CSF

Protein binding: Valacyclovir: 13.5% to 17.9% bound to human plasma proteins

Metabolism: Valacyclovir: Rapidly and nearly completely converted to acyclovir and elvalene by first-pass intestinal and/or hepatic metabolism; acyclovir is hepatically metabolized to a very small extent

Bioavailability: Acyclovir: ~55%

Half-life: Adults: 2.5-3.3 hours (acyclovir), approximately 30 minutes (valacyclovir); acyclovir in end stage renal disease: 14-20 hours

Elimination: Acyclovir: Primarily eliminated by kidney

Usual Dosage Adults: Oral:

Shingles: 1 g 3 times/day for 7 days

Genital herpes:

Episodic treatment: 500 mg twice daily for 5 days

Prophylaxis: 500-1000 mg once daily

Dosing interval in renal impairment:

Cl_{cr} 30-49 mL/minute: 1 g every 12 hours

Cl_{cr} 10-29 mL/minute: 1 g every 24 hours

Cl_{cr} <10 mL/minute: 500 mg every 24 hours

Hemodialysis: 33% removed during 4-hour session

Monitoring Parameters Urinalysis, BUN, serum creatinine, liver enzymes, and CBC

Patient Information Take with plenty of water

Herpes zoster: Therapy is most effective when started within 48 hours of onset of zoster rash

Recurrent genital herpes: Therapy should be initiated within 24 hours after the onset of signs or symptoms

Nursing Implications Observe for CNS changes; avoid dehydration; begin therapy at the earliest sign of zoster infection (within 48 hours of the rash)

Dosage Forms Caplets: 500 mg

Selected Readings

Acosta EP and Fletcher CV, "Valacyclovir," *Ann Pharmacother*, 1997, 31(2):185-91.

Alrabiah FA and Sacks SL, "New Antiherpesvirus Agents. Their Targets and Therapeutic Potential," *Drugs*, 1996, 52(1):17-32.

Perry CM and Faulds D, "Valaciclovir. A Review of Its Antiviral Activity, Pharmacokinetic Properties and Therapeutic Efficacy in Herpesvirus Infections," *Drugs*, 1996, 52(5):754-72.

"Valacyclovir," *Med Lett Drugs Ther*, 1996, 38(965):3-4.

Weller S, Blum MR, Doucette M, et al, "Pharmacokinetics of the Acyclovir Pro-Drug Valaciclovir After Escalating Single- and Multiple-Dose Administration to Normal Volunteers," *Clin Pharmacol Ther*, 1993, 54(6):595-605.

Valtrex® *see Valacyclovir on previous page*

Vancocin® *see Vancomycin on next page*

Vancocin® CP *see Vancomycin on next page*

Vancoled® *see Vancomycin on next page*

Vancomycin (van koe MYE sin)

Related Information

Antimicrobial Activity Against Selected Organisms *on page 983*

U.S. Brand Names Lyphocin®; Vancocin®; Vancoled®

Canadian Brand Names Vancocin® CP

Synonyms Vancomycin Hydrochloride

Generic Available Yes

Use Treatment of patients with infections caused by staphylococcal species and streptococcal species; used orally for staphylococcal enterocolitis or for antibiotic-associated pseudomembranous colitis produced by *C. difficile*

Drug of Choice or Alternative for

Disease/Syndrome(s)

Catheter Infection, Intravascular *on page 21*
Endocarditis, Acute, I.V. Drug Abuse *on page 26*
Endocarditis, Acute Native Valve *on page 26*
Endocarditis, Prosthetic Valve, Early *on page 27*
Endocarditis, Prosthetic Valve, Late *on page 28*
Endocarditis, Subacute Native Valve *on page 28*
Fever, Neutropenic *on page 30*
Joint Replacement, Early Infection *on page 32*
Joint Replacement, Late Infection *on page 33*
Meningitis, Community-Acquired, Adult *on page 34*
Meningitis, Pediatric (>2 months of age) *on page 35*
Meningitis, Postsurgical *on page 36*
Meningitis, Neonatal (<2 months of age) *on page 35*
Meningitis, Post-traumatic *on page 37*
Osteomyelitis, Healthy Adult *on page 39*
Osteomyelitis, Pediatric *on page 39*
Pneumonia, Hospital-Acquired *on page 46*
Sepsis *on page 48*
Sinusitis, Hospital-Acquired *on page 49*
Skin and Soft Tissue *on page 50*
Thrombophlebitis, Suppurative *on page 50*
Toxic Shock Syndrome *on page 51*
Urinary Tract Infection, Catheter-Associated *on page 52*
Wound Infection, Surgical *on page 54*

Organism(s)

Bacillus cereus on page 74
Clostridium difficile on page 105
Corynebacterium jeikeium on page 113
Enterococcus Species *on page 137*
Rhodococcus Species *on page 242*
Staphylococcus aureus, Methicillin-Resistant *on page 256*
Staphylococcus aureus, Methicillin-Susceptible *on page 258*
Staphylococcus epidermidis, Methicillin-Resistant *on page 261*
Staphylococcus epidermidis, Methicillin-Susceptible *on page 263*
Streptococcus agalactiae on page 266
Streptococcus bovis on page 267
Streptococcus pneumoniae on page 268
Streptococcus pneumoniae, Drug-Resistant *on page 270*
Streptococcus pyogenes on page 274
Streptococcus-Related Gram-Positive Cocci *on page 278*
Streptococcus, Viridans Group *on page 279*

Pregnancy Risk Factor C

Contraindications Hypersensitivity to vancomycin or any component; avoid in patients with previous severe hearing loss

Warnings/Precautions Use with caution in patients with renal impairment or those receiving other nephrotoxic or ototoxic drugs; dosage modification required in patients with impaired renal function (especially elderly)

Adverse Reactions

Oral:

>10%: Gastrointestinal: Bitter taste, nausea, vomiting

1% to 10%:

Central nervous system: Chills, drug fever
Hematologic: Eosinophilia

(Continued)

Vancomycin *(Continued)*

<1%: Vasculitis, thrombocytopenia, ototoxicity, renal failure, interstitial nephritis

Parenteral:

>10%:

Cardiovascular: Hypotension accompanied by flushing

Dermatologic: Erythematous rash on face and upper body (red neck or red man syndrome - infusion rate related)

1% to 10%:

Central nervous system: Chills, drug fever

Dermatologic: Rash

Hematologic: Eosinophilia, reversible neutropenia

<1%: Vasculitis, Stevens-Johnson syndrome, ototoxicity (especially with large doses), thrombocytopenia, renal failure (especially with renal dysfunction or pre-existing hearing loss)

Overdosage/Toxicology

Symptoms of overdose include ototoxicity, nephrotoxicity

There is no specific therapy for an overdosage with vancomycin. Care is symptomatic and supportive in nature. Peritoneal filtration and hemofiltration (not dialysis) have been shown to reduce the serum concentration of vancomycin; high flux dialysis may remove up to 25%.

Drug Interactions Increased toxicity: Anesthetic agents; other ototoxic or nephrotoxic agents

Stability

Vancomycin reconstituted intravenous solutions are stable for 14 days at room temperature or refrigeration

Stability of parenteral admixture at room temperature (25°C) or refrigeration temperature (4°C): 7 days

Standard diluent: 500 mg/150 mL D_5W; 750 mg/250 mL D_5W; 1 g/250 mL D_5W

Minimum volume: Maximum concentration is 5 mg/mL to minimize thrombophlebitis

Incompatible with heparin, phenobarbital

After the oral solution is reconstituted, it should be refrigerated and used within 2 weeks

Mechanism of Action Inhibits bacterial cell wall synthesis by blocking glycopeptide polymerization through binding tightly to D-alanyl-D-alanine portion of cell wall precursor

Pharmacodynamics/Kinetics

Absorption:

Oral: Poor

I.M.: Erratic

Intraperitoneal: Can result in 38% absorption systemically

Distribution: Widely distributed in body tissues and fluids except for CSF

Relative diffusion of antimicrobial agents from blood into cerebrospinal fluid (CSF): Good only with inflammation (exceeds usual MICs)

Ratio of CSF to blood level (%):

Normal meninges: Nil

Inflamed meninges: 20-30

Protein binding: 10%-50%

Half-life (biphasic): Terminal:

Newborns: 6-10 hours

Infants and Children 3 months to 4 years: 4 hours

Children >3 years: 2.2-3 hours

Adults: 5-11 hours, prolonged significantly with reduced renal function

End stage renal disease: 200-250 hours

Time to peak serum concentration: I.V.: Within 45-65 minutes

Elimination: As unchanged drug in the urine via glomerular filtration (80% to 90%); oral doses are excreted primarily in the feces

Usual Dosage Initial dosage recommendation: I.V.:

Neonates:

Postnatal age ≤7 days:

<1200 g: 15 mg/kg/dose every 24 hours

1200-2000 g: 10 mg/kg/dose every 12 hours

>2000 g: 15 mg/kg/dose every 12 hours

Postnatal age >7 days:

    <1200 g: 15 mg/kg/dose every 24 hours

    ≥1200 g: 10 mg/kg/dose divided every 8 hours

Infants >1 month and Children:

    40 mg/kg/day in divided doses every 6 hours

    Prophylaxis for bacterial endocarditis:

        Dental, oral, or upper respiratory tract surgery: 20 mg/kg 1 hour prior to the procedure

        GI/GU procedure: 20 mg/kg plus gentamicin 2 mg/kg 1 hour prior to surgery

Infants >1 month and Children with staphylococcal central nervous system infection: 60 mg/kg/day in divided doses every 6 hours

Adults:

    With normal renal function: 1 g **or** 10-15 mg/kg/dose every 12 hours

    Prophylaxis for bacterial endocarditis:

        Dental, oral, or upper respiratory tract surgery: 1 g 1 hour before surgery

        GI/GU procedure: 1 g plus 1.5 mg/kg gentamicin 1 hour prior to surgery

Dosing interval in renal impairment (vancomycin levels should be monitored in patients with any renal impairment):

    Cl_{cr} >60 mL/minute: Start with 1 g or 10-15 mg/kg/dose every 12 hours

    Cl_{cr} 40-60 mL/minute: Start with 1 g or 10-15 mg/kg/dose every 24 hours

    Cl_{cr} <40 mL/minute: Will need longer intervals; determine by serum concentration monitoring

Hemodialysis: Not dialyzable (0% to 5%); generally not removed; exception minimal-moderate removal by some of the newer high-flux filters; dose may need to be administered more frequently; monitor serum concentrations

Continuous ambulatory peritoneal dialysis (CAPD): Not significantly removed; administration via CAPD fluid: 15-30 mg/L (15-30 mcg/mL) of CAPD fluid

Continuous arteriovenous or venovenous hemofiltration (CAVH/CAVHD): Dose as for Cl_{cr} 10-40 mL/minute

Antibiotic lock technique (for catheter infections): 2 mg/mL in SWI/NS or D_5W; instill 3-5 mL into catheter port as a flush solution instead of heparin lock **(Note:** Do not mix with any other solutions)

Intrathecal: Vancomycin is available as a powder for injection and may be diluted to 1-5 mg/mL concentration in preservative-free 0.9% sodium chloride for administration into the CSF

    Neonates: 5-10 mg/day

    Children: 5-20 mg/day

    Adults: Up to 20 mg/day

Oral: Pseudomembranous colitis produced by *C. difficile*:

    Neonates: 10 mg/kg/day in divided doses

    Children: 40 mg/kg/day in divided doses, added to fluids

    Adults: 125 mg 4 times/day for 10 days

Monitoring Parameters Periodic renal function tests, urinalysis, serum vancomycin concentrations, WBC, audiogram

Reference Range

    Timing of serum samples: Draw peak 1 hour after 1-hour infusion has completed; draw trough just before next dose

    Therapeutic levels: Peak: 25-40 µg/mL; Trough: 5-12 µg/mL

    Toxic: >80 µg/mL (SI: >54 µmol/L)

Patient Information Report pain at infusion site, dizziness, fullness or ringing in ears with I.V. use; nausea or vomiting with oral use

Nursing Implications Obtain drug levels after the third dose unless otherwise directed; peaks are drawn 1 hour after the completion of a 1- to 2-hour infusion; troughs are obtained just before the next dose; slow I.V. infusion rate if maculopapular rash appears on face, neck, trunk, and upper extremities (Red man reaction)

Dosage Forms

    Capsule, as hydrochloride: 125 mg, 250 mg

    Powder for oral solution, as hydrochloride: 1 g, 10 g

    Powder for injection, as hydrochloride: 500 mg, 1 g, 2 g, 5 g, 10 g

Selected Readings

Cantú TG, Yamanaka-Yuen NA, and Lietman PS, "Serum Vancomycin Concentrations: Reappraisal of Their Clinical Value," *Clin Infect Dis*, 1994, 18(4):533-43.

Cunha BA, "Vancomycin," *Med Clin North Am*, 1995, 79(4):817-31.

French GL, "Enterococci and Vancomycin Resistance," *Clin Infect Dis*, 1998, 27(Suppl 1):S75-83.

Kelly CP, Pothoulakis C, and LaMont JT, "*Clostridium difficile* colitis," *N Engl J Med*, 1994, 330(4):257-62.

(Continued)

Vancomycin *(Continued)*

Lundstrom TS and Sobel JD, "Vancomycin, Trimethoprim-Sulfamethoxazole, and Rifampin," *Infect Dis Clin North Am*, 1995, 9(3):747-67.

Wilhelm MP, "Vancomycin," *Mayo Clin Proc*, 1991, 66(11):1165-70.

Vancomycin Hydrochloride *see Vancomycin on page 967*

Vansil™ *see Oxamniquine on page 851*

Vantin® *see Cefpodoxime on page 647*

VAQTA® *see Hepatitis A Vaccine on page 759*

Varicella Virus Vaccine *(var i SEL a VYE rus vak SEEN)*

U.S. Brand Names Varivax®

Synonyms Chicken Pox Vaccine; Varicella-Zoster Virus (VZV) Vaccine

Use The American Association of Pediatrics recommends that the chickenpox vaccine should be given to all healthy children between 12 months and 18 years; children between 12 months and 13 years who have not been immunized or who have not had chickenpox should receive 1 vaccination while children 13-18 years of age require 2 vaccinations 4-8 weeks apart; the vaccine has been added to the childhood immunization schedule for infants 12-28 months of age and children 11-12 years of age who have not been vaccinated previously or who have not had the disease; it is recommended to be given with the measles, mumps, and rubella (MMR) vaccine

Drug of Choice or Alternative for Organism(s)

Varicella-Zoster Virus *on page 294*

Pregnancy Risk Factor C

Pregnancy/Breast-Feeding Implications

Clinical effects on the fetus: Varivax® should not be administered to pregnant females and pregnancy should be avoided for 3 months following vaccination

Breast-feeding/lactation: Use during breast-feeding should be avoided

Contraindications Hypersensitivity to any component of the vaccine, including gelatin; a history of anaphylactoid reaction to neomycin; individuals with blood dyscrasias, leukemia, lymphomas, or other malignant neoplasms affecting the bone marrow or lymphatic systems; those receiving immunosuppressive therapy; primary and acquired immunodeficiency states; a family history of congenital or hereditary immunodeficiency; active untreated tuberculosis; febrile illness; pregnancy; I.V. injection

Warnings/Precautions

Children and adolescents with acute lymphoblastic leukemia in remission can receive the vaccine under an investigational protocol (215-283-0897); no clinical data are available on efficacy in children <12 months of age

Immediate treatment for anaphylactoid reaction should be available during vaccine use; defer vaccination for at least 5 months following blood or plasma transfusions, immune globulin (IgG), or VZIG (avoid IgG or IVIG use for 2 months following vaccination); salicylates should be avoided for 5 weeks after vaccination; vaccinated individuals should not have close association with susceptible high risk individuals (newborns, pregnant women, immunocompromised persons) following vaccination

Adverse Reactions All serious adverse reactions must be reported to the U.S. Department of Health and Human Services (DHHS) Vaccine Adverse Event Reporting System (VAERS) 1-800-822-7967.

Percentages are listed for children ≤12 years of age

>10%:

Central nervous system: Fever (14.7%)

Local: Induration/stiffness at the injection site (19.3%)

1% to 10%:

Central nervous system: Pain, irritability/nervousness, fatigue, disturbed sleep, headache, malaise, chills

Dermatologic: Redness, rash (at injection site - 3.4%), pruritus, generalized varicella-like rash (generalized - 3.8%)

Gastrointestinal: Diarrhea, loss of appetite, vomiting, abdominal pain, nausea

Hematologic: Hematoma

Neuromuscular & skeletal: Myalgia, arthralgia

Otic: Otitis

Respiratory: Upper respiratory illness, cough

Miscellaneous: Lymphadenopathy, allergic reactions

<1%: Febrile seizures (causality not established), pneumonitis

Drug Interactions Clinical studies show that Varivax® can be administered concomitantly with MMR and limited data indicate that DTP and PedvaxHIB™ may also be administered together (using separate sites and syringes)

Decreased effect: The effect of the vaccine may be decreased and the risk of varicella disease in individuals who are receiving immunosuppressant drugs may be increased

Increased effect: Salicylates may increase the risk of Reye's following varicella vaccination

Stability Store in freezer (-15°C), store diluent separately at room temperature or in refrigerator; discard if reconstituted vaccine is not used within 30 minutes

Mechanism of Action As a live, attenuated vaccine, varicella virus vaccine offers active immunity to disease caused by the varicella-zoster virus

Pharmacodynamics/Kinetics

Onset of action: Approximately 4-6 weeks postvaccination

Duration: Lowest breakthrough rates (0.2% to 2.9%) exist in the first 2 years following postvaccination, with slightly higher rates in the third through the fifth year

Usual Dosage S.C.:

Children 12 months to 12 years: 0.5 mL

Children 12 years to Adults: 2 doses of 0.5 mL separated by 4-8 weeks

Administration Inject S.C. into the outer aspect of the upper arm, if possible

Monitoring Parameters Rash, fever

Patient Information Report any adverse reactions to the healthcare provider or Vaccine Adverse Event Reporting System (1-800-822-7967); avoid pregnancy for 3 months following vaccination; avoid salicylates for 5 weeks after vaccination; avoid close association with susceptible high risk individuals following vaccination

Nursing Implications Obtain the previous immunization history (including allergic reactions) to previous vaccines; do not inject into a blood vessel; use the supplied diluent only for reconstitution; inject immediately after reconstitution

Additional Information Minimum potency level: 1350 plaque forming units (PFU)/0.5 mL

Dosage Forms Powder for injection, lyophilized powder, preservative free: 1350 plaque forming units (PFU)/0.5 mL (0.5 mL single-dose vials)

Varicella-Zoster Immune Globulin (Human)

(var i SEL a-ZOS ter i MYUN GLOB yoo lin HYU man)

Synonyms VZIG

Generic Available No

Use Passive immunization of susceptible immunodeficient patients after exposure to varicella; most effective if begun within 96 hours of exposure; there is no evidence VZIG modifies established varicella-zoster infections

Restrict administration to those patients meeting the following criteria:

Neoplastic disease (eg, leukemia or lymphoma)

Congenital or acquired immunodeficiency

Immunosuppressive therapy with steroids, antimetabolites or other immunosuppressive treatment regimens

Newborn of mother who had onset of chickenpox within 5 days before delivery or within 48 hours after delivery

Premature (≥28 weeks gestation) whose mother has no history of chickenpox

Premature (<28 weeks gestation or ≤1000 g VZIG) regardless of maternal history

One of the following types of exposure to chickenpox or zoster patient(s) may warrant administration:

Continuous household contact

Playmate contact (>1 hour play indoors)

Hospital contact (in same 2-4 bedroom or adjacent beds in a large ward or prolonged face-to-face contact with an infectious staff member or patient)

Susceptible to varicella-zoster

Age <15 years; administer to immunocompromised adolescents and adults and to other older patients on an individual basis

(Continued)

Varicella-Zoster Immune Globulin (Human) *(Continued)*

An acceptable alternative to VZIG prophylaxis is to treat varicella, if it occurs, with high-dose I.V. acyclovir

Age is the most important risk factor for reactivation of varicella zoster; persons <50 years of age have incidence of 2.5 cases per 1000, whereas those 60-79 have 6.5 cases per 1000 and those >80 years have 10 cases per 1000

Pregnancy Risk Factor C

Contraindications Not for prophylactic use in immunodeficient patients with history of varicella, unless patient's immunosuppression is associated with bone marrow transplantation; **not** recommended for nonimmunodeficient patients, including pregnant women, because the severity of chickenpox is much less than in immunosuppressed patients; allergic response to gamma globulin or anti-immunoglobulin; sensitivity to thimerosal; persons with IgA deficiency; do not administer to patients with thrombocytopenia or coagulopathies

Warnings/Precautions VZIG is not indicated for prophylaxis or therapy of normal adults who are exposed to or who develop varicella; it is not indicated for treatment of herpes zoster. Do not inject I.V.

Adverse Reactions

1% to 10%: Local: Discomfort at the site of injection (pain, redness, edema)

<1%: Malaise, headache, rash, angioedema, GI symptoms, respiratory symptom, anaphylactic shock

Drug Interactions Decreased effect: Live virus vaccines (do not administer within 3 months of immune globulin administration)

Stability Refrigerate at 2°C to 8°C (36°F to 46°F)

Mechanism of Action The exact mechanism has not been clarified but the antibodies in varicella-zoster immune globulin most likely neutralize the varicella-zoster virus and prevent its pathological actions

Usual Dosage High-risk susceptible patients who are exposed again more than 3 weeks after a prior dose of VZIG should receive another full dose; there is no evidence VZIG modifies established varicella-zoster infections.

I.M.: Administer by deep injection in the gluteal muscle or in another large muscle mass. Inject 125 units/10 kg (22 lb); maximum dose: 625 units (5 vials); minimum dose: 125 units; do not administer fractional doses. Do not inject I.V. See table.

VZIG Dose Based on Weight

Weight of Patient		Dose	
kg	lb	Units	No. of Vials
0-10	0-22	125	1
10.1-20	22.1-44	250	2
20.1-30	44.1-66	375	3
30.1-40	66.1-88	500	4
>40	>88	625	5

Administration Do not inject I.V.; administer deep I.M. into the gluteal muscle or other large muscle mass. For patients ≤10 kg, administer 1.25 mL at a single site; for patients >10 kg, administer no more than 2.5 mL at a single site. Administer entire contents of each vial.

Dosage Forms Injection: 125 units of antibody in single dose vials

Varicella-Zoster Virus (VZV) Vaccine *see Varicella Virus Vaccine on page 970*

Varivax® *see Varicella Virus Vaccine on page 970*

Vasocidin® Ophthalmic *see Sulfacetamide Sodium and Prednisolone on page 928*

Vasosulf® Ophthalmic *see Sulfacetamide Sodium and Phenylephrine on page 928*

V-Cillin K® *see Penicillin V Potassium on page 865*

Veetids® *see Penicillin V Potassium on page 865*

Velosef® *see Cephradine on page 666*

Venoglobulin®-I *see Immune Globulin, Intravenous on page 771*

Venoglobulin®-S *see Immune Globulin, Intravenous on page 771*

Vermizine® *see Piperazine on page 873*

Vermox® see Mebendazole on page 808
Vibramycin® see Doxycycline on page 713
Vibramycin® IV see Doxycycline on page 713
Vibra-Tabs® see Doxycycline on page 713

Vidarabine (vye DARE a been)
U.S. Brand Names Vira-A®
Synonyms Adenine Arabinoside; Ara-A; Arabinofuranosyladenine; Vidarabine Monohydrate
Generic Available No
Use Treatment of acute keratoconjunctivitis and epithelial keratitis due to herpes simplex virus type 1 and 2; superficial keratitis caused by herpes simplex virus
Pregnancy Risk Factor C
Contraindications Hypersensitivity to vidarabine or any component; sterile trophic ulcers
Warnings/Precautions Not effective against RNA virus, adenoviral ocular infections, bacterial fungal or chlamydial infections of the cornea, or trophic ulcers; temporary visual haze may be produced; neoplasia has occurred with I.M. vidarabine-treated animals; although in vitro studies have been inconclusive, they have shown mutagenesis
Adverse Reactions Percentage unknown: Burning eyes, lacrimation, keratitis, photophobia, foreign body sensation, uveitis
Overdosage/Toxicology No untoward effects anticipated with ingestion
Mechanism of Action Inhibits viral DNA synthesis by blocking DNA polymerase
Usual Dosage Children and Adults: Ophthalmic: Keratoconjunctivitis: Instill ½" of ointment in lower conjunctival sac 5 times/day every 3 hours while awake until complete re-epithelialization has occurred, then twice daily for an additional 7 days
Patient Information Do not use eye make-up when on this medication for ophthalmic infection; use sunglasses if photophobic reaction occurs; may cause blurred vision; notify physician if improvement not seen after 7 days or if condition worsens
Dosage Forms Ointment, ophthalmic, as monohydrate: 3% [30 mg/mL = 28 mg/mL base] (3.5 g)
Selected Readings
"Drugs for Non-HIV Viral Infections," Med Lett Drugs Ther, 1994, 36(919):27.
Whitley R, Arvin A, Prober C, et al, "A Controlled Trial Comparing Vidarabine With Acyclovir in Neonatal Herpes Simplex Virus Infection. Infectious Diseases Collaborative Antiviral Study Group," N Engl J Med, 1991, 324(7):444-9.

Vidarabine Monohydrate see Vidarabine on this page
Videx® see Didanosine on page 704
Vioform® [OTC] see Clioquinol on page 686
Vira-A® see Vidarabine on this page
Viracept® see Nelfinavir on page 831
Viramune® see Nevirapine on page 839
Virazole® Aerosol see Ribavirin on page 899
Viroptic® Ophthalmic see Trifluridine on page 957
Vistide® see Cidofovir on page 676
Vitrasert® see Ganciclovir on page 745
Vitravene™ see Fomivirsen on page 738
Vivotif Berna™ Oral see Typhoid Vaccine on page 963
VōSol® HC Otic see Acetic Acid, Propylene Glycol Diacetate, and Hydrocortisone on page 581
V.V.S.® see Sulfabenzamide, Sulfacetamide, and Sulfathiazole on page 927
Vytone® Topical see Iodoquinol and Hydrocortisone on page 782
VZIG see Varicella-Zoster Immune Globulin (Human) on page 971
WinRho SD® see Rh₀(D) Immune Globulin (Intravenous-Human) on page 897
Wycillin® see Penicillin G Procaine on page 862
Wymox® see Amoxicillin on page 592

Yellow Fever Vaccine (YEL oh FEE ver vak SEEN)
U.S. Brand Names YF-VAX®
Generic Available No
(Continued)

Yellow Fever Vaccine *(Continued)*

Use Induction of active immunity against yellow fever virus, primarily among persons traveling or living in areas where yellow fever infection exists. (Some countries require a valid international Certification of Vaccination showing receipt of vaccine; if a pregnant woman is to be vaccinated only to satisfy an international requirement, efforts should be made to obtain a waiver letter.) The WHO requires revaccination every 10 years to maintain traveler's vaccination certificate.

Pregnancy Risk Factor D

Contraindications Sensitivity to egg or chick embryo protein; pregnant women, children <6 months of age unless in high risk area

Warnings/Precautions Do not use in immunodeficient persons or patients receiving immunosuppressants (eg, steroids, radiation); have epinephrine available in persons with previous history of egg allergy if the vaccine must be used. Avoid use in infants <6 months and pregnant women unless travel to high-risk areas are unavoidable; avoid use in infants <4 months of age.

Adverse Reactions All serious adverse reactions must be reported to the U.S. Department of Health and Human Services (DHHS) Vaccine Adverse Event Reporting System (VAERS) 1-800-822-7967.

>10%: Central nervous system: Fever, malaise (7-14 days after administration - ~10%)

1% to 10%:
Central nervous system: Headache (2% to 5%)
Neuromuscular & skeletal: Myalgia (2% to 5%)

<1%: Encephalitis in very young infants (rare), anaphylaxis

Drug Interactions Administer yellow fever vaccine at least 1 month apart from other live virus vaccines; defer vaccination for 3 weeks following immune globulin; concurrent cholera and yellow fever and concurrent hepatitis B vaccine and yellow fever vaccines may decrease immune response; separate vaccinations by 1 month, if possible; defer vaccination for 8 weeks following blood or plasma transfusion

Stability Yellow fever vaccine is shipped with dry ice; do not use vaccine unless shipping case contains some dry ice on arrival; maintain vaccine continuously at a temperature between 0°C to 5°C (32°F to 41°F)

Usual Dosage One dose (0.5 mL) S.C. 10 days to 10 years before travel, booster every 10 years; see Warnings/Precautions

Administration Do not reconstitute the powder for injection with a diluent that has preservatives since they may inactivate the live virus

Patient Information Immunity develops by the tenth day and **WHO** requires revaccination every 10 years to maintain travelers' vaccination certificates

Nursing Implications Sterilize and discard all unused rehydrated vaccine and containers after 1 hour; avoid vigorous shaking

Additional Information Federal law requires that the date of administration, the vaccine manufacturer, lot number of vaccine, and the administering person's name, title and address be entered into the patient's permanent medical record

Dosage Forms Injection: Not less than 5.04 Log_{10} Plaque Forming Units (PFU) per 0.5 mL

YF-VAX® *see Yellow Fever Vaccine on page 973*

Yodoxin® *see Iodoquinol on page 781*

Zagam® *see Sparfloxacin on page 921*

Zalcitabine *(zal SITE a been)*

Related Information
HIV Therapeutic Information *on page 1008*

U.S. Brand Names Hivid®

Synonyms ddC; Dideoxycytidine

Generic Available No

Use Used in combination with at least two other antiretrovirals in the treatment of patients with HIV infection

It is not recommended that zalcitabine be given in combination with didanosine, stavudine, or lamivudine due to overlapping toxicities, virologic interactions, or lack of clinical data

Drug of Choice or Alternative for
Organism(s)
Human Immunodeficiency Virus *on page 177*

Pregnancy Risk Factor C

Pregnancy/Breast-Feeding Implications

Clinical effects on the fetus: Administer during pregnancy only if benefits to mother outweigh risks to the fetus

Breast-feeding/lactation: HIV-infected mothers are discouraged from breast-feeding to decrease potential transmission of HIV

Contraindications Hypersensitivity to the drug or any component of the product

Warnings/Precautions Careful monitoring of pancreatic enzymes and liver function tests in patients with a history of pancreatitis, increased amylase, those on parenteral nutrition or with a history of ethanol abuse; discontinue use immediately if pancreatitis is suspected; lactic acidosis and severe hepatomegaly and failure have rarely occurred with zalcitabine resulting in fatality; some cases may possibly be related to underlying hepatitis B; use with caution in patients on digitalis, congestive heart failure, renal failure, hyperphosphatemia; zalcitabine can cause severe peripheral neuropathy; avoid use, if possible, in patients with pre-existing neuropathy

Adverse Reactions

>10%:

Central nervous system: Fever (5% to 17%), malaise (2% to 13%)

Neuromuscular & skeletal: Peripheral neuropathy (28.3%)

1% to 10%:

Central nervous system: Headache (2.1%), dizziness (1.1%), myalgia (1% to 6%), foot pain, fatigue (3.8%), seizures (1.3%)

Dermatologic: Rash (2% to 11%), pruritus (3% to 5%)

Endocrine & metabolic: Hypoglycemia (1.8% to 6.3%), hyponatremia (3.5%), hyperglycemia (1% to 6%)

Gastrointestinal: Nausea (3%), dysphagia (1% to 4%), anorexia (3.9%), abdominal pain (3% to 8%), vomiting (1% to 3%), diarrhea (0.4% to 9.5%), weight loss, oral ulcers (3% to 7%), increased amylase (3% to 8%)

Hematologic: Anemia (occurs as early as 2-4 weeks), granulocytopenia (usually after 6-8 weeks)

Hepatic: Abnormal hepatic function (8.9%), hyperbilirubinemia (2% to 5%)

Respiratory: Pharyngitis (1.8%), cough (6.3%), nasal discharge (3.5%)

<1%: Edema, hypertension, palpitations, syncope, atrial fibrillation, tachycardia, heart racing, chest pain, night sweats, pain, hypocalcemia, constipation, pancreatitis, jaundice, hepatitis, hepatomegaly, hepatic failure, myositis, weakness, epistaxis

Overdosage/Toxicology

Symptoms of overdose include delayed peripheral neurotoxicity; following oral decontamination

Treatment is supportive

Drug Interactions

Decreased effect: Magnesium/aluminum-containing antacids and metoclopramide may reduce zalcitabine absorption

Increased toxicity:

Amphotericin, foscarnet, cimetidine, probenecid, and aminoglycosides may potentiate the risk of developing peripheral neuropathy or other toxicities associated with zalcitabine by interfering with the renal elimination of zalcitabine

Other drugs associated with peripheral neuropathy which should be avoided, if possible, include chloramphenicol, cisplatin, dapsone, disulfiram, ethionamide, glutethimide, didanosine, gold, hydralazine, iodoquinol, isoniazid, metronidazole, nitrofurantoin, phenytoin, ribavirin, and vincristine

It is not recommended that zalcitabine be given in combination with didanosine, stavudine, or lamivudine due to overlapping toxicities, virologic interactions, or lack of clinical data

Stability Tablets should be stored in tightly closed bottles at 59°F to 86°F

Mechanism of Action Purine nucleoside analogue, zalcitabine or 2',3'-dideoxycytidine (ddC) is converted to active metabolite ddCTP; lack the presence of the 3'-hydroxyl group necessary for phosphodiester linkages during DNA replication. As a result viral replication is prematurely terminated. ddCTP acts as a competitor for binding sites on the HIV-RNA dependent DNA polymerase (reverse transcriptase) to further contribute to inhibition of viral replication.

(Continued)

Zalcitabine (Continued)

Pharmacodynamics/Kinetics

Absorption: Well but variably absorbed from GI tract; food decreases absorption by 39%

Distribution: Minimal data available; CSF penetration is variable

Protein binding: Minimal, <4%

Metabolism: Intracellularly to active triphosphorylated agent

Bioavailability: >80%

Half-life: 2.9 hours, may be prolonged to 8.5 hours in patients with renal impairment

Elimination: Mainly renal, >70% unchanged

Usual Dosage Oral:

Children <13 years: Safety and efficacy have not been established

Adults: Daily dose: 0.75 mg every 8 hours

Dosing adjustment in renal impairment: Adults:

Cl_{cr} 10-40 mL/minute: 0.75 mg every 12 hours

Cl_{cr} <10 mL/minute: 0.75 mg every 24 hours

Moderately dialyzable (20% to 50%)

Dietary Considerations Food: Extent and rate of absorption may be decreased with food

Monitoring Parameters Renal function, viral load, liver function tests, CD4 counts, CBC, serum amylase, triglycerides, calcium

Patient Information Zalcitabine is not a cure; if numbness or tingling occurs, or if persistent, severe abdominal pain, nausea, or vomiting occur, notify physician. Women of childbearing age should use effective contraception while on zalcitabine; take on an empty stomach, if possible.

Additional Information Potential compliance problems, frequency of administration and adverse effects should be discussed with patients before initiating therapy to help prevent the emergence of resistance.

Dosage Forms Tablet: 0.375 mg, 0.75 mg

Selected Readings

"Drugs for AIDS and Associated Infections," Med Lett Drugs Ther, 1993, 35(904):79-86.

Hirsch MS and D'Aquila RT, "Therapy for Human Immunodeficiency Virus Infection," N Engl J Med, 1993, 328(23):1686-95.

Shelton MJ, O'Donnell AM, and Morse GD, "Zalcitabine," Ann Pharmacother, 1993, 27(4):480-9.

Skowron G, Bozzette SA, Lim L, et al, "Alternating and Intermittent Regimens of Zidovudine and Dideoxycytidine in Patients With AIDS or AIDS-Related Complex," Ann Intern Med, 1993, 118(5):321-30.

Zanamivir (za NA mi veer)

Use Investigational use as of 3/1/99; prophylaxis and treatment of influenza A and B

Adverse Reactions Percentage unknown: Epistaxis (similar to placebo), flu-like syndrome (same as placebo)

Mechanism of Action Zanamivir is an analogue of sialic acid; it inhibits influenza A- and B-specific neuroaminidases. Neuroaminidases allow the release of virus from infected cells by cleaving terminal sialic acid residues from glycoconjugates and may prevent aggregation of virus and inactivation of virus by respiratory mucus. These enzymes may also be essential for viral replication.

Pharmacodynamics/Kinetics

Distribution: Inhalation: 13% in lungs, 80% in oropharynx

Metabolism: Slightly by glucuronidation

Bioavailability: Intranasal: 10%; inhalation: 25%

Half-life: Inhalation: 2.9 hours; nasal: 3.4 hours

Elimination: Mostly unchanged in the urine

Usual Dosage Drug is most effective when administered within 48 hours of onset of symptoms.

Inhalation: 10 mg 2-6 times/day for 4-5 days

Intranasal: 6.4 mg 2-6 times/day for 4-5 days

Additional Information Product information not available at the time of this writing.

Selected Readings

Hayden FG, Osterhaus AD, Treanor JJ, et al, "Efficacy and Safety of the Neuroaminidase Inhibitor Zanamivir in the Treatment of Influenzavirus Infections. GG167 Influenza Study Group," N Engl J Med, 1997, 337(13):874-80.

Waghorn SL and Goa KL, "Zanamivir," Drugs, 1998, 55(5):721-5.

Zeasorb-AF® Powder [OTC] *see* Miconazole *on page 822*

Zeasorb-AF® Powder [OTC] *see* Tolnaftate *on page 956*

Zefazone® *see* Cefmetazole *on page 638*

Zerit™ *see* Stavudine *on page 923*

Ziagen® *see* Abacavir *on page 580*

Zidovudine (zye DOE vyoo deen)

Related Information
HIV Therapeutic Information *on page 1008*

U.S. Brand Names Retrovir®

Canadian Brand Names Apo®-Zidovudine; Novo-AZT

Synonyms Azidothymidine; AZT; Compound S

Generic Available No

Use
Management of patients with HIV infections in combination with at least two other antiretroviral agents; for prevention of maternal/fetal HIV transmission as monotherapy

Drug of Choice or Alternative for
Organism(s)
Human Immunodeficiency Virus *on page 177*

Pregnancy Risk Factor C

Pregnancy/Breast-Feeding Implications
Clinical effect on the fetus: Administer during pregnancy only if benefits to mother outweigh risks to the fetus

Breast-feeding/lactation: HIV-infected mothers are discouraged from breast-feeding to decrease potential transmission of HIV

Contraindications
Life-threatening hypersensitivity to zidovudine or any component

Warnings/Precautions
Often associated with hematologic toxicity including granulocytopenia and severe anemia requiring transfusions; zidovudine has been shown to be carcinogenic in rats and mice

Adverse Reactions
>10%:
Central nervous system: Severe headache (42%), fever (16%)

Dermatologic: Rash (17%)

Gastrointestinal: Nausea (46% to 61%), anorexia (11%), diarrhea (17%), pain (20%), vomiting (6% to 25%)

Hematologic: Anemia (23% in children), leukopenia, granulocytopenia (39% in children)

Neuromuscular & skeletal: Weakness (19%)

1% to 10%:
Central nervous system: Malaise (8%), dizziness (6%), insomnia (5%), somnolence (8%)

Dermatologic: Hyperpigmentation of nails (bluish brown)

Gastrointestinal: Dyspepsia (5%)

Hematologic: Changes in platelet count

Neuromuscular & skeletal: Paresthesia (6%)

<1%: Neurotoxicity, confusion, mania, seizures, bone marrow suppression, granulocytopenia, thrombocytopenia, pancytopenia, hepatotoxicity, cholestatic jaundice, tenderness, myopathy

Overdosage/Toxicology
Symptoms of overdose include nausea, vomiting, ataxia, granulocytopenia

Erythropoietin, thymidine, and cyanocobalamin have been used experimentally to treat zidovudine-induced hematopoietic toxicity, yet none are presently specified as the agent of choice. Treatment is supportive.

Drug Interactions
Decreased effect: Acetaminophen may decrease AUC of zidovudine as can the rifamycins

Increased toxicity: Coadministration with drugs that are nephrotoxic (amphotericin B), cytotoxic (flucytosine, Adriamycin®, vincristine, vinblastine, doxorubicin, interferon), inhibit glucuronidation or excretion (acetaminophen, cimetidine, indomethacin, lorazepam, probenecid, aspirin), or interfere with RBC/WBC number or function (acyclovir, ganciclovir, pentamidine, dapsone); although the AUC was unaffected, the rate of absorption and peak plasma concentrations were increased significantly when zidovudine was administered with clarithromycin (n=18); valproic acid increased AZT's AUC by 80%
(Continued)

Zidovudine *(Continued)*

and decreased clearance by 38% (believed due to inhibition first pass metabolism); fluconazole may increase zidovudine's AUC and half-life, concomitant interferon alfa may increase hematologic toxicities and phenytoin, trimethoprim, and interferon beta-1b may increase zidovudine levels

Stability After dilution to ≤4 mg/mL, the solution is physically and chemically stable for 24 hours at room temperature and 48 hours if refrigerated; attempt to administer diluted solution within 8 hours, if stored at room temperature or 24 hours if refrigerated to minimize potential for microbially contaminated solutions; store undiluted vials at room temperature and protect from light

Mechanism of Action Zidovudine is a thymidine analog which interferes with the HIV viral RNA dependent DNA polymerase resulting in inhibition of viral replication; nucleoside reverse transcriptase inhibitor

Pharmacodynamics/Kinetics

Absorption: Oral: Well absorbed (66% to 70%)

Distribution: Significant penetration into the CSF; crosses the placenta

Metabolism: Extensive first-pass metabolism; metabolized in the liver via glucuronidation to inactive metabolites

Half-life: Terminal: 60 minutes

Time to peak serum concentration: Within 30-90 minutes

Elimination: Urinary excretion (63% to 95%); following oral administration, 72% to 74% of the drug excreted in urine as metabolites and 14% to 18% as unchanged drug; following I.V. administration, 45% to 60% excreted in urine as metabolites and 18% to 29% as unchanged drug

Usual Dosage

Prevention of maternal-fetal HIV transmission:

Neonatal: Oral: 2 mg/kg/dose every 6 hours for 6 weeks beginning 8-12 hours after birth; infants unable to receive oral dosing may receive 1.5 mg/kg I.V. infused over 30 minutes every 6 hours

Maternal (>14 weeks gestation): Oral: 100 mg 5 times/day until the start of labor; during labor and delivery, administer zidovudine I.V. at 2 mg/kg over 1 hour followed by a continuous I.V. infusion of 1 mg/kg/hour until the umbilical cord is clamped

Children 3 months to 12 years for HIV infection:

Oral: 160 mg/m^2/dose every 8 hours; dosage range: 90 mg/m^2/dose to 180 mg/m^2/dose every 6-8 hours; some Working Group members use a dose of 180 mg/m^2 every 12 hours when using in drug combinations with other antiretroviral compounds, but data on this dosing in children is limited

I.V. continuous infusion: 20 mg/m^2/hour

I.V. intermittent infusion: 120 mg/m^2/dose every 6 hours

Adults:

Oral: 300 mg twice daily or 200 mg 3 times/day

I.V.: 1-2 mg/kg/dose (infused over 1 hour) administered every 4 hours around-the-clock (6 doses/day)

Prevention of HIV following needlesticks: 200 mg 3 times/day plus lamivudine 150 mg twice daily; a protease inhibitor (eg, indinavir) may be added for high risk exposures; begin therapy within 2 hours of exposure if possible

Patients should receive I.V. therapy only until oral therapy can be administered

Dosing interval in renal impairment: Cl$_{cr}$ <10 mL/minute: May require minor dose adjustment

Hemodialysis: At least partially removed by hemo- and peritoneal dialysis; administer dose after hemodialysis or administer 100 mg supplemental dose; during CAPD, dose as for Cl$_{cr}$ <10 mL/minute

Continuous arteriovenous or venovenous hemodiafiltration (CAVH) effects: Administer 100 mg every 8 hours

Dosing adjustment in hepatic impairment: Reduce dose by 50% or double dosing interval in patients with cirrhosis

Dietary Considerations Food: Administration with a fatty meal decreased zidovudine's AUC and peak plasma concentration

Monitoring Parameters Monitor CBC and platelet count at least every 2 weeks, MCV, serum creatinine kinase, viral load, and CD4 cell count; observe for appearance of opportunistic infections

Patient Information Take 30 minutes before or 1 hour after a meal with a glass of water; take zidovudine exactly as prescribed; take around-the-clock; limit acetaminophen-containing analgesics; report all side effects to you physician; zidovudine therapy has not been shown to reduce the risk of transmission of HIV to others nor will is cure HIV infections; opportunistic infections and other illnesses may still occur; maternal/fetal transmission may appear in some cases despite therapy; transfusion, dose modifications and even drug discontinuation may be needed if blood disorders such as anemia occur.

Additional Information Potential compliance problems, frequency of administration and adverse effects should be discussed with patients before initiating therapy to help prevent the emergence of resistance.

Dosage Forms
Capsule: 100 mg
Injection: 10 mg/mL (20 mL)
Syrup (strawberry flavor): 50 mg/5 mL (240 mL)
Tablet: 300 mg

Selected Readings
"Drugs for AIDS and Associated Infections," *Med Lett Drugs Ther*, 1993, 35(904):79-86.
Hirsch MS and D'Aquila RT, "Therapy for Human Immunodeficiency Virus Infection," *N Engl J Med*, 1993, 328(23):1686-95.
McLeod GX and Hammer SM, "Zidovudine: Five Years Later," *Ann Intern Med*, 1992, 117(6):487-501.
Skowron G, Bozzette SA, Lim L, et al, "Alternating and Intermittent Regimens of Zidovudine and Dideoxycytidine in Patients With AIDS or AIDS-Related Complex," *Ann Intern Med*, 1993, 118(5):321-30.

Zidovudine and Lamivudine
(zye DOE vyoo deen & la MI vyoo deen)

Related Information
Lamivudine *on page 793*
Zidovudine *on page 977*

U.S. Brand Names Combivir®

Synonyms AZT + 3TC

Use Treatment of HIV infection; given twice daily provides an alternative regimen to lamivudine 150 mg twice daily plus zidovudine 600 mg/day in divided doses; this drug form reduces capsule/tablet intake for these two drugs to 2 per day instead of up to 8. The antiviral activity/safety has been shown to be equivalent to that of Epivir® and Retrovir® taken together as dual therapy and as part of triple combination therapy with a protease inhibitor.

Usual Dosage Oral: 1 tablet twice daily

Dosage Forms Tablet: Zidovudine 300 mg and lamivudine 150 mg

Zinacef® Injection *see* Cefuroxime *on page 658*
Zithromax™ *see* Azithromycin *on page 613*
Zolicef® *see* Cefazolin *on page 632*
Zosyn™ *see* Piperacillin and Tazobactam Sodium *on page 871*
Zovirax® *see* Acyclovir *on page 581*

APPENDIX TABLE OF CONTENTS

ANTIMICROBIAL ACTIVITY AGAINST SELECTED ORGANISMS

KEY TO TABLE

A Recommended drug therapy

B Alternate drug therapy

C Organism is usually or always sensitive to this agent

D Organism portrays variable sensitivity to this agent

(Blank) This drug should not be used for this organism or insufficient data is available

GRAM-POSITIVE AEROBES

Column headers — Bacilli: Listeria monocytogenes; Corynebacterium jeikeium; Corynebacterium sp. — Cocci: Streptococcus, Viridans Group; Streptococcus pneumoniae; Streptococcus bovis (Group D); Enterococcus sp. (Group D); Streptococcus agalactiae (Group B); Streptococcus pyogenes (Group A); Staphylococcus epidermidis: Methicillin-Susceptible; Staphylococcus epidermidis: Methicillin-Resistant; Staphylococcus aureus: Methicillin-Susceptible; Staphylococcus aureus: Methicillin-Resistant

		Bacilli			Cocci									
	Drug	L. monocytogenes	C. jeikeium	Corynebacterium sp.	Strep. Viridans Grp	S. pneumoniae	S. bovis (Grp D)	Enterococcus (Grp D)	S. agalactiae (Grp B)	S. pyogenes (Grp A)	Staph epi. Meth-Susc.	Staph epi. Meth-Resist.	Staph aureus Meth-Susc.	Staph aureus Meth-Resist.
Penicillins	Amoxicillin				C	C	C		C	C				
	Ampicillin	A			C	C	C	A	C	C				
	Penicillin G	A	B	B	A	A	A	A	A	A				
	Penicillin V				C	C	C	C	C	C				
	Azlocillin													
	Mezlocillin				D	C	D	D	C	C	C			
	Piperacillin				D	C	D	C	C	C	C			
	Ticarcillin				D	C	D		C	C				
	Cloxacillin				D						A		A	
	Dicloxacillin				D						A		A	
	Methicillin				D						A		A	
	Nafcillin				D						A		A	
	Oxacillin				D						A		A	
Penicillin-Related Antibiotics	Amoxicillin/Clavulanate	C			C	C	C	C	C	C	C		C	
	Ampicillin/Sulbactam	C			C	C	C	C	C	C	C		C	
	Ticarcillin/Clavulanate				C	C	C	D	C	C	C		C	
	Aztreonam													
	Imipenem/Cilastatin				C	C	C	D	C	C	C		C	
	Meropenem				C	C					C		C	
	Piperacillin/Tazobactam				C	C	C	C	C	C	C		C	
Other Antibiotics	Chloramphenicol	C				B		D						
	Clindamycin				D	D	C	D	C	C	B		B	
	Co-trimoxazole	B				C					B	C	B	C
	Metronidazole													
	Rifampin			D							A	C	A	C
	Sulfonamides													
	Tetracyclines	C			C	C				C			A	D
	Vancomycin	D	A		B	B	B	B	B	B	A	B	A	B
UTI Agents	Indanyl Carbenicillin							D						
	Nitrofurantoin							D						

ANTIMICROBIAL ACTIVITY AGAINST SELECTED ORGANISMS (Continued)

KEY TO TABLE

- **A** Recommended drug therapy
- **B** Alternate drug therapy
- **C** Organism is usually or always sensitive to this agent
- **D** Organism portrays variable sensitivity to this agent
- (Blank) This drug should not be used for this organism or insufficient data is available

GRAM-POSITIVE AEROBES

Class	Drug	Listeria monocytogenes	Corynebacterium jeikeium	Corynebacterium sp.	Streptococcus, Viridans Group	Streptococcus pneumoniae	Streptococcus bovis (Group D)	Streptococcus sp. (Group D)	Enterococcus (Group D)	Streptococcus agalactiae (Group B)	Streptococcus pyogenes (Group A)	Staph. epidermidis: Methicillin-Susceptible	Staph. epidermidis: Methicillin-Resistant	Staph. aureus: Methicillin-Susceptible	Staph. aureus: Methicillin-Resistant
1st Generation	Cefadroxil				B	B	C			B	B	B		B	
	Cefazolin				B	B	C			B	B	B		B	
	Cephalexin				B	B	C			B	B	B		B	
	Cephalothin				B	B	C			B	B	B		B	
	Cephapirin				B	B	C			B	B	B		B	
	Cephradine				B	B	C			B	B	B		B	
2nd Generation and others	Cefaclor				C	C	C			C	C	D		D	
	Cefamandole				C	C	C			C	C	C		C	
	Cefmetazole				C	C	C			C	C	C		C	
	Cefonicid				C	C	C			C	C	D		D	
	Cefotetan				C	C	C			C	C	D		D	
	Cefoxitin				C	C	C			C	C	D		D	
	Cefpodoxime Proxetil				C	C	C			C	C	D		D	
	Cefprozil				C	C	D			C	C			D	
	Ceftibuten					D				C	C				
	Cefuroxime				C	C	C			C	C	D		D	
	Cefuroxime Axetil				C	C				C	C	C		C	
	Loracarbef				C	C	D			C	C	C		C	
3rd Generation	Cefepime				C	C				C	C	C		C	
	Cefixime				D	D				C	C				
	Cefoperazone				D	D	C			C	C	D		D	
	Cefotaxime				D	D	C			C	C	D		D	
	Ceftazidime					D				D		D		D	
	Ceftizoxime				D	D	C			C	C	D		D	
	Ceftriaxone				C	C	C			C	C	D		D	
Aminoglycosides	Amikacin	C	C					D	D						
	Gentamicin	A	B		A			D	A			A	D	A	D
	Netilmicin	C	C						C						
	Streptomycin							D	C						
	Tobramycin	C	C						D						D
Macrolides	Azithromycin	C			C	C				C	C				C
	Clarithromycin	C			C	C				C	C				C
	Dirithromycin	C			C	C				C	C				C
	Erythromycin	C	C		A	C	B			B	B				C
Quinolones	Ciprofloxacin		D		D	D	D	D	D	D	D	D	D	D	D
	Grepafloxacin		D				C	D	C	C					
	Levofloxacin				C	C	C	C	D	C	C	C	D	C	D
	Lomefloxacin		D		D	D	D	D	D	D	D	D	D	D	D
	Norfloxacin							D	D						
	Ofloxacin		D		D	D	D	D	D	D	D	D	D	D	D
	Sparfloxacin		D				C	D	C	C					
	Trovafloxacin				C	C	C	C	D	C	C	C	D	C	D

Penicillins, Penicillin-Related Antibiotics & Other Antibiotics

KEY TO TABLE

- **A** Recommended drug therapy
- **B** Alternate drug therapy
- **C** Organism is usually or always sensitive to this agent
- **D** Organism portrays variable sensitivity to this agent
- (Blank) This drug should not be used for this organism or insufficient data is available

GRAM-NEGATIVE AEROBES — Enteric bacilli and Cocci

Drug	Yersinia enterocolitica	Shigella sp.	Serratia sp.	Salmonella sp.	Providencia sp.	Proteus sp.	Proteus mirabilis	Klebsiella pneumoniae	Escherichia coli	Enterobacter sp.	Citrobacter sp.[1]	Neisseria meningitidis	Neisseria gonorrhoeae	Moraxella (Branhamella) catarrhalis
Penicillin														
Amoxicillin				B			A		C			C	D	
Ampicillin		A		B			A		A			C	D	
Penicillin G												A	D	
Penicillin V													D	
Azlocillin														
Mezlocillin			A		B	B	C	B	C	A	A		D	
Piperacillin			A		B	B	C	B	C	A	A		D	
Ticarcillin			A		B	B	C	D	C	A	A		D	
Cloxacillin														
Dicloxacillin														
Methicillin														
Nafcillin														
Oxacillin														
Penicillin-Related Antibiotics														
Amoxicillin/Clavulanate				C			C	C	C			C	C	A
Ampicillin/Sulbactam	C			C			C	C	C			C	C	C
Ticarcillin/Clavulanate	C	A	C	C	B	C	B	C	A	A	C	C	C	C
Aztreonam	C	B	C	C	C	C	B	C	A	C			C	C
Imipenem/Cilastatin	B	B	C	B	B	B	C	B	C	B	B	D	C	C
Piperacillin/Tazobactam	C	A	C	C	B	C	B	C	A	A	C	C	C	C
Other Antibiotics														
Chloramphenicol		C		B					C			B		
Clindamycin														
Co-trimoxazole	C	A	C	B	A	C	B	C	A	C	C			A
Metronidazole														
Rifampin												D		
Sulfonamides		C		C				C	C	C		D		
Tetracyclines	C	C						C	C		D	C	B	C
Vancomycin														
UTI Agents														
Indanyl Carbenicillin			C		C	C	C	C	C	C	C			
Nitrofurantoin								C	C	C	C			

[1] *Citrobacter freundii, Citrobacter diversus, Enterobacter cloacae* and *Enterobacter aerogenes* often have significantly different antibiotic sensitivity patterns. Speciation and susceptibility testing are particularly important

ANTIMICROBIAL ACTIVITY AGAINST SELECTED ORGANISMS (Continued)

KEY TO TABLE

- **A** Recommended drug therapy
- **B** Alternate drug therapy
- **C** Organism is usually or always sensitive to this agent
- **D** Organism portrays variable sensitivity to this agent
- ☐ (Blank) This drug should not be used for this organism or insufficient data is available

GRAM-NEGATIVE AEROBES — Enteric bacilli and Cocci

Class	Drug	Yersinia enterocolitica	Shigella sp.	Serratia sp.	Salmonella sp.	Providencia sp.	Proteus sp.	Proteus mirabilis	Klebsiella pneumoniae	Escherichia coli	Enterobacter sp.[1]	Citrobacter sp.[1]	Neisseria meningitidis	Neisseria gonorrhoeae	Moraxella (Branhamella) catarrhalis
1st Generation	Cefadroxil							A	A	B					D
1st Generation	Cefazolin							A	A	B					D
1st Generation	Cephalexin							A	A	B					D
1st Generation	Cephalothin							A	A	B					D
1st Generation	Cephapirin							A	A	B					D
1st Generation	Cephradine							A	A	B					D
2nd Generation and others	Cefaclor							C	A	B				C	B
2nd Generation and others	Cefamandole						D	C	A	B				C	B
2nd Generation and others	Cefmetazole	D	C	C		C	D	C	A	B				C	B
2nd Generation and others	Cefonicid							C	A	B				C	B
2nd Generation and others	Cefotetan	C	C	C		C	D	C	A	B				C	B
2nd Generation and others	Cefoxitin			D		C	D	C	A	B				C	B
2nd Generation and others	Cefpodoxime Proxetil							C	A	B				C	B
2nd Generation and others	Cefprozil		C					C	D	B				C	B
2nd Generation and others	Ceftibuten														
2nd Generation and others	Cefuroxime	C	C				D	C	A	B				C	B
2nd Generation and others	Cefuroxime Axetil							C	A	B			C	C	B
2nd Generation and others	Loracarbef							C	C	B				C	B
3rd Generation	Cefepime			C	C	C	C	C	C	C	C	C			C
3rd Generation	Cefixime	C	C					C	C	A	A			C	B
3rd Generation	Cefoperazone		B	A	A	A	A	C	A	A	A	A			B
3rd Generation	Cefotaxime	A	B	A	A	A	A	C	A	A	A	A	B	C	B
3rd Generation	Ceftazidime	B	A			A	A	C	A	A	A	A			B
3rd Generation	Ceftizoxime	A	B	A	A	A	A	C	A	A	A	A	B	C	B
3rd Generation	Ceftriaxone	A	B	A	A	A	A	C	A	A	A	A	B	C	B
Aminoglycosides	Amikacin	A		C		C	C	C	C	C	C	C			
Aminoglycosides	Gentamicin	A	D	C	D	D	C	C	C	C	C	C			
Aminoglycosides	Netilmicin	A	D	C	D	D	C	C	C	C	C	C			
Aminoglycosides	Streptomycin				D										
Aminoglycosides	Tobramycin	A		C	D	D	C	C	C	C	C	C			
Macrolides	Azithromycin													C	C
Macrolides	Clarithromycin													C	C
Macrolides	Dirithromycin														
Macrolides	Erythromycin													D	C
Quinolones	Ciprofloxacin	C	B	C	B	C	C	C	C	C	C	C	C	A	C
Quinolones	Grepafloxacin						C	C	C	C	C	C	C	C	C
Quinolones	Levofloxacin	C	C	C	C	C	C	C	C	C	C	D	C	C	C
Quinolones	Lomefloxacin		C	C	C	C	C	C	C	C	C	C	C	C	
Quinolones	Norfloxacin	C	C	C	C	C	C	C	C	C	C	C		C	
Quinolones	Ofloxacin	C	C	C	C	C	C	C	C	C	C	C	C	A	C
Quinolones	Sparfloxacin						C	C	C	C	C	C	C	C	C
Quinolones	Trovafloxacin			C	C	C	C	C	C	C	C	C	C	C	C

[1] Citrobacter freundii, Citrobacter diversus, Enterobacter cloacae and Enterobacter aerogenes often have significantly different antibiotic sensitivity patterns. Speciation and susceptibility testing are particularly important

KEY TO TABLE

- **A** Recommended drug therapy
- **B** Alternate drug therapy
- **C** Organism is usually or always sensitive to this agent
- **D** Organism portrays variable sensitivity to this agent
- (Blank) This drug should not be used for this organism or insufficient data is available

GRAM-NEGATIVE AEROBES — Other bacilli

Drug	Vibrio cholerae	Stenotrophomonas maltophilia	Pseudomonas aeruginosa	Pasteurella multocida	Legionella pneumophila	Haemophilus influenzae	Haemophilus ducreyi	Gardnerella vaginalis	Francisella tularensis	Campylobacter jejuni	Brucella sp.	Bordetella pertussis	Alcaligenes	Acinetobacter sp.
Penicillin														
Amoxicillin				C		B		C						
Ampicillin				C		B		B		D				
Penicillin G				A										
Penicillin V				C										
Azlocillin														
Mezlocillin			A	C		D								A
Piperacillin			A	C		D								A
Ticarcillin			A	C		D								A
Cloxacillin														
Dicloxacillin														
Methicillin														
Nafcillin														
Oxacillin														
Penicillin-Related Antibiotics														
Amoxicillin/Clavulanate				B		B	B	C						C
Ampicillin/Sulbactam				B		C	C	C						C
Ticarcillin/Clavulanate		B	A	C		C								A
Aztreonam			C			C								B
Imipenem/Cilastatin			A			C								B
Meropenem			C	C		C					C			C
Piperacillin/Tazobactam			A	C		C								A
Other Antibiotics														
Chloramphenicol		C		C		B			A	C	C			
Clindamycin										C		C		
Co-trimoxazole	A	A				A	B					B	A	
Metronidazole										A				
Rifampin						A	D				D		A	
Sulfonamides				C					C			C		
Tetracyclines	A			C		C	C				B	A	C	
Vancomycin														
UTI Agents														
Indanyl Carbenicillin			D											C
Nitrofurantoin														

ANTIMICROBIAL ACTIVITY AGAINST SELECTED ORGANISMS (Continued)

KEY TO TABLE

- **A** Recommended drug therapy
- **B** Alternate drug therapy
- **C** Organism is usually or always sensitive to this agent
- **D** Organism portrays variable sensitivity to this agent
- (Blank) This drug should not be used for this organism or insufficient data is available

GRAM-NEGATIVE AEROBES — Other bacilli

Class	Drug	Vibrio cholerae	Stenotrophomonas maltophilia	Pseudomonas aeruginosa	Pasteurella multocida	Legionella pneumophila	Haemophilus influenzae	Haemophilus ducreyi	Gardnerella vaginalis	Francisella tularensis	Campylobacter jejuni	Brucella sp.	Bordetella pertussis	Alcaligenes	Acinetobacter sp.
1st Generation	Cefadroxil						D								
	Cefazolin						D								
	Cephalexin						D								
	Cephalothin						D								
	Cephapirin						D								
	Cephradine						D								
2nd Generation and others	Cefaclor						B								
	Cefamandole				C		B								
	Cefmetazole				D		C								
	Cefonicid						C								
	Cefotetan				D		C								
	Cefoxitin				D		C			D					
	Cefpodoxime Proxetil						B								
	Cefprozil						B								
	Ceftibuten														
	Cefuroxime						B								
	Cefuroxime Axetil				D		B								
	Loracarbef						B								
3rd Generation	Cefepime			C			C								C
	Cefixime						A								D
	Cefoperazone		D	D	C		A	C							D
	Cefotaxime		D		C		C	C							A
	Ceftazidime		D	A			C	C							A
	Ceftizoxime		D				C	C							A
	Ceftriaxone		D		C		A			D					A
Aminoglycosides	Amikacin		C	A			C			C					C
	Gentamicin		C	A			C			A	C	C			C
	Netilmicin		C	A			C			C					C
	Streptomycin									A		C			
	Tobramycin		C	A			C			C					C
Macrolides	Azithromycin				D	B	C	C			C		C		
	Clarithromycin				D	B	C				C		C		
	Dirithromycin														
	Erythromycin				D	A		C		C	A		A		
Quinolones	Ciprofloxacin	C	B	A	C	B	C	B		C	C	B	C		C
	Grepafloxacin	C				C									
	Levofloxacin	C				C									
	Lomefloxacin	C	C	D	C		C	C	D			B	C		D
	Norfloxacin			C								B			D
	Ofloxacin	C	B	D	C	C	C	C		C	C	C	B		C
	Sparfloxacin	C				C									
	Trovafloxacin	C				C									

Penicillins, Penicillin-Related Antibiotics & Other Antibiotics

KEY TO TABLE

A — Recommended drug therapy

B — Alternate drug therapy

C — Organism is usually or always sensitive to this agent

D — Organism portrays variable sensitivity to this agent

(Blank) This drug should not be used for this organism or insufficient data is available

		OTHERS									ANAEROBES			
											Gram -	Gram +		
		Treponema pallidum	Leptospira sp.	Borrelia burgdorferi (Lyme disease)	Rickettsia sp.	Ureaplasma urealyticum	Mycoplasma pneumoniae	Chlamydia trachomatis	Chlamydia psittaci	Chlamydia pneumoniae (TWAR)	Bacteroides sp.	Clostridium perfringens	Streptococcus, anaerobic	Clostridium difficile²
Penicillin	Amoxicillin			B							D	C	D	
	Ampicillin			B							C	C	D	
	Penicillin G	A	A	B							C	A	A	
	Penicillin V	C	C	B							C	C	C	
	Azlocillin													
	Mezlocillin										C	C	C	
	Piperacillin										C	C	C	
	Ticarcillin										C	C	C	
	Cloxacillin													
	Dicloxacillin													
	Methicillin													
	Nafcillin													
	Oxacillin													
Penicillin-Related Antibiotics	Amoxicillin/Clavulanate										C	C	C	
	Ampicillin/Sulbactam										C	C	C	
	Ticarcillin/Clavulanate										C	C	C	
	Aztreonam													
	Imipenem/Cilastatin										C	C	B	
	Piperacillin/Tazobactam										C	C	C	
Other Antibiotics	Chloramphenicol				A						C	C	C	D
	Clindamycin										A	B	B	
	Co-trimoxazole													
	Metronidazole										A	D	A	A
	Rifampin													
	Sulfonamides								D					
	Tetracyclines	B	B	A	A	A	A	A	B	B	D	C	C	
	Vancomycin												B	B
UTI Agents	Indanyl Carbenicillin													
	Nitrofurantoin										·			

² Vancomycin is effective orally only.

ANTIMICROBIAL ACTIVITY AGAINST SELECTED ORGANISMS *(Continued)*

KEY TO TABLE

- **A** Recommended drug therapy
- **B** Alternate drug therapy
- **C** Organism is usually or always sensitive to this agent
- **D** Organism portrays variable sensitivity to this agent
- (Blank) This drug should not be used for this organism or insufficient data is available

Column groups: **OTHERS** = Treponema pallidum; Leptospira sp.; Borrelia burgdorferi (Lyme disease); Rickettsia sp.; Ureaplasma urealyticum; Mycoplasma pneumoniae; Chlamydia trachomatis; Chlamydia psittaci; Chlamydia pneumoniae (TWAR). **ANAEROBES** = Gram − : Bacteroides sp.; Gram + : Streptococcus, anaerobic; Clostridium perfringens; Clostridium difficile [2].

Drug	Trep. pallidum	Leptospira sp.	Borrelia burgdorferi (Lyme)	Rickettsia sp.	Ureaplasma urealyticum	Mycoplasma pneumoniae	Chlamydia trachomatis	Chlamydia psittaci	Chlamydia pneumoniae (TWAR)	Bacteroides sp.	Streptococcus, anaerobic	Clostridium perfringens	Clostridium difficile [2]
1st Generation													
Cefadroxil											B		
Cefazolin											B		
Cephalexin											B		
Cephalothin											B		
Cephapirin											B		
Cephradine											B		
2nd Generation and others													
Cefaclor													
Cefamandole													
Cefmetazole										C	C	C	
Cefonicid													
Cefotetan										B	C	C	
Cefoxitin										B	C	C	
Cefpodoxime Proxetil													
Cefprozil													
Ceftibuten													
Cefuroxime											C	C	
Cefuroxime Axetil													
Loracarbef													
3rd Generation													
Cefepime													
Cefixime													
Cefoperazone												D	
Cefotaxime			C							D	C	C	
Ceftazidime												D	
Ceftizoxime			C							D	C	C	
Ceftriaxone	C		A								C		
Aminoglycosides													
Amikacin													
Gentamicin													
Netilmicin													
Streptomycin													
Tobramycin													
Macrolides													
Azithromycin	D		C		B	C	C	C	C		D	D	
Clarithromycin	D		D		B	C	C	C	C		D	D	
Dirithromycin					C	C	C	C	C		D	D	
Erythromycin	D		C		A	A	A	A	A		D	D	
Quinolones													
Ciprofloxacin				D	D	D	D						
Grepafloxacin								C	C	D	D	D	D
Levofloxacin							C	C	C				
Lomefloxacin					D	D	D						
Norfloxacin													
Ofloxacin					D	D	D	C					
Sparfloxacin								C	C	D	D	D	D
Trovafloxacin							C	C	C	C	C	C	

[2] Vancomycin is effective orally only.

BODY SURFACE AREA OF ADULTS AND CHILDREN

Calculating Body Surface Area in Children

In a child of average size, find weight and corresponding surface area on the boxed scale to the left, or use the nomogram to the right. Lay a straightedge on the correct height and weight points for the child, then read the intersecting point on the surface area scale.

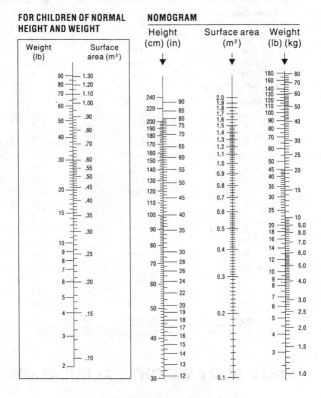

FOR CHILDREN OF NORMAL HEIGHT AND WEIGHT

NOMOGRAM

BODY SURFACE AREA FORMULA
(Adult and Pediatric)

$$BSA\ (m^2) = \sqrt{\frac{Ht\ (in) \times Wt\ (lb)}{3131}} \quad \text{or, in metric: } BSA\ (m^2) = \sqrt{\frac{Ht\ (cm) \times Wt\ (kg)}{3600}}$$

References
Lam TK and Leung DT, "More on Simplified Calculation of Body Surface Area," *N Engl J Med*, 1988, 318(17):1130 (Letter).
Mosteller RD, "Simplified Calculation of Body Surface Area", *N Engl J Med*, 1987, 317(17):1098 (Letter).

AVERAGE WEIGHTS AND SURFACE AREAS

Average Weight and Surface Area of Preterm Infants, Term Infants, and Children

Age	Average Weight (kg)*	Approximate Surface Area (m²)
Weeks Gestation		
26	0.9-1	0.1
30	1.3-1.5	0.12
32	1.6-2	0.15
38	2.9-3	0.2
40	3.1-4	0.25
(term infant at birth)		
Months		
3	5	0.29
6	7	0.38
9	8	0.42
Year		
1	10	0.49
2	12	0.55
3	15	0.64
4	17	0.74
5	18	0.76
6	20	0.82
7	23	0.90
8	25	0.95
9	28	1.06
10	33	1.18
11	35	1.23
12	40	1.34
Adult	70	1.73

*Weights from age 3 months and over are rounded off to the nearest kilogram.

IDEAL BODY WEIGHT CALCULATION

Adults (18 years and older) (IBW is in kg)

IBW (male) = 50 + (2.3 x height in inches over 5 feet)

IBW (female) = 45.5 + (2.3 x height in inches over 5 feet)

Children (IBW is in kg; height is in cm)

a. 1-18 years

$$IBW = \frac{(height^2 \times 1.65)}{1000}$$

b. 5 feet and taller

IBW (male) = 39 + (2.27 x height in inches over 5 feet)

IBW (female) = 42.2 + (2.27 x height in inches over 5 feet)

CREATININE CLEARANCE ESTIMATING METHODS IN PATIENTS WITH STABLE RENAL FUNCTION

The following formulas provide an acceptable estimate of the patient's creatinine clearance except when:

    a.   patient's serum creatinine is changing rapidly (either up or down)

    b.   patients are markedly emaciated

In these situations (a and b above), certain assumptions have to be made.

    c.   In patients with rapidly rising serum creatinines (ie, >0.5-0.7 mg/dL/day), it is best to assume that the patient's creatinine clearance is probably <10 mL/minute.

    d.   In emaciated patients, although their actual creatinine clearance is less than their calculated creatinine clearance (because of decreased creatinine production), it is not possible to easily predict how much less.

Adults (18 years and older)

Method 1: (Cockroft DW and Gault MH, *Nephron*, 1976, 16:31-41)

Estimated creatinine clearance (Cl_{cr}):
(mL/min)

$$\text{Male} = \frac{(140 - \text{age}) \text{ IBW (kg)}}{72 \times S_{cr}}$$

$$\text{Female} = \text{Estimated } Cl_{cr} \text{ male} \times 0.85$$

Note: The use of the patient's ideal body weight (IBW) is recommended for the above formula except when the patient's actual body weight is less than ideal. Use of the IBW is especially important in obese patients.

Method 2: (Jelliffe RW, *Ann Intern Med*, 1973, 79:604)

Estimated creatinine clearance (Cl_{cr}):
(mL/min/1.73 m^2)

$$\text{Male} = \frac{98 - 0.8 (\text{age} - 20)}{S_{cr}}$$

$$\text{Female} = \text{Estimated } Cl_{cr} \text{ male} \times 0.90$$

Children (1-18 years)

Method 1: (Traub SL, Johnson CE, *Am J Hosp Pharm*, 1980, 37:195-201)

$$Cl_{cr} = \frac{0.48 \times (\text{height}) \times BSA}{S_{cr} \times 1.73}$$

where

    BSA = body surface area in m^2
    Cl_{cr} = creatinine clearance in mL/min
    S_{cr} = serum creatinine in mg/dL
    Height = in cm

CREATININE CLEARANCE ESTIMATING METHODS IN PATIENTS WITH STABLE RENAL FUNCTION *(Continued)*

Method 2: Nomogram (Traub SL and Johnson CE, *Am J Hosp Pharm*, 1980, 37:195-201)

Children 1-18 Years

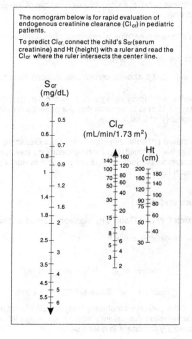

The nomogram below is for rapid evaluation of endogenous creatinine clearance (Cl_{cr}) in pediatric patients.

To predict Cl_{cr} connect the child's S_{cr} (serum creatinine) and Ht (height) with a ruler and read the Cl_{cr} where the ruler intersects the center line.

S_{cr}
(mg/dL)

Cl_{cr}
(mL/min/1.73 m²)

Ht
(cm)

TEMPERATURE CONVERSION

Celsius to Fahrenheit = (°C x 9/5) + 32 = °F
Fahrenheit to Celsius = (°F -32) x 5/9 = °C

°C	= °F	°C	= °F	°C	= °F
100.0	212.0	39.0	102.2	36.8	98.2
50.0	122.0	38.8	101.8	36.6	97.9
41.0	105.8	38.6	101.5	36.4	97.5
40.8	105.4	38.4	101.1	36.2	97.2
40.6	105.1	38.2	100.8	36.0	96.8
40.4	104.7	38.0	100.4	35.8	96.4
40.2	104.4	37.8	100.1	35.6	96.1
40.0	104.0	37.6	99.7	35.4	95.7
39.8	103.6	37.4	99.3	35.2	95.4
39.6	103.3	37.2	99.0	35.0	95.0
39.4	102.9	37.0	98.6	0	32.0
39.2	102.6				

DESENSITIZATION PROTOCOLS

PENICILLIN DESENSITIZATION PROTOCOL

Acute penicillin desensitization should only be performed in an intensive care setting. Any remedial risk factor should be corrected. All β-adrenergic antagonists such as propranolol or even timolol ophthalmic drops should be discontinued. Asthmatic patients should be under optimal control. An intravenous line should be established, baseline electrocardiogram (EKG) and spirometry should be performed, and continuous EKG monitoring should be instituted. Premedication with antihistamines or steroids is not recommended, as these drugs have not proven effective in suppressing severe reactions but may mask early signs of reactivity that would otherwise result in a modification of the protocol.

Protocols have been developed for penicillin desensitization using both the oral and parenteral route. As of 1987 there were 93 reported cases of oral desensitization, 74 of which were done by Sullivan and his collaborators. Of these 74 patients, 32% experienced a transient allergic reaction either during desensitization (one-third) or during penicillin treatment after desensitization (two-thirds). These reactions were usually mild and self-limited in nature. Only one IgE-mediated reaction (wheezing and bronchospasm) required discontinuation of the procedure before desensitization could be completed. It has been argued that oral desensitization may be safer than parenteral desensitization, but most patients can also be safely desensitized by the parenteral route.

During desensitization any dose that causes mild systemic reactions such as pruritus, fleeting urticaria, rhinitis, or mild wheezing should be repeated until the patient tolerates the dose without systemic symptoms or signs. More serious reactions such as hypotension, laryngeal edema, or asthma require appropriate treatment, and if desensitization is continued, the dose should be decreased by at least tenfold and withheld until the patient is stable.

Once desensitized, the patient's treatment with penicillin must not lapse or the risk of an allergic reaction increases. If the patient requires a β-lactam antibiotic in the future and still remains skin test-positive to penicillin reagents, desensitization would be required again.

Several patients have been maintained on long-term, low-dose penicillin therapy (usually bid-tid) to sustain a chronic state of desensitization. Such individuals usually require chronic desensitization because of continuous occupationally related exposure to β-lactam drugs.

Order for placement/availability at the bedside in the event of a hypersensitivity reaction during scratch/skin testing and desensitization:

> Hydrocortisone: 100 mg IVP
> Diphenhydramine: 50 mg IVP
> Epinephrine: 1:1000 S.C.

Several investigators have demonstrated that penicillin can be administered to history-positive, skin test-positive patients if initially small but gradually increasing doses are given. However, patients with a history of exfoliative dermatitis secondary to penicillin should not be re-exposed to the drug, even by desensitization.

Desensitization is a potentially dangerous procedure and should be only performed in an area where immediate access to emergency drugs and equipment can be assured.

Begin between 8-10 AM in the morning.

Follow desensitization as indicated for penicillin G or ampicillin.

AMPICILLIN
Oral Desensitization Protocol

1. Begin 0.03 mg of ampicillin
2. Double the dose administered every 30 minutes until complete
3. Example of oral dosing regimen:

Dose #	Ampicillin (mg)
1	0.03
2	0.06
3	0.12
4	0.23
5	0.47
6	0.94
7	1.87
8	3.75
9	7.5
10	15
11	30
12	60
13	125
14	250
15	500

PENICILLIN G PARENTERAL
Desensitization Protocol: Typical Schedule

Injection No.	Benzylpenicillin Concentration (units/mL)	Volume and Route (mL)*
1†	100	0.1 I.D.
2	↓	0.2 S.C.
3		0.4 S.C.
4		0.8 S.C.
5†	1,000	0.1 I.D.
6	↓	0.3 S.C.
7		0.6 S.C.
8†	10,000	0.1 I.D.
9	↓	0.2 S.C.
10		0.4 S.C.
11		0.8 S.C.
12†	100,000	0.1 I.D.
13	↓	0.3 S.C.
14		0.6 S.C.
15†	1,000,000	0.1 I.D.
16	↓	0.2 S.C.
17		0.2 I.M.
18		0.4 I.M.
19	Continuous I.V. infusion (1,000,000 units/h)	

*Administer progressive doses at intervals of not less than 20 minutes.

†Observe and record skin wheal and flare response to intradermal dose.

Abbreviations: I.D. = intradermal, S.C. = subcutaneous, I.M. = intramuscular, I.V. = intravenous.

DESENSITIZATION PROTOCOLS *(Continued)*

PENICILLIN
Oral Desensitization Protocol

Step*	Phenoxymethyl Penicillin (units/mL)	Amount (mL)	Dose (units)	Cumulative Dosage (units)
1	1000	0.1	100	100
2	1000	0.2	200	300
3	1000	0.4	400	700
4	1000	0.8	800	1500
5	1000	1.6	1600	3100
6	1000	3.2	3200	6300
7	1000	6.4	6400	12,700
8	10,000	1.2	12,000	24,700
9	10,000	2.4	24,000	48,700
10	10,000	4.8	48,000	96,700
11	80,000	1	80,000	176,700
12	80,000	2	160,000	336,700
13	80,000	4	320,000	656,700
14	80,000	8	640,000	1,296,700
	Observe patient for 30 minutes			
Change to benzylpenicillin G I.V.				
15	500,000	0.25	125,000	
16	500,000	0.50	250,000	
17	500,000	1	500,000	
18	500,000	2.25	1,125,000	

*Interval between steps, 15 min

AMPHOTERICIN B

Challenge and Desensitization Protocol

1. Procedure supervised by physician

2. Epinephrine, 1:1000 wt/vol, multidose vial at bedside

3. Premixed albuterol solution at bedside for nebulization

4. Endotracheal intubation supplies at bedside with anesthesiologist on standby

5. Continuous cardiac telemetry with electronic monitoring of blood pressure

6. Continuous pulse oximetry

7. Premedication with methylprednisolone, 60 mg, I.V. and diphenhydramine, 25 mg I.V.

8. Amphotericin B (Fungizone®)* administration schedule

   a. 10^{-6} dilution, infused over 10 minutes

   b. 10^{-5} dilution, infused over 10 minutes

   c. 10^{-4} dilution, infused over 10 minutes

   d. 10^{-3} dilution, infused over 10 minutes

   e. 10^{-2} dilution, infused over 10 minutes

   f. 10^{-1} dilution (1 mg), infused over 30 minutes

   g. 30 mg in 250 mL 5% dextrose, infused over 4 hours

*Mixtures were prepared in 10 mL 5% dextrose by hospital intensive care unit pharmacy, unless otherwise noted.

From Kemp SF and Lockey RF, "Amphotericin B: Emergency Challenge in a Neutropenic, Asthmatic Patient With Fungal Sepsis," *J Allergy Clin Immunol*, 1995, 96(3):425-7.

BACTRIM™ ORAL DESENSITIZATION PROTOCOL

(Adapted from Gluckstein D and Ruskin J, "Rapid Oral Desensitization to Trimethoprim-Sulfamethoxazole (TMP-SMZ): Use in Prophylaxis for *Pneumocystis carinii* Pneumonia in Patients With AIDS Who Were Previously Intolerant to TMP-SMZ," *Clin Infect Dis*, 1995, 20:849-53.)

Please read the directions carefully before starting the protocol!

1. There must be a clear cut need for a sulfa drug or a sulfa drug combination product such as Bactrim™. The decision to use sulfa must be made prior to skin testing.
2. Informed consent from the patient or an appropriate relative must have been obtained.
3. A trained individual, physician, nurse, or aide, **must be with the patient** at all times.
4. A physician **must** be on the floor at all times.
5. Injectable epinephrine 0.3 mL 1:1000, diphenhydramine (Benadryl®) 50 mg, corticosteroids and oral ibuprofen 400 mg solution should be drawn up and available at the bedside.
6. Appropriate resuscitative equipment must be available.
7. All dilution of oral Bactrim™ should be made up prior to beginning procedure.
8. Patient should drink 180 mL of water after each Bactrim™ dose.

Dilution for Bactrim™ Desensitization

Final Concentration	Bottle #	Procedure
Oral Bactrim™ 40/200 mg/5 mL	A	Conventional oral Bactrim™ suspension 5 mL = 40/200 mg
Oral Bactrim™ 0.4/2 mg/mL	B	1. Add 5 mL conventional oral Bactrim™ suspension or A (concentration = 40/200 mg/5 mL) to 95 mL of sterile water 2. Shake well. This will give 100 mL of 40/200 mg Bactrim™; each mL = 0.4/2 mg Bactrim™. 3. Dispense 20 mL for use
Oral Bactrim™ 0.004/0.02 mg/mL	C	1. Add 1 mL of the 0.4/2 mg/mL Bactrim™ or B to 99 mL of sterile water 2. Shake well. This will give 100 mL of 0.4/2 mg Bactrim™; each mL = 0.004/0.02 mg Bactrim™. 3. Dispense 20 mL for use

Adverse Reactions and Response During the Protocol

Types of Reactions	Alteration of Protocol
Mild reactions (rash, fever, nausea)	I.V. diphenhydramine (Benadryl®) 50 mg and oral ibuprofen suspension 400 mg
Urticaria, dyspnea, severe vomiting, or hypotension	**STOP** the protocol IMMEDIATELY

- If patient tolerates up to Bactrim™ DS, he/she is desensitized.
- Assuming that there was no complications, the procedure will take up to 6 hours.

DESENSITIZATION PROTOCOLS (Continued)

Sample Bactrim™ Desensitization Flow Sheet

Patient Name _____

Diagnosis _____ Physician _____

Age _____ Gender _____ Hospital # _____

Pager _____ History of sulfa reaction _____

# Hour	Actual Time	Suggested Dose	Form	Suggested Volume	Actual Dose	Form	Actual Volume	Reaction/ Notes	Initial
0		Bactrim™ 0.004/0.02 mg (use **0.004/0.02 mg/mL** bottle or bottle C)	Susp (C)	1 mL					
1		Bactrim™ 0.04/0.2 mg (use 0.004/0.02 mg/mL bottle or bottle C)	Susp (C)	10 mL					
2		Bactrim™ 0.4/2 mg (use **0.4/2 mg/mL bottle** or bottle B)	Susp (B)	1 mL					
3		Bactrim™ 4/20 mg (use 0.4/2 mg/mL bottle or bottle B)	Susp (B)	10 mL					
4		Bactrim™ 40/200 mg (use **40/200 mg/5 mL unit dose** Bactrim™ or A)	Susp (A)	5 mL					
5		Bactrim™ 80/400 mg (use 40/200 mg/5 mL unit dose Bactrim™ or A)	Susp (A)	10 mL					
6		Bactrim™ DS tablet	Tablet	1 DS pill					

Note: Drink 180 mL of water after each Bactrim™ dose.

CIPROFLOXACIN DESENSITIZATION

Modified from *J Allergy Clin Immunol*, 1996, 97:1426-7.

Premedicated with diphenhydramine hydrochloride, ranitidine, and prednisone 1 hour before the desensitization.

The individual doses were administered at 15-minute intervals. Because the patient was intubated in the intensive care unit, vital signs were continually monitored. The patient's skin was inspected for development of urticaria, and his chest was auscultated every 10 minutes for wheezing. No rash, hypotension, or wheezing developed during desensitization. The procedure took 4 hours, and once finished, the patient had received an equivalent to his first scheduled dose (400 mg twice daily). The second dose was given 4 hours later, followed by routine administration of 400 mg every 12 hours, with a small dose (25 mg intravenously) between therapeutic doses to maintain a drug level in the blood. The patient subsequently received 4 weeks of ciprofloxacin treatment without difficulty.

Desensitization Regimen for Ciprofloxacin

Ciprofloxacin Concentration (mg/mL)	Volume Given (mL)	Absolute Amount (mg)	Cumulative Total Dose (mg)
0.1	0.1	0.01	0.01
0.1	0.2	0.02	0.03
0.1	0.4	0.04	0.07
0.1	0.8	0.08	0.15
1	0.16	0.16	0.31
1	0.32	0.32	0.63
1	0.64	0.64	1.27
2	0.6	1.2	2.47
2	1.2	2.4	4.87
2	2.4	4.8	9.67
2	5	10	19.67
2	10	20	39.67
2	20	40	79.67
2	40	80	159.67
2	120	240	399.67

Drug volumes <1 mL were mixed with normal saline solution to a final volume of 3 mL and then slowly infused; the other doses were administered over 10 minutes, except the last dose (240 mg in 120 mL), which was given with an infusion pump over 20 minutes.

RIFAMPIN and ETHAMBUTOL
Oral Desensitization in Mycobacterial Disease

Time from Start (h:min)	Rifampin (mg)	Ethambutol (mg)
0	0.1	0.1
00:45	0.5	0.5
01:30	1	1
02:15	2	2
03:00	4	4
03:45	8	8
04:30	16	16
05:15	32	32
06:00	50	50
06:45	100	100
07:30	150	200
11:00	300	400
Next day		
6:30 AM	300 twice daily	400 three times/day

From *Am J Respir Crit Care Med*, 1994, 149:815-7.

SKIN TESTS

Delayed Hypersensitivity (Anergy)

Delayed cutaneous hypersensitivity (DCH) is a cell-mediated immunological response which has been used diagnostically to assess previous infection (eg, purified protein derivative (PPD), histoplasmin, and coccidioidin) or as an indicator of the status of the immune system by using mumps, *Candida*, tetanus toxoid, or trichophyton to test for anergy. Anergy is a defect in cell-mediated immunity that is characterized by an impaired response, or lack of a response to DCH testing with injected antigens. Anergy has been associated with several disease states, malnutrition, and immunosuppressive therapy, and has been correlated with increased risk of infection, morbidity, and mortality.

Many of the skin test antigens have not been approved by the FDA as tests for anergy, and so the directions for use and interpretation of reactions to these products may differ from that of the product labeling. There is also disagreement in the published literature as to the selection and interpretation of these tests for anergy assessment, leading to different recommendations for use of these products.

General Guidelines

Read these guidelines before using any skin test.

Administration

1. Use a separate sterile TB syringe for each antigen. Immediately after the antigen is drawn up, make the injection intradermally in the flexor surface of the forearm.
2. A small bleb 6-10 mm in diameter will form if the injection is made at the correct depth. If a bleb does not form or if the antigen solution leaks from the site, the injection must be repeated.
3. When applying more than one skin test, make the injections at least 5 cm apart.
4. Do any serologic blood tests before testing or wait 48-96 hours.

Reading

1. Read all tests at 24, 48, and 72 hours. Reactions occurring before 24 hours are indicative of an immediate rather than a delayed hypersensitivity.
2. Measure the diameter of the induration in two directions (at right angles) with a ruler and record each diameter in millimeters. Ballpoint pen method of measurement is the most accurate.
3. Test results should be recorded by the nurse in the Physician's Progress Notes section of the chart, and should include the millimeters of induration present, and a picture of the arm showing the location of the test(s).

Factors Causing False-Negative Reactions

1. Improper administration, interpretation, or use of outdated antigen
2. Test is applied too soon after exposure to the antigen (DCH takes 2-20 weeks to develop.)
3. Concurrent viral illnesses (eg, rubeola, influenza, mumps, and probably others) or recent administration of live attenuated virus vaccines (eg, measles)
4. Anergy may be associated with:
   a. Immune suppressing chronic illnesses such as diabetes, uremia, sarcoidosis, metastatic carcinomas, Hodgkin's, acute lymphocytic leukemia, hypothyroidism, chronic hepatitis, and cirrhosis.
   b. Some antineoplastic agents, radiation therapy, and corticosteroids. If possible, discontinue steroids at least 48 hours prior to DCH skin testing.
   c. Congenital immune deficiencies.
   d. Malnutrition, shock, severe burns, and trauma.
   e. Severe disseminated infections (miliary or cavitary TB, cocci granuloma, and other disseminated mycotic infections, gram-negative bacillary septicemia).
   f. Leukocytosis (>15,000 cells/mm^3).

Factors Causing False-Positive Reactions

1. Improper interpretation
2. Patient sensitivity to minor ingredients in the antigen solutions such as the phenol or thimerosal preservatives
3. Cross-reactions between similar antigens

Candida 1:1000

Dose = 0.1 mL intradermally (30% of children <18 months of age and 50% >18 months of age respond)

Can be used as a control antigen

Coccidioidin 1:1000

Dose = 0.1 mL intradermally (apply with PPD **and** a control antigen)

Mercury derivative used as a preservative for spherulin.

Histoplasmin 1:1000

Dose = 0.1 mL intradermally (yeast derived)

Multitest CMI (*Candida*, diphtheria toxoid, tetanus toxoid, *Streptococcus*, old tuberculin, *Trichophyton*, *Proteus* antigen, and negative control)

Press loaded unit into the skin with sufficient pressure to puncture the skin and allow adequate penetration of all points.

Mumps 40 cfu per mL

Dose = 0.1 mL intradermally (contraindicated in patients allergic to eggs, egg products, or thimerosal)

Dosage as Part of Disease Diagnosis

Tuberculin Testing

Purified Protein Derivative (PPD)

Preparation	Dilution	Units/0.1 mL
First strength	1:10,000	1
Intermediate strength	1:2000	5
Second strength	1:100	250

The usual initial dose is 0.1 mL of the intermediate strength. The first strength should be used in the individuals suspected of being highly sensitive. The second strength is used only for individuals who fail to respond to a previous injection of the first or intermediate strengths.

A positive reaction is 10 mm induration or greater except in HIV-infected individuals where a positive reaction is ≥5 mm of induration.

Adverse Reactions

In patients who are highly sensitive, or when higher than recommended doses are used, exaggerated local reactions may occur, including erythema, pain, blisters, necrosis, and scarring. Although systemic reactions are rare, a few cases of lymph node enlargement, fever, malaise, and fatigue have been reported.

To prevent severe local reactions, never use second test strengths as the initial agent. Use diluted first strengths in patients with known or suspected hypersensitivity to the antigen.

Have epinephrine and antihistamines on hand to treat severe allergic reactions that may occur.

Treatment of Adverse Reactions

Severe reactions to intradermal skin tests are rare and treatment consists of symptomatic care.

Skin Testing

All skin tests are given intradermally into the flexor surface of one arm.

Purified protein derivative (PPD) is used most often in the diagnosis of tuberculosis. *Candida, Trichophyton*, and mumps skin tests are used most often as controls for anergy.

SKIN TESTS *(Continued)*

Dose: The usual skin test dose is as follows:

Antigen		Standard Dose	Concentration
PPD	1 TU	0.1 mL	1 TU – highly sensitive patients
	5 TU	0.1 mL	5 TU – standard dose
	250 TU	0.1 mL	250 TU – anergic patients in whom TB is suspected
Candida		0.02 mL	
Histoplasmin		0.1 mL	Seldom used. Serology is preferred method to diagnose histoplasmosis.
Mumps		0.1 mL	
Trichophyton		0.02 mL	

Interpretation:

Skin Test	Reading Time	Positive Reaction
PPD	48-72 h	**≥5 mm considered positive for:** • close contacts to an infectious case • persons with abnormal chest x-ray indicating old healed TB • persons with known or suspected HIV infection **≥10 mm considered positive for:** • other medical risk factors • foreign born from high prevalence areas • medically underserved, low income populations • alcoholics and intravenous drug users • residents of long-term care facilities (including correctional facilities and nursing homes) • staff in settings where disease would pose a hazard to large number of susceptible persons **≥15 mm considered positive for:** • persons without risk factors for TB
Candida	24-72 h	5 mm induration or greater
Histoplasmin	24-72 h	5 mm or greater
Mumps	24-36 h	5 mm or greater
Trichophyton	24-72 h	5 mm induration or greater

Recommended Interpretation of Skin Test Reactions

Reaction	Local Reaction	
	After Intradermal Injections of Antigens	After Dinitrochlorobenzene
1+	Erythema >10 mm and/or induration >1-5 mm	Erythema and/or induration covering <½ area of dose site
2+	Induration 6-10 mm	Induration covering >½ area of dose site
3+	Induration 11-20 mm	Vesiculation and induration at dose site or spontaneous flare at days 7-14 at the site
4+	Induration >20 mm	Bulla or ulceration at dose site or spontaneous flare at days 7-14 at the site

Penicillin Allergy

The recommended battery of major and minor determinants used in penicillin skin testing will disclose those individuals with circulating IgE antibodies. This procedure is therefore useful to identify patients at risk for immediate or accelerated reactions. Skin tests are of no value in predicting the occurrence of non-IgE-mediated hypersensitivity reactions to penicillin such as delayed exanthem, drug fever, hemolytic anemia, interstitial nephritis, or exfoliative dermatitis. Based on large scale trials, skin testing solutions have been standardized.

Antihistamines, tricyclic antidepressants, and adrenergic drugs, all of which may inhibit skin test results, should be discontinued at least 24 hours prior to skin testing. Antihistamines with long half-lives (hydroxyzine, terfenadine, astemizole, etc) may attenuate skin test results up to a week, or longer after discontinuation.

When properly performed with due consideration for preliminary scratch tests and appropriate dilutions, skin testing with penicillin reagents can almost always be safely accomplished. Systemic reactions accompany about 1% of positive skin tests; these are usually mild but can be serious. **Therefore skin tests should be done in the presence of a physician and with immediate access to medications and equipment needed to treat anaphylaxis.**

History of Penicillin Allergy

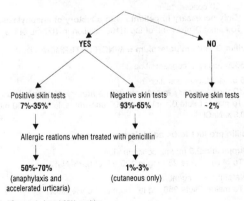

*One study found 65% positive

Prevalence of positive and negative skin tests and subsequent allergic reactions in patients treated with penicillin (based on studies using both penicilloyl-polylysine and minor determinant mixture as skin test reagents).

SKIN TESTS *(Continued)*

Penicillin Skin Testing Protocol

Skin tests evaluate the patient for the presence of penicillin IgE-sensitive mast cells which are responsible for anaphylaxis and other immediate hypersensitivity reactions. Local or systemic allergic reactions rarely occur due to skin testing, therefore, a tourniquet, I.V., and epinephrine should be at the bedside. The breakdown products of penicillin provide the antigen which is responsible for the allergy. Testing is performed with benzylpenicilloyl-polylysine (Pre-Pen®), the major determinant, penicillin G which provides the minor determinants and the actual penicillin which will be administered.

Controls are important if the patient is extremely ill or is taking antihistamines, codeine, or morphine. Normal saline is the negative control. Morphine sulfate, a mast cell degranulator, can be used as a positive control, if the patient is not on morphine or codeine. Histamine is the preferred positive control, however, is not manufactured in a pharmaceutical formulation anymore. A false-positive or false-negative will make further skin testing invalid.

Control Solutions

Normal saline = negative control
Morphine sulfate (10 mg/100 mL 0.9% NaCl, 0.1 mg/mL) = positive control

Test Solutions

Order the necessary solutions as 0.5 mL in a tuberculin syringe. **Note:** May need to order two syringes of each – one for scratch testing and one for intradermal skin testing.

I.   **Pre-Pen®: Benzylpenicilloyl-polylysine (0.25 mL ampul) = MAJOR DETERMINANT**

    A.   Undiluted Pre-Pen®

    B.   1:100 concentration
        To make: Dilute 0.1 mL of Pre-Pen® in 10 mL of 0.9% NaCl

    C.   1:10,000 concentration
        (Only necessary in patients with a history of anaphylaxis)
        To make: Dilute 1 mL of the 1:100 solution in 100 mL of 0.9% NaCl

II. **Penicillin G sodium/potassium = MINOR DETERMINANT**

    A.   5000 units/mL concentration

    B.   5 units/mL concentration
        (Only necessary in patients with a history of anaphylaxis)
        To make: Dilute 0.1 mL of a 5000 units/mL solution in 100 mL of 0.9% NaCl

III. **Penicillin product to be administered – if not penicillin G**

    A.   **Ampicillin** 2.5 mg/mL concentration
        To make: Dilute 250 mg in 100 mL of 0.9% NaCl

    B.   ·**Nafcillin** 2.5 mg/mL concentration
        To make: Dilute 250 mg in 100 mL of 0.9% NaCl

Order for placement/availability at the bedside in the event of a hypersensitivity reaction during scratch/skin testing and desensitization:

Hydrocortisone: 100 mg IVP
Diphenhydramine: 50 mg IVP
Epinephrine: 1:1000 S.C.

Scratch/Skin Testing Protocol: Must Be Done by Physician!

1. Begin with the control solutions (ie, normal saline and morphine).

2. Administer **scratch tests** in the following order (beginning with the most dilute solution):

Pre-Pen®	Syringes: C,B,A
Penicillin G	Syringes: E,D
Ampicillin/Nafcillin	Syringe: F

    The inner volar surface of the forearm is usually used.

    A nonbleeding scratch of 3-5 mm in length is made in the epidermis with a 20-gauge needle.

    If bleeding occurs, another site should be selected and another scratch made using less pressure.

    A small drop of the test solution is then applied and rubbed gently into the scratch using an applicator, toothpick, or the side of the needle.

    The scratch test site should be observed for the appearance of a wheal, erythema, and pruritis.

    A positive reaction is signified by the appearance within 15 minutes of a pale wheal (usually with pseudopods) ranging from 5-15 mm or more in diameter.

    As soon as a positive response is elicited, or 15 minutes has elapsed, the solution should be wiped off the scratch.

    If the scratch test is negative or equivocal (ie, a wheal <5 mm in diameter with little or no erythema or itching appears), an intradermal test may be performed.

    If significant reaction, treat and proceed to desensitization.

3. Administer **intradermal tests** in the following order (beginning with the most dilute solution):

Pre-Pen®	Syringes: C,B,A
Penicillin G	Syringes: E,D
Ampicillin/Nafcillin	Syringe: F

    Intradermal tests are usually performed on a sterilized area of the upper outer arm at a sufficient distance below the deltoid muscle to permit proximal application of a tourniquet if a severe reaction occurs.

    Using a tuberculin syringe with a 3/8-5/8 inch 26- to 30-gauge needle, an amount of each tet solution sufficient to raise the smallest perceptible bleb (usually 0.01-0.02 mL) is injected immediately under the surface of the skin.

    A separate needle and syringe must be used for each solution.

    Each test and control site should be at least 15 cm apart.

    Positive reactions are manifested as a wheal at the test site with a diameter at least 5 mm larger than the saline control, often accompanied by itching and a marked increase in the size of the bleb.

    Skin responses to penicillin testing will develop within 15 minutes.

    If no significant reaction, may challenge patient with reduced dosage of the penicillin to be administered.

    Physician should be at the bedside during this challenge dose!

    If significant reaction, treat and begin desensitization.

ANTIRETROVIRAL AGENTS

Renal Dosing Adjustment, Dosage Forms, and Adverse Reactions

Chemical and Generic Names	Brand Name (company)	Dose (renal adjustment)	Dosage Forms	Adverse Reaction
NRTIs (Nucleoside Reverse Transcriptase Inhibitors)				
Zidovudine (AZT)	Retrovir® (Glaxo-Wellcome)	200 mg tid or 300 mg bid on empty stomach (ESRD: 100 mg q6-8 h)	Tablet: 300 mg. Capsule: 100 mg. Syrup: 50 mg/mL (240 mL). Injection: 10 mg/mL (20 mL)	Anemia, neutropenia, thrombocytopenia, headache, nausea, vomiting, myopathy, hepatitis, hyperpigmentation of nails
Zidovudine/ lamivudine	Combivir® (Glaxo-Wellcome)	1 tablet bid (see lamivudine for dose adjustment)	Tablet: 300 mg zidovudine, 150 mg lamivudine	See individual agents
Didanosine (ddI)	Videx® (Bristol-Myers Squibb)	>60 kg: 200 mg bid on empty stomach. <60 kg: 125 mg bid (adjust for Cl_{cr} <60)	Tablet, chewable: 25 mg, 50 mg, 100 mg, 150 mg. Powder, oral: 100 mg, 167 mg, 250 mg, 375 mg. Powder, pediatric: 2 g, 4 g	Peripheral neuropathy, pancreatitis, abdominal pain, nausea, diarrhea, retinal depigmentation, anxiety, insomnia
Zalcitabine (ddC)	Hivid® (Roche)	0.75 mg tid on empty stomach. Cl_{cr} 10-40: bid. Cl_{cr} <10: qd	Tablet: 0.375 mg, 0.75 mg	Peripheral neuropathy, oral/esophageal ulceration, rash, nausea, vomiting, diarrhea, abdominal pain, myalgia, pancreatitis
Stavudine (d4T)	Zerit® (Bristol-Myers Squibb)	≥60 kg: 40 mg bid. Cl_{cr} 26-50: 20 mg bid. Cl_{cr} 10-25: 20 mg qd. <60 kg: 30 mg bid. Cl_{cr} 26-50: 15 mg bid. Cl_{cr} 10-25: 15 mg qd	Capsule: 15 mg, 20 mg, 30 mg, 40 mg. Solution, oral: 1 mg/mL (200 mL)	Peripheral neuropathy, headache, abdominal or back pain, asthenia, nausea, vomiting, diarrhea, myalgia, anxiety, depression, pancreatitis, less frequently hepatotoxicity
Lamivudine (3TC)	Epivir® (Glaxo-Wellcome)	≥50 kg: 150 mg bid. <50 kg: 2 mg/kg bid. Cl_{cr} 30-49: 150 mg qd. Cl_{cr} 15-29: 150 mg first dose, then 100 mg qd. Cl_{cr} 5-14: 150 mg first dose, then 50 mg qd. Cl_{cr} <5: 50 mg first dose, then 25 mg qd	Tablet: 150 mg. Solution, oral: 10 mg/mL (240 mL)	Headache, insomnia, nausea, vomiting, diarrhea, abdominal pain, myalgia, arthralgia, pancreatitis in children
Abacavir	Ziagen® (Glaxo-Wellcome)	300 mg bid	Tablet: 300 mg. Solution, oral: 20 mg/mL (240 mL)	Hypersensitivity syndrome (fever, fatigue, GI symptoms, ±rash); **do not restart abacavir in patients who have experienced this**; GI symptoms

Renal Dosing Adjustment, Dosage Forms, and Adverse Reactions *(continued)*

Chemical and Generic Names	Brand Name (company)	Dose (renal adjustment)	Dosage Forms	Adverse Reaction
		NNRTIs (Non-nucleoside Reverse Transcriptase Inhibitors)		
Nevirapine	Viramune® (Roxane)	200 mg qd for 14 days, then 200 mg bid	Tablet: 200 mg	Rash (severe), abnormal liver function tests, fever, nausea, headache
Delavirdine	Rescriptor® (Pharmacia/Upjohn)	400 mg tid	Tablet: 100 mg	Rash
Efavirenz	Sustiva™ (DuPont)	600 mg qd	Capsule: 50 mg, 100 mg, 200 mg	Dizziness, psychiatric symptoms (hallucinations, confusion, depersonalization, others), agitation, vivid dreams, rash, GI intolerance
		PIs (Protease Inhibitors)		
Saquinavir	Invirase® (Roche) Fortovase® (Roche)	600 mg tid with a full meal 1200 mg tid with a full meal	Capsule: 200 mg Gelcap: 200 mg	Diarrhea, abdominal discomfort, nausea, headache, hyperglycemia (and sometimes diabetes), dyslipidemia including fat redistribution ("buffalo hump," "protease paunch"), hyperlipidemia, hypercholesterolemia
Ritonavir	Norvir® (Abbott)	600 mg bid with food (titrate)	Capsule: 100 mg Solution, oral: 80 mg/mL (240 mL)	Asthenia, nausea, diarrhea, vomiting, anorexia, abdominal pain, circumoral and peripheral paresthesia, taste perversion, headache, hyperglycemia (and sometimes diabetes), dyslipidemia including fat redistribution ("buffalo hump," "protease paunch"), hyperlipidemia, hypercholesterolemia
Indinavir	Crixivan® (Merck)	800 mg q8h with water (Hepatic insufficiency: 600 mg tid)	Capsule: 200 mg, 400 mg	Hyperbilirubinemia, nephrolithiasis, elevated AST/ALT, abdominal pain, nausea, vomiting, diarrhea, taste perversion, hyperglycemia (and sometimes diabetes), dyslipidemia including fat redistribution ("buffalo hump," "protease paunch"), hyperlipidemia, hypercholesterolemia
Nelfinavir	Viracept® (Agouron)	750 mg tid with food	Tablet: 250 mg Powder, oral: 50 mg/g (144 g)	Diarrhea, nausea, hyperglycemia (and sometimes diabetes), dyslipidemia including fat redistribution ("buffalo hump," "protease paunch"), hyperlipidemia, hypercholesterolemia
Amprenavir	Agenerase (Glaxo-Wellcome)	1200 mg bid (avoid high fat meal)	Capsule: 150 mg Solution, oral: 15 mg/mL (240 mL)	Rash (life-threatening), paresthesias (perioral), depression, nausea, diarrhea, vomiting, hyperglycemia (and sometimes diabetes), dyslipidemia including fat redistribution ("buffalo hump," "protease paunch"), hyperlipidemia, hypercholesterolemia

ANTIRETROVIRAL AGENTS *(Continued)*

Antiretroviral Drug Interactions

Antiretroviral Agent	Interacting Agent	Severity*	Additional Comments
Zidovudine	Ganciclovir	1	Increased toxicity (hematologic)
	Interferon	2	Dose reduction or interruption may be necessary or change to foscarnet
	Probenecid	2	Increased zidovudine levels
Didanosine	Tetracycline, itraconazole, ketoconazole, indinavir	2	Decreased absorption with didanosine
	Dapsone	3	Administer 2 hours before didanosine
	Ciprofloxacin/norfloxacin (quinolones)	2	Administer didanosine 6 hours before or 2 hours after quinolone
Zalcitabine	Antacids (aluminum-, magnesium-containing)	2	Decreased zalcitabine absorption by 25%; do not administer simultaneously
	Pentamidine	2	Increased risk of pancreatitis; avoid concomitant use
Stavudine	None		
Lamivudine	Trimethoprim/ sulfamethoxazole	3	Increased lamivudine AUC by 44%
	Zidovudine	3	Increased zidovudine C_{max} by 39%
Abacavir	Ethanol	3	Increased abacavir AUC
Nevirapine	Oral contraceptives	1	Decreased oral contraceptives concentration
	Protease inhibitors	1	Decreased concentrations of protease inhibitors; avoid concomitant use
	Rifabutin/rifampin	2	Decreased nevirapine concentrations
Delavirdine	Protease inhibitors	2	Increased levels of protease inhibitors; start indinavir at 600 mg every 8 hours; nelfinavir may decrease delavirdine levels by 50%
	Terfenadine, astemizole, cisapride, alprazolam, midazolam, triazolam	1	Delavirdine may significantly increase concentrations of these drugs
	Dihydropyridine calcium channel blockers, ergot derivatives, quinidine	2	Delavirdine may increase concentrations of these drugs
	Warfarin	2	Delavirdine may increase warfarin concentrations
	Rifampin/rifabutin, phenytoin, carbamazepine	1	Avoid concomitant use; decreased delavirdine concentration
	Antacids, H_2-antagonists, didanosine	2	Decreased delavirdine absorption; administer antacids or didanosine at least 1 hour apart from delavirdine
	Clarithromycin, dapsone	2	Delavirdine may increase levels of these drugs; clarithromycin may increase delavirdine levels
	Ketoconazole, fluoxetine	3	May increase delavirdine concentration by 50%
Efavirenz	Astemizole, cisapride, ergot derivatives, midazolam, triazolam	1	Contraindicated. Avoid concomitant use.
	Indinavir	2	Decreased indinavir AUC by 31% and Cp_{max} by 16%. Increase indinavir dose to 1000 mg every 8 hours.
	Ritonavir	3	Increased AUC by ~20% for each drug
	Saquinavir	2	Decreased saquinavir AUC by 62% and Cp_{max} by 50%. Not recommended as sole protease inhibitor with efavirenz.
	Rifampin	2	Decreased efavirenz AUC by 26% and Cp_{max} by 20%
	Clarithromycin	2	Decreased clarithromycin AUC by 39% and Cp_{max} by 49%; increased hydroxy metabolite of clarithromycin AUC by 34% and Cp_{max} by 49%
	Ethinyl estradiol	2	Increased ethinyl estradiol AUC by 37%
	Warfarin	2	Decreased or increased warfarin effects

Antiretroviral Drug Interactions *(continued)*

Antiretroviral Agent	Interacting Agent	Severity*	Additional Comments
Saquinavir	Carbamazepine, dexamethasone, phenobarbital, phenytoin	2	May decrease saquinavir levels
	Rifampin	1	Decreased saquinavir level by 80%
	Rifabutin	2	Decreased saquinavir level by 40%
Ritonavir	Meperidine	1	Contraindicated. Alternative: Acetaminophen
	Piroxicam	1	Contraindicated. Alternative: Aspirin
	Propoxyphene	1	Contraindicated. Alternative: Oxycodone
	Amiodarone, encainide, flecainide, propafenone, quinidine/quinine	1	Contraindicated
	Rifabutin	1	Contraindicated. Alternatives: Clarithromycin, ethambutol
	Bepridil	1	Contraindicated
	Astemizole/terfenadine	1	Contraindicated. Alternatives: Loratadine
	Cisapride	1	Contraindicated
	Bupropion	1	Contraindicated. Alternative: Fluoxetine, desipramine
	Clozapine	1	Contraindicated
	Alprazolam, clorazepate, diazepam, estazolam, flurazepam, midazolam, triazolam, zolpidem	1	Contraindicated. Alternatives: Temazepam, lorazepam
	Clarithromycin	2	Increased clarithromycin AUC by 77%; decrease dose of clarithromycin by 50% if Cl_{cr} is 30-60 mL/minute and by 75% if Cl_{cr} is <30 mL/minute
	Erythromycin	2	>3 times increase in AUC of erythromycin
	Desipramine	2	Increased desipramine AUC by 145%
	Disulfiram/metronidazole	2	Disulfiram-like reaction
	Oral contraceptives	1	Decreased ethinyl estradiol AUC by 40%
	Theophylline	2	Decreased theophylline AUC by 43%
	Antiarrhythmics, anticoagulants, anticonvulsants, tricyclic antidepressants, neuroleptics	2	1.5 to >3 times increase in AUC of interacting drug
	Phenytoin, phenobarbital, rifampin/rifabutin	2	May decrease ritonavir levels
Indinavir	Rifabutin	1	Increased rifabutin AUC by 204%; decrease rifabutin dose to one-half
	Ketoconazole	2	Increased indinavir AUC by 68%; decrease indinavir dose to 600 mg every 8 hours
	Didanosine	2	Decreased indinavir absorption; administer 1 hour apart on an empty stomach
	Rifampin	1	Avoid concomitant use due to decreased indinavir concentration
	Terfenadine/astemizole, cisapride, triazolam/midazolam	1	Indinavir may increase toxicity of these drugs; avoid concomitant use
Nelfinavir	Astemizole, cisapride, midazolam, rifampin, terfenadine, triazolam	1	Contraindicated. Avoid concomitant use.
	Rifabutin	2	Increased rifabutin concentrations; reduce rifabutin dose
	Anticonvulsants	1	May decrease nelfinavir concentrations
	Oral contraceptives	1	Decreased oral contraceptive concentrations
	Delavirdine	2	Nelfinavir concentration doubled; delavirdine level decreased by 50%

ANTIRETROVIRAL AGENTS *(Continued)*

Antiretroviral Drug Interactions *(continued)*

Antiretroviral Agent	Interacting Agent	Severity*	Additional Comments
Amprenavir	Astemizole, rifampin, midazolam, bepridil, dihydroergotamine, ergotamine, cisapride	1	Contraindicated. Avoid concomitant use.
	Abacavir, clarithromycin, indinavir, ritonavir?, cimetidine?	2	Increased amprenavir C_{max} and AUC
	Saquinavir	1	Decreased amprenavir AUC and C_{max}
	Rifabutin	1	Increased rifabutin AUC by 193%; administer one-half usual rifabutin dose
	Amiodarone, lidocaine, quinidine, warfarin, tricyclic antidepressants	1	Increased toxic effect of these agents; must have concentration monitoring
	HMGCoA reductase inhibitors, diltiazem, nicardipine, nifedipine, nimodipine, alprazolam, clarzepate, diazepam, flurazepam, itraconazole, dapsone, erythromycin, loratadine, silfenafil, carbamazepine, pimozide	2	Increased serum concentrations of these agents, potential for increased toxic effects
	Oral contraceptives	1	Decreased oral contraceptive concentrations

*Severity: 1 = major; 2 = moderate; 3 = minor.

ANTIRETROVIRAL AGENTS IN PEDIATRIC HIV INFECTION

Indications for Initiation of Antiretroviral Therapy in Children With Human Immunodeficiency Virus (HIV) Infection*

- Clinical symptoms associated with HIV infection
- Evidence of immune suppression, indicated by CD4+ T-lymphocyte absolute number or percentage
- Age <12 months - regardless of clinical, immunologic, or virologic status
- For asymptomatic children ≥1 year with normal immune status, two options can be considered:

  - Preferred approach: Initiate therapy - regardless of age or symptom status

  - Alternative approach: Defer treatment in situations in which the risk for clinical disease progression is low and other factors (eg, concern for the durability of response, safety, and adherence) favor postponing treatment. In such cases, the healthcare provider should regularly monitor virologic, immunologic, and clinical status. Factors to be considered in deciding to initiate therapy include the following:

    - High or increasing HIV RNA copy number
    - Rapidly declining CD4+ T-lymphocyte number or percentage to values approaching those indicative of moderate immune suppression
    - Development of clinical symptoms

Adapted from Guidelines for the Use of Antiretroviral Agents in Pediatric HIV Infection, *MMWR Morb Mortal Wkly Rep*, 1998, 47(RR-4):16. Updated from website www.hivatis.org.

ANTIRETROVIRAL AGENTS *(Continued)*

Recommended Antiretroviral Regimens for Initial Therapy for Human Immunodeficiency Virus (HIV) Infection in Children

Strongly Recommended

Clinical trial evidence of clinical benefit and/or sustained suppression of HIV replication in adults and/or children.

- One highly active protease inhibitor plus two nucleoside analogue reverse transcriptase inhibitors (NRTIs)

  - Preferred protease inhibitor for infants and children who cannot swallow pills or capsules: nelfinavir or ritonavir. Alternative for children who can swallow pills or capsules: indinavir.

  - Recommended dual NRTI combinations: The most data on use in children are available for the combinations of zidovudine (ZDV) and dideoxyinosine (ddI) and for ZDV and lamivudine (3TC). More limited data are available for the combinations of stavudine (d4T) and ddI, d4T and 3TC, and ZDV and zalcitabine (ddC).*

- Alternative for children who can swallow capsules: Efavirenz (Sustiva)† plus two NRTIs (see above) or efavirenz (Sustiva) plus nelfinavir and one NRTI.

Recommended as an Alternative

Clinical trial evidence of suppression of HIV replication, but 1) durability may be less in adults and/or children than with strongly recommended regimens; or 2) the durability of suppression is not yet defined; or 3) evidence of efficacy may not outweigh potential adverse consequences (eg, toxicity, drug interactions, cost, etc).

- Nevirapine and two NRTIs
- Abacavir in combination with ZDV and 3TC

Offer only in Special Circumstances

Clinical trial evidence of 1) limited benefit for patients; or 2) data are inconclusive, but may be reasonably offered in special circumstances.

- Two NRTIs

Not Recommended

Evidence against use because of 1) overlapping toxicity; and/or 2) because use may be virologically undesirable.

- Any monotherapy¶
- d4T and ZDV
- ddC and ddI
- ddC and d4T
- ddC and 3TC

---

*ddC is not available in a liquid preparation commercially, although a liquid formulation is available through a compassionate use program of the manufacturer (Hoffman-LaRoche Inc, Nutley, NJ). ZDV and ddC is a less preferred choice for use in combination with a protease inhibitor.

†Efavirenz is currently available only in capsule form, but liquid preparation is currently being evaluated. There are currently no data on appropriate dosage of efavirenz in children under age 3 years.

¶Except for ZDV chemoprophylaxis administered to HIV-exposed infants during the first 6 weeks of life to prevent perinatal HIV transmission; if an infant is identified as HIV-infected while receiving ZDV prophylaxis, therapy should be changed to a combination antiretroviral drug regimen.

Adapted from Guidelines for the Use of Antiretroviral Agents in Pediatric HIV Infection, *MMWR Morb Mortal Wkly Rep*, 1998, 47(RR-4):19. Updated from website www.hivatis.org.

Considerations for Changing Antiretroviral Therapy for Human Immunodeficiency Virus (HIV)-Infected Children

Virologic Considerations*

- Less than a minimally acceptable virologic response after 8-12 weeks of therapy. For children receiving antiretroviral therapy with two nucleoside analogue reverse transcriptase inhibitors (NRTIs) and a protease inhibitor, such a response is defined as a less than tenfold (1.0 $\log_{10}$) decrease from baseline HIV RNA levels. For children who are receiving less potent antiretroviral therapy (ie, dual NRTI combinations), an insufficient response is defined as a less than fivefold (0.7 $\log_{10}$) decrease in HIV RNA levels from baseline.

- HIV RNA not suppressed to undetectable levels after 4-6 months of antiretroviral therapy.†

- Repeated detection of HIV RNA in children who initially responded to antiretroviral therapy with undetectable levels.§

- A reproducible increase in HIV RNA copy number among children who have had a substantial HIV RNA response but still have low levels of detectable HIV RNA. Such an increase would warrant change in therapy if, after initiation of the therapeutic regimen, a greater than threefold (0.5 $\log_{10}$) increase in copy number for children ≥2 years of age and a greater than fivefold (0.7 $\log_{10}$) increase is observed for children <2 years of age.

Immunologic Considerations*

- Change in immunologic classification.¶

- For children with CD4+ T-lymphocyte percentages <15%, a persistent decline of five percentiles or more in CD4+ cell percentage (eg, from 15% to 10%)

- A rapid and substantial decrease in absolute CD4+ T-lymphocyte count (eg, a >30% decline in <6 months).

Clinical Considerations

- Progressive neurodevelopmental deterioration.

- Growth failure defined as persistent decline in weight-growth velocity despite adequate nutritional support and without other explanation.

- Disease progression defined as advancement from one pediatric clinical category to another.**

---

*At least two measurements (taken 1 week apart) should be performed before considering a change in therapy.

†The initial HIV RNA level of the child at the start of therapy and the level achieved with therapy should be considered when contemplating potential drug changes. For example, an immediate change in therapy may not be warranted if there is a sustained 1.5-2.0 $\log_{10}$ decrease in HIV RNA copy number, even if RNA remains detectable at low levels.

§More frequent evaluation of HIV RNA levels should be considered if the HIV RNA increase is limited (eg, if when using an HIV RNA assay with a lower limit of detection of 1000 copies/mL, there is a ≤0.7 $\log_{10}$ increase from undetectable to approximately 5000 copies/mL in an infant <2 years of age).

¶Minimal changes in CD4+ T-lymphocyte percentile that may result in change in immunologic category (eg, from 26% to 24%, or 16% to 14%) may not be as concerning as a rapid substantial change in CD4+ percentile within the same immunologic category (eg, a drop from 35% to 25%).

**In patients with stable immunologic and virologic parameters, progression from one clinical category to another may not represent an indication to change therapy. Thus, in patients whose disease progression is not associated with neurologic deterioration or growth failure, virologic and immunologic considerations are important in deciding whether to change therapy.

Adapted from Guidelines for the Use of Antiretroviral Agents in Pediatric HIV Infection, *MMWR Morb Mortal Wkly Rep*, 1998, 47(RR-4):22.

ANTIRETROVIRAL AGENTS *(Continued)*

ANTIRETROVIRAL USE GUIDELINES IN ADULTS AND ADOLESCENTS INFECTED WITH HIV

(From "Report of the NIH Panel to Define Principles of Therapy of HIV Infection and Guidelines for the Use of Antiretroviral Agents in HIV-Infected Adults and Adolescents," *MMWR Morb Mortal Wkly Rep*, 1998, 47(RR-5).)

Indications for Plasma HIV RNA Testing*

Clinical Indication	Information	Use
Syndrome consistent with acute HIV infection	Establishes diagnosis when HIV antibody test is negative or indeterminate	Diagnosis†
Initial evaluation of newly diagnosed HIV infection	Baseline viral load "set point"	Decision to start or defer therapy
Every 3-4 months in patients not on therapy	Changes in viral load	Decision to start therapy
4-8 weeks after initiation of antiretroviral therapy	Initial assessment of drug efficacy	Decision to continue or change therapy
3-4 months after start of therapy	Maximal effect of therapy	Decision to continue or change therapy
Every 3-4 months in patients on therapy	Durability of antiretroviral effect	Decision to continue or change therapy
Clinical event or significant decline in CD4+ T cells	Association with changing or stable viral load	Decision to continue, initiate, or change therapy

* Acute illness (eg, bacterial pneumonia, tuberculosis, HSV, PCP, etc) and immunizations can cause increases in plasma HIV RNA for 2-4 weeks; viral load testing should not be performed during this time. Plasma HIV RNA results should usually be verified with a repeat determination before starting or making changes in therapy. HIV RNA should be measured using the same laboratory and the same assay.

†Diagnosis of HIV infection made by HIV RNA testing should be confirmed by standard methods such as Western blot serology performed 2-4 months after the initial indeterminate or negative test.

Risks and Benefits of Early Initiation of Antiretroviral Therapy in the Asymptomatic HIV-Infected Patient

Potential Benefits

Control of viral replication and mutation; reduction of viral burden

Prevention of progressive immunodeficiency; potential maintenance or reconstitution of a normal immune system

Delayed progression to AIDS and prolongation of life

Decreased risk of selection of resistant virus

Decreased risk of drug toxicity

Potential Risks

Reduction in quality of life from adverse drug effects and inconvenience of current maximally suppressive regimens

Earlier development of drug resistance

Limitation in future choices of antiretroviral agents due to development of resistance

Unknown long-term toxicity of antiretroviral drugs

Unknown duration of effectiveness of current antiretroviral therapies

Indications for the Initiation of Antiretroviral Therapy in the Chronically HIV-Infected Patient

Clinical Category	CD4+ T Cell Count and HIV RNA	Recommendation
Symptomatic (ie, AIDS, thrush, unexplained fever)	Any value	Treat
Asymptomatic	CD4+ T cells <500/mm³ **or** HIV RNA >10,000 (bDNA) or >20,000 (RT-PCR)	Treatment should be offered. Strength of recommendation is based on prognosis for disease-free survival and willingness of the patient to accept therapy.*
Asymptomatic	CD4+ T cells >500/mm³ **and** HIV RNA <10,000 (bDNA) or <20,000 (RT-PCR)	Many experts would delay therapy and observe; however, some experts would treat.

*Some experts would observe patients whose CD4+ T-cell counts are between 350-500/mm³ and HIV RNA levels <10,000 (bDNA) or <20,000 (RT-PCR).

ANTIRETROVIRAL AGENTS *(Continued)*

Prognostic Value of Viral RNA Counts

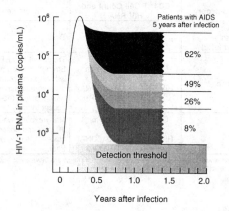

From Ho DD *Science 272*:1124-1125, 1996

Surrogate End Points Reflect Clinical Course

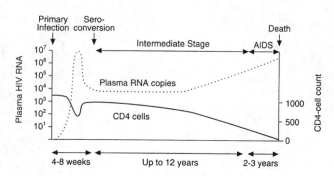

Adapted from Piatak M Jr et al *Science 259*:1749-1753, 1993; Weiss RA *Science 260*: 1273-1279, 1993

Recommended Antiretroviral Agents for Treatment of Established HIV Infection

Preferred: Strong evidence of clinical benefit and/or sustained suppression of plasma viral load. One choice each from column A and column B. Drugs are listed in random, not priority, order.

Column A	Column B
Indinavir (AI)	ZDV + ddl (AI)
Nelfinavir (AII)	d4T + ddl (AII)
Ritonavir (AI)	ZDV + ddC (AI)
Saquinavir - SGC* (AII)	ZDV + 3TC† (AI)
Ritonavir + Saquinavir-SGC or HGC* (BII)	d4T + 3TC† (AII)
Efavirenz (AII)	ddl + 3TC† (BII)

Alternative: Less likely to provide sustained virus suppression, or data inadequate

Nevirapine or delavirdine + 2 NRTIs (Column B, above)‡ (BII)

Abacavir + ZDV + 3TC# (BII)

Not generally recommended: Strong evidence of clinical benefit, but initial virus suppression is not sustained in most patients

Two NRTIs (Column B, above) (CI)

Saquinavir-HGC + two NRTIs (Column B, above)§ (CI)

Not recommended: Evidence against use, virologically undesirable, or overlapping toxicities

All monotherapies¶ (DI)

d4T + ZDV (DI)

ddC + ddl• (DII)

ddC + d4T• (DII)

ddC + 3TC (DII)

---

*Use of ritonavir 400 mg twice daily with saquinavir-SGC (Fortovase™) 400 mg twice daily results in similar drug exposure and antiretroviral activity as when using 400 mg twice daily of saquinavir-HGC (Invirase®) in combination with ritonavir. However, this combination with Fortovase™ has not been extensively studied, and gastrointestinal toxicity may be greater when using Fortovase™.

†High-level resistance to 3TC develops within 2-4 weeks in partially suppressive regimens; optimal use is in 3-drug antiretroviral combinations that reduce viral load to undetectable levels.

‡The combination of any of the three available NRTIs + two NNRTI can suppress viremia to undetectable levels in the majority of patients remaining on treatment for >28 weeks. An efavirenz-containing regimen has been shown to compare favorably to a PI-containing regimen with regard to suppression of viremia through 48 weeks; such head-to-head comparative trials have not been performed with nevirapine or delavirdine. Of note, use of efavirenz, nevirapine, or delavirdine may result in resistance that precludes efficacy of any other member of this drug class.

#Virologic and immunologic responses obtained with abacavir + ZDV + 3TC are similar to those obtained with indinavir + ZDV + 3TC at 48 weeks. The durability of viral load suppression with this regimen that includes drugs from a single drug class (ie, NRTIs) is uncertain; in addition, abacavir is associated with a potentially life-threatening hypersensitivity reaction. For these reasons, a PI-containing or efavirenz-containing regimen is preferred until longer-term data are available for an abacavir-containing three NRTI regimen.

§Use of saquinavir-HGC (Invirase®) is generally not recommended, except in combination with ritonavir.

¶Zidovudine monotherapy may be considered for prophylactic use in pregnant women with low viral load and high CD4+T cell counts to prevent perinatal transmission.

•This combination of NRTIs is not recommended based on lack of clinical data using the combination and/or overlapping toxicities.

Updated from website www.hivatis.org.

ANTIRETROVIRAL AGENTS (Continued)

Drugs That Should Not Be Used With Protease Inhibitors

Drug Category	Indinavir	Ritonavir*	Saquinavir#	Nelfinavir	Alternatives
Analgesics	None	Meperidine, piroxicam, propoxyphene	None	None	ASA, oxycodone, acetaminophen
Cardiac	None	Amiodarone, encainide, flecainide, propafenone, quinidine	None	None	Limited experience
Antimycobacterial	Rifampin	Rifabutin†	Rifampin, rifabutin	Rifampin	For rifabutin (as alternative for MAI treatment): clarithromycin, ethambutol (treatment; not prophylaxis), or azithromycin
Calcium channel blocker	None	Bepridil	None	None	Limited experience
Antihistamine	Astemizole, terfenadine	Astemizole, terfenadine	Astemizole, terfenadine	Astemizole, terfenadine	Loratadine
Gastrointestinal	Cisapride	Cisapride	Cisapride	Cisapride	Limited experience
Antidepressant	None	Bupropion	None	None	Fluoxetine, desipramine
Neuroleptic	None	Clozapine, pimozide	None	None	Limited experience
Psychotropic	Midazolam, triazolam	Clorazepate, diazepam, estazolam, flurazepam, midazolam, triazolam, zolpidem	Midazolam, triazolam	Midazolam, triazolam	Temazepam, lorazepam
Ergot alkaloid (vasoconstrictor)		Dihydroergotamine (D.H.E. 45), ergotamine§ (various forms)		Dihydroergotamine (D.H.E. 45), ergotamine§ (various forms)	

*The contraindicated drugs listed are based on theoretical considerations. Thus, drugs with low therapeutic indices yet with suspected major metabolic contribution from cytochrome P-450 3A, CYP2D6, or unknown pathways are included in this table. Actual interactions may or may not occur in patients.
#Given as Invirase® or Fortovase™
†Reduce rifabutin dose to one-fourth of the standard dose.
§This is likely a class effect.

Guidelines for Changing an Antiretroviral Regimen
for Suspected Drug Failure

- Criteria for changing therapy include a suboptimal reduction in plasma viremia after initiation of therapy, reappearance of viremia after suppression to unde-tectable, significant increases in plasma viremia from the nadir of suppression, and declining CD4+ T-cell numbers.

- When the decision to change therapy is based on viral load determination, it is preferable to confirm with a second viral load test.

- Distinguish between the need to change a regimen due to drug intolerance or inability to comply with the regimen versus failure to achieve the goal of sustained viral suppression; single agents can be changed or dose reduced in the event of drug intolerance.

- In general, do not change a single drug or add a single drug to a failing regimen; it is important to use at least two new drugs and preferably to use an entirely new regimen with at least three new drugs.

- Many patients have limited options for new regimens of desired potency; in some of these cases, it is rational to continue the prior regimen if partial viral suppression was achieved.

- In some cases, regimens identified as suboptimal for initial therapy are rational due to limitations imposed by toxicity, intolerance, or nonadherence. This especially applies in late stage disease. For patients with no rational alternative options who have virologic failure with return of viral load to base-line (pretreatment levels) and a declining CD4+ T-cell count, there should be consideration for discontinuation of antiretroviral therapy.

- Experience is limited with regimens using combinations of two protease inhibi-tors or combinations of protease inhibitors with nevirapine or delavirdine; for patients with limited options due to drug intolerance or suspected resistance, these regimens provide possible alternative treatment options.

- There is limited information about the value of restarting a drug that the patient has previously received. The experience with zidovudine is that resistant strains are often replaced with "wild-type" zidovudine-sensitive strains when zidovudine treatment is stopped, but resistance recurs rapidly if zidovudine is restarted. While there is primary evidence that this occurs with indinavir, it is not known if similar problems apply to other nucleoside analogues, protease inhibitors, or NNRTIs, but a conservative stance is that they probably do.

- Avoid changing from ritonavir to indinavir or vice-versa for drug failure, since high-level cross-resistance is likely.

- Avoid changing from nevirapine to delavirdine or vice-versa for drug failure, since high-level cross-resistance is likely.

- The decision to change therapy and the choice of a new regimen requires that the clinician have considerable expertise in the care of people living with HIV. Physicians who are less experienced in the care of persons with HIV infection are strongly encouraged to obtain assistance through consultation with or referral to a clinician with considerable expertise in the care of HIV-infected patients.

ANTIRETROVIRAL AGENTS *(Continued)*

Possible Regimens for Patients Who Have Failed Antiretroviral Therapy: A Work in Progress*†

Prior Regimen	New Regimen (Not Listed in Priority Order)
2 NRTIs +	2 new NRTIs +
Nelfinavir	RTV; or IDV; or SQV + RTV; or NNRTI†† + RTV; or NNRTI + IDV§
Ritonavir	SQV + RTV§; NFV + NNRTI; or NFV + SQV
Indinavir	SQV + RTV; NFV + NNRTI; or NFV + SQV
Saquinavir	RTV + SQV; or NFV + IDV
2 NRTIs + NNRTI	2 new NRTIs + a protease inhibitor
2 NRTIs	2 new NRTIs + a protease inhibitor
	2 new NRTIs + RTV + SQV
	1 new NRTI + 1 NNRTI + a protease inhibitor
	2 protease inhibitors + NNRTI
1 NRTI	2 new NRTIs + a protease inhibitor
	2 new NRTIs + NNRTI
	1 new NRTI + 1 NNRTI + a protease inhibitor

* These alternative regimens have not been proven to be clinically effective and were arrived at through discussion by the Panel of theoretically possible alternative treatments and the elimination of those alternatives with evidence of being ineffective. Clinical trials in this area are urgently needed.

†RTV = ritonavir; IDV = indinavir; SQV = saquinavir; NVP = nevirapine; NFV = nelfinavir; DLV = delavirdine

§ There are some clinical trials with viral burden data to support this recommendation.

††Of the two available NNRTIs, clinical trials support a preference for nevirapine over delavirdine based on results of viral load assays. These two agents have opposite effects on the CYP450 pathway, and this must be considered in combining these drugs with other agents.

Acute Retroviral Syndrome: Associated Signs and Symptoms and Expected Frequency*

- Fever (96%)
- Lymphadenopathy (74%)
- Pharyngitis (70%)
- Rash (70%)
    - Erythematous maculopapular with lesions on face and trunk and sometimes extremities, including palms and soles
    - Mucocutaneous ulceration involving mouth, esophagus, or genitals
- Myalgia or arthralgia (54%)
- Diarrhea (32%)
- Headache (32%)
- Nausea and vomiting (27%)
- Hepatosplenomegaly (14%)
- Thrush (12%)
- Weight loss
- Neurologic symptoms (12%)
    - Meningoencephalitis or aseptic meningitis
    - Peripheral neuropathy or radiculopathy
    - Facial palsy
    - Guillain-Barré syndrome
    - Brachial neuritis
    - Cognitive impairment or psychosis

Preclinical and Clinical Data Relevant to Use of Antiretrovirals During Pregnancy

Antiretroviral Drug	FDA Pregnancy Category*	Placental Passage (Newborn:Maternal Drug Ratio)	Long-Term Animal Carcinogenicity Studies	Rodent Teratogen
Zidovudine†	C	Yes (human) [0.85]	Positive (rodent, vaginal tumors)	Positive (near lethal dose)
Zalcitabine	C	Yes (rhesus) [0.30–0.50]	Positive (rodent, thymic lymphomas)	Positive (hydrocephalus at high dose)
Didanosine	B	Yes (human) [0.5]	Negative (no tumors, lifetime rodent study)	Negative
Stavudine	C	Yes (rhesus) [0.76]	Not completed	Negative (but sternal bone calcium decreases)
Lamivudine	C	Yes (human) [~1.0]	Negative (no tumors, lifetime rodent study)	Negative
Saquinavir	B	Unknown	Not completed	Negative
Indinavir	C	Yes (rats) [significant in rats, low in rabbits]	Not completed	Negative (but extra ribs in rats)
Ritonavir	B	Yes (rats) [midterm fetus, 1.15; late-term fetus, 0.15–0.64]	Not completed	Negative (but cryptorchidism in rats)††

ANTIRETROVIRAL AGENTS (Continued)

Preclinical and Clinical Data Relevant to Use of Antiretrovirals During Pregnancy (continued)

Antiretroviral Drug	FDA Pregnancy Category*	Placental Passage (Newborn:Maternal Drug Ratio)	Long-Term Animal Carcinogenicity Studies	Rodent Teratogen
Nelfinavir	B	Unknown	Not completed	Negative
Nevirapine	C	Yes (human) [~1.0]	Not completed	Negative
Delavirdine	C	Yes (rats) [late-term fetus, blood, 0.15; late-term fetus, liver 0.04]	Not completed	Ventricular septal defect

*FDA Pregnancy Categories: A - Adequate and well-controlled studies of pregnant women fail to demonstrate a risk to the fetus during the first trimester of pregnancy (and there is no evidence of risk during later trimesters); B - Animal reproduction studies fail to demonstrate a risk to the fetus and adequate but well-controlled studies of pregnant women have not been conducted; C - Safety in human pregnancy has not been determined, animal studies are either positive for fetal risk or have not been conducted, and the drug should not be used unless the potential benefit outweighs the potential risk to the fetus; D - Positive evidence of human fetal risk based on adverse reaction data from investigational or marketing experiences, but the potential benefits from the use of the drug in pregnant women may be acceptable despite its potential risks; X - Studies in animals or reports of adverse reactions have indicated that the risk associated with the use of the drug for pregnant women clearly outweighs any possible benefit.

†Despite certain animal data showing potential teratogenicity of ZDV when near lethal doses are given to pregnant rodents, considerable human data are available to date indicating that the risk to the fetus, if any, is extremely small when given to the pregnant mother beyond 14 weeks gestation. Follow-up for up to 6 years of age for 734 infants born to HIV-infected women who had *in utero* exposure to ZDV has not demonstrated any tumor development. However, no data is available on longer follow-up for late effects.

††These effects seen only at maternally toxic doses.

Adapted from "Public Health Service Task Force Recommendations for the Use of Antiretroviral Drugs in Pregnant Women Infected With HIV-1 for Maternal Health and for Reducing Perinatal HIV-1 Transmission in the United States," *MMWR Morb Mortal Wkly Rep*, 1998, 47(RR-2):16-7.

MANAGEMENT OF OCCUPATIONAL EXPOSURE TO HIV

RECOMMENDATIONS FOR POSTEXPOSURE PROPHYLAXIS

Adapted from "Public Health Service Guidelines for the Management of Health-Care Worker Exposures to HIV and Recommendations for Postexposure Prophylaxis," *MMWR Morb Mortal Wkly Rep*, 1998, 47(RR-7)

Figure 1. Determining the need for HIV postexposure prophylaxis (PEP) after an occupational exposure*

Step 1: Determine the Exposure Code (EC)

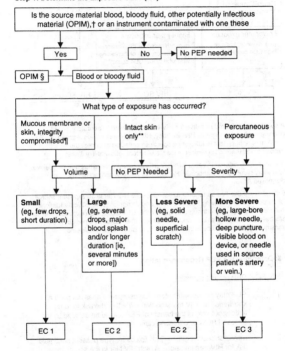

* This algorithm is intended to guide initial decisions about PEP and should be used in conjunction with other guidance provided in this report.

† Semen or vaginal secretions; cerebrospinal, synovial, pleural, peritoneal, pericardial, or amniotic fluids; or tissue

§ Exposure to OPIM must be evaluated on a case-by-case basis. In general, these body substances are considered a low risk for transmission in health-care settings. Any unprotected contact to concentrated HIV in a research laboratory or production facility is considered an occupational exposure that requires clinical evaluation to determine the need for PEP.

¶ Skin integrity is considered compromised if there is evidence of chapped skin, dermatitis, abrasion, or open wound.

** Contact with intact skin is not normally considered a risk for HIV transmission. However, if the exposure was to blood, and the circumstance suggests a higher volume exposure (eg, an extensive area of skin was exposed or there was prolonged contact with blood), the risk for HIV transmission should be considered.

†† The combination of these severity factors (eg, large-bore, hollow needle and deep puncture) contribute to an elevated risk for transmission if the source person is HIV-positive.

MANAGEMENT OF OCCUPATIONAL EXPOSURE TO HIV
(Continued)

Figure 1. Determining the need for HIV postexposure prophylaxis (PEP) after an occupational exposure* — Continued

Step 2: Determine the HIV Status Code (HIV SC)

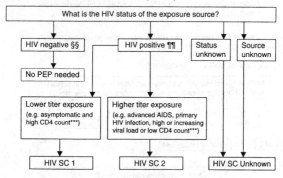

§§ A source is considered negative for HIV infection if there is laboratory documentation of a negative HIV antibody, HIV polymerase chain reaction (PCR), or HIV p24 antigen test result from a specimen collected at or near the time of exposure and there is no clinical evidence of recent retroviral-like illness.

¶¶ A source is considered infected with HIV (HIV positive) if there has been a positive laboratory result for HIV antibody, HIV PCR, or HIV p24 antigen or physician-diagnosed AIDS.

*** Examples are used as surrogates to estimates the HIV titer in an exposure source for purposes of considering PEP regimens and do not reflect all clinical situations that may be observed. Although a high HIV titer (HIV SC 2) in an exposure source has been associated with an increased risk for transmission, the possibility of transmission from a source with a low HIV titer also must be considered.

Step 3: Determine the PEP Recommendation

EC	HIV SC	PEP recommendation
1	1	PEP may not be warranted. Exposure type does not pose a known risk for HIV transmission. Whether the risk for drug toxicity outweighs the benefit of PEP should be decided by the exposed HCW and treating clinician.
1	2	Consider basic regimen. ††† Exposure type poses a negligible risk for HIV transmission. A high HIV titer in the source may justify consideration of PEP. Whether the risk for drug toxicity outweighs the benefit of PEP should be decided by the exposed HCW and treating clinician.
2	1	Recommended basic regimen. Most HIV exposures are in thes category; no increased risk for HIV transmission has been observed but use of PEP is appropriate.
2	1	Recommended expanded regimen. §§§ Exposure type represents an increased HIV transmission risk.
3	1 or 2	Recommended expanded regimen. Exposure type represents an increased HIV transmission risk.

††† Basic regimen is four weeks of zidovudine, 600 mg per day in two or three divided doses, and lamivudine, 150 mg twice daily.

§§§ Expanded regimen is the basic regimen plus either indinavir, 800 mg every 8 hours, or nelfinavir, 750 mg three times a day.

Basic and Expanded Postexposure Prophylaxis Regimens

Regimen Category	Application	Drug Regimen
Basic	Occupational HIV exposures for which there is a recognized transmission risk.	4 weeks (28 days) of both zidovudine 600 mg every day in divided doses (ie, 300 mg twice daily, 200 mg 3 times/day, or 100 mg every 4 hours) **and** lamivudine 150 mg twice daily.
Expanded	Occupational HIV exposures that pose an increased risk for transmission (eg, larger volume of blood and/or higher virus titer in blood)	Basic regimen plus **either** indinavir 800 mg every 8 hours **or** nelfinavir 750 mg 3 times/day.*

*Indinavir should be taken on an empty stomach (ie, without food or with a light meal) and with increased fluid consumption (ie, drinking six 8 oz glasses of water throughout the day); nelfinavir should be taken with meals.

RECOMMENDATIONS FOR REDUCING PERINATAL HIV TRANSMISSION

Clinical Scenarios and Recommendations for the Use of Antiretroviral Drugs to Reduce Perinatal Human Immunodeficiency Virus (HIV) Transmission

Clinical Scenario	Recommendations*
Scenario #1 HIV-infected pregnant women who have not received prior antiretroviral therapy	HIV-1-infected pregnant women must receive standard clinical, immunologic, and virologic evaluation. Recommendations for initiation and choice of antiretroviral therapy should be based on the same parameters used for persons who are not pregnant, although the known and unknown risks and benefits of such therapy during pregnancy must be considered and discussed. The three-part zidovudine (ZDV) chemoprophylaxis regimen should be recommended for all HIV-infected pregnant women to reduce the risk for perinatal transmission. The combination of ZDV chemoprophylaxis with additional antiretroviral drugs for treatment of HIV infection should be a) discussed with the woman; b) recommended for infected women whose clinical, immunologic, and virologic status indicates the need for treatment; and c) offered to other infected women (although in the latter circumstance, it is not known if the combination of antenatal ZDV chemoprophylaxis with other antiretroviral drugs will provide additional benefits or risks for the infant). Women who are in the first trimester of pregnancy may consider delaying initiation of therapy until after 10-12 weeks gestation.
Scenario #2 HIV-infected women receiving antiretroviral therapy during the current pregnancy	HIV-1-infected women receiving antiretroviral therapy in whom pregnancy is identified after the first trimester should continue therapy. For women receiving antiretroviral therapy in whom pregnancy is recognized during the first trimester, the woman should be counseled regarding the benefits and potential risks of antiretroviral administration during this period and continuation of therapy should be considered. If therapy is discontinued during the first trimester, all drugs should be stopped and reintroduced simultaneously to avoid the development of resistance. If the current therapeutic regimen does not contain ZDV, the addition of ZDV or substitution of ZDV for another nucleoside analogue antiretroviral is recommended after 14 weeks gestation. ZDV administration is recommended for the pregnant woman during the intrapartum period and for the newborn - regardless of the antepartum antiretroviral regimen.
Scenario #3 HIV-infected women in labor who have had no prior therapy	Administration of intrapartum intravenous ZDV should be recommended along with the 6-week ZDV regimen for the newborn. In the immediate postpartum period, the woman should have appropriate assessments (eg, CD4+ count and HIV-1 RNA copy number) to determine whether antiretroviral therapy is recommended for her own health.
Scenario #4 Infants born to mothers who have received no antiretroviral therapy during pregnancy or intrapartum	The 6-week neonatal ZDV component of the ZDV chemoprophylactic regimen should be discussed with the mother and offered for the newborn. ZDV should be initiated as soon as possible after delivery - preferably within 12-24 hours of birth.

Clinical Scenarios and Recommendations for the Use of Antiretroviral Drugs to Reduce Perinatal Human Immunodeficiency Virus (HIV) Transmission *(continued)*

Clinical Scenario	Recommendations*
	Some clinicians may choose to use ZDV in combination with other antiretroviral drugs, particularly if the mother is known or suspected to have ZDV-resistant virus. However, the efficacy of this approach for prevention of transmission is unknown, and appropriate dosing regimens for neonates are incompletely defined.
	In the immediate postpartum period, the woman should undergo appropriate assessment (eg, CD4⁺ count and HIV-1 RNA copy number) to determine if antiretroviral therapy is required for her own health.

*Discussion of treatment options and recommendations should be noncoercive, and the final decision regarding the use of antiretroviral drugs is the responsibility of the woman. A decision to not accept treatment with ZDV or other drugs should not result in punitive action or denial of care. Use of ZDV should not be denied to a woman who wishes to minimize exposure of the fetus to other antiretroviral drugs and who, therefore, chooses to receive only ZDV during pregnancy to reduce the risk for perinatal transmission.

Adapted from "Public Health Service Task Force Recommendations for the Use of Antiretroviral Drugs in Pregnant Women Infected With HIV-1 for Maternal Health and for Reducing Perinatal HIV-1 Transmission in the United States," *MMWR Morb Mortal Wkly Rep*, 1998, 47(RR-2):16-7.

TREATMENT FOR AIDS WASTING

Generic (Trade Name)	Adult Dose	Available Dosage Forms
Dronabinol (Marinol®)	Initial: 2.5 mg twice daily (before lunch and dinner); titrate up to a maximum of 20 mg/day	Capsule: 2.5 mg, 5 mg, 10 mg
Fluoxymesterone (Halotestin®)	10 mg twice daily	Tablet: 2 mg, 5 mg, 10 mg
Megesterol (Megace®)	Initial: 800 mg/day; daily doses of 400 and 800 mg/day were found to be clinically effective	Suspension, oral: 40 mg/mL with alcohol 0.06% Tablet: 20 mg, 40 mg
Nandrolone (Androlone®, Androlone®-D, Deca-Durabolin®, Durabolin®. Hybolin™ Decanoate, Hybolin™ Improved; Neo-Durabolic)	100 mg/week; up to 600 mg/week may be used	Injection: In oil, as phenproprionate: 25 mg/mL; 50 mg/mL In oil, as decanoate: 50 mg/mL; 100 mg/mL; 200 mg/mL Repository, as decanoate: 50 mg/mL; 100 mg/mL; 200 mg/mL
Oxandrolone (Oxandrin®)	10 mg twice daily	Tablet: 2.5 mg
Oxymetholone (Anadrol®)	50 mg 3 times/day	Tablet: 50 mg
Somatropin (r-DNA origin for injection) (Serostim®)	S.C.: >55 kg: 6 mg/day; 45-55 kg: 5 mg/day; 35-45 kg: 4 mg/day	Injection: 4 mg, 5 mg, 6 mg
Testosterone (various)	I.M.: 200-400 mg every 2 weeks	Injection: Aqueous suspension: 25 mg/mL, 50 mg/mL, 100 mg/mL In oil, as cypionate: 100 mg/mL, 200 mg/mL In oil, as enanthate: 100 mg/mL, 200 mg/mL In oil, as propionate: 50 mg/mL, 100 mg/mL
Thalidomide	300 mg/day	Tablet: 50 mg

USPHS/IDSA GUIDELINES FOR THE PREVENTION OF OPPORTUNISTIC INFECTIONS IN PERSONS INFECTED WITH HIV

(From "1997 USPHS/IDSA Guidelines for the Prevention of Opportunistic Infections in Persons Infected With Human Immunodeficiency Virus. USPHS/IDSA Prevention of Opportunistic Infections Working Group," *MMWR Morb Mortal Wkly Rep*, 1997, 46(RR-12):1-46. Updated from website www.hivatis.org.)

DRUG REGIMENS FOR ADULTS AND ADOLESCENTS

Prophylaxis for First Episode of Opportunistic Disease in HIV-Infected Adults and Adolescents

Pathogen	Indication	Preventive Regimens	
		First Choice	Alternatives
I. Strongly Recommended as Standard of Care			
Pneumocystis carinii*	CD4+ count <200/µL *or* oropharyngeal candidiasis *or* unexplained fever for ≥2 weeks	TMP-SMZ, 1 DS P.O. once daily (AI); TMP-SMZ, 1 SS P.O. once daily (AI)	Dapsone, 50 mg P.O. twice daily *or* 100 mg P.O. once daily (BI); dapsone, 50 mg P.O. once daily *plus* pyrimethamine, 50 mg P.O. weekly *plus* leucovorin, 25 mg P.O. weekly (BI); dapsone, 200 mg P.O. *plus* pyrimethamine, 75 mg P.O. *plus* leucovorin, 25 mg P.O. weekly (BI); aerosolized pentamidine, 300 mg monthly via Respirgard II™ nebulizer (BI); atovaquone, 1500 mg P.O. once daily (BI); TMP-SMZ, 1 DS P.O. 3 times/week (CI)
Mycobacterium tuberculosis			
Isoniazid-sensitive†	TST reaction ≥5 mm *or* prior positive TST result without treatment *or* contact with case of active tuberculosis	Isoniazid, 300 mg P.O. *plus* pyridoxine, 50 mg P.O. once daily x 9 months (AII) *or* isoniazid, 900 mg P.O. *plus* pyridoxine, 100 mg P.O. twice a week x 9 months (BI); rifampin 600 mg *plus* pyrazinamide 20 mg/kg P.O. once daily x 2 months (AI)	Rifampin, 300 mg P.O. once daily *plus* pyrazinamide 20 mg/kg P.O. once daily x 2 months (BIII); rifampin, 600 mg P.O. once daily x 4 months (BIII)
Isoniazid-resistant	Same; high probability of exposure to isoniazid-resistant tuberculosis	Rifampin, 600 mg *plus* pyrazinamide 20 mg/kg P.O. once daily x 2 months (AI)	Rifabutin, 300 mg *plus* pyrazinamide 20 mg/kg P.O. once daily x 2 months (BIII); rifampin, 600 mg P.O. once daily x 4 months (BIII) *plus* rifabutin, 300 mg P.O. once daily x 4 months (CIII)
Multidrug (isoniazid and rifampin)-resistant	Same; high probability of exposure to multidrug-resistant tuberculosis	Choice of drugs requires consultation with public health authorities	None

USPHS/IDSA GUIDELINES FOR THE PREVENTION OF OPPORTUNISTIC INFECTIONS IN PERSONS INFECTED WITH HIV *(Continued)*

Prophylaxis for First Episode of Opportunistic Disease in HIV-Infected Adults and Adolescents *(continued)*

Pathogen	Indication	Preventive Regimens	
		First Choice	Alternatives
Toxoplasma gondii§	IgG antibody to *Toxoplasma* and CD4⁺ count <100/µL	TMP-SMZ, 1 DS P.O. once daily (AII)	TMP-SMZ, 1 SS P.O. once daily (BIII); dapsone, 50 mg P.O. once daily *plus* pyrimethamine, 50 mg P.O. once weekly *plus* leucovorin, 25 mg P.O. once weekly (BI); atovaquone, 1500 mg P.O. once daily (CIII)
Mycobacterium avium complex¶	CD4⁺ count <50/µL	Azithromycin, 1200 mg P.O. once weekly (AI) or clarithromycin, 500 mg P.O. twice daily (AI)	Rifabutin, 300 mg P.O. once daily (BI); azithromycin, 1200 mg P.O. once weekly *plus* rifabutin, 300 mg P.O. once daily (CI)
Varicella zoster virus (VZV)	Significant exposure to chickenpox or shingles for patients who have no history of either condition or, if available, negative antibody to VZV	Varicella zoster immune globulin (VZIG), 5 vials (1.25 mL each) I.M., administered ≤96 hours after exposure, ideally within 48 hours (AIII)	
II. Generally Recommended			
Streptococcus pneumoniae**	All patients	Pneumococcal vaccine, 0.5 mL I.M. (CD4⁺ ≥200/µL [BII]; CD4⁺ <200/µL [CIII]) — may reimmunize if initial immunization was given when CD4⁺ <250/µL and if CD4⁺ increases to >200/µL on HAART (CIII)	None
Hepatitis B virus††	All susceptible (anti-HBc- and anti-HBs-negative) patients	Hepatitis B vaccine: 3 doses (BII)	None
Influenza virus††	All patients (annually, before influenza season)	Whole or split virus, 0.5 µL/year I.M. (BIII)	Rimantadine, 100 mg P.O. twice daily (CIII) *or* amantadine, 100 mg P.O. twice daily (CIII)
Hepatitis A virus ††	All susceptible (anti-HAV-negative) patients with chronic hepatitis C	Hepatitis A vaccine: 2 doses (BIII)	None
III. Not Routinely Indicated			
Bacteria	Neutropenia	Granulocyte-colony-stimulating factor (G-CSF), 5-10 mcg/kg S.C. once daily x 2-4 weeks *or* granulocyte-macrophage colony-stimulating factor (GM-CSF), 250 mcg/m² I.V. over 2 hours once daily x 2-4 weeks (CII)	None

Prophylaxis for First Episode of Opportunistic Disease in HIV-Infected Adults and Adolescents *(continued)*

Pathogen	Indication	Preventive Regimens	
		First Choice	Alternatives
Cryptococcus neoformans§§	CD4⁺ count <50/μL	Fluconazole, 100-200 mg P.O. once daily (CI)	Itraconazole, 200 mg P.O. once daily (CIII)
Histoplasma capsulatum§§	CD4⁺ count <100/μL, endemic geographic area	Itraconazole, 200 mg P.O. once daily (CI)	None
Cytomegalovirus (CMV)¶¶	CD4⁺ count <50/μL and CMV antibody positivity	Oral ganciclovir, 1 g P.O. 3 times/day (CI)	None

Note: Information included in these guidelines may not represent Food and Drug Administration (FDA) approval or approved labeling for the particular products or indications in question. Specifically, the terms "safe" and "effective" may not be synonymous with the FDA-defined legal standards for product approval. Anti-HBc = antibody to hepatitis B core antigen; CMV = cytomegalovirus; DS = double-strength tablet; SS = single-strength tablet; TMP-SMZ = trimethoprim-sulfamethoxazole; and TST = tuberculin skin test. The Respirgard II™ nebulizer is manufactured by Marquest, Englewood, CO. Letters and Roman numerals in parentheses after regimens indicate the strength of the recommendation and the quality of evidence supporting it.

*Prophylaxis should also be considered for persons with a CD4⁺ percentage <14%, for persons with a history of an AIDS-defining illness, and possibly for those with CD4⁺count >200 but <250 cells/μL. TMP-SMZ also reduces the frequency of toxoplasmosis and some bacterial infections. Patients receiving dapsone should be tested for glucose-6-phosphate dehydrogenase deficiency. A dosage of 50 mg once daily is probably less effective than that of 100 mg once daily. The efficacy of parenteral pentamidine (eg, 4 mg/kg/month) is uncertain. Fansidar® (sulfadoxine-pyrimethamine) is rarely used because of severe hypersensitivity reactions. Patients who are being administered therapy for toxoplasmosis with sulfadiazine-pyrimethamine are protected against *Pneumocystis carinii* pneumonia and do not need additional prophylaxis against PCP.

†Directly observed therapy recommended for isoniazid (INH), 900 mg twice weekly; INH regimens should include pyridoxine to prevent peripheral neuropathy. Rifampin should not be administered concurrently with protease inhibitors or non-nucleoside reverse transcriptase inhibitors. Rifabutin should not be given with hard-gel saquinavir, ritonavir, or delavirdine; caution is also advised when the drug is coadministered with soft-gel saquinavir. Rifabutin may be administered at a reduced dose (150 mg once daily) with indinavir, nelfinavir, or amprenavir, or at an increased dose (450 mg once daily) with efavirenz; information is lacking regarding coadministration of rifabutin and nevirapine. Exposure to multidrug-resistant tuberculosis may require prophylaxis with two drugs; consult public health authorities. Possible regimens include pyrazinamide plus either ethambutol or a fluoroquinolone.

§Protection against *Toxoplasma* is provided by TMP-SMZ, dapsone plus pyrimethamine, and possibly by atovaquone. The latter may be used with or without pyrimethamine. Pyrimethamine alone probably provides little, if any, protection.

¶See footnote above (†) regarding use of rifabutin with protease inhibitors or non-nucleoside reverse transcriptase inhibitors.

**Vaccination should be offered to persons who have a CD4⁺T-lymphocyte count <200 cells/μL, although the efficacy may be diminished. Revaccination ≥5 years after the first dose or sooner if the initial immunization was given when the CD4⁺ count was <200 cells/μL and if the CD4⁺ count has increased to >200 cells/μL on HAART is considered optional. Some authorities are concerned that immunizations may stimulate the replication of HIV. However, one study showed no adverse effect of pneumococcal vaccination on patient survival.

††These immunizations or chemoprophylactic regimens do not target pathogens traditionally classified as opportunistic but should be considered for use in HIV-infected patients as indicated. Data are inadequate concerning clinical benefit of these vaccines in this population, although it is logical to assume that those patients who develop antibody responses will derive some protection. Some authorities are concerned that immunizations may stimulate HIV replication, although, for influenza vaccination, a large observational study of HIV-infected persons in clinical care showed no adverse effect of this vaccine, including multiple doses, on patient survival (J. Ward, CDC, personal communication). Hepatitis B vaccine has been recommended for all children and adolescents and for all adults with risk factors for hepatitis B infection. Rimantadine/amantadine are appropriate during outbreaks of influenza A. Because of the theoretical concern that increases in HIV plasma RNA following vaccination during pregnancy might increase the risk of perinatal transmission of HIV, providers may wish to defer vaccination until after antiretroviral therapy is initiated.

§§There may be a few unusual occupational or other circumstances under which to consider prophylaxis; consult a specialist.

¶¶Acyclovir is not protective against CMV. Valacyclovir is not recommended because of an unexplained trend toward increased mortality observed in persons who have AIDS who were being administered this drug for prevention of CMV disease.

USPHS/IDSA GUIDELINES FOR THE PREVENTION OF OPPORTUNISTIC INFECTIONS IN PERSONS INFECTED WITH HIV (Continued)

Prophylaxis for Recurrence of Opportunistic Disease (After Chemotherapy for Acute Disease) in HIV-Infected Adults and Adolescents

Pathogen	Indication	Preventive Regimens	
		First Choice	Alternatives
I. Recommended for Life as Standard of Care			
Pneumocystis carinii	Prior P. carinii pneumonia	TMP-SMZ, 1 DS P.O. once daily (AI); TMP-SMZ, 1 SS P.O. once daily (AI)	Dapsone, 50 mg P.O. twice daily or 100 mg P.O. once daily (BI); dapsone, 50 mg P.O. once daily plus pyrimethamine, 50 mg P.O. weekly plus leucovorin, 25 mg P.O. weekly (BI); dapsone, 200 mg P.O. plus pyrimethamine, 75 mg P.O. plus leucovorin, 25 mg P.O. weekly (BI); aerosolized pentamidine, 300 mg monthly via Respirgard II™ nebulizer (BI); atovaquone, 1500 mg P.O. once daily (BI); TMP-SMZ, 1 DS P.O. 3 times/week (CI)
Toxoplasma gondii*	Prior toxoplasmic encephalitis	Sulfadiazine, 500-1000 mg P.O. 4 times/day plus pyrimethamine 25-75 mg P.O. once daily plus leucovorin, 10 mg P.O. once daily (AI)	Clindamycin, 300-450 mg P.O. every 6-8 hours plus pyrimethamine, 25-75 mg P.O. once daily plus leucovorin, 10-25 mg P.O. once daily (BI)
Mycobacterium avium complex†	Documented disseminated disease	Clarithromycin, 500 mg P.O. twice daily (AI) plus ethambutol, 15 mg/kg P.O. once daily (AII); with or without rifabutin, 300 mg P.O. once daily (CI)	Azithromycin, 500 mg P.O. once daily (AII) plus ethambutol, 15 mg/kg P.O. once daily (AII); with or without rifabutin, 300 mg P.O. once daily (CI)
Cytomegalovirus	Prior end-organ disease	Ganciclovir, 5-6 mg/kg I.V. 5-7 days/week or 1000 mg P.O. 3 times/day (AI); or foscarnet, 90-120 mg/kg I.V. once daily (AI); or (for retinitis) ganciclovir sustained-release implant, every 6-9 months plus ganciclovir, 1.0-1.5 g P.O. 3 times/day (AI)	Cidofovir, 5 mg/kg I.V. every other week (AI); fomivirsen, 1 vial injected into the vitreous, then repeated every 2-4 weeks (AI)
Cryptococcus neoformans	Documented disease	Fluconazole, 200 mg P.O. once daily (AI)	Amphotericin B, 0.6-1 mg/kg I.V. weekly to 3 times/week (AI); itraconazole, 200 mg P.O. once daily (BI)
Histoplasma capsulatum	Documented disease	Itraconazole, 200 mg P.O. twice daily (AI)	Amphotericin B, 1 mg/kg I.V. weekly (AI)
Coccidioides immitis	Documented disease	Fluconazole, 400 mg P.O. once daily (AII)	Amphotericin B, 1 mg/kg I.V. weekly (AI); itraconazole, 200 mg P.O. twice daily (AII)
Salmonella species (non-typhi)§	Bacteremia	Ciprofloxacin, 500 mg P.O. twice daily for several months (BII)	None
II. Recommended Only if Subsequent Episodes Are Frequent or Severe			
Herpes simplex virus	Frequent/severe recurrences	Acyclovir, 200 mg P.O. 3 times/day or 400 mg P.O. twice daily (AI); famciclovir, 500 mg P.O. twice daily (AI)	None
Candida (oropharyngeal or vaginal)	Frequent/severe recurrences	Fluconazole, 100-200 mg P.O. once daily (CI)	Itraconazole solution, 200 mg P.O. once daily (CI); ketoconazole, 200 mg P.O. once daily (CIII)

Prophylaxis for Recurrence of Opportunistic Disease (After Chemotherapy for Acute Disease) in HIV-Infected Adults and Adolescents *(continued)*

Pathogen	Indication	Preventive Regimens	
		First Choice	Alternatives
Candida (esophageal)	Frequent/ severe recurrences	Fluconazole, 100-200 mg P.O. once daily (BI)	Itraconazole solution, 200 mg P.O. once daily (BI); ketoconazole, 200 mg P.O. once daily (CIII)

Note: Information included in these guidelines may not represent Food and Drug Administration (FDA) approval or approved labeling for the particular products or indications in question. Specifically, the terms "safe" and "effective" may not be synonymous with the FDA-defined legal standards for product approval. DS = double-strength tablet; SS = single-strength tablet; and TMP-SMZ = trimethoprim-sulfamethoxazole. The Respirgard II™ nebulizer is manufactured by Marquest, Englewood, CO. Letters and Roman numerals in parentheses after regimens indicate the strength of the recommendation and the quality of the evidence supporting it.

* Pyrimethamine/sulfadiazine confers protection against PCP as well as toxoplasmosis; clindamycin-pyrimethamine does not.

† Many multiple-drug regimens are poorly tolerated. Drug interactions (eg, those seen with clarithromycin/rifabutin) can be problematic; rifabutin has been associated with uveitis, especially when administered at daily doses of >300 mg or concurrently with fluconazole or clarithromycin. Rifabutin should not be administered concurrently with hard-gel saquinavir, ritonavir, or delavirdine; caution is also advised when the drug is coadministered with soft-gel saquinavir. Rifabutin may be administered at reduced dose (150 mg once daily) with indinavir, nelfinavir, or amprenavir, or at increased dose (450 mg once daily) with efavirenz. Information is lacking regarding coadministration of rifabutin with nevirapine.

§ The efficacy of eradication of *Salmonella* has been demonstrated only for ciprofloxacin.

USPHS/IDSA GUIDELINES FOR THE PREVENTION OF OPPORTUNISTIC INFECTIONS IN PERSONS INFECTED WITH HIV *(Continued)*

Criteria for Discontinuing and Restarting Opportunistic Infection Prophylaxis for Adult Patients With HIV Infection*

Opportunistic Illness	Discontinuation Criteria for Prophylaxis		Criteria for Restarting Prophylaxis
	Primary	Secondary	
Pneumocystis carinii pneumonia	CD4+>200 cells/µL for >3-6 months (CII)	No criteria recommended for stopping	Same as criteria for initiating (CIII)
Disseminated *Mycobacterium avium* complex	CD4+ >100 cells/µL for >3-6 months; sustained suppression of HIV plasma RNA (CIII)	No criteria recommended for stopping	Same as criteria for initiating (CIII)
Toxoplasmosis	No criteria recommended for stopping	No criteria recommended for stopping	NA
Cryptococcosis	NA	No criteria recommended for stopping	NA
Histoplasmosis	NA	No criteria recommended for stopping	NA
Coccidioidomycosis	NA	No criteria recommended for stopping	NA
Cytomegalovirus	NA	• CD4 >100-150 cells/µL for >3-6 months • Nonsite-threatening lesion • Adequate vision in contralateral eye • Regular ophthalmic examination • No extraocular disease (CIII)	Restart maintenance when CD4 <50-100 cells/µL (CIII)

*The safety of discontinuing prophylaxis in children whose CD4+ counts have increased in response to HAART has not been studied.

DRUG REGIMENS FOR INFANTS AND CHILDREN

Prophylaxis for First Episode of Opportunistic Disease in HIV-Infected Infants and Children

Pathogen	Indication	Preventive Regimens	
		First Choice	Alternatives
I. Strongly Recommended as Standard of Care			
Pneumocystis carinii*	HIV-infected or HIV-indeterminate infants 1-12 months old; HIV-infected children 1-5 years of age with CD4⁺ count <500/µL or CD4⁺ percentage <15%; HIV-infected children 6-12 years of age with CD4⁺ count <200/µL or CD4⁺ percentage <15%	TMP-SMZ, 150/750 mg/m²/d in 2 divided doses P.O. 3 times/week on consecutive days (AII); acceptable alternative dosage schedules: (AII); single dose P.O. 3 times/week on consecutive days; 2 divided doses P.O. once daily; 2 divided doses P.O. 3 times/week on alternate days	Dapsone (children ≥1 month old), 2 mg/kg (max: 100 mg) P.O. once daily or 4 mg/kg (max: 200 mg) P.O. once weekly (CII); aerosolized pentamidine (children ≥5 years of age), 300 mg/month via Respirgard II™ nebulizer (CIII); atovaquone (children 1-3 months and >24 months old, 30 mg/kg P.O. once daily; children 4-24 months old, 45 mg/kg P.O. once daily) (CII)
Mycobacterium tuberculosis†			
Isoniazid-sensitive	TST reaction ≥5 mm or prior positive TST result without treatment or contact with case of active tuberculosis	Isoniazid, 10-15 mg/kg (max: 300 mg) P.O. once daily x 9 months (AI), or 20-30 mg/kg (max: 900 mg) P.O. twice weekly x 9 months (BIII)	Rifampin, 10-20 mg/kg (max: 600 mg) P.O. once daily x 4-6 months (BIII)
Isoniazid-resistant	Same as above; high probability of exposure to isoniazid-resistant tuberculosis	Rifampin, 10-20 mg/kg (max: 600 mg) P.O. once daily x 4-6 months (BIII)	Uncertain
Multidrug (isoniazid and rifampin)-resistant	Same as above; high probability of exposure to multidrug-resistant tuberculosis	Choice of drug requires consultation with public health authorities	None
Mycobacterium avium complex†	For children ≥6 years of age, CD4⁺ count <50/µL; 2-6 years of age, CD4⁺ count <75/µL; 1-2 years of age, CD4⁺ count <500/µL; <1 year of age, CD4⁺ count <750/µL	Clarithromycin, 7.5 mg/kg (max: 500 mg) P.O. twice daily (AII), or azithromycin, 20 mg/kg (max: 1200 mg) P.O. weekly (AII)	Azithromycin, 5 mg/kg (max: 250 mg) P.O. once daily (AII); children ≥6 years of age, rifabutin, 300 mg P.O. once daily (BI)
Varicella zoster virus§	Significant exposure to varicella with no history of chickenpox or shingles	Varicella zoster immune globulin (VZIG), 1 vial (1.25 mL)/10 kg (max: 5 vials) I.M., administered ≤96 hours after exposure, ideally within 48 hours (AII)	None
Vaccine-preventable pathogens¶	HIV exposure/infection	Routine immunizations	None
II. Generally Recommended			
Toxoplasma gondii*	IgG antibody *Toxoplasma* and severe immunosuppression	TMP-SMZ, 150/750 mg/m²/d in 2 divided doses P.O. once daily (BIII)	Dapsone (children ≥1 month old), 2 mg/kg or 15 mg/m² (max: 25 mg) P.O. once daily plus pyrimethamine, 1 mg/kg P.O. once daily plus leucovorin, 5 mg P.O. every 3 days (BIII); atovaquone (children 1-3 months and >24 months old, 30 mg/kg P.O. once daily; children 14-24 months old, 45 mg/kg P.O. once daily) (CIII)

USPHS/IDSA GUIDELINES FOR THE PREVENTION OF OPPORTUNISTIC INFECTIONS IN PERSONS INFECTED WITH HIV *(Continued)*

Prophylaxis for First Episode of Opportunistic Disease in HIV-Infected Infants and Children *(continued)*

Pathogen	Indication	Preventive Regimens	
		First Choice	Alternatives
Varicella zoster virus¶	HIV-infected children who are asymptomatic and not immunosuppressed	Varicella zoster vaccine (see vaccine-preventable pathogens) (BII)	None
Influenza virus¶	All patients (annually, before influenza season)	Influenza vaccine (see vaccine-preventable pathogens) (BIII)	Rimantadine or amantadine (during outbreaks of influenza A); children 1-9 years of age, 5 mg/kg in 2 divided doses P.O. once daily; ≥10 years of age, use adult doses (CIII)
III. Not Recommended for Most Children; Indicated for Use Only in Unusual Circumstances			
Invasive bacterial infections††	Hypogamma-globulinemia	IVIG (400 mg/kg/month) (AI)	None
Cryptococcus neoformans	Severe immunosuppression	Fluconazole, 3-6 mg/kg P.O. once daily (CII)	Itraconazole, 2-5 mg/kg P.O. every 12-24 hours (CIII)
Histoplasma capsulatum	Severe immunosuppression, endemic geographic area	Itraconazole, 2-5 mg/kg P.O. every 12-24 hours (CII)	None
Cytomegalovirus (CMV)§§	CMV antibody positivity and severe immunosuppression	Oral ganciclovir 30 mg/kg P.O. 3 times/day (CII)	None

Note: Information included in these guidelines may not represent Food and Drug Administration (FDA) approval or approved labeling for the particular products or indications in question. Specifically, the terms "safe" and "effective" may not be synonymous with the FDA-defined legal standards for product approval. CMV = cytomegalovirus; IVIG = intravenous immune globulin; TMP-SMZ = trimethoprim-sulfamethoxazole; and VZIG = varicella zoster immune globulin. The Respirgard II™ nebulizer is manufactured by Marquest, Englewood, CO. Letters and Roman numerals in parentheses after regimens indicate the strength of the recommendation and the quality of the evidence supporting it.

*Daily TMP-SMZ reduces the frequency of some bacterial infections. TMP-SMZ, dapsone-pyrimethamine, and possibly atovaquone (with or without pyrimethamine) appear to protect against toxoplasmosis, although data have not been prospectively collected. When compared with weekly dapsone, a recent study suggested that daily dapsone is associated with lower incidence of PCP but higher hematologic toxicity and mortality ( ). The efficacy of parenteral pentamidine (eg, 4 mg/kg/ every 2-4 weeks) is controversial. Patients receiving therapy for toxoplasmosis with sulfadiazine-pyrimethamine are protected against *Pneumocystis carinii* pneumonia (PCP) and do not need TMP-SMZ.

†Significant drug interactions may occur between rifamycins (rifampin and rifabutin) and protease inhibitors and non-nucleoside reverse transcriptase inhibitors. Consult a specialist.

§Children routinely being administered intravenous immune globulin (IVIG) should receive VZIG if the last dose of IVIG was administered >21 days before exposure.

¶HIV-infected and HIV-exposed children should be immunized according to the following childhood immunization schedule, which has been adapted from the January-December 1999 schedule recommended for immunocompetent children by the Advisory Committee on Immunization Practices, the American Academy of Pediatrics, and the American Academy of Family Physicians. This schedule differs from that for immunocompetent children in that IPV replaces OPV, and vaccination against influenza (BIII) and *S. pneumoniae* (BII) should be offered. MMR should not be administered to severely immunocompromised children (DIII). Vaccination against varicella is indicated only for asymptomatic nonimmunosuppressed children (BII), and rotavirus vaccine is contraindicated in all HIV-infected children (EIII). Once an HIV-exposed child is determined not to be HIV infected, the schedule for immunocompetent children applies.

**Protection against *Toxoplasma* is provided by the preferred antipneumocystis regimens and possibly by atovaquone. The latter may be used with or without pyrimethamine. Pyrimethamine alone probably provides little, if any, protection.

††Respiratory syncytial virus (RSV) IVIG, not monoclonal RSV antibody, may be substituted for IVIG during the RSV season to provide broad anti-infective protection, if this product is available.

§§Oral ganciclovir results in reduced CMV shedding in CMV-infected children. Acyclovir is not protective against CMV.

Prophylaxis for Recurrence of Opportunistic Disease (After Chemotherapy for Acute Disease) in HIV-Infected Infants and Children

Pathogen	Indication	Preventive Regimens	
		First Choice	Alternatives
I. Recommended for Life as Standard of Care			
Pneumocystis carinii	Prior P. carinii pneumonia	TMP-SMZ, 150/750 mg/m²/d in 2 divided doses P.O. 3 times/week on consecutive days (AII); or 4 mg/kg (max: 200 mg) P.O. weekly (CII); aerosolized pentamidine (children ≥5 years of age), 300 mg monthly via Respirgard II™ nebulizer (CIII); atovaquone (children 1-3 months and >24 months old, 30 mg/kg P.O. once daily; children 4-24 months, 45 mg/kg P.O. once daily) (CII)	Dapsone (children ≥1 month of age), 2 mg/kg (max: 100 mg) P.O. once daily
		Acceptable alternative schedules for same dosage (AII)	
		Single dose P.O. 3 times/week on consecutive days; 2 divided doses P.O. once daily; 2 divided doses P.O. 3 times/week on alternate days	
Toxoplasma gondii*	Prior toxoplasmic encephalitis	Sulfadiazine, 85-120 mg/kg/d in 2-4 divided doses P.O. once daily plus pyrimethamine, 1 mg/kg or 15 mg/m² (max: 25 mg) P.O. once daily plus leucovorin, 5 mg P.O. every 3 days (AI)	Clindamycin, 20-30 mg/kg/d in 4 divided doses P.O. once daily plus pyrimethamine, 1 mg/kg P.O. once daily plus leucovorin, 5 mg P.O. every 3 days (BI)
Mycobacterium avium complex†	Prior disease	Clarithromycin, 7.5 mg/kg (max: 500 mg) P.O. twice daily (AII) plus ethambutol, 15 mg/kg (max: 900 mg) P.O. once daily (AII); with or without rifabutin, 5 mg/kg (max: 300 mg) P.O. once daily (CII)	
Cryptococcus neoformans	Documented disease	Fluconazole, 3-6 mg/kg P.O. once daily (AII)	Amphotericin B, 0.5-1 mg/kg I.V. 1-3 times/week (AI); itraconazole, 2-5 mg/kg P.O. every 12-24 hours (BII);
Histoplasma capsulatum	Documented disease	Itraconazole, 2-5 mg/kg P.O. every 12-48 hours (AIII)	Amphotericin B, 1 mg/kg I.V. weekly (AIII)
Coccidioides immitis	Documented disease	Fluconazole, 6 mg/kg P.O. once daily (AIII)	Amphotericin B, 1 mg/kg I.V. weekly (AII); itraconazole, 2-5 mg/kg P.O. every 12-48 hours (AIII)
Cytomegalovirus	Prior end-organ disease	Ganciclovir, 5 mg/kg I.V. once daily, or foscarnet, 90-120 mg/kg I.V. once daily (AI)	(For retinitis) — ganciclovir sustained-release implant, every 6-9 months plus ganciclovir, 30 mg/kg P.O. 3 times/d (BIII)
Salmonella species (non-typhi)§	Bacteremia	TMP-SMZ, 150/750 mg/m² in 2 divided doses P.O. once daily for several months (CIII)	Antibiotic chemoprophylaxis with another active agent (CIII)
II. Recommended Only if Subsequent Episodes Are Frequent or Severe			
Invasive bacterial infections¶	>2 infections in 1-year period	TMP-SMZ, 150/750 mg/m² in 2 divided doses P.O. once daily (BI); or IVIG, 400 mg/kg monthly (BI)	Antibiotic chemoprophylaxis with another active agent (BIII)

USPHS/IDSA GUIDELINES FOR THE PREVENTION OF OPPORTUNISTIC INFECTIONS IN PERSONS INFECTED WITH HIV *(Continued)*

Prophylaxis for Recurrence of Opportunistic Disease (After Chemotherapy for Acute Disease) in HIV-Infected Infants and Children *(continued)*

Pathogen	Indication	Preventive Regimens	
		First Choice	Alternatives
Herpes simplex virus	Frequent/severe recurrences	Acyclovir, 80 mg/kg/d in 3-4 divided doses P.O. once daily (AII)	
Candida (oropharyngeal)	Frequent/severe recurrences	Fluconazole, 3-6 mg/kg P.O. once daily (CIII)	
Candida (esophageal)	Frequent/severe recurrences	Fluconazole, 3-6 mg/kg P.O. once daily (BIII)	Itraconazole pill, 5-10 mg/kg P.O. every 24 hours (CIII); ketoconazole, 5-10 mg/kg P.O. every 12-24 hours (CIII)

Note: Information included in these guidelines may not represent Food and Drug Administration (FDA) approval or approved labeling for the particular products or indications in question. Specifically, the terms "safe" and "effective" may not be synonymous with the FDA-defined legal standards for product approval. IVIG = intravenous immune globulin and TMP-SMZ = trimethoprim-sulfamethoxazole. The Respirgard II™ nebulizer is manufactured by Marquest, Englewood, CO. Letters and Roman numerals in parentheses after regimens indicate the strength of the recommendations and the quality of the evidence supporting it.

* Only pyrimethamine plus sulfadiazine confers protection against PCP as well as toxoplasmosis. Although the clindamycin plus pyrimethamine regimen is the preferred alternative in adults, it has not been tested in children. However, these drugs are safe and are used for other infections.

†Significant drug interactions may occur between rifabutin and protease inhibitors and non-nucleoside reverse transcriptase inhibitors. Consult an expert.

§ Drug should be determined by susceptibilities of the organism isolated. Alternatives to TMP-SMZ include ampicillin, chloramphenicol, or ciprofloxacin. However, ciprofloxacin is not approved for use in persons aged <18 years; therefore, it should be used in children with caution and only if no alternatives exist.

¶ Antimicrobial prophylaxis should be chosen based on the microorganism and antibiotic sensitivities. TMP-SMZ, if used, should be administered daily. Providers should be cautious about using antibiotics solely for this purpose because of the potential for development of drug-resistant microorganisms. IVIG may not provide additional benefit to children receiving daily TMP-SMZ, but may be considered for children who have recurrent bacterial infections despite TMP-SMZ prophylaxis. Choice of antibiotic prophylaxis vs IVIG should also involve consideration of adherence, ease of intravenous access, and cost. If IVIG is used, RSV-IVIG, not monoclonal RSV antibody, may be substituted for IVIG during the RSV season to provide broad anti-infective protection, if this product is available.

ADVERSE EVENTS AND VACCINATION

Reportable Events Following Vaccination*

These events are reportable by law to the Vaccine Adverse Event Reporting System (VAERS) (1-800-822-7967). In addition, individuals are encouraged to report any clinically significant or unexpected events (even if uncertain whether the vaccine caused the event) for any vaccine, whether or not it is listed in the table. Manufacturers also are required to report to the VAERS program all adverse events made known to them for any vaccine.

Vaccine/Toxoid		Event	Interval From Vaccination
Tetanus in any combination; DTaP, DTP, DTP-Hib, DT, Td, TT	A.	Anaphylaxis or anaphylactic shock	7 d
	B.	Brachial neuritis	28 d
	C.	Any sequela (including death) of above	No limit
	D.	Events described in manufacturer's package events insert as contraindications to additional doses of vaccine	See package insert
Pertussis in any combination; DTaP, DTP, DTP-Hib, P	A.	Anaphylaxis or anaphylactic shock	7 d
	B.	Encephalopathy (or encephalitis)	7 d
	C.	Any sequela (including death) of above events	No limit
	D.	Events described in manufacturer's package insert as contraindications to additional doses of vaccine	See package insert
Measles, mumps, and rubella in any combination; MMR, MR, M, R	A.	Anaphylaxis or anaphylactic shock	7 d
	B.	Encephalopathy (or encephalitis)	15 d
	C.	Any sequela (including death) of above events	No limit
	D.	Events described in manufacturer's package insert as contraindications to additional doses of vaccine	See package insert
Rubella in any combination; MMR, MR, R	A.	Chronic arthritis	42 d
	B.	Any sequela (including death) of above events	No limit
	C.	Events described in manufacturer's package insert as contraindications to additional doses of vaccine	See package insert
Measles in any combination; MMR, MR, M	A.	Thrombocytopenic purpura	30 d
	B.	Vaccine-strain measles viral infection in an immunodeficient recipient	6 mo
	C.	Any sequela (including death) of above events	No limit
	D.	Events described in manufacturer's package insert as contraindications to additional doses of vaccine	See package insert
Oral polio (OPV)	A.	Paralytic polio	
		• in a nonimmunodeficient recipient	30 d
		• in an immunodeficient recipient	6 mo
		• in a vaccine-associated community case	No limit
	B.	Vaccine-strain polio viral infection	
		• in a nonimmunodeficient recipient	30 d
		• in an immunodeficient recipient	6 mo
		• in a vaccine-associated community case	No limit
	C.	Any sequela (including death) of above events	No limit
	D.	Events described in manufacturer's package insert as contraindications to additional doses of vaccine	See package insert
Inactivated polio (IPV)	A.	Anaphylaxis or anaphylactic shock	7 d
	B.	Any sequela (including death) of above events	No limit
	C.	Events described in manufacturer's package insert as contraindications to additional doses of vaccine	See package insert
Hepatitis B	A.	Anaphylaxis or anaphylactic shock	7 d
	B.	Any sequela (including death) of above events	No limit
	C.	Events described in manufacturer's package insert as contraindications to additional doses of vaccine	See package insert
Haemophilus influenzae type b	A.	Early onset Hib disease	7 d
	B.	Any sequela (including death) of above events	No limit
	C.	Events described in manufacturer's package insert as contraindications to additional doses of vaccine	See package insert
Varicella	A.	No condition specified for compensation	Not applicable
	B.	Events described in manufacturer's package insert as contraindications to additional doses of vaccine	See package insert

*Effective March 24, 1997.

Adapted from "Report of the Committee on Infectious Diseases," *1997 Red Book®*, 24th ed.

IMMUNIZATION RECOMMENDATIONS

Standards for Pediatric Immunization Practices

Standard 1.	Immunization services are readily available.
Standard 2.	There are no barriers or unnecessary prerequisites to the receipt of vaccines.
Standard 3.	Immunization services are available free or for a minimal fee.
Standard 4.	Providers utilize all clinical encounters to screen and, when indicated, immunize children.
Standard 5.	Providers educate parents and guardians about immunizations in general terms.
Standard 6.	Providers question parents or guardians about contraindications and, before immunizing a child, inform them in specific terms about the risks and benefits of the immunizations their child is to receive.
Standard 7.	Providers follow only true contraindications.
Standard 8.	Providers administer simultaneously all vaccine doses for which a child is eligible at the time of each visit.
Standard 9.	Providers use accurate and complete recording procedures.
Standard 10.	Providers co-schedule immunization appointments in conjunction with appointments for other child health services.
Standard 11.	Providers report adverse events following immunization promptly, accurately, and completely.
Standard 12.	Providers operate a tracking system.
Standard 13.	Providers adhere to appropriate procedures for vaccine management.
Standard 14.	Providers conduct semiannual audits to assess immunization coverage levels and to review immunization records in the patient populations they serve.
Standard 15.	Providers maintain up-to-date, easily retrievable medical protocols at all locations where vaccines are administered.
Standard 16.	Providers operate with patient-oriented and community-based approaches.
Standard 17.	Vaccines are administered by properly trained individuals.
Standard 18.	Providers receive ongoing education and training on current immunization recommendations.

Recommended by the National Vaccine Advisory Committee, April 1992.

Approved by the United States Public Health Service, May 1992.

Endorsed by the American Academy of Pediatrics, May 1992.

The Standards represent the consensus of the National Vaccine Advisory Committee (NVAC) and of a broad group of medical and public health experts about what constitutes the most desirable immunization practices. It is recognized by the NVAC that not all of the current immunization practices of public and private providers are in compliance with the Standards. Nevertheless, the Standards are expected to be useful as a means of helping providers to identify needed changes, to obtain resources if necessary, and to actually implement the desirable immunization practices in the future.

Recommended Childhood Immunization Schedule
United States, January - December 1999

Vaccines [1] are listed under the routinely recommended ages. ⬚Bars⬚ indicate range of recommended ages for immunization. Any dose not given at the recommended age should be given as a "catch up" immunization at any subsequent visit when indicated and feasible. ◯Ovals◯ indicate vaccines to be given if previously recommended doses were missed or given earlier than the recommended minimum age.

Age ► Vaccine ▼	Birth	1 mo	2 mo	4 mo	6 mo	12 mo	15 mo	18 mo	4-6 y	11-12 y	14-16 y
Hepatitis B [2]	Hep B									(Hep B)	
		Hep B			Hep B						
Diphtheria, Tetanus, Pertussis [3]			DTaP	DTaP	DTaP		DTaP[3]		DTaP	Td	
H. influenzae type b [4]			Hib	Hib	Hib	Hib					
Polio [5]			IPV	IPV		Polio[5]			Polio		
Rotavirus [6]			Rv [6]	Rv [6]	Rv [6]						
Measles, Mumps, Rubella [7]						MMR			MMR[7]	(MMR[7])	
Varicella [8]						Var				(Var[8])	

[1] This schedule indicates the recommended ages for routine administration of currently licensed childhood vaccines. Combination vaccines may be used whenever any components of the combination are indicated and its other components are not contraindicated. Providers should consult the manufacturers' package inserts for detailed recommendations.

[2] Infants born to HBsAg-negative mothers should receive the second dose of hepatitis B vaccine at least 1 month after the first dose. The third dose should be administered at least 4 months after the first dose and at least 2 months after the second dose, but not before 6 months of age for infants.

Infants born to HBsAg-positive mothers should receive hepatitis B vaccine and 0.5 mL hepatitis B immune globulin (HBIG) within 12 hours of birth at separate sites. The second dose is recommended at 1-2 months of age and the third dose at 6 months of age.

Infants born to mothers whose HBsAg status is unknown should receive hepatitis B vaccine within 12 hours of birth. Maternal blood should be drawn at the time of delivery to determine the mother's HBsAg status; if the HBsAg test is positive, the infant should receive HBIG as soon as possible (no later than 1 week of age).

All children and adolescents (through 18 years of age) who have not been immunized against hepatitis B may begin the series during any visit. Special efforts should be made to immunize children who were born in or whose parents were born in areas of the world with moderate or high endemicity of HBV infection.

[3] DTaP (diphtheria and tetanus toxoids and acellular pertussis vaccine) is the preferred vaccine for all doses in the immunization series, including completion of the series in children who have received 1 or more doses of whole-cell DTP vaccine. Whole-cell DTP is an acceptable alternative to DTaP. The fourth dose (DTP or DTaP) may be administered as early as 12 months of age, provided 6 months have elapsed since the third dose and if the child is unlikely to return at age 15-18 months. Td (tetanus and diphtheria toxoids) is recommended at 11-12 years of age if at least 5 years have elapsed since the last dose of DTP, DTaP, or DT. Subsequent routine Td boosters are recommended every 10 years.

[4] Three H. influenzae type b (Hib) conjugate vaccines are licensed for infant use. If PRP-OMP (PedvaxHIB® and COMVAX® [Merck]) is administered at 2 and 4 months of age, a dose at 6 months is not required. Because clinical studies in infants have demonstrated that using some combination products may induce a lower immune response to the Hib vaccine component, DTaP/Hib combination products should not be used for primary immunization in infants at 2, 4, or 6 months of age, unless FDA-approved for these ages.

[5] Two poliovirus vaccines currently are licensed in the United States: Inactivated poliovirus vaccine (IPV) and oral poliovirus vaccine (OPV). The ACIP, AAP, and AAFP now recommend that the first two doses of poliovirus vaccine should be IPV. The ACIP continues to recommend a sequential schedule of two doses of IPV administered at ages 2 and 4 months, followed by two doses of OPV at 12-18 months and 4-6 years. Use of IPV for all doses also is acceptable and is recommended for immunocompromised persons and their household contacts. OPV is no longer recommended for the first two doses of the schedule and is acceptable only for special circumstances such as: Children of parents who do not accept the recommended number of injections, late initiation of immunization which would require an unacceptable number of injections, and imminent travel to polio-endemic areas. OPV remains the vaccine of choice for mass immunization campaigns to control outbreaks due to wild poliovirus.

[6] Rotavirus vaccine(Rv) is italicized to indicate: 1) Health care providers may require time and resources to incorporate this new vaccine into practice; and 2) the AAFP feels that the decision to use rotavirus vaccine should be made by the parent or guardian in consultation with their physician or other health care provider. The first dose of Rv vaccine should not be administered before 6 weeks of age, and the minimum interval between doses is 3 weeks. The Rv vaccine series should not be initiated at 7 months of age or older, and all doses should be completed by the first birthday.

[7] The second dose of measles, mumps, and rubella vaccine (MMR) is recommended routinely at 4-6 years of age but may be administered during any visit, provided at least 4 weeks have elapsed since receipt of the first dose and that both doses are administered beginning at or after 12 months of age. Those who have not previously received the second dose should complete the schedule by the 11- to 12-year-old visit.

[8] Varicella vaccine is recommended at any visit on or after the first birthday for susceptible children, ie, those who lack a reliable history of chickenpox (as judged by a health care provider) and who have not been immunized. Susceptible persons 13 years of age or older should receive 2 doses, given at least 4 weeks apart.

Adapted from Advisory Committee on Immunization Practices (ACIP), the American Academy of Pediatrics (AAP), and the American Academy of Family Physicians (AAFP).

IMMUNIZATION RECOMMENDATIONS *(Continued)*

RECOMMENDATIONS OF THE ADVISORY COMMITTEE ON IMMUNIZATION PRACTICES (ACIP)

Recommended Poliovirus Vaccination Schedules for Children

Vaccine	Child's Age			
	2 mo	4 mo	12-18 mo	4-6 y
Sequential IPV*/OPV*/ OPV†	IPV	IPV	OPV	OPV
OPV*	OPV	OPV	OPV‡	OPV
IPV†	IPV	IPV	IPV	OPV

*Inactivated poliovirus vaccine.

†Live, oral poliovirus vaccine.

‡For children who receive only OPV, the third dose of OPV may be administered as early as 6 months of age.

Adapted from "Poliomyelitis Prevention in the United States: Introduction of a Sequential Vaccination Schedule of Inactivated Poliovirus Vaccine Followed by Oral Poliovirus Vaccine" *MMWR Morb Mortal Wkly Rep*, 1997, 46(RR-3).

Recommendations for Measles Vaccination*

Category	Recommendations
Unvaccinated, no history of measles (12-15 mo)	A 2-dose schedule (with MMR) is recommended if born after 1956. The first dose is recommended at 12-15 mo; the second is recommended at 4-6 y
Children 12 mo in areas of recurrent measles transmission	Vaccinate; a second dose is indicated at 4-6 y (at school entry)
Children 6-11 mo in epidemic situations†	Vaccinate (with monovalent measles vaccine or, if not available, MMR); revaccination (with MMR) at 12-15 mo is necessary and a third dose is indicated at 4-6 y
Children 11-12 y who have received 1 dose of measles vaccine at ≥12 mo	Revaccinate (1 dose)
Students in college and other posthigh school institutions who have received 1 dose of measles vaccine at ≥12 mo	Revaccinate (1 dose)
History of vaccination before the first birthday	Consider susceptible and vaccinate (2 doses)
Unknown vaccine, 1963-1967	Consider susceptible and vaccinate (2 doses)
Further attenuated or unknown vaccine given with IG	Consider susceptible and vaccinate (2 doses)
Egg allergy	Vaccinate; no reactions likely
Neomycin allergy, nonanaphylactic	Vaccinate; no reactions likely
Tuberculosis	Vaccinate; vaccine does not exacerbate infection
Measles exposure	Vaccinate or give IG, depending on circumstances
HIV-infected	Vaccinate (2 doses) unless severely compromised
Immunoglobulin or blood product received	Vaccinate at the appropriate interval

*See text for details. MMR indicates measles-mumps-rubella vaccine; IG, immune globulin.

†See Outbreak Control.

Adapted from "Report of the Committee on Infectious Diseases," *1997 Red Book*®, 24th ed.

Recommended Immunization Schedules for Children Not Immunized in the First Year of Life*

Recommended Time/Age	Immunization(s)[1,2,3]	Comments
Younger Than 7 Years		
First visit	DTaP (or DTP), Hib, HBV, MMR, OPV[3]	If indicated, tuberculin testing may be done at same visit.
		If child is ≥5 y of age, Hib is not indicated in most circumstances.
Interval after first visit		
1 mo (4 wk)	DTaP (or DTP), HBV, Var[4]	The second dose of OPV may be given if accelerated poliomyelitis vaccination is necessary, such as for travelers to areas where polio is endemic.
2 mo	DTaP (or DTP), Hib, OPV[3]	Second dose of Hib is indicated only if the first dose was received when <15 mo.
≥8 mo	DTaP (or DTP), HBV, OPV[3]	OPV and HBV are not given if the third doses were given earlier.
Age 4-6 y (at or before school entry)	DTaP (or DTP), OPV,[3] MMR[5]	DTaP (or DTP) is not necessary if the fourth dose was given after the fourth birthday; OPV is not necessary if the third dose was given after the fourth birthday.
Age 11-12 y	See Childhood Immunization Schedule	
7-12 Years		
First visit	HBV, MMR, Td, OPV[3]	
Interval after first visit		
2 mo (8 wk)	HBV, MMR,[5] Var,[4] Td, OPV[3]	OPV also may be given 1 mo after the first visit if accelerated poliomyelitis vaccination is necessary.
8-14 mo	HBV,[6] Td, OPV[3]	OPV is not given if the third dose was given earlier.
Age 11-12 y	See Childhood Immunization Schedule	

*Table is not completely consistent with all package inserts. For products used, also consult manufacturer's package insert for instructions on storage, handling, dosage, and administration. Biologics prepared by different manufacturers may vary, and package inserts of the same manufacturer may change from time to time. Therefore, the physician should be aware of the contents of the current package insert.

Vaccine abbreviations: HBV indicates hepatitis B virus vaccine; Var, varicella vaccine; DTP, diphtheria and tetanus toxoids and pertussis vaccine; DTaP, diphtheria and tetanus toxoids and acellular pertussis vaccine; Hib, *Haemophilus influenzae* type b conjugate vaccine; OPV, oral poliovirus vaccine; IPV, inactivated poliovirus vaccine; MMR, live measles-mumps-rubella vaccine; Td, adult tetanus toxoid (full dose) and diphtheria toxoid (reduced dose), for children ≥7 years and adults.

[1] If all needed vaccines cannot be administered simultaneously, priority should be given to protecting the child against those diseases that pose the greatest immediate risk. In the United States, these diseases for children <2 years usually are measles and *Haemophilus influenzae* type b infection; for children >7 years, they are measles, mumps, and rubella. Before 13 years of age, immunity against hepatitis B and varicella should be ensured.

[2] DTaP, HBV, Hib, MMR, and Var can be given simultaneously at separate sites if failure of the patient to return for future immunizations is a concern.

[3] IPV is also acceptable. However, for infants and children starting vaccination late (ie, after 6 months of age), OPV is preferred in order to complete an accelerated schedule with a minimum number of injections.

[4] Varicella vaccine can be administered to susceptible children any time after 12 months of age. Unvaccinated children who lack a reliable history of chickenpox should be vaccinated before their 13th birthday.

[5] Minimal interval between doses of MMR is 1 month (4 weeks).

[6] HBV may be given earlier in a 0-, 2-, and 4-month schedule.

Adapted from "Report of the Committee on Infectious Diseases," *1997 Red Book®*, 24th ed.

IMMUNIZATION RECOMMENDATIONS *(Continued)*

Minimum Age for Initial Vaccination and Minimum Interval Between Vaccine Doses, by Type of Vaccine

Vaccine	Minimum *Age* for First Dose*	Minimum *Interval* From Dose 1 to 2*	Minimum *Interval* From Dose 2 to 3*	Minimum *Interval* From Dose 3 to 4*
DTP (DT)†	6 wk‡	4 wk	4 wk	6 mo
Combined DTP-Hib	6 wk	1 mo	1 mo	6 mo
DTaP*	6 wk			6 mo
Hib (primary series)				
HbOC	6 wk	1 mo	1 mo	§
PRP-T	6 wk	1 mo	1 mo	§
PRP-OMP	6 wk	1 mo	§	
OPV			6 wk	
IPV¶	6 wk	4 wk	6 mo#	
MMR	12 mo•	1 mo		
Hepatitis B	Birth	1 mo	2 mo♦	
Varicella-zoster	12 mo	4 wk		

DTP = diphtheria-tetanus-pertussis.

DTaP = diphtheria-tetanus-acellular pertussis.

Hib = *Haemophilus influenzae* type b conjugate.

IPV = inactivated poliovirus vaccine.

MMR = measles-mumps-rubella.

OPV = poliovirus vaccine, live oral, trivalent.

*These minimum acceptable ages and intervals may not correspond with the optimal recommended ages and intervals for vaccination. See tables for the current recommended routine and accelerated vaccination schedules.

†DTaP can be used in place of the fourth (and fifth) dose of DTP for children who are at least 15 months of age. Children who have received all four primary vaccination doses before their fourth birthday should receive a fifth dose of DTP (DT) or DTaP at 4-6 years of age before entering kindergarten or elementary school **and** at least 6 months after the fourth dose. The total number of doses of diphtheria and tetanus toxoids should not exceed six each before the seventh birthday.

‡The American Academy of Pediatrics permits DTP to be administered as early as 4 weeks of age in areas with high endemicity and during outbreaks.

§The booster dose of Hib vaccine which is recommended following the primary vaccination series should be administered no earlier than 12 months of age **and** at least 2 months after the previous dose of Hib vaccine.

¶See text to differentiate conventional inactivated poliovirus vaccine from enhanced-potency IPV.

#For unvaccinated adults at increased risk of exposure to poliovirus with <3 months but >2 months available before protection is needed, three doses of IPV should be administered at least 1 month apart.

•Although the age for measles vaccination may be as young as 6 months in outbreak areas where cases are occurring in children <1 year of age, children initially vaccinated before the first birthday should be revaccinated at 12-15 months of age and an additional dose of vaccine should be administered at the time of school entry or according to local policy. Doses of MMR or other measles-containing vaccines should be separated by at least 1 month.

♦This final dose is recommended no earlier than 4 months of age.

Modified from *MMWR Morb Mortal Wkly Rep*, 1994, 43(RR-1).

LIVERPOOL
JOHN MOORES UNIVERSITY
AVRIL ROBARTS LRC
TEL. 0151 231 4022

Recommended Immunization Schedule For HIV-Infected Children[1]

Age ▶ Vaccine ▼	Birth	1 mo	2 mos	4 mos	6 mos	12 mos	15 mos	18 mos	24 mos	4-6 yrs	11-12 yrs	14-16 yrs
Recommendations for these vaccines are the same as those for immunocompetent children												
Hepatitis B[2]	HepB-1											
		Hep B-2			Hep B-3						Hep B[3]	
Diphtheria, Tetanus, Pertussis[4]			DTaP or DTP	DTaP or DTP	DTaP or DTP		DTaP or DTP			DTaP or DTP	Td	
Haemophilus influenzae type b[5]			Hib	Hib	Hib	Hib						
Recommendations for these vaccines differ from those for immunocompetent children												
Polio[6]			IPV	IPV		IPV				IPV		
Measles, Mumps, Rubella[7]						MMR			MMR			
Influenza[8]						Influenza (a dose is required every year)						
Streptococcus pneumoniae[9]									pneumo-coccal			
Varicella						**CONTRAINDICATED in all HIV-infected persons**						

Note: Modified from the immunization schedule for immunocompetent children. This schedule also applies to children born to HIV-infected mothers whose HIV infection status has not been determined. Once a child is known not to be HIV-infected, the schedule for immunocompetent children applies. This schedule indicates the recommended age for routine administration of currently licensed childhood vaccines. Some combination vaccines are available and may be used whenever administration of all components of the vaccine is indicated. Providers should consult the manufacturers' package inserts for detailed recommendations.

[1] Vaccines are listed under the routinely recommended ages. Bars indicate range of acceptable ages for vaccination. Shaded bars indicate catch-up vaccination: at 11-12 years of age, hepatitis B vaccine should be administered to children not previously vaccinated.

[2] *Infants born to HBsAg-negative mothers* should receive 2.5 µg of Merck vaccine (Recombivax HB®) or 10 µg of Smith Kline Beecham (SB) vaccine (Engerix-B®). The 2nd dose should be administered >1 mo after the 1st dose.

Infants born to HBsAg-positive mothers should receive 0.5 mL of hepatitis B immune globulin (HBIG) within 12 h of birth and either 5 µg of Merck vaccine (Recombivax HB®) or 10 µg of SB vaccine (Engerix-B®) at a separate site. The 2nd dose is recommended at 1-2 months of age and the 3rd dose at 6 months of age.

Infants born to mothers whose HBsAg status is unknown should receive either 5 µg of Merck vaccine (Recombivax HB®) or 10 µg of SB vaccine (Engerix-B®) within 12 h of birth. The 2nd dose of vaccine is recommended at 1 month of age and the 3rd dose at 6 of age. Blood should be drawn at the time of delivery to determine the mother's HBsAg status; if it is positive, the infant should receive HBIG as soon as possible (no later than 1 week of age). The dosage and timing of subsequent vaccine doses should be based upon the mother's HBsAg status.

[3] Children and adolescents who have not been vaccinated against hepatitis B in infancy may begin the series during any childhood visit. Those who have not previously received 3 doses of hepatitis B vaccine should initiate or complete the series during the 11 to 12 years of age visit. The 2nd dose should be administered at least 1 month after the 1st dose and at least 2 months after the 2nd dose.

[4] DTaP (diphtheria and tetanus toxoids and acellular pertusssis vaccine) is the preferred vaccine for all doses in the vaccination series, including copletion of the series in children who have received >1 dose of whole-cell DtP vaccine. Whole-cell DTP is an acceptable alternative to DTaP. The 4th dose of DTaP may be administered as early as 12 months of age, provided 6 months have elapsed since the 3rd dose, and if the child is considered unlikely to return at 15-18 months of age. Td (tetanus and diphtheria toxoids, absorbed for adult use) is recommended at 11-12 years of age if at least 5 years have elapsed since the last dose of DTP, DTaP, or DT. Subsequent routine Td boosters are recommended every 10 years.

[5] Three H. influenzae type b (Hib) conjugate vaccines are licensed for infant use. If PRP-OMP (PedvaxHIB® [Merck]) is administered at 2 and 4 months of age, a dose at 6 months is not required. After the primary series has been completed, any Hib conjugate vaccine may be used as a booster.

[6] Inactivated poliovirus vaccine (IPV) is the only poliovirus vaccine recommended for HIV-infected persons and their household contacts. Although the third dose for IPV is generally administered at 12-18 months, the 3rd dose of IPV has been approved to be administered as early as 6 months of age. Oral poliovirus vaccine (OPV) should NOT be administered to HIV-infected persons or their household contacts.

[7] MMR should not be administered to severely immunocompromised children. HIV-infected children without severe immunosuppression should routinely receive their first dose of MMR as soon as possible upon reaching the first birthday. Consideration should be given to administering the 2nd dose of MMR vaccine as soon as one month (ie, minimum 28 days) after the first dose, rather than waiting until school entry.

[8] Influenza virus vaccine should be administered to all HIV-infected children >6 months of age each year. Children aged 6 months to 8 years who are receiving influenza vaccine for the first time should receive two doses of split virus vaccine separated by at least one month. In subsequent years, a single dose is administered each year. The dose of vaccine for children aged 6-35 months is 0.25 mL; the dose for children aged ≥3 years is 0.5 mL.

[9] The 23-valent pneumococcal vaccine should be administered to HIV-infected children at 24 months of age. Revaccination should generally be offered to HIV-infected children vaccinated 3-5 years (children aged ≤10 years) or >5 years (children aged >10 years) earlier.

Adapted from the American Academy of Pediatrics and American Academy of Family Practice Physicians, Advisory Committee on Immunization Practices and the Centers for Disease Control.

IMMUNIZATION RECOMMENDATIONS *(Continued)*

Licensed Vaccines and Toxoids Available in the United States, by Type and Recommended Routes of Administration

	Type	Route
Adenovirus*	Live virus	Oral
Anthrax†	Inactivated bacteria	Subcutaneous
Bacillus of Calmette and Guerin (BCG)	Live bacteria	Intradermal/percutaneous
Cholera	Inactivated bacteria	Subcutaneous, intramuscular, or intradermal‡
Diphtheria-tetanus-pertussis (DTP)	Toxoids and inactivated whole bacteria	Intramuscular
DTP-*Haemophilus influenzae* type b conjugate (DTP-Hib)	Toxoids, inactivated whole bacteria, and bacterial polysaccharide conjugated to protein	Intramuscular
Diphtheria-tetanus-acellular pertussis (DTaP)	Toxoids and inactivated bacterial components	Intramuscular
Hepatitis A	Inactivated virus	Intramuscular
Hepatitis B	Purified viral antigen	Intramuscular
Haemophilus influenzae type b conjugate (Hib)§	Bacterial polysaccharide conjugated to protein	Intramuscular
Influenza	Inactivated virus or viral components	Intramuscular
Japanese encephalitis	Inactivated virus	Subcutaneous
Measles	Live virus	Subcutaneous
Measles-mumps-rubella (MMR)	Live virus	Subcutaneous
Meningococcal	Bacterial polysaccharides of serotypes A/C/Y/W-135	Subcutaneous
Mumps	Live virus	Subcutaneous
Pertussis†	Inactivated whole bacteria	Intramuscular
Plague	Inactivated bacteria	Intramuscular
Pneumococcal	Bacterial polysaccharides of 23 pneumococcal types	Intramuscular or subcutaneous
Poliovirus vaccine		
Inactivated (IPV)	Inactivated viruses of all 3 serotypes	Subcutaneous
Oral (OPV)	Live viruses of all 3 serotypes	Oral
Rabies	Inactivated virus	Intramuscular or intradermal¶
Rubella	Live virus	Subcutaneous
Tetanus	Inactivated toxin (toxoid)	Intramuscular#
Tetanus-diphtheria (Td or DT)•	Inactivated toxins (toxoids)	Intramuscular#
Typhoid		
Parenteral	Inactivated bacteria	Subcutaneous♦
Ty21a oral	Live bacteria	Oral
Varicella	Live virus	Subcutaneous
Yellow fever	Live virus	Subcutaneous

*Available only to the U.S. Armed Forces.

†Distributed by the Division of Biologic Products, Michigan Department of Public Health.

‡The intradermal dose is lower than the subcutaneous dose.

§The recommended schedule for infants depends on the vaccine manufacturer; consult the package insert and ACIP recommendations for specific products.

¶The intradermal dose of rabies vaccine, human diploid cell (HDCV), is lower than the intramuscular dose and is used only for pre-exposure vaccination. **Rabies vaccine, adsorbed (RVA) should not be used intradermally.**

#Preparations with adjuvants should be administered intramuscularly.

•Td-tetanus and diphtheria toxoids for use among persons ≥7 years of age. Td contains the same amount of tetanus toxoid as DTP or DT, but contains a smaller dose of diphtheria toxoid. DT = tetanus and diphtheria toxoids for use among children <7 years of age.

♦Booster doses may be administered intradermally unless vaccine that is acetone-killed and dried is used.

Modified from *MMWR Morb Mortal Wkly Rep*, 1994, 43(RR-1).

Immune Globulins and Antitoxins* Available in the United States, by Type of Antibodies and Indications for Use

Immunobiologic	Type	Indication(s)
C. botulinum antitoxin	Specific equine antibodies	Treatment of botulism
Cytomegalovirus immune globulin, intravenous (CMV-IGIV)	Specific human antibodies	Prophylaxis for bone marrow and kidney transplant recipients
Diphtheria antitoxin	Specific equine antibodies	Treatment of respiratory diphtheria
Immune globulin (IG)	Pooled human antibodies	Hepatitis A pre- and postexposure prophylaxis; measles postexposure prophylaxis
Immune globulin, intravenous (IGIV)	Pooled human antibodies	Replacement therapy for antibody deficiency disorders; immune thrombocytopenic purpura (ITP); hypogammaglobulinemia in chronic lymphocytic leukemia; Kawasaki disease
Hepatitis B immune globulin (HBIG)	Specific human antibodies	Hepatitis B postexposure prophylaxis
Rabies immune globulin (HRIG)†	Specific human antibodies	Rabies postexposure management of persons not previously immunized with rabies vaccine
Tetanus immune globulin (TIG)	Specific human antibodies	Tetanus treatment; postexposure prophylaxis of persons not adequately immunized with tetanus toxoid
Vaccinia immune globulin (VIG)	Specific human antibodies	Treatment of eczema vaccinatum, vaccinia necrosum, and ocular vaccinia
Varicella-zoster immune globulin (VZIG)	Specific human antibodies	Postexposure prophylaxis of susceptible immunocompromised persons, certain susceptible pregnant women, and perinatally exposed newborn infants

*Immune globulin preparations and antitoxins are administered intramuscularly unless otherwise indicated.

†HRIG is administered around the wounds in addition to the intramuscular injection.

Modified from *MMWR Morb Mortal Wkly Rep*, 1994, 43(RR-1).

IMMUNIZATION RECOMMENDATIONS *(Continued)*

Suggested Intervals Between Administration of Immune Globulin Preparations for Various Indications and Vaccines Containing Live Measles Virus*

Indication	Dose (including mg IgG/kg)	Time Interval (mo) Before Measles Vaccination
Tetanus (TIG) prophylaxis	I.M.: 250 units (10 mg IgG/kg)	3
Hepatitis A (IG) prophylaxis		
Contact prophylaxis	I.M.: 0.02 mL/kg (3.3 mg IgG/kg)	3
International travel	I.M.: 0.06 mL/kg (10 mg IgG/kg)	3
Hepatitis B prophylaxis (HBIG)	I.M.: 0.06 mL/kg (10 mg IgG/kg)	3
Rabies immune globulin (HRIG)	I.M.: 20 IU/kg (22 mg IgG/kg)	4
Varicella prophylaxis (VZIG)	I.M.: 125 units/10 kg (20-40 mg IgG/kg) (max: 625 units)	5
Measles prophylaxis (IG) Standard (ie, nonimmunocompromised contact)	I.M.: 0.25 mL/kg (40 mg IgG/kg)	5
Immunocompromised contact	I.M.: 0.50 mL/kg (80 mg IgG/kg)	6
Blood transfusion		
RBCs, washed	I.V.: 10 mL/kg (negligible IgG/kg)	0
RBCs, adenine-saline added	I.V.: 10 mL/kg (10 mg IgG/kg)	3
Packed RBCs (Hct 65%)†	I.V.: 10 mL/kg (60 mg IgG/kg)	6
Whole blood cells (Hct 35%-50%)†	I.V.: 10 mL/kg (80-100 mg IgG/kg)	6
Plasma/platelet products	I.V.: 10 mL/kg (160 mg IgG/kg)	7
Replacement therapy for immune deficiencies	I.V.: 300-400 mg/kg (as IGIV)‡	8
Treatment of Immune thrombocytopenic purpura§	I.V.: 400 mg/kg (as IGIV)	8
Immune thrombocytopenic purpura§	I.V.: 1000 mg/kg (as IGIV)	10
Kawasaki disease	I.V.: 2 g/kg (as IGIV)	11

*This table is not intended for determining the correct indications and dosage for the use of immune globulin preparations. Unvaccinated persons may not be fully protected against measles during the entire suggested time interval, and additional doses of immune globulin and/or measles vaccine may be indicated after measles exposure. The concentration of measles antibody in a particular immune globulin preparation can vary by lot. The rate of antibody clearance after receipt of an immune globulin preparation also can vary. The recommended time intervals are extrapolated from an estimated half-life of 30 days of passively acquired antibody and an observed interference with the immune response to measles vaccine for 5 months after a dose of 80 mg IgG/kg.

†Assumes a serum IgG concentration of 16 mg/mL.

‡Measles vaccination is recommended for most HIV-infected children who do not have evidence of severe immunosuppression, but it is contraindicated for patients who have congenital disorders of the immune system.

§Formerly referred to as idiopathic thrombocytopenic purpura.

Modified from *MMWR Morb Mortal Wkly Rep*, 1996, 45(RR-12).

HAEMOPHILUS INFLUENZAE VACCINATION

Recommendations for *Haemophilus influenzae* Type b Conjugate Vaccination in Children Immunized Beginning at 2-6 Months of Age

Vaccine Product at Initiation*	Total No. of Doses to Be Administered	Currently Recommended Vaccine Regimens
HbOC or PRP-T	4	3 doses at 2-month intervals When feasible, same vaccine for doses 1-3 Fourth dose at 12-15 months of age Any conjugate vaccine for dose 4
PRP-OMP	3	2 doses at 2-month intervals When feasible, same vaccine for doses 1 and 2 Third dose at 12-15 months of age Any conjugate vaccine for dose 3†

*See text. The HbOC, PRP-T, or PRP-OMP should be given in a separate syringe and at a separate site from other immunizations unless specific combinations are approved by the FDA. HbOC is also available as a combination vaccine with DTP (HbOC-DTP). This combination can be used in infants scheduled to receive separate injections of DTP and HbOC. PRP-T may be reconstituted with DTP, made by Connaught Laboratories; other licensed formulations of DTP may not be used for this purpose.

†The safety and efficacy of PRP-OMP, PRP-D, PRP-T, and HbOC are likely to be equivalent in children 12 months and older.

Adapted from "Report of the Committee on Infectious Diseases," *1994 Red Book®*, 23rd ed, Montvale, NJ: Medical Economics Co, Inc.

Recommendations for *Haemophilus influenzae* Type b Conjugate Vaccination in Children in Whom Initial Vaccination Is Delayed Until 7 Months of Age or Older

Age at Initiation of Immunization (mo)	Vaccine Product at Initiation	Total No. of Doses to Be Administered	Currently Recommended Vaccine Regimens*
7-11	HbOC, PRP-T, or PRP-OMP	3	2 doses at 2-month intervals† When feasible, same vaccine for doses 1 and 2 Third dose at 12-18 months, given at least 2 months after dose 2 Any conjugate vaccine for dose 3‡
12-14	HbOC, PRP-T, PRP-OMP, or PRP-D	2	2-month interval between doses† Any conjugate vaccine for dose 2‡
15-59	HbOC, PRP-T, PRP-OMP, or PRP-D	1	Any conjugate vaccine
60 and older§	HbOC, PRP-T, PRP-OMP, or PRP-D	1 or 2¶	Any conjugate vaccine

*See text. HbOC, PRP-T, or PRP-OMP should be given in a separate syringe and at a separate site from other immunizations unless specific combinations are approved by the FDA. HbOC is also available as a combination vaccine with DTP (HbOC-DTP). This combination can be used in infants scheduled to receive separate injections of DTP and HbOC. PRP-T may be reconstituted with DTP, made by Connaught Laboratories; other licensed formulations of DTP may not be used for this purpose. In children 15 months or older eligible to receive DTaP (containing acellular pertussis vaccine), however, separate injections of conjugate vaccine and DTaP are acceptable because of the lower rate of febrile, minor local and systemic reactions associated with DTaP.

†For "catch up," a minimum of a 1-month interval between doses may be used.

‡The safety and efficacy of PRP-OMP, PRP-D, PRP-T, and HbOC are likely to be equivalent for use as a booster dose in children 12 months or older.

§Only for children with chronic illness known to be associated with an increased risk for *H. influenzae* type b disease (see text).

¶Two doses separated by 2 months are recommended by some experts for children with certain underlying diseases associated with increased risk of disease and impaired antibody responses to *H. influenzae* type conjugate vaccination (see text).

Adapted from "Report of the Committee on Infectious Diseases," *1994 Red Book®*, 23rd ed, Montvale, NJ: Medical Economics Co, Inc.

IMMUNIZATION RECOMMENDATIONS *(Continued)*

Recommendations for *Haemophilus influenzae* Type b Conjugate Vaccination in Children With a Lapse in Vaccination

Age at Presentation (mo)	Previous Vaccination History	Recommended Regimen
7-11	1 dose*	1 dose of conjugate at 7-11 months, with a booster dose given at least 2 months later, at 12-15 months†
	2 doses of HbOC or PRP-T	Same as above
12-14	2 doses before 12 months*	A single dose of any licensed conjugate‡
	1 dose before 12 months*	2 additional doses of any licensed conjugate, separated by 2 months‡
15-59	Any incomplete schedule	A single dose of any licensed conjugate‡

*PRP-OMP, PRP-T, or HbOC. HbOC is also available as a combination vaccine with DTP (HbOC-DTP), which may be used in infants scheduled to receive separate injections of DTP and HbOC. PRP-T may be reconstituted with DTP, made by Connaught Laboratories; other licensed formulations of DTP may not be used for this purpose. In children 15 months or older eligible to receive DTaP (containing acellular pertussis), however, separate injections of conjugate vaccine and DTaP may be given because of the lower rate of febrile, minor local and systemic reactions associated with DTaP.

†For the dose given at 7-11 months, when feasible, the same vaccine should be given as was used for the dose given at 2-6 months. For the dose given at 12-15 months, any licensed conjugate can be used.

‡The Academy considers that safety and efficacy of PRP-OMP, PRP-D, PRP-T, or HbOC are likely to be equivalent when used in children ≥12 months of age.

Adapted from "Report of the Committee on Infectious Diseases," *1994 Red Book*®, 23rd ed, Montvale, NJ: Medical Economics Co, Inc.

LYME DISEASE VACCINE GUIDELINES

Recommendations for Use of Recombinant Outer-Surface Protein A Vaccine for the Prevention of Lyme Disease (Advisory Committee on Immunization Practices, 1999)

	Vaccination Recommendation
Persons who reside, work, or recreate in areas of high or moderate risk	
Persons 15-70 years of age whose exposure to tick-infested habitat is frequent or prolonged	Should be considered
Persons 15-70 years of age who are exposed to tick-infested habitat, but whose exposure is not frequent or prolonged	May be considered
Persons whose exposure to tick-infested habitat is minimal or none	Not recommended
Persons who reside, work, or recreate in areas of low or no risk	Not recommended
Travelers to areas of high or moderate risk	
Travelers 15-70 years of age whose exposure to tick-infested habitat is frequent or prolonged	Should be considered
Children <15 years of age	Not recommended
Pregnant women	
Healthcare providers are encouraged to register vaccinations of pregnant women by calling SmithKline Beecham, toll free, at (800) 366-8900, ext 5231	Not recommended
Persons with immunodeficiency	No available data
Persons with musculoskeletal disease	Limited data available
Persons with previous history of Lyme disease	
Persons 15-70 years of age with previous umcomplicated Lyme disease who are at continued high risk	Should be considered
Persons with treatment-resistant Lyme arthritis	Not recommended
Persons with chronic joint or neurologic illness related to Lyme disease and persons with second or third degree atrioventricular block	No available data

Other Recommendations

Vaccine schedule

Three doses administered by intramuscular infection as follows:

Initial dose, followed by a second dose 1 month later, followed by a third dose 12 months after the first dose

Second dose (year 1) and third dose (year 2) administered several weeks before the beginning of the disease-transmission season, which is usually April

Boosters

Existing data indicate that boosters might be needed, but additional data are required before recommendations can be made regarding booster schedules

Simultaneous administration with other vaccines

Additional data needed

If simultaneous administration is necessary, use separate syringes and separate injection sites

From "Recommendations for the Use of Lyme Disease Vaccine. Recommendations of the Advisory Committee on Immunization Practices (ACIP)," *MMWR Morb Mortal Wkly Rep*, 1999, 48(RR-7):25.

IMMUNIZATION RECOMMENDATIONS *(Continued)*

POSTEXPOSURE PROPHYLAXIS FOR HEPATITIS B*

Exposure	Hepatitis B Immune Globulin	Hepatitis B Vaccine
Perinatal	0.5 mL I.M. within 12 h of birth	0.5 mL† I.M. within 12 h of birth (no later than 7 d), and at 1 and 6 mo‡; test for HB$_s$Ag and anti-HB$_s$ at 12-15 mo
Sexual	0.06 mL/kg I.M. within 14 d of sexual contact; a second dose should be given if the index patient remains HB$_s$Ag-positive after 3 mo and hepatitis B vaccine was not given initially	1 mL I.M. at 0, 1, and 6 mo for homosexual and bisexual men and regular sexual contacts of persons with acute and chronic hepatitis B
Percutaneous; exposed person unvaccinated		
Source known HB$_s$Ag-positive	0.06 mL/kg I.M. within 24 h	1 mL I.M. within 7 d, and at 1 and 6 mo§
Source known, HB$_s$Ag status not known	Test source for HB$_s$Ag; if source is positive, give exposed person 0.06 mL/kg I.M. once within 7 d	1 mL I.M. within 7 d, and at 1 and 6 mo§
Source not tested or unknown	Nothing required	1 mL I.M. within 7 d, and at 1 and 6 mo
Percutaneous; exposed person vaccinated		
Source known HB$_s$Ag-positive	Test exposed person for anti-HB$_s$¶. If titer is protective, nothing is required; if titer is not protective, give 0.06 mL/kg within 24 h	Review vaccination status#
Source known, HB$_s$Ag status not known	Test source for HB$_s$Ag and exposed person for anti-HB$_s$. If source is HB$_s$Ag-negative, or if source is HB$_s$Ag-positive but anti-HB$_s$ titer is protective, nothing is required. If source is HB$_s$Ag-positive and anti-HB$_s$ titer is not protective or if exposed person is a known nonresponder, give 0.06 mL/kg I.M. within 24 h. A second dose of hepatitis B immune globulin can be given 1 mo later if a booster dose of hepatitis B vaccine is not given.	Review vaccination status#
Source not tested or unknown	Test exposed person for anti-HB$_s$. If anti-HB$_s$ titer is protective, nothing is required. If anti-HB$_s$ titer is not protective, 0.06 mL/kg may be given along with a booster dose of hepatitis B vaccine	Review vaccination status#

*HB$_s$Ag = hepatitis B surface antigen; anti-HB$_s$ = antibody to hepatitis B surface antigen; I.M. = intramuscularly; SRU = standard ratio units.

†Each 0.5 mL dose of plasma-derived hepatitis B vaccine contains 10 μg of HB$_s$Ag; each 0.5 mL dose of recombinant hepatitis B vaccine contains 5 μg (Merck Sharp & Dohme) or 10 μg (SmithKline Beecham) of HB$_s$Ag.

‡If hepatitis B immune globulin and hepatitis B vaccine are given simultaneously, they should be given at separate sites.

§If hepatitis B vaccine is not given, a second dose of hepatitis B immune globulin should be given 1 month later.

¶Anti-HB$_s$ titers <10 SRU by radioimmunoassay or negative by enzyme immunoassay indicate lack of protection. Testing the exposed person for anti-HB$_s$ is not necessary if a protective level of antibody has been shown within the previous 24 months.

#If the exposed person has not completed a three-dose series of hepatitis B vaccine, the series should be completed. Test the exposed person for anti-HB$_s$. If the antibody level is protective, nothing is required. If an adequate antibody response in the past is shown on retesting to have declined to an inadequate level, a booster dose (1 mL) of hepatitis B vaccine should be given. If the exposed person has inadequate antibody or is a known nonresponder to vaccination, a booster dose can be given along with one dose of hepatitis B immune globulin.

PREVENTION OF HEPATITIS A THROUGH ACTIVE OR PASSIVE IMMUNIZATION

Recommendations of the Advisory Committee on Immunization Practices (ACIP)

PROPHYLAXIS AGAINST HEPATITIS A VIRUS INFECTION

Recommended Doses of Immune Globulin (IG) for Hepatitis A Pre-exposure and Postexposure Prophylaxis

Setting	Duration of Coverage	IG Dose*
Pre-exposure	Short-term (1-2 months)	0.02 mL/kg
	Long-term (3-5 months)	0.06 mL/kg†
Postexposure	—	0.02 mL/kg

*IG should be administered by intramuscular injection into either the deltoid or gluteal muscle. For children <24 months of age, IG can be administered in the anterolateral thigh muscle.

†Repeat every 5 months if continued exposure to HAV occurs.

Recommended Dosages of Havrix®*

Vaccinee's Age (y)	Dose (EL.U.)†	Volume (mL)	No. Doses	Schedule (mo)‡
2-18	720	0.5	2	0, 6-12
>18	1440	1.0	2	0, 6-12

*Hepatitis A vaccine, inactivated, SmithKline Beecham Biologicals

†ELISA units

‡0 months represents timing of the initial dose; subsequent numbers represent months after the initial dose.

Recommended Dosages of VAQTA®*

Vaccinee's Age (y)	Dose (units)	Volume (mL)	No. Doses	Schedule (mo)†
2-17	25	0.5	2	0, 6-18
>17	50	1.0	2	0, 6

*Hepatitis A vaccine, inactivated, Merck & Company, Inc

†0 months represents timing of the initial dose; subsequent numbers represent months after the initial dose.

From *MMWR Morb Mortal Wkly Rep*, 1996, 45(RR-15).

IMMUNIZATION RECOMMENDATIONS *(Continued)*

RECOMMENDATIONS FOR TRAVELERS

Recommended Immunizations for Travelers to Developing Countries*

Immunizations	Length of Travel[1]		
	Brief, <2 wk	Intermediate, 2 wk - 3 mo	Long-term Residential, >3 mo
Review and complete age-appropriate childhood schedule	+	+	+
• DTaP (or DTP) may be given at 4 wk intervals[2]			
• Poliovirus vaccine may be given at 4-8 wk intervals[2]			
• Measles: extra dose given if 6-11 mo old at 1st dose			
• Varicella			
• Hepatitis B[3]			
Yellow fever[4]	+	+	+
Typhoid fever[5]	±	+	+
Meningococcal meningitis[6]	±	±	±
Rabies[7]	+	+	+
Japanese encephalitis[4]	−	±	+

*See disease-specific chapters for details. For further sources of information, see text.

[1]+ indicates recommended; ± consider; and −, not recommended.

[2]If necessary to complete the recommended schedule before departure.

[3]If insufficient time to complete 6-month primary series, accelerated series can be given (see *Red Book*® for details).

[4]For endemic regions see *Health Information for International Travel*, page 2 of *Red Book*®.

[5]Indicated for travelers who will consume food at nontourist facilities.

[6]For endemic regions of central Africa and during local epidemics.

[7]Indicated for persons with high risk of wild animal exposure and for spelunkers.

Adapted from "Report of the Committee on Infectious Diseases," *1997 Red Book*®, 24th ed.

Recommendations for Pre-exposure Immunoprophylaxis of Hepatitis A Infection for Travelers*

Age (y)	Likely Exposure (mo)	Recommended Prophylaxis
<2	<3	IG 0.02 mL/kg†
	3-5	IG 0.06 mL/kg†
	Long term	IG 0.06 mL/kg at departure and every 5 mo thereafter†
≥2	<3‡	HAV vaccine§¶
		or
		IG 0.02 mL/kg†
	3-5‡	HAV vaccine§¶
		or
		IG 0.06 mL/kg†
		HAV vaccine§¶

*HAV, hepatitis A virus; IG, immune globulin.

†IG should be administered deep into a large muscle mass. Ordinarily no more than 5 mL should be administered in one site in an adult or large child; lesser amounts (maximum 3 mL) should be given to small children and infants.

‡Vaccine is preferable, but IG is an acceptable alternative.

§To ensure protection in travelers whose departure is imminent, IG also may be given (see text).

¶Dose and schedule of HAV vaccine as recommended according to age.

Adapted from "Report of the Committee on Infectious Diseases," *1997 Red Book*®, 24th ed.

Prevention of Malaria*

Drug†	Adult Dosage	Pediatric Dosage
Chloroquine-Sensitive Areas		
Chloroquine phosphate	P.O.: 300 mg base (500 mg salt), once/week beginning 1 week before exposure, and continuing for 4 weeks after last exposure	5 mg/kg base (8.3 mg/kg salt) once/week (maximum 300 mg base)
Chloroquine-Resistant Areas		
Mefloquine‡	P.O.: 250 mg salt (228 mg base), once/week, beginning 1 week before travel and continuing for 4 weeks after last exposure	15-19 kg: ¼ tablet/wk 20-30 kg: ½ tablet/wk 31-45 kg: ¾ tablet/wk >45 kg: 1 tablet/wk
Alternatives		
Doxycycline§	100 mg/d, starting 1-2 days before exposure and continuing for 4 weeks after last exposure	>8 y: P.O.: 2 mg/kg/d (maximum 100 mg/d)
or		
Chloroquine phosphate	Same as above	Same as above
with or without		
Proguanil#	200 mg daily during exposure and for 4 weeks after last exposure	<2 y: 50 mg/d 2-6 y: 100 mg/d 7-10 y: 150 mg/d >10 y: 200 mg/d
plus		
Pyrimethamine-sulfadoxine (Fansidar®) for presumptive treatment¶	Carry a single dose (3 tablets) for self-treatment of febrile illness when medical care is not immediately available	Used as for adults in the following doses: <1 y: ¼ tablet 1-3 y: ½ tablet 4-8 y: 1 tablet 9-14 y: 2 tablets >14 y: 3 tablets

*Currently, no drug regimen guarantees protection against malaria. Travelers to countries with risk of malaria should be advised to avoid mosquito bites by using personal protective measures (see text).
†All drugs should be continued for 4 weeks after last exposure.
‡Mefloquine is not licensed by the Food and Drug Administration for children weighing <15 kg, but recent recommendations from the Centers for Disease Control and Prevention allow use of the drug to be considered in children without weight restrictions when travel to chloroquine-resistant *P. falciparum* areas cannot be avoided. Mefloquine is **contraindicated** for use by travelers with a known hypersensitivity to mefloquine and travelers with a history of epilepsy or severe psychiatric disorders. A review of available data suggests that a mefloquine may be administered to persons concurrently receiving β-blockers if they have no underlying arrhythmia. However, mefloquine is not recommended for persons with cardiac conduction abnormalities until additional data are available. Caution may be advised for persons involved in tasks requiring fine coordination and spatial discrimination, such as airline pilots. Quinidine or quinine may exacerbate the known side effects or mefloquine; patients not responding to mefloquine therapy or failing mefloquine prophylaxis should be closely monitored if they are treated with quinidine or quinine.
§Physicians who prescribe doxycycline as malaria chemoprophylaxis should advise patients to limit the exposure to direct sunlight to minimize the possibility of photosensitivity reaction. Use of doxycycline is contraindicated in pregnant women and usually in children <8 years. Physicians must weight the benefits of doxycycline therapy against the possibility of dental staining in children <8 years (see Antimicrobial and Related Therapy).
#Proguanil (chloroguanide hydrochloride) is not available in the United States but is widely available overseas. It is recommended primarily for use in Africa south of the Sahara. Failures in prophylaxis with chloroquine and chloroguanide have been reported commonly, however, as they are only 40% to 60% effective.
¶Use of Fansidar®, which contains 25 mg pyrimethamine and 500 mg sulfadoxine per tablet, is contraindicated in patients with a history of sulfonamide or pyrimethamine intolerance, in infants <2 months, and in pregnant women at term. Resistance to pyrimethamine-sulfadoxine has been reported from Southeast Asia and the Amazon Basin and therefore should not be used for treatment of malaria acquired in these area.
Adapted from "Report of the Committee on Infectious Diseases," *1997 Red Book®*, 24th ed.

AMINOGLYCOSIDE DOSING AND MONITORING

All aminoglycoside therapy should be individualized for specific patients in specific clinical situation. The following are guidelines for initiating therapy.

1. Loading dose based on estimated ideal body weight (IBW). **All patients require a loading dose independent of renal function.**

Agent	Dose
Gentamicin	2 mg/kg
Tobramycin	2 mg/kg
Amikacin	7.5 mg/kg

Significantly higher loading doses may be required in severely ill intensive care unit patients.

2. Initial maintenance doses as a percent of loading dose according to desired dosing interval and creatinine clearance (Cl_{cr}):

$$\text{Male } Cl_{cr} \text{ (mL/min)} = \frac{(140 - \text{age}) \times \text{IBW}}{72 \times \text{serum creatinine}}$$

$$\text{Female} = 0.85 \times Cl_{cr} \text{ males}$$

Cl_{cr} (mL/min)	Dosing Interval (h)		
	8	12	24
90	84%	—	—
80	80%	—	—
70	76%	88%	—
60	—	84%	—
50	—	79%	—
40	—	72%	92%
30	—	—	86%
25	—	—	81%
20	—	—	75%

Patients older than 65 years of age should not receive initial aminoglycoside maintenance dosing more often than every 12 hours.

3. Serum concentration monitoring

    a. Serum concentration monitoring is necessary for **safe** and **effective** therapy, particularly in patients with serious infections and those with risk factors for toxicity.

    b. Peak serum concentrations should be drawn 30 minutes after the completion of a 30-minute infusion. Trough serum concentrations should be drawn within 30 minutes prior to the administered dose.

    c. Serum concentrations should be drawn after 5 half-lives, usually around the third dose or thereafter.

4. Desired measured serum concentrations

	Peak (μg/mL)	Trough (μg/mL)
Gentamicin	6-10	0.5-2.0
Tobramycin	6-10	0.5-2.0
Amikacin	20-30	<5
Netilmicin	4-10	<2

5. For patients receiving hemodialysis:

- administer the **same** loading dose
- administer $2/3$ of the loading dose after each dialysis
- **serum concentrations must be monitored**
- watch for ototoxicity from accumulation of drug

6. For individual clinical situations the prescribing physician should feel free to consult Infectious Disease, the Pharmacology Service, or the Pharmacy.

"Once Daily" Aminoglycosides

High dose, "once daily" aminoglycoside therapy for treatment of gram-negative bacterial infections has been studied and remains controversial. The pharmacodynamics of aminoglycosides reveal dose-dependent killing which suggests an efficacy advantage of "high" peak serum concentrations. It is also suggested that allowing troughs to fall to unmeasurable levels decreases the risk of nephrotoxicity without detriment to efficacy. Because of a theoretical saturation of tubular cell uptake of aminoglycosides, decreasing the number of times the drug is administered in a particular time period may play a role in minimizing the risk of nephrotoxicity. Ototoxicity has not been sufficiently formally evaluated through audiometry or vestibular testing comparing "once daily" to standard therapy. Over 100 letters, commentaries, studies and reviews have been published on the topic of "once daily" aminoglycosides with varying dosing regimens, monitoring parameters, inclusion and exclusion criteria, and results (most of which have been favorable for the "once daily" regimens). The caveats of this simplified method of dosing are several, including assurance that creatinine clearances be calculated, that all patients are not candidates and should not be considered for this regimen, and that "once daily" is a semantic misnomer.

Because of the controversial nature of this method, it is beyond the scope of this book to present significant detail and dosing regimen recommendations. Considerable experience with two methods warrants mention. The Hartford Hospital has experience with over 2000 patients utilizing a 7 mg/kg dose, a dosing scheme for various creatinine clearance estimates, and a serum concentration monitoring nomogram.[1] Providence Medical Center utilizes a 5 mg/kg dosing regimen but only in patients with excellent renal function; serum concentrations are monitored 4-6 hours prior to the dose administered.[2] Two excellent reviews discuss the majority of studies and controversies regarding these dosing techniques.[3,4] An editorial accompanies one of the reviews and is worth examination.[5]

"Once daily" dosing may be a safe and effective method of providing aminoglycoside therapy to a large number of patients who require these efficacious yet toxic agents. As with any method of aminoglycoside administration, dosing must be individualized and the caveats of the method considered.

Footnotes

1. Nicolau DP, Freeman CD, Belliveau PP, et al, "Experience With a Once-Daily Aminoglycoside Program Administered to 2,184 Patients," *Antimicrob Agents Chemother*, 1995, 39:650-5.

2. Gilbert DN, "Once-Daily Aminoglycoside Therapy," *Antimicrob Agents Chemother*, 1991, 35:399-405.

3. Preston SL and Briceland LL, "Single Daily Dosing of Aminoglycosides," *Pharmacotherapy*, 1995, 15:297-316.

4. Bates RD and Nahata MC, "Once-Daily Administration of Aminoglycosides," *Ann Pharmacother*, 1994, 28:757-66.

5. Rotschafer JC and Rybak MJ,"Single Daily Dosing of Aminoglycosides: A Commentary," *Ann Pharmacother*, 1994, 28:797-801.

AMINOGLYCOSIDE DOSING AND MONITORING *(Continued)*

Aminoglycoside Penetration Into Various Tissues

Site	Extent of Distribution
Eye	Poor
CNS	Poor (<25%)
Pleural	Excellent
Bronchial secretions	Poor
Sputum	Fair (10%-50%)
Pulmonary tissue	Excellent
Ascitic fluid	Variable (43%-132%)
Peritoneal fluid	Poor
Bile	Variable (25%-90%)
Bile with obstruction	Poor
Synovial fluid	Excellent
Bone	Poor
Prostate	Poor
Urine	Excellent
Renal tissue	Excellent

From Neu HC, "Pharmacology of Aminoglycosides," *The Aminoglycosides*, Whelton E, Neu HC, eds, New York, NY: Marcel Dekker, Inc, 1981.

ANIMAL AND HUMAN BITES GUIDELINES

Wound Management

Irrigation: Critically important; irrigate all penetration wounds using a 20 mL syringe, 19-gauge needle and >250 mL 1% povidone iodine solution. This method will reduce wound infection by a factor of 20. When there is high risk of rabies, use viricidal 1% benzalkonium chloride in addition to the 1% povidone iodine. Irrigate wound with normal saline after antiseptic irrigation.

Debridement: Remove all crushed or devitalized tissue remaining after irrigation; minimize removal on face and over thin skin areas or anywhere you would create a worse situation than the bite itself already has; do not extend puncture wounds surgically — rather, manage them with irrigation and antibiotics.

Suturing: Close most dog bites if <8 hours (<12 hours on face); do not routinely close puncture wounds, or deep or severe bites on the hands or feet, as these are at highest risk for infection. Cat and human bites should not be sutured unless cosmetically important. Wound edge freshening, where feasible, reduces infection; minimize sutures in the wound and use monofilament on the surface.

Immobilization: Critical in all hand wounds; important for infected extremities.

Hospitalization/I.V. Antibiotics: Admit for I.V. antibiotics all significant human bites to the hand, especially closed fist injuries, and bites involving penetration of the bone or joint (a high index of suspicion is needed). Consider I.V. antibiotics for significant established wound infections with cellulitis or lymphangitis, any infected bite on the hand, any infected cat bite, and any infection in an immunocompromised or asplenic patient. Outpatient treatment with I.V. antibiotics may be possible in selected cases by consulting with infectious disease.

Laboratory Assessment

Gram's Stain: Not useful prior to onset of clinically apparent infection; examination of purulent material may show a predominant organism in established infection, aiding antibiotic selection; not warranted unless results will change your treatment.

Culture: Not useful or cost-effective prior to onset of clinically apparent infection.

X-ray: Whenever you suspect bony involvement, especially in craniofacial dog bites in very small children or severe bite/crush in an extremity; cat bites with their long needle like teeth may cause osteomyelitis or a septic joint, especially in the hand or wrist.

Immunizations

Tetanus: All bite wounds are contaminated. If not immunized in last 5 years, or if not current in a child, give DPT, DT, Td, or TT as indicated. For absent or incomplete primary immunization, give 250 units tetanus immune globulin (TIG) in addition.

Rabies: In the U.S., 30,000 persons are treated each year in an attempt to prevent 1-5 cases. Domestic animals should be quarantining for 10 days to prove need for prophylaxis. High-risk animal bites (85% of cases = bat, skunk, raccoon) usually receive treatment consisting of:
- human rabies immune globulin (HRIG): 20 units/kg I.M. (unless previously immunized with HDCV)
- human diploid cell vaccine (HDCV): 1 mL I.M. on days 0, 3, 7, 14, and 28 (unless previously immunized with HDCV - then give only first 2 doses)

Consult with Infectious Disease before ordering rabies prophylaxis.

Bite Wounds and Prophylactic Antibiotics

Parenteral vs Oral: If warranted, consider an initial I.V. dose to rapidly establish effective serum levels, especially if high risk, delayed treatment, or if patient reliability is poor.

ANIMAL AND HUMAN BITES GUIDELINES *(Continued)*

Dog Bite:

1. Rarely get infected (~5%)

2. Infecting organisms: Coagulase-negative *Staphylococcus*, coagulase-positive *Staphylococcus*, alpha strep, diphtheroids, beta strep, *Pseudomonas aeruginosa*, gamma strep, *Pasteurella multocida*

3. Prophylactic antibiotics are seldom indicated. Consider for high risk wounds such as distal extremity puncture wounds, severe crush injury, bites occurring in cosmetically sensitive areas (eg, face), or in immunocompromised or asplenic patients.

Cat Bite:

1. Often get infected (~25% to 50%)

2. Infecting organisms: *Pasteurella multocida* (first 24 hours), coagulase-positive *Staphylococcus*, anaerobic cocci (after first 24 hours)

3. Prophylactic antibiotics are indicated in all cases.

Human Bite:

1. Intermediate infection rate (~15% to 20%)

2. Infecting organisms: Coagulase-positive *Staphylococcus*; alpha, beta, or gamma strep; *Haemophilus*; *Eikenella corrodens*; anaerobic streptococci; *Fusobacterium*; *Veillonella*; *Bacteroides*.

3. Prophylactic antibiotics are indicated in almost all cases except superficial injuries.

Bite Wound Antibiotic Regimens

	Dog Bite	Cat Bite	Human Bite
Prophylactic Antibiotics			
Prophylaxis	No routine prophylaxis, consider if involves face or hand, or immunosuppressed or asplenic patients	Routine prophylaxis	Routine prophylaxis
Prophylactic antibiotic	Amoxicillin	Amoxicillin	Amoxicillin
Penicillin allergy	Doxycycline if >10 y or co-trimoxazole	Doxycycline if >10 y or co-trimoxazole	Doxycycline if >10 y or erythromycin and cephalexin*
Outpatient Oral Antibiotic Treatment (mild to moderate infection)			
Established infection	Amoxicillin and clavulanic acid	Amoxicillin and clavulanic acid	Amoxicillin and clavulanic acid
Penicillin allergy (mild infection only)	Doxycycline if >10 y	Doxycycline if >10 y	Cephalexin* or clindamycin
Outpatient Parenteral Antibiotic Treatment (moderate infections – single drug regimens)			
	Ceftriaxone	Ceftriaxone	Cefotetan
Inpatient Parenteral Antibiotic Treatment			
Established infection	Ampicillin + cefazolin	Ampicillin + cefazolin	Ampicillin + clindamycin
Penicillin allergy	Cefazolin*	Ceftriaxone*	Cefotetan* or imipenem

Duration of Prophylactic and Treatment Regimens
Prophylaxis: 5 days
Treatment: 10-14 days

*Contraindicated if history of immediate hypersensitivity reaction (anaphylaxis) to penicillin.

Antibiotic Dosages

Antibiotic	Adult Dosage	Pediatric Dosage
Oral Regimens		
Amoxicillin	500 mg P.O. tid	50 mg/kg/d with tid dosing
Amoxicillin/clavulanate	500/125 P.O. tid (750 mg P.O. qid if >180 lb)	50 mg/kg/d based on amoxicillin content with tid dosing
Cephalexin	500 mg P.O. qid (750 mg P.O. qid if >180 lb)	50 mg/kg/d with qid dosing
Clindamycin	450 mg P.O. tid	25-30 mg/kg/d with tid-qid dosing
Co-trimoxazole	2 tabs P.O. bid	8 mg/kg/d based on trimethoprim content with bid dosing
Dicloxacillin	500 mg P.O. qid	50 mg/kg/d with qid dosing
Doxycycline	100 mg P.O. bid	5 mg/kg/d with bid dosing
Erythromycin	500 mg P.O. qid	50 mg/kg/d with qid dosing
Penicillin VK	500 mg P.O. qid	75-100 mg/kg/d with qid dosing
Parenteral Regimens		
Ampicillin	2 g I.V. q4-6h	250-300 mg/kg/d I.V. given q6h
Ampicillin/sulbactam	2 g I.V. q6h based on ampicillin component	250-300 mg/kg/d I.V. based on ampicillin component given q6h
Cefazolin	2 g I.V. q8h	100 mg/kg/d I.V. given q8h
Cefotetan	2 g I.V. q12h	60-80 mg/kg/d I.V. given q12h
Ceftriaxone	2 g I.V. or I.M. q24h	75 mg/kg/d I.M./I.V. given q24h
Clindamycin	900 mg I.V. q8h	25-30 mg/kg/d I.V. given q8h
Imipenem	500 mg I.V. q6h	

ANTIBIOTIC TREATMENT OF ADULTS WITH INFECTIVE ENDOCARDITIS

Table 1. Suggested Regimens for Therapy of Native Valve Endocarditis Due to Penicillin-Susceptible Viridans Streptococci and *Streptococcus bovis*
(Minimum Inhibitory Concentration ≤0.1 µg/mL)*

Antibiotic	Dosage and Route	Duration (weeks)	Comments
Aqueous crystalline penicillin G sodium or	12-18 million units/24 h I.V. either continuously or in 6 equally divided doses	4	Preferred in most patients older than 65 y and in those with impairment of the eighth nerve or renal function
Ceftriaxone sodium	2 g once daily I.V. or I.M.†	4	
Aqueous crystalline penicillin G sodium	12-18 million units/24 h I.V. either continuously or in 6 equally divided doses	2	When obtained 1 hour after a 20- to 30-minute I.V. infusion or I.M. injection, serum concentration of gentamicin of approximately 3 µg/mL is desirable; trough concentration should be <1 µg/mL
With gentamicin sulfate‡	1 mg/kg I.M. or I.V. every 8 hours	2	
Vancomycin hydrochloride§	30 mg/kg/24 h I.V. in 2 equally divided doses, not to exceed 2 g/24 h unless serum levels are monitored	4	Vancomycin therapy is recommended for patients allergic to β-lactams; peak serum concentrations of vancomycin should be obtained 1 hour after completion of the infusion and should be in the range of 30-45 µg/mL for twice-daily dosing

*Dosages recommended are for patients with normal renal function. For nutritionally variant streptococci, see Table 3. I.V. indicates intravenous; I.M., intramuscular.

†Patients should be informed that I.M. injection of ceftriaxone is painful.

‡Dosing of gentamicin on a mg/kg basis will produce higher serum concentrations in obese patients that in lean patients. Therefore, in obese patients, dosing should be based on ideal body weight. (Ideal body weight for men is 50 kg + 2.3 kg per inch over 5 feet, and ideal body weight for women is 45.5 kg + 2.3 kg per inch over 5 feet.) Relative contraindications to the use of gentamicin are age >65 years, renal impairment, or impairment of the eighth nerve. Other potentially nephrotoxic agents (eg, nonsteroidal anti-inflammatory drugs) should be used cautiously in patients receiving gentamicin.

§Vancomycin dosage should be reduced in patients with impaired renal function. Vancomycin given on a mg/kg basis will produce higher serum concentrations in obese patients than in lean patients. Therefore, in obese patients, dosing should be based on ideal body weight. Each dose of vancomycin should be infused over at least 1 h to reduce the risk of the histamine-release "red man" syndrome.

Table 2. Therapy for Native Valve Endocarditis Due to Strains of Viridans Streptococci and *Streptococcus bovis* Relatively Resistant to Penicillin G
(Minimum Inhibitory Concentration >0.1 µg/mL and <0.5 µg/mL)*

Antibiotic	Dosage and Route	Duration (week)	Comments
Aqueous crystalline penicillin G sodium	18 million units/24 h I.V. either continuously or in 6 equally divided doses	4	Cefazolin or other first-generation cephalosporins may be substituted for penicillin in patients whose penicillin hypersensitivity is not of the immediate type.
With gentamicin sulfate†	1 mg/kg I.M. or I.V. every 8 h	2	
Vancomycin hydrochloride§	30 mg/kg/24 h I.V. in 2 equally divided doses, not to exceed 2 g/24 h unless serum levels are monitored	4	Vancomycin therapy is recommended for patients allergic to β-lactams

*Dosages recommended are for patients with normal renal function. I.V. indicates intravenous; I.M., intramuscular.

†For specific dosing adjustment and issues concerning gentamicin (obese patients, relative contraindications), see Table 1 footnotes.

‡For specific dosing adjustment and issues concerning vancomycin (obese patients, length of infusion), see Table 1 footnotes.

Table 3. Standard Therapy for Endocarditis Due to Enterococci*

Antibiotic	Dosage and Route	Duration (week)	Comments
Aqueous crystalline penicillin G sodium	18-30 million units/24 h I.V. either continuously or in 6 equally divided doses	4-6	4-week therapy recommended for patients with symptoms <3 months in duration; 6-week therapy recommended for patients with symptoms >3 months in duration.
With gentamicin sulfate†	1 mg/kg I.M. or I.V. every 8 h	4-6	
Ampicillin sodium	12 g/24 h I.V. either continuously or in 6 equally divided doses	4-6	
With gentamicin sulfate†	1 mg/kg I.M. or I.V. every 8 hours	4-6	
Vancomycin hydrochloride†‡	30 mg/kg/24 h I.V. in 2 equally divided doses, not to exceed 2 g/24 h unless serum levels are monitored	4-6	Vancomycin therapy is recommended for patients allergic to β-lactams; cephalosporins are not acceptable alternatives for patients allergic to penicillin
With gentamicin sulfate†	1 mg/kg I.M. or I.V. every 8 h	4-6	

*All enterococci causing endocarditis must be tested for antimicrobial susceptibility in order to select optimal therapy. This table is for endocarditis due to gentamicin- or vancomycin-susceptible enterococci, viridans streptococci with a minimum inhibitory concentration >0.5 µg/mL, nutritionally variant viridans streptococci, or prosthetic valve endocarditis caused by viridans streptococci or *Streptococcus bovis*. Antibiotic dosages are for patients with normal renal function. I.V. indicates intravenous; I.M., intramuscular.

†For specific dosing adjustment and issues concerning gentamicin (obese patients, relative contraindications), see Table 1 footnotes.

‡For specific dosing adjustment and issues concerning vancomycin (obese patients, length of infusion), see Table 1 footnotes.

ANTIBIOTIC TREATMENT OF ADULTS WITH INFECTIVE ENDOCARDITIS *(Continued)*

Table 4. Therapy for Endocarditis Due to Staphylococcus in the Absence of Prosthetic Material*

Antibiotic	Dosage and Route	Duration	Comments
Methicillin-Susceptible Staphylococci			
Regimens for non-β-lactam-allergic patients			
Nafcillin sodium or oxacillin sodium	2 g I.V. every 4 h	4-6 wk	Benefit of additional aminoglycosides has not been established
With optional addition of gentamicin sulfate†	1 mg/kg I.M. or I.V. every 8 h	3-5 d	
Regimens for β-lactam-allergic patients			
Cefazolin (or other first-generation cephalosporins in equivalent dosages)	2 g I.V. every 8 h	4-6 wk	Cephalosporins should be avoided in patients with immediate-type hypersensitivity to penicillin
With optional addition of gentamicin†	1 mg/kg I.M. or I.V. every 8 hours	3-5 d	
Vancomycin hydrochloride‡	30 mg/kg/24 h I.V. in 2 equally divided doses, not to exceed 2 g/24 h unless serum levels are monitored	4-6 wk	Recommended for patients allergic to penicillin
Methicillin-Resistant Staphylococci			
Vancomycin hydrochloride‡	30 mg/kg/24 h I.V. in 2 equally divided doses; not to exceed 2 g/24 h unless serum levels are monitored	4-6 wk	

*For treatment of endocarditis due to penicillin-susceptible staphylococci (minimum inhibitory concentration ≤0.1 µg/mL), aqueous crystalline penicillin G sodium (Table 1, first regimen) can be used for 4-6 weeks instead of nafcillin or oxacillin. Shorter antibiotic courses have been effective in some drug addicts with right-sided endocarditis due to *Staphylococcus aureus*. I.V. indicates intravenous; I.M., intramuscular.

†For specific dosing adjustment and issues concerning gentamicin (obese patients, relative contraindications), see Table 1 footnotes.

‡For specific dosing adjustment and issues concerning vancomycin (obese patients, length of infusion), see Table 1 footnotes.

Table 5. Treatment of Staphylococcal Endocarditis in the Presence of a Prosthetic Valve or Other Prosthetic Material*

Antibiotic	Dosage and Route	Duration (week)	Comments
Regimen for Methicillin-Resistant Staphylococci			
Vancomycin hydrochloride†	30 mg/kg/24 h I.V. in 2 or 4 equally divided doses, not to exceed 2 g/24 h unless serum levels are monitored	≥6	
With rifampin‡	300 mg orally every 8 h	≥6	Rifampin increases the amount of warfarin sodium required for antithrombotic therapy.
And with gentamicin sulfate§¶	1 mg/kg I.M. or I.V. every 8 h	2	
Regimen for Methicillin-Susceptible Staphylococci			
Nafcillin sodium or oxacillin sodium†	2 g I.V. every 4 h	≥6	First-generation cephalosporins or vancomycin should be used in patients allergic to β-lactam. Cephalosporins should be avoided in patients with immediate-type hypersensitivity to penicillin or with methicillin-resistant staphylococci.
With rifampin‡	300 mg orally every 8 h	≥6	
And with gentamicin sulfate§¶	1 mg/kg I.M. or I.V. every 8 h	2	

*Dosages recommended are for patients with normal renal function. I.V. indicates intravenous; I.M., intramuscular.

†For specific dosing adjustment and issues concerning gentamicin (obese patients, relative contraindications), see Table 1 footnotes.

‡Rifampin plays a unique role in the eradication of staphylococcal infection involving prosthetic material; combination therapy is essential to prevent emergence of rifampin resistance.

§For specific dosing adjustment and issues concerning gentamicin (obese patients, relative contraindications), see Table 1 footnotes.

¶Use during initial 2 weeks.

Table 6. Therapy for Endocarditis Due to HACEK Microorganisms (*Haemophilus parainfluenzae, Haemophilus aphrophilus, Actinobacillus actinomycetemcomitans, Cardiobacterium hominus, Eikenella corrodens,* and *Kingella kingae*)*

Antibiotic	Dosage and Route	Duration (week)	Comments
Ceftriaxone sodium†	2 g once daily I.V. or I.M.†	4	Cefotaxime sodium or other third-generation cephalosporins may be substituted
Ampicillin sodium‡	12 g/24 h I.V. either continuously or in 6 equally divided doses	4	
With gentamicin sulfate§	1 mg/kg I.M. or I.V. every 6 h	4	

*Antibiotic dosages are for patients with normal renal function. I.V. indicates intravenous; I.M. intramuscular.

†Patients should be informed that I.M. injection of ceftriaxone is painful.

‡Ampicillin should not be used if laboratory tests show β-lactamase production.

§For specific dosing adjustment and issues concerning gentamicin (obese patients, relative contraindications), see Table 1 footnotes.

Note: Tables 1-6 are from Wilson WR, Karchmer AW, Dajani AS, et al, "Antibiotic Treatment of Adults With Infective Endocarditis Due to Streptococci, Enterococci, Staphylococci, and HACEK Microorganisms," *JAMA*, 1995, 274(21):1706-13, with permission.

CLINICAL SYNDROMES ASSOCIATED WITH FOODBORNE DISEASES

Clinical Syndromes	Incubation Period (h)	Causes	Commonly Associated Vehicles
Nausea and vomiting	<1-6	*Staphylococcus aureus* (preformed toxins, A, B, C, D, E)	Ham, poultry, cream-filled pastries, potato and egg salad, mushrooms
		Bacillus cereus (emetic toxin)	Fried rice, pork
		Heavy metals (copper, tin, cadmium, zinc)	Acidic beverages
Histamine response and gastrointestinal (GI) tract	<1	Histamine (scombroid)	Fish (bluefish, bonito, mackerel, mahi-mahi, tuna)
Neurologic, including paresthesia and GI tract	0-6	Tetrodotoxin, ciguatera	Puffer fish
			Fish (amberjack, barracuda, grouper, snapper)
		Paralytic compounds	Shellfish (clams, mussels, oysters, scallops, other mollusks)
		Neurotoxic compounds	Shellfish
		Domoic acid	Mussels
		Monosodium glutamate	Chinese food
Neurologic and GI tract manifestations	0-2	Mushroom toxins (early onset)	Mushrooms
Moderate-to-severe abdominal cramps and watery diarrhea	8-16	*B. cereus* enterotoxin	Beef, pork, chicken, vanilla sauce
		Clostridium perfringens enterotoxin	Beef, poultry, gravy
	16-48	Caliciviruses	Shellfish, salads, ice
		Enterotoxigenic *E. coli*	Fruits, vegetables
		Vibrio cholerae 01 and 0139	Shellfish
		V. cholerae non-01	Shellfish
Diarrhea, fever, abdominal cramps, blood and mucus in stools	16-72	*Salmonella*	Poultry, pork, eggs, dairy products, including ice cream, vegetables, fruit
		Shigella	Egg salad, vegetables
		Campylobacter jejuni	Poultry, raw milk
		Invasive *E. coli*	
		Yersinia enterocolitica	Pork chitterlings, tofu, raw milk
		Vibrio parahaemolyticus	Fish, shellfish
Bloody diarrhea, abdominal cramps	72-120	Enterohemorrhagic *E. coli*	Beef (hamburger), raw milk, roast beef, salami, salad dressings
Methemoglobin poisoning	6-12	Mushrooms (late onset)	Mushrooms
Hepatorenal failure	6-24	Mushrooms (late onset)	Mushrooms
Gastrointestinal then blurred vision, dry mouth, dysarthria, diplopia, descending paralysis	18-36	*Clostridium botulinum*	Canned vegetables, fruits and fish, salted fish, bottled garlic
Extraintestinal manifestations	Varied	Brainerd disease	Unpasteurized milk
		Brucella	Cheese, raw milk
		Group A streptococcus	Egg and potato salad
		Listeria monocytogenes	Cheese, raw milk, hot dogs, cole slaw, cold cuts
		Trichinella spiralis	Pork
		Vibrio vulnificus	Shellfish

Adapted from "Report of the Committee on Infectious Diseases," *1997 Red Book®*, 24th ed.

Timing of Food Poisoning

Symptoms	Time from Ingestion			
	<2 h	2-7 h	8-14 h	>14 h
Nausea/vomiting	—	S. aureus B. cereus	—	—
Diarrhea	—	—	C. perfringens B. cereus	V. cholerae Enterotoxic or invasive E. coli Shigella sp Vibrio sp
Both upper and lower gastrointestinal	—	—	—	Salmonella Vibrio sp
Extragastrointestinal (ie, some gastrointestinal plus other symptoms, usually paresthesias or other abnormal sensory complaints)	Scombrotoxin Shellfish toxin Mushroom toxin	Ciguatoxin	Mushroom toxin	C. botulinum

From Altman DF, "Food Poisoning," *Cecil's Textbook of Medicine*, 19th ed, ch 110, Wyngaarden JB, Smith LH Jr, and Bennett JC, eds, Philadelphia, PA: WB Saunders Co, 1992.

COMMUNITY-ACQUIRED PNEUMONIA IN ADULTS

GUIDELINES FOR MANAGEMENT

(Adapted from the Guidelines From the Infectious Diseases Society of America, *Clin Infect Dis*, 1998, 26:811-38.)

Algorithm

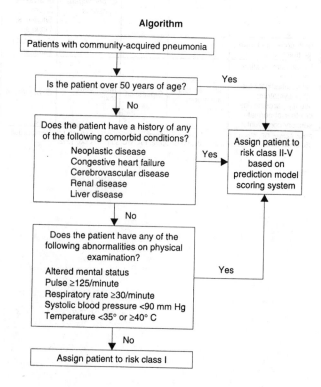

Stratification of Risk Score

Risk	Risk class	Based on
	I	Algorithm
Low	II	≤ 70 total points
	III	71-90 total points
Moderate	IV	91-130 total points
High	V	> 130 total points

The table below is the prediction model for identification of patient risk for persons with community-acquired pneumonia. This model may be used to help guide the initial decision on site of care; however, its use may not be appropriate for all patients with this illness and, therefore, should be applied in conjunction with physician judgment.

Scoring System

Patient Characteristic	Points Assigned*
Demographic factors	
Age: Male	age (in years)
Female	age (in years) - 10
Nursing home resident	+10
Comorbid illnesses	
Neoplastic disease	+30
Liver disease	+20
Congestive heart failure	+10
Cerebrovascular disease	+10
Renal disease	+10
Physical examination findings	
Altered mental status	+20
Respiratory rate ≥30/minute	+20
Systolic blood pressure <90 mm Hg	+20
Temperature <35°C or ≥40°C	+15
Pulse ≥125/minute	+10
Laboratory findings	
pH <7.35	+30
BUN >10.7 mmol/L	+20
Sodium <130 mEq/L	+20
Glucose >13.9 mmol/L	+10
Hematocrit <30%	+10
PO_2 <60 mm Hg†	+10
Pleural effusion	+10

*A risk score (reset point score) for a given patient is obtained by summing the patient age in years (age -10 for females) and the points for each applicable patient characteristic.

†Oxygen saturation <90% also was considered normal.

Risk-Class Mortality Rates for Patients With Pneumonia

Risk Class	No. of Points	Validation Cohort		Recommendations for Site of Care
		No. of Patients	Mortality (%)	
I	No predictors	3,034	0.1	Outpatient
II	≤70	5,778	0.6	Outpatient
III	71-90	6,790	2.8	Inpatient (briefly)
IV	91-130	13,104	8.2	Inpatient
V	>130	9,333	29.2	Inpatient

COMMUNITY-ACQUIRED PNEUMONIA IN ADULTS
(Continued)

Epidemiological and Underlying Conditions Related to Specific Pathogens in Selected Patients With Community-Acquired Pneumonia

Conditions	Commonly Encountered Pathogens
Alcoholism	*Streptococcus pneumoniae*, anaerobes, gram-negative bacilli
COPD/smoker	*Streptococcus pneumoniae, Haemophilus influenzae, Moraxella catarrhalis, Legionella* species
Nursing home residency	*Streptococcus pneumoniae*, gram-negative bacilli, *Haemophilus influenzae, Staphylococcus aureus*, anaerobes, *Chlamydia pneumoniae*
Poor dental hygiene	Anaerobes
Epidemic Legionnaires' disease	*Legionella* species
Exposure to bats or soil enriched with bird droppings	*Histoplasma capsulatum*
Exposure to birds	*Chlamydia psittaci*
Exposure to rabbits	*Francisella tularensis*
HIV infection (early stage)	*Streptococcus pneumoniae, Haemophilus influenzae, Mycobacterium tuberculosis*
Travel to the southwestern United States	*Coccidioides immitis*
Exposure to farm animals or parturient cats	*Coxiella burnetii**
Influenza active in community	Influenza, *Streptococcus pneumoniae, Staphylococcus aureus, Streptococcus pyogenes, Haemophilus influenzae*
Suspected large-volume aspiration	Anaerobes, chemical pneumonitis
Structural disease of the lung (bronchiectasis or cystic fibrosis)	*Pseudomonas aeruginosa, Burkholderia (Pseudomonas) cepacia*, or *Staphylococcus aureus*
Injection drug use	*Staphylococcus aureus*, anaerobes, *Mycobacterium tuberculosis*
Airway obstruction	Anaerobes

*Agent of Q fever

COPD = chronic obstructive pulmonary disease

Flow Chart Approach to Treating Outpatients and Inpatients with Community-Acquired Pneumonia

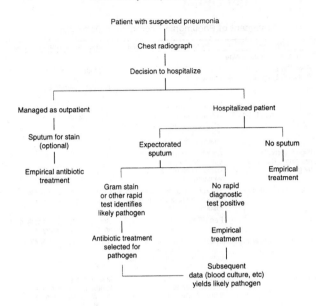

Patient with suspected pneumonia

Chest radiograph

Decision to hospitalize

Managed as outpatient

Sputum for stain (optional)

Empirical antibiotic treatment

Hospitalized patient

Expectorated sputum

No sputum

Empirical treatment

Gram stain or other rapid test identifies likely pathogen

No rapid diagnostic test positive

Antibiotic treatment selected for pathogen

Empirical treatment

Subsequent data (blood culture, etc) yields likely pathogen

Community-Acquired Pneumonia

Possible reasons for failure of empirical treatment in patients with community-acquired pneumonia.

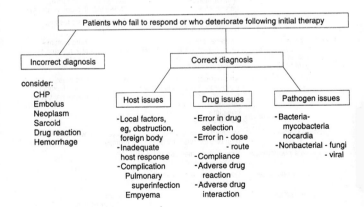

Patients who fail to respond or who deteriorate following initial therapy

Incorrect diagnosis

consider:
CHP
Embolus
Neoplasm
Sarcoid
Drug reaction
Hemorrhage

Correct diagnosis

Host issues

-Local factors, eg, obstruction, foreign body
-Inadequate host response
-Complication
  Pulmonary superinfection
  Empyema

Drug issues

-Error in drug selection
-Error in - dose
           - route
-Compliance
-Adverse drug reaction
-Adverse drug interaction

Pathogen issues

-Bacteria-
  mycobacteria
  nocardia
-Nonbacterial - fungi
              - viral

COMMUNITY-ACQUIRED PNEUMONIA IN ADULTS
(Continued)

Treatment of Pneumonia According to Pathogen

Pathogen	Preferred Antimicrobial	Alternative Antimicrobial
Streptococcus pneumoniae		
Penicillin susceptible (MIC, <0.1 µg/mL)	Penicillin G or penicillin V, amoxicillin	Cephalosporins,* macrolides,† clindamycin, fluoroquinolones,‡ doxycycline
Intermediately penicillin resistant (MIC, 0.1-1 µg/mL)	Parenteral penicillin G, ceftriaxone or cefotaxime, amoxicillin, fluoroquinolones,‡ other agents based on *in vitro* susceptibility test results	Clindamycin, doxycycline, oral cephalosporins*
Highly penicillin-resistant¤ (MIC, ≥2 mcg/mL)	Agents based on *in vitro* susceptibility results, fluoroquinolones,‡ vancomycin	
Empirical selection	Fluoroquinolones,‡ selection based on susceptibility test results in community§	Clindamycin, doxycycline, vancomycin
	Penicillin¶	Cephalosporins,* macrolides,† amoxicillin, clindamycin
Haemophilus influenzae	Second- or third-generation cephalosporins, doxycycline, beta-lactam - beta-lactamase inhibitor, fluoroquinolones‡	Azithromycin, TMP-SMZ
Moraxella catarrhalis	Second- or third-generation cephalosporins, TMP-SMZ, amoxicillin/clavulanate	Macrolides,† fluoroquinolones,‡ beta-lactam - beta-lactamase inhibitor
Anaerobes	Clindamycin, penicillin plus metronidazole, beta-lactam - beta-lactamase inhibitor	Penicillin G or penicillin V, ampicillin/amoxicillin with or without metronidazole
Staphylococcus aureus¤		
Methicillin-susceptible	Nafcillin/oxacillin with or without rifampin or gentamicin¤	Cefazolin or cefuroxime, vancomycin, clindamycin, TMP-SMZ, fluoroquinolones‡
Methicillin-resistant	Vancomycin with or without rifampin or gentamicin	Requires *in vitro* testing; TMP-SMZ
Enterobacteriaceae (coliforms: *Escherichia coli, Klebsiella, Proteus, Enterobacter*)¤	Third-generation cephalosporin with or without an aminoglycoside, carbapenems**	Aztreonam, beta-lactam - beta-lactamase inhibitor, fluoroquinolones‡
Pseudomonas aeruginosa¤	Aminoglycoside plus antipseudomonal beta-lactam: ticarcillin, piperacillin, mezlocillin, cefazidime, cefepime, aztreonam, or carbapenems**	Aminoglycoside plus ciprofloxacin, ciprofloxacin plus antipseudomonal beta-lactam
Legionella species	Macrolides† with or without rifampin, fluoroquinolones‡	Doxycycline with or without rifampin
Mycoplasma pneumoniae	Doxycycline, macrolides,† fluoroquinolones‡	
Chlamydia pneumoniae	Doxycycline, macrolides,† fluoroquinolones‡	
Chlamydia psittaci	Doxycycline	Erythromycin, chloramphenicol

Treatment of Pneumonia According to Pathogen *(continued)*

Pathogen	Preferred Antimicrobial	Alternative Antimicrobial
Nocardia species	Sulfonamide with or without minocycline or amikacin, TMP-SMZ	Imipenem with or without amikacin, doxycycline, or minocycline
Coxiella burnetii#	Tetracycline	Chloramphenicol
Influenza A	Amantadine or rimantadine	
Hantavirus	None††	

Note: TMP-SMZ = trimethoprim-sulfamethoxazole

* Intravenous: Cefazolin, cefuroxime, cefotaxime, ceftriaxone; oral: cefpodoxime, cefprozil, cefuroxime

† Erythromycin, clarithromycin, or azithromycin

‡ Levofloxacin, sparfloxacin, grepafloxacin, trovafloxacin, or another fluoroquinolone with enhanced activity against *S. pneumoniae*; ciprofloxacin is appropriate for *Legionella* species, fluoroquinolone-susceptible *S. aureus*, and most gram-negative bacilli.

¤ *In vitro* susceptibility tests are required for optimal treatment; for *Enterobacter* species, the preferred antibiotics are fluoroquinolones and carbapenems.

§ High rates of high-level penicillin resistance, susceptibility of community strains unknown, and/or patient is seriously ill

¶ Low rates of penicillin resistance in community and patient is at low risk for infection with resistant *S. pneumoniae*

** Imipenem and meropenem

Agent of Q fever

†† Provide supportive care

Empirical Antibiotic Selection for Patients With Community-Acquired Pneumonia

Outpatients

  Generally preferred: Macrolides,* fluoroquinolones,† or doxycycline

  Modifying factors

    Suspected penicillin-resistant *Streptococcus pneumoniae*: fluoroquinolones†

    Young adult (>17-40 y): Doxycycline

Hospitalized patients

  General medical ward

    Generally preferred: Beta-lactam‡ with or without a macrolide* or a fluoroquinolone† (alone)

    Alternatives: Cefuroxime with or without a macrolide* or azithromycin (alone)

  Hospitalized in the intensive care unit for serious pneumonia

    Generally preferred: Erythromycin, azithromycin, or a fluoroquinolone† plus cefotaxime, ceftriaxone, or a beta-lactam - beta-lactamase inhibitor§

  Modifying factors

    Structural disease of the lung: Antipseudomonal penicillin, a carbapenem, or cefepime plus a macrolide* or a fluoroquinolone† plus an aminoglycoside

    Penicillin allergy: A fluoroquinolone† with or without clindamycin

    Suspected aspiration: A fluoroquinolone plus either clindamycin or metronidazole or a beta-lactam - beta-lactamase inhibitor§

*Azithromycin, clarithromycin, or erythromycin

†Levofloxacin, sparfloxacin, grepafloxacin, trovafloxacin, or another fluoroquinolone with enhanced activity against *S. pneumoniae*

‡Cefotaxime, ceftriaxone, or a beta-lactam - beta-lactamase inhibitor

§Ampicillin/sulbactam, or ticarcillin/clavulanate, or piperacillin/tazobactam (for structural disease of the lung, ticarcillin/clavulanate or piperacillin)

HELICOBACTER PYLORI TREATMENT

Multiple Drug Regimens for the Treatment of *H. pylori* Infection

Drug	Dosages*	Duration of Therapy
Regimen 1†		
Bismuth subsalicylate (Pepto-Bismol®)	Two 262 mg tablets 4 times/day	2 weeks
plus		
Metronidazole (Flagyl®)	250 mg 3 or 4 times/day	2 weeks
plus		
Tetracycline (various) or amoxicillin (Amoxil®, others)	250-500 mg 4 times/day	2 weeks
plus		
Histamine H_2-receptor antagonist	Full dose‡ at bedtime	4-6 weeks
Regimen 2		
Metronidazole (Flagyl®)	500 mg 3 times/day	12-14 days
plus		
Amoxicillin (Amoxil®, others)	750 mg 3 times/day	12-14 days
plus		
Histamine H_2-receptor antagonist	Full dose† at bedtime	6-10 weeks
Regimen 3		
Bismuth subsalicylate (Pepto-Bismol®)	Two 262 mg tablets 4 times/day	2 weeks
plus		
Tetracycline (various)	500 mg 4 times/day	2 weeks
plus		
Clarithromycin (Biaxin™)	500 mg 3 times/day	2 weeks
plus		
Histamine H_2-receptor antagonist	Full dose† after evening meal	6 weeks
Regimen 4		
Omeprazole (Prilosec™)	20 mg twice daily	2 weeks
plus		
Amoxicillin (Amoxil®, others)	1 g twice daily or 500 mg 4 times/day	2 weeks
Regimen 5		
Omeprazole (Prilosec™)	20 mg twice daily	2 weeks
plus		
Clarithromycin (Biaxin™)	250 mg twice a day or 500 mg 2 or 3 times/day	2 weeks
Regimen 6		
Ranitidine bismuth citrate (Tritec™)	400 mg twice daily	4 weeks
plus		
Clarithromycin (Biaxin™)	500 mg 3 times/day	2 weeks

*All therapies are oral and begin concurrently.

†Marketed as Helidac®, a packet containing 262.4 mg bismuth subsalicylate, 250 mg metronidazole and 500 mg tetracycline; an H_2-antagonist must be purchased separately.

‡Full dose refers to the dosage used to treat acute ulcers, not to the maintenance dose.

IMPAIRED RENAL FUNCTION DOSING, ADULTS

Drug	Cl$_{cr}$ (mL/min)	Suggested Dosage Regimen	Supplement for Dialysis	
			Hemo-dialysis	Peritoneal Dialysis
Acyclovir (I.V.)	>50	5-10 mg/kg q8h	Yes	—
	25-50	5-10 mg/kg q12h		
	10-25	5-10 mg/kg q24h		
Amantadine (P.O.)	>80	100 mg bid	No	No
	60-80	200 mg/100 mg alternating daily		
	40-60	100 mg/d		
	30-40	200 mg 2 times/wk		
	20-30	100 mg 3 times/wk		
	10-20	200 mg/100 mg alternating weekly		
Amikacin (I.M., I.V.)	Individualize regimen with serum concentrations.		Yes	Yes
Aminosalicylate sodium (P.O.)	>50	150 mg/kg/day in 2-3 divided doses	—	—
	10-50	50%-75%		
	<10	50% of dose		
Amoxicillin (P.O.)	>50	250-500 mg q8h	Yes	No
	10-50	250-500 mg q12h		
	<10	250-500 mg q24h		
Amoxicillin clavulanate (P.O.)	>30	250-500 mg q6h	Yes	No
	15-30	250-500 mg q12h		
	5-15	250-500 mg q24h		
Amphotericin B (I.V.)	Usual dose: 0.3-0.7 mg/kg q24h; a 1 mg test dose may be administered over 30 minutes with vital sign monitoring over the next hour to assure no anaphylactoid reaction; then remaining full dose may be administered.			
Ampicillin (I.V.)	>50	1-2 g q4-6h	Yes	No
	10-30	1-2 g q8-12h		
	30-50	1-2 g q6-8h		
	<10	1-2 g q12-24h		
Ampicillin/sulbactam (I.V.)	≥30	1.5-3 g q6-8h	Yes	—
	15-29	1.5-3 g q12h		
	5-14	1.5-3 g q24h		
Amprenavir	—	1200 mg twice daily	—	—
Atovaquone (P.O.)*	—	750 mg tid	—	—
Azithromycin (P.O.)*	—	500 mg day 1 then 250 mg daily	—	—
Aztreonam (I.V.)	>50	500 mg-2 g q6-8h	Yes	Yes
	10-50	50% to 75% of usual dosage		
	<10	25% of usual dosage		
Bismuth (P.O.)	See specific indication. Avoid use in renal failure.			
Capreomycin (I.M.)	>100	13-15 mg/kg q24h	—	—
	80-100	10-13 mg/kg q24h		
	60-80	7-10 mg/kg q24h		
	40-60	11-14 mg/kg q48h		
	20-40	10-14 mg/kg q72h		
	<20	4-7 mg/kg q72h		
Carbenicillin (P.O.)	>50	382-764 mg q8-12h	Yes	—
	10-50	382-764 mg q12-24h		
	<10	382-764 mg q24-48h		
Cefaclor (P.O.)	>50	250-500 mg q8h	Yes	Yes
	10-50	125-500 mg q8h		
Cefadroxil (P.O.)	>25	500 mg-1 g q12h	Yes	No
	10-25	500 mg q24h		
	<10	500 mg q36h		

IMPAIRED RENAL FUNCTION DOSING, ADULTS *(Continued)*

Drug	Cl$_{cr}$ (mL/min)	Suggested Dosage Regimen	Supplement for Dialysis	
			Hemo-dialysis	Peritoneal Dialysis
Cefamandole (I.V.)	>50	1-2 g q4h	Yes	—
	25-50	1-2 g q8h		
	10-25	1 g q8h		
	<10	1 g q12h		
Cefazolin (I.V.)	>30	1-2 g q8h	Yes	No
	10-30	1 g q12h		
	<10	1 g q24h		
Cefepime (I.V.)	>60	500 mg - 2 g q12h		
	11-60	500 mg - 1 g q24h		
	<10	250-500 mg q24h		
Cefixime (P.O.)	>60	400 mg q24h	—	—
	21-60	300 mg q24h		
	≤20	200 mg q24h		
Cefmetazole (I.V.)	>50	1-2 g q12h	—	—
	30-49	1-2 g q16h		
	10-29	1-2 g q24h		
	<10	1-2 g q48h		
Cefonicid (I.M., I.V.)	>20	1 g q24h	No	No
	10-20	500 mg-1 g q48h		
	<10	250 mg-1 g q72h		
Cefoperazone (I.M., I.V.)*	—	1-2 g q8-12h	No	No
Cefotaxime (I.M., I.V.)	>50	1-2 g q6-8h	Yes	No
	10-50	1-2 g q8-12h		
	<10	1-2 g q24h		
Cefotetan (I.M., I.V.)	>30	1-2 g q12h	Yes	No
	10-30	1-2 g q24h		
	<10	1-2 g q48h		
Cefoxitin (I.M., I.V.)	>50	1-2 g q6-8h	Yes	No
	30-50	1-2 g q8-12h		
	10-30	1-2 g q12-24h		
	<10	500 mg-1 g q24-48h		
Cefpodoxime (P.O.)	>30	100-200 mg q12h	Yes	—
	<30	100-200 mg q24h		
Cefprozil (P.O.)	≥30	250-500 mg q12-24h	Yes	—
	<30	125-250 mg q12-24h		
Ceftazidime (I.V.)	>50	1-2 g q8-12h	Yes	Yes
	30-50	1 g q12h		
	15-30	1 g q24h		
	<15	500 mg-1 g q24h		
Ceftibuten (P.O.)	<50	Administer 9 mg/kg or 400 mg q24h	Yes	—
	30-49	4.5 mg/kg or 200 mg q24h		
	5-29	2.25 mg/kg or 100 mg q24h		
Ceftizoxime (I.V.)	>30	1-2 g q8-12h	Yes	—
	10-30	1 g q12h		
	<10	1 g q24h		
Ceftriaxone (I.M., I.V.)*	—	1-2 g q24h	—	—
Cefuroxime (I.V.)	>20	750 mg-1.5 g q8h	Yes	No
	10-20	750 mg q12h		
	<10	750 mg q24h		
Cephalexin (P.O.)	>40	250-500 mg q6h	Yes	Yes
	10-40	250-500 mg q8-12h		
	<10	250 mg q12-24h		
Cephalothin (I.M., I.V.)	>50	500 mg-2 g q4-6h	Yes	No
	10-50	500 mg-1 g q6h		
	<10	500 mg-1 g q8h		

Drug	Cl_{cr} (mL/min)	Suggested Dosage Regimen	Supplement for Dialysis	
			Hemo-dialysis	Peritoneal Dialysis
Cephapirin (I.M., I.V.)	>50	1 g q6h	Yes	No
	10-50	1 g q6-8h		
	<10	1 g q12h		
Cephradine (P.O.)	>50	500 mg q6h	Yes	Yes
	10-50	250 mg q6h		
	<10	125 mg q6h		
Chloramphenicol (I.V.)*	—	0.5-1 g q6h	No	No
Chloroquine (P.O.)	See monograph for dosing information		No	—
Cidofovir (I.V.)#	41-55	2 mg/kg weekly x2 doses	—	—
	30-40	1.5 mg/kg weekly x2 doses		
	20-29	1 mg/kg weekly x2 doses		
	<19	0.5 mg/kg weekly x2 doses		
Cinoxacin (P.O.)	>50	250 mg q6-12h	—	—
	20-50	250 mg bid		
	<20	250 mg/d		
Ciprofloxacin (P.O.)	>30	250 mg q12h, 500 mg q12h, or 750 mg q12h	No	No
	<30	500 mg q24h or 750 mg q24h		
Clarithromycin (P.O.)	>30	250-500 mg bid	—	—
	<30	500 mg loading dose, then 250 mg once daily or bid		
Clindamycin (I.V.)*	—	900 mg q8h	No	No
Clindamycin (P.O.)*	—	150-450 mg q6h	No	No
Clofazimine (P.O.)*	—	100 mg/d	—	—
Cloxacillin sodium (P.O.)*	—	250-500 mg q6h	—	—
Colistimethate (I.M., I.V.)	S_{cr} (mg/dL)		—	—
	0.7-1.2	100-125 mg bid-qid		
	1.3-1.5	75-115 mg bid		
	1.6-2.5	66-150 mg bid or once daily		
	2.6-4	100-150 mg q36h		
Co-trimoxazole (I.V.)†	Cl_{cr} (mL/min)		Yes	No
	>30	5 mg/kg q6-8h		
	15-30	2.5-5 mg/kg q12h		
	<15	2.5-5 mg/kg q24h		
Co-trimoxazole (P.O.)†	>50	1 DS tablet q12h	Yes	No
	30-50	1 DS tablet q12-18h		
	15-30	1 DS tablet q24h or 1 SS tablet q12h		
	<15	Not recommended		
Cycloserine (P.O.)	>50	250 mg q12h	—	—
	10-50	250 mg q24h		
	<10	250 mg q36-48h		
Dapsone (P.O.)*	—	100 mg q24h	No	No
Delavirdine (P.O.)	—	No renal dosage required	—	—
Demeclocycline (P.O.)	—	300 mg bid (do not use in renal impairment)		
Dicloxacillin (P.O.)*	—	500 mg q6h	No	—
Didanosine (P.O.)	>60	See individual dosing per body weight range	—	—
	<60	Consider dosage reduction		
Dirithromycin (P.O.)*	—	500 mg once daily for 7-14 d	—	—
Doxycycline (P.O., I.V.)	>10	100 mg q12h	No	—
	<10	100 mg q24h		
Efavirenz	—	600 mg once daily	—	—
Eflornithine (P.O.)	>60	100 mg/kg q6h	—	—
	<60	Consider dosage reduction		
Enoxacin (P.O.)	>30	400 mg bid	—	—
	<30	200 mg bid		

IMPAIRED RENAL FUNCTION DOSING, ADULTS *(Continued)*

Drug	Cl$_{cr}$ (mL/min)	Suggested Dosage Regimen	Supplement for Dialysis Hemo-dialysis	Supplement for Dialysis Peritoneal Dialysis
Erythromycin (I.V.)	>10	0.5-1 g q6h		
	<10	250-500 mg q6h	No	No
Erythromycin (P.O.)*	—	250-500 mg q6h	No	No
Erythromycin & sulfisoxazole (P.O.)	10-50	Give q8-12h	—	—
	<10	Give q12-24h		
Ethambutol (P.O.)	>50	15-25 mg/kg q24h		
	10-50	15 mg/kg q24-36h		
	<10	15 mg/kg q48h	Yes	Yes
	—	Max dose: 2.5 g/d		
Ethionamide (P.O.)	>50	250-500 mg q12h	—	—
	<50	125-250 mg q12h		
Famciclovir (P.O.)	≥60	500 mg q8h		
	40-59	500 mg q12h	—	—
	20-39	500 mg q24h		
Fluconazole (P.O., I.V.)	>50	100-400 mg loading dose x 1 then usual recommended dose q24h	Yes	—
	11-50	Loading dose then 50% of recommended dose		
Flucytosine (P.O.)	>40	12.5-37.5 mg/kg q6h		
	20-40	12.5-37.5 mg/kg q12h	Yes	—
	<20	12.5-37.5 mg/kg q24-48h		
Foscarnet (I.V.)# (induction)	(mL/min/kg)			
	≥1.6	60 mg/kg q8h		
	1.5	57 mg/kg q8h		
	1.4	53 mg/kg q8h		
	1.3	49 mg/kg q8h		
	1.2	46 mg/kg q8h		
	1.1	42 mg/kg q8h		
	1.0	39 mg/kg q8h	—	—
	0.9	35 mg/kg q8h		
	0.8	32 mg/kg q8h		
	0.7	28 mg/kg q8h		
	0.6	25 mg/kg q8h		
	0.5	21 mg/kg q8h		
	0.4	18 mg/kg q8h		
Fosfomycin	Cl$_{cr}$ (mL/min)			
	—	400-600 mg qd	—	—
Ganciclovir (I.V.)	>80	5 mg/kg q12h		
	50-80	2.5 mg/kg q12h	—	—
	25-50	2.5 mg/kg q24h		
	<25	1.25 mg/kg q24h		
Gentamicin (I.M., I.V.)	Individualize regimen with serum concentrations		Yes	Yes
Grepafloxacin (P.O.)	—	1 sachet once daily	—	—
Imipenem/cilastatin (I.V.)	>70	500 mg q6h		
	30-70	500 mg q8h	Yes	—
	20-30	500 mg q12h		
	0-20	250 mg q12h		
Isoniazid (P.O., I.V.)*	—	300 mg q24h	Yes	Yes
Itraconazole (P.O.)*	—	200 mg once daily	—	—
Kanamycin	Avoid I.V. administration		—	—
Ketoconazole (P.O.)*	—	200 mg q24h	No	No

Drug	Cl_{cr} (mL/min)	Suggested Dosage Regimen	Supplement for Dialysis	
			Hemo-dialysis	Peritoneal Dialysis
Lamivudine (P.O.)	≥50	150 mg twice daily	—	—
	30-49	150 mg once daily		
	15-29	150 mg first dose then 100 mg once daily		
	5-14	150 mg first dose then 50 mg once daily		
	<5	50 mg first dose then 25 mg once daily		
Levofloxacin (P.O., I.V.)	>50	250-500 mg q24h	—	—
	20-49	500 mg 1st dose, then 250 mg q24h		
	10-19	500 mg 1st dose, then 250 mg q48h		
Lomefloxacin (P.O.)	>40	400 mg q24h	—	—
	≤40	400 mg 1st dose, then 200 mg once daily		
Loracarbef (P.O.)	>50	200-400 mg q12h	—	—
	10-49	200-400 mg q24h		
	<10	200-400 mg q3-5d		
Mefloquine (P.O.)*	—	See individual dosing for prophylaxis vs treatment	—	—
Meropenem (I.V.)	26-50	1 g q12h	—	—
	10-25	500 mg q12h		
	<10	500 mg q24 h		
Methenamine (P.O.)	<50	Avoid use	—	—
Methicillin (I.M., I.V.)	>50	1-2 g q4-6h	No	No
	10-50	1-2 g q6-8h		
	<10	1-2 g q8-12h		
Metronidazole (P.O., I.V.)	>10	250-500 mg q6-8h	Yes	—
	<10	250-500 mg q8-12h		
Mezlocillin (I.M., I.V.)	>30	3-4 g q4-6h	No	No
	10-30	1-3 g q6-8h		
	<10	3 g q8h		
Miconazole (I.V.)*	—	400-1200 mg q8h	No	No
Minocycline (P.O., I.V.)	—	No renal dosage required	No	No
Nafcillin sodium (I.M., I.V.)*	—	1-2 g q4-6h	No	No
Nalidixic acid (P.O.)	<50	Avoid use	—	—
Nelfinavir (P.O.)	—	No renal dosage required	—	—
Neomycin sulfate (P.O.)	Avoid I.V. administration		—	—
Netilmicin (I.M., I.V.)	Individualize regimen with serum concentrations		Yes	Yes
Nevirapine	—	200 mg twice daily	—	—
Nitrofurantoin (P.O.)	>50	50-100 mg q6h	—	—
	<50	Avoid use		
Norfloxacin (P.O.)	>30	400 mg q12h	No	—
	<30	400 mg q24h		
Ofloxacin (P.O., I.V.)	>50	200-400 mg q12h	—	—
	10-50	200-400 mg q24h		
	<10	100-200 mg q24h		
Oxacillin (I.V.)*	—	1-2 g q4-6h	No	—
Oxytetracycline (P.O.)	>10	250-500 mg q6h	—	—
	<10	Avoid use		
Palivizumab (I.V.)	—	No renal dosage required	—	—
Penicillin G (I.V.)	>50	2-4 million units q2-4h	Yes	—
	10-50	1-2 million units q4-6h		
	<10	1-2 million units q8-12h or 0.5-1 million units q4-6h		
Penicillin V potassium (P.O.)	>10	250-500 mg q6h	Yes	—
	<10	250 mg q6h		

IMPAIRED RENAL FUNCTION DOSING, ADULTS *(Continued)*

Drug	Cl$_{cr}$ (mL/min)	Suggested Dosage Regimen	Supplement for Dialysis Hemo-dialysis	Supplement for Dialysis Peritoneal Dialysis
Pentamidine (I.V.)	>50	4 mg/kg q24h		
	10-50	4 mg/kg q24-36h	—	—
	<10	4 mg/kg q48h		
Piperacillin (I.V.)	>40	3-4 g q4-6h		
	20-40	3-4 g q8h	Yes	—
	<20	3-4 g q12h		
Piperacillin/tazobactam (I.V.)	>40	3.375 g q6h		
	20-40	2.25 g q6h	Yes	Yes
	<20	2.25 g q8h		
Polymyxin B		Avoid I.V. administration	—	—
Pyrazinamide (P.O.)	—	15-30 mg/kg q24h	—	—
	—	Max dose: 2 g/d		
Pyrimethamine (P.O.)*	—	100 mg q24h	—	—
Quinacrine (P.O.)	—	See individual dosing per disease	—	—
Quinidine*	—	See monograph	Yes	Yes
Quinine (P.O.)	>50	650 mg q6-8h		
	10-50	650 mg q8-12h	Yes	No
	<10	650 mg q24h		
Rifabutin*	—	300 mg/d	—	—
Rifampin (P.O., I.V.)*	—	600 mg/d	No	—
Rifapentine	—	No data on renal adjustment	—	—
Rimantadine (P.O.)	>10	100 mg q12h		
	<10	100 mg q24h	—	—
Ritonavir	—	600 mg twice daily	—	—
Saquinavir				
Fortovase®	—	1200 mg 3 times/day in combination with a nucleoside analog	—	—
Invirase®	—	600 mg 3 times/day in combination with a nucleoside analog	—	—
Sparfloxacin (P.O.)	>50	400 mg 1st day, then 200 mg qd		
	<50	400 mg 1st day, then 200 mg qod	—	—
Spectinomycin (I.M.)*	—	2-4 g q24h	Yes	Yes
Stavudine (P.O.) <60 kg	>50	30 mg q12 h		
	26-50	15 mg q12h	—	—
	10-25	15 mg q24h		
Stavudine (P.O.) ≥60 kg	>50	40 mg q12h		
	26-50	20 mg q12h	—	—
	10-25	20 mg q24h		
Streptomycin sulfate (I.M., I.V.)	—	See individual dosing per disease	Yes	—
Sulfadiazine (P.O.)*	—	1-2 g q6h	—	—
Sulfamethoxazole (P.O.)	>50	1 g q12h		
	10-50	1 g q12-24h	Yes	No
	<10	1 g q24h		
Sulfisoxazole (P.O.)	>50	1-2 g q6h		
	10-50	1 g q8-12h	Yes	No
	<10	1 g q12-24h		
Terbinafine	—	No renal dosage required	—	—
Tetracycline (P.O.)	>50	250-500 mg q6-12h		
	10-50	250-500 mg q12-24h	No	No
	<10	250-500 mg q24h		
Thiabendazole (P.O.)	—	See individual dosing per disease	—	—

Drug	Cl$_{cr}$ (mL/min)	Suggested Dosage Regimen	Supplement for Dialysis	
			Hemo-dialysis	Peritoneal Dialysis
Ticarcillin/clavulanate (I.V.)	>60	3.1 g q4-6h	Yes	Yes
	30-60	3.1 g q8h		
	10-30	2 g q8h or 3.1 g q12h		
Ticarcillin (I.M., I.V.)	>60	3 g q4h	Yes	No
	30-60	2 g q4h or 3.1 q8h		
	10-30	2 g q8h or 3.1 q12h		
	<10	2 g q12h		
Tobramycin	Individualize regimen with serum concentrations		Yes	Yes
Trimethoprim (P.O.)	>30	100 mg q12h	Yes	—
	15-30	50 mg q12h		
Trovafloxacin	—	See monograph	—	—
Valacyclovir (P.O.) (herpes zoster)	≥50	1 g q8h	—	—
	30-49	1 g q12h		
	10-29	1 g q24h		
	<10	500 mg q24h		
Valacyclovir (P.O.) (genital herpes)	≥50	500 mg q12h	—	—
	30-49	500 mg q12h		
	10-29	500 mg q24h		
	<10	500 mg q24h		
Vancomycin (I.V.)	Individualize dosing with serum concentrations; 1 g q12h is usual starting dose in patients with normal renal function; see monograph			
Vancomycin (P.O.)*	—	125-250 mg q6h	—	—
Zalcitabine (P.O.)	>40	0.75 mg q8h	—	—
	10-40	0.75 mg q12h		
	<10	0.75 mg q24h		
Zidovudine	—	100 mg 5 times/d	—	—

*No renal dose adjustment necessary.
†All doses based on trimethoprim.
#See monograph for maintenance dosing.

INTERPRETATION OF GRAM'S STAIN RESULTS GUIDELINES

These guidelines are not definitive but presumptive for the identification of organisms on Gram's stain. Treatment will depend on the quality of the specimen and appropriate clinical evaluation.

Gram-Negative Bacilli (GNB)	**Example**
Enterobacteriaceae	*Escherichia coli*
	Serratia sp
	Klebsiella sp
	Enterobacter sp
	Citrobacter sp
Nonfermentative GNB	*Pseudomonas aeruginosa*
	Stenotrophomonas maltophilia
	Haemophilus influenzae
	Bacteroides fragilis group
If fusiform (long and pointed)	*Fusobacterium* sp
	Capnocytophaga sp
Gram-Negative Cocci (GNC)	
Diplococci, pairs	*Neisseria meningitidis*
	Neisseria gonorrhoeae
	Moraxella (Branhamella) catarrhalis
Coccobacilli	*Acinetobacter* sp
Gram-Positive Bacilli (GPB)	
Diphtheroids (small pleomorphic)	*Corynebacterium* sp
	Propionibacterium
Large, with spores	*Clostridium* sp
	Bacillus sp
Branching, beaded, rods	*Nocardia* sp
	Actinomyces sp
Other	*Listeria* sp
	Lactobacillus sp
Gram-Positive Cocci (GPC)	
Pairs, chains, clusters	*Staphylococcus* sp
	Streptococcus sp
	Enterococcus sp
Pairs, lancet-shaped	*Streptococcus pneumoniae*

KEY CHARACTERISTICS OF SELECTED BACTERIA

Gram-Negative Bacilli (GNB)	**Example**
Lactose-positive	*Escherichia coli* *Klebsiella pneumoniae* *Enterobacter* sp* *Citrobacter* sp*
Lactose-negative/ oxidase-negative	*Proteus mirabilis:* indole-negative *Proteus vulgaris:* indole-positive *Providencia* sp *Morganella morganii* *Serratia* sp† *Salmonella* sp *Shigella* sp *Acinetobacter* sp *Stenotrophomonas maltophilia*
Lactose-negative/ oxidase-positive	*Pseudomonas aeruginosa* *Aeromonas hydrophila* (may be lactose-positive) Other *Pseudomonas* sp *Moraxella* sp‡ *Alcaligenes* sp *Flavobacterium* sp
Other	*Haemophilus influenzae* (coccobacillus)

Gram-Positive Bacilli (GPB)	
Often blood culture contaminants	Diphtheroids (may be *Corynebacterium* sp)
Resistant to many agents except vancomycin	*Corynebacterium jeikeium*
Anaerobic diphtheroids	*Propionibacterium acnes*
Bacillus sp	*Bacillus cereus, B. subtilis*
CSF, blood	*Listeria monocytogenes*
Vaginal flora, rarely blood	*Lactobacillus* sp
Branching, beaded; partial acid-fast positive	*Nocardia* sp
Rapidly growing mycobacteria	*Mycobacterium fortuitum* *Mycobacterium chelonei*

Gram-Positive Cocci (GPC)	
Catalase-positive	*Staphylococcus* sp
Catalase-negative	*Streptococcus* sp (chains) *Micrococcus* sp (usually insignificant)
Coagulase-positive	*Staphylococcus aureus*
Coagulase-negative	Coagulase-negative *Staphylococcus* (CNS)
Bloods	*Staphylococcus epidermidis* or CNS
Urine	*Staphylococcus saprophyticus* (CNS)

KEY CHARACTERISTICS OF SELECTED BACTERIA
(Continued)

Fungi

Yeast

> *Candida* sp (germ tube positive = *C. albicans*)
> *Cryptococcus* sp (no pseudohyphae)
> *C. neoformans*
> *Torulopsis glabrata*
> *Trichosporon* sp
> *Rhodotorula, Saccharomyces* sp

Molds

Sparsely septate hyphae

> Zygomycetes (eg, *Rhizopus* sp and *Mucor*)

Septate hyphae
brown pigment

> Phaeohyphomycetes, for example,
> *Bipolaris* sp
> *Exserohilum* sp
> *Alternaria* sp
> *Curvularia* sp

Nonpigmented (hyaline)

> Hyalophomycetes, for example,
> *Aspergillus* sp (*A. fumigatus, A. flavus*)
> *Fusarium* sp
> *Penicillium* sp
> *Paecilomyces* sp
> Dermatophytes

Thermally dimorphic (yeast in tissue; mold *in vitro*)

> *Histoplasma capsulatum* (slow growing)
> *Blastomyces dermatitidis*
> *Coccidioides immitis*
> *Sporothrix schenckii*
> *Paracoccidioides brasiliensis*

Anaerobes

Gram-positive bacilli

> *Propionibacterium acnes*
> *Clostridium* sp (spores)
> *Actinomyces* sp (branching, filamentous)
> *Lactobacillus* sp
> *Eubacterium* sp
> *Bifidobacterium* sp

Gram-positive cocci

> *Peptostreptococcus* sp

Gram-negative bacilli

> *Bacteroides* sp (*B. fragilis*)
> *Fusobacterium* sp

Gram-negative cocci

> *Veillonella* sp

Most Common Blood Culture Contaminants

Coagulase-negative staphylococci

Alpha-hemolytic streptococci

Diphtheroids

Micrococcus sp

Lactobacillus

Propionibacterium sp

Bacillus sp

*May be lactose-negative.

†May produce red pigment and appear lactose-positive initially.

‡May be either bacillary or coccoid.

NEUTROPENIC FEVER GUIDELINES

(From Hughes WT, Armstrong D, Bodey GP, et al, "1997 Guidelines for the Use of Antimicrobial Agents in Neutropenic Patients With Unexplained Fever," *Clin Infect Dis*, 1997, 25(3):551-73.

1997 GUIDELINES FOR THE USE OF ANTIMICROBIAL AGENTS IN NEUTROPENIC PATIENTS WITH UNEXPLAINED FEVER

EXECUTIVE SUMMARY

Definitions

Fever: A single oral temperature of >38.3°C (101°F) or ≥38.0°C (100.4°F) over at least 1 hour.

Neutropenia: Neutrophil count <500/mm^3 or <1000/mm^3 with predicted decline to ≤500/mm^3

Evaluation: Cultures of blood (peripheral and catheter), lesions, and diarrheal stools; chest radiograph; complete blood count; determination of levels of transaminases, sodium, potassium, creatinine, and blood urea nitrogen. Other tests as indicated.

Guidelines for Treatment

Initial antibiotic therapy: One of three regimens:

- If vancomycin is needed (criteria given):
  Vancomycin and ceftazidime

- If vancomycin is not needed:
  Monotherapy: Ceftazidime or imipenem (cefepime or meropenem)
  or
  Duotherapy: Aminoglycoside and antipseudomonal β-lactam

Afebrile within first 3 days of treatment:

- If no etiology identified:
  Low risk (defined): Change to oral antibiotic (cefixime or quinolone)
  High risk (defined): Continue same antibiotics

- If etiology identified, adjust to most appropriate treatment

Persistent fever during first 3 days of treatment:

- Reassess on day 4 or 5
  - If no change, continue antibiotics; consider stopping vancomycin if cultures are negative
  - If progressive disease, change antibiotics
  - If febrile on days 5-7, add amphotericin B with or without antibiotic changes

Duration of antibiotic therapy:

Afebrile by day 3:
- If absolute neutrophil count ≥500/mm^3 by day 7, stop after 7 days
- If absolute neutrophil count <500/mm^3 by day 7:
  Low risk: Stop when afebrile for 5-7 days
  High risk: Continue antibiotics

Persistent fever:
- If absolute neutrophil count ≥500/mm^3, stop after 4-5 days; if absolute count is >500/mm^3, reassess
- If absolute neutrophil count <500/mm^3, continue for 2 weeks, reassess and stop if no disease sites

Use of antivirals: Not routine

Use of colony-stimulating factors: Not routine; consider in certain cases with predicted worsening of course (defined)

Antibiotic prophylaxis in afebrile neutropenic patients:

- Not routine, except for *Pneumocystis carinii* pneumonitis prophylaxis

Economic issues: Suggestions for cost containment

OCCUPATIONAL EXPOSURE TO BLOODBORNE PATHOGENS (UNIVERSAL PRECAUTIONS)

Overview and Regulatory Considerations

Every healthcare employee, from nurse to housekeeper, has some (albeit small) risk of exposure to HIV and other viral agents such as hepatitis B and Jakob-Creutzfeldt agent. The incidence of HIV-1 transmission associated with a percutaneous exposure to blood from an HIV-1 infected patient is approximately 0.3% per exposure.[1] In 1989, it was estimated that 12,000 United States healthcare workers acquired hepatitis B annually.[2] An understanding of the appropriate procedures, responsibilities, and risks inherent in the collection and handling of patient specimens is necessary for safe practice and is required by Occupational Safety and Health Administration (OSHA) regulations.

The Occupational Safety and Health Administration published its "Final Rule on Occupational Exposure to Bloodborne Pathogens" in the Federal Register on December 6, 1991. OSHA has chosen to follow the Center for Disease Control (CDC) definition of universal precautions. The Final Rule provides full legal force to universal precautions and requires employers and employees to treat blood and certain body fluids as if they were infectious. The Final Rule mandates that healthcare workers must avoid parenteral contact and must avoid splattering blood or other potentially infectious material on their skin, hair, eyes, mouth, mucous membranes, or on their personal clothing. Hazard abatement strategies must be used to protect the workers. Such plans typically include, but are not limited to, the following:

- safe handling of sharp items ("sharps") and disposal of such into puncture resistant containers
- gloves required for employees handling items soiled with blood or equipment contaminated by blood or other body fluids
- provisions of protective clothing when more extensive contact with blood or body fluids may be anticipated (eg, surgery, autopsy, or deliveries)
- resuscitation equipment to reduce necessity for mouth to mouth resuscitation
- restriction of HIV- or hepatitis B-exposed employees to noninvasive procedures

OSHA has specifically defined the following terms: **Occupational exposure** means reasonably anticipated skin, eye mucous membrane, or parenteral contact with blood or other potentially infectious materials that may result from the performance of an employee's duties. **Other potentially infectious materials** are human body fluids including semen, vaginal secretions, cerebrospinal fluid, synovial fluid, pleural fluid, pericardial fluid, peritoneal fluid, amniotic fluid, saliva in dental procedures, and body fluids that are visibly contaminated with blood, and all body fluids in situations where it is difficult or impossible to differentiate between body fluids; any unfixed tissue or organ (other than intact skin) from a human (living or dead); and HIV-containing cell or tissue cultures, organ cultures, and HIV- or HBV-containing culture medium or other solutions, and blood, organs, or other tissues from experimental animals infected with HIV or HBV. An **exposure incident** involves specific eye, mouth, other mucous membrane, nonintact skin, or parenteral contact with blood or other potentially infectious materials that results from the performance of an employee's duties.[3] It is important to understand that some exposures may go unrecognized despite the strictest precautions.

A written Exposure Control Plan is required. Employers must provide copies of the plan to employees and to OSHA upon request. Compliance with OSHA rules may be accomplished by the following methods.

- **Universal precautions (UPs)** means that all human blood and certain body fluids are treated as if known to be infectious for HIV, HBV, and other bloodborne pathogens. UPs do not apply to feces, nasal secretions, saliva, sputum, sweat, tears, urine, or vomitus unless they contain visible blood.

- **Engineering controls (ECs)** are physical devices which reduce or remove hazards from the workplace by eliminating or minimizing hazards or by isolating the worker from exposure. Engineering control devices include sharps disposal containers, self-resheathing syringes, etc.
- **Work practice controls (WPCs)** are practices and procedures that reduce the likelihood of exposure to hazards by altering the way in which a task is performed. Specific examples are the prohibition of two-handed recapping of needles, prohibition of storing food alongside potentially contaminated material, discouragement of pipetting fluids by mouth, encouraging handwashing after removal of gloves, safe handling of contaminated sharps, and appropriate use of sharps containers.
- **Personal protective equipment (PPE)** is specialized clothing or equipment worn to provide protection from occupational exposure. PPE includes gloves, gowns, laboratory coats (the type and characteristics will depend upon the task and degree of exposure anticipated), face shields or masks, and eye protection. Surgical caps or hoods and/or shoe covers or boots are required in instances in which gross contamination can reasonably be anticipated (eg, autopsies, orthopedic surgery). If PPE is penetrated by blood or any contaminated material, the item must be removed immediately or as soon as feasible. **The employer must provide and launder or dispose of all PPE at no cost to the employee.** Gloves must be worn when there is a reasonable anticipation of hand contact with potentially infectious material, including a patient's mucous membranes or nonintact skin. Disposable gloves must be changed as soon as possible after they become torn or punctured. Hands must be washed after gloves are removed. OSHA has revised the PPE standards, effective July 5, 1994, to include the requirement that the employer certify in writing that it has conducted a hazard assessment of the workplace to determine whether hazards are present that will necessitate the use of PPE. Also, verification that the employee has received and understood the PPE training is required.[4]

Housekeeping protocols: OSHA requires that all bins, cans, and similar receptacles, intended for reuse which have a reasonable likelihood for becoming contaminated, be inspected and decontaminated immediately or as soon as feasible upon visible contamination and on a regularly scheduled basis. Broken glass that may be contaminated must not be picked up directly with the hands. Mechanical means (eg, brush, dust pan, tongs, or forceps) must be used. Broken glass must be placed in a proper sharps container.

Employers are responsible for teaching appropriate clean-up procedures for the work area and personal protective equipment. A 1:10 dilution of household bleach is a popular and effective disinfectant. It is prudent for employers to maintain signatures or initials of employees who have been properly educated. If one does not have written proof of education of universal precautions teaching, then by OSHA standards, such education never happened.

Pre-exposure and postexposure protocols: OSHA's Final Rule includes the provision that employees, who are exposed to contamination, be offered the hepatitis B vaccine at no cost to the employee. Employees may decline; however, a declination form must be signed. The employee must be offered free vaccine if he/she changes his/her mind. Vaccination to prevent the transmission of hepatitis B in the healthcare setting is widely regarded as sound practice.[5] In the event of exposure, a confidential medical evaluation and follow-up must be offered at no cost to the employee. Follow-up must include collection and testing of blood from the source individual for HBV and HIV if permitted by state law if a blood sample is available. If a postexposure specimen must be specially drawn, the individual's consent is usually required. Some states may not require consent for testing of patient blood after accidental exposure. One must refer to state and/or local guidelines for proper guidance.

The employee follow-up must also include appropriate postexposure prophylaxis, counseling, and evaluation of reported illnesses. The employee has the right to decline baseline blood collection and/or testing. If the employee gives consent for the collection but not the testing, the sample must be preserved for 90 days in the event that the employee changes his/her mind within that time. Confidentiality related to blood testing must be ensured. **The employer does not have the right**

OCCUPATIONAL EXPOSURE TO BLOODBORNE PATHOGENS
(UNIVERSAL PRECAUTIONS) *(Continued)*

to know the results of the testing of either the source individual or the exposed employee.[3]

The Management of Occupational Exposure to HIV in the Workplace[6]

1. Likelihood of transmission of HIV-1 from occupational exposure is 0.2% per parenteral exposure (eg, needlestick) to blood from HIV-infected patients.

2. Factors that increase risk for occupational transmission include advanced stages of HIV in source patient, hollow bore needle puncture, a poor state of health, or inexperience of healthcare worker (HCW).

3. Immediate actions an exposed healthcare worker should take include aggressive first aid at the puncture site (eg, scrubbing site with povodone-iodine solution for 10 minutes) or at mucus membrane site (eg, saline irrigation of eye for 15 minutes), then immediate reporting to the hospital's occupational medical service. The authors indicate that there is no direct evidence for the efficacy of their recommendations. Other institutions suggest rigorous scrubbing with soap.

4. After first aid is initiated, the healthcare worker should report exposure to a supervisor and to the institution's occupational medical service for evaluation.

5. Occupational medicine should perform a thorough investigation including identifying the HIV and hepatitis B status of the source, type of exposure, volume of innoculum, timing of exposure, extent of injury, appropriateness of first aid, as well as psychological status of the healthcare worker. HIV serologies should be performed on the healthcare worker. HIV risk counselling should begin at this point.

6. All parenteral exposures should be treated equally until they can be evaluated by the occupational medicine service, who will then determine the actual risk of exposure. Follow-up counselling sessions may be necessary.

7. Although the data are not clear, antiviral prophylaxis may be offered to healthcare workers who are parenterally or mucous membrane exposed. If used, antiretroviral prophylaxis should be initiated within 1-2 hours after exposure.

8. Counselling regarding risk of exposure, antiviral prophylaxis, plans for follow up, exposure prevention, sexual activity, and providing emotional support and response to concerns are necessary to support the exposed healthcare worker. Follow-up should consist of periodic serologic evaluation and blood chemistries and counts if antiretroviral prophylaxis is initiated. Additional information should be provided to healthcare workers who are pregnant or planning to become pregnant.

See also Postexposure Prophylaxis for Hepatitis B in the Appendix.

Hazardous Communication

Communication regarding the dangers of bloodborne infections through the use of labels, signs, information, and education is required. Storage locations (eg, refrigerators and freezers, waste containers) that are used to store, dispose of, transport, or ship blood or other potentially infectious materials require labels. The label background must be red or bright orange with the biohazard design and the word biohazard in a contrasting color. The label must be part of the container or affixed to the container by permanent means.

Education provided by a qualified and knowledgeable instructor is mandated. The sessions for employees must include:[4]

- accessible copies of the regulation
- general epidemiology of bloodborne diseases
- modes of bloodborne pathogen transmission
- an explanation of the exposure control plan and a means to obtain copies of the written plan
- an explanation of the tasks and activities that may involve exposure
- the use of exposure prevention methods and their limitations (eg, engineering controls, work practices, personal protective equipment)

- information on the types, proper use, location, removal, handling, decontamination, and disposal of personal protective equipment)
- an explanation of the basis for selection of personal protective equipment
- information on the HBV vaccine, including information on its efficacy, safety, and method of administration and the benefits of being vaccinated (ie, the employee must understand that the vaccine and vaccination will be offered free of charge)
- information on the appropriate actions to take and persons to contact in an emergency involving exposure to blood or other potentially infectious materials
- an explanation of the procedure to follow if an exposure incident occurs, including the method of reporting the incident
- information on the postexposure evaluation and follow-up that the employer is required to provide for the employee following an exposure incident
- an explanation of the signs, labels, and color coding
- an interactive question-and-answer period

Record Keeping

The OSHA Final Rule requires that the employer maintain both education and medical records. The medical records must be kept confidential and be maintained for the duration of employment plus 30 years. They must contain a copy of the employee's HBV vaccination status and postexposure incident information. Education records must be maintained for 3 years from the date the program was given.

OSHA has the authority to conduct inspections without notice. Penalties for cited violation may be assessed as follows.

Serious violations. In this situation, there is a substantial probability of death or serious physical harm, and the employer knew, or should have known, of the hazard. A violation of this type carries a mandatory penalty of up to $7000 for each violation.

Other-than-serious violations. The violation is unlikely to result in death or serious physical harm. This type of violation carries a discretionary penalty of up to $7000 for each violation.

Willful violations. These are violations committed knowingly or intentionally by the employer and have penalties of up to $70,000 per violation with a minimum of $5000 per violation. If an employee dies as a result of a willful violation, the responsible party, if convicted, may receive a personal fine of up to $250,000 and/or a 6-month jail term. A corporation may be fined $500,000.

Large fines frequently follow visits to laboratories, physicians' offices, and healthcare facilities by OSHA Compliance Safety and Health Offices (CSHOS). Regulations are vigorously enforced. A working knowledge of the final rule and implementation of appropriate policies and practices is imperative for all those involved in the collection and analysis of medical specimens.

Effectiveness of universal precautions in averting exposure to potentially infectious materials has been documented.[7] Compliance with appropriate rules, procedures, and policies, including reporting exposure incidents, is a matter of personal professionalism and prudent self-preservation.

Footnotes

1. Henderson DK, Fahey BJ, Willy M, et al, "Risk for Occupational Transmission of Human Immunodeficiency Virus Type 1 (HIV-1) Associated With Clinical Exposures. A Prospective Evaluation," *Ann Intern Med*, 1990, 113(10):740-6.
2. Niu MT and Margolis HS, "Moving Into a New Era of Government Regulation: Provisions for Hepatitis B Vaccine in the Workplace, *Clin Lab Manage Rev*, 1989, 3:336-40.
3. Bruning LM, "The Bloodborne Pathogens Final Rule — Understanding the Regulation," *AORN Journal*, 1993, 57(2):439-40.
4. "Rules and Regulations," *Federal Register*, 1994, 59(66):16360-3.
5. Schaffner W, Gardner P, and Gross PA, "Hepatitis B Immunization Strategies: Expanding the Target," *Ann Intern Med*, 1993, 118(4):308-9.
6. Fahey BJ, Beekmann SE, Schmitt JM, et al, "Managing Occupational Exposures to HIV-1 in the Healthcare Workplace," *Infect Control Hosp Epidemiol*, 1993, 14(7):405-12.
7. Wong ES, Stotka JL, Chinchilli VM, et al, "Are Universal Precautions Effective in Reducing the Number of Occupational Exposures Among Healthcare Workers?" *JAMA*, 1991, 265:1123-8.

OCCUPATIONAL EXPOSURE TO BLOODBORNE PATHOGENS
(UNIVERSAL PRECAUTIONS) *(Continued)*

References

Buehler JW and Ward JW, "A New Definition for AIDS Surveillance," *Ann Intern Med*, 1993, 118(5):390-2.

Brown JW and Blackwell H, "Complying With the New OSHA Regs, Part 1: Teaching Your Staff About Biosafety," *MLO*, 1992, 24(4)24-8. Part 2: "Safety Protocols No Lab Can Ignore," 1992, 24(5):27-9. Part 3: "Compiling Employee Safety Records That Will Satisfy OSHA," 1992, 24(6):45-8.

Department of Labor, Occupational Safety and Health Administration, "Occupational Exposure to Bloodborne Pathogens; Final Rule (29 CFR Part 1910.1030),"*Federal Register*, December 6, 1991, 64004-182.

Gold JW, "HIV-1 Infection: Diagnosis and Management," *Med Clin North Am*, 1992, 76(1):1-18.

"Hepatitis B Virus: A Comprehensive Strategy for Eliminating Transmission in the United States Through Universal Childhood Vaccination," *MMWR Morb Mortal Wkly Rep*, 1991, 40(RR-13):1-25.

"Mortality Attributable to HIV Infection/AIDS — United States", *MMWR Morb Mortal Wkly Rep*, 1991, 40(3):41-4.

National Committee for Clinical Laboratory Standards, "Protection of Laboratory Workers From Infectious Disease Transmitted by Blood, Body Fluids, and Tissue," NCCLS Document M29-T, Villanova, PA: NCCLS, 1989, 9(1).

"Nosocomial Transmission of Hepatitis B Virus Associated With a Spring-Loaded Fingerstick Device — California," *MMWR Morb Mortal Wkly Rep*, 1990, 39(35):610-3.

Polish LB, Shapiro CN, Bauer F, et al, "Nosocomial Transmission of Hepatitis B Virus Associated With the Use of a Spring-Loaded Fingerstick Device," *N Engl J Med*, 1992, 326(11):721-5.

"Recommendations for Preventing Transmission of Human Immunodeficiency Virus and Hepatitis B Virus to Patients During Exposure-Prone Invasive Procedures," *MMWR Morb Mortal Wkly Rep*, 1991, 40(RR-8):1-9.

"Update: Acquired Immunodeficiency Syndrome — United States," *MMWR Morb Mortal Wkly Rep*, 1992, 41(26):463-8.

"Update: Transmission of HIV Infection During an Invasive Dental Procedure — Florida," *MMWR Morb Mortal Wkly Rep*, 1991, 40(2):21-7, 33.

"Update: Universal Precautions for Prevention of Transmission of Human Immunodeficiency Virus, Hepatitis B Virus, and Other Bloodborne Pathogens in Healthcare Settings," *MMWR Morb Mortal Wkly Rep*, 1988, 37(24):377-82, 387-8.

PHARMACOKINETICS, ADULTS

Drug	Half-life (h) Normal Renal Function	Half-life (h) Impaired Renal Function	V_d (L/kg)	Protein Binding (%)	Time to Peak (h)	Bioavail-ability (%)
Acyclovir	3	20	0.7-0.8	15-30	P.O.: 1.7	20
Albendazole	8.5			70		
Amantadine	10-28	7-10 d	4-5	60	1-4	90
Amikacin sulfate	1.6-96	17-150	0.22-0.29	<5	I.M.: 0.75-2	
Amoxicillin	0.7-1.4	7-21	0.26	15-25	2	85
Amphotericin B	15-48		4	90		
Ampicillin	1-1.8	7-20	0.17-0.31	8-20	I.M.: 1 P.O.: 2	50
Ampicillin/sulbactam	1	5-9		20-40		
Amprenavir				90		
Atovaquone	2.9 d			>99.9	1-8	~30
Azithromycin	35-40		31.1	7-51	3-4	37
Aztreonam	1.3-2.6	6-8	0.1-0.2	50-60	I.M.: 0.6-1.3	
Capreomycin	4-6	55			I.M.: 1-2	
Carbenicillin	1.5	10-20	0.12-0.2	30-60	1-3	30-50
Cefaclor	0.5-1	3	0.34-0.35	25	0.5-1	95
Cefadroxil	1-2	20-24	0.31	20	1.2-1.5	95
Cefamandole	0.5-1	3-18	0.16-0.25	75		
Cefazolin	1.5-2.4	40-70	0.13-0.22	80		
Cefepime	2-2.3	Up to 21	0.26	26	I.M.: 1.4-1.8	100
Cefixime	3-4	11.5	0.11	65-70	2-6	45
Cefmetazole	1.2-1.8		0.3	65	I.M.: 1.5	I.M.: 70
Cefonicid	3.5-4.5	17-56	0.11-0.13	90-98	I.M.: 1.3	
Cefoperazone	1.6-2.5	2.9	0.14-0.2	90		
Cefotaxime	1-1.5	15	0.15-0.55	37		
Cefotetan	3-5	13-25	0.15	85		
Cefoxitin	0.75-1	13-25	0.13-0.39	41-75		
Cefpodoxime	2-3	9.8	0.46	21-29	1	40-60
Cefprozil	1-2	5.2		36	1-2	95
Ceftazidime	1-2	13-25	0.28	17		
Ceftibuten			0.21	65		
Ceftizoxime	1.6	25	0.26-0.42	28-50		
Ceftriaxone	5-9	12-24	0.12-0.14	85-95		
Cefuroxime	1-2	17	0.13-1.8	33	P.O.: 3	52
Cephalexin	0.5-1.2	20-40	0.26	10-15	1	95
Cephalothin	0.5-1	20-40	0.18-0.33	15		
Cephapirin	0.5-1	2.4-2.7	45-60	0.5		
Cephradine	1-2	6-15	0.25-0.33	10	1-2	95
Chloramphenicol	1.6-3.3	3-7	0.6-1	60	P.O.: 0.5-3	80
Chloroquine phosphate	3-5 d	5-50 d	800*	50-65	1-2	89
Cidofovir	2.6		0.4	6		
Cinoxacin	1.5	>10	0.24-0.26	60-80	2-3	30-40
Ciprofloxacin	3-5	6-9	2.1	40	P.O.: 0.5-2	70-80
Clarithromycin	3-7	22		65-75	2-4	55
Clindamycin	2-3	3-5	0.6-1.2	60-95	P.O.: 1-3	90
Clofazimine	70 d				1-6	45-62
Cloxacillin	0.5-1.5	1	0.15-0.2	85-94	0.5-2	
Co-trimoxazole SMZ	9	20-50	0.21	60-70	P.O.: 2-4	90-100
Co-trimoxazole TMP	6-17	20-40	1.2-2	40-70	P.O.: 1-4	90-100
Cycloserine	10		0.11-0.26		3-4	
Delavirdine	2-11			98	1	85

PHARMACOKINETICS, ADULTS *(Continued)*

Drug	Half-life (h) Normal Renal Function	Half-life (h) Impaired Renal Function	V_d (L/kg)	Protein Binding (%)	Time to Peak (h)	Bioavail-ability (%)
Demeclocycline	10-17	40-60	1.79	91	3-6	41-50
Dicloxacillin	0.6-0.8	1-2	0.13-0.19	91-98	0.5-2	80
Didanosine	1.3-1.6		0.3-1.3	<5	0.6-1	23-43
Dirithromycin	~42		11.4	~19		
Doxycycline	12-15	24	22-24	80-93	P.O.: 1.5-4	90-100
Efavirenz	52-76			>99	3-8	
Eflornithine	3.0-3.5		0.3-0.35		4-6	54-58
Enoxacin	3-6	9.4		40	1-2	90
Erythromycin	1.5-2	5-6	0.72	75-90	P.O.: 1-4	Variable
Ethambutol	2.5-3.6	7-15	1.6-2.3	10-30	2-4	75-80
Ethionamide	3		2-8	10	1.8	100
Fluconazole	25-30		0.7-1	11	P.O.: 1-2	<90
Flucytosine	2.5-6	12-250	0.6	2-4	1-2	78-90
Foscarnet	3.3-6.8		0.3-0.7	14-17		
Fosfomycin	4-8	50	2	<3	2-2.5	34-65
Ganciclovir	1.7-5.8	5-28	0.15-0.31	1-2		
Gentamicin	1.5-3	36-70	0.23-0.26	0.5-1.5		
Grepafloxacin	15.7		~5	50	2-3	70
Griseofulvin ·	9-22				4	25-70
Halofantrine	23		570			
Imipenem/cilastatin						
imipenem	1	4	0.26	20	2	65-70
cilastatin	1	17		40	1	95-100
Indinavir	1.8			~60		
Interferon alfa-2b	6-8				3.8	
Isoniazide						
fast acetylizers	0.5-1.5		0.6	<10	1.2	
slow acetylizers	2-5	22-28				
Itraconazole	21		796	99	3-4	
Ivermectin	22-28		46.8	93	3.6	
Kanamycin	2-4	40-96	0.23-0.29	<5	3.6	
Ketoconazole	1.5-3		0.36	99	1-4	37-97
Lamivudine	5-7		1.3	36		~86
Levofloxacin	6		1.25	50	1	100
Lomefloxacin	7-8	21-45	1.8-2.5	10	1.5	95-98
Loracarbef	1	≤32		25	1.2	
Mebendazole	1-11.5	35		90-95	2-4	
Mefloquine	21-22		20	98	7-24	85
Meropenem	1		0.3	2		
Methenamine	3-6		0.56		2-8	
Methicillin	0.4-0.5	4	0.43	35-60		
Metronidazole	6-8	21	0.25-0.85	20	P.O.: 1-2	80
Mezlocillin	0.8-1.2	2.6-5.4	0.17-0.2	20-46		
Miconazole	0.8-2.1	20-24	2.1	90		
Minocycline	15	11-23	0.14-0.7	70-75	2-4	
Moxalactam disodium	2-3	18-23	0.18-0.4	35-50		
Nafcillin	0.5-1.5	1.2	0.31-0.38	80-90		
Nalidixic acid	6-7	21	0.25-0.35	90	1-2	90
Nelfinavir	3.5-5		2-7	98	2-4	
Neomycin	2-4	40-96	0.23-0.29	<5	3.6	
Netilmicin	2-3	24-52	0.6-1.3	<5		
Nevirapine	22-84		1.4	50-60		
Nitrofurantoin	0.3-0.6	1	0.8	40		60
Norfloxacin	4.8	6-9	3.2	10-15	1-2	30-70
Ofloxacin	5-7.5	30	0.9-1.8	20-25	P.O.: 1.2-2	95-100
Oxacillin	0.5-0.7	1-3	0.2	90-93		
Oxamniquine	1-2.5				1-1.5	50

Drug	Half-life (h) Normal Renal Function	Half-life (h) Impaired Renal Function	V_d (L/kg)	Protein Binding (%)	Time to Peak (h)	Bioavail-ability (%)
Oxytetracycline	8.5-9.6	47-66	0.9-1.6	35	2-4	
Palivizumab	18 d					
Penicillin G benzathine, parenteral	0.5	6-20	0.2	40-60	12-24	
Penicillin G, parenteral	0.3-0.9	6-20	0.2	40-60		
Penicillin G procaine, aqueous	0.3-0.9	6-20	0.2	40-60	1-4	
Pentamidine	6.4-9.4†	48	3	69		
Piperacillin	0.5-1.2	3.3-5.1	0.18-0.3	20-40	0.5-0.9	
Polymyxin B	4.6-6				I.M.: <2	
Praziquantel	0.8-1.5			80	1-3	80
Primaquine	3.7-9.6		3.5		<6	
Pyrazinamide	9-10	26	0.57-0.74	10-20	1-2	~100
Pyrimethamine	111		3	87	2	
Quinidine	6			70-80	I.M.: 1	
Quinine	8-14	8-14	0.7-3.7	70	1-3	
Ribavirin	24	1-40 d		0	1-1.5	45
Rifabutin	16-69		9.32	85	2-4	20
Rifampin	3-4	1.8-11	1.6	89	P.O.: 1.5-4	
Rifapentine	14-17		70.2	97.7	5-6	70
Ritonavir	3-5			98-99	2-4	
Saquinavir			700	~98		~4
Sparfloxacin	20		3.9	45		92
Spectinomycin	1.7	16-29	0.25	5-20	1-2	
Stavudine	1-1.6		0.5		1	82
Streptomycin	2-4.7	100	0.26	35	I.M.: 1	
Sulfadiazine	10	34	0.29	45	3-6	
Sulfadoxine	169			90	2.5-6	
Sulfamethoxazole	9-12	20-50	0.15	70	3-4	
Sulfisoxazole	4-7	6-12	0.14-0.28	85-88	2-3	
Terbinafine	200-400				2	40-70
Tetracycline	6-11	57-108	1.3-1.6	65	2-3 d	
Thiabendazole	1.2				1-2	
Ticarcillin	1.1-1.2	16	0.18-0.21	45-60		
Tobramycin	2.5	27-60	0.22-0.33	<5	I.M.: 0.5-1	
Trimetrexate	15-17		0.62	86-94	1.8	42
Trovafloxacin	9-12			76		88
Valacyclovir	3	14-20		13.5 to 17.9		~55
Vancomycin	6-8	200-250	0.47-1.25	55		
Vidarabine	1.5		0.7	20-30		
Zalcitabine	2-2.3	>8	0.53-0.64	<4	1.6	80
Zidovudine	0.8-1.2		1.4-1.7	30-38	0.5-1.5	

*In plasma.
†Multiphasic elimination.

PREVENTION OF BACTERIAL ENDOCARDITIS

Recommendations by the American Heart Association

(*JAMA*, 1997, 277:1794-801.)

Consensus Process - The recommendations were formulated by the writing group after specific therapeutic regimens were discussed. The consensus statement was subsequently reviewed by outside experts not affiliated with the writing group and by the Science Advisory and Coordinating Committee of the American Heart Association. These guidelines are meant to aid practitioners but are not intended as the standard of care or as a substitute for clinical judgment.

Table 1. Cardiac Conditions*

Endocarditis Prophylaxis Recommended

High-Risk Category

Prosthetic cardiac valves, including bioprosthetic and homograft valves

Previous bacterial endocarditis

Complex cyanotic congenital heart disease (eg, single ventricle states, transposition of the great arteries, tetralogy of Fallot)

Surgically constructed systemic pulmonary shunts or conduits

Moderate-Risk Category

Most other congenital cardiac malformations (other than above and below)

Acquired valvar dysfunction (eg, rheumatic heart disease)

Hypertrophic cardiomyopathy

Mitral valve prolapse with valvar regurgitation and/or thickened leaflets

Endocarditis Prophylaxis Not Recommended

Negligible-Risk Category (no greater risk than the general population)

Isolated secundum atrial septal defect

Surgical repair of atrial septal defect, ventricular septal defect, or patent ductus arteriosus (without residua beyond 6 months)

Previous coronary artery bypass graft surgery

Mitral valve prolapse without valvar regurgitation†

Physiologic, functional, or innocent heart murmurs

Previous Kawasaki disease without valvar dysfunction

Previous rheumatic fever without valvar dysfunction

Cardiac pacemakers (intravascular and epicardial) and implanted defibrillators

*This table lists selected conditions but is not meant to be all-inclusive.

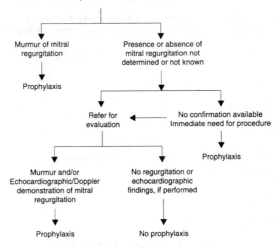

Patient With Suspected Mitral Valve Prolapse

Table 2. Dental Procedures and Endocarditis Prophylaxis

Endocarditis Prophylaxis Recommended*

Dental extractions

Periodontal procedures including surgery, scaling and root planing, probing, and recall maintenance

Dental implant placement and reimplantation of avulsed teeth

Endodontic (root canal) instrumentation or surgery only beyond the apex

Subgingival placement of antibiotic fibers or strips

Initial placement of orthodontic bands but not brackets

Intraligamentary local anesthetic injections

Prophylactic cleaning of teeth or implants where bleeding is anticipated

Endocarditis Prophylaxis Not Recommended

Restorative dentistry† (operative and prosthodontic) with or without retraction cord‡

Local anesthetic injections (nonintraligamentary)

Intracanal endodontic treatment; post placement and buildup

Placement of rubber dams

Postoperative suture removal

Placement of removable prosthodontic or orthodontic appliances

Taking of oral impressions

Fluoride treatments

Taking of oral radiographs

Orthodontic appliance adjustment

Shedding of primary teeth

*Prophylaxis is recommended for patients with high- and moderate-risk cardiac conditions.

†This includes restoration of decayed teeth (filling cavities) and replacement of missing teeth.

‡Clinical judgment may indicate antibiotic use in selected circumstances that may create significant bleeding.

PREVENTION OF BACTERIAL ENDOCARDITIS *(Continued)*

Table 3. Recommended Standard Prophylactic Regimen for Dental, Oral, or Upper Respiratory Tract Procedures in Patients Who Are at Risk*

Endocarditis Prophylaxis Recommended

Respiratory Tract
  Tonsillectomy and/or adenoidectomy
  Surgical operations that involve respiratory mucosa
  Bronchoscopy with a rigid bronchoscope
Gastrointestinal Tract*
  Sclerotherapy for esophageal varices
  Esophageal stricture dilation
  Endoscopic retrograde cholangiography with biliary obstruction
  Biliary tract surgery
  Surgical operations that involve intestinal mucosa
Genitourinary Tract
  Prostatic surgery
  Cystoscopy
  Urethral dilation

Endocarditis Prophylaxis Not Recommended

Respiratory Tract
  Endotracheal intubation
  Bronchoscopy with a flexible bronchoscope, with or without biopsy†
  Tympanostomy tube insertion
Gastrointestinal Tract
  Transesophageal echocardiography†
  Endoscopy with or without gastrointestinal biopsy†
Genitourinary Tract
  Vaginal hysterectomy†
  Vaginal delivery†
  Cesarean section
  In uninfected tissues:
    Urethral catheterization
    Uterine dilatation and curettage
    Therapeutic abortion
    Sterilization procedures
    Insertion or removal of intrauterine devices
Other
  Cardiac catheterization, including balloon angioplasty
  Implanted cardiac pacemakers, implanted defibrillators, and coronary stents
  Incision or biopsy or surgically scrubbed skin
  Circumcision

*Prophylaxis is recommended for high-risk patients, optional for medium-risk patients.
†Prophylaxis is optional for high-risk patients.

Table 4. Prophylactic Regimens for Dental, Oral, Respiratory Tract, or Esophageal Procedures

Situation	Agent	Regimen*	
		Adults	Children
Standard general prophylaxis	Amoxicillin	2 g P.O. 1 h before procedure	50 mg/kg P.O. 1 h before procedure
Unable to take oral medications	Ampicillin	2 g I.M./I.V. within 30 min before procedure	50 mg/kg I.M./I.V. within 30 min before procedure
Allergic to penicillin	Clindamycin or	600 mg P.O. 1 h before procedure	20 mg/kg P.O. 1 h before procedure
	Cephalexin† or cefadroxil† or	2 g P.O. 1 h before procedure	50 mg/kg P.O. 1 h before procedure
	Azithromycin or clarithromycin	500 mg P.O. 1 h before procedure	15 mg/kg P.O. 1 h before procedure
Allergic to penicillin and unable to take oral medications	Clindamycin or	600 mg I.V. within 30 min before procedure	20 mg/kg I.V. within 30 min before procedure
	Cefazolin†	1 g I.M./I.V. within 30 min before procedure	25 mg/kg I.M./I.V. within 30 min before procedure

*Total children's dose should not exceed adult dose.

†Cephalosporins should not be used in individuals with immediate-type hypersensitivity reaction (urticaria, angioedema, or anaphylaxis) to penicillins

Table 5. Prophylactic Regimens for Genitourinary/Gastrointestinal (Excluding Esophageal) Procedures*

Situation	Agents*	Regimen†	
		Adults	Children
High-risk‡ patients	Ampicillin plus gentamicin	Ampicillin 2 g I.M. or I.V. plus gentamicin 1.5 mg/kg (not to exceed 120 mg) within 30 min of starting the procedure; 6 h later, ampicillin 1 g I.M./I.V. or amoxicillin 1 g orally	Ampicillin 50 mg/kg I.M./I.V. (not to exceed 2 g) plus gentamicin 1.5 mg/kg within 30 min of starting the procedure; 6 h later, ampicillin 25 mg/kg I.M./I.V. or amoxicillin 25 mg/kg orally
High-risk‡ patients allergic to ampicillin/amoxicillin	Vancomycin plus gentamicin	Vancomycin 1 g I.V. over 1-2 h plus gentamicin 1.5 mg/kg I.M./I.V. (not to exceed 120 mg); complete injection/infusion within 30 min of starting the procedure	Vancomycin 20 mg/kg I.V. over 1-2 h plus gentamicin 1.5 mg/kg I.M./I.V.; complete injection/infusion within 30 min of starting the procedure
Moderate-risk§ patients	Amoxicillin or ampicillin	Amoxicillin 2 g orally 1 h before procedure, or ampicillin 2 g I.M./I.V within 30 min of starting the procedure	Amoxicillin 50 mg/kg orally 1 h before procedure, or ampicillin 50 mg/kg I.M./I.V. within 30 min of starting the procedure

PREVENTION OF BACTERIAL ENDOCARDITIS *(Continued)*

Table 5. Prophylactic Regimens for Genitourinary/Gastrointestinal (Excluding Esophageal) Procedures* *(continued)*

Situation	Agents*	Regiment	
		Adults	Children
Moderate-risk§ patients allergic to ampicillin/amoxicillin	Vancomycin	Vancomycin 1 g I.V. over 1-2 h; complete infusion within 30 min of starting the procedure	Vancomycin 20 mg/ kg I.V. over 1-2 h; complete infusion within 30 min of starting the procedure

*Total children's dose should not exceed adult dose

†No second dose of vancomycin or gentamicin is recommended

‡High-risk: Patients are those who have prosthetic valves, a previous history of endocarditis (even in the absence of other heart disease, complex cyanotic congenital heart disease, or surgically constructed systemic pulmonary shunts or conduits).

§Moderate-risk: Individuals with certain other underlying cardiac defects. Congenital cardiac conditions include the following uncorrected conditions: Patent ductus arteriosus, ventricular septal defect, primum atrial septal defect, coarctation of the aorta, and bicuspid aortic valve. Acquired valvar dysfunction and hypertrophic cardiomyopathy are also moderate risk conditions.

PREVENTION OF WOUND INFECTION AND SEPSIS IN SURGICAL PATIENTS

Nature of Operation	Likely Pathogens	Recommended Drugs	Adult Dosage Before Surgery[1]
Cardiac			
Prosthetic valve, coronary artery bypass, other open-heart surgery, pacemaker or defibrillator implant	*S. epidermidis, S. aureus, Corynebacterium*, enteric gram-negative bacilli	Cefazolin or cefuroxime or vancomycin[3]	1-2 g I.V.[2] 1-2 g I.V.[2] 1 g I.V.
Gastrointestinal			
Esophageal, gastroduodenal	Enteric gram-negative bacilli, gram-positive cocci	*High risk[4] only:* cefazolin	1-2 g I.V.
Biliary tract	Enteric gram-negative bacilli, enterococci, clostridia	*High risk[5] only:* cefazolin	1-2 g I.V.
Colorectal	Enteric gram-negative bacilli, anaerobes, enterococci	*Oral:* neomycin + erythromycin base[6]	1-2 g I.V.
		Parenteral:	
		Cefoxitin	1-2 g I.V.
		or cefotetan	1-2 g I.V.
Appendectomy, nonperforated	Enteric gram-negative bacilli, anaerobes, enterococci	Cefoxitin or cefotetan	1-2 g I.V. 1-2 g I.V.
Genitourinary	Enteric gram-negative bacilli, enterococci	*High risk[7] only:* Ciprofloxacin	500 mg P.O. or 400 mg I.V.
Gynecologic and Obstetric			
Vaginal or abdominal hysterectomy	Enteric gram-negatives, anaerobes, group B streptococci, enterococci	Cefazolin or cefotetan or cefoxitin	1-2 g I.V. 1-2 g I.V. 1 g I.V.
Cesarean section	Same as for hysterectomy	*High risk[8] only:* Cefazolin	1 g I.V. after cord clamping
Abortion	Same as for hysterectomy	*First trimester, high-risk[9] only:* Aqueous penicillin G	2 mill units I.V.
		or doxycycline	300 mg P.O.[10]
		Second trimester: Cefazolin	1 g I.V.
Head and Neck			
Entering oral cavity or pharynx	*S. aureus*, streptococci, oral anaerobes	Cefazolin or clindamycin ± gentamicin	1-2 g I.V. 600-900 mg I.V. 1.5 mg/kg I.V.
Neurosurgery			
Craniotomy	*S. aureus, S. epidermidis*	Cefazolin or vancomycin[3]	1-2 g I.V. 1 g I.V.
Ophthalmic	*S. aureus, S. epidermidis*, streptococci, enteric gram-negative bacilli, *Pseudomonas*	Gentamicin or tobramycin or neomycin-gramicidin-polymyxin B	Multiple drops topically over 2-24 h
		Cefazolin	100 mg subconjunctivally at end of procedure

PREVENTION OF WOUND INFECTION AND SEPSIS IN SURGICAL PATIENTS *(Continued)*

Nature of Operation	Likely Pathogens	Recommended Drugs	Adult Dosage Before Surgery[1]
Orthopedic			
Total joint replacement, internal fixation of fractures	S. aureus, S. epidermidis	Cefazolin	1-2 g I.V.
		or vancomycin[3]	1 g I.V.
Thoracic (Noncardiac)	S. aureus, S. epidermidis, streptococci, enteric gram-negative bacilli	Cefazolin	1-2 g I.V.
		or cefuroxime	1-2 g I.V.
		or vancomycin[3]	1 g I.V.
Vascular			
Arterial surgery involving the abdominal aorta, a prosthesis, or a groin incision	S. aureus, S. epidermidis, enteric gram-negative bacilli	Cefazolin	1-2 g I.V.
		or vancomycin[3]	1 g I.V.
Lower extremity amputation for ischemia	S. aureus, S. epidermidis, enteric gram-negative bacilli, clostridia	Cefazolin	1-2 g I.V.
		or vancomycin[3]	1 g I.V.
Contaminated Surgery[11]			
Ruptured viscus	Enteric gram-negative bacilli, anaerobes, enterococci	Cefoxitin	1-2 g I.V. q6h
		or cefotetan	1-2 g I.V. q12h
		± gentamicin	1.5 mg/kg I.V. q8h
		or clindamycin	600 mg I.V. q6h
		+ gentamicin	1.5 mg/kg I.V. q8h
Traumatic wound	S. aureus, group A strep, clostridia	Cefazolin[12]	1-2 g I.V. q8h

[1]Parenteral prophylactic antimicrobials can be given as a single intravenous dose just before the operation. For prolonged operations, additional intraoperative doses should be given every 4-8 hours for the duration of the procedure.

[2]Some consultants recommend an additional dose when patients are removed from bypass during open-heart surgery.

[3]For hospitals in which methicillin-resistant S. aureus and S. epidermidis are a frequent cause of postoperative wound infection, or for patients allergic to penicillins or cephalosporin. Rapid I.V. administration may cause hypotension, which could be especially dangerous during induction of anesthesia. Even if the drug is given over 60 minutes, hypotension may occur; treatment with diphenhydramine (Benadryl® and others) and further slowing of the infusion rate may be helpful (Maki DG, et al, *J Thorac Cardiovasc Surg*, 1992, 104:1423). For procedures in which enteric gram-negative bacilli are likely pathogens, such as vascular surgery involving a groin incision, cefazolin should be included in the prophylaxis regimen for patients not allergic to cephalosporins.

[4]Morbid obesity, esophageal obstruction, decreased gastric acidity or gastrointestinal motility.

[5]Age >70 years, acute cholecystitis, nonfunctioning gall bladder, obstructive jaundice or common duct stones.

[6]After appropriate diet and catharsis, 1 g of each at 1 PM, 2 PM, and 11 PM the day before an 8 AM operation.

[7]Urine culture positive or unavailable, preoperative catheter.

[8]Active labor or premature rupture of membranes.

[9]Patients with previous pelvic inflammatory disease, previous gonorrhea or multiple sex partners.

[10]Divided into 100 mg 1 hour before the abortion and 200 mg 30 minutes after.

[11]For contaminated or "dirty" surgery, therapy should usually be continued for about 5 days.

[12]For bite wounds, in which likely pathogens may also include oral anaerobes, *Eikenella corrodens* (human) and *Pasteurella multocida* (dog and cat), some *Medical Letter* consultants recommend use of amoxicillin/clavulanic acid (Augmentin®) or ampicillin/sulbactam (Unasyn®)

Adapted with permission from *The Medical Letter*, 1997, 39(1012).

PROPHYLAXIS FOR PATIENTS EXPOSED TO COMMON COMMUNICABLE DISEASES

Disease	Exposure	Prophylaxis/Management
Hepatitis A	Direct contact with an infected child, or sharing of food or utensils	Give 0.02 mL/kg immune globulin (IG) within 7 days of exposure.
Hepatitis B	Needlestick (used needle) Mucous membrane exposure with blood or body fluid Direct inoculation of blood or body fluid into open cut, lesion, or laceration	**Known source and employee status unknown: test patient for HB$_s$Ag and employee for anti-HB$_s$** If patient is HB$_s$Ag-negative and the patient does not have non-A, non-B hepatitis, do nothing. If patient is HB$_s$Ag-negative and has non-A, non-B hepatitis, offer ISG (optional). If patient is HB$_s$Ag-positive, give HBIG and hepatitis B vaccine within 48 hours of exposure. Employee antibody status may not be available for up to a week so the above should be given as soon as patient's antigen status is known. Occasionally, the patient's antigen status will be unavailable for more than 24 hours. In these cases, HBIG should be given if the patient is high risk (ie, Asian immigrant, institutionalized patient, homosexual, intravenous drug abuser, hemodialysis patient, patient with a history of hepatitis). If the employee is anti-HB$_s$-negative, give the second and third doses of hepatitis B vaccine. **Known source if employee documented anti-HB$_s$-positive:** If source has non-A, non-B hepatitis, offer ISG (optional). If employee is believed to be anti-HB$_s$-positive due to vaccination, has received 3 doses of vaccine, and has not had an anti-HB$_s$ test done, draw serum for anti-HB$_s$.
Invasive Haemophilus influenzae disease	Close contact with an infected child for >4 hours	Give rifampin 20 mg/kg orally once daily for 4 days (600 mg maximum daily dose) to entire family with at least one household contact younger than 48 months of age. Contraindication: Pregnant contacts.
Measles	15 minutes or more in the same room with a child with measles from 2 days before the onset of symptoms to 4 days after the appearance of the rash	Children who have not been vaccinated and have not had natural infection should be isolated from the 7th through the 18th day after exposure and/or for 4 days after the rash appears. Those who have not been vaccinated should be vaccinated within 72 hours of exposure if no contraindication exists, or receive immune globulin (IG) 0.25 mL/kg I.M. for immunocompetent individuals and 0.5 mL/kg (maximum 15 mL) for immunosuppressed individuals. Children who are younger than 15 months of age should be revaccinated at 15 months of age but at least 3 months after receipt of vaccine or IG. Older individuals who have received IG should be vaccinated 3 months later.

PROPHYLAXIS FOR PATIENTS EXPOSED TO COMMON COMMUNICABLE DISEASES *(Continued)*

Disease	Exposure	Prophylaxis/Management
Meningococcal disease	Household contact or direct contact with secretions	Household, day care center, and nursery school children should receive rifampin prophylaxis for 2 days. Dosages are given every 12 hours for a total of 4 doses. Dosage is 10 mg/kg/dose for children ages 1 month to 12 years (maximum: 600 mg/dose), 5 mg/kg/dose for infants less than 1 month of age, and 600 mg/dose for adults. Contraindication: Pregnant contacts. Because prophylaxis is not always effective, exposed children should be monitored for symptoms. Employee exposure: Anyone who develops a febrile illness should receive prompt medical evaluation. If indicated, antimicrobial therapy should be administered
Pertussis	Housed in the same room with an infected child or spent 15 minutes in a playroom with an infected child	**Prophylaxis:** Contacts <7 years of age who have had at least 4 doses of pertussis vaccine should receive a booster dose of DTP, unless a dose has been given within the past 3 years, and should receive erythromycin 40-50 mg/kg/day orally for 14 days. Contacts <7 years of age who are not immunized or who have received less than 4 doses of DTP should have DTP immunization initiated or continued according to the recommended schedule. Children who have received their third dose 6 months or more before exposure should be given their fourth dose at this time. Erythromycin should also be given for 14 days. Contacts ≥7 years of age should receive prophylactic erythromycin (maximum of 1 g/day) for 10-14 days. All exposed patients should be watched closely for respiratory symptoms for 14 days after exposure has stopped because immunity conferred by the vaccine is not absolute and the efficacy of erythromycin in prophylaxis has not been established.
Tuberculosis	Housed in the same room with a child with contagious tuberculosis (tuberculosis is contagious if the child has a cough plus AFB seen on smear plus cavitation on chest x-ray)	Place PPD immediately and 10 weeks after exposure. Start on INH. Consult Infectious Diseases if seroconversion occurs.

Disease	Exposure	Prophylaxis/Management
Varicella-zoster	1 hour or more in the same room with a contagious child from 24 hours before vesicles appear to when all vesicles are crusted, which is usually 5-7 days after vesicles appear. In household exposure, communicability is 48 hours before vesicles appear.	**Immunocompetent** children who have not been vaccinated or had natural infection should have titers drawn only if they will still be hospitalized for more than 10 days after exposure. If titers are negative, they should be isolated 10-21 days after exposure and/or until all lesions are crusted and dry. If VZIG was given, the child should be isolated 10-28 days after exposure. **Immunocompromised** children who have not been vaccinated or had natural infection should first have titers drawn, and then receive VZIG (varicella-zoster immune globulin) **1 vial/10 kg I.M.** up to a maximum of 5 vials as soon as possible but at most 96 hours after exposure. Fractional doses are not recommended. If titers are positive, nothing further need be done. If titers are negative, the child should be isolated 10-28 days after exposure and should be monitored very carefully for the appearance of vesicles so that treatment can be initiated. VZIG is available from the Blood Bank.

SODIUM CONTENT

Drug Name and Dosage Unit	Sodium	
	mg	mEq
Acyclovir, 1 g	96.6	4.2
Amikacin sulfate, 1 g	29.9	1.3
Aminosalicylate sodium, 1 g	108.1	4.7
Ampicillin, 1 g	66.7	3
Ampicillin sodium & sulbactam sodium, 1.5 g	115	5
Ampicillin, suspension, 250 mg/5 mL, 5 mL	10	0.4
Carbenicillin, 382 mg, tablet	23	1
Cefamandole nafate, 1 g	76	3.3
Cefazolin sodium, 1 g	47	2
Cefmetazole sodium, 1 g	47	2
Cefonicid sodium, 1 g	85.1	3.7
Cefoperazone sodium, 1 g	34.5	1.5
Cefotaxime sodium, 1 g	50.6	2.2
Cefotetan disodium, 1 g	80.5	3.5
Cefoxitin sodium, 1 g	53	2.3
Ceftazidime, 1 g	54	2.3
Ceftizoxime sodium, 1 g	59.8	2.6
Ceftriaxone sodium, 1 g	59.8	2.6
Cefuroxime, 1 g	55.2	2.4
Cephalothin sodium, 1 g	64.4	2.8
Cephapirin sodium, 1 g	55.2	2.4
Chloramphenicol, 1 g	51.8	2.25
Cloxacillin sodium, 125 mg/5 mL	11	0.48
Cloxacillin sodium, 250 mg, capsule	13.8	0.6
Colistimethate sodium, 150 mg	22.9	1
Dicloxacillin, 250 mg, capsule	13	0.6
Dicloxacillin, suspension, 65 mg/5 mL	27	1.2
Didanosine, buffered tablets	264.5	11.5
Erythromycin base Filmtab®, 250 mg	70	3
Erythromycin, ethyl succinate, suspension, 200 mg/5 mL	29	1.3
Ganciclovir, 500 mg vial	46	2
Imipenem/cilastatin, injection, 1 g, I.V.	73.6	3.2
Imipenem/cilastatin, injection, 1 g, I.M.	64.4	2.8
Meropenem, 1 g	90.2	3.92
Methicillin sodium, 1 g	59.8-71.3	2.6-3.1
Metronidazole, 500 mg, I.V.	322	14
Mezlocillin sodium, 1 g	42.6	1.85
Nafcillin sodium, 1 g	66.7	2.9
Oxacillin sodium, 1 g	64.4-71.3	2.8-3.1
Penicillin G potassium, 1 million units parenteral	7	0.3
Penicillin G sodium, 1 million units parenteral	46	2
Piperacillin sodium, 1 g	42.6	1.85
Piperacillin sodium & tazobactam sodium	54 mg	2.35
Ticarcillin and clavulanate potassium, 1 g	109.3	4.75
Ticarcillin disodium, 1 g	119.6-149.5	5.2-6.5

TREATMENT OF SEXUALLY TRANSMITTED DISEASES

Type or Stage	Drug of Choice	Dosage	Alternatives
CHLAMYDIA TRACHOMATIS			
Urethritis, cervicitis, conjunctivitis, or proctitis (except lymphogranuloma venereum)			
	Azithromycin or	1 g oral once	Ofloxacin[2] 300 mg oral bid x 7 d; erythromycin 500 mg oral qid x 7 d
	Doxycycline[1,2]	100 mg oral bid x 7 d	
Infection in pregnancy			
	Erythromycin[3]	500 mg oral qid x 7 d[4]	Amoxicillin 500 mg oral tid x 10 d; azithromycin[5] 1 g oral once
Neonatal			
Ophthalmia	Erythromycin	12.5 mg/kg oral or I.V. qid x 14 d	
Pneumonia	Erythromycin	12.5 mg/kg oral or I.V. qid x 14 d	Sulfisoxazole[6] 100 mg/kg/d oral or I.V. in divided doses x 14 d
Lymphogranuloma venereum			
	Doxycycline[1,2]	100 mg oral bid x 21 d	Erythromycin[3] 500 mg oral qid x 21 d
GONORRHEA[7]			
Urethral, cervical, rectal, or pharyngeal			
	Cefpodoxime 200 mg as a single dose; ceftriaxone	125 mg I.M. once	Cefixime 400 mg oral once; ciprofloxacin[2] 500 mg oral once; ofloxacin[2] 400 mg oral once; spectinomycin 2 g I.M. once[8]
Ophthalmia (adults)[9]			
	Ceftriaxone	1 g I.M. once, plus saline irrigation	
Bacteremia, arthritis, and disseminated[10,11]			
	Ceftriaxone	1 g I.V. daily x 7-10 days, or for 2-3 d, followed by cefixime 400 mg oral bid or ciprofloxacin 500 mg oral bid to complete 7-10 d total therapy	Ceftizoxime or cefotaxime, 1 g I.V. q8h for 2-3 days or until improved, followed by cefixime 400 mg oral bid or ciprofloxacin 500 mg oral bid to complete 7-10 d total therapy
Neonatal			
Ophthalmia	Cefotaxime or	25 mg/kg I.V. or I.M. q8-12h x 7 d, plus saline irrigation	Penicillin G[12] 100,000 units/kg/d I.V. in 4 doses x 7 d, plus saline irrigation
	Ceftriaxone	125 mg I.M. once, plus saline irrigation	
Bacteremia, arthritis, and disseminated	Cefotaxime	25-50 mg/kg I.V. q8-12h x 7-14 d	Penicillin G[12] 75,000-100,000 units/kg/d I.V. in 4 doses x 7-14 d
Children (<45 kg)			
Urogenital, rectal, and pharyngeal	Ceftriaxone	125 mg I.M. once	Spectinomycin[13] 40 mg/kg I.M. once; amoxicillin[12] 50 mg/kg oral once, plus probenecid 25 mg/kg (max: 1 g) oral once

TREATMENT OF SEXUALLY TRANSMITTED DISEASES
(Continued)

Type or Stage	Drug of Choice	Dosage	Alternatives
Bacteremia, arthritis, and disseminated	Ceftriaxone or	50-100 mg/kg/d (max: 2 g) I.V. x 7-14 d	Penicillin G[12] 150,000-250,000 units/kg/d I.V. x 7-14 d
	Cefotaxime	50-200 mg/kg/d I.V. in 2-4 doses x 7-14 d	

SEXUALLY-ACQUIRED EPIDIDYMITIS

	Ofloxacin	300 mg bid x 10 d	Ceftriaxone 250 mg I.M. once, followed by doxycycline[1] 100 mg oral bid x 10 d

PELVIC INFLAMMATORY DISEASE

Hospitalized patients	Cefoxitin or	2 g I.V. q6h	Clindamycin 900 mg I.V. q8h plus gentamicin 2 mg/kg I.V. once, followed by gentamicin 1.5 mg/kg I.V. q8h until improved, followed by doxycycline 100 mg oral bid to complete 14 days[14]
	Cefotetan either one, plus	2 g I.V. q12h	
	Doxycycline[2] followed by	100 mg I.V. q12h, until improved	
	Doxycycline[2]	100 mg oral bid to complete 14 days	
Outpatients	Cefoxitin, plus	2 g I.M. once	Ofloxacin[2] 400 mg oral bid x 14 d, plus metronidazole 500 mg oral bid x 14 d or clindamycin 450 mg oral qid x 14 d
	Probenecid or	1 g oral once	
	Ceftriaxone, either one followed by	250 mg I.M. once	
	Doxycycline[2]	100 mg oral bid x 14 d	

VAGINAL INFECTION

Trichomoniasis

	Metronidazole[15]	2 g oral once	Metronidazole 375 mg or 500 mg oral bid x 7 d

Bacterial vaginosis

	Metronidazole gel 0.75%	5 g intravaginally bid x 5 d	Metronidazole 500 mg oral bid x 7 d

Vulvovaginal candidiasis

	Topical butoconazole, clotrimazole, miconazole, terconazole, or tioconazole[17]		Metronidazole 2 g oral once[16]; fluconazole 150 mg oral once

SYPHILIS

Early (primary, secondary, or latent <1 y)

	Penicillin G benzathine	2.4 million units I.M. once[18]	Doxycycline[2] 100 mg oral bid x 14 d

Late (more than 1 year's duration, cardiovascular, gumma, late-latent)

	Penicillin G benzathine	2.4 million units I.M. weekly x 3 wk	Doxycycline[2] 100 mg oral bid x 4 wk

Neurosyphilis[19]

	Penicillin G	2-4 million units I.V. q4h x 10-14 d	Penicillin G procaine 2.4 million units I.M. daily, plus probenecid 500 mg qid oral, both x 10-14 d

Type or Stage	Drug of Choice	Dosage	Alternatives
Congenital			
	Penicillin G or	50,000 units/kg I.M. or I.V. q8-12h for 10-14 d	
	Penicillin G procaine	50,000 units/kg I.M. daily for 10-14 d	
CHANCROID[20]			
	Erythromycin[3] or	500 mg oral qid x 7 d	Ciprofloxacin[2] 500 mg oral bid x 3 d
	Ceftriaxone or	250 mg I.M. once	
	Azithromycin	1 g oral once	
HERPES SIMPLEX			
First episode genital			
	Acyclovir	400 mg oral tid x 7-10 d	Acyclovir 200 mg oral 5 times/d x 7-10 d
First episode proctitis			
	Acyclovir	800 mg oral tid x 7-10 d	Acyclovir 400 mg oral 5 times/d x 7-10 d
Recurrent			
	Acyclovir[21]	400 mg oral tid x 5 d	
Severe (hospitalized patients)			
	Acyclovir	5 mg/kg I.V. q8h x 5-7 d	
Prevention of recurrence[22]			
	Acyclovir	400 mg oral bid	Acyclovir 200 mg oral 2-5 times/d

[1] Or tetracycline 500 mg oral qid or minocycline 100 mg oral bid.
[2] Contraindicated in pregnancy.
[3] Erythromycin estolate is contraindicated in pregnancy.
[4] In the presence of severe gastrointestinal intolerance, decrease to 250 mg qid and extend duration to 14 days.
[5] Safety in pregnancy not established.
[6] Only for infants older than 4 weeks.
[7] All patients should also receive a course of treatment effective for *Chlamydia*.
[8] Recommended only for use during pregnancy in patients allergic to beta-lactams. Not effective for pharyngeal infection.
[9] An oral fluoroquinolone, such as ciprofloxacin for 3-5 days, probably would also be effective, but experience is limited.
[10] If the infecting strain of *N. gonorrhoeae* has been tested and is known to be susceptible to penicillin or the tetracyclines, treatment may be changed to penicillin G 10 million units I.V. daily, amoxicillin 500 mg orally qid, doxycycline 100 mg orally bid, or tetracycline 500 mg orally qid.
[11] Endocarditis requires at least 3-4 weeks of parenteral therapy.
[12] If infecting strain of *N. gonorrhoeae* has been tested and is known to be susceptible.
[13] Not effective for pharyngeal infection.
[14] Or clindamycin 450 mg oral qid to complete 14 days.
[15] Metronidazole should be avoided during the first trimester of pregnancy; 2 g oral (single dose) may be given after the first trimester.
[16] Higher relapse rate, but useful for patients who may not comply with multiple-dose therapy.
[17] For preparations and dosage, see *The Medical Letter*, 36:81, 1994; avoid single-dose therapy.
[18] Some experts recommend repeating this regimen after 7 days, especially in patients with HIV infection.
[19] Patients allergic to penicillin should be desensitized.
[20] All regimens, especially single-dose ceftriaxone, are less effective in HIV-infected patients.
[21] Not highly effective for treatment of recurrences, but may help some patients if started early.
[22] Preventive treatment should be discontinued for 1-2 months once a year to reassess the frequency of recurrence.

COMPATIBILITY INFORMATION

Compatibility of Medications With <u>Hyperalimentation</u> Solutions

The following is a list to be used as a quick reference guide. Drug compatibility is dependent on several factors such as drug concentration, the type, pH and volume of solutions used, and duration of mixing. These variations make it impossible to determine the compatibility of various medications at all times.

Antibiotics – Compatible	References
Amikacin sulfate‡	1,2,4
Azlocillin sodium	1,2,4
Aztreonam	7
Carbenicillin disodium	1,2
Cefamandole nafate	1,2,4
Cefazolin sodium	1,2
Cefoperazone sodium	1,2
Cefotaxime sodium	1,2
Cefoxitin sodium	1,2
Ceftazidime	7
Ceftriaxone sodium	7
Cefuroxime sodium	7
Cephalothin sodium	1,2,4
Chloramphenicol sodium succinate	1,2
Clindamycin phosphate	1,2
Dopamine	
Doxycycline hyclate*	1,2
Erythromycin gluceptate*‡	2
Erythromycin lactobionate*‡	1,2
Gentamicin sulfate‡	1,2
Kanamycin sulfate†‡	1,2
Methicillin sodium	1,2
Mezlocillin sodium	1,2,4
Miconazole*	1,2
Morphine	
Moxalactam disodium	1,2,4
Nafcillin sodium	1,2,4
Netilmicin sulfate‡	1,2
Oxacillin sodium	1,2,4
Penicillin G potassium	1,2,4
Piperacillin sodium	1,2,4
Polymyxin B sulfate	1,2
Tetracycline hydrochloride*§	1,2,5
Tobramycin sulfate‡	1,2,4
Ticarcillin disodium	1,2,4
Vancomycin hydrochloride‡	1,2,3

*Physically compatible – no chemical compatibility data.

†Reported physical compatibility with conflicting chemical compatibility data.

‡Heparin in various concentrations is incompatible with amikacin, erythromycin, gentamicin, kanamycin, netilmicin, tobramycin, and vancomycin at usual dosages.[1] The interaction may be drug concentration dependent and less likely to occur in more dilute concentrations. A TPN solution containing 1 unit/mL of heparin was physically compatible with vancomycin, tobramycin, gentamicin, and amikacin.[6]

§Chelation with magnesium and calcium ions has been documented. The degree of chelation is influenced by the concentration of magnesium and calcium ions as well as pH of the solution.

Ampicillin sodium was reported physically compatible and physically incompatible with precipitate formation in different studies (1,2). Reference number 4 states incompatible.

Antibiotics – Incompatible	References
Acyclovir	
Amphotericin B	1,5
Metronidazole	1,5
Trimethoprim-sulfamethoxazole	5

Other Medications – Compatible	
Albumin*	2,8
Aminophylline¶	1,2,9
Cimetidine HCl	1,2,9
Cyanocobalamin*	1
Cyclophosphamide*	1
Cytarabine*	1,9
Digoxin physically compatible for 4 h (Y-site)	1
Dobutamine physically compatible for 4 h (Y-site)	1
Dopamine HCl*	1,2
Famotidine*	9
Fluorouracil*	1,9
Folic acid*	1,2
Furosemide*	1,2
Heparin sodium*	1,2
Hydrocortisone sodium succinate*	9
Isoproterenol HCl	1,2
Levarterenol bitartrate*	2,9
Lidocaine HCl*	1,2
Meperidine HCl*	1,9
Metaraminol bitartrate*	1,2
Methotrexate sodium*	1
Methyldopate HCl*	1,2
Methylprednisolone sodium succinate*	1,2
Metoclopramide HCl	1,2
Morphine sulfate*	1,9
Nizatidine*	9
Norepinephrine bitartrate	1,2
Ranitidine HCl*	1,9
Urokinase (no loss of urokinase activity when assayed immediately after mixing)	1

*Physically compatible – no chemical compatibility data.

¶Precipitation is more likely to be seen in neonatal TPN solutions upon the addition of aminophylline, than adult solutions because of the lesser concentrations of amino acids and greater concentrations of calcium and phosphate. The high pH of aminophylline also contributes to the problem. With the administration of aminophylline by retrograde injection, TPN solutions of Travasol® 1% and dextrose 10% will show precipitation at levels of 10 mEq/L calcium and 10 mmol/L phosphorus. Solutions of Travasol® 2% and dextrose were compatible with the same levels of electrolytes.[4]

Other Medications – Incompatible	
Bleomycin sulfate	1
Blood (possible pseudoagglutination)	1

COMPATIBILITY INFORMATION *(Continued)*

Compatibility of Medications With Fat Emulsions

Antibiotics – Compatible	References
Ampicillin sodium	1
Cefamandole nafate	1
Cefazolin sodium	1
Cefoxitin sodium	1
Clindamycin phosphate	1
Erythromycin lactobionate	1
Gentamicin sulfate	1
Kanamycin sulfate	1
Penicillin G potassium	1
Ticarcillin sodium	1
Tobramycin sulfate	1

Above antibiotics are physically compatible via Y-site (1:1 mixture) for 4 hours at 25°C by visual observation.

Antibiotics – Incompatible

Tetracycline hydrochloride	1

Other Medications – Compatible

Aminophylline	
physically compatible for 48 h	4
conflicting data – states compatible and incompatible	1
Cimetidine HCl	1
physically compatible	
Digoxin	
physically compatible for 4 h (Y-site only)	1,4
Diphenhydramine HCL	1,4
physically compatible	
Dopamine HCl	1,4
physically compatible for 4 h (Y-site only)	
Furosemide	1,4
physically compatible for 4 h (Y-site only)	
Heparin	1,4
physically compatible	
Hydrocortisone sodium succinate	1
physically compatible	
Isoproterenol HCl	1,4
physically compatible for 4 h (Y-site only)	
Lidocaine HCl	1,4
physically compatible for 4 h (Y-site only)	
Methyldopate HCl	1
compatible when diluted with sodium chloride 0.9%; incompatible when diluted with dextrose 5% water	
Norepinephrine bitartrate	1,4
physically compatible for 4 h (Y-site only)	

Other Medications – Incompatible

Calcium gluconate	1,4
Phenytoin sodium	

References

1. Trissel LA, *Handbook on Injectable Drugs*, Bethesda, MD: American Society of Hospital Pharmacists, Inc, 1988.
2. Frey AM, "Taking the Confusion Out of Multiple Infusion: I.V. Medications and TPN," *NITA*, 1986, 9(6):460-3.
3. Schilling CG, Watson DM, McCoy HG, et al, "Stability and Delivery of Vancomycin Hydrochloride When Admixed in a Total Parenteral Nutrition Solution," *JPEN J Parenter Enteral Nutr*, 1989, 13(1):63-4.
4. Kamen BA, Gunther N, Sowinsky N, et al, "Analysis of Antibiotic Stability in a Parenteral Nutrition Solution," *Pediatr Infect Dis*, 1985, 4(4):387-9.
5. Stranz MH and Barfoot KS, "Total Parenteral Nutrition. Compatibility of Antibiotic Admixtures," *J Intraven Nurs*, 1988, 11(1):43-8.
6. Schilling CG, "Compatibility of Drugs With a Heparin-Containing Neonatal Total Parenteral Nutrient Solution," *Am J Hosp Pharm*, 1988, 45(2):313-4.
7. Fox AS, Boyer KM, and Sweeney HM, "Antibiotic Stability in a Pediatric Parenteral Alimentation Solution," *J Pediatr*, 1988, 112(5):813-7.
8. Niemiec PW Jr and Vanderveen TW, "Compatibility Considerations in Parenteral Nutrient Solutions," *Am J Hosp Pharm*, 1984, 41(5):893-911.
9. King J, *Guide to Parenteral Admixtures*, St Louis, MO: Pacemarq, Inc, 1989.

TUBERCULOSIS

Tuberculin Skin Test Recommendations*

Children for whom immediate skin testing is indicated:

- Contacts of persons with confirmed or suspected infectious tuberculosis (contact investigation); this includes children identified as contacts of family members or associates in jail or prison in the last 5 years

- Children with radiographic or clinical findings suggesting tuberculosis

- Children immigrating from endemic countries (eg, Asia, Middle East, Africa, Latin America)

- Children with travel histories to endemic countries and/or significant contact with indigenous persons from such countries

Children who should be tested annually for tuberculosis†:

- Children infected with HIV or living in household with HIV-infected persons

- Incarcerated adolescents

Children who should be tested every 2-3 years†:

- Children exposed to the following individuals: HIV-infected, homeless, residents of nursing homes, institutionalized adolescents or adults, users of illicit drugs, incarcerated adolescents or adults, and migrant farm workers. Foster children with exposure to adults in the preceding high-risk groups are included.

Children who should be considered for tuberculin skin testing at ages 4-6 and 11-16 years:

- Children whose parents immigrated (with unknown tuberculin skin test status) from regions of the world with high prevalence of tuberculosis; continued potential exposure by travel to the endemic areas and/or house-hold contact with persons from the endemic areas (with unknown tuber-culin skin test status) should be an indication for repeat tuberculin skin testing

- Children without specific risk factors who reside in high-prevalence areas; in general, a high-risk neighborhood or community does not mean an entire city is at high risk; rates in any area of the city may vary by neighborhood, or even from block to block; physicians should be aware of these patterns in determining the likelihood of exposure; public health officials or local tuberculosis experts should help clinicians identify areas that have appreciable tuberculosis rates

Children at increased risk of progression of infection to disease: Those with other medical risk factors, including diabetes mellitus, chronic renal failure, malnutri-tion, and congenital or acquired immunodeficiencies deserve special consideration. Without recent exposure, these persons are not at increased risk of acquiring tuber-culosis infection. Underlying immune deficiencies associated with these conditions theoretically would enhance the possibility for progression to severe disease. Initial histories of potential exposure to tuberculosis should be included on all of these patients. If these histories or local epidemiologic factors suggest a possibility of exposure, immediate and periodic tuberculin skin testing should be considered. An initial Mantoux tuberculin skin test should be performed before initiation of immuno-suppressive therapy in any child with an underlying condition that necessitates immunosuppressive therapy.

---

*BCG immunization is not a contraindication to tuberculin skin testing.

†Initial tuberculin skin testing is at the time of diagnosis or circumstance, beginning as early as at age 3 months.

Tuberculosis Therapy

Specific Circumstances/ Organism	Comments	Regimen
Category I. Exposure		
(Household members and other close contacts of potentially infectious cases) (Exposee tuberculin test negative)*		
Neonate	Rx essential	INH (10 mg/kg/d) for 3 months, then repeat tuberculin test (TBnT). If mother's smear negative and infant's TBnT negative and chest x-ray (CXR) are normal, stop INH. In the United Kingdom, BCG is then given (*Lancet*, 1990, 2:1479), unless mother is HIV-positive. If infants repeat TBnT is positive and/or CXR abnormal (hilar adenopathy and/or infiltrate), administer INH + RIF (10-20 mg/kg/d) (or streptomycin) for a total of 6 months. If mother is being treated, separation from mother is not indicated.
Children <5 y	Rx indicated	As for neonate first 3 months. If repeat TBnT is negative, stop. If repeat TBnT is positive, continue INH for a total of 9 months. If INH is not given initially, repeat TBnT at 3 months; if positive, treat with INH for 9 months (see Category II below).
Older children and adults	No Rx	Repeat TBnT at 3 months, if positive, treat with INH for 6 months (see Category II below)
Category II. Infection Without Disease		
(Positive tuberculin test)*		
Regardless of age (see INH Preventive Therapy)	Rx indicated	INH (5 mg/kg/d, maximum: 300 mg/d for adults, 10 mg/kg/d not to exceed 300 mg/d for children). Results with 6 months of treatment are nearly as effective as 12 months (65% vs 75% reduction in disease). *Am Thoracic Society* (6 months), *Am Acad Pediatrics*, 1991 (9 months). If CXR is abnormal, treat for 12 months. In HIV-positive patient, treatment for a minimum of 12 months, some suggest longer. Monitor transaminases monthly (*MMWR Morb Mortal Wkly Rep* 1989, 38:247).
Age <35 y	Rx indicated	Reanalysis of earlier studies favors INH prophylaxis for 6 months (if INH-related hepatitis case fatality rate is <1% and TB case fatality is ≥6.7%, which appears to be the case, monitor transaminases monthly (*Arch Int Med*, 1990, 150:2517).
INH-resistant organisms likely	Rx indicated	Data on efficacy of alternative regimens is currently lacking. Regimens include ETB + RIF daily for 6 months. PZA + RIF daily for 2 months, then INH + RIF daily until sensitivities from index case (if available) known, then if INH-CR, discontinue INH and continue RIF for 9 months, otherwise INH + RIF for 9 months (this latter is *Am Acad Pediatrics*, 1991 recommendation).
INH + RIF resistant organisms likely	Rx indicated	Efficacy of alternative regimens is unknown; PZA (25-30 mg/kg/d P.O.) + ETB (15-25 mg/kg/d P.O.) (at 25 mg/kg ETB, monitoring for retrobulbar neuritis required), for 6 months unless HIV-positive, then 12 months; PZA + ciprofloxacin (750 mg P.O. bid) or ofloxacin (400 mg P.O. bid) x 6-12 months (*MMWR Morb Mortal Wkly Rep*, 1992, 41(RR11):68).

INH = isoniazid; RIF = rifampin; KM = kanamycin; ETB = ethambutol
SM = streptomycin; CXR = chest x-ray; Rx = treatment
See also guidelines for interpreting PPD in "Skin Testing for Delayed Hypersensitivity" found in the Skin Tests section of the Appendix.
*Tuberculin test (TBnT). The standard is the Mantoux test, 5 TU PPD in 0.1 mL diluent stabilized with Tween 80. Read at 48-72 hours measuring maximum diameter of induration. A reaction ≥5 mm is defined as positive in the following: positive HIV or risk factors, recent close case contacts, CXR consistent with healed TBc. ≥10 mm is positive in foreign-born in countries of high prevalence, injection drug users, low income populations, nursing home residents, patients with medical conditions which increase risk (see above, preventive treatment). ≥15 mm is positive in all others (*Am Rev Resp Dis*, 1990, 142:725). Two-stage TBnT: Use in individuals to be tested regularly (ie, healthcare workers). TBn reactivity may decrease over time but be boosted by skin testing. If unrecognized, individual may be incorrectly diagnosed as recent converter. If first TBnT is reactive but <10 mm, repeat 5 TU in 1 week, if then ≥10 mm = positive, not recent conversion (*Am Rev Resp Dis*, 1979, 119:587).

TUBERCULOSIS *(Continued)*

TUBERCULOSIS TREATMENT GUIDELINES

Recommended Treatment Regimens for Drug-Susceptible Tuberculosis in Infants, Children, and Adolescents*

Infection or Disease Category	Regimen	Remarks
Asymptomatic infection (positive skin test, no disease):		If daily therapy is not possible, therapy twice a week may be used for 6-9 months. HIV-infected children should be treated for 12 months.
• Isoniazid-susceptible	6-9 months of isoniazid once a day	
• Isoniazid-resistant	6-9 months of rifampin once a day	
• Isoniazid-rifampin-resistant*	Consult a tuberculosis specialist	
Pulmonary	**6-Month Regimens** 2 months of isoniazid, rifampin, and pyrazinamide once a day, followed by 4 months of isoniazid and rifampin daily	If possible drug resistance is a concern (see text), another drug (ethambutol or streptomycin) is added to the initial drug therapy until drug susceptibilities are determined.
	or 2 months of isoniazid, rifampin, and pyrazinamide daily, followed by 4 months of isoniazid and rifampin twice a week	Drugs can be given 2 or 3 times per week under direct observation in the initial phase if nonadherence is likely.
	9-Month Alternative Regimens (for hilar adenopathy only) 9 months of isoniazid and rifampin once a day **or** 1 month of isoniazid and rifampin once a day, followed by 8 months of isoniazid and rifampin twice a week	Regimens consisting of 6 months of isoniazid and rifampin once a day, and 1 month of isoniazid and rifampin once a day, followed by 5 months of isoniazid and rifampin twice a week, have been successful in areas where drug resistance is rare.
Extrapulmonary meningitis, disseminated (miliary), bone/joint disease	2 months of isoniazid, rifampin, pyrazinamide, and streptomycin once a day, followed by 10 months of isoniazid and rifampin once a day (12 months total)	Streptomycin is given with initial therapy until drug susceptibility is known.
	or 2 months of isoniazid, rifampin, pyrazinamide, and streptomycin once a day, followed by 10 months of isoniazid and rifampin twice a week (12 months total)	For patients who may have acquired tuberculosis in geographic areas where resistance to streptomycin is common, capreomycin (15-30 mg/kg/d) or kanamycin (15-30 mg/kg/d) may be used instead of streptomycin.
Other (eg, cervical lymphadenopathy)	Same as for pulmonary disease	See Pulmonary.

*Duration of therapy is longer in HIV-infected persons and additional drugs may be indicated.

Adapted from "Report of the Committee on Infectious Diseases," *1997 Red Book*®, 24th ed.

Commonly Used Drugs for the Treatment of Tuberculosis in Infants, Children, and Adolescents

Drugs	Dosage Forms	Daily Dose (mg/kg/d)	Twice a Week Dose (mg/kg per dose)	Maximum Dose	Adverse Reactions
Ethambutol	Tablets 100 mg 400 mg	15-25	50	2.5 g	Optic neuritis (usually reversible), decreased visual acuity, decreased red-green color discrimination, gastrointestinal disturbances, hypersensitivity
Isoniazid*	Scored tablets 100 mg 300 mg Syrup 10 mg/mL	10-15†	20-30	Daily, 300 mg Twice a week, 900 mg	Mild hepatic enzyme elevation, hepatitis,† peripheral neuritis, hypersensitivity
Pyrazinamide*	Scored tablets 500 mg	20-40	50	2 g	Hepatotoxicity, hyperuricemia
Rifampin*	Capsules 150 mg 300 mg Syrup formulated in syrup from capsules	10-20	10-20	600 mg	Orange discoloration of secretions/urine, staining contact lenses, vomiting, hepatitis, flu-like reaction, and thrombocytopenia; may render birth-control pills ineffective
Streptomycin (I.M. administration)	Vials 1 g 4 g	20-40	20-40	1 g	Auditory and vestibular toxicity, nephrotoxicity, rash

*Rifamate® is a capsule containing 150 mg of isoniazid and 300 mg of rifampin. Two capsules provide the usual adult (>50 kg body weight) daily doses of each drug. Rifater® is a capsule containing 50 mg of isoniazid, 120 mg of rifampin, and 300 mg of pyrazinamide.

†When isoniazid in a dosage exceeding 10 mg/kg/day is used in combination with rifampin, the incidence of hepatotoxicity may be increased.

Adapted from "Report of the Committee on Infectious Diseases," *1997 Red Book®,* 24th ed.

Rifampin is a bactericidal agent. It is metabolized by the liver and affects the pharmacokinetics of many other drugs, affecting their serum concentrations. Mycobacterium tuberculosis, initially resistant to rifampin, remains relatively uncommon in most areas of the United States. Rifampin is excreted in bile and urine and can cause orange urine, sweat and tears. It can also cause discoloration of soft contact lenses and render oral contraceptives ineffective. Hepatotoxicity occurs rarely. Blood dyscrasia accompanied by influenza-like symptoms can occur if doses are taken sporadically.

TUBERCULOSIS *(Continued)*

Less Commonly Used Drugs for Treatment of Drug-Resistant Tuberculosis in Infants, Children, and Adolescents*

Drugs	Dosage Forms	Daily Dose (mg/kg/d)	Maximum Dose	Adverse Reactions
Capreomycin	Vials 1 g	15-30 (I.M. administration)	1 g	Ototoxicity, nephrotoxicity
Ciprofloxacin†	Tablets 250 mg 500 mg 750 mg	Adults 500-1500 mg total per day (twice a day)	1.5 g	Theoretical effect on growing cartilage, gastrointestinal tract disturbances, rash, headache
Cycloserine	Capsules 250 mg	10-20	1 g	Psychosis, personality changes, convulsions, rash
Ethionamide	Tablets 250 mg	15-20 given in 2 or 3 divided doses	1 g	Gastrointestinal tract disturbances, hepatotoxicity, hypersensitive reactions
Kanamycin	Vials 75 mg/2 mL 500 mg/2 mL 1 g/3 mL	15-30 (I.M. 1 g administration)	1 g	Auditory toxicity, nephrotoxicity, vestibular toxicity
Ofloxacin†	Tablets 200 mg 300 mg 400 mg	Adults 400-800 mg total per day (twice a day)	0.8 g	Theoretical effect on growing cartilage, gastrointestinal tract disturbances, rash, headache
Para-amino salicylic acid (PAS)	Tablets 500 mg	200-300 (3 or 4 times a day)	10 g	Gastrointestinal tract disturbances, hypersensitivity, hepatotoxicity

*These drugs should be used in consultation with a specialist in tuberculosis.

†Fluoroquinolones are not currently approved for use in persons younger than 18 years; their use in younger patients necessitates assessment of the potential risks and benefits (see Antimicrobials and Related Therapy).

Adapted from "Report of the Committee on Infectious Diseases," *1997 Red Book*®, 24th ed.

TB Drugs in Special Situations

Drug	Pregnancy	CNS TB Disease	Renal Insufficiency
Isoniazid	Safe	Good penetration	Normal clearance
Rifampin	Safe	Fair penetration Penetrates inflamed meninges (10% to 20%)	Normal clearance
Pyrazinamide	Avoid	Good penetration	Clearance reduced Decrease dose or prolong interval
Ethambutol	Safe	Penetrates inflamed meninges only (4% to 64%)	Clearance reduced Decrease dose or prolong interval
Streptomycin	Avoid	Penetrates inflamed meninges only	Clearance reduced Decrease dose or prolong interval
Capreomycin	Avoid	Penetrates inflamed meninges only	Clearance reduced Decrease dose or prolong interval
Kanamycin	Avoid	Penetrates inflamed meninges only	Clearance reduced Decrease dose or prolong interval
Ethionamide	Do not use	Good penetration	Normal clearance
Para-aminosalicylic acid	Safe	Penetrates inflamed meninges only (10% to 50%)	Incomplete data on clearance
Cycloserine	Avoid	Good penetration	Clearance reduced Decrease dose or prolong interval
Ciprofloxacin	Do not use	Fair penetration (5% to 10%) Penetrates inflamed meninges (50% to 90%)	Clearance reduced Decrease dose or prolong interval
Ofloxacin	Do not use	Fair penetration (5% to 10%) Penetrates inflamed meninges (50% to 90%)	Clearance reduced Decrease dose or prolong interval
Amikacin	Avoid	Penetrates inflamed meninges only	Clearance reduced Decrease dose or prolong interval
Clofazimine	Avoid	Penetration unknown	Clearance probably normal

Safe = the drug has not been demonstrated to have teratogenic effects.

Avoid = data on the drug's safety are limited, or the drug is associated with mild malformations (as in the aminoglycosides).

Do not use = studies show an association between the drug and premature labor, congenital malformations, or teratogenicity.

CLASSIFICATION OF ORGANISMS

CLASSIFICATION OF ORGANISMS

ALPHABETICAL INDEX

INTERNATIONAL BRAND NAME INDEX

The following countries are included in this index and are abbreviated as follows:

Australia (Astral)
Austria (Austria)
Belgium (Belg)
Canada (Can)
Denmark (Den)
France (Fr)
Germany (Ger)
Ireland (Irl)
Italy (Ital)
Japan (Jpn)

Mexico (Mex)
Monaco (Mon)
Netherlands (Neth)
Norway (Norw)
South Africa (S. Afr)
Spain (Spain)
Sweden (Swed)
Switzerland (Switz)
United Kingdom (UK)
United States (USA)

INTERNATIONAL BRAND NAME INDEX

NOTES

NOTES

NOTES

NOTES

Other titles offered by Lexi-Comp . . .

DRUG INFORMATION HANDBOOK 7th Edition 1999-2000

by Charles Lacy, PharmD; Lora L. Armstrong, BSPharm; Morton P. Goldman, PharmD; and Leonard L. Lance, BSPharm

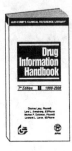

Specifically compiled and designed for the healthcare professional requiring quick access to concisely stated comprehensive data concerning clinical use of medications.

The Drug Information Handbook is an ideal portable drug information resource, containing 1250 drug monographs. Each monograph typically provides the reader with up to 29 key points of data concerning clinical use and dosing of the medication. Material provided in the Appendix section is recognized by many users to be, by itself, well worth the purchase of the handbook.

DRUG INFORMATION HANDBOOK POCKET 1999-2000

by Charles Lacy, PharmD; Lora L. Armstrong, BSPharm; Morton P. Goldman, PharmD; and Leonard L. Lance, BSPharm

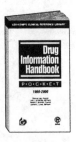

All medications found in the Drug Information Handbook, 7th Edition are included in this abridged pocket edition. It is specifically compiled and designed for the healthcare professional requiring quick access to concisely stated comprehensive data concerning clinical use of medications.

The outstanding cross-referencing allows the user to quickly locate the brand name, generic name, synonym, and related information found in the Appendix making this a useful quick reference for medical professionals at any level of training or experience.

GERIATRIC DOSAGE HANDBOOK 4th Edition 1998/99

by Todd P. Semla, PharmD; Judith L. Beizer, PharmD; and Martin D. Higbee, PharmD

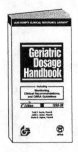

Many physiologic changes occur with aging, some of which affect the pharmacokinetics or pharmacodynamics of medications. Strong consideration should also be given to the effect of decreased renal or hepatic functions in the elderly as well as the probability of the geriatric patient being on multiple drug regimens.

Healthcare professionals working with nursing homes and assisted living facilities will find the 745 drug monographs contained in this handbook to be an invaluable source of helpful information.

To order call toll free: 1-800-837-LEXI (5394)

PEDIATRIC DOSAGE HANDBOOK 6th Edition 1999-2000
by Carol K. Taketomo, PharmD; Jane Hurlburt Hodding, PharmD; and Donna M. Kraus, PharmD

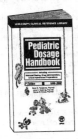

Special considerations must frequently be taken into account when dosing medications for the pediatric patient. This highly regarded quick reference handbook is a compilation of recommended pediatric doses based on current literature as well as the practical experience of the authors and their many colleagues who work every day in the pediatric clinical setting.

The Pediatric Dosage Handbook 6th Edition includes neonatal dosing, drug administration, and extemporaneous preparations for 640 medications used in pediatric medicine.

DRUG INFORMATION HANDBOOK FOR NURSING 2nd Edition 1999/2000
by Beatrice B. Turkoski, RN, PhD; Brenda R. Lance, RN, MSN; Mark F. Bonfiglio, PharmD

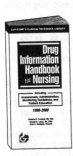

Registered Professional Nurses and upper-division nursing students involved with drug therapy will find this handbook provides quick access to drug data in a concise easy-to-use format.

Over 4750 U.S., Canadian, and Mexican medications are covered with up to 43 key points of information in each monograph. The handbook contains basic pharmacology concepts and nursing issues such as patient factors that influence drug therapy (ie, pregnancy, age, weight, etc) and general nursing issues (ie, assess-ment, administration, monitoring, and patient education). The Appendix contains over 220 pages of valuable information.

DRUG INFORMATION HANDBOOK FOR ADVANCED PRACTICE NURSING 1999/2000
by Beatrice B. Turkoski, RN, PhD; Brenda R. Lance, RN, MSN; Mark F. Bonfiglio, PharmD

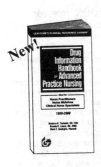

This handbook was designed specifically to meet the needs of Nurse Practitioners, Clinical Nurse Specialists, Nurse Midwives and graduate nursing students. The handbook is a unique resource for detailed, accurate information, which is vital to support the advanced practice nurse's role in patient drug therapy management.

A concise introductory section reviews topics related to Pharmacotherapeutics.

Over 4750 U.S., Canadian, and Mexican medications are covered in the 1055 monographs. Drug data is presented in an easy-to-use, alphabetically organized format covering up to 46 key points of information including Adult, Pediatric and Geriatric Dosing (with adjustments for renal/hepatic impairment), Laboratory Tests used to monitor drug therapy, Pregnancy/Breast-feeding Implications, Physical Assessment/Monitoring Guidelines and Patient Education/Instruction. Monographs are cross-referenced to an Appendix of over 230 pages of valuable comparison tables and additional information. Also included are two indices, Pharmacologic Category and Controlled Substance, which facilitate comparison between agents.

To order call toll free: 1-800-837-LEXI (5394)

ANESTHESIOLOGY & CRITICAL CARE DRUG HANDBOOK
2nd Edition 1999-2000
by Andrew J. Donnelly, PharmD; Francesca E. Cunningham, PharmD; and Verna L. Baughman, MD

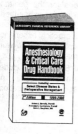

Contains over 512 generic medications with up to 25 fields of information presented in each monograph. It also contains the following Special Issues and Topics: Allergic Reaction, Anesthesia for Cardiac Patients in Noncardiac Surgery, Anesthesia for Obstetric Patients in Nonobstetric Surgery, Anesthesia for Patients With Liver Disease, Chronic Pain Management, Chronic Renal Failure, Conscious Sedation, Perioperative Management of Patients on Antiseizure Medication, Substance Abuse and Anesthesia.

The Appendix includes Abbreviations & Measurements, Anesthesiology Information, Assessment of Liver & Renal Function, Comparative Drug Charts, Infectious Disease-Prophylaxis & Treatment, Laboratory Values, Therapy Recommendation, Toxicology, *and much more . . .*

DRUG INFORMATION HANDBOOK FOR ONCOLOGY 1999-2000
by Dominic A. Solimando, Jr, MA; Linda R. Bressler, PharmD, BCOP; Polly E. Kintzel, PharmD, BCPS, BCOP; Mark C. Geraci, PharmD, BCOP

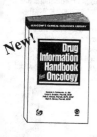

This comprehensive and easy-to-use oncology handbook was designed specifically to meet the needs of anyone who provides, prescribes, or administers therapy to cancer patients.

Presented in a concise and uniform format, this book contains the most comprehensive collection of oncology-related drug information available. Organized like a dictionary for ease of use, drugs can be found by looking up the *brand or generic name!*

This book contains 253 monographs, including over 1100 Antineoplastic Agents and Ancillary Medications.

It also contains up to 33 fields of information per monograph including Use, U.S. Investigational, Bone Marrow/Blood Cell Transplantation, Vesicant, Emetic Potential. A Special Topics Section, Appendix, and Therapeutic Category & Key Word Index are valuable features to this book, as well.

DRUG-INDUCED NUTRIENT DEPLETION HANDBOOK 1999-2000
by Ross Pelton, RPh, PhD, CCN; James B. LaValle, RPh, DHM, NMD, CCN; Ernest B. Hawkins, RPh, MS; Daniel L. Krinsky, RPh, MS

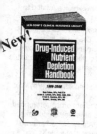

A complete and up-to-date listing of all drugs known to deplete the body of nutritional compounds.

This book is alphabetically organized and provides extensive cross-referencing to related information in the various sections of the book. Nearly 150 generic drugs that cause nutrient depletion are identified and are cross-referenced to more detailed descriptions of the nutrients depleted and their actions. Symptoms of deficiencies, and sources of repletion are also included. This book also contains a Studies and Abstracts section, a valuable Appendix, and Alphabetical & Pharma-cological Indices.

To order call toll free: 1-800-837-LEXI (5394)

DRUG INFORMATION HANDBOOK FOR PHYSICIAN ASSISTANTS
1999-2000 by Michael J. Rudzinski, RPA-C, RPh; J. Fred Bennes, RPA, RPh

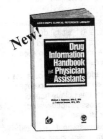

This comprehensive and easy-to-use handbook covers over 3600 drugs and also includes monographs on commonly used herbal products. There are up to 24 key fields of information per monograph, such as Pediatric And Adult Dosing With Adjustments for Renal/hepatic Impairment, Labeled And Unlabeled Uses, Pregnancy & Breast-feeding Precautions, and Special PA issues. Brand (U.S. and Canadian) and generic names are listed alphabetically for rapid access. It is fully cross-referenced by page number and includes alphabetical and pharmacologic indices.

DRUG INFORMATION HANDBOOK FOR DENTISTRY 5th Ed 1999-2000
by Richard L. Wynn, BSPharm, PhD; Timothy F. Meiller, DDS, PhD; and Harold L. Crossley, DDS, PhD

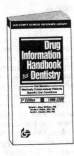

This handbook presents dental management and therapeutic considerations in medically compromised patients. Issues covered include oral manifestations of drugs, pertinent dental drug interactions, and dosing of drugs in dental treatment.

Selected oral medicine topics requiring therapeutic intervention include managing the patient with acute or chronic pain including TMD, managing the patient with oral bacterial or fungal infections, current therapeutics in periodontal patients, managing the patient receiving chemotherapy or radiation for the treatment of cancer, managing the anxious patient, managing dental office emergencies, and treatment of common oral lesions.

DRUG INFORMATION HANDBOOK FOR PSYCHIATRY 1999-2000
by Matthew A. Fuller, PharmD; Martha Sajatovic, MD

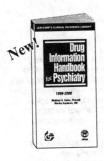

As a source for comprehensive and clinically relevant drug information for the mental health professional, this handbook is alphabetically arranged by generic and brand name for ease-of-use. It contains monographs on 1063 generic drugs and up to 34 key fields of information including effect on mental status and effect on psychiatric treatment.

A special topics/issues section includes psychiatric assessment, overview of selected major psychiatric disorders, clinical issues in the use of major classes of psychotropic medications, psychiatric emergencies, special populations, diagnostic and statistical manual of mental disorders (DSM-IV), and suggested readings. Also contains a valuable Appendix section, as well as, a Therapeutic Category Index and an Alphabetical Index.

To order call toll free: 1-800-837-LEXI (5394)

DRUG INFORMATION HANDBOOK FOR THE ALLIED HEALTH PROFESSIONAL 6th Edition 1999-2000

by Leonard L. Lance, BSPharm; Charles Lacy, PharmD; and Morton P. Goldman, PharmD

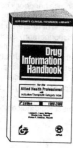

Working with clinical pharmacists, hospital pharmacy and therapeutics committees, and hospital drug information centers, the authors have assisted hundreds of hospitals in developing institution specific formulary reference documentation.

The most current basic drug and medication data from those clinical settings have been reviewed, coalesced, and cross-referenced to create this unique handbook. The handbook offers quick access to abbreviated monographs for 1384 generic drugs.

This is a great tool for physician assistants, medical records personnel, medical transcriptionists and secretaries, pharmacy technicians, and other allied health professionals.

DRUG INFORMATION HANDBOOK FOR THE CRIMINAL JUSTICE PROFESSIONAL

by Marcelline Burns, PhD; Thomas E. Page, MA; and Jerrold B. Leikin, MD

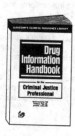

Compiled and designed for police officers, law enforcement officials, and legal professionals who are in need of a reference which relates to information on drugs, chemical substances, and other agents that have abuse and/or impairment potential. This handbook covers over 450 medications, agents, and substances. Each monograph is presented in a consistent format and contains up to 33 fields of information including Scientific Name, Commonly Found In, Abuse Potential, Impairment Potential, Use, When to Admit to Hospital, Mechanism of Toxic Action, Signs & Symptoms of Acute Overdose, Drug Interactions, Warnings/Precautions, and Reference Range. There are many diverse chapter inclusions as well as a glossary of medical terms for the layman along with a slang street drug listing. The Appendix contains Chemical, Bacteriologic, and Radiologic Agents - Effects and Treatment; Controlled Substances - Uses and Effects; Medical Examiner Data; Federal Trafficking Penalties, *and much more.*

POISONING & TOXICOLOGY COMPENDIUM

by Jerrold B. Leikin, MD and Frank P. Paloucek, PharmD

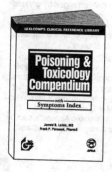

A six-in-one reference wherein each major entry contains information relative to one or more of the other sections. This handbook offers comprehensive concisely-stated monographs covering 645 medicinal agents, 256 nonmedicinal agents, 273 biological agents, 49 herbal agents, 254 laboratory tests, 79 antidotes, and 222 pages of exceptionally useful appendix material.

A truly unique reference that presents signs and symptoms of acute overdose along with considerations for overdose treatment. Ideal reference for emergency situations.

To order call toll free: 1-800-837-LEXI (5394)

LABORATORY TEST HANDBOOK 4th Edition

by David S. Jacobs MD, FACP; Wayne R. DeMott, MD, FACP; Harold J. Grady, PhD; Rebecca T. Horvat, PhD; Douglas W. Huestis, MD; and Bernard L. Kasten Jr., MD, FACP

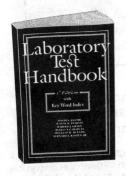

Contains over 900 clinical laboratory tests and is an excellent source of laboratory information for physicians of all specialties, nurses, laboratory professionals, students, medical personnel, or anyone who needs quick access to most the routine and many of the more specialized testing procedures available in today's clinical laboratory.

Including updated AMA CPT coding, each monograph contains test name, synonyms, patient care, specimen requirements, reference ranges, and interpretive information with footnotes and references.

LABORATORY TEST HANDBOOK CONCISE version

by David S. Jacobs MD, FACP; Wayne R. DeMott, MD, FACP; Harold J. Grady, PhD; Rebecca T. Horvat, PhD; Douglas W. Huestis, MD; and Bernard L. Kasten Jr., MD, FACP

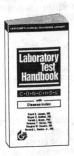

The authors of Lexi-Comp's highly regarded *Laboratory Test Handbook, 4th Edition* have selected and extracted key information for presentation in this portable abridged version.

The *Laboratory Test Handbook Concise* contains more than 800 tests entries for quick reference and is ideal for residents, nurses, and medical students or technologists requiring information concerning patient preparation, specimen collection and handling, and test result interpretation.

DIAGNOSTIC PROCEDURE HANDBOOK

by Joseph A. Golish, MD

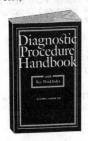

An ideal companion to the Laboratory Test Handbook this publication details 295 diagnostic procedures including Allergy, Immunology/Rheumotology, Infectious Disease, Cardiology, Critical Care, Gastro-enterology, Nephrology, Urology, Hematology, Neurology, Ophthalmology, Pulmonary Function, Pulmonary Medicine, Computed Tomography, Diagnostic Radiology, Invasive Radiology, Magnetic Resonance Imaging, Nuclear Medicine, and Ultra-sound. A great reference handbook for healthcare professionals at any level of training and experience.

To order call toll free: 1-800-837-LEXI (5394)

NEW titles soon to be released in print and on CD-ROM will include:

- *Natural Therapeutics Pocket Guide*
- *Natural Products Information Handbook*
- *Drug Information Handbook for Cardiology*

"*Lexi-Comp's Clinical Reference Library™ (CRL)* has established the new standard for quick reference information"

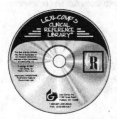

Lexi-Comp offers the Clinical Reference Library™ (CRL™), a series of clinical databases, as portable handbooks or integrated as part of a CD-ROM that also includes clinical decision support modules. CRL™ is delivered with a powerful search engine on a single CD-ROM and can be used with Microsoft® Windows™ release 3.1 or higher. In addition to our CD-ROM for Windows™, Lexi-Comp's databases can also be licensed for distribution on your Intranet, or used with your palmtop, Newton, or Windows™ CE device.

Clinical Decision Support Modules

The Clinical Decision Support Modules are unique and significant to the power offered by Lexi-Comp's Clinical Reference Library™ on CD-ROM. These modules are also directly linked to CRL™'s databases.

 Patient Analysis - Users can specify a patient's drug profile and automatically analyze the data for drug interactions, duplicate therapy, and drug allergy alerts. Printing this medication summary report for review by the physician will help decrease adverse drug events, increase productivity, and improve patient care.

 Stedman's Electronic Medical Dictionary™ - Instant access to the full functionality of a medical dictionary, including over 100,000 medical definitions, phrases, pronunciations, and related terms.

 Calculations - Instant access to the following calculations: Body Surface Area, Ideal Body Mass for Pediatrics and Adults, Estimated Creatinine Clearance (Cockroft & Gault), and Temperature Conversion.

 Drug Identification - This powerful module allows rapid identification of medications based on one or more of the following descriptors: use, pattern, shape, scoring, markings, form, coatings, color, generic name, and manufacturer name. Color images are displayed for visual verification.

 Symptoms Analysis - Enter symptoms presented by a patient to receive separate lists of medicinal, nonmedicinal, and biological agents associated with the selected symptoms.

To order call toll free: 1-800-837-LEXI (5394)